49⁹⁵

Practical Strategies in Outpatient Medicine

BRENDAN M. REILLY, M.D.

Associate Professor of Clinical Medicine,
Section of General Internal Medicine,
Department of Medicine,
Dartmouth-Hitchcock Medical Center,
Hanover, New Hampshire

ILLUSTRATIONS BY BRUCE FARRELL

1984

W. B. SAUNDERS COMPANY

Philadelphia • London • Toronto • Mexico City • Rio de Janeiro • Sydney • Tokyo

W. B. Saunders Company: West Washington Square
Philadelphia, PA 19105

1 St. Anne's Road
Eastbourne, East Sussex BN21 3UN, England

1 Goldthorne Avenue
Toronto, Ontario M8Z 5T9, Canada

Apartado 26370—Cedro 512
Mexico 4, D.F., Mexico

Rua Coronel Cabrita, 8
Sao Cristovao Caixa Postal 21176
Rio de Janeiro, Brazil

9 Waltham Street
Artarmon, N.S.W. 2064, Australia

Ichibancho, Central Bldg., 22-1 Ichibancho
Chiyoda-Ku, Tokyo 102, Japan

Library of Congress Cataloging in Publication Data

Reilly, Brendan M.

Practical strategies in outpatient medicine.

1. Ambulatory medical care.   I. Title. [DNLM: 1. Ambulatory care—Methods. WX 205 R362c]

RC48.R44 1984   616   83–14342

ISBN 0–7216–7539–5

Practical Strategies in Outpatient Medicine   ISBN   0-7216-7539-5

Last digit is the print number: 9   8   7   6   5   4   3   2   1

To my wife,
Janice Dickerson Reilly

PREFACE

This book describes one internist's approach to a variety of common adult medical problems. It was written to help medical students and house officers learn the ways of ambulatory medical care. It does not pretend to be a comprehensive textbook; relatively few diseases or specific syndromes are discussed in detail, and epidemiology, pathophysiology, and pharmacology receive little attention. The encyclopedic textbooks of medicine already admirably address these issues. This book was written to supplement those textbooks because, for the novice physician, those weighty tomes are sometimes not so helpful as they might be. Ready access to the wisdom of famous subspecialists regarding the diagnosis and treatment of specific diseases is valuable primarily when patients' symptoms and signs have already been translated into a specific diagnosis. It is this latter process that is the subject of this book. Given a patient with a common complaint, how does the clinician make a correct specific diagnosis and help the patient in a pragmatic and cost-conscious manner?

Clinical medicine, not just "outpatient medicine," is the subject of this book: how to recognize common diseases in their usual and unusual disguises; how to maintain vigilance for those uncommon but serious disorders that require emergency action, consultation, and/or hospitalization; how to treat common diseases "correctly" but pragmatically; what to do when the "correct" treatment is either impossible or ineffective; and how to do all these things while remaining the patient's advocate in a health care system threatening to become frankly adversarial. These clinical responsibilities are a tall order, even for the experienced physician, and this book pays inadequate tribute to the generalist ("primary care") practitioners who fill that order every day for countless patients with an intimidating array of problems and complaints. Those practitioners will object, rightfully, that such things are learned by doing, not by reading. This book readily acknowledges that fact but tries to serve as one practical guide for the physician-in-training who aspires to that goal.

Such aspirations demand attention not only to the scientific capabilities and technologic advances of modern medicine but also to other aspects of the physician-patient relationship: patients' attitudes towards illness, physicians' shortcomings as humane decision-makers, and cost-benefit trade-offs in providing medical care that is both intelligent and practical. Such "non-scientific" matters relate importantly to all patient care, whether in a physician's office or an intensive care unit.

The clinical strategies suggested in this book, however, are specifically directed toward helping the ambulatory patient. Each year, students and house officers in most training programs are exposed to a variety of outpatient educational experiences in ambulatory clinics, emergency rooms, local physicians' offices, and family practice training units. Even under the best of circumstances, for many novice physicians this can be a frustrating experience. More than a few well-intentioned and knowledgeable house officers, brimming with the confidence gleaned from their increasing mastery of "high-tech" hospital medicine, have been known to slink back to the wards to escape a clinic filled with "boring" (translate: complex) patients complaining of dizziness or headache or low back pain. But it is not just the psychologic drain of sorting out undifferentiated subjective symptoms that wears down the novice clinician. There is also a broad body of knowledge that pertains to "ambulatory medicine" in particular and that until recently has not received its due attention in medical education. For the physician-in-training who confronts his first patient with a sore shoulder or a swollen knee, for example, the study of gross anatomy suddenly becomes very "relevant" indeed. Several recently published "primary care" textbooks have begun to address this pertinent "core curriculum." This book summarizes only part of that curriculum, but my equal purpose is to suggest strategies to lighten still other burdens that conspire against the "outpatient" clinician: the burdens imposed by time, financial constraints, and unavoidable diagnostic uncertainties. For example:

1. Early clinical training of most physicians emphasizes the critical importance of thorough patient evaluation—detailed history, pertinent socio-cultural questions, and complete physical examination. Such thoroughness is always desirable but is only sometimes essential in the ambulatory patient with one specific complaint. The clamor from the waiting room does not allow time for funduscopic examination in all patients with acute diarrhea, for example. For the patient with headaches, that time must be found. The efficient use of physicians' time is a significant issue in ambulatory medicine. The physician-in-training must learn to interview and examine patients in a concise, directed manner appropriate to the specific complaint. This takes practice, and lots of it.

2. The physician-in-training must learn to formulate diagnostic hypotheses on the basis of purely clinical information—the history and physical examination—before he or she can utilize (expensive) laboratory testing purposefully and cost effectively. The cost of medical care can no longer be ignored. The unbridled proliferation of high-powered technologic tertiary care is not the only economic scandal in medicine today; it is clear that abuse of "low-level technology"—routine tests and x-rays and medications that don't work—also spends too much of the nation's health dollar. Ironically, the skills most crucial to the practice of cost-conscious clinical medicine—listening, looking, talking, touching, and thinking—are the very skills de-emphasized by the recent technologic revolution in medicine. This need not be so, but especially in ambulatory care, expensive technology must be relegated to its proper place. A major thesis throughout this book is that a careful, directed history and physical examination are always the most important (and often the only necessary) "tests" in evaluating the ambulatory patient.

3. What is most disconcerting for many well-trained but inexperienced physicians is the unavoidable fact that we must learn sometimes to treat symptoms, rather than specific diseases. Especially in ambulatory care, many

patients cannot be assigned a specific patho-anatomic diagnosis, no matter how thorough our evaluation of the problem. Although we often talk about "viral" labyrinthitis with the dizzy patient or musculoligamentous "strains" with the back pain victim or "vasospasm" with the headache sufferer, much of this is presumptive speculation calling for presumptive treatments. Living with such uncertainties is a fact of life for the generalist physician. The inherent dangers are difficult to escape: missing specific diseases requiring specific treatment when symptoms and signs are nonspecific; or acceding to tempting "shotgun therapy" for all superficially similar syndromes—in short, losing (or never attaining) that sharp edge of clinical acumen honed by success and failure with clearly defined problems. Such clarity, however, is often elusive among many ambulatory patients with vague and/or self-limited illness. This fact of life contributes to clinicians' anxiety and is often the cause of costly and inappropriate testing and/or inefficient use of time.

Thus, the sometimes conflicting impulses to be fast, cost-effective, and sure must be reconciled every time the clinician confronts an ambulatory patient. This dilemma is the raison d'être for this book, and the specific problems discussed in each chapter have thus been chosen for two major reasons. First, each problem is extremely common—the aggregate of problems discussed in the book does comprise a substantial part of the daily burden borne by the generalist physician. Second, the problems discussed here are difficult, for a variety of reasons. Many are multidisciplinary in scope—they impinge on different "subspecialty territories"—and a broad perspective, not available in much literature directed at subspecialists, is essential for the generalist physician. Dizziness, chest pain, and abdominal pain are examples of such problems. Other chapters describe common problems that are more difficult from a procedural point of view—given a particular problem patient, what is the most efficient and effective strategy for reaching a satisfactory outcome? Urinary infections, sore throat, and diarrhea are examples of these. Still other problems are difficult because a satisfactory outcome depends on patient compliance with a variety of non-technologic, nonpharmacologic measures—exercise, behavioral modification, home remedies, and the simple "watch and wait" approach so appropriate to management of many minor illnesses. Low back pain, cough, and headache are examples of these.

As such, different chapters have different emphases. Throughout the book, however, the prevailing emphasis tries to reflect the concerns of the primary care practitioner. None of these chapters is meant to be a definitive treatment of a complicated issue—many large volumes elsewhere have been devoted to each of these individual problems. Nevertheless, each chapter tries at least to touch upon much of what the generalist physician needs to learn to be an effective practitioner when dealing with patients with these problems.

A few caveats about the text deserve brief emphasis:

1. Each chapter focuses on one or two hypothetical patients whose illness is analyzed in detail. This is not intended to be a "case studies" book, however. The sample patients are used here as stylistic devices to exemplify very specific diagnostic and therapeutic approaches to specific problems. In some chapters, this device is more cumbersome than in others. Nevertheless, it is used throughout the book in order to focus on an essential fact of ambulatory medicine: the patient must be followed after the initial encounter. Many important diagnostic and therapeutic decisions in medicine evolve as

the patient's illness evolves over time. Any attempt to teach a practical approach to ambulatory medicine must recognize this principle.

For example, only by following patients through to the conclusion (or stabilization) of their illness does the clinician learn the natural history of disease and the spectrum of complications that may attend it. Thus, several of the patients in the text do not respond to treatment as expected or develop illnesses whose evolution over time invalidates or complicates the original diagnosis. Such events are common in medicine, no matter how skilled the clinician, and only by following the patient is the clinician's experience and skill enhanced.

In addition, a central theme throughout this text is the notion that following the patient allows most cost-effective use of laboratory (and radiologic) testing. After careful clinical evaluation of many of these problems, testing can often be deferred or avoided entirely, pending the patient's response to "presumptive" treatment.

Finally, the clinical practice of medicine is not just a series of problem-solving exercises. It is also a unique human experience. The physician-in-training who limits himself or herself to a series of isolated "patient encounters" and simply "solves problems" is not fully participating in the privileged opportunity that medicine (especially primary care) provides: to observe the human condition and to learn about "human nature." Only by observing and sharing patients' experience with illness, recovery, and wellness will the novice clinician begin to appreciate the art of medicine, without which the science loses some of its power and much of its purpose.

2. Some attention is devoted to the economic cost of evaluating and treating these clinical problems. Thus, most chapters include the cost of various tests that may be necessary to evaluate the problem, depending on the specific circumstances. The costs of these tests are derived from the 1983 fee schedule at the Dartmouth-Hitchcock Medical Center. (Fees include technical and physician's fees.) Testing fees vary extraordinarily among different practice settings and geographic locations. They also change (almost yearly and ever upward) and may thus already be out of date. Nevertheless, these costs are included here primarily to illustrate the *relative* costs of diagnostic strategies: each clinician should know the local cost of the test he or she performs.

Similarly, the costs of various medications are often noted. Medication prices in the text are derived from average retail prices at several pharmacies in my own locale—wherever possible, generic drug prices are listed preferentially. As such, the cost to the patient of the least expensive drug preparation is emphasized. Again, the purpose here is to emphasize *relative* costs of (often equally effective) drugs. In addition, the variations in costs of medications even among neighboring pharmacies can be preposterous: the clinician should be aware of not only what drugs cost but where to buy them. If patients are so informed, the local drugstores will get the message soon enough.

3. Some of the bibliographies are extensive, and some readers may object that too many references are worse than none. Again, this book is meant to be a guide, not a comprehensive text. As such, many very important issues are only lightly touched upon in some chapters. Often, references are provided simply to direct the interested reader elsewhere. In addition, much of what is written here is simply a distillation of what I have learned from more expert clinicians—the references only begin to acknowledge that debt.

Finally, there is often no one correct approach to these problems. An attempt is made here to support at least some of the specific recommendations with references from the research literature. The "scientific" basis of primary care is growing but remains shallow—its research literature is still in its infancy. The strategies recommended here, even when reinforced with extensive references, may raise as many questions as they answer.

4. The text includes suggestions about how to "make use of" our subspecialist colleagues. I realize that the working relationships among generalist and specialist physicians vary greatly in different settings. Thus, the relationships suggested here are not meant to be rigidly defined. Only the individual practitioner can decide when he or she needs help. Nevertheless, suggestions are often quite specific here in order to underline my own bias about our "health care system": too many high-priced and overtrained subspecialists provide general medical care according to clinical strategies appropriate to consultative subspecialty practices but inadequate (and even counterproductive) in the primary care setting. Just because the many domains of general (primary care) medicine encroach upon the territory of various subspecialties does not mean that the available subspecialist should be consulted whenever we trespass on his "turf." Far from it. My chauvinism here extends to the belief that the practice of "general medicine" is the most fulfilling specialty in medicine today, but only in proportion to the breadth of clinical responsibilities assumed by the generalist physician. Yes, we generalists must know our own limitations, and those limitations must be clearly defined if we are to best help our patients, but we will remain vital in our efforts and proud of our work if we heed our patients' plea: *Be my doctor.*

5. Much of the current emphasis on "strategies" and "decision-making" in clinical medicine today incorporates the methods of quantitative decision analysis, especially the uses and corollaries of Bayes' theorem. I am an admirer of these methods and believe that such quantitative training is essential for the modern clinician. This book contains very little formal mathematical decision analysis, but not because of my lack of enthusiasm for those methods. Rather, I personally am able to apply these concepts to only a few of the problems discussed here. As "primary care" research about practical clinical strategies continues, such approaches will, I think, be forthcoming, and I will welcome them. For now, what follows is the best that this nonmathematical practitioner can do.

BRENDAN M. REILLY

ACKNOWLEDGMENTS

This book surely would not have been completed were it not for the help and encouragement of many fine people. I am fully responsible for the book's inadequacies, but the credit for whatever herein is worthwhile must be shared.

My special thanks go to Dr. George Bernier, Chairman of the Department of Medicine at Dartmouth, who encouraged me to begin and who has sustained me throughout the writing of the book. Without him, this book would never have happened.

I am also very lucky to have had from the beginning the support, suggestions, and chastisements of two exceptionally perceptive internists—my brother, Dr. Phillip C. Reilly, Jr., and my father, Dr. Philip C. Reilly, Sr. Their embarrassingly objective criticisms helped immeasurably.

My own patients suffered some inconvenience—but little harm, I think—during the long time it took to finish this book. Their well-being and my peace of mind were possible only because I work with a group of general internists here at Dartmouth who every day exemplify the professional quality to which I aspire and which I try to communicate in this book. To Drs. Paul Gerber, Wayne Kniffin, Eric Manheimer, Lou Matthews, John Milne, Rob Smith, and Dick Whiting—thank you.

So many other members of the faculty here have helped me that I dare not try to mention all for fear of forgetting one. The physicians of the Hitchcock Clinic have been my teachers, colleagues, and friends, and in a very real sense, this book was written by all of them. I am fortunate to be among them.

The Dartmouth Medical House Staff have stimulated and cajoled me throughout the writing of this book—their energy and friendship and dedication to patient care continue to make it all worthwhile.

Thanks also go to the Hitchcock Foundation, which underwrote some of the initial expenses; to Pierre Bastianelli, whose photographs and x-ray reproductions are so painstakingly well done; to Joan Thomson, who helped with the drawings in the sore throat chapter; to Bruce Farrell, whose exceptional original drawings fill this book—without him, I don't know what I would have done; to Joy Lacagnina Williams, Maureen Campbell, Joanne LeBaron Rice, and Linda Strong Greene, who transcribed each chapter more times than they would like to remember but who were always willing to do more; and to my medical secretaries, Dianne Heath Hartwell and Patty Guitar, who were always so helpful and cheerful when I was not.

It has been a special pleasure to work with Jack Hanley and John Dyson, who have been instrumental in the conception, development, and production of this text; little wonder that Saunders has no peer in the medical publishing business.

More than anyone, my own family knows what it took to write this book. The time I took from them can never be replaced. To my son BJ and my daughter Caitie, I send my love and promises of better times ahead. My wife Janice, to whom this book is dedicated, has somehow kept us all together and happy and growing closer every day, despite the demands of her own busy life. Alongside that accomplishment, this book pales in comparison.

CONTENTS

1

LOW BACK PAIN 1

Acute Low Back Pain 1
   Initial Approach 1
   Physical Examination 5
Simple Mechanical Low Back Pain 16
   Tests? 18
   Treatment 20
Radicular Low Back Pain 29
   Practical Neurology of the Low Back and Leg 29
   Diagnosis and Treatment 34
Chronic Low Back Pain 42
   Diagnosis 43
   Treatment 51
Appendix I: When Back Pain is Dangerous 54
Appendix II: Compression Fractures, Osteopenia, and Osteoporosis 57
Appendix III: Back Pain and Back Anatomy 61
Appendix IV: Back Manipulation 66
References 68

2

SORE THROAT 71

An Overview 71
Streptococcal or Nonstreptococcal Pharyngitis? 76
Treatment of Pharyngitis 79
Special Cases: Complicated Sore Throat 82
   Peritonsillar Abscess 83
   Epiglottitis 84
   Diphtheria 86
   Retropharyngeal Abscess 86
   Ludwig's Angina 88
   Unusual Pathogens 90
Chronic or Recurrent Sore Throat 92
Appendix: Throat Cultures, Streptococcal Infections and the
Cost-Benefit Debate 94
References 98

3

DIARRHEA 100

   Acute Diarrhea 100
      Symptoms and Signs 100
      Tests 106
      Treatment.. 108
      Acute Dysentery 111
      When Acute Diarrhea Persists 115
      Lactose Intolerance 119
   Chronic Diarrhea 121
      The Initial Approach... 121
      Sequence of Investigation....................................... 121
      Chronic Bloody Diarrhea 129
      Therapeutic Trials... 133
      Steatorrhea 138
      Hospitalization.. 142
    Appendix I: Acute Proctitis 145
    Appendix II: Food-Borne Diarrhea................................. 148
      Food Poisoning 148
      Food Intolerance 150
      Traveler's Diarrhea ("Turista") 151
    Appendix III: Postoperative Diarrhea 152
    Appendix IV: Diets: Diagnostic and Therapeutic................ 155
    Appendix V: Pancreatic Enzyme Replacement 158
    References 160

4

HEADACHE 164

   New (Acute) Headache 165
      Intracranial Hemorrhage.. 166
      Ocular Headache.. 169
      Post-traumatic Headache 172
      Headache in the Elderly 173
      Infectious Headache... 175
   Physical Examination of the Headache Patient 176
   Headache in Special Circumstances.................................... 181
   Chronic, Recurrent Headache 184
      Classic Migraine 186
      Cluster Headache 188
      Trigeminal Neuralgia... 189
      Common Migraine versus Tension Headache 191
   Diagnostic Tests in Headache... 196
   Analgesics and Headache 202
   Treatment of Migraine 202
      Pharmacologic Therapy 203
         Symptomatic Treatment 203
         Preventive Therapy 205
   Treatment of Tension Headache.. 209
   References 213

5

KNEE PAIN 216

The History 216
Physical Examination of the Knee 221
Localized Swellings and Tenderness 229
Patellofemoral Syndromes 233
    Treatment of Patellofemoral Syndromes 239
Traumatic Knee Pain 241
The Swollen Knee 255
    Arthrocentesis and Synovial Fluid Analysis 256
Monarthritis of the Knee 258
Appendix: Functional Knee Anatomy 265
References 271

6

FEMALE URINARY TRACT INFECTIONS 272

The Traditional Approach 272
Common UTI Syndromes 275
The Empiric Approach 280
The Individualized Approach 282
Initial Treatment of Suspected UTI 285
    Urine Cultures 288
    When the Patient with Acute UTI Does Not Improve 290
    Follow-up after Treatment 293
Recurrent UTI 293
    Prophylactic Antibiotics in Recurrent UTI 298
Appendix I: Acute Pyelonephritis 300
Appendix II: Localizing the Site of Infection 303
Appendix III: Economics of UTI 305
References 306

7

VULVOVAGINAL DISORDERS 310

Symptoms and Signs 310
The Initial Approach 311
Differential Diagnosis 313
Infectious Vaginitis 318
    Treatment of Trichomoniasis 324
    Treatment of Vaginal Candidiasis 327
    Recurrent Vaginal Candidiasis 329
Atrophic Vaginitis 333
Vulvar Pruritus 334
Appendix: Nonspecific Vaginitis 337
References 339

8

MALE GENITOURINARY INFECTIONS 341

Symptoms and Signs 342
Urethritis 349
    Gonococcal versus Nongonococcal Urethritis 350
    Treatment of Gonococcal Urethritis 353
    Treatment of Nongonococcal Urethritis 357
    Recurrent Nongonococcal Urethritis 360
Bacterial Urinary Infections 363
Recurrent Urinary Infections 365
    Prostatitis 366
        Localization Studies 367
    Summary 374
Appendix I: Urinary Symptoms and Fever 375
Appendix II: Syphilis: Tests and Treatment 378
Appendix III: "Personal" Diseases are Public Problems 382
References 384

9

SHOULDER PAIN 387

Initial Approach 387
Symptoms and Signs 388
    Examination of the Shoulder 393
Periarticular Shoulder Disorders 407
    Diagnosis 410
    Treatment 416
        Pain Relief 416
        Anti-Inflammatory Measures 417
        Injections 418
        Exercise Therapy 418
        When the Patient Does Not Improve 423
The Shoulder and the Hand 426
Practical Neurology of the Upper Extremity 431
Appendix I: Shoulder Biomechanics and Anatomy 441
Appendix II: Traumatic Shoulder Pain 447
Appendix III: Thoracic Outlet Syndromes 451
References 454

10

DIZZINESS 456

Classifying Dizziness 456
Dizziness Simulation Tests 461
Disequilibrium 463
(Pre)Syncope 471
    Common Causes 471
    General Approach 473
    Orthostatic Hypotension 478
    Diagnostic Categories of Syncope 480
    Neurologic Causes 481
    Cardiac Causes 483
Vertigo 486

Peripheral Versus Central Vertigo 486
Peripheral Vestibular Disease 493
Light-Headedness.. 502
Appendix I: Syncope: Is the Cause a Cardiac Arrhythmia?............... 509
Appendix II: Evaluation of Vestibular Function 512
Nystagmus 512
Nylen-Bárány Test 515
Caloric Testing 516
Appendix III: Auditory Testing.. 519
Bedside Hearing Tests 519
Technologic Testing.. 522
Appendix IV: Costs of Tests That May Be Useful in Evaluating
Dizziness.. 524
References 525

11

ABDOMINAL PAIN 528

Acute Abdominal Pain 530
History.. 530
Physical Examination 539
Tests 549
Acute Right Lower Quadrant Pain...................................... 560
Acute Right Upper Quadrant Pain...................................... 568
Chronic/Recurrent Abdominal Pain 575
Chronic/Recurrent Lower Abdominal Pain........................... 577
Presumptive Diagnosis and Treatment of Chronic
Lower Abdominal Pain 583
Chronic/Recurrent Upper Abdominal Pain........................... 594
Severe Central Abdominal Pain 608
Appendix: Ambulatory Treatment of Peptic Ulcer Disease............... 619
References 624

12

COUGH.. 628

Acute Cough.. 629
Initial Approach.. 629
Bronchitis versus Pneumonia 631
Treatment of Acute Bronchitis 638
When the Patient Does Not Improve......................... 640
Hemoptysis 642
Diagnosis of Pneumonia 643
Treatment of Pneumonia 657
Follow-up... 664
Chronic Cough.. 667
Appendix: The Worried Well 672
References 674

13

CHEST PAIN 677

Episodic (Recurrent) Chest Pain... 678
Typical Angina Pectoris... 682

Nonangina 687

"Compatible" Chest Pain... 693

Physical Examination 694

Chest Wall Syndromes 698

Tests and Chest Pain.. 705

Management of Angina Pectoris... 713

Drug Therapy 713

Coronary Artery Surgery 718

Patient Education 720

When to Worry, When to Refer, When to Hospitalize 725

Acute Severe Chest Pain.. 727

Acute Pleuritic Chest Pain 741

Appendix I: Exercise Testing and Chest Pain: Populations and
Persons 754

Appendix II: Esophageal Chest Pain 766

Appendix III: Psychosomatic Chest Pain 770

Appendix IV: Lung Scans and Pulmonary Embolism.................... 772

Reference 780

INDEX 785

1

LOW
BACK
PAIN

ACUTE LOW BACK PAIN........................... 1
    Initial Approach 1
    Physical Examination........................... 5
SIMPLE MECHANICAL BACK PAIN.................. 16
    Tests? 18
    Treatment 20
RADICULAR BACK PAIN 29
    Practical Neurology of the Low Back and Leg... 29
    Diagnosis and Treatment 34
CHRONIC LOW BACK PAIN 42
    Diagnosis...................................... 43
    Treatment 51
APPENDIX I: WHEN BACK PAIN IS DANGEROUS 54
APPENDIX II: COMPRESSION FRACTURES,
OSTEOPENIA, AND OSTEOPOROSIS 57
APPENDIX III: BACK PAIN AND BACK ANATOMY.... 61
APPENDIX IV: BACK MANIPULATION 66
REFERENCES....................................... 68

ACUTE LOW BACK PAIN

Initial Approach

> Dick Disc, a 42-year-old janitor, limps into the clinic complaining of back pain. The day before, while loading trash cans on a truck, he felt "something give way" in the lower back. The pain occurred immediately, and Dick could not straighten up for several minutes without severe pain. He was unable to continue working, had to be driven home, but rested comfortably in a reclining chair for the rest of the day and night. Upon arising this morning, he noted stiffness and persistent pain in the lower back, such that walking is difficult.
>
> Past medical history is unremarkable, but Dick admits to one prior episode of back pain very similar to his current problem about 2 years before, which resolved after several days of bedrest. Dick did not seek medical attention at that time, but does note mild intermittent back discomfort and stiffness, especially after a long day's work.

In every patient complaining of low back pain, three initial questions must be answered:

1. Where is the pain?

Low back pain means different things to different people. Always ask the patient to point with one finger to the area where he or she feels pain and to describe any spread or radiation of the pain. Most patients with low back pain localize their major discomfort to the lumbosacral area, in the midline or to one side. Such pain may "spread" to the thoracic (or cervical) spine as well as to the buttocks, abdomen, groin, or legs. When this is so, it

1

is usually easy to determine that the primary site of discomfort is the lumbosacral area, but specific areas of pain radiation should also raise specific differential diagnostic possibilities (see below and Fig. 1–1).

A primary pain site above the level of the T12 vertebra suggests disease processes different from those discussed here.

2. Is the back pain acute or chronic?

The sudden onset of acute low back pain may result from disorders as diverse as a dissecting aortic aneurysm or a herniated intervertebral disc. Careful history and physical examination will always narrow the differential diagnosis (see below).

Chronic or intermittently recurrent low back pain deserves a different emphasis (see "Chronic Low Back Pain" below).

3. Is the pain mechanical or nonmechanical?

Most low back pain is due to disorders of the spine or the paraspinal structures. Disease of the intervertebral discs, spinal articulations (facet

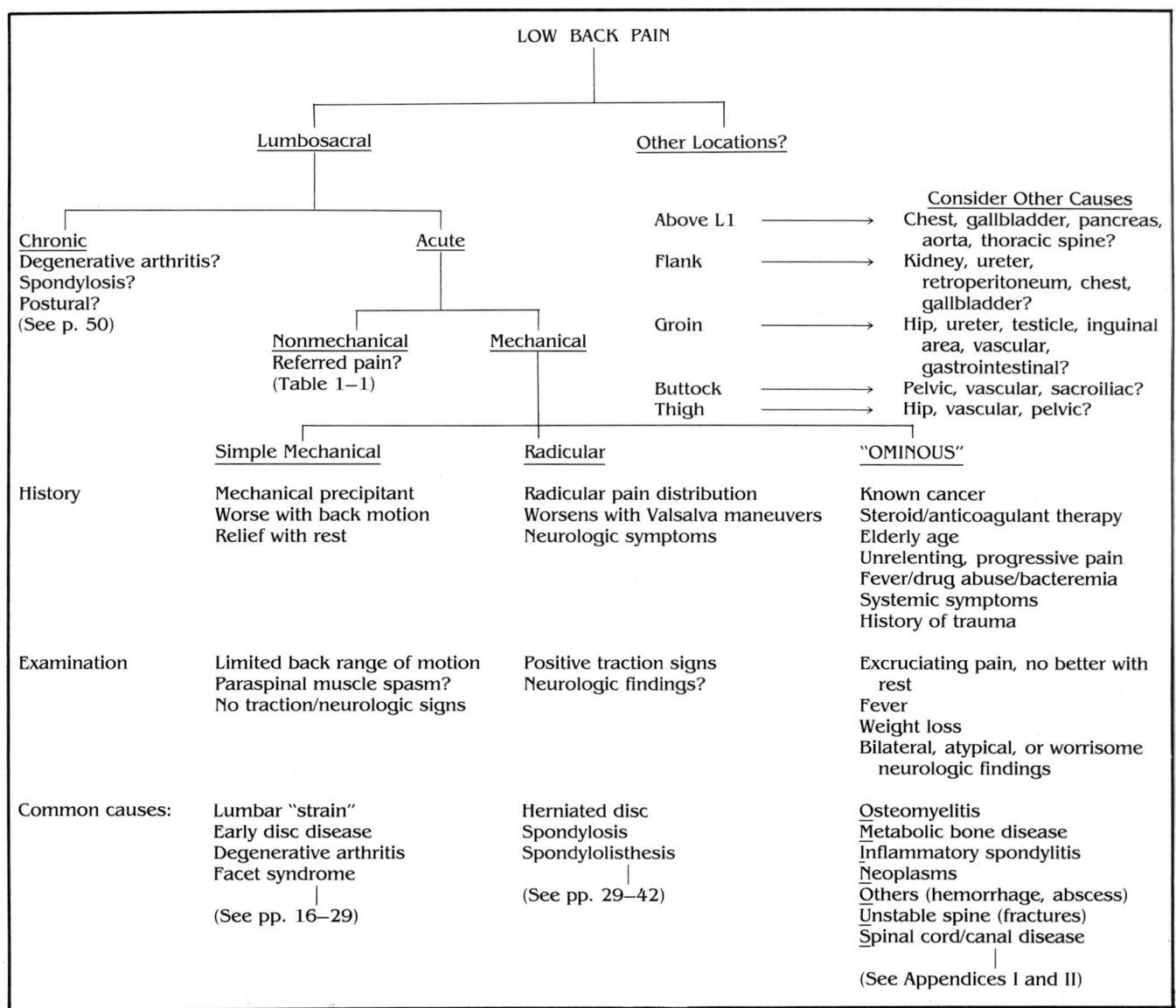

FIGURE 1–1. Diagnosis of low back pain.

joints), spinal ligaments, or paraspinal musculature, singly or combined, comprises the great majority. Occasionally, however, back pain is the initial manifestation of extraspinal disorders—the back pain is "referred" from a variety of intra-abdominal, pelvic, or other sites. In general, pelvic disorders refer pain to the sacral area; intra-abdominal and retroperitoneal disorders refer pain to the lumbar area.

Most local (spinal) back pain disorders are mechanical, i.e., are symptomatically related to the mechanical function of the lower spine: The pain begins after a specific mechanical event (bending, lifting, falling, twisting); the pain is aggravated by mechanical stress, i.e., back movements; or the pain improves by preventing mechanical stress, i.e., bedrest. On the other hand, most referred low back pain is not mechanical. As seen in Table 1–1, many of the causes of referred low back pain are serious, even life-threatening, diseases; hence the crucial importance of early suspicion that acute back pain is not mechanical but referred.

(This distinction between mechanical and nonmechanical back pain is somewhat artificial. Not all mechanical back disorders are precipitated by an identifiable mechanical event, nor is such back pain always reproduced by mechanical testing of the lower back (see page 7). Similarly, nonmechanical disorders may have superficially mechanical features: Diseases of the pancreas, kidney, hip, or pelvis may cause symptoms that vary in different bodily positions or that may cause secondary paraspinal muscle spasm, thus mimicking mechanical disease. Most of the time, however, this distinction between mechanical and nonmechanical back pain is both obvious and useful.)

Once acute low back pain is recognized to be mechanical, the diagnostic and therapeutic approach is simplified because the history and examination

TABLE 1–1. NONMECHANICAL OR REFERRED LOW BACK PAIN

Gastrointestinal disorders
  Colorectal carcinoma
  Gastric carcinoma
  Pancreatic carcinoma
  Retrocecal (or pelvic) appendicitis
  Pancreatitis
  Diverticulitis
  Irritable bowel
  Peptic ulcer (posterior penetration)

Retroperitoneal disorders
  Aortic dissection
  Abdominal aortic aneurysm
  Retroperitoneal tumor, bleeding, abscess
  Renal or ureteral colic/carcinoma

Gynecologic
  Endometriosis
  Uterine myomas
  Gynecologic carcinomas
  Uterine or ectopic pregancy
  Pelvic infection
  Ovarian cyst/torsion
  Menstruation

Others
  Prostatitis, acute or chronic
  Prostatic carcinoma
  Incipient herpes zoster

alone will usually then distinguish among the three general subsets of mechanical low back pain (Fig. 1–1). These include:

I. "OMINOUS" low back pain.

This heterogeneous group of "serious spinal" disorders can be remembered by the mnemonic OMINOUS: Osteomyelitis, Metabolic bone disease, Inflammatory disease (spondylitis, sacroiliitis), Neoplasm, Others (abscess, local hemorrhage), Unstable spine (for example, due to fractures or spondylolisthesis), and Spinal canal disease (cord compression, cauda equina lesions, primary neurologic tumors). Historical clues that should suggest OMINOUS disease include:

A. A history of prior malignant disease or systemic symptoms suggestive of cancer (weight loss, anorexia, hemoptysis, and the like).
B. A history of fever, bacteremia, or parenteral drug abuse—pyogenic vertebral osteomyelitis may occur without any of these features (see Appendix I), but this history is important.
C. Corticosteroid therapy (or other predispositions to metabolic bone disease or compression fractures (see Appendix II).
D. Anticoagulant therapy (see Appendix I).
E. Elderly age—serious disease is found more commonly among the elderly with low back pain[1] (and only rarely in the young).
F. Back pain that is very severe, unrelenting, progressively worsening, and unrelieved by bedrest.
G. Severe trauma.

II. Radicular back pain.

Back pain that is associated with leg or foot pain or both, especially when pain is described as shooting, sharp and dysesthetic (numb, tingling, "electric"); or that worsens with Valsalva maneuvers (cough, sneeze, strain); or that is associated with lower extremity weakness, sensory disturbances, or bowel and bladder dysfunction must suggest back pain with accompanying neurologic impairment. The neurologic examination is obviously crucial here. There are many types of radicular back pain—often called sciatica; these are discussed below (see page 29).

III. Simple mechanical back pain.

Simple mechanical back pain is by far the most common subset of problems. Such patients have acute "mechanical" back pain without neurologic symptoms or signs and without evidence for OMINOUS diseases. Most patients suffer from lumbar strains (musculoligamentous tears or sprains), early disc disease (without nerve root involvement), or disorders of the facet joints (usually due to degenerative arthritis). It is often impossible to distinguish clinically among these various types of simple mechanical back pain, but their treatment is usually similar (see page 16).

CONSIDER AGAIN OUR PATIENT

Dick localizes his pain in the midline at the level of the lumbosacral junction. There is associated discomfort in the left buttock and upper posterior area of the thigh but no neurologic symptoms, radiation of pain below the knees, other symptoms referable to the abdomen, or genitourinary or gastrointestinal symptoms. Dick has always been healthy, takes no medications, and denies trauma, fever, or any constitutional symptoms. Cough and Valsalva maneuvers do not affect the pain.

Dick's prior episode of back pain 2 years before was similar but not so severe and remitted after several days without treatment. Intermittently since then, he notes occasional (perhaps monthly) vague "tiredness" in the lower back after a long day's work, but he denies chronic low back pain.

Dick's major concern is "how to get back on my feet as soon as possible since they won't pay me if I am laid up, and I can't work like this." There is no history of medical disability, compensation litigation, alcoholism, or frequent work absences.

NOTE

1. The pain is acute, localized to the lumbosacral area, and appears to have been precipitated by mechanical stress. These features suggest a simple mechanical lumbosacral disorder.

Sudden severe low back pain that occurs at rest and without any obvious mechanical cause merits great caution: Pathologic compression fractures, abdominal aortic aneurysms, ruptured intra-abdominal viscus, spinal vascular accidents, and ectopic pregnancy must be remembered in this setting.

2. The pain worsens with mechanical stress (walking, bending) and is better with bedrest. Again, mechanical back pain is likely. Referred or nonmechanical low back pain will either remain constant or vary with gastrointestinal, genitourinary, or other functions, depending on the precise source of pain. Occasionally, vascular claudication or "neurogenic claudication" (see page 49) will cause symptoms that episodically recur with exertion and remit with rest, but the character and distribution of this pain are distinctive from those of most mechanical back pain.

Acute low back pain that does not improve with bedrest, or that progressively worsens in spite of bedrest, must raise one's clinical suspicion of either referred pain or OMINOUS mechanical pain.

3. The history does not otherwise suggest either neurologic involvement or OMINOUS disease. The pain does involve the buttock and thigh, but back pain that does not compromise any neurologic structures is often referred into these areas; however, such referred muscular pain rarely, if ever, extends below the knee. True radicular pain tends to be sharp, lancinating, or electric, often is associated with numbness and paresthesias, and usually travels below the knee.

Similarly, there are no historical clues that suggest OMINOUS disease (see Fig. 1–1).

Thus the history here suggests simple mechanical back pain. Physical examination must now confirm or refute this impression.

Physical Examination

There are five components in the examination of the patient with low back pain. These include:

I. Observation
II. Back range of motion
III. Palpation of the spine and paraspinal structures
IV. Traction maneuvers
V. Neurologic examination

I. Observation.

The examination begins when the patient first confronts the clinician. Much can be learned simply by observing the patient's posture, general appearance, and gait.

The patient who sits comfortably and calmly discusses his back pain is unlikely to be suffering from an acute mechanical disorder. Many patients with acute mechanical pain are least comfortable when seated, so much so that one authority believes that "arrival in a wheelchair should inspire caution."[2] The supine position is usually most comfortable.

Patients with severe muscle spasm or radicular back pain often move cautiously, sometimes listing awkwardly to one side, and yet often pace the examining room, unable to sit still in spite of their obvious discomfort when standing or walking. When sitting, such patients may sprawl in peculiar positions—one or both legs extended at the hip, the buttocks at the edge of the seat.

The patient should be completely undressed. Evidence of weight loss or chronic illness should be noted. Obesity, paunchiness, poor muscle tone or posture, and the presence or absence of back/pelvic tilting or asymmetry should be recorded. Figure 1–2 illustrates normal posture and the postures that increase lumbar lordosis due to weakened abdominal musculature, obesity, or both. Figure 1–2 also illustrates the

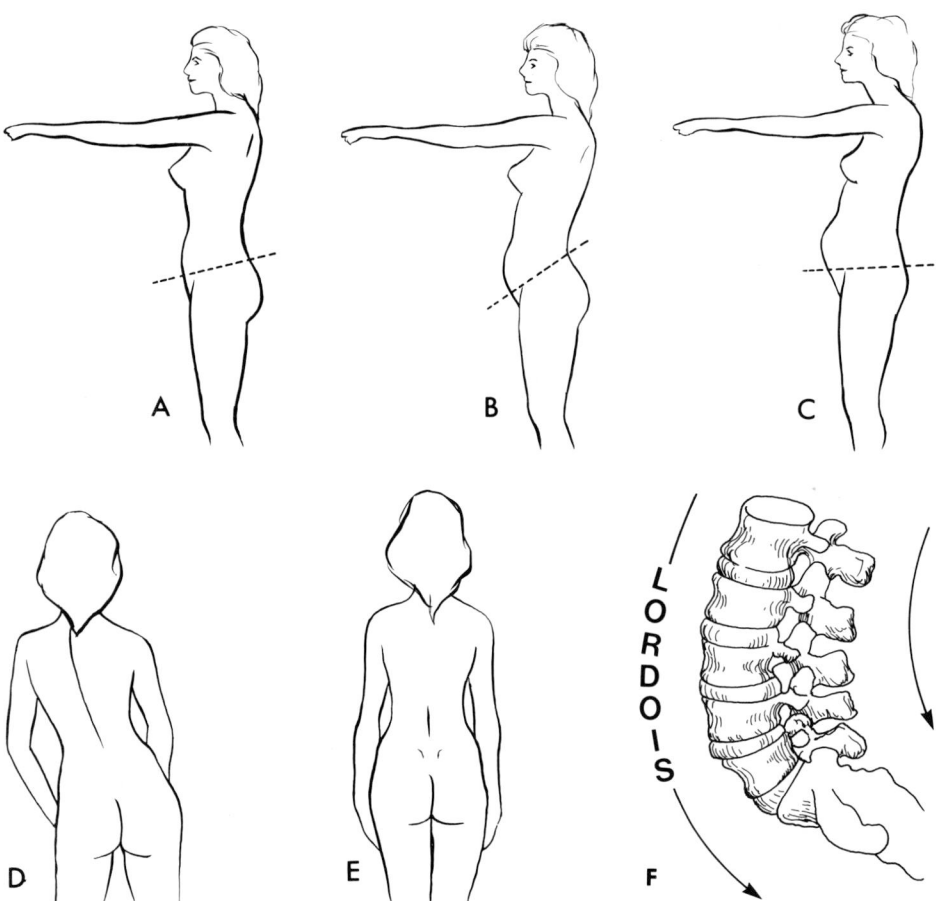

FIGURE 1–2. *A,* Normal posture with normal lumbar lordosis. *B,* Exaggerated lumbar lordosis due to pelvic tilting. *C,* "Paunchy" posture. *D,* Spastic scoliosis due to muscle spasm. *E,* Normal posture without scoliosis. *F,* The <u>normal orientation</u> of the lumbar spine is that of mild lordosis. Exaggerated lordosis may predispose the patient to mechanical back pain.

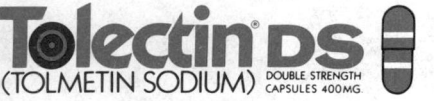

Tolectin® DS
(TOLMETIN SODIUM) DOUBLE STRENGTH CAPSULES 400MG.

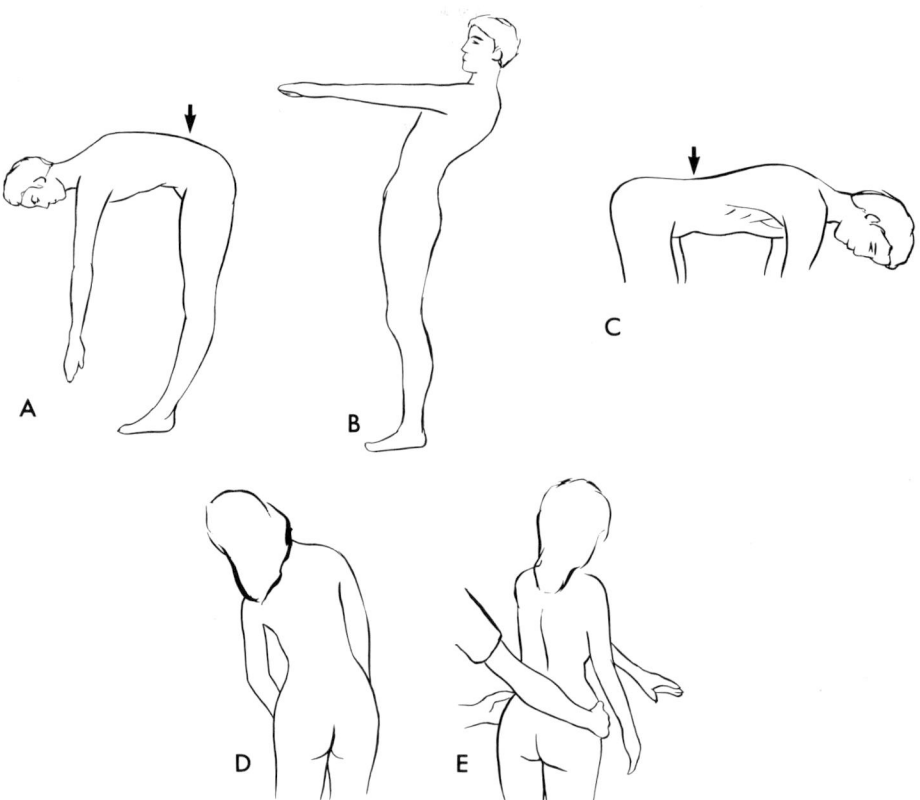

FIGURE 1–3. Back range of motion. A, Flexion—note the normal reversal of lumbar lordosis during flexion (arrow). B, Extension. C, Persistent lordosis during back flexion due to muscle spasm (arrow). D, Lateral flexion. E, Lateral torsion (rotation).

"spastic scoliosis"* due to asymmetric paraspinal muscle spasm, which may be caused by any of a variety of mechanical back disorders.

The patient's attitude toward his own complaint deserves attention. Recognition that the patient is stoical, dramatically overreactive, worried, anxious, depressed, or afraid will be helpful in assessing the patient's response to illness and pain. Most patients with acute mechanical back pain describe their symptoms concisely and precisely; patients whose symptoms are vague, inconsistent, or histrionic may have more complicated problems, but careful examination and repeated questioning will usually distinguish significant "organic" problems from "functional" disorders[3] (see below and page 51).

II. Back range of motion (Fig. 1–3).

Assessing the mobility of the back is the most important "test" for mechanical back disorders. Because there is such wide variation among individuals of different ages in the flexibility of low back movements, the exact quantitation of motion in different planes of movement is not as helpful as is this simple observation: Is back pain precipitated or exacerbated during back range of motion? If so, there is usually at least some "mechanical" component to the problem. If not, the mechanical disorder is either very mild (or has resolved) or the back pain is not mechanical at all—here referred pain or functional back pain should be considered again.

*"Spastic scoliosis"—due to muscle spasm—is very different from structural scoliosis of the spine.

With the patient standing, flexion of the back with the knees extended should be observed: Motion limited by stiffness or pain must be noted, as must failure to reverse the normal lumbar lordosis (Fig. 1–3C) during flexion (usually implying paravertebral muscle spasm or excessive anatomic spinal lordosis or both). If measurement is desirable, the distance from the patient's outstretched fingers to the floor is easy to record. (The Schober test is conveniently performed here as well, but this is a test more often helpful in patients with chronic low back pain—see page 43 and Fig. 1–21).

Back extension simply further tenses paralumbar musculature and thus usually intensifies simple mechanical back pain. Back extension may occasionally exacerbate specific disorders and thus suggest specific diseases. Referred pain from the retroperitoneum (retroperitoneal hemorrhage or abscess, appendicitis) may worsen with back extension, as may mechanical back pain due to facet joint disease (page 47) or (rarely) a high lumbar disc (above L3).

Lateral flexion and torsion may also be restricted by simple paralumbar muscle spasm, but usually less so than are flexion and extension.

(When radicular pain is present—usually due to disc disease [see page 35]—some examiners suggest that the location of a herniated intervertebral disc can be suspected on the basis of the response of the patient's radicular back pain to the direction of lateral flexion or torsion which worsens that pain. Disc herniations medial to the affected nerve root tend to produce more pain as the patient bends away from the affected side (see Fig. 1–20B); discs that herniate lateral to the nerve root tend to worsen as the patient bends toward the affected side.)

Most patients with acute mechanical back disorders have limited (or painful) back range of motion.

III. Palpation of the spine and paraspinal structures (Fig. 1–4).

Often palpation is not very enlightening. Nevertheless, familiarity with the palpable anatomy is important because:

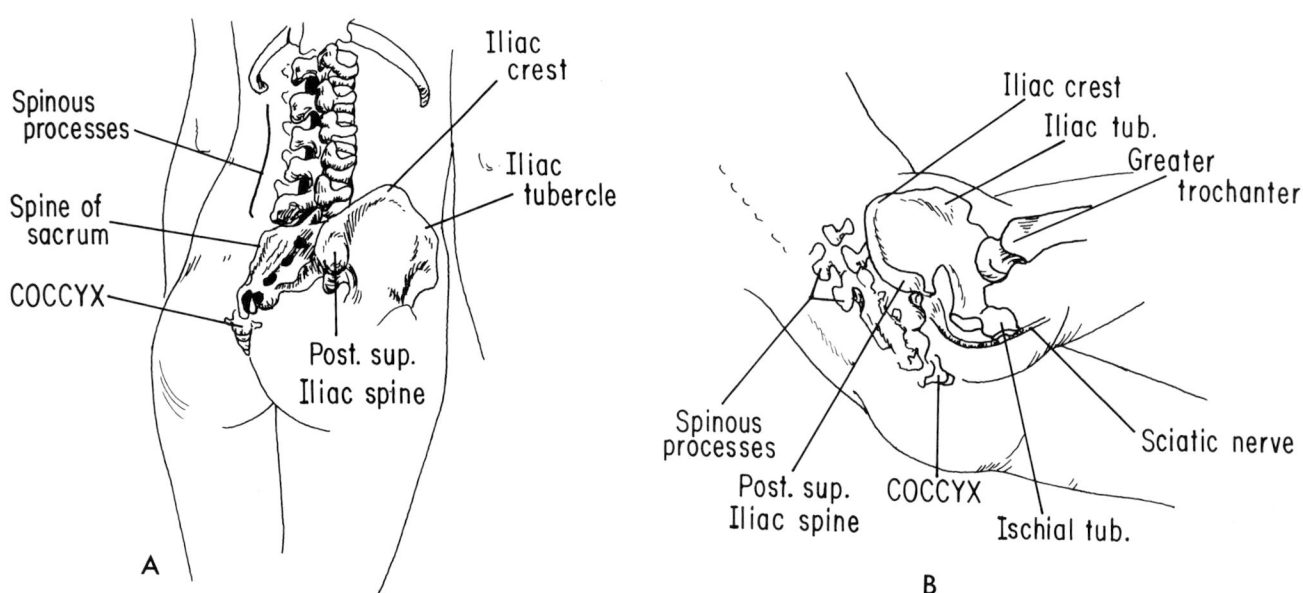

FIGURE 1–4. Palpable structures of the lumbosacral spine and pelvis. *A*, Patient upright. *B*, Patient recumbent on left side.

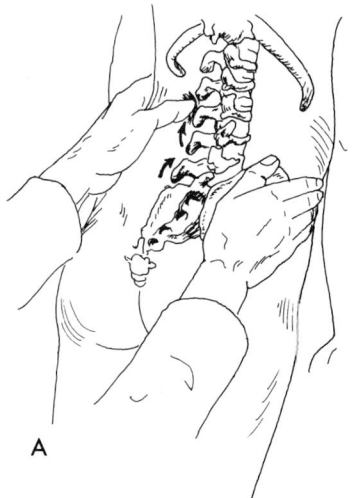
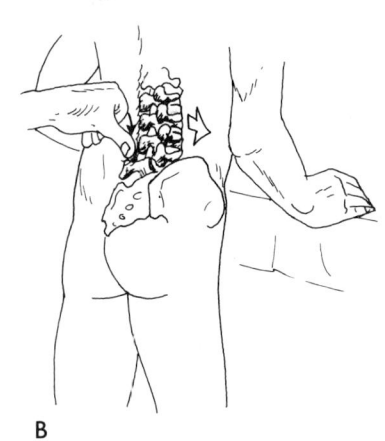
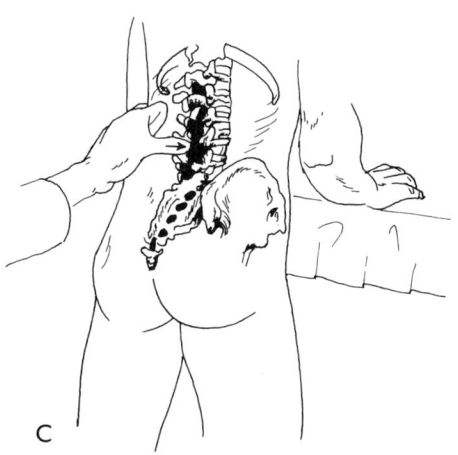

A   B   C

FIGURE 1–5. *A,* Palpation of normal spinous processes. *B,* Spondylolisthesis—the lower spinous process appears posteriorly displaced. *C,* The palpable "gap" sometimes apparent in patients with spina bifida. (See also Fig. 1–25).

A. Occasionally, specific diseases will be suggested by palpable abnormalities (Fig. 1–5).

Palpation of the spinous processes may reveal: a "shelf" where the superior spinous process seems anteriorly displaced on the subjacent inferior process—suggesting spondylolisthesis; an unexplained widening or "gap" between processes—suggesting spina bifida; or an angular lumbar kyphosis—suggesting a compression fracture with anterior concavity of the lumbar spine (the reverse of Fig. 1–2*F*).

Excruciating point tenderness of a bony process of the spine may suggest an inflammatory or destructive process (fracture, neoplasm, infection), but local tenderness is a nonspecific finding frequently seen in patients without such OMINOUS disease.

Palpable paravertebral muscle spasm (unilateral or bilateral) is usually evidence of a local mechanical back derangement.

Some authorities[4] believe that "trigger points" are common and therapeutically important findings in mechanical back pain. These trigger points are areas of reproducible point tenderness that may feel hard or nodular and that are located in deep subcutaneous or muscular tissues. Palpation of these areas is said to trigger the patient's pain, which may then be ameliorated by local injections or massage. Trigger points are rarely prominent findings in acute mechanical back pain in my experience (but may be more important in the patient with chronic back pain).

B. Other "nonspinal" structures should be palpated, especially when back pain is accompanied by buttock, hip, or leg pain.

The coccyx, pelvic bones, ischial tuberosity, hip trochanter, sciatic notch, and rectum should be examined (Fig. 1–4*B*).

Coccydynia refers to pain and tenderness of the coccyx, which most often follows a fall on the buttocks. Manipulation of the coccyx reproduces the pain.

Rarely, neoplasms or inflammatory lesions of the pelvic bones will cause back pain.

Ischial bursitis (weaver's bottom) causes back, buttock, and leg pain but is reproduced by palpation of the ischial tuberosity and improves with anti-inflammatory drugs or local injections or both.

Trochanteric bursitis is a common cause of hip and back pain, especially in the middle-aged or older patient—pain is worse with sudden movements of the leg or the initiation of walking, but the greater trochanter is usually tender and either oral or injectable anti-inflammatory measures are curative.

The sciatic notch runs between the ischial tuberosity and greater trochanter—various forms of "sciatica" may be associated with tenderness here.

Rectal (or pelvic) examination (or both) should always be performed whenever back pain is puzzling, not clearly mechanical, or when the patient is elderly. Prostate, rectal, and gynecologic malignancies will occasionally present with low back/buttock pain.

C. Sometimes x-rays of a specifically localized area are needed (when pain or tenderness is extremely localized).

Familiarity with local palpable anatomy will facilitate intelligent x-ray requests: Note that the L4-5 interspace lies at the same level as the tops of the iliac crests, while the S2 spinous process lies on the middle of a line drawn between the two posterior superior iliac spines (Fig. 1–4).

Most patients with acute mechanical back disorders will have no palpable abnormality beyond (perhaps) paravertebral muscle spasm.

IV. Traction maneuvers.

Straight leg raising (Fig. 1–6) is a maneuver that attempts to demonstrate or exclude disorders that produce lumbosacral nerve root compression.[5-8] This test is diagnostically valuable only when performed, recorded, and interpreted according to stringent guidelines.

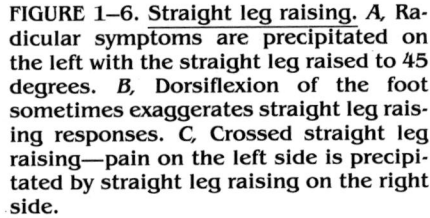

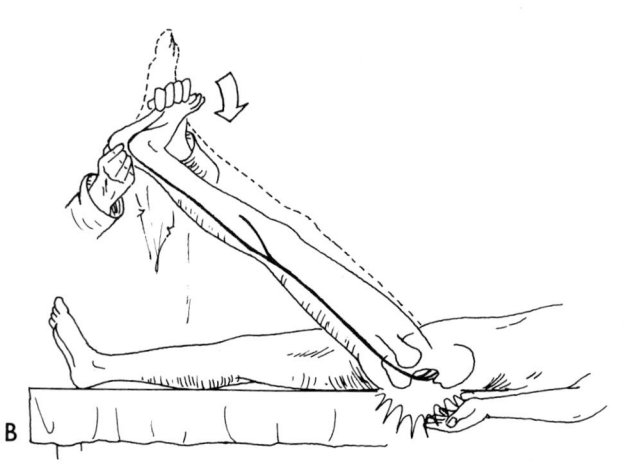

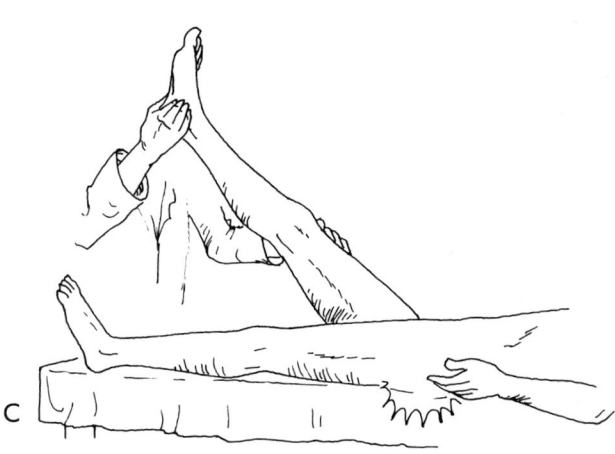

FIGURE 1–6. Straight leg raising. *A,* Radicular symptoms are precipitated on the left with the straight leg raised to 45 degrees. *B,* Dorsiflexion of the foot sometimes exaggerates straight leg raising responses. *C,* Crossed straight leg raising—pain on the left side is precipitated by straight leg raising on the right side.

With the patient supine and the opposite leg flat to the examining table (to prevent pelvic rotation during the maneuver), each leg is passively elevated (flexed at the hip) with the knee fully extended. This maneuver elicits traction on lower lumbosacral nerve roots (primarily L5 and S1), which are themselves lined by pain-sensitive dura mater as they exit the spinal canal via the intervertebral foramina (see Fig. 1–38). When these nerve roots are compressed, inflamed, or otherwise irritated, straight leg traction will induce pain along the distribution of these nerve roots.

Positive straight leg raising refers to the reproducible induction of radicular (leg or foot) pain when the straight leg is raised to between 30 degrees and 60 degrees of elevation. Each leg should be tested and compared with the other. Positive straight leg raising, when so defined, is highly suggestive of nerve root compression (and positive "crossed straight leg raising"—Fig. 1–6C—is virtually diagnostic). When straight leg raising appears to worsen local back pain but does not induce radicular pain involving the leg or foot, no specific conclusions can be drawn.

NOTE

A. Straight leg raising "stretches" many structures other than nerve roots.

Spinal extensor muscles, spinal ligaments, pelvic structures, and the hamstring muscles and tendons may also be sources of discomfort during (or limitation of) straight leg raising. The assumption that positive straight leg raising indicates nerve root involvement depends on: the radicular nature of the pain elicited (shooting, burning, tingling pain extending below the knee) and the precipitation of pain primarily at leg elevations between 30 and 60 degrees. Pain that begins beyond 60 degrees of leg elevation is nonspecific (hamstring tightness is common here), while leg elevation to less than 30 degrees does not usually significantly stretch nerve roots (thus, for example, pain at only 10 degrees elevation is "peculiar").*

Remember that nerve root pain may occur at any or all points along the course of the nerve. For example, L5 nerve root pain may be felt along the entire course of the nerve (from the buttock and thigh into the lateral aspect of the calf and foot) or (occasionally) only at one distal location without intervening pain (for example, only in the calf and foot—see Table 1–6 and Fig. 1–10). Reproducible precipitation of lateral calf and foot pain on straight leg raising (between 30 degrees and 60 degrees) is a "positive" finding, even if back pain per se does not worsen.

The main distinction that must be made is between true radicular pain and referred muscular pain. Referred muscular pain "never" extends below the knee, tends to be most prominent beyond 60 degrees of leg elevation, and usually "sounds" nonradicular ("tight" and "stretched" rather than sharp, shooting, or tingling).

B. In general, it is best not to equivocate about the results of straight leg raising: Attempt to categorize the maneuver as positive or negative in all patients.

---

*A few patients with severe sciatica (especially those with very large disc herniations or free fragments) will develop pain between 0 and 30° elevation, but this is not common.

Additional maneuvers that stretch the nerve roots may be helpful here. Simultaneous dorsiflexion of the foot or flexion of the neck during straight leg raising may further stretch the involved nerve roots (Fig. 1–6B). Voluntary Valsalva maneuvers during straight leg raising may be helpful in a few equivocal cases.

The "flip sign" should always be elicited. Here, straight leg raising is performed with the patient in a sitting position (and unaware of the examiner's intent). Figure 1–7 illustrates positive and negative flip signs. While apparently examining the patient's foot, pulses, or calves, the examiner gradually passively extends the patient's knee and notes the patient's postural response while sitting. Achievement of 60 to 90 degrees back/hip flexion with the knee fully extended and without postural adjustment constitutes a negative flip sign and casts doubt on "positive" straight leg raising elicited in the supine position (Fig. 1–7B). When the patient is forced to fall back to prevent such full straight leg raising in the sitting position, this positive flip sign adds credence to a positive straight leg raising test in the supine position (Fig. 1–7A).

C. Negative straight leg raising does not always mean that nerve roots are spared.

Unusual nerve root lesions above the level of L4 will not be associated with positive straight leg raising. In such instances, reverse straight leg raising (Fig. 1–7C) may elicit radicular pain in the anterior part of the thigh. Such atypical radicular pain is discussed further below (and is always a cause for concern—see Table 1–6).

Young patients with nerve root compression due to disc herniation (by far, the most common cause of lumbosacral root disease—Table 1–6) almost always demonstrate positive traction signs.[5] This is not always so in the elderly, perhaps in part because lumbosacral

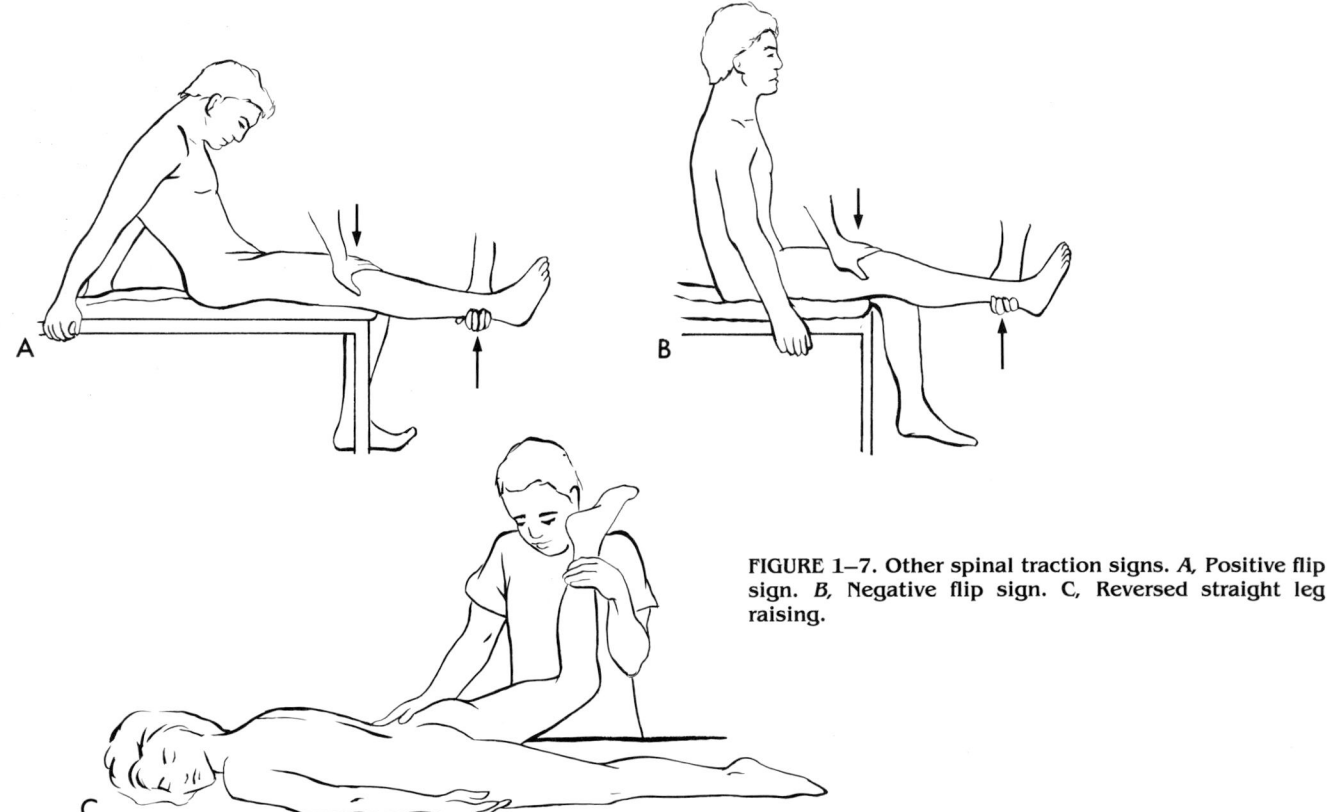

FIGURE 1–7. Other spinal traction signs. A, Positive flip sign. B, Negative flip sign. C, Reversed straight leg raising.

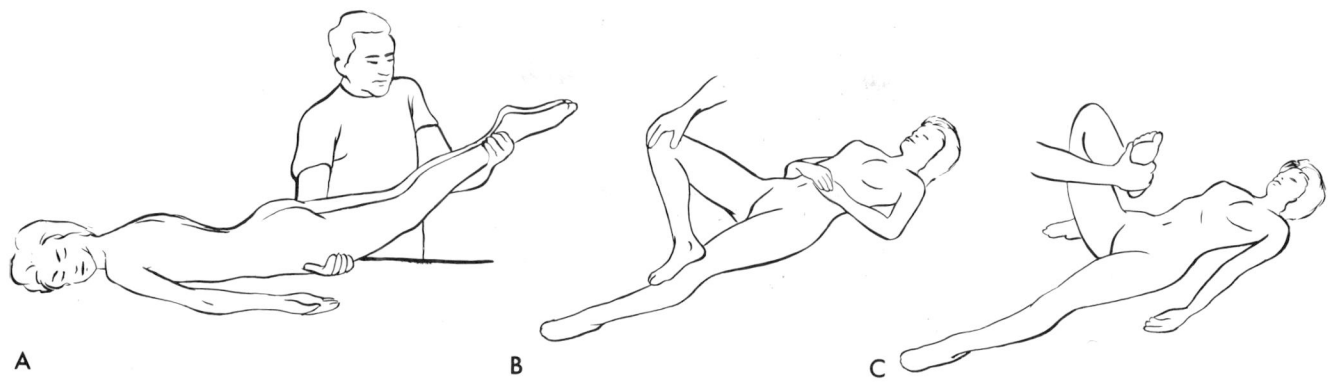

A   B   C

FIGURE 1–8. A, Yeoman's test. B, Patrick's test. C, Laguerre's test.

spondylosis (see page 47) may cause root involvement without positive traction signs, and spondylosis is a more common cause of radicular back pain in the elderly than is simple disc herniation.

Before the neurologic examination is discussed, a few other "traction maneuvers" should be noted (Figs. 1–8 and 1–9).

Yeoman's test involves stabilizing the pelvis and extending each hip in turn, with the patient in the prone position (similar to reverse straight leg raising—Fig. 1–7C). Unilateral hyperextension usually just exacerbates the discomfort of lumbosacral mechanical disorders. When mechanical back pain is mild or when other ranges of motion appear normal, simultaneous bilateral hip extension (Fig. 1–8A) will reproduce pain—this is helpful since one hopes to confirm on examination that back pain is indeed "mechanical" (page 3).

Patrick's test requires placement of the heel on the opposite knee, and then lateral force is exerted on both leg and knee toward the examining table (hip abduction). This maneuver usually is painful when hip or sacroiliac disease is present.

Laguerre's test is more specific for hip disease than Patrick's test. Here the heel is held by the examiner who rotates the hip internally and externally with the knee flexed.

Gaenslen's test is more specific for sacroiliac disease. Here, the supine patient is asked to draw both legs up to the chest and then to

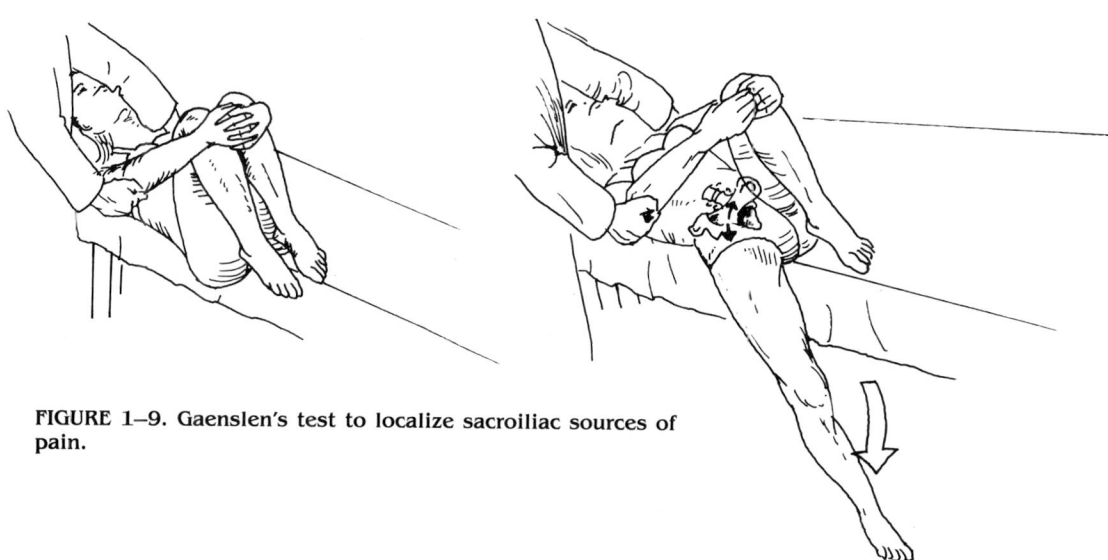

FIGURE 1–9. Gaenslen's test to localize sacroiliac sources of pain.

allow one unsupported leg to hang over the edge of the table. This is then repeated on the opposite side. Resulting pain is usually localized to the sacroiliac joint on the side of the extended hip (the sacroiliac joint is "opened up"—Fig. 1–9, arrows).

V. Neurologic Examination

A neurologic examination of the lower extremities should be performed on all patients with low back pain.

When radicular pain is present, or neurologic dysfunction is suspected for other reasons, the neurologic examination obviously must be careful and thorough. A complete (but time-consuming) neurologic examination is discussed in greater detail below (page 29).

Extensive neurologic examination is almost never fruitful if the history and traction maneuvers do not suggest nerve root or other neurologic compromise. Even when this is the case, however, a brief screening neurologic examination is simple and well worth the effort. The screening examination should include:

A. Rule out "long tract signs"—extensor plantar responses (Babinski reflexes) or spasticity does not result from spinal lesions below the L1-2 level since the spinal cord ends at L1 or L2. Such long tract signs, then, imply different problems from those discussed here.

B. Rule out cauda equina involvement—this serious problem may be quite subtle (see page 37), but perineal and sacral sensation (and anorectal tone) should be quickly tested, especially in patients with low back pain that involves both buttocks or both legs.

C. Since the great majority of neurologic problems associated with low back pain involve the roots of the sciatic nerve, familiarity with the pattern of radicular pain, sensorimotor impairment, and reflex changes appropriate to lesions of the L4, L5, and S1 nerve roots is essential.

Figure 1–10 summarizes these findings (see also page 29). Since objective findings may be subtle, extensive experience with the normal neurologic examination is crucial if significant neurologic lesions are to be discovered early. (Note, for example, that the very common L4-5 disc protrusion may result in minimal or no reflex or sensory changes and that motor weakness may be confined entirely to the extensor muscle of the big toe.)

All patients with low back pain, then, should undergo a screening neurologic examination that includes testing of the knee and ankle jerk reflexes; Babinski reflexes; gross sensory testing (touch) of the perineum; and brief motor testing of dorsiflexion, eversion, and inversion of the foot, and dorsiflexion of the big toe. This brief examination can be done very quickly in most patients.

CONSIDER NOW THE EXAMINATION OF OUR PATIENT

Dick is clearly uncomfortable and prefers not to sit down. He stands while he describes his problem, slightly bent at the waist, his left knee slightly flexed and not bearing full weight. He tries to suppress visible facial expressions of discomfort and tends to minimize his pain. He is afebrile, looks healthy but is paunchy.

While he is standing, the lumbar spine is straight (without normal lordosis), and flexion of the back is limited, painful, and does not "round out" the lower back (there is no reversal of the lumbar lordosis—see Fig.

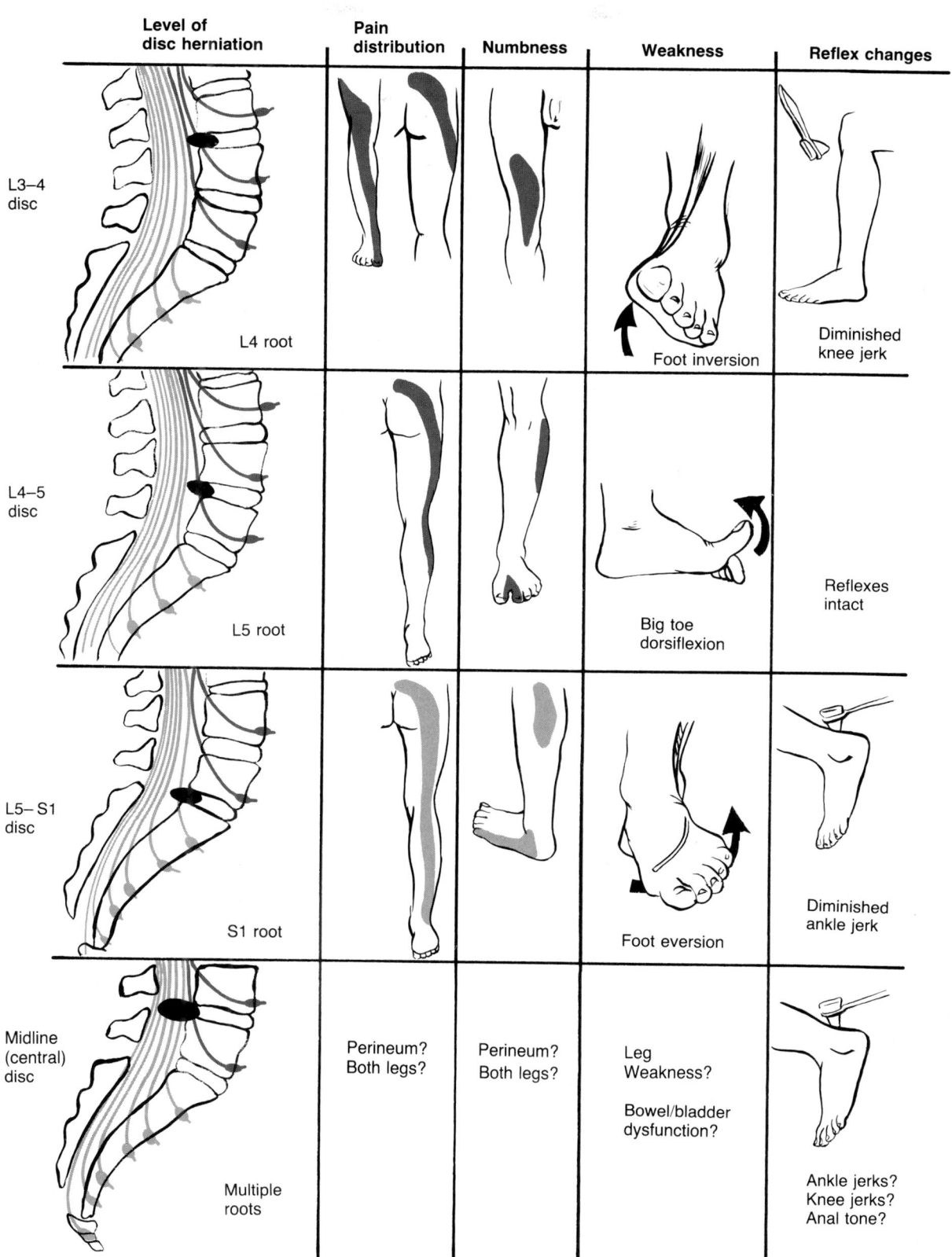

Level of disc herniation	Pain distribution	Numbness	Weakness	Reflex changes
L3–4 disc / L4 root			Foot inversion	Diminished knee jerk
L4–5 disc / L5 root			Big toe dorsiflexion	Reflexes intact
L5–S1 disc / S1 root			Foot eversion	Diminished ankle jerk
Midline (central) disc / Multiple roots	Perineum? Both legs?	Perineum? Both legs?	Leg Weakness? Bowel/bladder dysfunction?	Ankle jerks? Knee jerks? Anal tone?

FIGURE 1–10. Common disc syndromes: neurologic findings.

1–3C). Back and left buttock pain limits back flexion at about 30 degrees; lateral flexion and torsion are less uncomfortable, and back extension is limited, but "feels even a little better that way."

Palpation of the spine, pelvis, and hips is unremarkable, except for palpable paravertebral muscle spasm, more prominent on the left. In the supine position, Dick "feels a little better," and brief examination of the abdomen, groin, pulses, and hips is normal.

Straight leg raising is normal to 60 degrees bilaterally, beyond which point back and thigh discomfort occur, and the hamstrings "feel tight." The flip sign is negative in the sitting position, Yeoman's test "makes it feel a little better." A screening neurologic examination is normal.

What does this mean?

Physical examination confirms the initial impression that this is simple mechanical low back pain, i.e., the pain "sounds mechanical," it is aggravated by back range of motion and is associated with paravertebral muscle spasm. There are no suspicions of OMINOUS disease. The neurologic examination and traction signs are unremarkable, thus excluding radiculopathy.

This is by far the most common type of low back pain and is in fact a major public health problem.[9-13]

SIMPLE MECHANICAL LOW BACK PAIN

For many years following Mixter and Barr's report in 1934[14] of successful surgical repair in patients with the syndrome of disc herniation, lumbosacral disc disease dominated clinical perspectives on low back pain.[15] Most early studies of patients with low back pain, however, dealt with hospitalized patients whose illness was severe or refractory enough to warrant the attention of orthopaedic or neurologic specialists. Several more recent studies in primary care settings emphasize that most acute low back pain is diagnostically nonspecific and is either self-limited or responds well to simple conservative treatment.[16-20] (These studies emphasize that we have much to learn about low back pain—most such "soft tissue injuries" are difficult to study.) Some orthopaedists or chiropractors of long experience may have the clinical acumen to distinguish among musculoligamentous strains, facet joint imbalances, and "non-neurologic" disc herniations (see below)—which together probably comprise the majority of simple mechanical acute back pains—but most of us are not so capable. A "nonspecific" clinical diagnosis of simple mechanical back pain is often the best we can do, but this is usually adequate to institute effective treatment (see below).

A few clinical points may be of interest:

1. The young or middle-aged person whose first episode of acute low back pain follows some obvious mechanical event (lifting, for example) usually suffers from a musculoligamentous "strain" (see Appendix III). Occasionally such a patient will describe a sudden unilateral "catch" in the lower back such that further back motion is suddenly restricted and painful. This, too, is most often a simple strain but may at times be the result of a subluxated facet joint—while this diagnosis is difficult to confirm, back manipulation may be worth a try in this setting (see Appendix IV).

2. Acute disc herniations[21-23] usually afflict the young or middle-aged. Intradiscal pressure studies[24] suggest that the nucleus pulposus acts as a liquid

confined within the disc by fibers of the surrounding anulus fibrosus (see Appendix III). The lumbosacral spine is subjected to great mechanical stresses during daily living, such that intradiscal pressures may exceed the retentive forces of the anulus fibrosus. Figure 1–11 illustrates that this may result in disc "bulges" (concealed herniations) that remain confined within the anulus fibrosus, or disc "prolapses" in which nuclear material, fragments of the anulus itself, or both actually rupture (usually posterolaterally—toward the spinal cord and nerve roots—since the posterior anulus is most vulnerable to high intradiscal pressures. See also Figs. 1–20 and 1–38).

Disc herniation is thus a heterogeneous set of problems—some only bulge, some prolapse, some compress neural structures, but some do not. Many disc herniations are probably entirely asymptomatic.[26] The syndrome (if any) produced by disc herniation will depend on the type, size, and location of disc bulge or prolapse, as well as on the integrity of surrounding ligamentous support, local anatomy of exiting nerve roots, and the size of the spinal canal (Appendix III). While most clinical studies of disc herniations deal with neurologically compromised patients, these pathoanatomic features emphasize that disc herniations may cause local back pain without radiculopathy. In fact, many patients who ultimately develop radicular back pain due to disc disease give a history of prior episodes of simple mechanical back pain. Invasive diagnostic studies (for example, myelography) are rarely performed in the absence of neurologic findings, but it is likely that such prior mechanical episodes represent tears of the anulus or bulges of the disc that temporarily resolve (clinically) but antedate the eventual full-blown disc syndrome with neurologic impairment (see page 35).

3. The elderly patient is not often afflicted by uncomplicated disc herniations, probably because the liquid nucleus pulposus usually desiccates and solidifies with age. The new onset of simple mechanical back pain in the elderly patient should raise the question(s) of compression fractures (even after very minor or no traumatic events), various OMINOUS diseases (see

Concealed

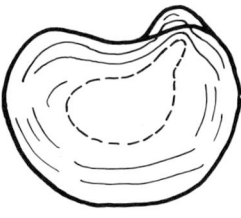 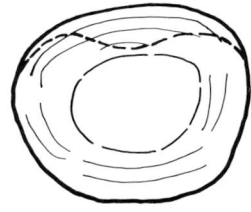

localized bulge diffuse bulge

FIGURE 1–11. A classification of disc herniations. (From Kelley, WN, Harris, ED, Jr, Ruddy, S, and Sledge, CB: Textbook of Rheumatology. WB Saunders, Philadelphia, 1981, p. 462.)

Prolapsed

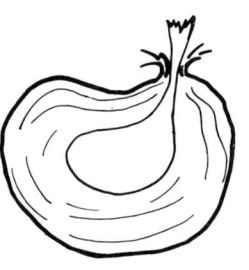 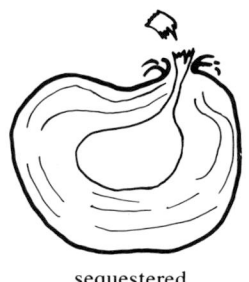

sequestered

above and Appendix I), and mechanical exacerbations of (previously asymptomatic) chronic spinal disease—spondylosis, facet joint arthritis, osteoporosis, for example. (See "Chronic Back Pain.") Disc disease with acute herniation may, however, afflict patients of all ages.

Tests?

With few exceptions, most patients with acute simple mechanical low back pain do not require x-rays.

Lumbosacral spine x-rays are expensive (Table 1–2) and their diagnostic or prognostic value in this type of patient is minimal at best.[17, 27] On the one hand, the common causes of simple mechanical back pain—musculoligamentous strains, uncomplicated disc disease, facet joint malalignments—are usually not identifiable by x-ray. On the other hand, many abnormal x-ray findings are so common in asymptomatic individuals that it is often difficult to correlate such findings (disc space narrowing, osteophyte formation, and the like) with symptoms in the patient who does have back pain.[28-31]

When one considers that most acute simple mechanical back pain resolves spontaneously,[32] that OMINOUS disease is usually strongly suspected on the basis of the history and examination alone, and that therapeutically significant radiographic abnormalities are rarely found in "low-risk" patients, routine x-ray examination is wasteful.

It is true that various radiographic abnormalities may predispose certain patients to recurrent low back pain—the various "malalignment disorders" (page 44)—but these are usually not important to document in the patient with one or two episodes of acute simple mechanical back pain. Thus, when back pain is recurrent or chronic (see "Chronic Back Pain"), x-rays should be obtained. When x-rays are obtained, anteroposterior and lateral views are usually enough:[33, 34] Spot films, oblique films, and other special

TABLE 1–2. LABORATORY TESTS FOR LOW BACK PAIN

Test	Cost	When to Order
Lumbosacral spine x-rays (AP and lateral)	$75	Recurrent back pain OMINOUS suspicions
Plus obliques	$85	Trauma
Plus coned-down views (tomograms)	$150	Failure to improve with conservative therapy
Bone scan	$220	Suspected neoplasm, osteomyelitis, inapparent fracture (when x-ray is normal)
Gallium scan	$240	Neoplasm vs. infection vs. spondylosis
CT scan (lumbar spine)	$330	Neurologic findings: disc, spinal stenosis, spinal neoplasm?
Myelogram	$210	Same as for CT scan
Sedimentation rate	$6	In elderly patient with new back pain or when back pain is puzzling or OMINOUS
Serum protein electrophoresis	$32	
Calcium, phosphate	$6, $9	
Alkaline phosphatase	$6	
Acid phosphatase	$27	

TABLE 1–3. CAUSES OF ABNORMAL RADIOTRACER UPTAKE ON A BONE SCINTISCAN

Focal increase in uptake
  Congenital
    Fibrous dysplasia
    Osteochondromatosis
  Acquired
    Neoplasia—primary malignant bone tumors: some benign bone tumors, for example, osteoid osteoma, aneurysmal bone cyst
    Infection—acute and chronic osteomyelitis
    Trauma—bone surgery; fracture; subperiosteal haematoma; repair, for example after ischemic necrosis
    Vascular disease—bone infarct
    Metabolic disease—"brown tumors" of hyperparathyroidism
    Degenerative disease—adjacent to sites of arthropathy
    Other disease—Paget's disease of bone
Diffuse increase in uptake
  Rickets and osteomalacia
  Hyperparathyroidism, primary, secondary, and tertiary
  Diffuse metastatic malignant involvement of bone
  Myelosclerosis
Focal decrease in uptake
  Ischemic or dead bone
  Radiation-induced osteoblastic suppression
  Metastatic malignant tumors (very rarely) and eosinophilic granuloma
  "Prosthesis," or other artifact

From Lentle, B. C., et al.: Bone scintiscanning update. Ann Intern Med 84:297–303, 1976.

views only rarely add additional information and always add to the cost (Table 1–2).

Other laboratory tests are not usually necessary either. While "screening" blood tests will detect many of the potentially serious causes of low back pain[1]—ESR, protein electrophoresis, calcium and phosphate levels, alkaline phosphatase and acid phosphatase—these will rarely be helpful in the uncomplicated case of simple mechanical back pain.

Radionuclide bone scans[35] may be helpful in specific (uncommon) situations, but these tests are probably much overutilized. Table 1–3 illustrates the range of conditions that may result in abnormal bone scans and emphasizes the relative nonspecificity of various abnormal findings. In general, a bone scan is most helpful when plain spine x-rays are normal but serious disease is nonetheless strongly suspected: for example, vertebral osteomyelitis, spinal neoplasms, or inapparent fractures (see Appendices I and II). Early metastatic disease to the spine may not be apparent on routine radiographs,[36] but the majority of patients with low back pain due to neoplastic disease will have abnormal spine films.[37] Rarely both plain films and bone scans will be equivocal: here, gallium scans may help support the clinical suspicion of neoplastic or infectious disease of the spine when abnormal gallium uptake correlates with abnormal bone scan uptake (but the gallium scan may also be nonspecific[25]).

X-rays and laboratory tests should then usually be reserved for situations that are worrisome. Such worrisome situations include:

1. When back pain is excruciating, constant, and unrelenting, or when OMINOUS disease is suspected for other reasons (see above).

2. Back pain following trauma always deserves x-rays. Compression fractures or fractures of transverse or posterior spinous processes must be excluded (in the latter situation, retroperitoneal hemorrhage can occur).

3. The elderly patient with new back pain.

4. When apparently simple mechanical back pain does not improve (or worsens) in spite of appropriate therapy (see below).

Treatment

Hospitalization is indicated in general only when the patient is seriously disabled by pain and limitation of motion and is thus unable to care for himself or herself at home (most often, the elderly patient who lives alone). In all other instances, the key to successful treatment is guaranteeing strict compliance with a precisely defined regimen of conservative therapy at home. Such conservative home therapy involves three sequential stages:

1. The acutely painful stage. Strict bedrest is the essential step here, while various adjunctive measures may help, too (see page 21).

2. The recovery stage. As pain resolves, progressive back exercises and careful resumption of ambulation are emphasized.

3. The preventive stage. After substantial (or complete) improvement, various prophylactic measures will ensure long-term success.

While the duration of each stage of treatment must be individualized, this overall approach should be used for all patients with (acute) simple mechanical back pain. This approach will be successful in 99 percent of such cases if the physician takes the time to educate the patient. Patients must be taught the rationale for the various treatment stages if patient compliance is to be expected. Hurried, vague talk about aspirin, "rest," and "time heals all wounds" is rarely reassuring or helpful to patients with acute back pain who are uncomfortable, often irritable, and understandably demanding of some active therapeutic intervention. Because the conservative home treatment of acute low back pain is at least initially passive in nature (bedrest is the key), such patient education is a challenge. The following outline of the stages of treatment includes a few practical explanations of the various treatment modalities.

Usually one or two follow-up office visits should punctuate the overall treatment schedule (see Fig. 1–12); each successive stage of treatment should be carefully explained during each visit, but a general overview of the entire treatment should be outlined during the initial patient encounter.

I. The Acutely Painful Stage.

Bedrest

> To get better quickly, you must rest your back completely. A sprained back is like a sprained ankle—you must not use your back at all for a few days so that the internal swelling will resolve and the muscle spasm will relax. With a sprained ankle, you can get around on crutches. You now know as well as anyone that you use your back for everything—sitting, standing, walking—everything. The only way to rest your back is to stay flat on your back and do nothing at all.

The patient should be instructed to lie in bed, preferably on a firm mattress or bedboard. The most comfortable (and beneficial) positions involve lying supine with hips and knees flexed, with a few pillows under the knees; and lying on one side with both knees moderately flexed (semifetal position). As illustrated on page 25 (under "How to Put Your Back to Bed"), each of these positions flattens the lumbar spine (reverses lumbar lordosis). The patient must understand that lying absolutely flat or prone is not desirable nor is modified sitting (in a reclining chair or on a couch with many pillows under the shoulders and lower spine).

Complete bedrest is advocated. The patient should be told specifically that the benefit of 22 hours in bed may be offset by 2 hours of ambulation. The patient rises from bed only to use the bathroom. Meals should be taken in bed.

Many patients do not comply with such severe restrictions, but these instructions at least emphasize to the patient the importance of complete bedrest. It is also worthwhile to explain to the patient how to get out of bed—see Table 1–5, No. 5.

During this painful stage, several adjunctive measures help:
A. Topical heat or cold.

A heating pad, hot water bottle, or topical salve (Ben-Gay) applied to the area of maximal pain, tenderness, and spasm is a soothing measure whose mechanism of action may be more as a sedative than as a true skeletal muscle antispasmodic. Some patients find that local application of ice provides more relief—especially in the first 24 hours following a specific injury. A homemade ice applicator[38] is easy to prepare by filling a paper cup with water, standing a tongue blade upright in the cup, and placing the cup in the freezer until the ice is solid.

In general, heat is easier to use than ice, and more often effective.

B. Drug therapy.

Most cases of simple mechanical back pain will resolve without any drug therapy. Nevertheless, anti-inflammatory drugs may have a temporary role in reducing local edema and inflammation in injured "soft tissue" and will have moderate analgesic effects as well. Aspirin is usually the first drug of choice: Two aspirin every 4 hours while awake (to be taken whether in pain or not) will exert anti-inflammatory effects and provide effective analgesia for most. If aspirin is contraindicated or not tolerated, other nonsteroidal anti-inflammatory agents may be substituted, but these drugs are all much more expensive (see Table 1–4) and probably no more beneficial than aspirin.

Patients with severe muscle spasm may actually worsen during the first 24 hours of bedrest as muscle tension decelerates. Especially in the first 24 to 48 hours of bedrest, more potent analgesics (codeine, oxycodone [Percodan], pentazocine [Talwin], oxycodone and acetaminophen [Tylox]) may be needed by some. When used at all, potent analgesics should be given in small numbers (10 to 15) without refills. The patient who complains that potent narcotics are required beyond the first few days should be suspected of noncompliance with bedrest, OMINOUS disease, or analgesic abuse. Occasionally, such demands are appropriate, but avoiding narcotics in the first place is a good general rule.

Muscle relaxants—diazepam (Valium), cyclobenzaprine HCl (Flexeril), or methocarbamol (Robaxin)—are recommended as skeletal muscle antispasmodics, but there is some controversy about their mechanism of action. Whether these agents act directly on

TABLE 1–4. ANTI-INFLAMMATORY AGENTS

	DOSE AVG./MAX.	PATIENT COST/MONTH
Aspirin	650 mg qid	$4
Indomethacin (Indocin)	25 mg qid 50 mg qid	$20 $32
Sulindac (Clinoril)	150 mg bid 250 mg bid	$19 $23
Naproxen (Naprosyn)	250 mg bid 375 mg bid	$22 $29
Ibuprofen (Motrin)	400 mg qid 600 mg qid	$21 $29
Fenoprofen calcium (Nalfon)	300 mg qid	$29
Tolmetin sodium (Tolectin)	200 mg qid 400 mg tid	$19 $25
Meclofenamate sodium (Meclomen)	50 mg qid 100 mg tid	$18 $19
Piroxicam (Feldene)	10 mg qd 20 mg qd	$27 $33

skeletal muscle or not, their effectiveness as mild sedatives should not be disregarded, since compliance with complete bedrest may be improved by mild sedation.

In general, polypharmacy should be avoided. Aspirin, with or without a few days' supply of sedatives and codeine, is usually sufficient.

These medicines will help relieve the pain of your muscle spasms and you should not hesitate to use them for the first few days, if you need them. Taking these pills will not help you if you do not stay in bed—they may even hurt you by masking the pain as you move around. Usually, if you rest your back properly, you won't need pills at all.

C. Bed Exercises.

Even during the acutely painful stage, a few exercises in bed should be recommended. These are gentle flexion exercises that reverse lumbar lordosis and relax paraspinal muscles (exercises Nos. 1 to 3 in Table 1–5). Some patients, especially the elderly, are unable to easily perform even these exercises. For these patients, isometric back exercises are helpful. The patient is instructed to contract—in sequence—the abdominal muscles for 5 to 15 seconds and then relax; the gluteus (buttocks) for 5 to 15 seconds and then relax; and then the abdominal and gluteus together for 5 to 15 seconds. These exercises are performed in bed while supine. (After recovery, they may also be performed prophylactically—see "Exercise Without Attracting Attention" on page 25).

The duration of this first "bedrest stage" of therapy must be individualized. Most patients benefit from at least 48 to 72 hours of bedrest, but some may require a week or more of bedrest. (When back pain is very mild and there is minimal or no restriction of back

TABLE 1–5. BACK EXERCISES

General Instructions: These exercises are to be done once or twice a day lying in bed or on the floor. Begin with 5 repetitions, adding 5 repetitions each day until you are doing each exercise 25 times.

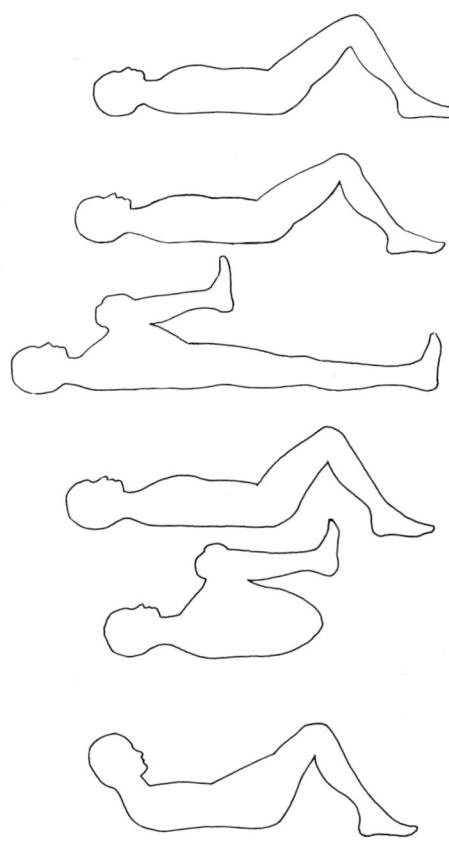

1. Pelvic Tilt
   A. Position —Lie flat on your back, knees bent.
   B. Exercise —Tighten abdominal muscles and buttocks, flattening the small of your back to the floor—hold for count of 10. (If done properly, abdominal muscles will feel tight.)

2. Hip Flexor Stretch
   A. Position —Lie flat on your back, knees bent.
   B. Exercise —Lift right knee toward your chest as far as possible; hold right knee to chest and stretch left leg to floor by tightening leg muscles and pushing down; return to original position and repeat on opposite side. Maintain a pelvic tilt while doing this exercise.

3. Low Back Stretch
   A. Position —Place small pillow under your head, lie flat on your back, arms at sides, knees bent.
   B. Exercise —Bring both knees to your chest, one at a time; clasp them and pull toward chest—hold for count of 10. Keep shoulders on the floor. Repeat pulling and holding 3 times, then return to original position.

4. Partial Sit-up
   A. Position —Lie flat on your back, arms at sides, knees bent.
   B. Exercise —Do a pelvic tilt, bring chin to chest, reach hands toward knees, curl to a partial sitting position, bringing shoulders off floor. Relax and repeat.

5. Getting Out of Bed
   Turn on one side with your hips and knees bent (fetal position). Allow the lower legs to swing over the edge of the bed as you gently push against the bed with one arm—this will bring you to a sitting position, feet flat on the floor. Push with the arms, straighten the knees and stand. Return to the bed by reversing this process.

motion on examination, bedrest can be omitted entirely.) Usually the patient can tell when he or she is improved enough to move on to the next stage. When rising from bed to go to the bathroom is not a difficult, painful maneuver and when bed exercises are tolerated easily, it is usually time to move on to the "recovery stage."

II. The Recovery Stage.

These exercises will both relax and strengthen your lower back and abdominal muscles—the back and abdominal muscles work together to protect the spine—and so these exercises will allow you to resume your full activities sooner.

At this stage, simple ambulation is encouraged, but all lifting, improper bending, and physical work should be avoided. Daily back exercises should include simple bed exercises as well as "recovery stage exercises"—primarily abdominal muscle strengthening in the form of partial sit-ups (see Table 1–5). Medications can be discontinued.

In general, back supports in the form of lumbosacral corsets or braces should be avoided. Occasionally these are useful in the elderly patient in whom ambulation must be encouraged but who is unlikely to

Your back and how to care for it

Whatever the cause of low back pain, part of its treatment is the correction of faulty posture. But good posture is not simply a matter of "standing tall." It refers to correct use of the body at all times. In fact, for the body to function in the best of health it must be so used that no strain is put upon muscles, joints, bones, and ligaments. To prevent low back pain, avoiding strain must become a way of life, practiced while lying, sitting, standing, walking, working, and exercising. When body position is correct, internal organs have enough room to function normally and blood circulates more freely.

With the help of this guide, you can begin to correct the positions and movements which bring on or aggravate backache. Particular attention should be paid to the positions recommended for resting, since it is possible to strain the muscles of the back and neck even while lying in bed. By learning to live with good posture, under all circumstances, you will gradually develop the proper carriage and stronger muscles needed to protect and support your hard-working back.

HOW TO STAY ON YOUR FEET WITHOUT TIRING YOUR BACK

To prevent strain and pain in everyday activities, it is restful to change from one task to another before fatigue sets in. Housewives can lie down between chores; others should check body position frequently, drawing in the abdomen, flattening the back, bending the knees slightly.

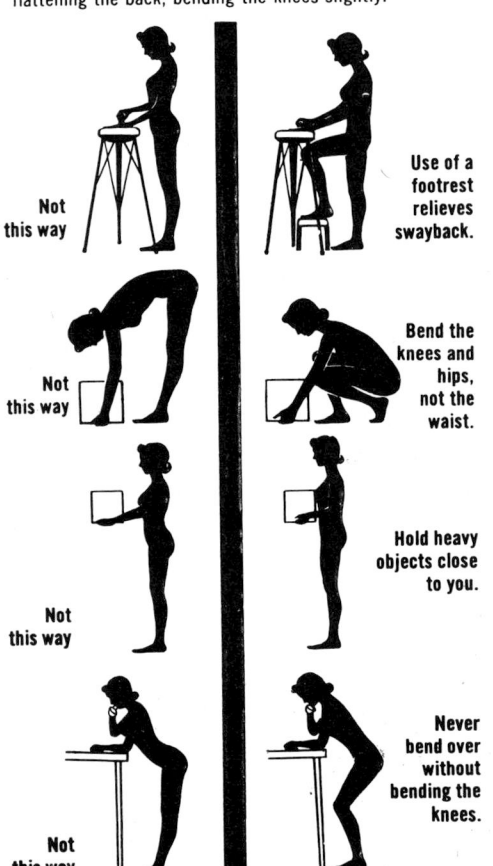

Not this way

Use of a footrest relieves swayback.

Not this way

Bend the knees and hips, not the waist.

Not this way

Hold heavy objects close to you.

Not this way

Never bend over without bending the knees.

CHECK YOUR CARRIAGE HERE

In correct, fully erect posture, a line dropped from the ear will go through the tip of the shoulder, middle of hip, back of kneecap, and front of anklebone.

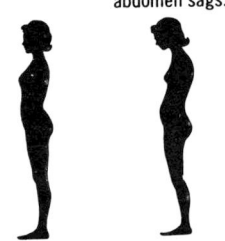

Incorrect:
Lower back is arched or hollow.

Incorrect:
Upper back is stooped, lower back is arched, abdomen sags.

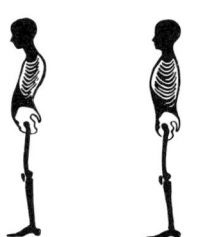

Incorrect:
Note how, in strained position, pelvis tilts forward, chin is out, and ribs are down, crowding internal organs.

Correct:
In correct position, chin is in, head up, back flattened, pelvis held straight.

To find the correct standing position: Stand one foot away from wall. Now sit against wall, bending knees slightly. Tighten abdominal and buttock muscles. This will tilt the pelvis back and flatten the lower spine. Holding this position, inch up the wall to standing position, by straightening the legs. Now walk around the room, maintaining the same posture. Place back against wall again to see if you have held it.

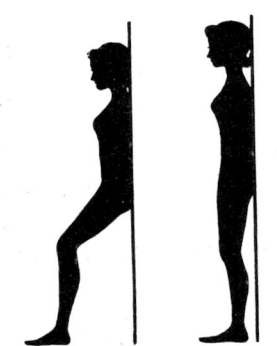

HOW TO SIT CORRECTLY

A back's best friend is a straight, hard chair. If you can't get the chair you prefer, learn to sit properly on whatever chair you get. To correct sitting position from forward slump: Throw head well back, then bend it forward to pull in the chin. This will straighten the back. Now tighten abdominal muscles to raise the chest. Check position frequently.

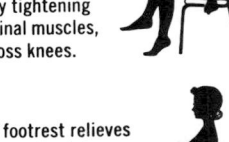

Relieve strain by sitting well forward, flatten back by tightening abdominal muscles, and cross knees.

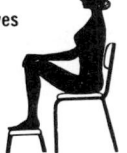

Use of footrest relieves swayback. Aim is to have knees higher than hips.

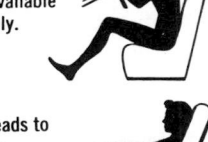

Correct way to sit while driving, close to pedals. Use seat belt or hard backrest, available commercially.

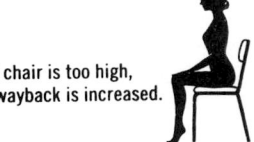

TV slump leads to "dowager's hump," strains neck and shoulders.

If chair is too high, swayback is increased.

Keep neck and back in as straight a line as possible with the spine. Bend forward from hips.

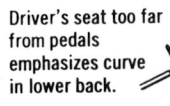

Driver's seat too far from pedals emphasizes curve in lower back.

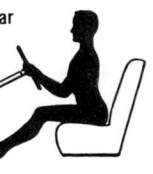

Strained reading position. Forward thrusting strains muscles of neck and head.

HOW TO PUT YOUR BACK TO BED

For proper bed posture, a firm mattress is essential. Bedboards, sold commercially, or devised at home, may be used with soft mattresses. Bedboards, preferably, should be made of ¾ inch plywood. Faulty sleeping positions intensify swayback and result not only in backache but in numbness, tingling, and pain in arms and legs.

Incorrect:	Correct:
Lying flat on back makes swayback worse.	Lying on side with knees bent effectively flattens the back. Flat pillow may be used to support neck, especially when shoulders are broad.

Use of high pillow strains neck, arms, shoulders.	Sleeping on back is restful and correct when knees are properly supported.

 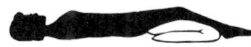

Sleeping face down exaggerates swayback, strains neck and shoulders.	Raise the foot of the mattress eight inches to discourage sleeping on the abdomen.

 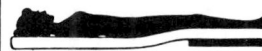

Bending one hip and knee does not relieve swayback.	Proper arrangement of pillows for resting or reading in bed.

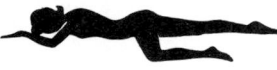 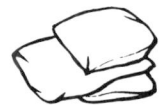

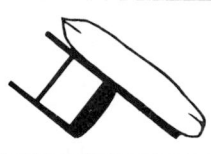

A straight-back chair used behind a pillow makes a serviceable backrest.

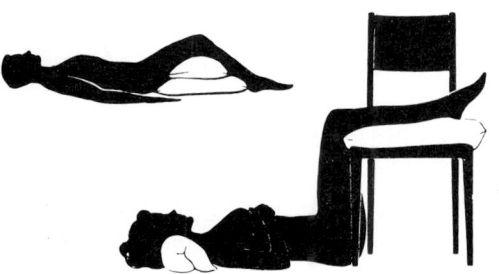

WHEN DOING NOTHING, DO IT RIGHT

Rest is the first rule for the tired, painful back. The following positions relieve pain by taking all pressure and weight off the back and legs.

Note pillows under knees to relieve strain on spine.

For complete relief and relaxing effect, these positions should be maintained from 5 to 25 minutes.

EXERCISE—WITHOUT GETTING OUT OF BED

Exercises to be performed while lying in bed are aimed not so much at strengthening muscles as at teaching correct positioning. But muscles used correctly become stronger and in time are able to support the body with the least amount of effort.

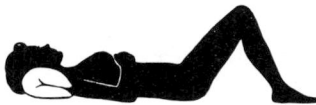

Do all exercises in this position. Legs should not be straightened.

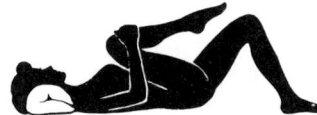

Bring knee up to chest. Lower slowly but do not straighten leg. Relax. Repeat with each leg 10 times.

Bring both knees slowly up to chest. Tighten muscles of abdomen, press back flat against bed. Hold knees to chest 20 seconds, then lower slowly. Relax. Repeat 5 times. This exercise gently stretches the shortened muscles of the lower back, while strengthening abdominal muscles. Clasp knees, bring them up to chest, at the same time coming to a sitting position. Rock back and forth.

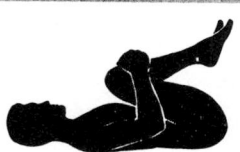

EXERCISE—WITHOUT ATTRACTING ATTENTION

Use these inconspicuous exercises whenever you have a spare moment during the day, both to relax tension and improve the tone of important muscle groups.

1. Rotate shoulders, forward and backward.
2. Turn head slowly side to side.
3. Watch an imaginary plane take off, just below the right shoulder. Stretch neck, follow it slowly as it moves up, around and down, disappearing below the other shoulder. Repeat, starting on left side.
4. Slowly, slowly, touch left ear to left shoulder; right ear to right shoulder. Raise both shoulders to touch ears, drop them as far down as possible.
5. At any pause in the day—waiting for an elevator to arrive, for a specific traffic light to change—pull in abdominal muscles, tighten, hold it for the count of eight without breathing. Relax slowly. Increase the count gradually after the first week, practice breathing normally with the abdomen flat and contracted. Do this sitting, standing, and walking.

RULES TO LIVE BY—FROM NOW ON

1. Never bend from the waist only; bend the hips and knees.
2. Never lift a heavy object higher than your waist.
3. Always turn and face the object you wish to lift.
4. Avoid carrying unbalanced loads; hold heavy objects close to your body.
5. Never carry anything heavier than you can manage with ease.
6. Never lift or move heavy furniture. Wait for someone to do it who knows the principles of leverage.
7. Avoid sudden movements, sudden "overloading" of muscles. Learn to move deliberately, swinging the legs from the hips.
8. Learn to keep the head in line with the spine, when standing, sitting, lying in bed.
9. Put soft chairs and deep couches on your "don't sit" list. During prolonged sitting, cross your legs to rest your back.
10. Your doctor is the only one who can determine when low back pain is due to faulty posture. He is the best judge of when you may do general exercises for physical fitness. When you do, omit any exercise which arches or overstrains the lower back: backward bends, or forward bends, touching the toes with the knees straight.
11. Wear shoes with moderate heels, all about the same height. Avoid changing from high to low heels.
12. Put a footrail under the desk, and a footrest under the crib.
13. Diaper the baby sitting next to him or her on the bed.
14. Don't stoop and stretch to hang the wash; raise the clothesbasket and lower the washline.
15. Beg or buy a rocking chair. Rocking rests the back by changing the muscle groups used.
16. Train yourself vigorously to use your abdominal muscles to flatten your lower abdomen. In time, this muscle contraction will become habitual, making you the envied possessor of a youthful body-profile!
17. Don't strain to open windows or doors.
18. For good posture, concentrate on strengthening "nature's corset"—the abdominal and buttock muscles. The pelvic roll exercise is especially recommended to correct the postural relation between the pelvis and the spine.

SCHERING CORPORATION • KENILWORTH, N.J.

PRINTED IN U S A   CE-504/11656900 8-78

improve rapidly or who simply cannot perform progressive back exercises. Sometimes the young or middle-aged patient who is obese or has weakened abdominal muscles will require temporary back support until exercise therapy improves the situation. Most often, however, these "aids" should be avoided, since dependency on such devices is common and this will hinder compliance with subsequent exercise therapy. (The patient with severe chronic back pain is another matter—see "Chronic Low Back Pain.")

The timing of resumption of work must be individualized. The manual laborer, for example, has different needs from the sedentary office worker.

All patients should be encouraged to read and practice the advice provided on pages 24 and 25 about proper posture, bending, and lifting.

III. The Preventive Stage.

> If you sprain your back once, you may be troubled by it again unless you take the time to prevent it. This can be done very simply by spending 5 minutes a day on your back exercises and by using a little common sense!

When back pain has resolved, most patients fail to continue exercises and other prophylactic measures that will help prevent recurrent episodes of back pain (which are very common). Daily back exercises, especially partial sit-ups, should be continued indefinitely—these can be done in fewer than 5 minutes per day. Again, instructions on "How to Take Care of Your Back" should be reviewed (pages 24 and 25).

General exercise—especially walking, swimming (the backstroke is best!), and bicycle riding—help maintain physical fitness without overly stressing the lower spine. The role of obesity and poor posture as contributing factors to chronic back pain (page 50) must be repeatedly emphasized.

Dick is told that he is suffering from a "sprain" of the muscles and ligaments of the lower spine and that much of his pain is caused by the tightness and spasm of those muscles. He is told that simple treatment at home will help him, but only if he follows the treatment plan completely. Dick is told that strict bedrest is the only way to fully relax the strained muscles and ligaments and that this is the most important part of therapy. He is told to go home and get out of bed only to go to the bathroom. Proper positioning, methods of getting out of bed, and copies of "Painful Stage" back exercises are provided. Aspirin 8 to 10 per day is recommended and prescriptions for codeine 30 mg, 10 tablets; and diazepam (Valium) 5 mg, 15 tablets (without refills) are provided. Local heat is recommended, and Dick is told that he probably will need at least 3 days and nights in bed but that he can get out of bed when walking is not painful and when bed exercises are easily performed.

Dick complains that he will not be paid while he is out of work, and "Can't you give me a shot or massage those muscles to get me on my feet quicker?" We explain there is no easier and safer way to get better faster, and that he may need up to a couple of weeks before he can resume any heavy lifting. Dick is given a note of explanation for his employer and is asked to return in 7 days.

NOTE

A. A simple (however simplistic) explanation of the mechanism of back pain ("muscle spasm") is always helpful in allowing the patient to understand the rationale of treatment. Compliance will be enhanced if the patient realizes that conservative therapy is almost always effective but that failure to improve (usually due to noncompliance) will necessitate expensive testing and maybe even hospitalization.

B. This treatment approach deemphasizes the chiropractic model.[39, 40] Appendix IV illustrates one manipulation technique that I have personally observed to be effective on some occasions. This and other types of spinal manipulation should be subjected to careful controlled clinical study, if only because so many patients "swear by" these techniques. Manipulation is not avidly recommended here for several reasons:

1. The few clinical studies available do not corroborate any long-term benefit of spinal manipulation, even in highly selected patients; some such patients are more likely to "feel better faster," but this important benefit must be balanced by the fact that:

2. There are at least a few reports of serious complications (for example, paraparesis[41]) associated with back manipulations. Traditional conservative therapy at home may be slow, but it is never dangerous.

3. Most manipulators are careful to obtain x-rays before initiating treatment, and several (10 to 20) repeat treatments are often deemed necessary. Since our conservative treatment approach described above attempts to be economical, we usually try to omit expensive x-rays and keep repetitive office visits to a minimum (Fig. 1–12).*

4. Nevertheless, follow-up examination of patients with acute low back pain is always worthwhile. Figure 1–12 illustrates a typical schedule. Most patients are much improved after 7 to 10 days and should then be instructed about further exercise and preventive therapy (or should be subjected to further investigation if

---

*These cost-conscious considerations must be balanced against the possible economic value of chiropractic manipulations in returning the patient to work more quickly.

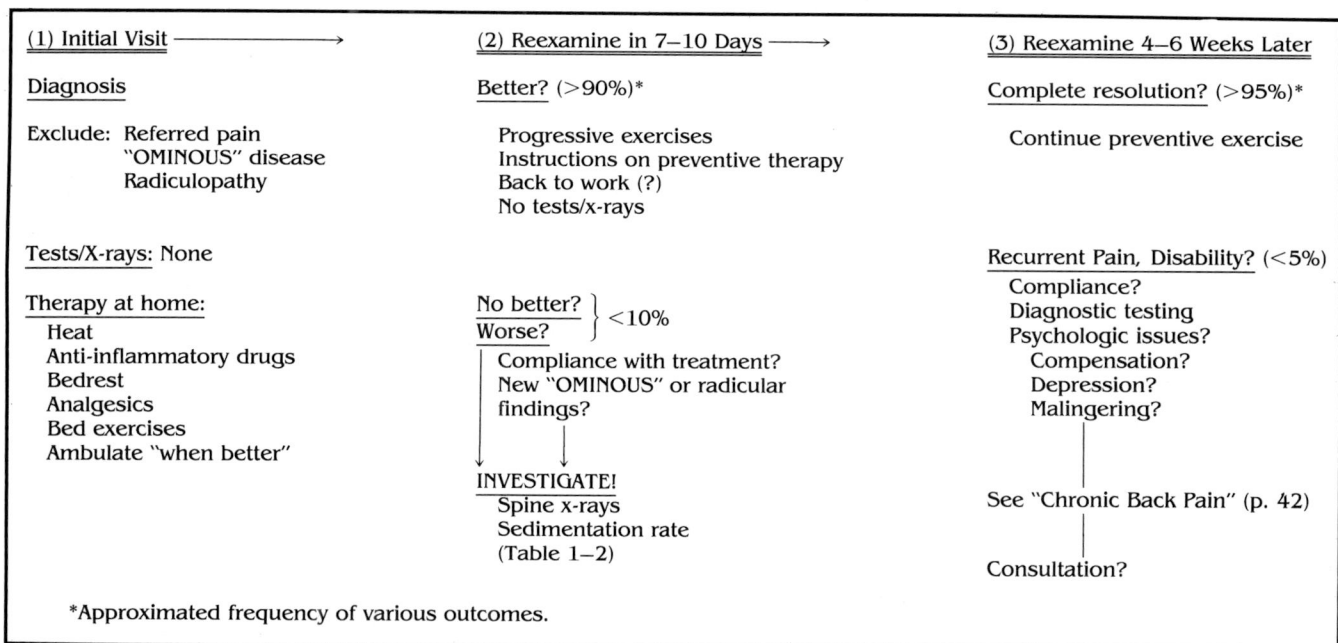

FIGURE 1–12. Acute simple mechanical back pain.

they are not improved or are worse). Final follow-up in several weeks is an opportunity to review the patient's progress and emphasize ongoing preventive measures, but this last (third) visit may be omitted if the patient is doing well after 7 to 10 days and seems receptive to a preventive exercise program.

One week later, Dick limps into the clinic saying "I'm a little better." He remained in bed for 5 days because he still "hurt quite a lot" after 72 hours, but admits, "I just had to get out of that bed."

The lumbar spine remains straightened with continued visible lordosis (Fig. 1–3C) during back flexion. Back range of motion is fuller, but still limited, and there is still some paravertebral muscle spasm (Fig. 1–2D). Straight leg raising, sitting and supine, is unchanged: There remains some back and buttock discomfort at 60 degrees on the left. Neurologic examination is normal.

Several more days of bedrest are recommended. Lumbosacral spine films are obtained (and are normal).

Dick is obviously unhappy about further bedrest and medication, but reluctantly agrees. He is told to remain in bed for the next 3 to 7 days, depending on his progress, and to return 10 days hence.

Most patients with acute simple mechanical back pain will be better after a week of conservative home therapy. (Some patients will still be disabled, but almost all will be improved.) Failure to improve at all should suggest an incorrect diagnosis (an OMINOUS sign), patient noncompliance, or malingering.

The timing of laboratory investigations must, then, be individualized. In Dick's case, only minimal improvement after 1 week of conservative therapy with the history of prior intermittent back pain suggests that at least x-rays should be obtained.

Other treatments are occasionally helpful for simple mechanical back pain. These include manipulation (see Appendix IV), epidural or intradural steroid injections, percutaneous nerve blocks, facet joint injections, and even oral corticosteroids. These methods are advocated by various practitioners in different circumstances—most often in the treatment of chronic back pain or acute radicular back pain (see below)—but are almost never necessary for simple mechanical back pain.

Ten days later, Dick does not return for his appointment. His wife calls and says, "Dick had to go back to work. He is doing all right, but he still has pain." She is told to bring him back if he does not improve more.

Another 10 days later, Dick's wife calls to say that Dick is worse but must keep working because "the company doctor finds nothing wrong." The following day, after work, Dick limps into the clinic, holding his left hip, clearly in pain. He apologizes for not keeping his prior appointment, but says his back was "much better" after a few days' more bedrest, and he was able to work without much difficulty until the pain in his hip and leg began. His pain is now sharp and "shooting," involves the left buttock and posterolateral thigh area (without "much" back pain). Dick admits that the side and front of his lower leg hurt sometimes, too, but, "I figured I just strained my leg by favoring my back."

Examination is unchanged, except that pain in the buttock, lateral portion of the thigh and lateral portion of the calf is precipitated by straight leg raising at 40 degrees on the left. Crossed straight leg raising is normal. Sensory examination, all reflexes, and Babinski responses are normal, but there is definite weakness of dorsiflexion of the left big toe, which is reproducible on repetitive testing.

What does this mean?

Dick now has radicular low back pain.

RADICULAR LOW BACK PAIN

The approach to this type of problem is quite different from the approach to simple mechanical back pain. Here, the neurologic examination is most important—in establishing the fact that the pain is, in fact, radicular (neurologic), in assessing the location of the "lesion" in the nervous system (spinal cord, nerve roots, plexus, or peripheral nerve), and thereafter in achieving a more specific anatomic and pathologic diagnosis. Treatment (or the need for hospitalization) is based largely on the neurologic findings.

Practical Neurology of the Low Back and Leg

The neurologic examination of the lower extremity may be quite complex, but understanding several general concepts will usually make evaluation less formidable.

CONSIDER

I. The motor examination is often the best objective clinical indicator of the site of the neurologic lesion.

Three basic facts are worth remembering:

A. Most muscle groups of the lower extremity are supplied by more than one nerve root.
As Keim has noted,[42]

In general, any movement of a joint is innervated by nerves from two adjoining segments. The four segments concerned in two opposing movements (for example, hip flexion—L2-3 and hip extension—L4-5) are in numerical sequence. In the lower limb, each joint distal to the preceding one is innervated by one segment lower in the spinal cord. Thus, four spinal segments control the hip, knee and ankle (the hip L2-5; knee L3-S1; ankle L4-S1).

Figure 1–13 illustrates this segmental innervation of lower limb movements.
B. A few motor functions of the foot are primarily innervated by a single nerve root. L4 supplies foot inversion, L5 dorsiflexion of the great toe, S1 foot eversion.
These are easily remembered when one considers the dermatomal sensory distribution of these roots in the foot—L4 supplies the inner foot (and inversion), S1 the outer foot (and eversion), L5 the dorsum of the foot (and toe dorsiflexion)—see Figs. 1–10 and 1–14. Even when motor weakness is inapparent to the patient, these motor functions should always be carefully tested in the patient with radicular back pain.
C. Prominent motor weakness thus usually indicates involvement of multiple roots, a peripheral nerve, or both, rather than a lesion of a single nerve root.

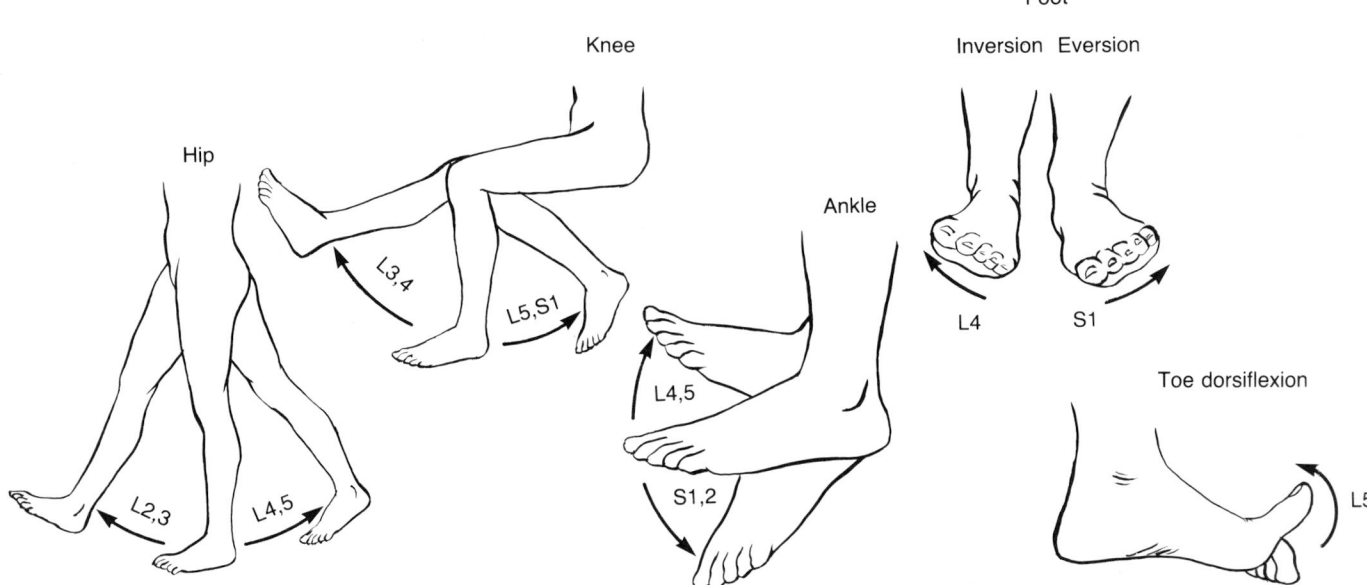

FIGURE 1–13. Motor control of the lower extremity.

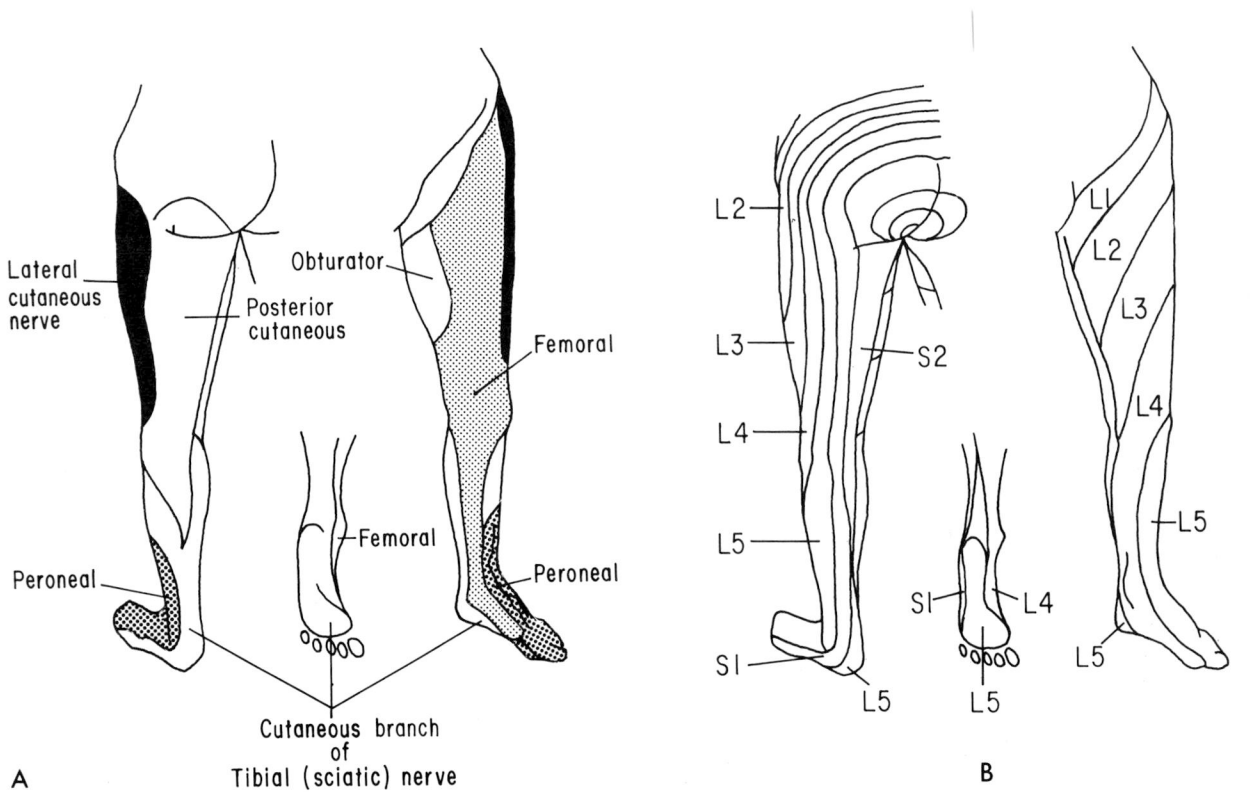

FIGURE 1–14. Sensory innervation of the lower extremity. *A*, Peripheral nerve innervation. *B*, Dermatomal (root) innervation.

Tables 1–6 and 1–7 demonstrate typical neurologic findings associated with disorders of nerve roots and peripheral nerves respectively.[43] While weakness of the foot is a common finding in patients with radicular back pain due to disc disease, careful motor testing of the foot will usually distinguish a single root lesion from a peripheral nerve lesion.* Complete footdrop (absence of foot dorsiflexion), for example, may result from simultaneous root lesions involving both L4 and L5 but is much more commonly caused by peripheral lesions of the peroneal branch of the peripheral sciatic nerve.

Most disorders of peripheral nerves are not associated with back pain per se—the neurologic symptoms predominate instead. However, pelvic masses or buttock trauma may be the cause of peripheral nerve lesions and cause local back pain as well. Usually the combination of the clinical history and a careful physical and neurologic examination will distinguish root from peripheral nerve lesions.

II. The sensory examination is often normal, even when a dermatomal distribution of pain or (less commonly) motor weakness localizes the problem to a single nerve root.

Dermatomes overlap; disorders of a single nerve root often do not cause loss of sensation because the adjacent roots, which are not involved, help supply the same sensory area. In most patients with radicular back pain, only a single nerve root is involved—thus the distribution of sensory symptoms is much more helpful than is the formal sensory neurologic examination. Nevertheless, sensory symptoms and objective sensory losses must be carefully analyzed.

REMEMBER

A. Sacral (perineal) sensation must always be tested since loss of sacral sensation (especially when bilateral) must suggest a lesion of the cauda equina (see page 37).

---

*Familiarity with the anatomic course of the various peripheral nerves will also be helpful (Fig. 1–15). Tapping the peroneal nerve, for example, as it encircles the neck of the fibula will often indicate the site of peripheral nerve compression—pain or dysesthesias in the anterior portion of the leg and dorsal aspect of the foot constitute a positive Tinel's sign.

TABLE 1–6. ISOLATED NERVE ROOT LESIONS

Root	Sensory Supply (Fig. 1–14)	Sensory Loss	Motor Loss	Reflex Change	Lesion
L2	Upper anterior thigh	Often none	Often none ± hip flexion	None	
L3	Lower anterior thigh	Often none	Often none ± knee extension	None	Neurofibroma Meningioma Malignant neoplasm Disc, rarely
L4*	Anterior knee, medial leg	Often none ± medial leg	Foot inversion	Diminished knee jerk	
L5*	Posterior thigh, lateral leg, dorsal foot, and sole of foot	Often none ± dorsal foot and sole	Dorsiflexion great toe ± foot dorsiflexion	None	Disc, usually (see Table 1–8)
S1*	Posterior thigh and leg, lateral foot	Often none ± lateral foot	Foot eversion ± foot plantar flexion	Diminished ankle jerk	Disc, usually (see Table 1–8)

*See also Figure 1–10.

TABLE 1–7. PERIPHERAL NERVE LESIONS

Nerve (Root Derivation)	Sensory Supply (Fig. 1–14)	Sensory Loss	Motor Loss	Reflex Change	Lesion
Lateral cutaneous nerve of thigh (L2, 3)	Lateral thigh	Lateral thigh; often intermittent	None	None	Lateral inguinal entrapment
Posterior cutaneous nerve of thigh (S1, S2)	Posterior thigh	Posterior thigh	None (N.B. Sciatic nerve often involved, too)	None	Local (buttock) trauma Pelvic mass Hip fracture
Saphenous branch of femoral nerve (L2, 3, 4)	Anteromedial knee and medial leg	Medial leg	None (N.B. Positive Tinel sign 5–10 cm above medial femoral epicondyle of knee)	None	Local trauma Entrapment above medial epicondyle
Obturator nerve (L2, 3, 4)	Medial thigh	Often none ± medial thigh	Thigh adduction	None	Pelvic mass?
Femoral nerve (L2, 3, 4)	Anteromedial thigh and leg	Anteromedial thigh and leg	Knee extension ± hip flexion	Diminished knee jerk	Retroperitoneal or pelvic mass Femoral artery aneurysm (or puncture) Diabetic mononeuritis
Sciatic nerve (L4, 5; S1)	Anterior and posterior leg Sole and dorsum of foot	Entire foot	Foot dorsiflexion Foot inversion ± plantar flexion ± knee flexion	Diminished ankle jerk	Pelvic mass Hip fracture Pyriform entrapment Misplaced buttock injection
Peroneal nerve (division of sciatic)	Anterior leg, dorsum of foot	None or dorsal foot	Foot dorsiflexion, inversion, and eversion (N.B. Positive Tinel sign at lateral fibular neck)	None	Entrapment pressure at neck of fibula Rarely, diabetes, vasculitis, leprosy

B. The most common causes of objective sensory loss in the lower extremity are peripheral nerve lesions, not root lesions.

The most common sensory disturbance in the leg—called meralgia paresthetica—is caused by entrapment of the lateral cutaneous nerve of the thigh in which dysesthesias involve the lateral surface of the thigh (this may superficially resemble root lesions, especially L2 through L4 (Fig. 1–14). Almost as common is peroneal nerve entrapment at the knee—here, dysesthesias of the lower leg and weakness of the foot may mimic root lesions. Femoral neuropathy (probably most commonly caused by diabetes mellitus[44, 45]) is less common but will produce sensory disturbances along the anterior aspect of the thigh and medial part of the leg (this may also resemble

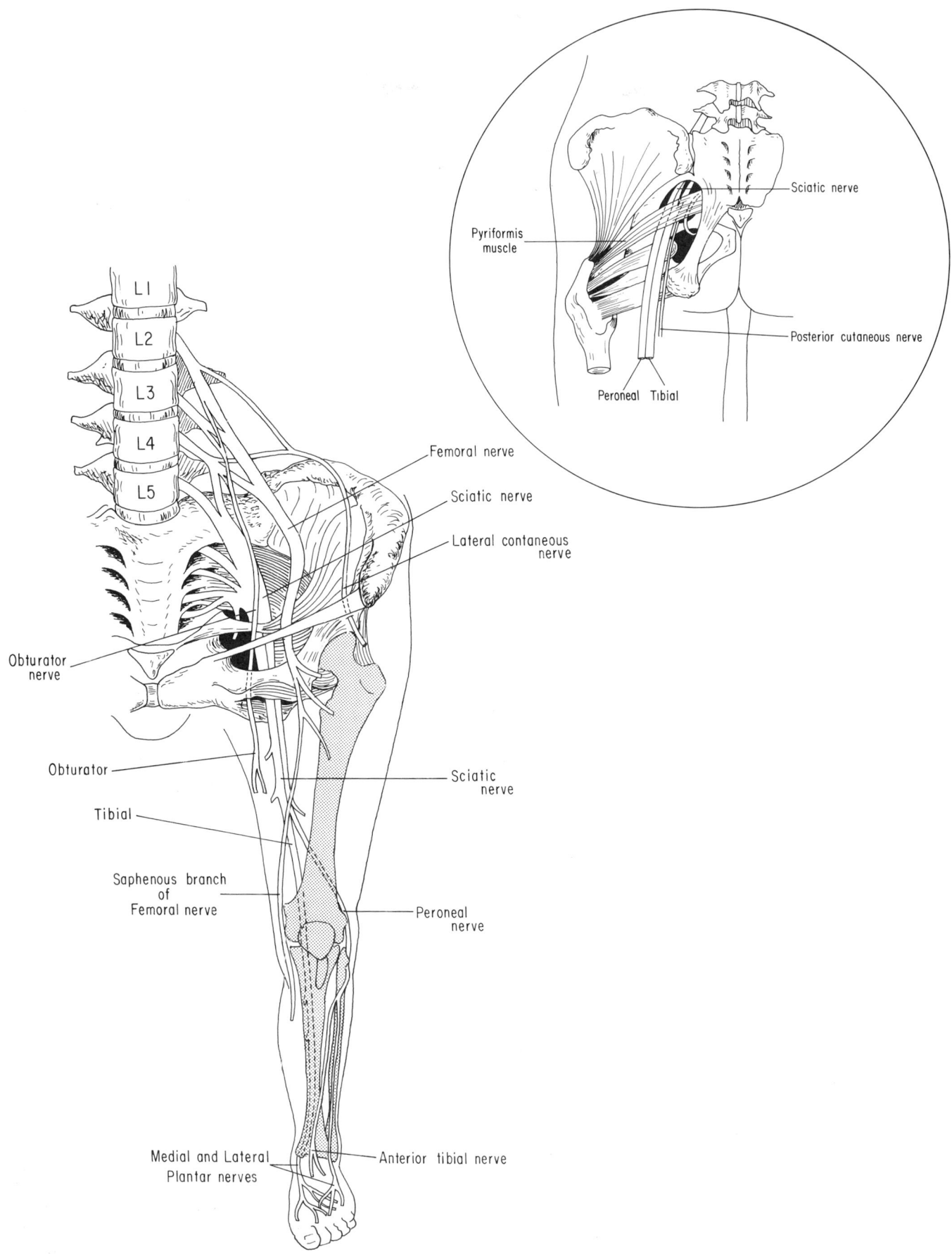

FIGURE 1–15. The course of nerve roots and peripheral nerves to the lower extremity. *Inset:* Course of the sciatic nerve as it exits the pelvis posteriorly.

root lesions at L2 through L4). Tables 1–6 and 1–7 and Figure 1–14 illustrate the overlap of sensory innervation of the leg by nerve roots and peripheral nerves. Figure 1–15 describes the anatomic course of peripheral nerves.

C. Pain or sensory loss involving the anterior portion of the thigh is most unlikely to be due to disc disease—other diagnoses must be strongly considered (see Tables 1–6 through 1–8).

Surgically proven disc herniation usually causes pain in a dermatomal distribution, but more than 90 percent involve the L5 or S1 nerve roots or both.[46-49] (Even when disc disease is responsible for lesions at or above the L4 level, the diagnosis is often difficult because myelography may miss extreme "lateral" disc herniations in this location.[50]) As Table 1–6 illustrates, the differential diagnosis of "high" lumbar root lesions is very different from the differential diagnosis of typical "low" lumbosacral lesions (the typical disc syndromes—Fig. 1–10).

III. Reflexes on one side should always be compared with those of the opposite leg. Bilateral loss of ankle jerks, for example, is much more often due to diffuse peripheral neuropathy (for example, in the diabetic) than to bilateral root or nerve lesions.

REMEMBER

A. Since the spinal cord ends at L1 or L2, "long tract signs" (Babinski reflexes, spasticity—suggesting spinal cord compression) in the patient with back pain always imply processes different from those discussed here.

Lumbosacral disc disease never causes long tract signs.

B. Classic root lesions may or may not impair reflexes. The knee jerk is primarily supplied by L4; the ankle jerk, by S1. Isolated L5 root lesions usually do not cause any reflex changes.

Unilateral diminution of the knee jerk should suggest processes that involve L4 (discs only uncommonly) or the femoral nerve. Unilateral loss of the ankle jerk is usually due to lesions of S1 or the sciatic nerve—other features must then distinguish S1 root lesions from peripheral sciatic nerve lesions (Tables 1–6 and 1–7).

Diagnosis and Treatment

As noted in Figure 1–16, after the history and the general and neurologic examination, patients with radicular back pain will fall into one of several categories:

I. Pseudosciatica.

Sciatica is a diagnostic label often hastily applied to pain that simultaneously involves the low back and various locations in the leg—the buttock, thigh, calf, shin, or foot. While it is true that various components of the sciatic nerve are usually involved in radicular back pain, the term "sciatica" is often misleading for two reasons. First, sciatica is not a diagnosis but is rather the headline for a lengthy differential diagnosis (Table 1–8). Second, many causes of non-neuro-

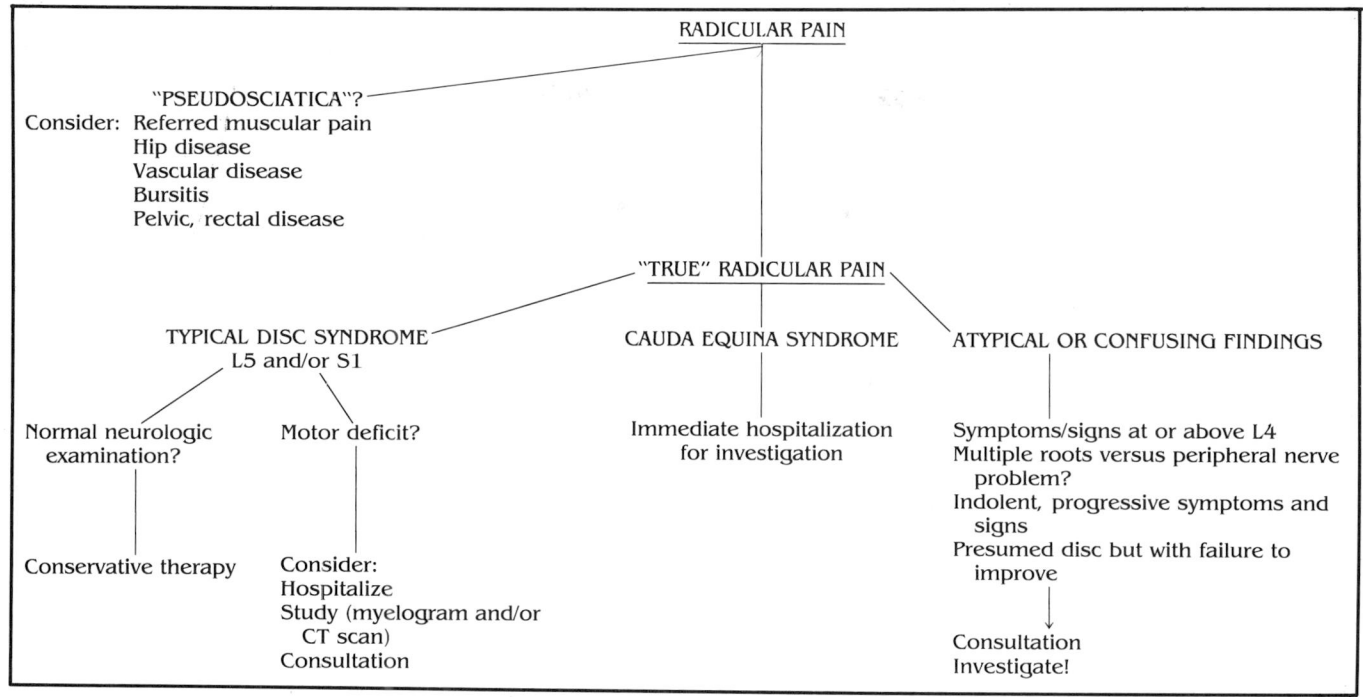

FIGURE 1–16. Radicular pain.

genic back, buttock, and leg pain effect symptoms that superficially resemble sciatica. Such pseudosciatica is very common. Usually pseudosciatica is easy to distinguish from true radicular back pain—the neurologic examination is normal, pain is only superficially similar to neurogenic pain in quality and radiation, traction signs are negative, and other non-neurogenic sources of pain can be discovered by careful history and examination. For example:

As noted previously, simple mechanical back pain without nerve root involvement often refers pain into the buttocks or posterior thighs or both. Such referred muscular pain rarely involves the leg below the knee, and this is a valuable maxim in differential diagnosis.

Disorders of the hip (degenerative arthritis, trochanteric bursitis, psoas bursitis) may superficially resemble sciatica, especially when the lateral or posterior area of the thigh is painful. Manipulation of the hip and palpation of the greater trochanter (see Figs. 1–4 and 1–8) will help here.

Coccydynia (pain and tenderness of the coccyx) is usually easy to exclude by manual palpation of the coccyx (see Fig. 1–4).

Vascular claudication may resemble sciatica when leg exertion induces back, hip, and leg symptoms; usually the history and vascular examination will be characteristic, however. Occasionally vascular claudication will be confused with neurogenic claudication,[54] a specific type of sciatica (see page 49, "Chronic Low Back Pain").

Disorders of the pelvis or rectum may be mistaken for sciatica when buttock pain is prominent—pelvic or rectal neoplastic or inflammatory disease must be remembered. Ischial bursitis can usually be diagnosed by simple palpation (see Fig. 1–4).

II. "True" radicular back pain with clinical findings typical of disc disease.

Dick's case illustrates the typical clinical picture of L5 nerve root irritation due to disc herniation. The description of qualitative "neuritic"

TABLE 1-8. "SCIATICA"[51-53]

CAUSE	WHEN TO SUSPECT	DIAGNOSIS
Nerve Root Disease		
Herniated disc	L5 and/or S1 Traction signs Typical history	Presumptive and/or CT scan (Fig. 1-19) and/or myelography (page 41)
Degenerative spondylosis (and/or spinal stenosis)	X-ray changes (page 48) May be bilateral, multiple roots Neurogenic claudication? Typical history (page 49)	X-ray and/or CT scan and/or myelography
Spondylolisthesis	X-ray (Fig. 1-25)	
Facet syndrome Pedicle kinking Extraforaminal disc	Disc syndrome with "negative" myelogram	CT scan, surgical exploration
Paget's disease	X-rays (Fig. 1-22)	
Compression fracture (Fig. 1-33) Vertebral neoplasm (Fig. 1-23)	History	X-rays, bone scan Find the cause!
Herpes zoster	Dermatomal rash	Visual
Arachnoiditis	Prior surgery and/or myelography	
Primary spinal neoplasm (Fig. 1-18)	Insidious, progressive, nocturnal pain Often multiple root and/or cauda equina syndrome	Myelography, CT scan, exploration
Epidural/subdural metastases or abscess	History (Appendix I)	Myelography/CT scan, and/or exploration
Osteomyelitis	History, ESR (Appendix I)	Bone scan, x-rays (Fig. 1-32)
Lumbosacral Plexus Disease		
Multiple nerve root involvement unilaterally	Cancer Anticoagulation Aortoiliac aneurysm Pelvic disease Diabetic amyotrophy[44, 45]	Abdominal/pelvic CT scan, and/or ultrasound EMG/nerve conduction studies?
Peripheral Nerve Disease		
Pyriform syndrome	Female with dyspareunia Pain worse with extension/ abduction of hip	Clinical findings, EMG/nerve conduction study
Femoral or sciatic mononeuritis (See Table 1-7)	Diabetes mellitus[44, 45] Vasculitis Traumatic	Nerve conduction studies
Meralgia paresthestica	History	Clinical
Peroneal nerve entrapment	+ Tinel sign at fibular head	Clinical, EMG/nerve conduction study

(electric, tingling) pain in a classic L5 dermatomal distribution (see case page 28 and Fig. 1–14), demonstration of unequivocally positive straight leg raising traction maneuvers, and the presence of weakness of motor function supplied solely by the L5 nerve root (big toe dorsiflexion) are all consistent with this conclusion. A middle-aged man with preceding bouts of mechanical back pain who then develops such an acute syndrome (and has normal spinal x-rays) will almost always be found to have a herniated (bulging/prolapsing) disc.

It must be remembered, however, that when clinical findings point to nerve root compression, many diverse disorders may be responsible. When L5 or S1 roots are involved in the young or middle-aged patient with back pain, disc disease is usually the problem. Nevertheless, the clinical setting and x-ray findings must be carefully reviewed,[51, 55] since spondylolisthesis, compression fractures, degenerative spondylosis, Paget's disease, and many other entities may also be responsible for sciatica (Table 1–8). True sciatica is only rarely caused by peripheral nerve or lumbosacral plexus disease. As Table 1–8 suggests, involvement of *multiple* nerve roots simultaneously on one side should suggest lumbosacral plexus compression by neoplasm, hemorrhage, aneurysm, or other masses. Various causes of mononeuritis (Table 1–7) may superficially resemble sciatica. The pyriform syndrome[56] is an unusual problem in young women who describe dyspareunia and sciatic pain that is exacerbated by tension on the pyriformis muscle (Fig. 1–15), which entraps the sciatic nerve — extension and abduction of the hip tense this muscle (and worsen the pain).

Definitive diagnosis thus sometimes requires more sophisticated or invasive studies (computed tomography [CT], myelography, nerve conductions studies), but it is often apparent after clinical and x-ray examination alone. Unlike most patients with simple mechanical back pain, all patients with radicular back pain require x-ray examination of the lumbosacral spine. Other laboratory testing must be individualized.

III. Suspected cauda equina syndromes.

In adults, there are three general types of cauda equina syndrome.[57]

"Conus" lesions (Fig. 1–17A) cause ascending, progressive, bilateral involvement of sacral nerve roots—tumors[58] are the most common cause of this syndrome, which is characterized by insidiously worsening rectal/back/perineal pain with disturbance of perineal sensation (saddle anesthesia), loss of sphincter control (bowel/bladder incontinence) or constipation/urinary retention, and sexual impotence in the male. Motor loss is inapparent until the lesion rises to the S1 or L5 level, and thus the diagnosis is often too long delayed.[59]

Lateral cauda equina lesions (Fig. 1–17B) may produce an atypical "disc syndrome": Involvement of "high" (L4 and above) lumbar roots causes pain and sensory loss over the *anterior* aspect of the thigh, weakness (and atrophy) of thigh muscles, and loss of knee reflexes, sometimes with long tract signs if the neurofibroma (a common cause) also compresses the spinal cord above.

Other "midline" cauda equina lesions cause bilateral lumbar or sacral root lesions in varying combinations: central disc herniations (see Fig. 1–20) are usually the cause when roots L5 through S2 are involved, but other serious (usually neoplastic) diseases must be excluded, especially when high lumbar or low sacral roots are impaired. When a cauda

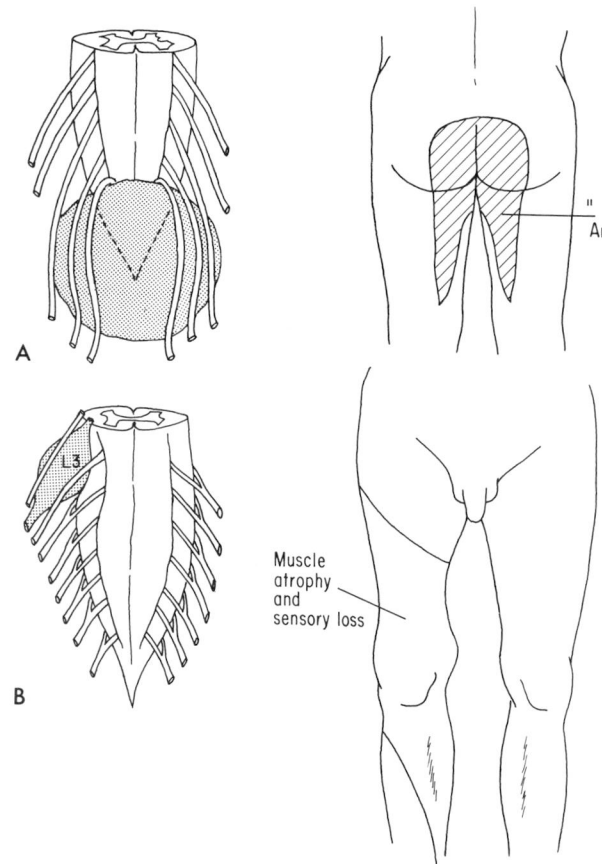

"Saddle" Anesthesia

Muscle atrophy and sensory loss

FIGURE 1–17. Cauda equina syndromes. *A,* A "conus" lesion—gradual expansion of the tumor from below causes ascending bilateral symptoms and signs. *B,* A lateral cauda equina lesion—the upper lumbar roots are involved by a neurofibroma of the third lumbar root.

equina lesion is suspected, the patient should be hospitalized and investigation begun immediately.

IV. Radicular pain with atypical or confusing findings.
Such findings include:

A. Symptoms/signs at or above the L4 level.

B. When the distinction between multiple root involvement and peripheral nerve disease is difficult.

C. When symptoms or signs are insidious in onset, progressive, or both.

D. When other OMINOUS clues are present. Those clues (Fig. 1–1) apply as much to radicular back pain as to simple mechanical back pain.

E. When a presumed disc syndrome does not improve with conservative therapy (see page 40).

Such atypical or confusing findings always merit further investigation (Fig. 1–18). For example, the various tumors that often cause cauda equina syndromes may be "neurologically silent" for a long time[59] or quite closely mimic disc lesions.[60, 61] The urgency of consultation, the need for hospitalization and further invasive studies will vary with the specific situation.

Dick is told that his examination has changed and that it is very likely now that a herniated disc is causing his back and leg pain; there is now evidence of pressure on a particular nerve and weakness of a muscle in the toe. He is told that occasionally this can be a serious problem requiring surgery, especially if there are signs of progressive "nerve damage," but that usually the problem will resolve without surgery if strict bedrest and therapy are

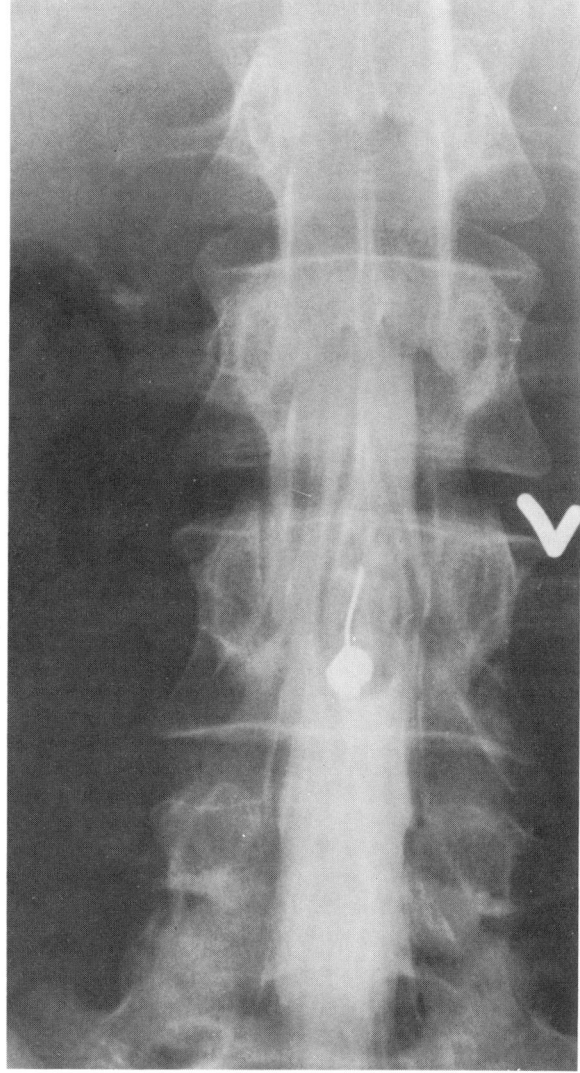

FIGURE 1–18. Primary tumor of the cauda equina. This 22-year-old man complained of 7 weeks of low back pain. Initially, examination was unremarkable. Conservative therapy failed to produce improvement. X-rays of the lumbosacral spine (followed by CT scan of the lumbosacral spine) were normal. Worsening of back pain and the development of bilateral buttock and leg dysesthesias prompted the performance of this myelogram. At the level of the L3–4 interspace, there is an ovoid mass lesion that is deflecting the nerve roots as they pass down the cauda equina. Surgical exploration revealed an ependymoma. (The tumor is located right at the level of the spinal needle.)

followed. This is so important now that hospitalization will be necessary if he does not improve by complying with treatment.

Strict bedrest is ordered for the next 10 days, and conservative measures are reemphasized.

NOTE

I. The clinical picture here is so typical of disc herniation that the diagnosis can be presumed, at least temporarily. Because most patients (perhaps 80 percent) with radicular back pain due to disc herniation will improve with conservative medical therapy (see Table 1–9), further diagnostic studies are not necessary at this time.[63, 66, 67]

   Myelography or CT of the spine or both are indicated in general only when the clinical picture is OMINOUS or atypical (see above) or when surgical intervention is planned. Note that each of these circumstances mandates subspecialty consultation anyway—most such invasive testing decisions should thus be left to the subspecialist, when possible.

II. Immediate hospitalization or urgent referral to a subspecialist is indicated when a cauda equina lesion is suspected, when there are long tract signs,

TABLE 1–9. LONG-TERM RESULTS OF
TREATMENT OF LUMBAR DISC DISEASE

SERIES	PATIENTS	FOLLOW-UP, yr	RESULTS (%)			
			Excellent	*Good*	*Fair*	*Poor*
Conservative						
Friedenberg, Shoemaker,[62]	36	2–10	47	31	11	11
Pearce, Moll[63]	91	0–13	27	41	17	15
	Summary		**37**	**36**	**14**	**13**
Surgical						
Spurling, Grantam[48]	378	0–8	40	39	14	7
Gurdjian, et al[47]	772	3–13	20	54	20	7
Barr, et al[64]	644	10–20	68	22	5	5
Rosen[49]	300	0.5–1.0	82	11	4	2
Shannon, Paul[46]	323	3.1	85	12	—	3
	Summary		**50**	**33**	**10**	**7**

Adapted from reference 65.

and (perhaps) when there is prominent focal motor weakness (for example, footdrop).

The former two situations require emergency study and (often) surgery; there is some controversy about the urgency of extreme focal motor weakness,[68–71] but certainly a specialist should be consulted in such circumstances. Dermatomal sensory loss and diminution of segmental reflexes (for example, absence of ankle jerk) are helpful diagnostic findings but do not necessarily mandate consultation, testing, or hospitalization.

III. Conservative therapy of[66] presumed disc herniation is similar to that for simple mechanical back pain,[72] with a few exceptions:

A. Complete bedrest is often needed for more prolonged periods (1 to 3 weeks).

Since many patients (especially active wage earners) are unhappy about such prolonged immobilization, various adjunctive measures are often proposed. These include:

B. Epidural corticosteroid injections.[73, 74] Such injections often produce dramatic and prompt improvement in selected patients.

C. Systemic (oral) corticosteroids in huge doses (64 mg of dexamethasone [Decadron] per day—the equivalent of more than 300 mg of prednisone) have been found useful by some.[75] Whether lower doses of oral prednisone (40 to 60 mg a day) are helpful is unproven, but they are commonly used in this situation.

D. Gravity traction,[69] usually in hospital.

E. Chemonucleolysis[76, 77]—the injection of chymopapain[133] under fluoroscopic guidance directly into a disc—appears to be effective in selected patients, but its use remains controversial.

(These and other adjunctive measures must be remembered for what they are: Strict bedrest, pain control, and careful follow-up are usually much more important.)

One week later, Dick reports that his back and leg "feel fine" when he remains in bed, but arising just to go to the bathroom causes recurrent radicular pain. Examination is unchanged—there is no further neurologic impairment, but straight leg raising remains positive at 40 degrees on the left, and the left big toe is weak on dorsiflexion.

Dick is admitted to the hospital. CT scan confirms the presence of a posterolaterally protruding disc at the L4-5 level without other abnormalities. A neurosurgical consultant recommends further conservative treatment. Epidural steroid injections provide moderate pain relief over the next few days; gravity traction for the next 10 days results in marked improvement. After 2 weeks of such treatment and complete bedrest (with simple back flexion bed exercises) radicular pain is absent on ambulation, straight leg raising is negative, and toe weakness can no longer be demonstrated.

Dick is discharged from the hospital, is begun on gradual back exercises, and is told to avoid any physical work/lifting for the next month.

One month later, Dick is ambulating without difficulty. There is very mild low back pain without hip or leg pain. Dick is allowed to return to work after 2 more weeks of daily exercise therapy.

REMEMBER

1. Hospitalization for further aggressive conservative therapy is often preferable to hasty surgery. Most patients with disc disease and radiculopathy do not require surgery.[78, 79] The consulting surgeon's approach should reflect this attitude if the primary care physician (who requests the consultation) is to be an effective advocate for the patient (see also Table 1–9). Fortunately, the "failed back syndrome"[53, 80] that follows unsuccessful (or unnecessary) back surgery is decreasing in incidence precisely because experienced spinal surgeons are highly conservative. Greater awareness of the differential diagnosis of sciatica[53] (Table 1–8) and a greater array of sensitive diagnostic studies (especially the CT scan) have also contributed to recent improvement in diagnosis and treatment.

2. While myelography is the traditional diagnostic procedure in such situations, CT scanning has achieved impressive results in recent studies and may now be the procedure of choice (Fig. 1–19).[81-83] The CT scan is especially valuable in detecting disorders that may clinically mimic disc herniation but

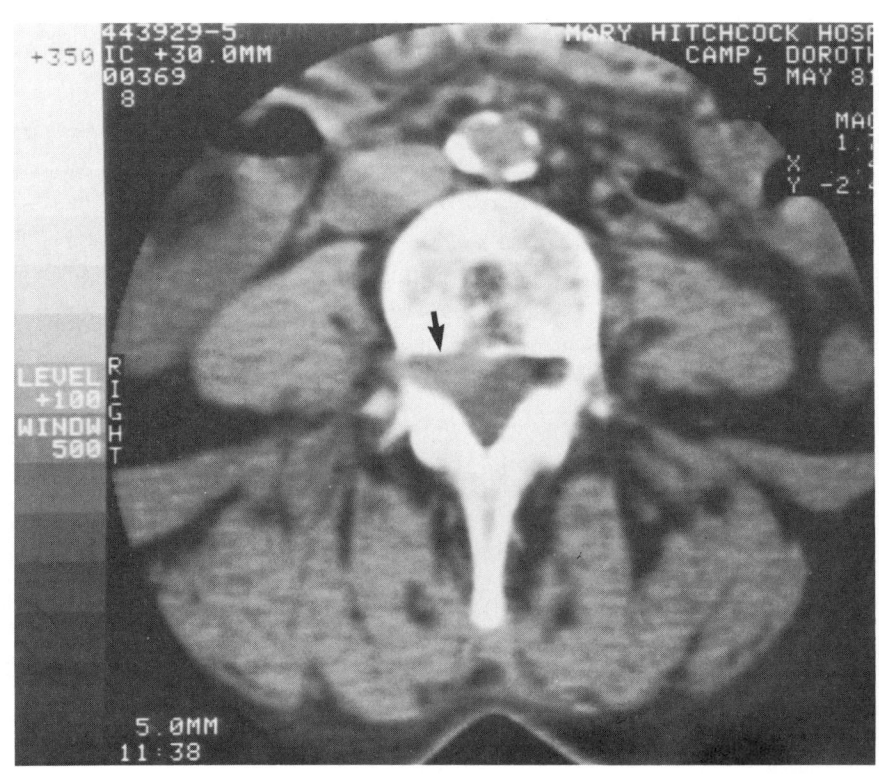

FIGURE 1–19. This 45-year-old woman described severe low back pain radiating into her right leg and foot (L5 distribution), which began while straining to lift a television set from the floor. Examination revealed impaired range of back motion, positive straight leg raising (at 40 degrees), and mild weakness of big toe dorsiflexion. Reflexes were normal. Conservative treatment at home for 10 days was unsuccessful. This CT scan demonstrates a large disc protrusion at the L4–5 level on the right (arrow). Surgical discectomy relieved all symptoms and signs.

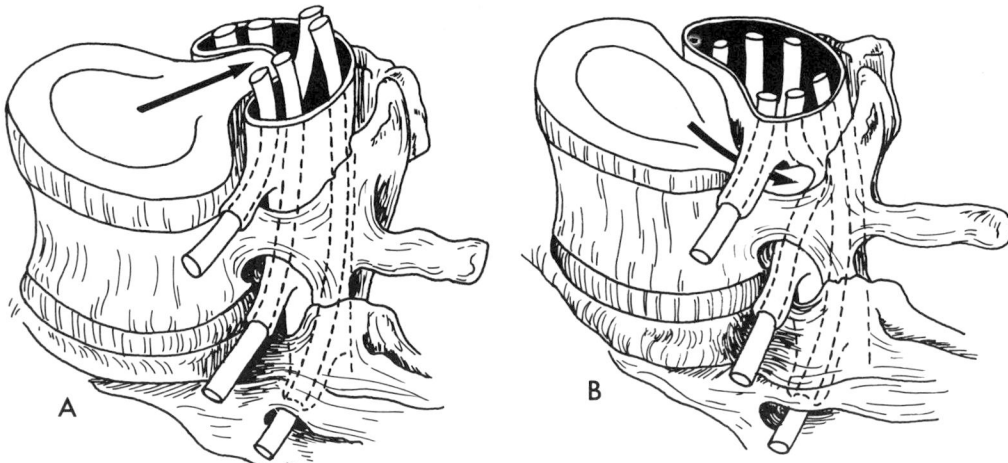

FIGURE 1–20. *A,* An L4–5 disc herniating centrally. This event might result in compression of multiple roots—a cauda equina syndrome. *B,* An L4–5 disc herniating posterolaterally. This event will usually compress only one nerve root, most often L5, but not always.

that cause nerve root entrapment by other mechanisms (which may be missed by myelography[53]).

Occasionally, epidural venography[84] will help when the myelogram is equivocal (and the patient has not undergone prior back surgery), but the CT scan will probably render this procedure a rarity. Electromyograms and nerve conduction studies may be difficult to perform (and interpret) in the lower extremity but are especially useful when peripheral nerve lesions are difficult to distinguish clinically from root lesions.

Even when disc herniation is almost certainly the clinical diagnosis, myelography or CT scanning (or both) is necessary for the surgeon to plan his approach because, while clinical examination accurately defines nerve root entrapment, the intervertebral level of disc herniation cannot be confidently predicted by the clinical findings.[85, 86] In Dick's case, an L4-5 disc is causing L5 root compression (a common situation: see Fig. 1–10), but disc herniations at all levels below L2 may compress any of the lumbosacral nerve roots, depending on the size, direction, and location of the disc prolapse (see Fig. 1–20).

3. Disc disease tends to cause recurrent, relapsing illness. Prophylactic exercise therapy should be recommended indefinitely. Daily exercises and preventive measures (see pages 24 and 25) should be stressed for all patients with disc disease.

Chronic low back pain tends not to be due to recurrent disc herniation, however. A different diagnostic and therapeutic emphasis is usually needed for patients with chronic low back pain.

CHRONIC LOW BACK PAIN

The distinction between acute and chronic low back pain must be somewhat arbitrary because chronic back pain must begin sometime, and thus those disorders commonly responsible for chronic pain may obviously cause acute symptoms. Nevertheless, the patient whose low back has been painful for months or years requires a different approach. A few general principles will help in most cases:

Diagnosis

I. How long has the back pain been present?

As noted previously, many serious diseases of the spine and extraspinal organs may cause low back pain. Subacute, insidious onset of progressively worsening back pain over several weeks or months is always worrisome. Pain present for many years is much less likely to be due to serious disease (or referred pain). Usually degenerative or postural disorders of the spine are the causes of longstanding back pain (see pages 47 to 51).

II. Are there clues that point to uncommon but therapeutically important diseases?

A careful history is the key here.

Pain and stiffness of the lower back, which are prominent when first arising from bed (morning stiffness) but which improve gradually throughout the day only to recur the following morning (or after prolonged rest), are common in simple postural disorders or in degenerative spondylosis. However, prominent morning stiffness in the young patient should suggest ankylosing spondylitis and other spondyloarthropathies (due to rheumatoid arthritis, inflammatory bowel disease, Reiter's syndrome, and the like). (Schober testing—Fig. 1–21—and sacroiliac joint films—Fig. 1–24—are helpful here.) Such symptoms in the older patient should raise the question of polymyalgia rheumatica (usually associated with neck/shoulder stiffness and an elevated sedimentation rate).

Weight loss associated with chronic back pain should suggest neoplasms, vertebral osteomyelitis (see Appendix I), and certain endocrine or systemic diseases (hyperthyroidism, or malabsorption, for example) that may induce metabolic bone disease (see Appendix II).

Chronic low back pain that "sounds nonmechanical" (see page 3) requires a search for referred pain. Other concomitant complaints must always be assessed: pelvic disease (especially uterine myomas and

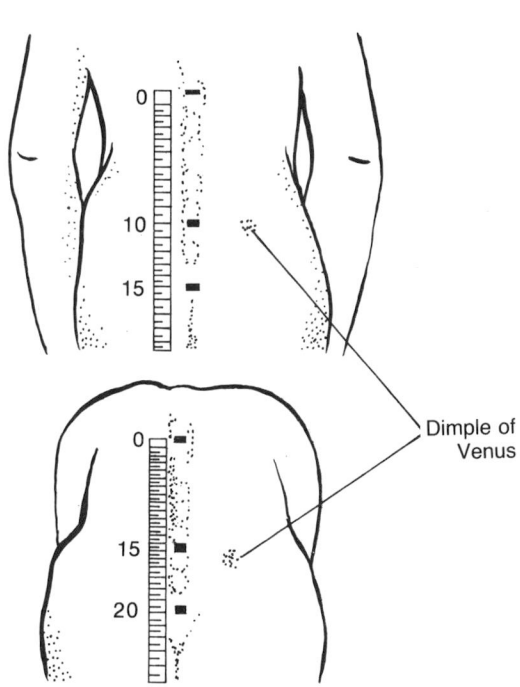

FIGURE 1–21. Schöber testing. The Schöber test is performed by aligning a tape measure vertically along the spine, beginning at 10 cm above an imaginary horizontal line which joins the "dimples of Venus," which are the small hollows located at either side of the lumbosacral spine as noted in the figure. Marks are then made at 0, 10, and 15 cm, with the tape measure still aligned. The patient is then asked to flex the back (touch the toes) fully, and the amount of mobility of the spine is measured, as noted in the lower figure. A normal range of motion is 5 cm, that is, from a total of 15 cm to a total of at least 20 cm. Many patients will apparently be able to perform full back flexion and yet have markedly limited range of motion of the lumbar spine when specifically tested. This "pseudoflexion" is accomplished primarily by changes in the motion of the hips and the pelvis, rather than in the lumbar spine itself. This measurement is a particularly good way to follow patients with ankylosing spondylitis.

Dimple of Venus

TABLE 1–10. CHRONIC LOW BACK PAIN WITH NORMAL LUMBOSACRAL SPINE X-RAYS

PROGRESSIVE WORSENING FOR WEEKS/MONTHS?	WEIGHT LOSS?	MORNING STIFFNESS?	NON-MECHANICAL?	NEUROLOGIC SYMPTOMS/ SIGNS?	INTRACTABLE DISC DISEASE?	POSTURAL?	PSYCHOGENIC?
↓	↓	↓	↓	↓	↓	↓	↓
OMINOUS	Neoplasm? Subacute osteomyelitis? Metabolic bone disease	Polyarthritis? Sacroiliitis? Polymyalgia rheumatica?	Referred pain? ↓ Endometriosis? Uterine myomas? Prostatitis? GI Ca? Retroperitoneal process?	Disc? Cauda equina? Spinal tumor?	CONSIDER: CT scan Myelogram	Obese Paunchy Postpartum Lordosis Pelvic tilt Unequal leg lengths Muscle weakness	Litigation? Disability? Depression? Psychosis? Malingering?
↓			↓				
Bone scan ESR	Bone scan ESR	ESR Sacroiliac films	Pelvic/rectal exam, etc.	CONSIDER: CT scan Myelogram			

endometriosis) in the female and prostate disease (chronic prostatitis) in the male should be remembered especially. Associated abdominal pain, fever, or other genitourinary complaints raise many other questions (see Table 1–1 and Appendix I).

Chronic low back pain in association with neurologic symptoms is usually related to recurrent disc disease, spondylosis with nerve root compression, or (rarely) spinal cord tumors.

III. X-rays and screening laboratory tests should always be performed.

Unlike the patient with acute simple mechanical back pain, in the patient with chronic back pain, x-rays and blood tests are usually helpful. This is so for three reasons:

A. When x-rays are normal (or nonspecific), but other clinical features are OMINOUS (progressive worsening, fever, elevated sedimentation rate, anemia), further studies are always necessary. Bone scans (osteomyelitis, neoplasm), bone marrow aspiration (multiple myeloma), CT scans or myelography (spinal canal neoplasm or abscess), or bone biopsy (metabolic bone disease) may then be needed, depending upon the clinical suspicion. Table 1–10 illustrates that a variety of disorders may cause chronic low back pain in the presence of normal x-rays.

Most OMINOUS causes of back pain can be excluded by a normal sedimentation rate, blood count, alkaline phosphatase, acid phosphatase, calcium, phosphate, and BUN determinations (see Appendices I and II).

B. Sometimes the x-ray and "screening" laboratory tests provide a specific diagnosis (Table 1–11). Most patients with Paget's disease (Fig. 1–22), metastatic neoplasm (Fig. 1–23), chronic sacroiliitis (Fig. 1–24) or inflammatory spondyloarthritis, severe metabolic bone disease (Fig. 1–33), or chronic osteomyelitis (Fig. 1–32) will demonstrate abnormal x-ray findings.

C. Sometimes the x-ray uncovers spinal abnormalities that may or may not cause the patient's pain, but that are worth noting.[87]

Spinal malalignment disorders are the most common examples. These include entities such as idiopathic (mild) scoliosis, spina bifida occulta, and symmetric transitional vertebrae (lumbarization of the first sacral vertebra, sacralization of the fifth lumber vertebra)—these are usually incidental radiographic findings. On the other hand, asymmetric transitional vertebrae (only unilaterally sacralized or

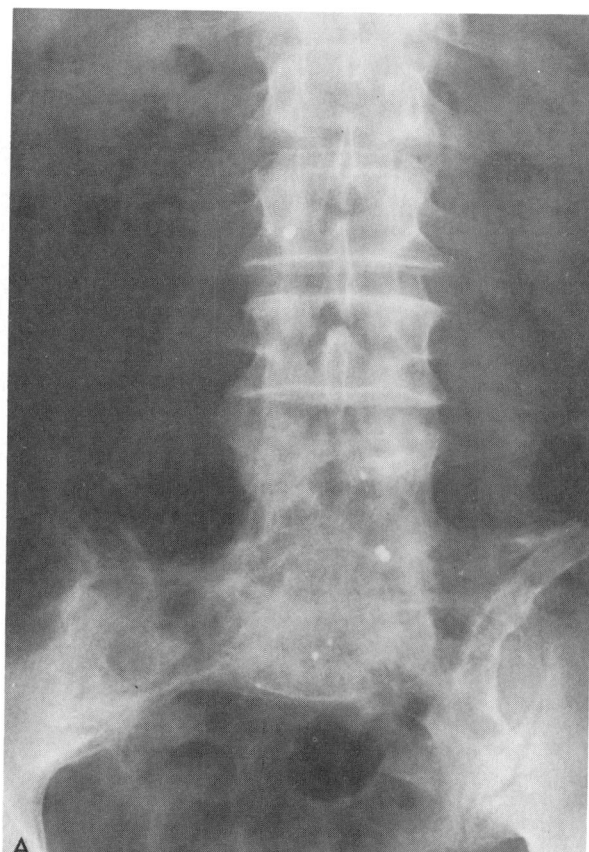

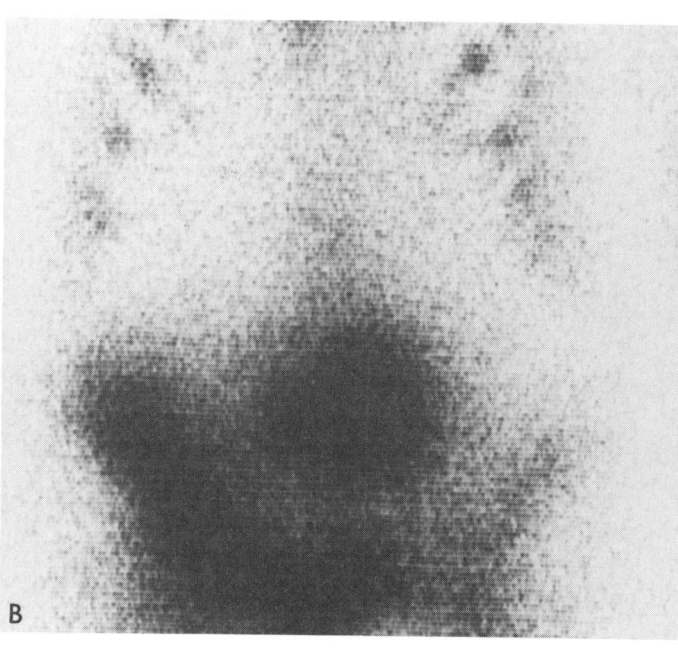

FIGURE 1–22. Paget's disease. This 74-year-old male described severe, progressive lower back pain for the previous 8 months. *A,* X-rays demonstrate extensive Paget's disease of the lumbosacral spine and pelvis. *B,* The bone scan illustrates the extent of involvement, primarily the lumbosacral spine and right pelvic bones.

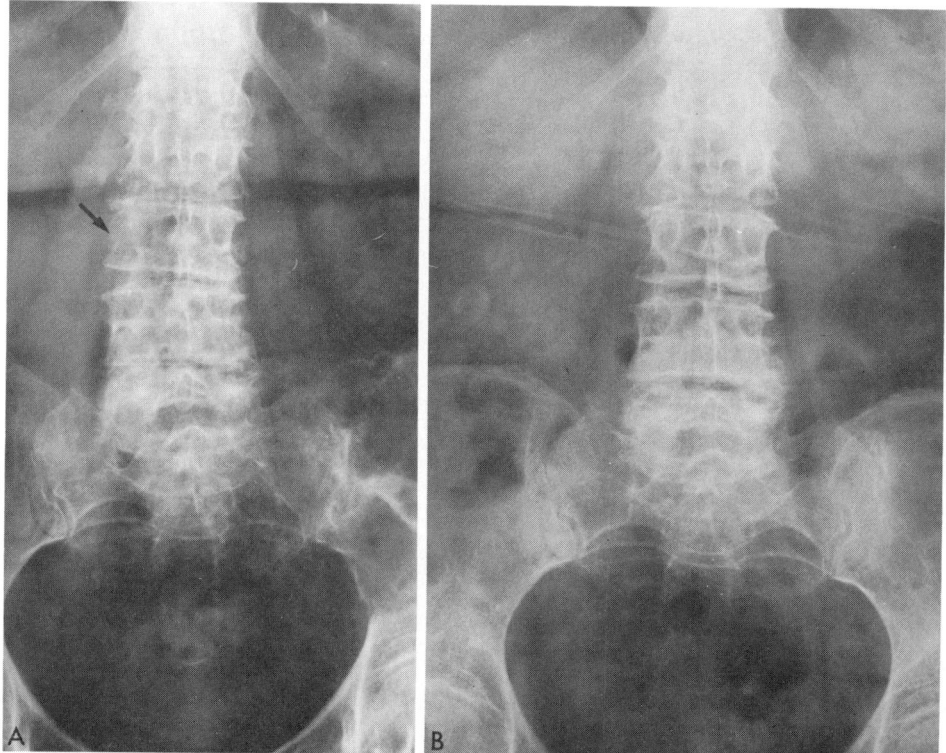

FIGURE 1–23. Metastatic breast carcinoma. This 57-year-old woman developed persistent low back pain 9 years following a radical mastectomy for breast carcinoma. Comparison of current lumbosacral spine films (*A*) with films taken previously (*B*) demonstrated destruction of the right half of the third lumbar vertebral body (*arrow*).

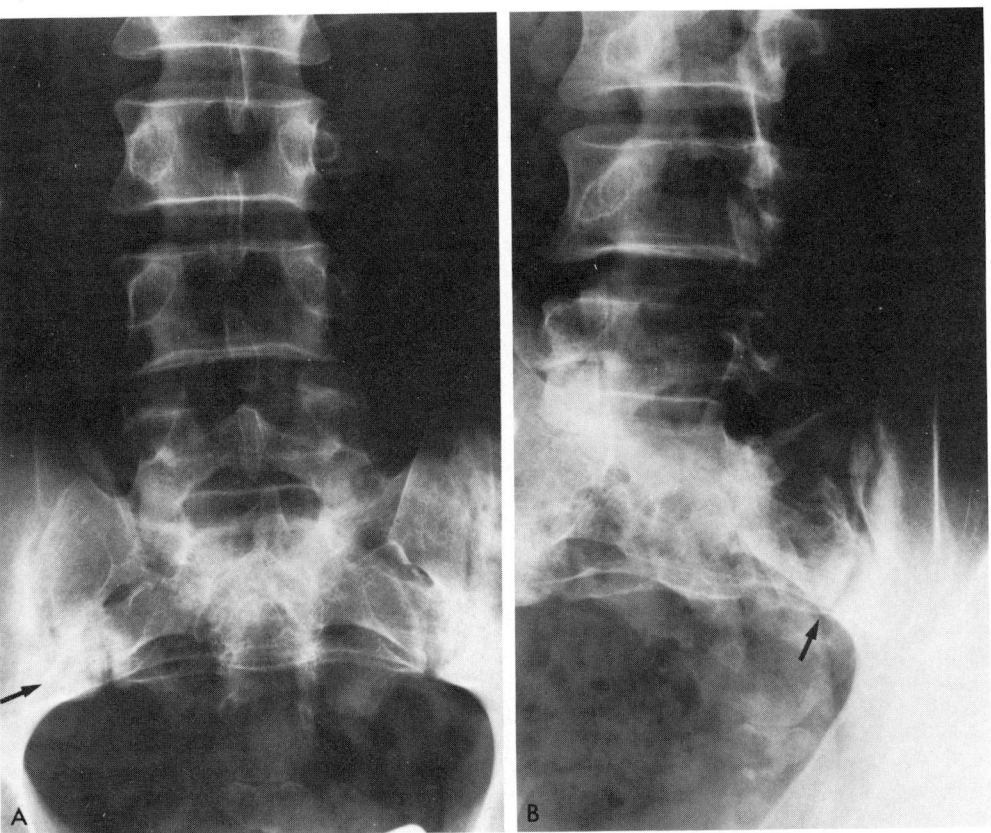

FIGURE 1–24. This 33-year-old male with longstanding psoriasis complained of chronic low back pain with pronounced morning stiffness. Back range of motion was slightly limited but Gaenslen's tests (Fig. 1–9) were markedly positive, more prominently on the left. X-rays reveal narrowing and irregularity of the sacroiliac joints bilaterally (A), with prominent involvement of the lower thirds (arrows). Oblique views of the left sacroiliac joint (B) confirm this finding.

lumbarized), spondylolysis with or without spondylolisthesis[88, 89] (Fig. 1–25A and B), and facet tropism—see Appendix III and Figure 1–34—(asymmetry of the planes of orientation of facet joints articulating at a particular vertebral level) may well be (at least partly) responsible for back pain.

Most of these disorders probably cause symptoms primarily by predisposing the patient to postural imbalances or accelerated progression of degenerative spine disease or both (see below). An exception is spondylolisthesis, which may require surgical correction under certain circumstances.[88]

TABLE 1–11. CHRONIC LOW BACK PAIN WITH ABNORMAL LUMBOSACRAL SPINE X-RAY

SPONDYLOSIS	OSTEOPENIA	PAGET'S DISEASE	MALALIGNMENT	METASTATIC NEOPLASM	PRIMARY BONY NEOPLASM	DISC SPACE INFECTION
↓	↓		↓	↓	↓	↓
Local back pain?	Compression fracture(s)?	Exclude osteoblastic metastatic disease (Fig. 1–26E)	Scoliosis Spina bifida Transitional vertebra Hemivertebra Spondylolysis Spondylolisthesis Facet tropism	Breast Ca Lung Ca Prostate Ca Kidney Ca Thyroid Ca Lymphoma Pelvic neoplasm	Osteoid osteoma Hemangioma Osteoblastoma Osteosarcoma Multiple myeloma	Bacterial Tuberculous Fungal
or						
Sciatica?	↓					
	Find causes! Osteoporosis? Osteomalacia? Multiple myeloma? Hyperparathyroidism?					
or						
Spinal stenosis			↓			
↓	↓					
Associated disc disease?	Appendix II		Related to back pain or not?			

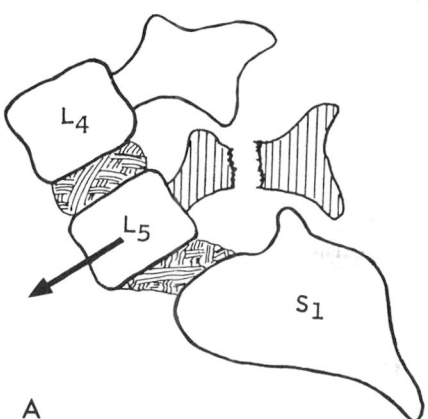

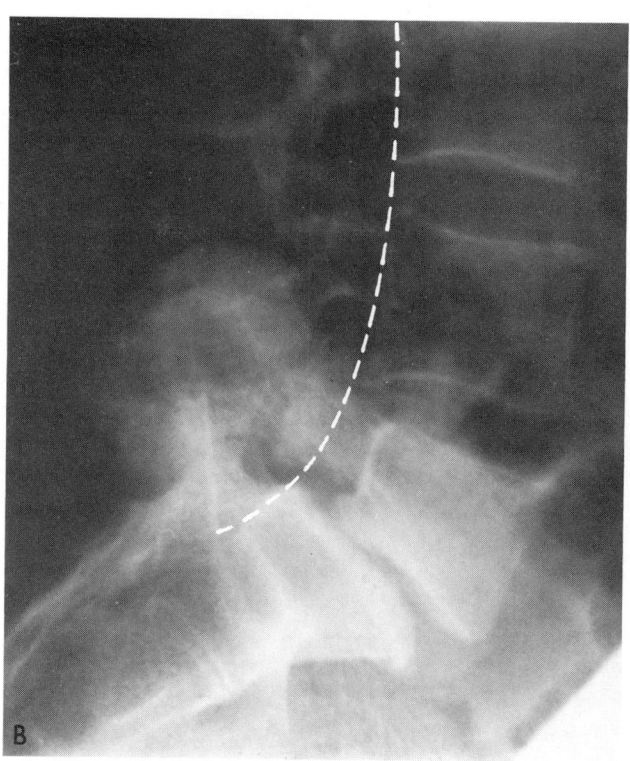

FIGURE 1–25. *A*, Spondylolysis refers to disruption of the posterior articulation so that continuity between the superior and inferior articular processes at one vertebral level (L5) is lost. Spondylolysis per se is rarely a problem unless it results in spondylolisthesis, in which the vertebral body subluxes forward on its subjacent vertebra.

B, This 42-year-old man presented with acute bilateral back and posterior leg pain. There had been a prior history of recurrent low back pain but no neurologic symptoms. Examination revealed evidence of bilateral L5 root dysfunction. X-ray demonstrates slippage of the fifth lumbar vertebra forward on the first sacral vertebra (dotted lines trace the normal vertebral positions). There is chronic degenerative change at the L5–S1 interspace as well. Surgical correction was required to alleviate symptoms.

The most common causes of chronic low back pain are spinal degenerative disease and chronic postural imbalance.

Degeneration of the intervertebral disc is probably a "normal" aging phenomenon, and this process results in various compensatory but pathologic reactions in the bones (reactive osteophyte formation) and joints (facet joint arthritis) of the lumbosacral spine, the end result of which is lumbosacral spondylosis (Fig. 1–26).

Degenerative spondylosis probably begins early in life but usually becomes symptomatic only in middle age (or after). (Younger patients with spondylosis often come to attention because of intercurrent disc herniations, and the combination of disorders contributes to the clinical events.[90]) The history is usually that of intermittently relapsing, chronic back pain over the course of many years that is often aggravated by the lordotic position (kneeling, standing, reaching overhead, for example—hyperextending the back) and that is characteristically improved by sitting or bending forward (the severely afflicted will walk "bent over" to reduce symptoms).

Spondylosis may cause several different clinical syndromes (Fig. 1–26, *A* through *D*). Local back pain may be due to: facet joint osteoarthritis (here, steroid-anesthetic facet joint injections may be therapeutic); irritation of local pain-sensitive structures (see Appendix III) by osteophytes; and associated musculoligamentous or facet joint instability.[91] Nerve root compression may cause sciatica when hypertrophied facets or reactive osteophytes impinge on the nerve root exiting the intervertebral foramen.[92–94] Spinal stenosis[95] (Fig. 1–26D) may result when disc space narrowing, vertebral instability, hypertrophic osteophytes, and facet arthritis conspire to narrow the internal area of the spinal canal (especially when the spinal canal is congenitally or developmentally narrowed to begin with). Such spinal stenosis may result in single nerve root compressions (rarely), cauda equina syndromes, or "neurogenic claudication."

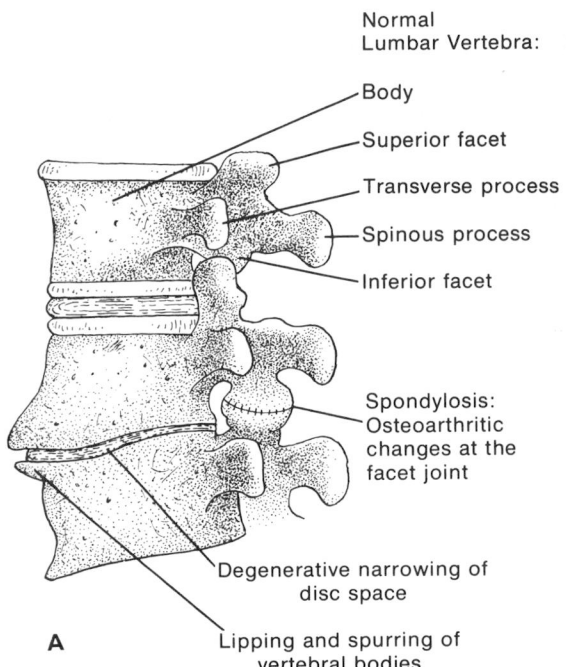

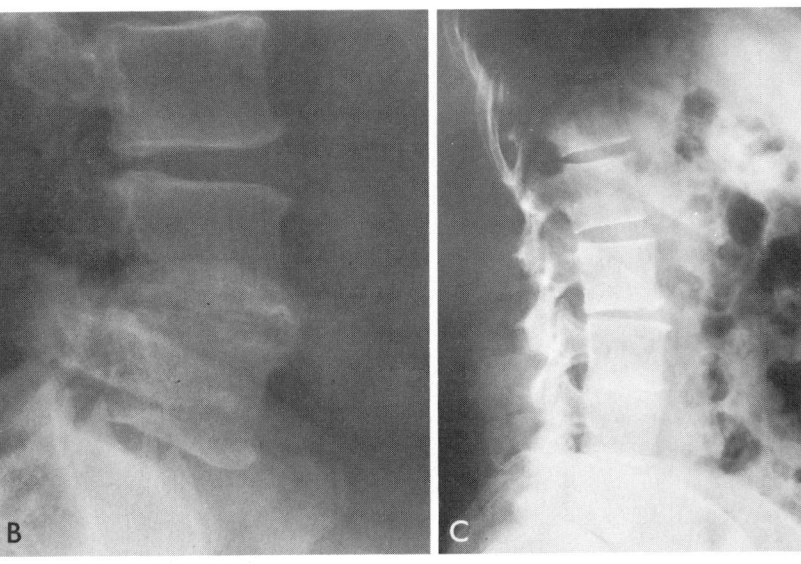

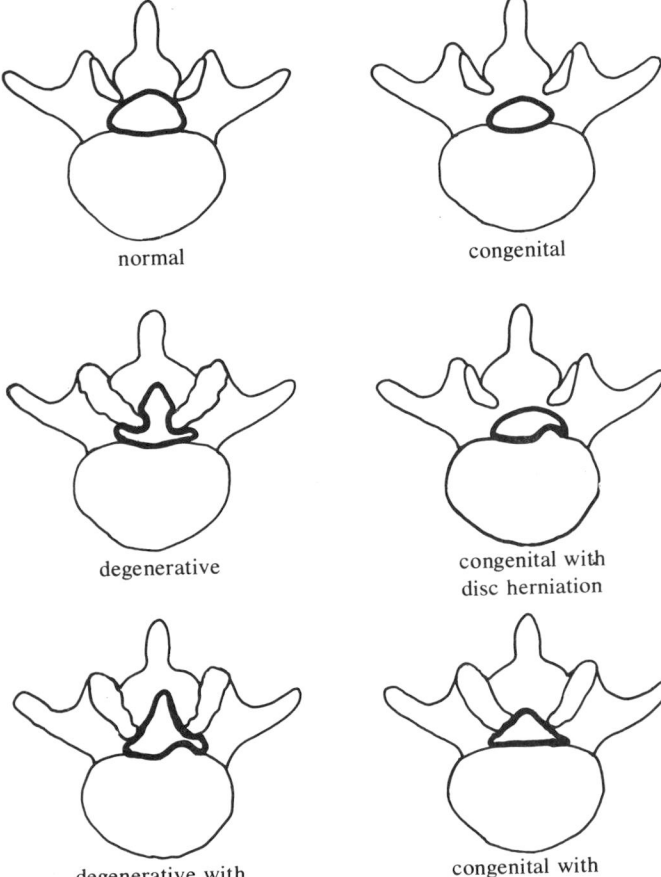

FIGURE 1–26. Degenerative spondylosis and spinal stenosis.

A, Degenerative spondylosis. Narrowing of the disc interspace accompanied by lipping and spurring of the adjacent vertebral bodies and by osteoarthritis of the facet joints.

B, This 64-year-old man described chronic recurrent low back pain for the previous 4 years. Physical examination was unremarkable except for back limitation of motion. X-rays demonstrate severe degenerative spondylosis with fusion of the L4 and L5 vertebrae.

C, This 60-year-old woman described progressively worsening low back pain over a period of 4 weeks. There had been intermittent low back pain in the past. Physical examination was normal with the exception of back limitation of motion. X-rays revealed degenerative spondylosis with narrowing of the interspaces at the L3–4, L4–5, and L5–S1 levels. There is near fusion of the L3–4 interspace.

D, Outlines of the cross section of the spinal canal in different types of spinal stenosis.

Illustration continued on following page

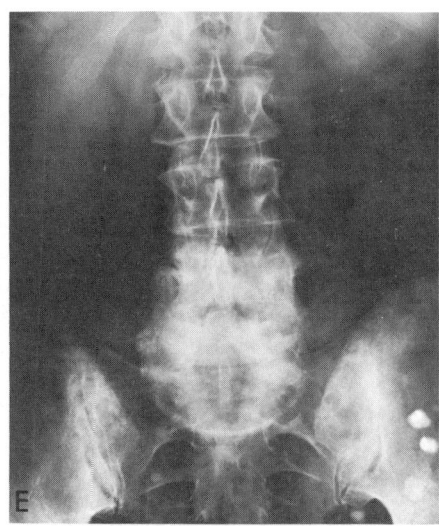

FIGURE 1–26 *Continued*

E–G, Spinal stenosis. This 77-year-old man described progressively worsening low back pain over the previous 6 months. Two months before these x-rays were obtained, he developed classic neurogenic claudication. Physical examination was unremarkable except for a hard, nodular prostate.

E, X-rays of the spine revealed extensive osteoblastic metastases in the lower lumbosacral spine.

F, CT scan shows extreme spinal stenosis with hypertrophy of the lamina and articular facets. There is marked expansion of the vertebral body by osteoblastic metastatic tumor (*arrows*).

G, Myelogram reveals complete block of the spinal canal at the L3–4 interspace (*arrow*). Laminectomy partially relieved the patient's neurogenic claudication. (Metastatic prostate carcinoma was documented histologically.) (*A* reproduced with permission from Branch, WT: Office Practice of Medicine. Philadelphia, W.B. Saunders Co., 1982; *D* reproduced with permission from Kelley, NN, Harris, ED, Jr, Ruddy, S, and Sledge, CB: Textbook of Rheumatology. Philadelphia, W.B. Saunders Co., 1981.)

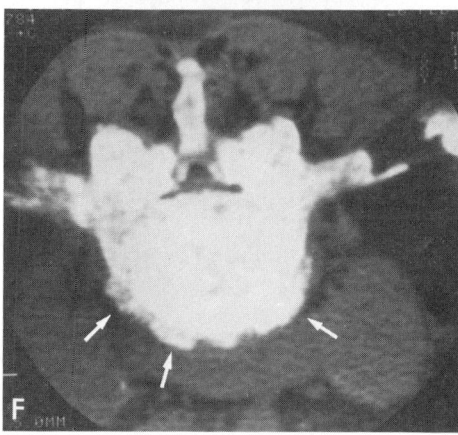

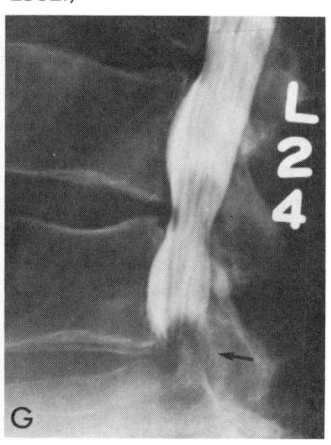

Neurogenic claudication refers to intermittent low back and (often bilateral) leg pain and dysesthesias, a syndrome sometimes confused with aortoiliac vascular claudication because exercise appears to induce symptoms. Closer questioning (and a normal vascular examination) usually distinguishes vascular from neurogenic claudication: Neurogenic claudication is often induced by prolonged standing, bending, or hyperextending the back as well as by walking; vascular claudication is precipitated by leg exercise and is relieved with (even standing) rest. Whether the symptoms of neurogenic claudication are caused by actual compression of neural structures or by positional neural ischemia is controversial, but spondylotic spinal stenosis is the usual cause of such symptoms (but not always—see Fig. 1–26E through G).

Radiographic spondylosis—disc space narrowing, osteophytosis, facet joint sclerosis, and foraminal narrowing—may be seen on x-rays (Fig. 1–26B and C) of many *asymptomatic* patients. Hence, while the diagnosis of spondylosis is supported by such x-ray findings, the diagnosis of symptomatic spondylosis is primarily clinical.

When symptomatic spinal stenosis is suspected clinically (and especially if surgery is contemplated), myelography or CT scans or both are needed to confirm the diagnosis (Fig. 1–26F through G).

When neurologic compromise is not a problem, the treatment of spondylosis usually involves anti-inflammatory drugs, back exercises, and other conservative measures (see above). Surgery is usually a last resort (but will be very successful in carefully selected patients).

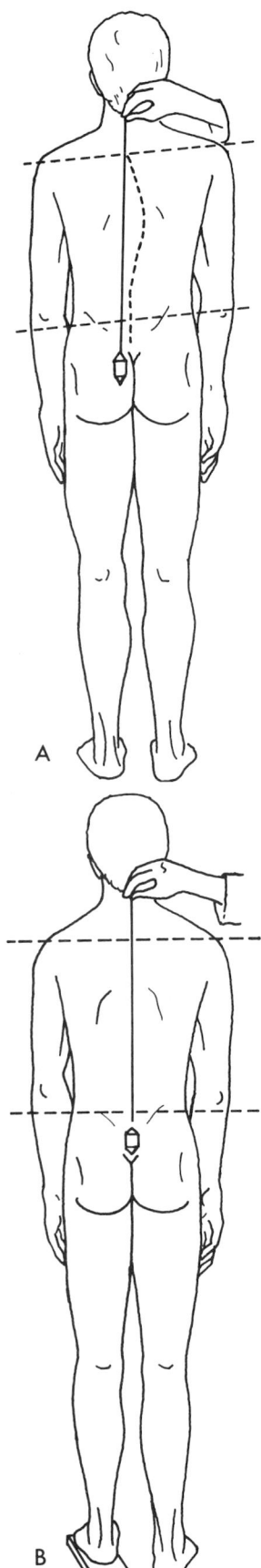

Chronic postural disorders are probably the most common initiating or contributory cause of chronic back pain. Here, often avoidable and remediable biomechanical stresses induce musculoligamentous strains, functional scoliosis, and excessive lumbar lordosis. These mechanical stresses are also common additive causes of disability in the patient with structural back disease (spondylosis, for example)—in fact, it is likely that such postural disorders play a role in the etiology of spondylosis.

Some postural disorders are both easy to detect and to correct:

1. Simple poor posture. The typical patient is obese with lax abdominal musculature (the middle-aged multiparous mother, for example) whose excessive lumbar lordosis is obvious on examination (see Fig. 1–2). Pregnancy and frequent use of high-heeled shoes (both of which exaggerate lumbar lordosis) often worsen matters. Weight loss, daily back flexion exercises, abdominal muscle strengthening, and general preventive health measures (diet, cardiovascular exercise, and back pain prophylaxis) will help most here.

2. Pelvic tilting. Asymmetric "tilt" of the pelvis results in asymmetric mechanical back actions when walking, bending, and lifting, and may result in "functional" kyphoscoliosis (due to muscle spasm) and facet joint imbalances. There are many causes of pelvic tilting—mild structural scoliosis, unequal leg lengths, and contracted iliotibial band or fascia lata in the hip are among the common causes.

Pelvic tilting that is present with the patient standing, but not apparent with the patient sitting, is usually due to leg problems—most often, unequal leg lengths or tensed fasciae latae or both (see below). Pelvic tilting that persists in all positions usually implies spinal malalignments (scoliosis, for example) or disorders of the lumbosacral junction. Pelvic tilting will usually be apparent on simple observation (see Fig. 1–2) when severe, but more subtle, pelvic tilting can be demonstrated by plumb-line testing. Figure 1–27 demonstrates the use of a plumb line to detect pelvic tilting and illustrates that the insertion of foot pads will relieve the problem.

Unequal leg lengths are common in the general population without back pain—discrepancies up to 1 to 2 inches may, in fact, be well tolerated. However, when recurrent back pain is associated with such discrepancies (Fig. 1–28 illustrates how to measure leg lengths), shoe lifts may be dramatically effective treatment.

Tensed fasciae latae or hamstring tendons may be corrected with simple exercises. The tensed fasciae latae can be demonstrated by Ober's test (Fig. 1–29).

3. Muscle weakness or imbalance. Kraus[4] has suggested that careful muscle testing of abdominal, back, and leg muscles may identify specific muscle groups in individual patients whose relative weakness may predispose the patient to remediable back pain. Patients who are obese, postoperative, postpartum, elderly, or sedentary are commonly so afflicted, but so may be

FIGURE 1–27. Plumb line testing for pelvic tilting. *A,* The plumb line does not fall in the midline. *B,* A small leg lift corrects the tilt.

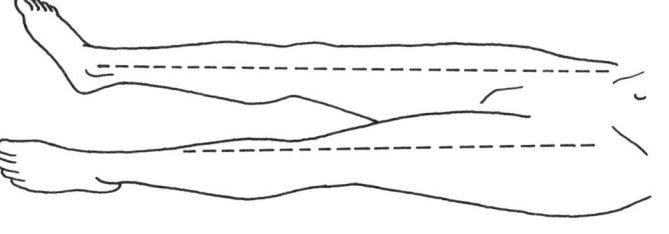

FIGURE 1–28. Leg lengths are measured by placing one end of a tape measure on the point of the anterior iliac crest and measuring the distance from this point to the medial malleolus.

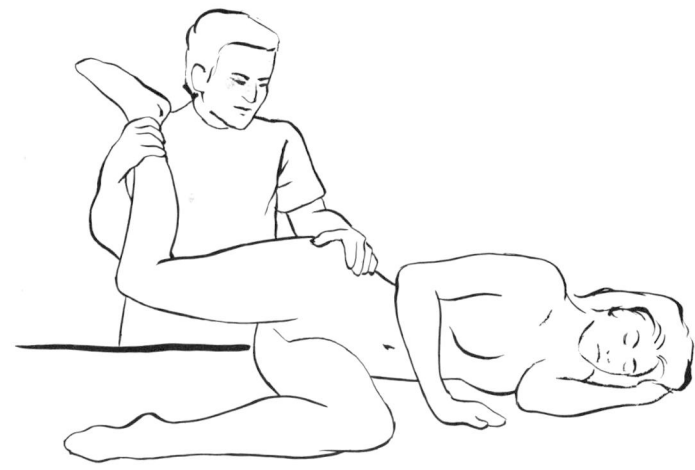

FIGURE 1–29. Ober's test. The patient attempts to maintain abduction of the hip, which has been passively elevated by the examiner. Pain or inability to do so suggests inflammation or contracture of the fasciae latae of the hip.

apparently healthy, vigorous patients. Calisthenics, muscle strengthening and stretching, and general physical conditioning are helpful here.

4. Failure to understand proper care of the lower back. Many patients will benefit simply from reading and practicing the common sense advice provided on pages 24 and 25 above.

Treatment

The symptomatic and preventive measures discussed under "Acute Back Pain" also apply to the patient with chronic back pain. Periods of bedrest, anti-inflammatory drugs, and exercise therapy usually play an important role. Several other considerations are also of great importance:

1. Proper treatment requires a specific diagnosis. While we have seen that acute simple mechanical back pain may defy a specific pathologic diagnosis, chronic back pain should be diagnosed specifically. Obviously, different diseases—tumors, infection, degenerative spondylosis—require different therapy. When a specific diagnosis is unclear, a consultation with a specialist is indicated.

2. Dependence on artificial means of support should be avoided when possible. Narcotic analgesics, tranquilizers, back braces, and repeated nerve blocks should be avoided as a general rule. Occasionally such measures may be necessary, but other approaches should be attempted first. Again, subspecialty consultations should be obtained before initiating such chronic therapies. Transcutaneous electrical nerve stimulation (TENS)[72] and other "pain clinic" procedures may be helpful in selected patients.

3. The patient's psychologic state, character, and motivation must be understood.

Compliance with conservative therapy is as essential in the treatment of chronic low back pain as in acute low back pain. Often a multidisciplinary approach is required for the patient with chronic low back pain in whom specific therapy (for example, surgery) is unsuccessful or inadvisable. The passive or otherwise uncooperative patient should be identified early and followed closely,[96] because success is less likely with such people. (In fact, the depressed patient sometimes will develop back pain precisely *because of* the postural stance that accompanies severe depression—the "morose, slumped shoulders" look). Some degree of depression is so common among patients with chronic pain of any kind that signs of depression should not be taken as evidence that back pain is feigned or functional.

Equally difficult are cases in which litigation or contested worker's disability claims confuse the situation. Such situations merit detailed evaluation, and referral to a specialist is usually wise.[97] Low back pain is so common, especially among wage-earning adults, that it is a leading cause of (temporary and permanent) employment disability.[9] While true hysteria and frank malingering are not common, both the economic "facts of life" and the diagnostic nonspecificity of much low back pain often entangle the physician in a knotty problem: Is the back pain real?

Many tests have been suggested to distinguish "real" from "functional" complaints. While these tests may indeed be helpful when other evidence points to such suspicions, the danger of excessive reliance on such tests as definitive diagnostic maneuvers cannot be overemphasized. The individual reaction to pain is so varied and so poorly understood that the examiner must remember: Real pain is often exaggerated by functional overlay; pain induces anxiety much more often than anxiety induces pain; placebo treatments are remarkably effective even among patients with unequivocally (for example, postoperative) "organic" pain.[98]

"Tests" that have been advocated in this situation include:

1. The floor touch test (Fig. 1–30). Even the patient with severe back disease can bend to touch the floor when kneeling on a low chair (unless severe hip disease or extreme acute muscle spasm is present). Protestation of inability to even try this maneuver is suspicious.

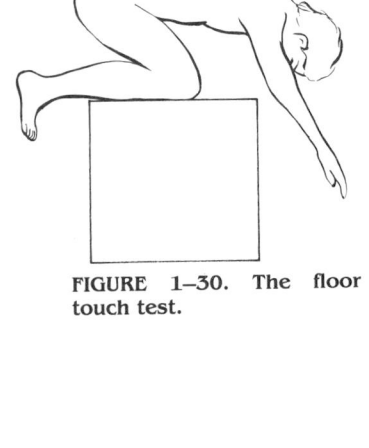

FIGURE 1–30. The floor touch test.

2. The flip sign (see Fig. 1–7). Prominent back and leg symptoms during supine straight leg raising that are not reproduced with straight leg raising in the sitting position should also be cause for suspicion.

3. The toe flexion test. The patient lies prone on the examining table with legs flexed at the knee to 90 degrees (i.e., heels facing the ceiling). If the patient complains of increased back pain or sciatica during flexion and extension of the toes (against resistance) in this position, at least exaggeration is likely.

4. Many patients with functional disease complain of tenderness to very superficial palpation in peculiar and inconsistent locations; they are "jumpy." These patients must be distinguished from those with fibrositis and "trigger points"—such areas of tenderness are highly localized, consistent areas of tenderness that are usually improved with local anesthetic infiltration and/or tricyclic antidepressants.

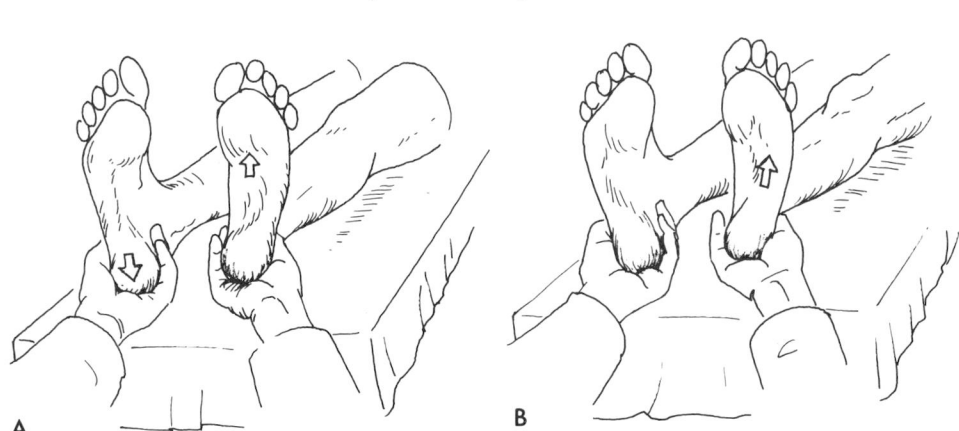

FIGURE 1–31. The Hoover test. A, Normally, attempts to elevate one leg will be accompanied by downward pressure by the opposite leg. B, When the "weak" leg attempts to elevate, but the opposite (asymptomatic) leg does not "help," suspect that at least some of the weakness is feigned.

A   B

5. Feigned motor loss. The Hoover test (Fig. 1–31) is helpful in detecting feigned leg weakness.

6. Nonanatomic sensory deficits. Paresthesias and alleged hypesthesias of the entire leg or both legs (anteriorly and posteriorly) are a common functional complaint and are only rarely due to definable organic disease, but obviously a careful neurologic examination is crucial.

Note: When physical findings are present that cannot be voluntarily created (for example, palpable muscle spasm), the back pain must be assumed to be "real."

Patients suspected of exaggerating their back pain (for whatever reason) should be treated in the same way as other patients, since appropriate treatment may relieve anxiety as well as pain. Such patients who do not improve are always entitled to a second opinion, preferably from a specialist experienced in disorders of the back, even when all tests and suspicions point to malingering or elaboration. While the careful examiner and historian is usually right when such suspicions are strong, confirmation of those findings by another examiner is essential.

Thus, referral to a specialist (usually, an orthopedist or neurosurgeon) should be considered in the patient with chronic back pain when:

1. As in acute low back pain, there is evidence of neurologic compromise—especially motor weakness or cauda equina symptoms and signs.

2. A specific diagnosis is unclear, in spite of x-rays and laboratory tests.

3. The patient fails to respond to primary conservative therapy (page 20).

4. X-ray abnormalities of the spine (especially spondylolisthesis, hemivertebra, or asymmetric transitional vertebrae) are present, but it is unclear whether such disorders are responsible for or contributory to the patient's symptoms.

5. Litigation is involved or malingering is suspected—when the extent of disability seems disproportionate to clinical findings.

6. Surgery is to be considered. Patients with chronic low back pain who may benefit from surgery include those with severe symptomatic spondylolisthesis, spinal stenosis, degenerative spondylosis, or disc syndromes refractory to all conservative therapy. Occasionally, surgical exploration is required to make a specific diagnosis—for example, in vertebral osteomyelitis (see Appendix I).

APPENDIX I

When Back Pain Is Dangerous

Several clinical situations should cause concern about life-threatening disease in the patient with low back pain. Amid an unselected population of patients with back pain, all of these disorders are very uncommon or rare. Nevertheless, these diseases require immediate diagnosis and treatment. Hence, the great importance of the following circumstances:

1. Fever. All patients with low back pain should have temperatures recorded. When fever is present, several problems should be considered immediately. Meningitis or subarachnoid hemorrhage will usually also present with headache or mental status impairment or both, but back pain may be the presenting complaint. (Meningismus may sometimes be mistaken for positive straight leg raising.) Bacterial endocarditis[99, 100] not infrequently presents with back pain, for obscure reasons. All patients with fever and back pain require blood cultures for this and other (see below) reasons.

Vertebral osteomyelitis,[101, 102] (bacterial,[103–106] tuberculous,[107–109] or fungal[110, 111]) may be especially difficult to diagnose in its early stages. While acute pyogenic vertebral osteomyelitis may be a severe, rampant illness characterized by high fever, toxicity, and bacteremia (often from a distant primary source—for example, endocarditis), many cases of pyogenic vertebral osteomyelitis are remarkable for their indolent "nontoxic" presentation. Middle-aged or elderly males with refractory lumbar back pain for several weeks or months are typical victims (Fig. 1–32)—an elevated sedimentation rate is always present, but fever, leukocytosis, and bacteremia are often absent (50 per cent of the time). Staphylococcus aureus is the most common pathogenic organism, but intravenous drug abusers[112] and patients whose source of infection is the urinary tract (implicated about 30 percent of the time) may present with a variety of other (especially gram-negative) infectious organisms. Spine x-rays are often "normal" in the first several weeks of illness (see Fig. 1–32), and only a strong clinical suspicion will allow early diagnosis by appropriate further testing—bone scan or gallium scan or both, and ultimately open vertebral biopsy or needle aspiration. Failure to make this diagnosis may result in disastrous disability, permanent neurologic deficit, and even death.

Epidural abscess,[113] with or without contiguous osteomyelitis, is heralded by high fever and back pain with rapid progression of neurologic events through a typical temporal sequence: radicular back pain (first 3 days), motor weakness (within 4 days), and paraplegia or cauda equina compression within the first week. Local spinal tenderness is common. The abscess often extends over four to five vertebral segments and thus may involve multiple/bilateral nerve roots. *Staphylococcus aureus* is again the most common organism, but many other organisms have been reported. Myelography and CT scan will almost always define the lesion, and emergency surgery will improve prognosis if undertaken immediately. Subdural empyema[114] is difficult to distinguish from epidural abscess, but a preceding or concurrent local focus of infection is often present (for example, a furuncle or cellulitis of the back)— emergency surgery is also crucial here.

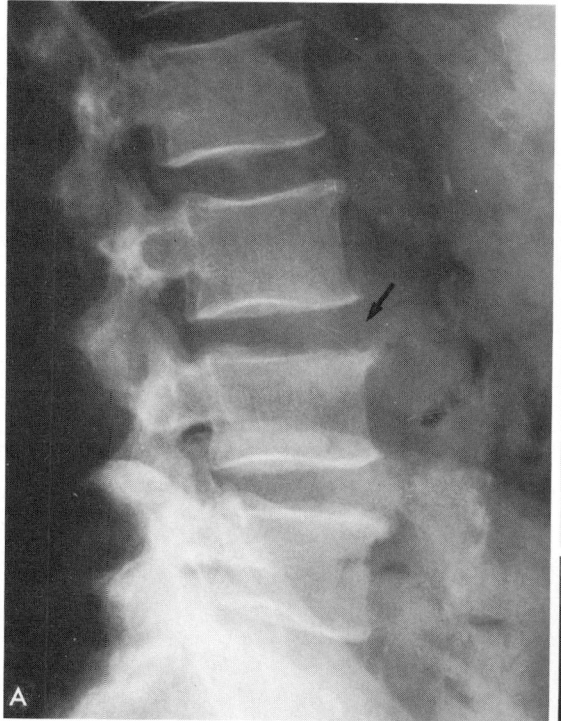

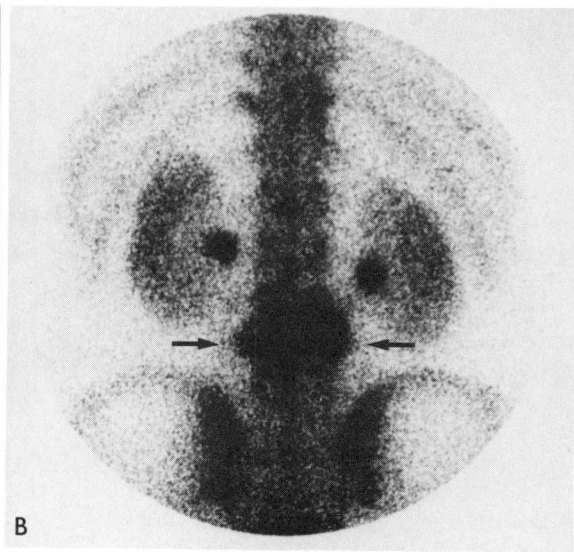

FIGURE 1–32. This 60-year-old man developed severe lower back pain while lifting a heavy box. Initial examination was unremarkable except for marked limitation of back movement and paralumbar muscle spasm. Conservative therapy provided no relief, and the patient's pain persisted in spite of 10 days of complete bed rest. Pain progressively worsened.

A, X-rays of the lumbar spine are unimpressive at this stage, but there is a suggestion of irregularity of the superior anterior border of the fourth lumbar vertebra (arrow).

B, Bone scan reveals marked isotope uptake at this level. A gallium scan was also "hot" at the L3–4 interspace. The patient was never febrile. Blood cultures were repeatedly normal. The sedimentation rate was, however, 74.

Percutaneous aspiration under fluoroscopy by the orthopaedist diagnosed staphylococcal (S. aureus) disc space infection with vertebral osteomyelitis.

Follow-up x-rays after 6 weeks of intravenous antibiotic therapy and 3 months of "body casting" (C) demonstrate the more classic x-ray changes of vertebral osteomyelitis. There is irregularity of the superior border of L4 and the inferior border of L3 with marked bony sclerosis on both sides of the disc space. (Residual barium in the colon partly obscures the anterior "bridge" of bone (arrow) fusing the disc space after healing.)

Acute back pain, fever, and rapidly progressive (1 to 3 days) neurologic impairment may also result from acute transverse myelitis.[115, 116] Here the neurologic events usually dominate the clinical picture.

In the patient with fever and mechanical low back pain, then, sedimentation rate, blood cultures, spinal x-rays, bone scans, and careful neurologic examination are usually necessary.

Many other "nonmechanical" disorders may produce fever with referred low back pain: Acute prostatitis, pelvic infections, pyelonephritis, perinephric abscess, renal infarction, pancreatitis or pancreatic abscess, aortic dissection, perforated duodenal ulcer, diverticulitis, retrocecal appendicitis, retroperitoneal hemorrhage or lymphoma, and splenic infarction or abscess are among such conditions.

2. When the patient is known or suspected to have cancer. Low back

pain (with or without sciatica) in the cancer patient should always alert the examiner to the possibility of vertebral metastases,[99] paravertebral tumor masses, epidural metastases, carcinomatous meningitis, and metastatic plexus lesions.

Vertebral metastases (most commonly from breast, lung, prostate, thyroid, and renal carcinomas) are usually apparent on spinal x-rays (Fig. 1–23), but isotope bone scans are more sensitive and should be done especially when the diagnosis is suspected but plain spinal films are nondiagnostic.[117, 118] (Bone scans may also be falsely negative,[119] but this is unusual.)

Associated neurologic findings (weakness, radiculopathy, cauda equina syndromes, cord compressions) necessitate immediate CT scans or myelography or both because epidural metastases are now a relatively common phenomenon,[120] and immediate treatment (radiation therapy and corticosteroids) is absolutely essential to a better prognosis.[121] Some authors suggest that back pain due to vertebral metastases that are apparent on plain films should be further investigated even when the neurologic examination is normal, since epidural metastases may be discovered at this critical early stage.[120] This approach is debatable, but at least frequent neurologic examinations are essential to detect early neurologic changes that would suggest epidural invasion by tumor.

Meningeal carcinomatosis[122] usually presents with a diversity of clinical findings through the neuraxis (headache, cranial nerve abnormalities, multiple nerve root findings) in the patient with known cancer or leukemia. Back pain without such findings is unlikely to be due to meningeal infiltration.

Systemic lymphomas[123, 124] may cause epidural tumor deposits with subsequent cord compression or cauda equina involvement, even in the absence of vertebral bony changes. Occasionally such neurologic disorders will be the presenting manifestation of lymphoma.

3. When the patient is receiving anticoagulation therapy. Back pain in the patient receiving anticoagulants may result from retroperitoneal hemorrhage or, rarely, from spinal epidural hematoma[125] (which usually produces a syndrome similar to that of epidural abscess but without fever). Demonstration that coagulation tests are within therapeutic range does not guarantee that bleeding has not occurred. CT scan or myelography may be necessary for correct diagnosis, but any patient receiving anticoagulant therapy who develops new back pain is cause for concern.

4. Even when fever, neurologic symptoms, or cancer is not (known to be) present, pain that is constant, unrelieved by bedrest, and unrelentingly progressive merits extensive investigation. Vertebral or epidural metastases may be present in patients without neurologic findings or known primary neoplasms.[120] As noted above, vertebral osteomyelitis often will not be associated with either fever or leukocytosis. Primary tumors of the spinal cord (meningiomas, neurofibromas, ependymomas, sarcomas, gliomas) may present with OMINOUS back pain, but sometimes without obvious neurologic findings.[59] Primary tumors of bone—osteoid osteomas, osteoblastoma, for example—may be missed on plain x-rays, but the bone scan will be helpful. Multiple myeloma may not be apparent on either plain x-rays or bone scan, but the clinical findings (persistent back pain, elevated sedimentation rate, anemia in an elderly patient) will usually be suggestive.

Careful attention to an OMINOUS history (and longitudinal follow-up of patients with "routine" back pain—a few of whom do not improve) will result in early diagnosis of most dangerous back pain.

Compression Fractures, Osteopenia, and Osteoporosis[126]

Compression fractures of the lumbosacral vertebrae are a common cause of low back pain. In most instances, acute, severe low back pain follows some traumatic or mechanical event—usually major trauma in the healthy young patient (for example, toboggan injuries), but quite minor trauma (a brief fall) may compress elderly vertebrae. Occasionally spontaneous compression fractures will occur—the elderly patient with severe osteoporosis is the usual victim (see below). Compression fractures are only rarely complicated by spinal cord or cauda equina involvement, nerve root involvement is unusual, and conservative therapy (bedrest, back braces)—often for several weeks—is usually successful.

The diagnosis of compression fractures is usually straightforward since the lumbar spine x-ray will be diagnostic (Fig. 1–33). Except in instances of

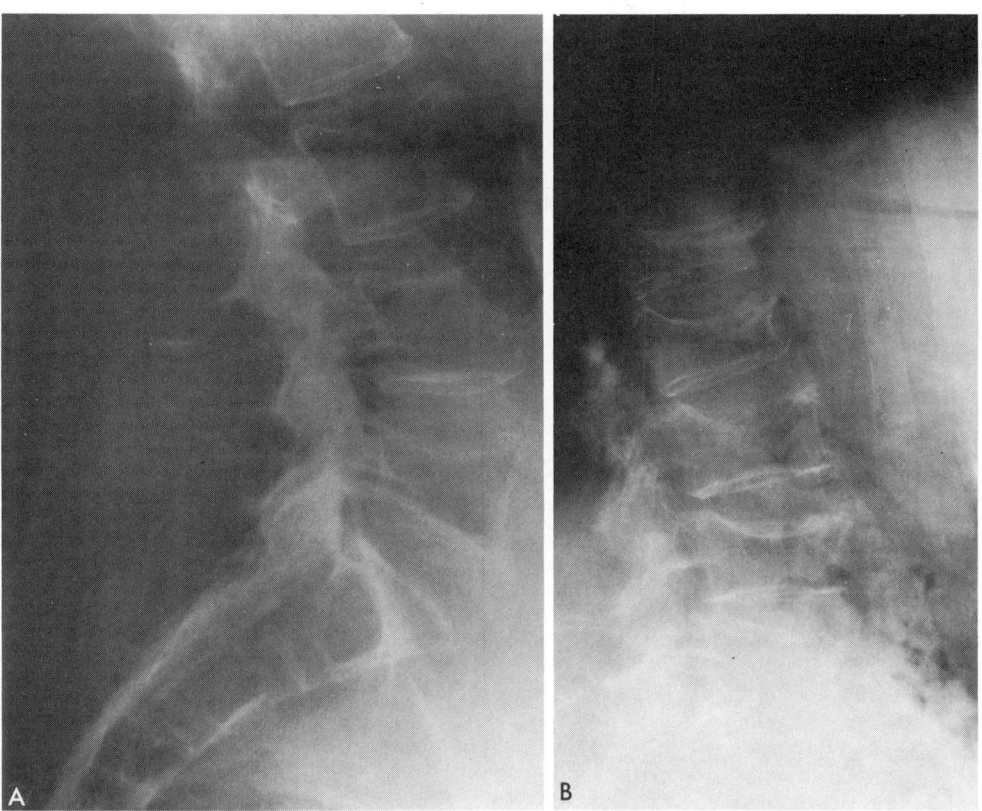

FIGURE 1–33. Osteopenia and compression fractures.

A, Osteoporosis. This 78-year-old woman complained of 2 days of severe lumbosacral back pain. There was no known injury or mechanical precipitant. X-rays reveal extraordinary undermineralization of all bony structures and multiple compression fractures of the vertebral bodies. (The film is not underpenetrated—the bones are, in fact, vanishing!)

B, Osteomalacia. This elderly woman developed severe low back pain 2 years after beginning phenytoin (Dilantin) therapy for trigeminal neuralgia. Bone biopsy revealed both osteoporosis and osteomalacia (the latter presumably due to phenytoin).

major trauma, compression fractures in one location are usually associated with other radiographic abnormalities of the spine. Metastatic or primary vertebral neoplasms may cause isolated compression fractures, and cancer should always be suspected when the radiographic abnormality is confined only to the level of the fracture (or when other systemic complaints coexist). Much more often, radiographic osteopenia is apparent throughout the bony skeleton. Osteopenia—radiographically diminished bone density—is usually the result of osteoporosis or osteomalacia or both. Achieving a specific diagnosis may be a frustrating and expensive undertaking: The various causes of osteoporosis and osteomalacia (Tables 1–12 and 1–13) suggest the potential complexity of the diagnostic problem. Nevertheless, an aggressive diagnostic and therapeutic approach is often warranted, since it is sometimes possible to prevent further bone loss, subsequent fractures, and disability due to these disorders.

TABLE 1–12. CLASSIFICATION OF OSTEOMALACIA AND RICKETS

1. Reduction of circulating vitamin D metabolites
   a. Vitamin D deficiency due to inadequate ultraviolet light and dietary lack
   b. Vitamin D malabsorption
      (1) Postgastrectomy?
      (2) Small intestinal disease
      (3) Pancreatic insufficiency
      (4) Insufficient bile salts
   c. Abnormal vitamin D metabolism
      (1) Liver disease
      (2) Chronic renal failure
      (3) Systemic acidosis
      (4) Vitamin D dependent rickets (25-hydroxyvitamin D-1α-hydroxylase deficiency)
      (5) Mesenchymal tumors
      (6) Anticonvulsant drugs
      (7) Glutethimide
   d. Renal loss
      Nephrotic syndrome
2. Peripheral resistance to vitamin D
      (1) Chronic renal failure
      (2) Anticonvulsant drugs
      (3) Vitamin D dependent rickets Type II
3. Hypophosphatemia
   a. Malnutrition
   b. Malabsorption due to gastrointestinal disease or phosphate binding antacids
   c. Chronic dialysis
   d. Renal phosphate wasting
      (1) Hypophosphatemic rickets
         (a) Familial X-linked
         (b) Autosomal recessive
         (c) Sporadic
      (2) Hypophosphatemic osteomalacia
         (a) Familial X-linked
         (b) Sporadic
      (3) Fanconi syndrome
      (4) Mesenchymal tumors, fibrous dysplasia, and epidermal nevus syndrome
      (5) Primary hyperparathyroidism
4. Miscellaneous
   a. Inhibitors of calcification
      (1) Sodium fluoride
      (2) Disodium etidronate
   b. Calcium
   c. Hypophosphatasia
   c. Fibrogenesis imperfecta ossium

From Kelley, WN, Harris, ED, Jr, Ruddy, S, and Sledge, CB: Textbook of Rheumatology. Philadelphia: W.B. Saunders, 1981, p. 1730.

TABLE 1–13. CLASSIFICATION OF OSTEOPOROSIS

1. Endocrine abnormality
   a. Estrogen deficiency
   b. Testosterone deficiency
   c. Glucocorticoid excess
   d. Thyrotoxicosis
   e. Diabetes mellitus
2. Immobilization or weightlessness
3. Genetic
   a. Osteogenesis imperfecta
   b. Homocystinuria
   c. Ehlers-Danlos syndrome
   d. Menkes syndrome
   e. Marfan syndrome
4. Scurvy
5. Juvenile osteoporosis
6. Heparin therapy
7. Systemic mastocytosis
8. Rheumatoid arthritis
9. Hematologic malignancy
   a. Multiple myeloma
   b. Leukemia
   c. Lymphoma
10. Liver disease

From Kelley, WN, Harris, ED, Jr, Ruddy, S, and Sledge, CB: Textbook of Rheumatology. Philadelphia: W.B. Saunders, 1981, p. 1722.

REMEMBER

1. Osteoporosis is by far the most common cause of osteopenia (and compression fractures) and the idiopathic or postmenopausal variety is responsible for most cases. Osteoporosis—a decreased mass of normally mineralized bone—results from the cumulative failure to replace bone mass resorbed over time during normal (or accelerated) catabolic bone turnover. Loss of bone mass is especially common in the female and greatly accelerates following the menopause. Unfortunately, osteoporosis becomes clinically apparent only after the development of radiographic osteopenia, at which time substantial (30 to 50 per cent) bone mass has been irrevocably lost. Treatment of osteoporosis remains controversial,[127–130] but it is probably possible at least to retard further bone loss by treatment with estrogens, calcium, vitamin D, or fluoride, singly or in combination. Treatment, however, depends on a specific diagnosis.

NOTE

2. Osteomalacia, a condition in which total bone mass is normal but bone mineralization is defective, may be radiographically indistinguishable from osteoporosis (and, in fact, the two disorders may coexist). As seen in Table 1–12, the causes of osteomalacia are many. Nevertheless, since most osteomalacia is related to disorders of vitamin D metabolism or hypophosphatemia, the clinical history and a few simple laboratory tests will at least suggest the presence of osteomalacia in most instances. As suggested in Table 1–12, reclusive life styles, malnutrition, known gastrointestinal, liver, or renal disease, and various medications must be reviewed. Determinations of serum calcium and phosphate, renal function tests, alkaline phosphatase, and 25-hydroxyvitamin D levels will help to exclude (or suggest) most disorders that initiate osteomalacia.

3. The only absolute proof of the cause of osteopenia is bone biopsy. The necessary expertise to perform and interpret such biopsies is now available in most medical centers. Preparation of undecalcified bone (usually obtained by relatively painless iliac crest biopsy), with or without "tetracycline labeling," will reveal the correct diagnosis most of the time. Bone biopsy

should be considered when the history, x-rays, and laboratory findings are atypical for simple postmenopausal osteoporosis. Some authorities recommend more liberal use of bone biopsies, since osteomalacia may coexist with postmenopausal osteoporosis in a minority of cases and may thus dictate more specific therapy.

As can be inferred from Tables 1–12 and 1–13, the clinical history, a thorough examination, complete blood count, "chemistry profile" (including determinations of BUN, calcium/phosphate, alkaline phosphatase), thyroid function tests, serum protein electrophoresis, and determination of 25-hydroxyvitamin D levels are reasonable outpatient "screening" procedures in the patient with radiographic osteopenia or compression fractures.

Back Pain and Back Anatomy

The lumbosacral spine is the structural foundation of the weight-bearing human. It is subjected daily to enormous mechanical stresses. These stresses are borne by the lumbar vertebrae, which are large cubes of bone, normally arranged in mild lordosis (bowing anteriorly, concave posteriorly). These vertebrae sit atop each other, forming amphiarthrodial joints: Each intervertebral space is occupied by a fibrocartilaginous disc (which serves as a shock absorber) interposed between the hyaline cartilage plates at top and bottom of each vertebral body (Fig. 1–34). This disc is composed of a central nucleus pulposus and a circumferential anulus fibrosus. The anulus is a matrix of concentric elastic lamellae that run obliquely between adjacent vertebral endplates and hold together the vertebrae while permitting necessary flexion, rotation, and extension of the spine. The nucleus "spring loads" the vertebrae (Fig. 1–35)—deforming itself with compression during weight bearing, regaining its resting form with release of compressive forces. Over the years, this disc tends to degenerate—the disc space narrows as the anular fibers fragment and the nucleus "spreads" into (and sometimes beyond) the anular

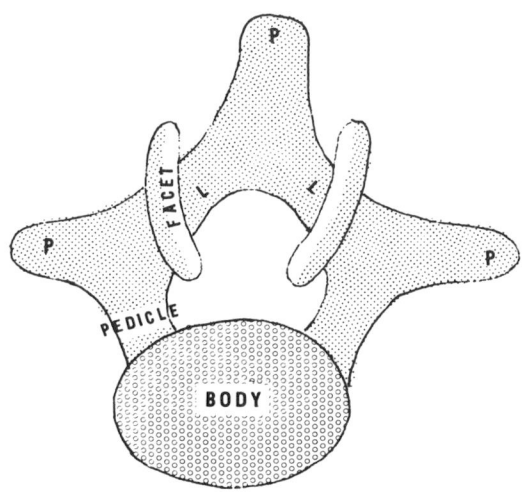

FIGURE 1–34. Functional vertebral unit. *Above,* View of the vertebral body, the posterior articulations (facets), the pedicles, the processes (P), and the lamina (L). *Below,* Lateral view demonstrating the intervertebral disk and its relationship to the components of the unit. (From Cailliet, R.: Soft Tissue Pain and Disability. Philadelphia, F.A. Davis Co., 1977.)

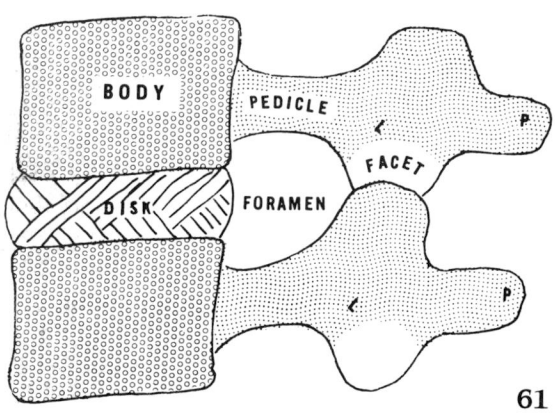

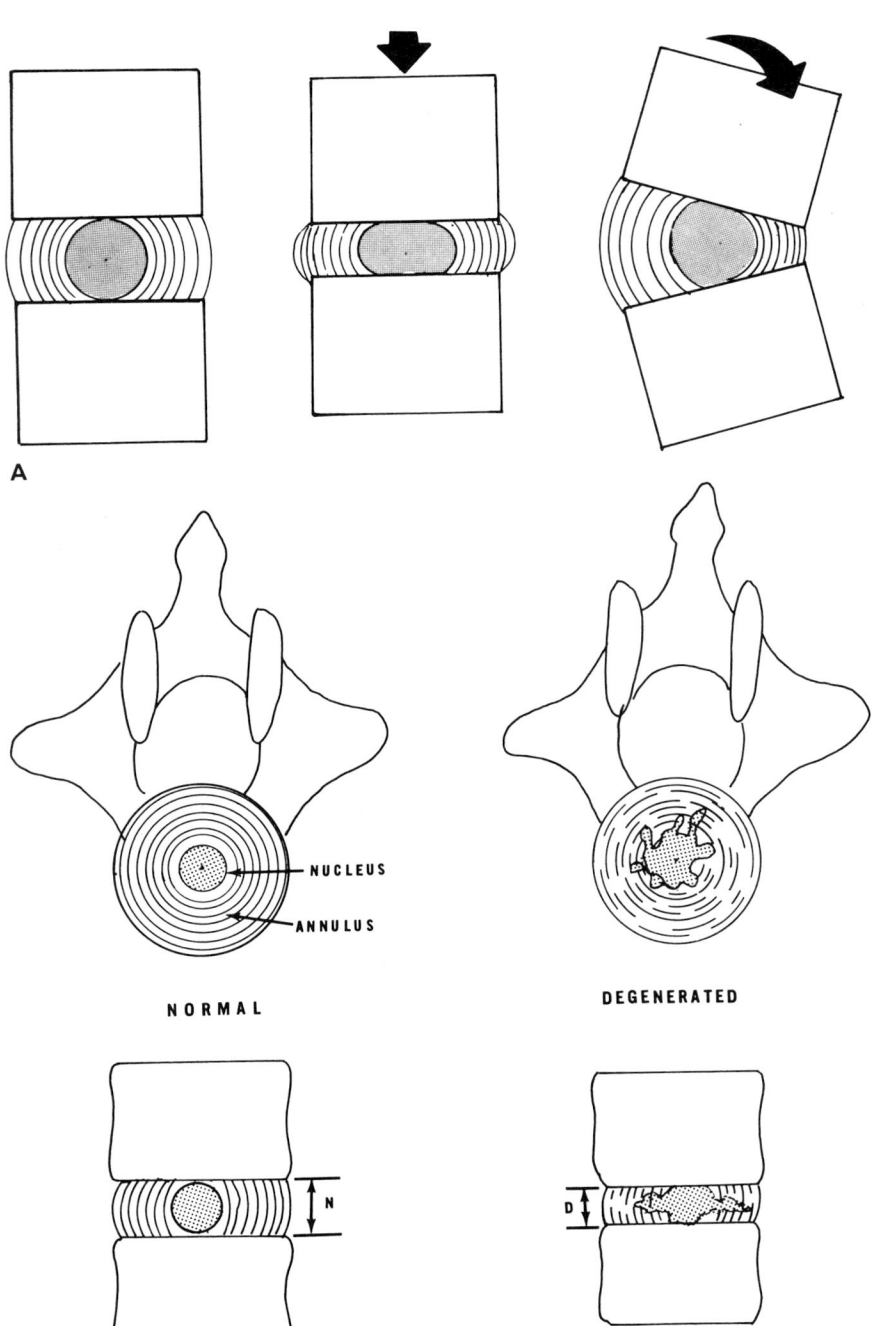

FIGURE 1–35. *A,* Deformation of the normal disc during weight bearing and spinal movement. *B,* Disc degeneration. *Left,* Normal disc with intact nucleus and annular fibers. The space is normal (N). *Right,* Degenerated disc with the nucleus outside its boundary and fragmented fibers and narrowed space (D). (From Cailliet, R: Soft Tissue Pain and Disability. Philadelphia, F.A. Davis Co., 1977.)

confines. Sudden "rupture" of the nucleus causes an acute disc syndrome (see Fig. 1–11); gradual deterioration of the disc is the forerunner of spondylosis (see Fig. 1–26).

Other bony structures of the lumbosacral spine form the circular (or triangular) spinal canal within which descends the spinal cord and cauda equina (Fig. 1–34). The pedicles are short, bony projections arising from either side of each vertebral body—the intervertebral foramina (through which exit the spinal nerve roots) are formed by the inferior surface of the superior pedicle and the superior surface of the inferior pedicle. The laminae complete the bony arch posteriorly, while the transverse processes and posterior spinous processes extend laterally and posteriorly, respectively—these serve as points of insertion for the various ligaments and muscles that support the bony spine.

The facet joints are diarthrodial joints, composed of apposing surfaces of cartilage (complete with synovium, joint capsule, and synovial fluid) that line the adjacent superior articular process of the inferior vertebra and the inferior articular process of the superior vertebra on both sides of each intervertebral articulation. Each facet joint is normally aligned in a plane identical with its fellow—asymmetric planar orientation of facet joints at the same vertebral level is termed facet tropism (which may predispose to various mechanical problems). Figure 1–36 illustrates normal facet alignment and an example of facet tropism.

These different bony structures are stabilized by a series of supporting ligaments and muscles (Fig. 1–36). The vertebral bodies are joined anteriorly by the very strong anterior longitudinal ligament (which separates the spine from the aorta) and posteriorly by the weaker posterior longitudinal ligament (which separates the vertebrae and intervertebral discs from the anterior aspect of the spinal canal). The posterior bony arch includes the ligamentum flavum, which interconnects the laminae and which extends laterally to the facet joints. The supraspinal ligaments join the tips of the posterior spinous processes, while the interspinal ligaments join the bodies of those processes.

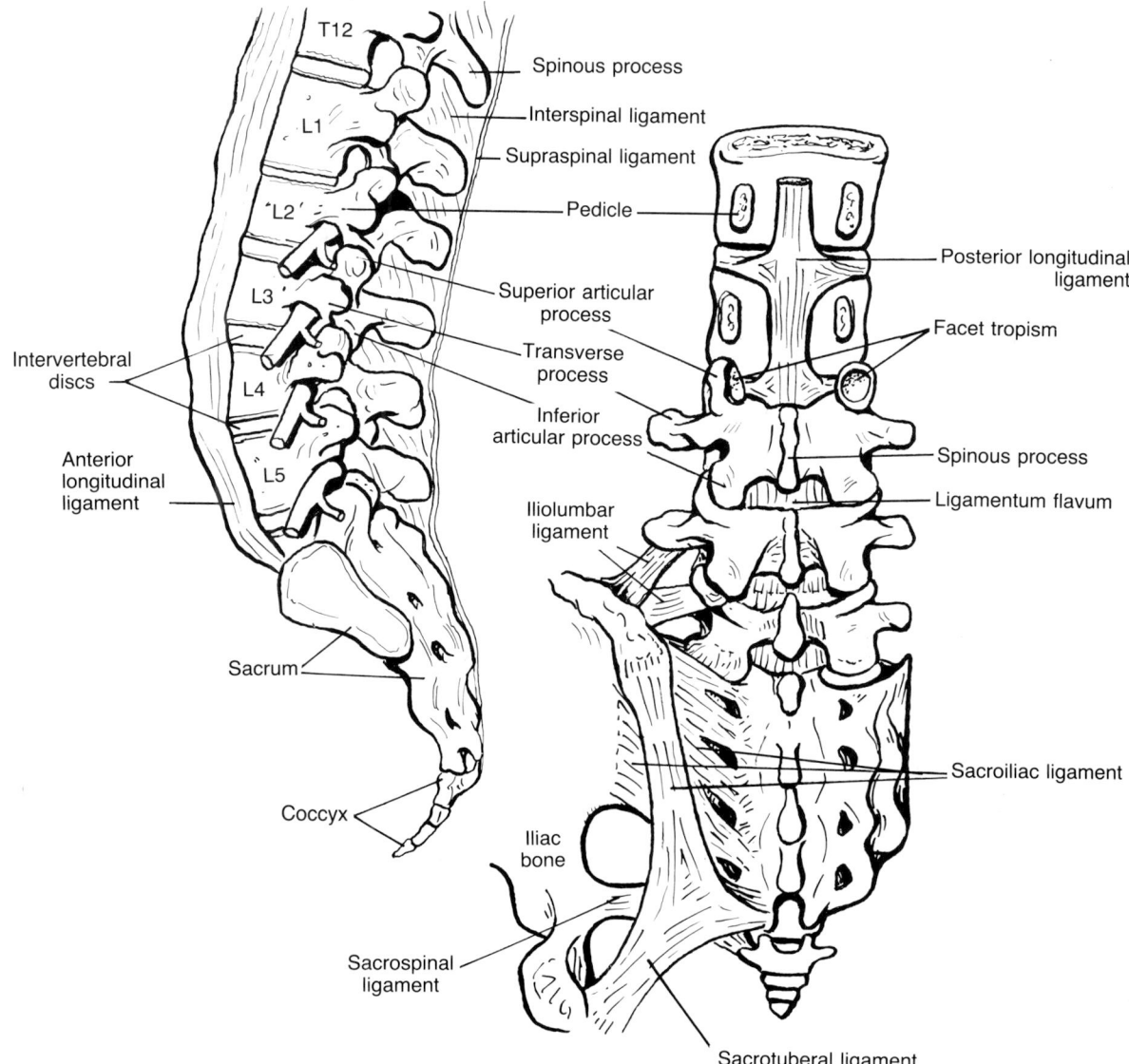

FIGURE 1–36. Gross anatomy of the lumbosacral spine. A, A lateral view. B, A posterior view— the upper two vertebrae have been cut (coronally) to demonstrate the posterior longitudinal ligament (which lies anterior to the spinal canal) and the articulating surfaces of the facet joints (which demonstrate facet tropism).

A series of larger, powerful ligaments attach the lumbosacral spine to both the ilium (iliolumbar and sacroiliac ligaments) and other pelvic structures (sacrospinal and sacrotuberal ligaments).

The muscular support of the lumbosacral spine includes two sets of opposing but complementary muscle groups.

The extensor muscle group includes primarily the sacrospinalis and the multifidis. The sacrospinalis muscle extends from the pelvis to the skull, connecting the lumbosacral spine (via its transverse and posterior spinous processes) with the remainder of the axial skeleton. The multifidis muscles are short muscles arising from the sacrum and transverse lumbar spinous processes to insert into all posterior spinous processes. (The smaller interspinalis muscles unite adjacent transverse spinous processes.)

The flexor muscle group includes the psoas, iliacus, and quadratus lumborum. The psoas muscle originates from the lateral vertebral bodies and discs of the lumbar vertebrae to insert into the lesser trochanter of the femur distal to the hip joint. The iliacus originates from the fan-shaped iliac fossa and inserts into the psoas tendon. The quadratus lumborum originates from the posterior iliac crest, inserts into the lower border of the twelfth rib, and also attaches to the transverse processes of the lumbar vertebrae.

The extensor and flexor muscle groups both support and antagonize each other. For example, weakened flexor muscles will allow excessive lumbar lordosis and create excessive strain on the extensor muscle group—a common cause of postural back pain.

Movements of the lower back stress these various structures in different ways.

Back flexion reverses the normal lumbar lordosis—adjacent anterior vertebral surfaces move closer, posterior surfaces separate—as illustrated in Figure 1–37. Flexion thus "stretches" the posterior longitudinal ligament, the ligamentum flavum, the supraspinal and intraspinal ligaments, as well as the extensor muscles of the back. Simultaneously the pelvis rotates anteriorly and intervertebral foramina widen as the facet joints separate. (Lateral rotation and lateral flexion of the back can be performed only in tandem with back flexion, since the facet joints are normally "locked" during extension, preventing rotatory and lateral motion.)

Return to the erect position derotates the pelvis, reapproximates the facet joints, narrows the intervertebral foramina, and restores the normal

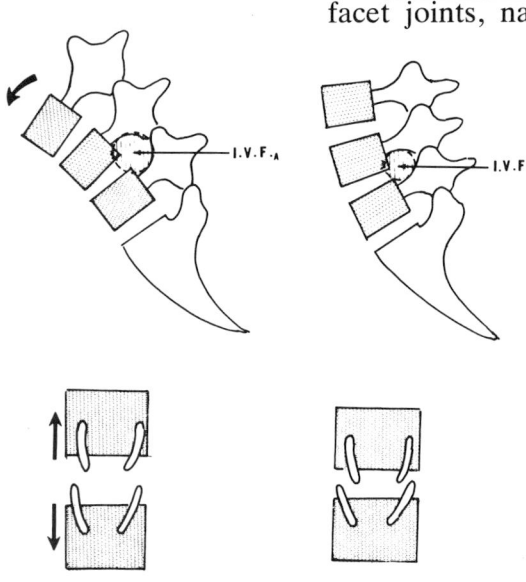
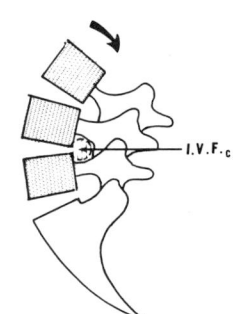
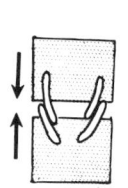

FIGURE 1–37. Facets in the lumbar spine. A, Separation of the facets in forward flexion; B, Opposition of the facets in the physiologic lordotic posture; C, Approximation and opposition of the facets on extension and hyperextension. (From Cailliet, R: Soft Tissue Pain and Disability. Philadelphia, F.A. Davis Co., 1977.)

lumbar lordosis. Further back extension exaggerates lordosis and further approximates facet joints.

These basic anatomic and mechanical features of the lower back shed some light on certain types of mechanical back pain. Not all of these structures are pain sensitive. Those that are, and thus may directly contribute to back pain, include:[131]

1. The vertebral bodies, the outermost fibers of the anulus fibrosus, and the posterior longitudinal ligament are innervated by the sinu-vertebral nerve. Pain then may result from vertebral inflammation or destruction or from displacement of the anulus or posterior ligament by a protruding intervertebral disc (even when spinal nerve roots are not compressed).

2. The facet joints are innervated by the articular nerve—malalignment, inflammation, or degeneration of these joints will cause local back pain. Similarly the supporting ligaments and muscles of the spine may cause pain when traumatized (torn, strained) or when tightened/imbalanced by underlying structural changes.

3. The dura mater, which lines the spinal canal and the proximal nerve roots as they exit the intervertebral foramina, causes pain when compressed, irritated, or inflamed.

Figure 1–38 illustrates these various pain-sensitive structures and their innervation at a single vertebral level (cauda equina).

Local mechanical low back pain, then, may be mediated through one or more of these pathways; some involve spinal nerve root compression, others do not. Disc herniations, for example, may cause pain in several ways (see text): by deforming the pain-sensitive posterior longitudinal ligament or outer anulus fibrosus; by compressing the structures of the cauda equina; or by compressing a spinal nerve root as it exits the intervertebral foramen. Spondylosis causes degenerative changes in facet joints. Muscular or ligamentous strains—the most common cause of acute back pain—probably do not directly affect any of the structures in Figure 1–38.

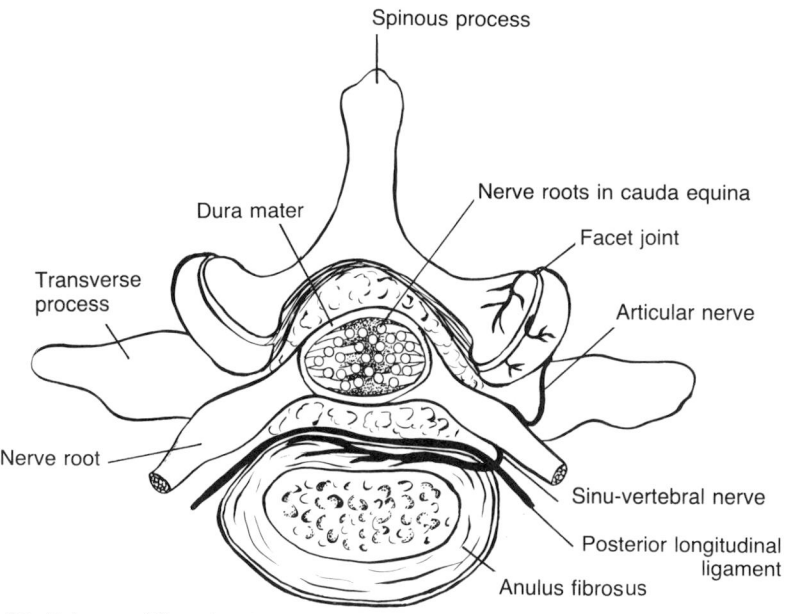

FIGURE 1–38. Pain-sensitive structures at a single vertebral level (below the termination of the spinal cord). (Adapted from Burton, C: Conservative management of low back pain. Postgrad Med 70:167–183, 1981.)

APPENDIX IV

Back Manipulation

As noted in the text proper, there is some controversy about the economy, efficacy, and safety of spinal manipulation in the patient with low back pain. Experienced manipulators claim success with a wide spectrum of back disorders from simple strain to herniated disc with neurologic deficits,[2, 132] and an extraordinary variety of techniques are available. For a number of reasons (see page 27), manipulation is not generally advocated here. The manipulation of elderly patients, those with neurologic deficits, and those with known structural spine disease cannot be recommended here under any circumstances (although such manipulations are performed sometimes by experienced therapists).

Whether manipulations per se are valuable therapeutic techniques is largely unproven. Whatever their scientific value, there is a lesson to be learned from chiropractic manipulations: The "therapeutic relationship" between physician and patient is essential to success. Even advocates of manipulation would probably agree that the "laying on of hands" in an active physical interaction, the attention to patient education, and ongoing longitudinal care* are as important as the manipulation maneuvers themselves.

There is at least one clinical situation in which manipulation is worth a try: the young, healthy patient who *suddenly* develops a "catch" with low back pain and restricted back motion during specific mechanical stress—usually bending or lifting—and who has no radicular symptoms or neurologic abnormality. Usually there is "spastic scoliosis." Especially when the physician is consulted immediately and the patient "needs" to improve more quickly than bedrest will usually allow (for example, the athlete or the manual laborer), the following procedure may help (see Fig. 1–39):

1. The patient lies on one side. The patient is asked to flex (90 degrees) the hip and knee of the uppermost leg such that the knee slides over the side of the examining table; at the same time the torso is voluntarily twisted backward, such that the uppermost shoulder is rotated down toward the table in the opposite direction from where the knee is pointing. The patient is thus in a twisted position—the upper trunk rotating back toward the examiner (who stands behind the patient), the lower body rotating forward, away from the examiner (Fig. 1–39A).

The manipulator then pushes downward forcefully on the upturned hip and shoulder, completing the rotational twisting of the torso already begun by the patient's initial position. While downward force is applied, the hip is simultaneously pushed forward (toward the knee) and the shoulder is pushed backward (toward the table and the examiner). The effect is that of forced lateral rotation of the lumbosacral spine. Sometimes an audible click with

---

*Follow-up is useful not simply for further manipulation but also for reinforcement of compliance with other conservative measures.

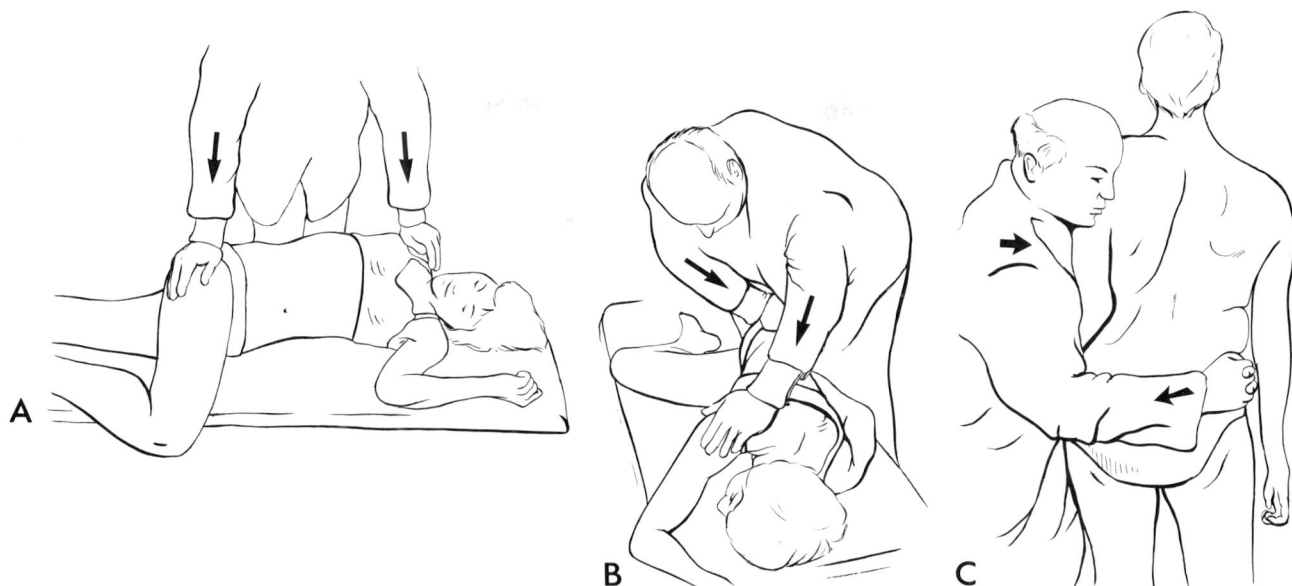

FIGURE 1–39. Spinal manipulation (see text).

relief of symptoms will result. Precisely what is happening here is unclear, but realignment of displaced facet joints may be one possible mechanism.

2. Repeating the maneuver on the opposite side, or reversing the body position (hip rotated back toward the examiner, shoulder rotated forward—see Fig. 1–39B), may also be tried if the initial manipulation does not help.

3. Another helpful maneuver can be done with the patient standing. The patient stands (with feet about 12 inches apart) with one elbow held in 90 degrees' flexion at the lower lateral rib cage. Figure 1–39C illustrates that the examiner then encircles the patient's pelvic area with both hands, such that the examiner's hands are clasped laterally over the patient's opposite iliac crest, while the examiner pushes with the chest and shoulder against the patient's flexed elbow and lateral area of the chest. Thus the patient's pelvis is pulled toward the examiner with the examiner's clasped hands, while the upper part of the patient's body is simultaneously pushed away. The effect of the manuever is that of "pulling" the lower spine and pelvis toward the manipulator while simultaneously pushing the upper spine in the opposite direction. This strenuous position is maintained for 1 to 2 minutes and may need to be repeated several times.

REFERENCES

1. Fernbach, JC, et al.: The significance of low back pain in older adults. Can Med Assoc J 115:898–900, 1976.
2. Cyriax, J: Textbook of Orthopaedic Medicine, Vol. I, 6th ed. Baltimore: Williams and Wilkins, 1977, p. 370.
3. Leavitt, F., et al.: Low back pain in patients with and without demonstrable organic disease. Pain 6:191–200, 1979.
4. Kraus, H: Clinic Treatment of Back and Neck Pain. New York: McGraw-Hill, 1970.
5. Sprangfort, E: Lasegue's sign in patients with lumbar disc herniation. Acta Orthop 42:459–460, 1971.
6. Cailliet, R: Soft Tissue Pain and Disability. Philadelphia: F. A. Davis, 1977, pp. 76–81.
7. Edgar, MA, Park, WM: Induced pain patterns on passive straight leg raising in lower lumbar disc protrusion. J Bone Joint Surg 56B:658–667, 1974.
8. Falconer, MA, et al.: Observations on the cause and mechanism of symptom production in sciatica and low back pain. J Neurol Neurosurg Psychiatry 11:13–26, 1948.
9. Quarterly Project Report 11a. Report of the Ambulatory Care Project. Lexington, Massachusetts Lincoln Laboratory, MIT. Boston, Mass.: Beth Israel Hospital, 1974.
10. Benn, RT, Wood P: Pain in the back: An attempt to estimate the size of the problem. Rheumatol Rehabil 14:121, 1975.
11. Steiner, SD: Incidence of neck pain and back pain in an industrial group. In Gurdjian, ES, Thomas, LM (eds): Neckache and Backache. Springfield, Ill.: Charles C Thomas, 1979, pp. 42–47.
12. Hayes, LF: Neckache and Backache: What do they cost? In Gurdjian, ES, Thomas, LM (eds): Neckache and Backache. Springfield, Ill.: Charles C Thomas, 1979, pp. 35–41.
13. Hadler, NM: Industrial rheumatology. Clinical investigation into the influence of the pattern of usage on the pattern of regional musculoskeletal disease. Arthritis Rheum 20:1019–1025, 1977.
14. Mixter, WJ, Barr, JS: Rupture of the intervertebral disc with involvement of the spinal canal. N Engl J Med 211:210–215, 1934.
15. Key, J: Intervetebral disc lesions as the most common cause of back pain with or without sciatica. Ann Surg 121:534–544, 1945.
16. Barton, JE, et al.: Low back pain in the primary care setting. J Fam Pract 3:363–366, 1976.
17. Rockey, PH, et al.: The usefulness of x-ray examinations in the evaluation of patients with back pain. J Fam Pract 7:455–465, 1978.
18. Greenfeld, S, et al.: Nurse-protocol management of low back pain. Outcome, patient satisfaction and efficiency of primary care. West J Med 123:350–359, 1975.
19. Hirsch, C: Etiology and pathogenesis of low back pain. Isr J Med Sci 2:362, 1966.
20. Wood, PHN: Epidemiology of back pain. In Jayson, M (ed): The Lumbar Spine and Back Pain. New York: Grune and Stratton, 1976, pp. 13–27.
21. Rothman, RH: The clinical syndrome of lumbar disc disease. Orthop Clin North Am 2:463–475, 1971.
22. Rothman, RH, Simeone, FA: The Spine. Philadelphia: W. B. Saunders, 1975, pp. 443–513.
23. Brown, MD: The pathophysiology of disc disease. Orthop Clin North Am 2(2):359–370, 1971.
24. Nachemson, A: The lumbar spine. An orthopaedic challenge. Spine 1:59, 1976.
25. Ebright, JR, et al.: The gallium scan. Arch Intern Med 142:246–262, 1982.
26. Hitselberger, WA, Witten, RM: Abnormal myelogram in asymptomatic patients. J Neurosurg 28:204–206, 1968.
27. Scavone, JG, et al.: Use of lumbar spine films. Statistical evaluation at a university teaching hospital. JAMA 246:1105–1108, 1981.
28. Kellgren, JH, Lawrence, JS: Osteoarthrosis and disc degeneration in an urban population. Ann Rheum Dis 17:388–397, 1958.
29. Splitoff, CA: Lumbosacral junction roentgenographic comparison of patients with and without backaches. JAMA 152:1610, 1953.
30. LaRocca, H, MacNab, J: Value of pre-employment radiographic assessment of the lumbar spine. Ind Med Surg 39:253, 1970.
31. Torgerson, WR, Dotter, WE: Comparative roentgenographic study of the asymptomatic and symptomatic lumbar spine. J Bone Joint Surg 58A:850, 1976.
32. Sims-Williams, H, et al.: Controlled trial of mobilization and manipulation for patients with low back pain in general practice. Br Med J 2:1338–1340, 1978.
33. Eisenberg, RL, et al.: Single well-centered lateral view of lumbosacral spine: Is coned view necessary? AJR 133:711–713, 1979.
34. Scavone, JG, et al.: Anteroposterior and lateral radiographs: An adequate lumbar spine examinaton. AJR 136:715–717, 1981.
35. Lentle, BC, et al.: Bone scintiscanning updated. Ann Intern Med 84:297–303, 1976.
36. Fornasier, VL, Horne, JG: Metastases to the vertebral column. Cancer 36:590–594, 1975.
37. Rodichok, L, et al.: Early diagnosis of spinal epidural metastases. Am J Med 70:1181–1187, 1981.
38. Cailliet, R: Soft Tissue Pain and Disability. Philadelphia: F. A. Davis, 1977, pp. 83–84.
39. Marshall, LL: Conservative management of low back pain. Med J Aust 1:266–267, 1967.
40. Hoehler, FK, et al.: Spinal manipulation for low back pain. JAMA 245:1835–1838, 1981.
41. Hooper, J: Low back pain and manipulation. Paraparesis after treatment of low back pain by physical methods. Med J Aust 1:549–551, 1973.
42. Keim, H: Low Back Pain. CIBA Clinical Symposia, Vol. 25, no. 3, 1973.
43. Patton, J: Neurological Differential Diagnosis. New York: Springer-Verlag, 1977.
44. Raff, MC, et al.: Ischemic mononeuropathy multiplex associated with diabetes mellitus. Arch Neurol 18:487–499, 1968.

45. Bastron, JA, Thomas, JE: Diabetic polyradiculopathy. Clinical and EMG findings in 105 patients. Mayo Clin Proc 56:725–732, 1981.
46. Shannon, N, Paul, EA: L4–5 and L5–S1 disc protrusions: Analysis of 323 cases operated on over 12 years. J Neurol Neurosurgy Psychiatry 42:804–809, 1979.
47. Gurdjian, ES, et al.: Results of operative treatment of protruded and ruptured lumbar discs based on 1,176 operative cases with 82% follow-up over 3 to 13 years. J Neurosurg 18:783–391, 1961.
48. Spurling, RG, Grantham EG: The end results of surgery for ruptured lumbar intervertebral discs. A follow-up study of 327 cases. J Neurosurg 6:57, 1949.
49. Rosen, HJ: Lumbar intervertebral disc surgery: Review of 300 cases. Can Med Assoc J 101:317–323, 1969.
50. Abdullah, AF, et al.: Extreme lateral lumbar disc herniation. Clinical syndrome and special problems of diagnosis. J Neurosurg 41:229–234, 1974.
51. Elliott, FA, Scheutta, HS: The differential diagnosis of sciatica. Orthop Clin North Am 2:477–484, 1971.
52. Hakelius, A.: Prognosis in sciatica. A clinical follow-up of surgical and nonsurgical treatment. Acta Orthop. Scand. Supplement No. 129, 1970.
53. MacNab, I: Negative disc exploration. An analysis of the cause of nerve root involvement in 68 patients. J Bone Joint Surg 53A:891–903, 1971.
54. Hawkes, CH, Roberts, GM: Neurogenic and vascular claudication. J Neurol Sci 38:337–345, 1978.
55. Patton, J: Neurological Differential Diagnosis. New York: Springer-Verlag, 1977, Chap. 19.
56. Pace, JB, Nagle, D: Pyriform syndrome. West J Med 124:435–439, 1976.
57. Patton, J: Neurological Differential Diagnosis. New York: Springer-Verlag, 1977, pp. 164–167.
58. Elsberg, CA, Constable, K: Tumors of the cauda equina. The differential diagnosis between new growths and inflammatory lesions of the caudal roots. Arch Neurol Psychiatry 23:79–105, 1930.
59. Moersch, FP, et al.: Spinalcord tumors with minimal neurologic findings. Neurology 1:39–47, 1951.
60. Love, JG: The differential diagnosis of intraspinal tumors and protruded intervertebral discs and their surgical treatment. J Neurosurg 1:275–290, 1944.
61. Love, JG, Rivers, MH: Spinal cord tumors simulating protruded intervertebral discs. JAMA 179:878, 1962.
62. Friedenberg, ZB, Shoemaker, RC: The results of nonoperative treatment of ruptured lumbar discs. Am J Surg 88:933, 1954.
63. Pearce, J, Moll, JMH: Conservative treatment and natural history of acute lumbar disc lesions. J Neurol Neurosurg Psychiatry 30:13–17, 1967.
64. Barr, JS, et al.: Evaluation of the end results in treatment of ruptured lumbar intervertebral discs with protrusion of nucleus pulposus. Surg Gynecol Obstet 125:250, 1967.
65. Branch, WT, Jr: Low back pain. In Branch, WT (ed): Office Practice of Medicine. Philadelphia: W. B. Saunders, 1982, Chap. 32.
66. Key, JA: The conservative and operative treatment of lesions of the intervertebral discs in the low back. Surgery 17:291–301, 1945.
67. Colonna, PC, Friedenberg, ZB: The disc syndrome. Results of the conservative care of patients with positive myelograms. J Bone Joint Surg 31A:614–618, 1949.
68. Andersson, H, Carlsson, CA: Prognosis of operatively-treated lumbar disc herniations causing foot extensor paralysis. Acta Chir Scand 132:501, 1966.
69. Weber, H: An evaluation of conservative and surgical treatment of lumbar disc protrusion. J Oslo City Hosp 20:81, 1970.
70. Weber, H: The effect of delayed disc surgery on muscular paresis. Acta Orthop Scand 46:631–1975.
71. Wiltse, LL: Surgery for intervertebral disc disease of the lumbar spine. Clin Orthop 129:22, 1977.
72. Burton, CV: Conservative management of low back pain. Postgrad Med 70:168–183, 1981.
73. Cailliet, R: Soft Tissue Pain and Disability. Philadelphia: F. A. Davis, 1977, pp. 99.
74. Dilke, TFW, et al.: Extradural corticosteroid injections in management of lumbar nerve root compression. Br Med J 2:635–637, 1973.
75. Green, LN: Dexamethasone in the management of symptoms due to herniated lumbar disc. J Neurol Neurosurg Psychiatry 38:1211–1217, 1975.
76. Sussman, BJ, et al.: Injection of collagenase in the treatment of herniated lumbar discs. Initial clinical report. JAMA 245:730–732, 1981.
77. Gunby, P: What is intradiscal therapy, anyway? JAMA 249:1120–1123, 1983.
78. Hirsch, C: Reflections on the use of surgery in lumbar disc disease. Orthop Clin North Am 2:493–498, 1971.
79. Gartland, JJ: Judgement in lumbar disc surgery. Orthop Clin North Am 2:507–520, 1971.
80. Burton, CV, et al.: Cause of failure of surgery in the lumbar spine. Clin Orthop 159:191–199, 1981.
81. Meyer, GA, et al.: Diagnosis of herniated lumbar disc with CT scan. N Engl J Med 301:1166–1167, 1979.
82. Carrera, GE, et al.: Computed tomography in sciatica. Radiology 137:433–437, 1980.
83. Heithoff, KB: High-resolution computed tomography of the lumbar spine. Postgrad Med 70:193–213, 1981.
84. MacNab, I, et al.: Selective ascending lumbosacral venography in the assessment of lumbar disc herniation. J Bone Joint Surg 58A:1093–1098, 1976.
85. Hakelius, A, Hindmarsh, J: The comparative reliability of preoperative diagnostic methods in lumbar disc surgery. Acta Orthop Scand 43:234–238, 1972.
86. Hakelius, A, Hindmarsh, J: The significance of neurological signs and myelographic findings in the diagnosis of lumbar root compression. Acta Orthop Scand 43:239–246, 1972.
87. Wiltse, LL: The effect of common anomalies of the lumbar spine upon disc degeneration and low back pain. Orthop Clin North Am 2:569, 1971.
88. Newman, PH: Surgical treatment for spondylolisthesis in the adult. Clin Orthop 117:106–111, 1976.
89. Wiltse, LL: Classification of spondylolysis and spondylolisthesis. Clin Orthop 117:30, 1976.
90. Paine, KWE, Haung, PWH: Lumbar disc syndrome. J Neurosurg 37:75–82, 1972.

91. Weinstein, PR, et al.: Lumbar Spondylosis: Diagnosis, Management and Surgical Treatment. Chicago: Yearbook Medical Publishers, 1977.
92. Epstein, JA, et al.: Sciatica caused by nerve root entrapment in the lateral recess: The superior facet syndrome. J Neurosurg 36:584–589, 1972.
93. Mooney, V, Robertson, J: The facet syndrome. Clin Orthop 115:149–156, 1976.
94. Ciric, I, et al.: The lateral recess syndrome: A variant of spinal stenosis. J Neurosurg 53:433–443, 1980.
95. Paine, KWE: Clinical features of lumbar spinal stenosis. Clin Orthop 115:77–82, 1976.
96. Mooney, V, et al.: A system for evaluating and treating chronic back disability. West J Med 124:370–376, 1976.
97. Hadler, NM: Legal ramifications of the medical definition of back disease. Ann Intern Med 89:992–999, 1978.
98. Benson, H, McCallie, D: Angina pectoris and the placebo effect. N Engl J Med 300:1424–1429, 1979.
99. Holler, JW, Pecora, JS: Backache in bacterial endocarditis. NY State J Med 70:1903, 1970.
100. Churchill, MA et al.: Musculoskeletal manifestations of bacterial endocarditis. Ann Intern Med 87:754–759, 1977.
101. Waldvogel, FA, et al.: Osteomyelitis: A review of clinical features, therapeutic considerations, and unusual aspects (part III). N Engl J Med 282:316–322, 1970.
102. Sapico, FL, Montgomerie, JZ: Pyogenic vertebral osteomyelitis: Reported nine cases and review of the literature. Rev Infect Dis 1:754–766, 1979.
103. Stone, DB, Bonfiglio, M: Pyogenic vertebral osteomyelitis. A diagnostic pitfall for the internist. Arch Intern Med 112:491–500, 1963.
104. Griffiths, H, Jones, D: Pyogenic infections of the spine. J Bone Joint Surg 53B:383–391, 1971.
105. Musher, DM, et al.: Vertebral osteomyelitis. Still a diagnostic pitfall. Arch Intern Med 136:105–110, 1976.
106. Frederickson, B, et al.: Management and outcome of pyogenic vertebral osteomyelitis. Clin Orthop 131:160–167, 1978.
107. Davidson, PT, Horowitz, I: Skeletal tuberculosis. A review with patient presentation and discussion. Am J Med 48:77–84, 1970.
108. Editorial: Tuberculosis of the spine. Br Med J 2:613, 1974.
109. Third report of the Medical Research Council Working Party on tuberculosis of the spine. A controlled trial of debridement and ambulatory treatment in the management of tuberculosis of the spine and patients on standard chemotherapy: A study of Bulawayo, Rhodesia. J Trop Med Hyg 77:72, 1974.
110. Edwards, JE, et al.: Hematogenous Candida osteomyelitis: Report of three cases and review of the literature. Am J Med 59:89, 1975.
111. Simpson, MB, et al.: Opportunistic mycotic osteomyelitis: Bone infections due to Aspergillus and Candida species. Medicine 56:475, 1977.
112. Holzman, RS: Osteomyleitis in heroin addicts. Ann Intern Med 75:693, 1971.
113. Baker, AS, et al.: Spinal epidural abscess. N Engl J Med 293:463–468, 1975.
114. Fraser, RAR, et al.: Spinal subdural empyema. Arch Neurol 28:235–238, 1973.
115. Altrocchi, PH: Acute transverse myleopathy. Arch Neurol 9:111–119, 1963.
116. Lipton, HL, Teasdall, RD: Acute transverse myelopathy. Arch Neurol 28:252–257, 1973.
117. O'Mara, RE: Bone scanning in osseous metastatic disease. JAMA 229:1915–1917, 1974.
118. Pistenma, DA, et al.: Screening for bone metastases. Are only scans necessary? JAMA 231:46–50, 1975.
119. Covelli, HD, et al.: Evaluation of bone pain in carcinoma of the lung. Role of the localized false-negative scan. JAMA 244:2625–2627, 1980.
120. Rodichok, L, et al.: Early diagnosis of spinal epidural metastases. Am J Med 70:1181–1187, 1981.
121. Gilbert, RW, et al.: Epidural spinal cord compression from metastatic tumor: Diagnosis and treatment. Ann Neurol 3:40–51, 1978.
122. Olson, ME, et al.: Infiltration of the leptomeninges by systemic cancer. A clinical and pathologic study. Arch Neurol 30:122–137, 1974.
123. Haddad, P, et al.: Lymphoma of the spinal extradural space. Cancer 38:1862, 1976.
124. Friedman, M, et al.: Spinal cord compression in malignant lymphoma. Treatment and results. Cancer, 37:1485, 1976.
125. Markham, JW, et al.: The syndrome of spontaneous spinal epidural hematoma. J Neurosurg 26:334–342, 1967.
126. Singer, FR: Metabolic bone disease. In Kelley, WN, et al. (eds): Textbook of Rheumatology. Philadelphia: W. B. Saunders, 1981, Chap. 107.
127. Horsman, A, et al.: Prospective trial of estrogen and calcium in postmenopausal women. Br Med J 2:789, 1977.
128. Recker, RR, et al.: Effect of estrogen and calcium carbonate on bone loss in postmenopausal women. Ann Intern Med 87:649, 1977.
129. Avioli, LV: What to do with "postmenopausal osteoporosis." Am J Med 65:881, 1978.
130. Riggs, BL, et al.: Effects of fluoride/calcium regimen on vertebral fracture occurrence in postmenopausal osteoporosis. Comparison with conventional therapy. N Engl J Med 306:446–450, 1982.
131. Cailliet, R: Soft Tissue Pain and Disability. Philadelphia: F. A. Davis, 1977, pp. 62–67.
132. Cyriax, J, Russell, G: Textbook of Orthopaedic Medicine, 6th ed. Baltimore: Williams and Wilkins, 1977.
133. Javid, MJ, et al.: Safety and efficacy of chymopapain (Chymodiactin) in herniated nucleus pulposus with sciatica. JAMA 249:2489–2494, 1983.

2

SORE THROAT

AN OVERVIEW...................................... 71

STREPTOCOCCAL OR NONSTREPTOCOCCAL
PHARYNGITIS?..................................... 76

TREATMENT OF PHARYNGITIS..................... 79

SPECIAL CASES: COMPLICATED SORE THROAT .. 82
    Peritonsillar Abscess 83
    Epiglottitis..................................... 84
    Diphtheria..................................... 86
    Retropharyngeal Abscess....................... 86
    Ludwig's Angina............................... 88
    Unusual Pathogens............................. 90

CHRONIC OR RECURRENT SORE THROAT......... 92

APPENDIX: THROAT CULTURES, STREPTOCOCCAL
INFECTIONS AND THE COST-BENEFIT DEBATE.... 94

REFERENCES....................................... 98

AN OVERVIEW

Phil Pharyngitis, a 22-year-old male, comes to the clinic complaining of sore throat. For the past 2 days, he has noted painful swallowing with discomfort bilaterally in the posterior pharynx and under the angles of the jaw. He believes he has been febrile, but has not taken his temperature and has noted no cough, rhinorrhea, or myalgias. He says that his room-mate has had an undiagnosed sore throat for 6 days that seems to be getting better without treatment. There is no past history of acute rheumatic fever or diabetes mellitus.

The practical clinical approach to the patient with sore throat is usually straightforward and simple. Most such patients have nonstreptococcal pharyngitis that usually resolves in several days without specific treatment. A properly obtained throat culture distinguishes these patients from the minority with streptococcal pharyngitis who do require specific antibiotic therapy. Most often, then, clinical decisions regarding whether, when, and how to treat the patient with sore throat are based on the results of the throat culture. Thus, many clinicians obtain a throat culture from all patients complaining of sore throat and prescribe antibiotics accordingly. Before accepting this "cookbook approach," however, a few generalizations should be remembered:

1. Sore throat is not always synonymous with pharyngitis. The patient with pharyngitis usually describes bilateral internal discomfort in the posterior pharynx, often associated with painful swallowing. Physical examination of the mouth and pharynx usually reveals erythema of the posterior pharynx with or without other findings that sometimes suggest a more specific diagnosis. When the patient's description of "sore throat" is atypical of pharyngitis, and especially when examination of the pharynx is also completely normal, other causes of sore throat must be remembered. Table 2–1

illustrates examples of systemic, mediastinal and "head and neck" diseases that may cause the patient to complain of sore throat that is, in various ways, atypical of pharyngitis.

TABLE 2–1. SORE THROAT: OTHER CAUSES

HEAD AND NECK DISORDERS	SYSTEMIC DISEASES	MEDIASTINAL DISORDERS
Otitis	Viral hepatitis	Myocardial infarction
Sinusitis	Juvenile rheumatoid	Aortic dissection
Salivary gland infection	arthritis	Pneumomediastinum
Dental infection	Rubella	Mediastinitis
Thyroiditis	Poliomyelitis	Esophageal rupture
Carotidynia	Campylobacter enteritis	Angina pectoris
Neck muscle strain	Mycoplasma pneumonia	Esophagitis
Glossopharyngeal neuralgia	Acute leukemia	Esophageal spasm
Retropharyngeal abscess	Toxic shock syndrome	Jugular/subclavian
Epiglottitis	Temporal arteritis	thrombophlebitis
	Agranulocytosis	Aortitis

Sudden, very severe throat pain in a patient whose pharynx is normal on examination should recall the possibility of myocardial infarction, aortic dissection, pneumomediastinum, esophageal rupture, or mediastinitis. These patients are usually obviously ill. Recurrent episodes of brief throat pain may be due to angina pectoris, esophageal spasm, reflux esophagitis, glossopharyngeal neuralgia, or subacute thyroiditis. Various systemic illnesses may begin with prominent sore throat—juvenile rheumatoid arthritis in adults, viral hepatitis, temporal arteritis, and others.

Careful examination of the head and neck (Fig. 2–1A) is always important, since otitis, sinusitis, salivary gland or thyroid inflammation,[2] dental problems, strains of the neck muscles, carotidynia,[3] and some rare but life-threatening upper airway infections (for example, epiglottitis, retropharyngeal abscess—see below) will usually be thus suspected.

2. Visualization of the mouth and pharynx (Fig. 2–1B) sometimes reveals physical findings that are diagnostic of a specific disease.[4]

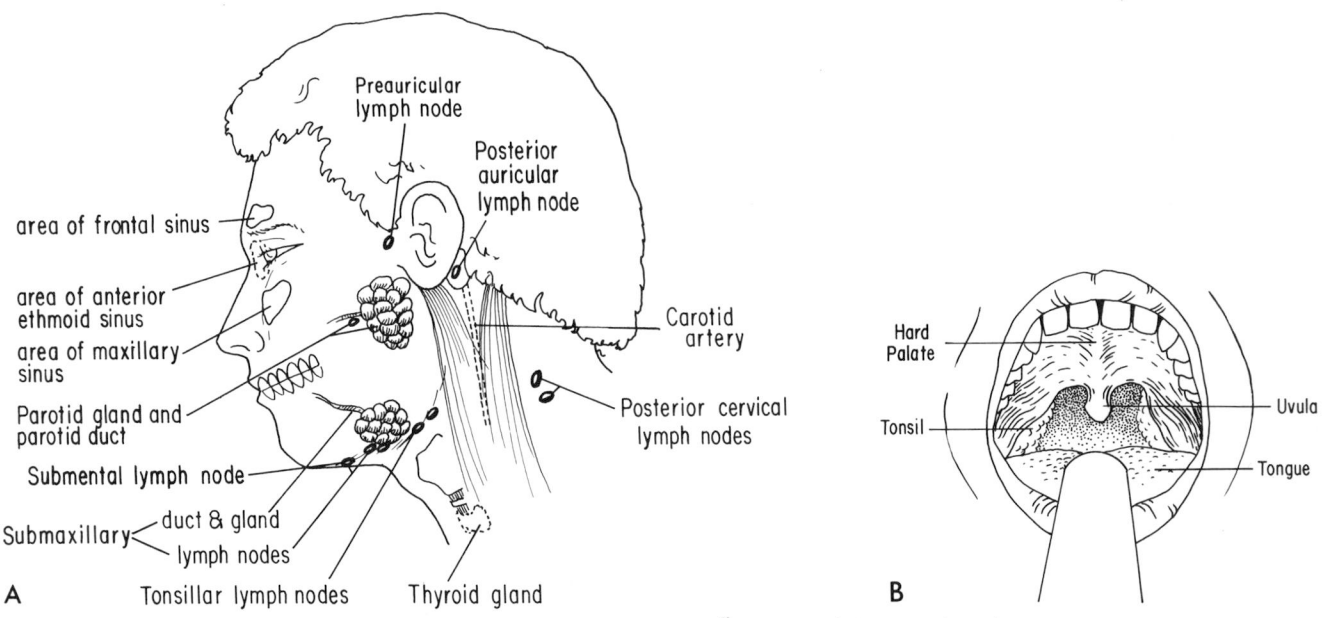

FIGURE 2–1. A, Normal structures of the head and neck. B, Normal structures of the mouth and pharynx.

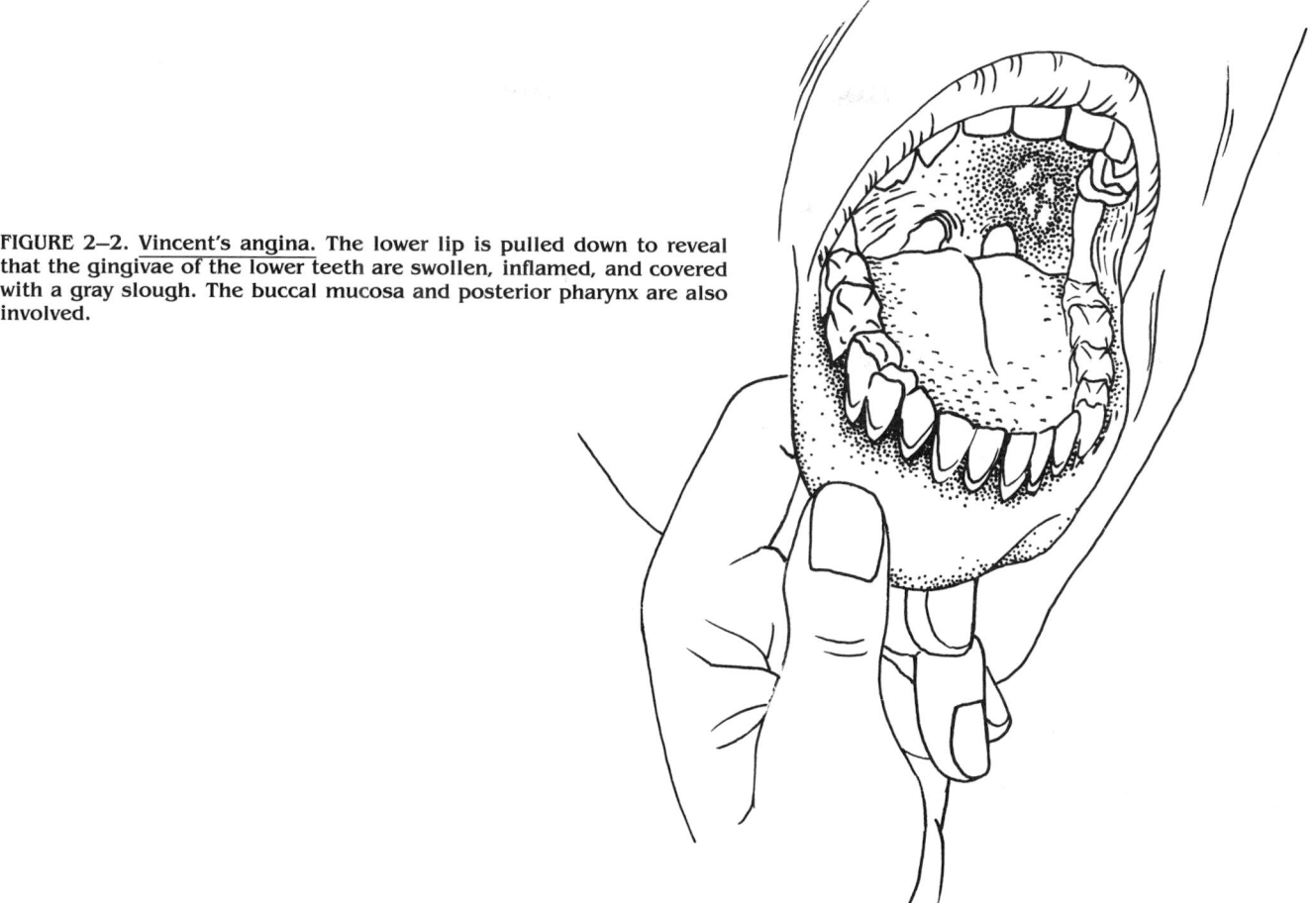

FIGURE 2–2. <u>Vincent's angina.</u> The lower lip is pulled down to reveal that the gingivae of the lower teeth are swollen, inflamed, and covered with a gray slough. The buccal mucosa and posterior pharynx are also involved.

<u>Vincent's angina</u> (necrotizing ulcerative gingivostomatitis) (Fig. 2–2) refers to infection with (usually) *Fusobacterium nucleatum* or *Borrelia vincentii* that begins as a characteristic gingivitis—the papillary gingivae are flattened and inflamed with typical gingival ulcerations, often covered with a fetid, grayish slough. The infection usually spreads to involve the oral mucosa or posterior pharynx with similar ulcerations. Fever, localized lymphadenitis, foul breath, and tonsillitis commonly coexist. Mouthwashes and broad-spectrum antibiotics (tetracycline), followed by continuing dental and peri-odontal care, will be curative.

<u>Herpes simplex</u> infection (Fig. 2–3) most often produces the typical cold sore or fever blister around the lips and external mouth but may also cause a vesicular eruption of the gingivae or oral mucosa or both, usually manifested by grouped, coalescing, superficial mucosal ulcerations. Fever and regional adenopathy are common. Rarely, early lesions will be confined to one or both tonsils and may thus be confused with streptococcal tonsillitis or even a peritonsillar abscess (when unilateral). Treatment is symptomatic only (see below).

<u>Herpangina</u> is a confusing name given to Coxsackie (not herpes) infections of the pharynx and oral mucosa. This diagnosis is usually suggested by multiple small ulcerations of the soft palate and pharynx. <u>Hand, foot, and mouth disease</u>, also caused by a Coxsackie virus, presents with similar oral lesions but is more aptly named since simultaneous lesions are found on the palms and soles. No treatment is necessary.

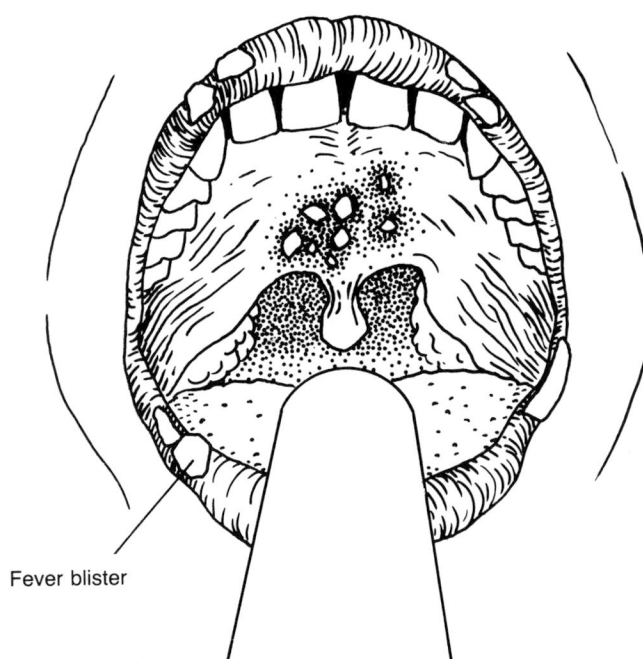

Fever blister

FIGURE 2–3. Herpes simplex infection. The grouped, inflamed vesicles and superficial ulcerations on the palate are typical. Herpangina (Coxsackie) will have a similar appearance, but lesions are usually more widespread and the "cold sore" is less apparent.

Aphthous stomatitis (canker sores) (Fig. 2–4) may be confused with herpes, Coxsackie, or other viral causes of gingivostomatitis, but it more often presents as discrete, shallow, ulcerations (with surrounding erythema) that are very tender, of varying size and location, and frequently recurrent. The etiology is unknown.

Treatment of viral or aphthous stomatitis is largely symptomatic. When painful lesions are few and well localized (as is usually the case with aphthous stomatitis), topical steroids in an Orabase vehicle (for example, triamcinolone acetonide [Kenalog] in Orabase) will often be soothing. More widespread eruptions are sometimes treated with tetracycline suspensions (the contents of a tetracycline capsule dissolved in water, gargled, and swallowed), but

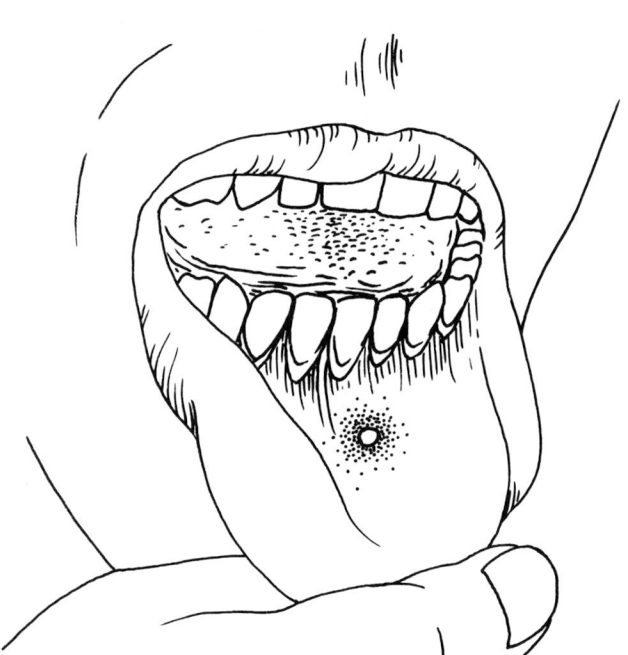

FIGURE 2–4. Aphthous stomatitis ("canker sore").

there are no strong clinical data supporting their efficacy. Topical anesthetics (for example, viscous lidocaine [Xylocaine]) may be helpful when pain is severe—these are only uncommonly necessary.

Oral candidiasis usually presents with white curd-like patches over the tongue and oral mucosa, which may bleed superficially as these patches are scraped from the mucosal surface. This infection may occur de novo, but is more common in diabetics, immunosuppressed or debilitated patients, or patients using antibiotics or corticosteroids (especially topical steroid preparations such as inhalers for asthma or allergic rhinitis) at the time of onset. Mycostatin mouthwash (swallowed after rinsing) 100,000 units three times a day is usually curative. Chronic atrophic candidiasis (denture stomatitis) is a more localized process resulting in an erythematous erosion underlying (usually) a poorly fitting denture.

Periodontal infection (or abscesses) present as acute gingivitis with or without localized fluctuance—broad-spectrum antibiotics and dental attention are indicated. Pericoronitis refers to acute inflammation of "gum flaps" overlying partly erupted wisdom teeth—dental surgery is often necessary.

Many rare or systemic diseases may also cause oral or pharyngeal ulcerations—systemic lupus erythematosus, Behçet's disease, syphilis, tuberculosis, neoplasms, pemphigus, pemphigoid, erythema multiforme, Reiter's syndrome, and many others.[87] Especially when lesions are recurrent or atypical of the common infectious processes discussed above, consultation or biopsy may be indicated.

3. Infectious mononucleosis is not an uncommon cause of sore throat in adolescents* but the diagnosis is usually suggested by physical examination. Infectious mononucleosis[6-9] is usually suspected for one of two reasons: (1) when a teenager's sore throat persists for more than 1 week, or relapses and recurs over many days (an unusual course in viral or streptococcal pharyngitis); or (2) when posterior cervical, postauricular, axillary, or inguinal adenopathy is palpable—such adenopathy is present in 80 to 90 per cent of mononucleosis patients. Malaise, persistent fever, generalized lymphadenopathy, splenomegaly, a foul-smelling tonsillar exudate, or palatal petechiae may also be prominent in some cases, but these are less common than are the classic findings: the teenager or young adult with fever, indolent and persistent sore throat with palpable posterior cervical or postauricular adenopathy. In older adults, the disease is rare, and the clinical features are often atypical.[10, 11]

The diagnosis of mononucleosis is confirmed by the peripheral blood count and the monospot test (the latter is less expensive and more convenient than the standard heterophil agglutination test).[12] The peripheral blood count will reveal atypical lymphocytosis in 80 per cent of patients during the first week of illness and in almost 100 per cent by the end of the second week.† The blood count and monospot test should both be performed when mononucleosis is suspected, because either test may be nondiagnostic at a particular point in time. Other more serious illnesses (toxoplasmosis, rubella, viral hepatitis, syphilis, drug reactions, leukemia, or lymphoma) may rarely produce a similar clinical illness as well as atypical lymphocytosis, but the

*Mononucleosis is uncommon among adults with sore throat—Aronson et al. found only a 2 per cent incidence among 709 patients (mean age 32 years).

†Lymphocytosis may be relative—greater than or equal to 50 per cent of the differential leukocyte count—or absolute—greater than or equal to 4500 per cu mm; more than 10 per cent of the lymphocytes will be atypical morphologically.

monospot test is quite specific. When the monospot test (or heterophil agglutination test) remains negative after 2 to 3 weeks of otherwise typical clinical mononucleosis ("heterophil negative mononucleosis"[13]), cytomegalovirus infection is more often responsible than the Epstein-Barr virus (the usual cause of mononucleosis).

Treatment of mononucleosis is usually expectant and symptomatic. Coexistent streptococcal pharyngitis should be excluded by throat culture. The use of ampicillin should be avoided because of the unexplained high incidence of reactions to this drug in patients with acute mononucleosis. Patients should be counseled to avoid contact sports or injuries to the abdomen for the first 2 to 3 weeks of illness, especially when there is palpable splenomegaly, because of the small (but real) risk of splenic rupture.

Corticosteroid therapy (40 to 60 mg of prednisone a day for 1 week) may produce prompt and dramatic clinical improvement,[14, 15] especially when fever and malaise are debilitating and tonsillar swelling and inflammation make eating and drinking difficult. ("Rebound" of symptoms may occur as steroids are quickly tapered, but this is rare.) Most patients do not require steroid therapy. Definite indications for steroid therapy, however, include pharyngeal obstruction with threatened upper airway closure due to tonsillar hyperplasia (the "kissing tonsil syndrome") and the very rare complications of hemolytic anemia, thrombocytopenia, or neurologic sequelae. Some such patients require hospitalization.

Routine testing for mononucleosis in all patients with sore throat is wasteful.[5] A careful clinical history and examination will usually suggest the diagnosis and allow selective (cost-effective) testing.

Thus a brief but careful history and examination will usually exclude nonpharyngeal causes of sore throat, infectious mononucleosis, and other obvious oral, dental, head, or neck infections.

CONSIDER AGAIN OUR PATIENT

Phil appears mildly ill. His oral temperature is 38°C. There is no respiratory difficulty. Phil localizes his discomfort to the posterior pharynx and complains of painful swallowing, but he is able to swallow food. The posterior pharynx is erythematous, but there are no pharyngeal exudates, oral mucosal lesions, tonsillar hypertrophy, or membranes. The teeth, gingivae, ears, and thyroid are normal. There are small but bilaterally tender upper anterior cervical lymph nodes. There are no posterior cervical or postauricular lymph nodes, splenomegaly, or axillary/inguinal lymphadenopathy.

What does this mean?

STREPTOCOCCAL OR NONSTREPTOCOCCAL PHARYNGITIS?

I. Phil appears to have uncomplicated pharyngitis.

Symptoms are typical of pharyngitis, and there is no specific reason to suspect mononucleosis, referred throat pain (Table 2–1), or other localized infections. Furthermore, Phil is not very ill—more extreme clinical toxicity, usually manifested by various worrisome symptoms and signs (see pages 82 to 90), warrants different considerations. Here the differential diagnosis involves primarily viral and streptococcal pharyngitis.

TABLE 2–2. CLINICAL FINDINGS IN 418 PATIENTS WITH POSITIVE
AND NEGATIVE THROAT CULTURES

	THROAT CULTURE: + (GROUP A) STREPTOCOCCUS (%)	THROAT CULTURE: NO STREPTOCOCCUS (%)
Total	64 (100)	354 (100)
Symptoms		
Rhinorrhea	17 (26)	169 (47)
Cough	11 (17)	169 (47)
Recent exposure to streptococcus	16 (25)	43 (12)
Hearing loss	9 (14)	29 (8)
Signs		
Pharyngeal erythema	63 (98)	299 (84)
Pharyngeal/tonsillar exudate	30 (47)	73 (21)
Swollen tonsils	41 (64)	131 (37)
Enlarged/tender cervical nodes	60 (93)	258 (72)
Temperature: under 37.2°C	33 (52)	238 (68)
37.2°–38.2°C	20 (31)	91 (26)
greater than 38.3°C	11 (17)	22 (6)

Incidence of streptococcal pharyngitis = 64/418 = 15%

Adapted from reference 16.

II. While certain clinical features suggest streptococcal pharyngitis the diagnosis is uncertain.

Table 2–2 enumerates clinical findings in 418 nonpediatric patients with sore throat, 15 percent of whom had streptococcal pharyngitis.[16] While a high temperature (greater than 38.3°C), pharyngeal exudate, tender anterior cervical adenopathy, and recent exposure to documented streptococcal infection should suggest streptococcal pharyngitis,[16] these findings are nonspecific because of the overall low prevalence of streptococcal infection among adults with pharyngitis.[17, 18] Even patients with all these findings are still more likely to have nonstreptococcal pharyngitis.[16] Since other upper respiratory symptoms (cough, rhinorrhea, and the like) are less common in patients with streptococcal pharyngitis (sore throat is their predominant and often only complaint), various combinations of positive and negative findings may be helpful—for example, high fever and pharyngitis with adenopathy but without other "viral symptoms" in the young patient should suggest streptococcal infection. Even this profile is not, however, highly predictive of streptococcal pharyngitis.[16]

III. A throat culture should be obtained.

As noted above, some clinicians routinely obtain throat cultures in all patients complaining of sore throat. As Table 2–2 and the Appendix illustrate, the throat culture is the only reliable, albeit imperfect, means of distinguishing streptococcal from nonstreptococcal pharyngitis.

Does this mean that every patient with a sore throat needs a throat culture? (The Appendix briefly discusses some of the epidemiologic, economic, and philosophic issues that relate to this question.)

If throat cultures are obtained, should antibiotics be given pending the results of the culture? Does it ever make sense to prescribe antibiotics without performing a culture? Can we ever avoid both the culture and antibiotics? These questions can be answered in most individual patients by considering a few clinical factors, as outlined in Figure 2–5:

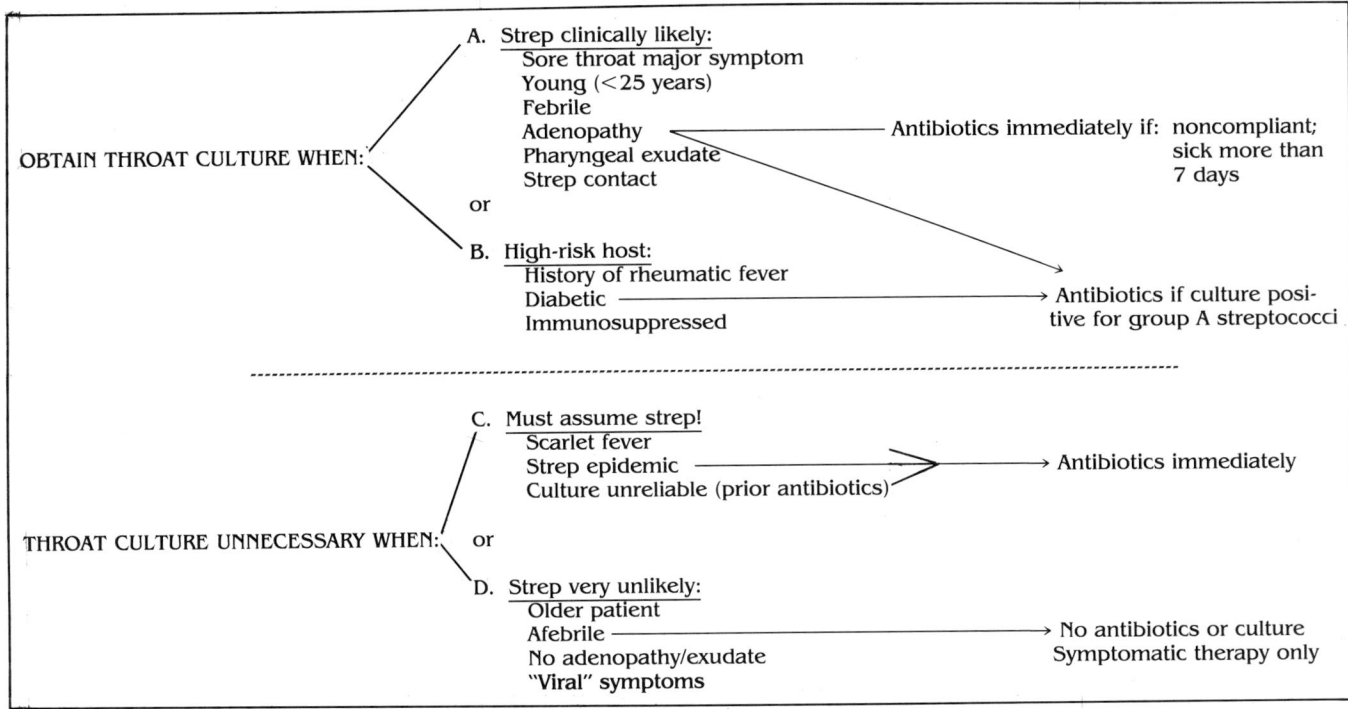

OBTAIN THROAT CULTURE WHEN:

A. Strep clinically likely:
   Sore throat major symptom
   Young (<25 years)
   Febrile
   Adenopathy ———————————— Antibiotics immediately if: noncompliant; sick more than 7 days
   Pharyngeal exudate
   Strep contact

or

B. High-risk host:
   History of rheumatic fever
   Diabetic ———————————→ Antibiotics if culture positive for group A streptococci
   Immunosuppressed

- -

THROAT CULTURE UNNECESSARY WHEN:

C. Must assume strep!
   Scarlet fever
   Strep epidemic ——————————→ Antibiotics immediately
   Culture unreliable (prior antibiotics)

or

D. Strep very unlikely:
   Older patient
   Afebrile ——————————————→ No antibiotics or culture Symptomatic therapy only
   No adenopathy/exudate
   "Viral" symptoms

FIGURE 2–5. Uncomplicated pharyngitis.

A. Do the clinical findings strongly suggest streptococcal pharyngitis?

As noted above, the young (under 25 years) patient whose predominant complaint is sore throat, who is in close contact with another patient with documented streptococcal infection, or who is febrile with tender anterior cervical adenopathy and a pharyngeal exudate (Fig. 2–6) should always be strongly suspected of having streptococcal pharyngitis. Throat cultures should be obtained. Antibiotics are then usually prescribed 24 to 48 hours later when cultures grow group A streptococci. Antibiotics should be begun immediately if the patient is unlikely to comply with subsequent follow-up or treatment (for example, the patient is leaving town) or if the patient has already been symptomatic for 7 or more days (since there is

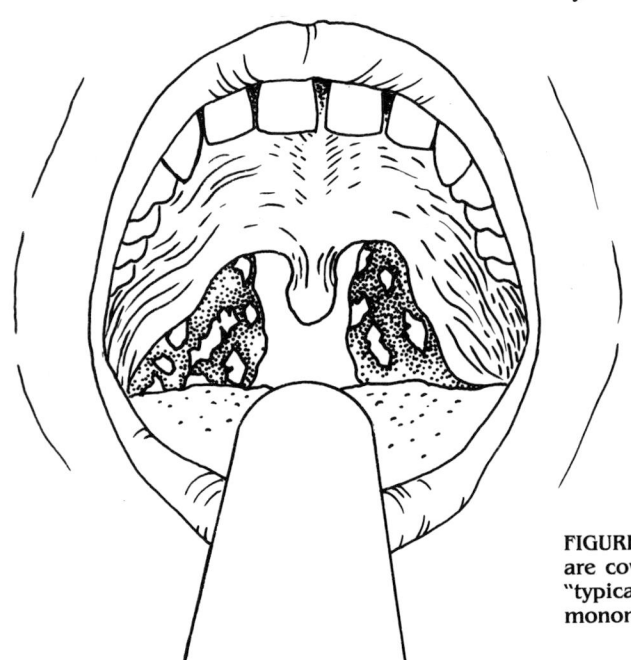

FIGURE 2–6. Tonsillar exudate. The tonsils are inflamed and swollen. They are covered with a loosely adherent, yellow exudate. Such an exudate is "typical" of streptococcal pharyngitis but may also be seen in infectious mononucleosis or viral pharyngitis (Table 2–2).

some evidence that antibiotics most effectively prevent acute rheumatic fever if prescribed within 10 days of the onset of pharyngitis).[19]

B. Is the patient a high-risk host, i.e., unusually prone to suppurative or nonsuppurative complications of streptococcal pharyngitis?

Cultures should always be obtained in patients with a past history of acute rheumatic fever or documented rheumatic heart disease, even if clinical suspicion is very low. Streptococcal pharyngitis is both more common and more dangerous in such patients.[20, 21] Diabetics combat bacterial infection poorly and may be more likely to develop suppurative complications (e.g., peritonsillar abscess). Other immunocompromised patients should also be cultured.

C. Is streptococcal pharyngitis so likely that the throat culture is superfluous?

This is the case only in the (currently) unusual situation in which a streptococcal epidemic is ongoing in the community or when the patient has scarlet fever (unusual in adults). The throat culture is also superfluous when antibiotics have been started (for example, by the patient) before cultures are obtained—here, the culture is much more likely to be "falsely negative" even if streptococcal infection is present. In all these circumstances, the patient should be treated for streptococcal pharyngitis without throat cultures.

D. Is streptococcal pharyngitis very unlikely, clinically? In general, throat cultures and antibiotics are unnecessary in the patient who is older, afebrile, has no lymphadenopathy or pharyngeal exudate, and whose sore throat is one of several other upper respiratory symptoms (cough, rhinitis, and hoarseness, among others). This subset comprises a large number of pharyngitis patients. The Appendix discusses some of the rationale for this "selective" testing and treatment approach.

Because Phil is young, febrile with cervical adenopathy, and has a roommate with a similar illness (which might be streptococcal pharyngitis), the throat culture makes sense in this case.

Phil is told that we are not sure whether his sore throat is due to streptococcal infection or a virus. We explain that he should be treated only if his throat culture is positive for streptococci and explain further that the rationale for antibiotic treatment is the prevention of acute rheumatic fever and that the earlier use of antibiotics will probably not make him better any more quickly. A throat culture is obtained; antipyretics, gargles, and rest are recommended, and Phil is provided with a 10-day prescription for oral penicillin and is told to fill that prescription 2 days from now if he is told over the phone at that time that his throat culture is positive.

Twenty-four hours later, Phil's throat culture is growing a few beta hemolytic streptococci. Forty-eight hours later, these few colonies have been typed and are described as not group A. When Phil calls back in 2 days, he admits that he still has the sore throat but thinks that he is now afebrile and may be feeling a little better while using aspirin and throat lozenges.

TREATMENT OF PHARYNGITIS

Symptomatic therapy of pharyngitis includes antipyretic medications, frequent gargles with warm salt water or nonprescription preparations (Cepacol, Chloraseptic), throat lozenges, cold drinks, or ice cream. Topical anesthetics (viscous lidocaine [Xylocaine]) are only rarely necessary. These various measures are useful in patients with either streptococcal or nonstreptococcal pharyngitis, i.e., whether antibiotics are prescribed or not.

The bulk of evidence supports current belief that streptococcal pharyngitis is a self-limited disease (averaging 5 days in duration) whose clinical course is not altered by antibiotic therapy.[22-24] Antibiotics are prescribed to prevent acute rheumatic fever (see Appendix)—antibiotics probably do not ameliorate the sore throat illness itself.

When antibiotics are prescribed—when streptococcal pharyngitis is documented by throat culture or is presumed for other reasons (Fig. 2–5)—a few practical points deserve emphasis:

1. Various treatment schedules for streptococcal pharyngitis have been studied.[22, 25-32] The eradication of the organism from the pharynx is the usual therapeutic end point in such studies, since the prevention of rheumatic fever depends on that factor.[33] It is the duration of appropriate antibiotic therapy that is the critical factor here—10 days of penicillin "activity" provides optimal benefit, either in daily oral form for 10 days or in the form of a long-acting penicillin preparation (benzathine penicillin, not procaine penicillin) given parenterally.

Oral penicillin G 250 mg (400,000 units) qid for 10 days is the usual recommended therapy for adults. Lesser doses, 125 mg qid or 250 mg bid, may be effective (but have been evaluated primarily in children); variables in compliance and minimal cost differences recommend the higher daily dose for adults.

A single dose of 1.2 million units intramuscular benzathine penicillin should be considered in patients unlikely to comply with prolonged oral therapy, although injections are painful and allergic reactions to penicillin are probably more common (but still rare) when the drug is given parenterally.[34, 35] Some patients prefer the single-dose parenteral injection, but, when treatment is based on culture results, this strategy requires a second visit (and usually an additional fee for the patient).

Erythromycin 250 mg qid for 10 days is the drug of choice in patients allergic to penicillin, while oral cephalosporins or clindamycin may be used in patients unable to tolerate either penicillin or erythromycin.* Tetracycline is never the drug of choice.

Only rarely will a patient with apparently typical streptococcal pharyngitis (documented by throat culture) not improve with one of these antibiotic regimens. While other disorders must always be considered in such circumstances (see "Special Cases" below), occasionally, higher-dose penicillin (500 mg qid) may apparently result in cure. This phenomenon has not been well studied, but the possibility that other pharyngeal bacteria may occasionally lessen the efficacy of usual doses of penicillin has been raised in patients with recurrent tonsillitis.[36]

2. The timing of antibiotic therapy is usually unimportant. As discussed above, since penicillin usually does not affect the severity or duration of the pharyngitis illness itself, antibiotics can usually be withheld until throat culture results are available. The few exceptions include those patients who

---

*Some authorities believe that erythromycin is the drug of choice for all pharyngitis because of its activity against streptococci *and* chlamydiae *and* mycoplasmas, but the last two infectious agents have not been proven to require any therapy at all.

Oral cephalosporins and clindamycin are much more expensive than penicillin or erythromycin.

will be treated regardless of culture results (Fig. 2–5, group C), those patients clinically suspected of having streptococcal pharyngitis who have already been symptomatic for 1 week or more (see page 79), and patients who are unlikely to comply with subsequent follow-up.

Occasionally, "two-stage" oral antibiotic therapy is worthwhile. Here, the patient is given two prescriptions: the first for 2 days of oral penicillin (8 tablets) to be taken while culture results are pending; the second prescription for 8 more days' treatment (32 tablets) to be filled only if the culture is positive. This is usually unnecessary and may not be more economical since many pharmacies have "minimal treatment charges"—8 penicillin tablets may be just as expensive as 40! Nevertheless, this may be worthwhile in patients (especially those with a history of acute rheumatic fever) who "want to get better sooner" (despite advice to the contrary) or "want to get started" on penicillin. This approach is of at least psychologic benefit to some.

3. Follow-up cultures are usually unnecessary. While even optimal antibiotic therapy with full compliance may still result in failure to eradicate streptococci from the pharynx in up to 20 per cent of patients,[32] it is likely that many such patients are "streptococcal carriers" (who are not at risk for acute rheumatic fever—see Appendix). Repeated courses of antibiotics and follow-up cultures in such patients can lead to "streptomania"[37] among both patients and physicians. Such a strategy should probably be limited to the very small number of high-risk patients with rheumatic heart disease or prior acute rheumatic fever in whom streptococci should be eradicated from the pharynx, whenever possible. Otherwise, post-treatment cultures are unnecessary.

In Phil's case, then, several possible strategies may now be considered:

1. Repeat the throat culture. Ten percent of throat cultures will be falsely negative in patients with streptococcal pharyngitis.[38] Repeat cultures may be indicated in patients with a highly likely clinical picture (Fig. 2–5A), those with a history of prior acute rheumatic fever, or other patients intensely anxious about "missing" a strep throat.
2. Treat Phil with antibiotics anyway. This contradicts the original strategy, but some clinicians would follow this course (see Appendix).
3. Simply reassure Phil that his "viral pharyngitis" will continue to resolve with symptomatic treatment.

> Phil agrees to wait to see. However, he asks if we can see his roommate who has now had his sore throat for 8 days and "seems worse" than he was 2 days before.

NOTE

The natural tendency here is to assume that the roommate has the same "viral illness" and to advise watchful waiting. That impulse should perhaps be overruled here because:

1. We do not have a specific diagnosis in Phil's case. If Phil had documented streptococcal pharyngitis, it might be reasonable to simply treat the roommate with antibiotics too. (Conversely, asymptomatic contacts of patients with streptococcal pharyngitis usually do not need cultures or antibiotics unless they are high-risk patients.) (Fig. 2–5B).

2. <u>Most pharyngitis resolves within a week.</u> Worsening of symptoms 1 week after onset is unusual with either viral or streptococcal pharyngitis and should suggest another diagnosis (mononucleosis, for example) or an unusual complication—a "Special Case" (see below).

> **Quentin Quinsy, the roommate, is told to come in. He is an ill-looking 17-year-old who describes in a vaguely muffled voice gradual worsening of sore throat over the past week. Quentin is unable to swallow any solids, has some difficulty swallowing even liquids, and says most of the pain is in the left ear, throat, and neck.**
>
> **Temperature is 39°C orally. There are enlarged bilateral anterior cervical lymph nodes, but the left are much larger and are exquisitely tender. The examining physician is irritated that Quentin barely opens his mouth at all when asked, but the patient, in fact, appears unable to do so. A less than optimal examination demonstrates marked erythema of the posterior pharynx with asymmetric tonsillar swelling, the left tonsil bulging and displacing the uvula slightly to the right. Teeth, gums, thyroid, and ears are normal. There is no meningismus. There is no respiratory stridor, but Quentin admits that he has had some difficulty breathing in the supine position over the last 24 hours. Cardiac examination is normal.**

This is a different problem altogether: a "Special Case."

SPECIAL CASES: COMPLICATED SORE THROAT

A very small minority of patients with sore throat have potentially serious (even life-threatening) illness. Several clinical findings can be important clues to the early diagnosis of such disorders. In Quentin's case, there are several:

1. <u>Trismus</u> (Fig. 2–7). Trismus refers to spasm or tightening of the facial and jaw muscles such that opening the mouth is difficult. The unwary examiner will often interpret mild to moderate trismus as a "functional" phenomenon in the patient with sore throat, i.e., as indicating fear of examination or excessive elaboration of milder symptoms. This can be a dangerous mistake. <u>Trismus</u>, especially when associated with <u>drooling</u> (inability to swallow even one's own secretions), <u>muffled voice</u>, and <u>severe</u> <u>dysphagia</u> or painful swallowing should always prompt suspicion of peritonsillar or retropharyngeal abscess, epiglottitis, or other "deep neck" infections[39] (see below).

Occasionally, severe streptococcal pharyngitis or infectious mononucleosis will cause trismus. Other clues are thus also important:

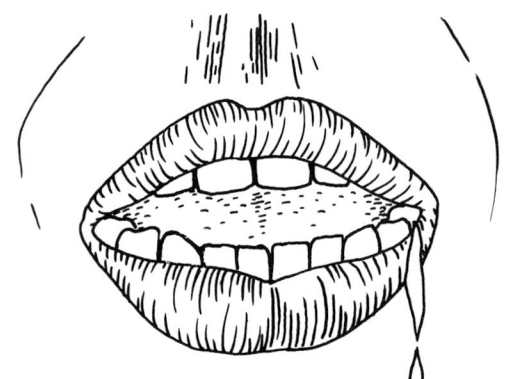

FIGURE 2–7. Trismus. The patient is unable to open the mouth fully. Drooling reflects difficulty in swallowing even one's own saliva.

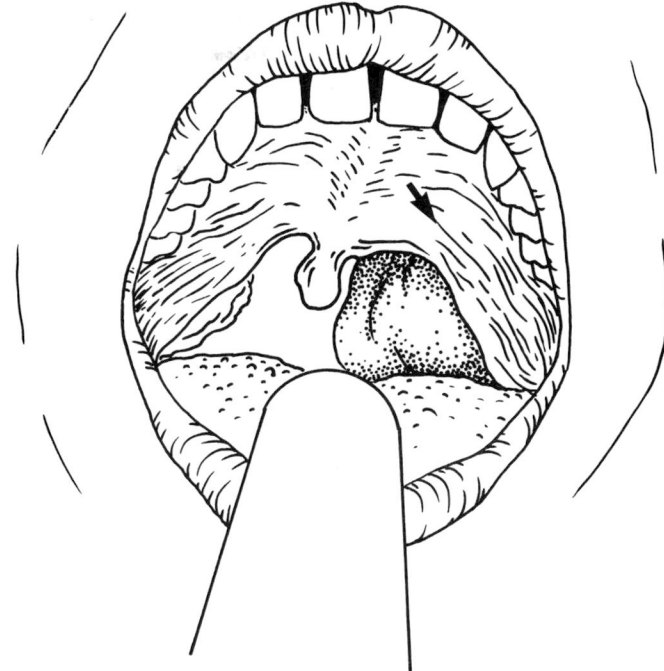

FIGURE 2–8. Peritonsillar abscess ("quinsy"). The left tonsil is asymmetrically inflamed and swollen—there is slight displacement of the uvula to the right. The supratonsillar space (arrow) is also swollen—here is the usual site of the surgical incision for drainage. Prominent unilateral adenopathy typically coexists.

2. Asymmetric tonsillar swelling or asymmetric cervical adenopathy.

Most "common" pharyngitis is bilateral. Peritonsillar abscess (quinsy)[39, 40] (Fig. 2–8) is a suppurative process in the peritonsillar space that may complicate acute pharyngotonsillitis. It usually presents with gradually increasing unilateral ear and throat pain (even in spite of standard penicillin treatment for "strep throat"), followed by trismus, dysphonia, drooling, and dysphagia. Examination usually reveals exquisitely tender ipsilateral upper anterior cervical lymphadenopathy and a bulging peritonsillar mass (sometimes displacing the uvula and soft palate to the contralateral side).

The cause of peritonsillar abscess is often anaerobic bacterial infection,[41] but group A beta hemolytic streptococci,[42] as well as other streptococci, *Hemophilus influenzae,* and *Staphylococcus aureus* may also be isolated from such patients. (Whether failure to respond to standard antistreptococcal penicillin treatment is due to relative resistance of anaerobes to low-dose penicillin or to interference with the eradication of group A streptococci by production of beta-lactamase by "innocent bystander organisms" is unknown.[36]) If unrecognized and untreated, serious complications may occur either locally—upper airway obstruction, lateral extension into the great vessels of the neck—or systemically—septicemia, contiguous mediastinitis, or even intracranial extension.

Treatment of peritonsillar abscess usually involves high-dose parenteral penicillin (10 to 20 million units intravenously per day) or semisynthetic penicillins or clindamycin, in hospital. Continuous irrigation of the edematous tonsillar area with warm saline is sometimes helpful,* and spontaneous rupture and drainage do then occasionally occur. However, a surgeon (preferably an otolaryngologist) must be consulted immediately, since immediate incision and drainage (usually under local anesthesia) is the treatment of choice for peritonsillar abscess. Tonsillectomy is usually performed 4 to 6 weeks later. (Immediate tonsillectomy is also an option.)[40]

---

*An intravenous bottle with warmed saline is hung and the patient irrigates the tonsillar area with continuous effluent from the IV tubing—obviously without a needle!

Pharyngeal or peritonsillar cellulitis, without frank abscess formation, may present in similar fashion, but usually without such pronounced asymmetry on examination (for example, displacement of the uvula). Most otolaryngologists distinguish between abscess formation (requiring surgical drainage) and severe cellulitis (requiring parenteral penicillin) by visualizing and palpating the supratonsillar space for demonstrable fluctuance. The peripheral white blood count is usually dramatically elevated (over 15,000) when frank abscess is present. Often, however, only attempted incision and drainage will distinguish abscess from cellulitis!

Carcinoma or lymphoma may occasionally present as unilateral tonsillar swelling with local adenopathy, but such severe systemic toxicity, trismus, and pain are unusual in such patients. Asymmetric tender anterior cervical adenopathy without any abnormalities in the pharynx should suggest deep neck infections (see below) when the patient is severely ill but is usually due to primary lymphadenitis—i.e., cat scratch disease, tuberculosis, or other local infections (such as otitis and dental infections).

3. Associated respiratory symptoms. Progressive respiratory distress, wheezing, or frank stridor in the patient with acute sore throat must always suggest epiglottitis, deep neck infections, and, rarely, diphtheria.

Epiglottitis[44-47] is uncommon in adults but is certainly not rare. Usually caused by infection with *Hemophilus influenzae* or other oral flora (streptococcus, staphylococcus, anaerobes), inflammatory swelling of the epiglottis leads to vague sore throat, difficulty in swallowing or phonating, fever, and signs of upper airway compromise (orthopnea, wheezing, stridor).* In children, epiglottitis is often a fulminant illness (progressing to respiratory failure in several hours), but in adults the onset may be more gradual (over 2 to 3 days).

Clinical suspicion is always crucial to early diagnosis. Only occasionally can the red and swollen epiglottis be visualized protruding above the posterior base of the tongue on examination of the oral cavity (Fig. 2–9). Much more often, the visual examination of the pharynx is unimpressive (or trismus limits the examination). In such circumstances, lateral "soft tissue" x-rays of the neck and upper airway should be obtained (Figs. 2–10 and 2–11). These are usually diagnostic. When x-rays are normal, indirect laryngoscopy can be performed (gently), but since laryngoscopy may precipitate fatal laryngospasm in the patient with acute epiglottitis, x-rays should always be obtained first (when possible).† Observation in an intensive care unit, full readiness for emergency tracheotomy, and intravenous ampicillin and chloramphenicol (pending the results of cultures) are usual in patients with acute epiglottitis. Epiglottitis may be fatal when treated suboptimally or diagnosed too late.

Severe bilateral tonsillar swelling due to infectious mononucleosis is a much more common cause of upper airway compromise with sore throat than is epiglottitis. (Mild orthopnea is usually the earliest warning symptom of impending airway obstruction.) Physical examination and laboratory findings usually distinguish mononucleosis from bacterial tonsillitis (see page 75), and high-dose oral or parenteral corticosteroids are often dramatically effective, reducing tonsillar swelling within 24 hours in most such cases of mononucleosis. Emergency tonsillectomy is rarely required, but it may be

---

*The absence of respiratory symptoms by no means excludes epiglottitis, however.

†Obviously, when the patient is severely and acutely ill with respiratory impairment, x-rays are not the first order of business. The patient should always be accompanied to the x-ray department, because clinical deterioration may occur very rapidly.

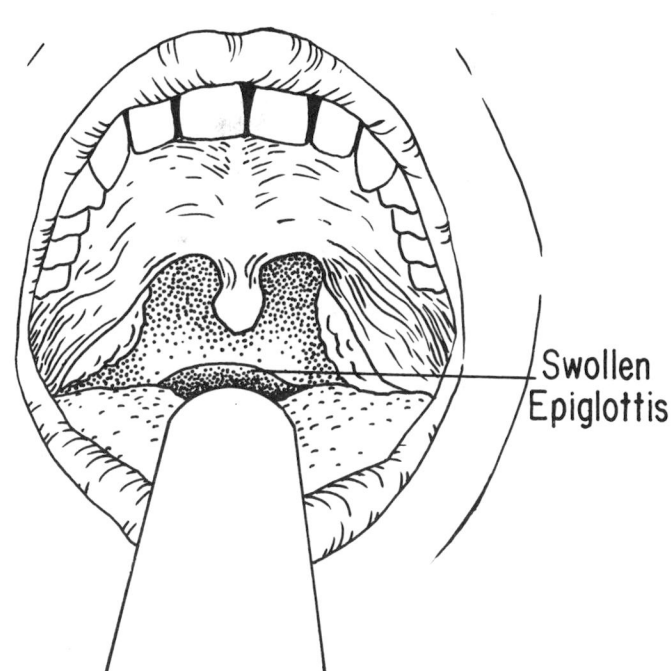

FIGURE 2–9. Acute epiglottitis. Only occasionally will the swollen epiglottis be visible on direct examination. More often, x-rays or laryngoscopy or both will be necessary.

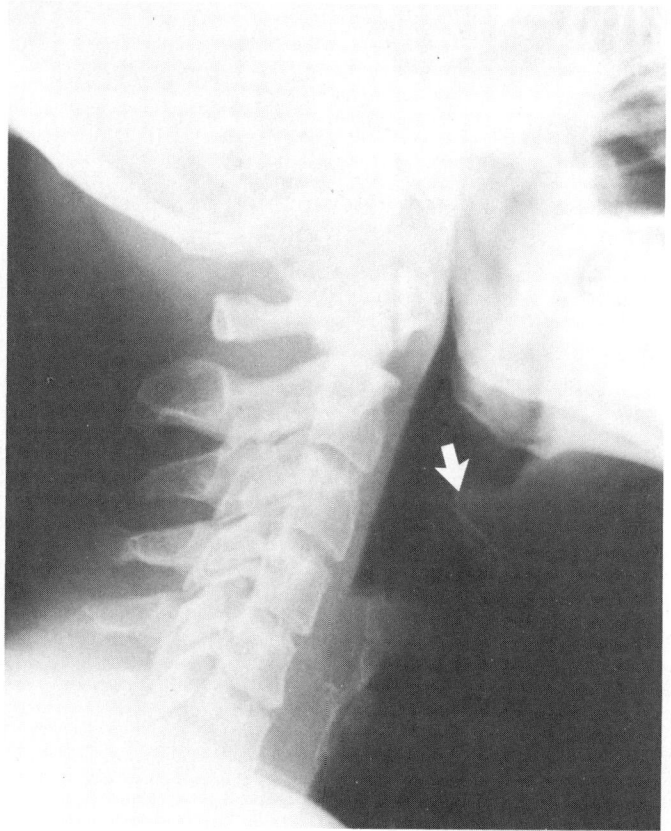

FIGURE 2–10. This 23-year-old man presented with 2 days of increasing sore throat, dysphagia, and fever. There were no respiratory symptoms, and physical examination of the pharynx was unremarkable, in spite of the patient's very dramatic subjective symptoms. The x-ray demonstrates the "thumb print sign" (arrow), indicative of swelling of the epiglottis. Intravenous antibiotics without intubation or tracheotomy resulted in cure.

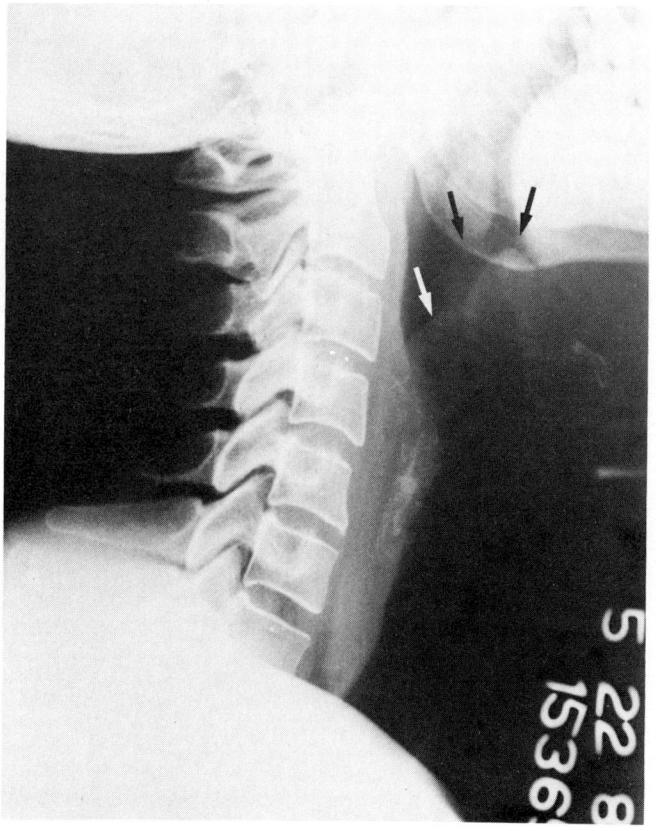

FIGURE 2–11. This 27-year-old man presented with 3 days of increasingly severe sore throat, high fever, extreme dysphagia, and increasing respiratory distress over the previous 6 hours. Examination revealed orthopnea and mild stridor, but examination of the pharynx and chest was normal. The x-ray demonstrates dramatic swelling of the epiglottis with a "triple thumb print sign" (arrows). Despite intravenous ampicillin and chloramphenicol (Hemophilus influenzae type B was the pathogen), tracheotomy was required 4 hours later. The patient recovered after a long and stormy course.

necessary in the patient with chronically enlarged tonsils with superimposed acute infectious pharyngitis who develops airway closure.

Diphtheria[48-50] is now rare in the United States, but both endemic and epidemic infections still occur. Recent exposés of inadequate immunization and adult susceptibility to diphtheria bear notice.[50]

The diphtheritic membrane is the hallmark of infection with *Corynebacterium diphtheriae*—the membrane is usually bluish white, sharply defined, and adherent to the posterior pharynx—and its appearance is usually distinctive from the more common "membrane" seen in infectious mononucleosis (a malodorous, yellow-gray "paste" covering the tonsil) or the pharyngeal exudate of streptococcal pharyngitis. Thus, the diphtheritic membrane is usually visible in the posterior pharynx, but it may be missed for one of two reasons: (1) In mild cases of diphtheria, the membrane is absent—such patients usually have a brief, self-limited illness, and, as such, the disease may be underdiagnosed today; (2) a few patients have only a laryngeal membrane—another reason to consider indirect laryngoscopy (following soft tissue neck x-rays) in the patient with sore throat and signs and symptoms of respiratory compromise. Respiratory compromise and the presence of the diphtheritic membrane are associated with a much worse prognosis in patients with diphtheria—fatalities are not rare in such circumstances. Treatment requires hospitalization, diphtheria antitoxin, parenteral antibiotics (penicillin or erythromycin), and occasionally tracheotomy. Systemic (especially cardiac and neurologic) complications are well-described, some of them life threatening.

> Quentin Quinsy is admitted to hospital. Large doses of intravenous penicillin are begun; the white blood count is 16,000 with 90 per cent polymorphonuclears, and the monospot test is negative. Throat and blood cultures are obtained (and are subsequently negative). Soft tissue x-rays of the neck demonstrate asymmetric pharyngeal edema but no evidence of airway compromise, swelling of the epiglottis, or retropharyngeal tissues.

> An otolaryngologist palpates a fluctuant swelling over the bulging tonsillar mass. Indirect laryngoscopy is otherwise normal. The abscess is incised and drained under local anesthesia. Subsequent cultures of purulent drainage reveal mixed anaerobic flora.

Figure 2–12 illustrates a general approach to patients suspected of "complicated sore throat."

Worrisome symptoms—trismus, asymmetric pain and swelling, or respiratory compromise—are usually associated with visible abnormalities on examination of the oral cavity. Most often, severe streptococcal pharyngotonsillitis, infectious mononucleosis, or peritonsillar abscess will be apparent (or suspected) on examination.

Occasionally, even more unusual physical findings will be noted. These include:

1. Retropharyngeal swelling.[51] Anterior bulging of the posterior pharyngeal wall may be seen in the very rare condition of retropharyngeal abscess. In adults this is seen primarily after extensive dental procedures, direct trauma, or in association with cervical vertebral osteomyelitis with contiguous abscess formation. Such patients are usually critically ill with high fever, headache, stiff neck, airway compromise, or associated complications due to spread of infection to the mediastinum, great neck vessels, meninges, or brain (Figs. 2–13 and 2–14). Broad-spectrum parenteral antibiotics (high-dose intravenous penicillin and an antistaphylococcal drug), intensive care, and surgical drainage are usually necessary.

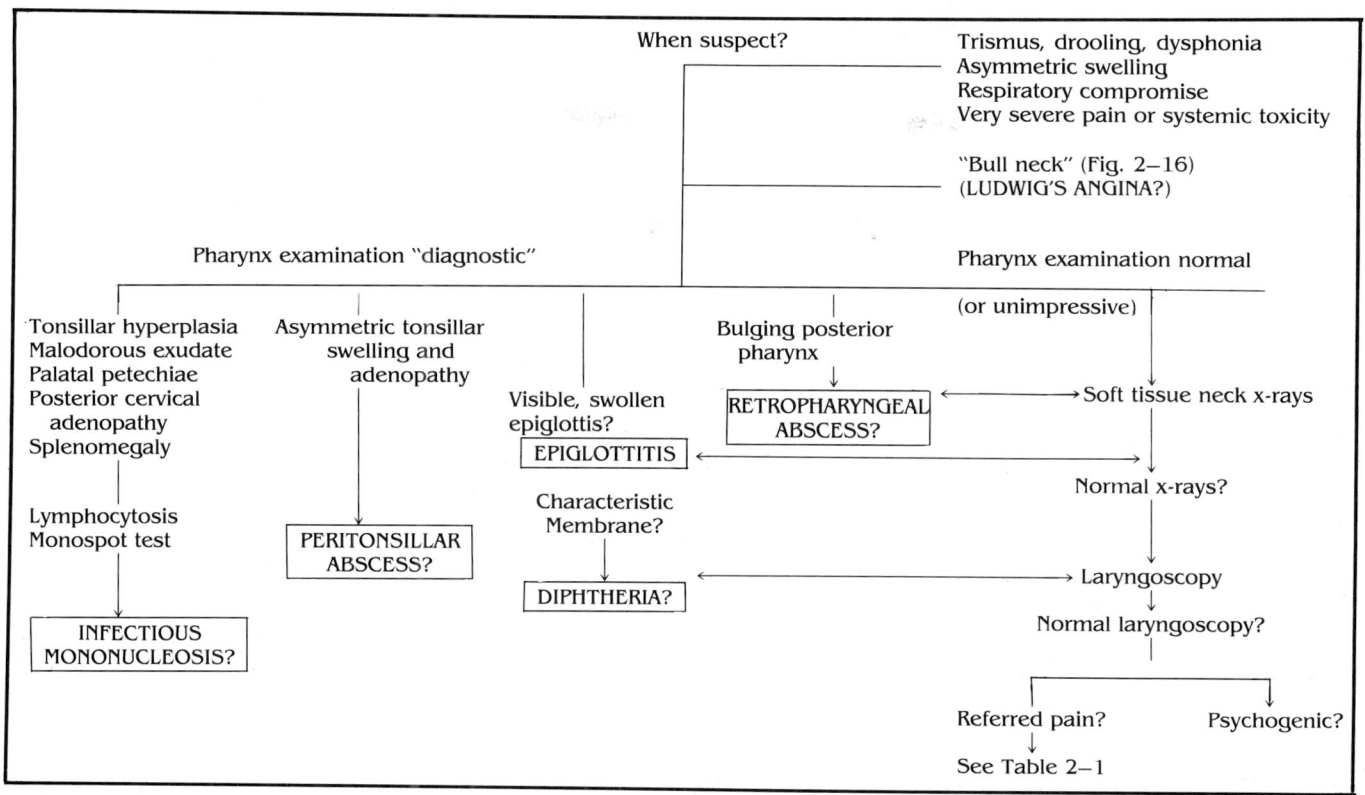

When suspect? — Trismus, drooling, dysphonia / Asymmetric swelling / Respiratory compromise / Very severe pain or systemic toxicity

"Bull neck" (Fig. 2–16) (LUDWIG'S ANGINA?)

Pharynx examination "diagnostic" | Pharynx examination normal (or unimpressive)

Tonsillar hyperplasia / Malodorous exudate / Palatal petechiae / Posterior cervical adenopathy / Splenomegaly → Lymphocytosis / Monospot test → **INFECTIOUS MONONUCLEOSIS?**

Asymmetric tonsillar swelling and adenopathy → **PERITONSILLAR ABSCESS?**

Visible, swollen epiglottis? → **EPIGLOTTITIS**

Characteristic Membrane? → **DIPHTHERIA?**

Bulging posterior pharynx → **RETROPHARYNGEAL ABSCESS?**

→ Soft tissue neck x-rays → Normal x-rays? → Laryngoscopy → Normal laryngoscopy? → Referred pain? (See Table 2–1) / Psychogenic?

FIGURE 2–12. Complicated sore throat.

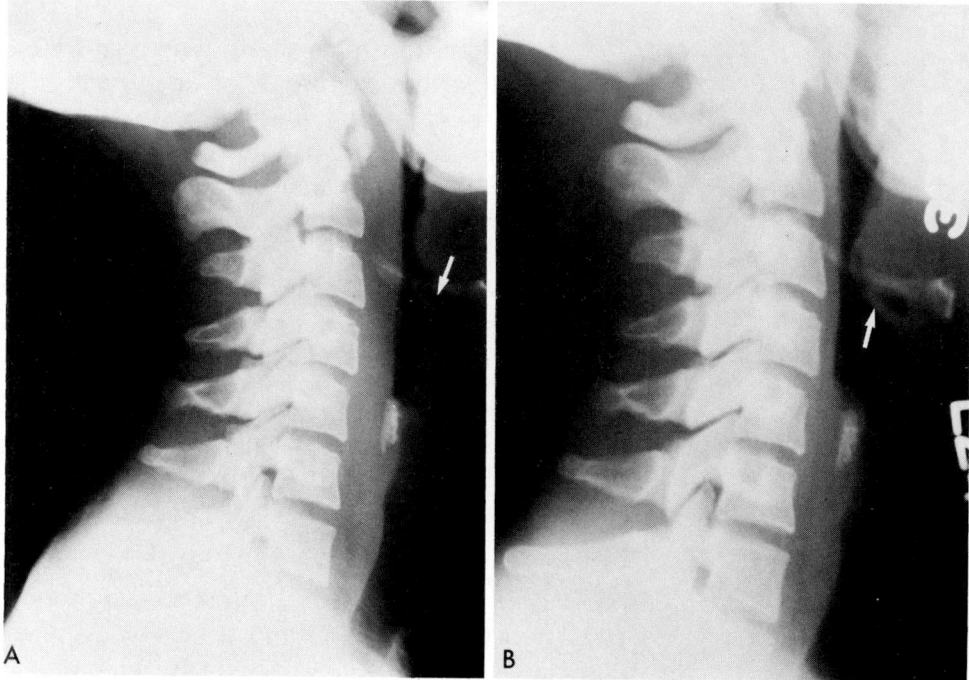

FIGURE 2–13. This 18-year-old woman developed a progressively severe sore throat 1 week after extensive dental work. She described severe headache, stiff neck, and an inability to swallow. Physical examination was unremarkable except for high fever and severe neck and throat pain. A, lateral neck x-ray demonstrates diffuse retropharyngeal soft tissue swelling. High-dose intravenous penicillin and nafcillin resulted in cure, without need for surgical drainage. (Note the normal epiglottis [*arrow*] compared with Figures 2–10 and 2–11.)

B, This x-ray demonstrates the patient's normal lateral neck x-ray 6 months later. (See also Figs. 2–14 and 2–15.)

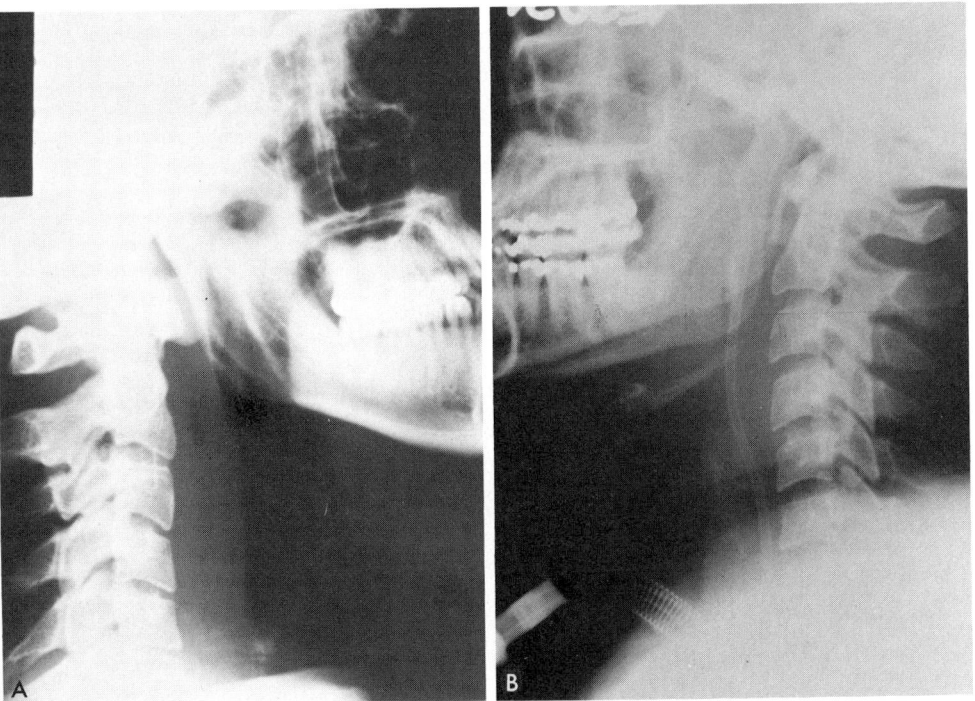

FIGURE 2–14. Three days following multiple wisdom teeth extractions, this 21-year-old man developed severe sore throat, dysphagia, and progressive respiratory distress. Physical examination was unremarkable except for high fever, severe neck and head pain, and a question of swelling of the posterior pharyngeal wall. The lateral neck x-ray demonstrates extensive soft tissue swelling of the entire precervical area. Surgical drainage of a retropharyngeal abscess (culture: a mixture of streptococci and staphylococci), as well as high-dose intravenous antibiotic therapy, ultimately resulted in cure, but only after a prolonged hospital course complicated by mediastinal, pulmonary, and pleural space infections.

A, X-ray on presentation.

B, Two days later.

Even when retropharyngeal swelling cannot be directly visualized in patients with severe symptoms of deep neck infections, this clinical presentation (severe symptoms without visible abnormalities in the oral cavity) should prompt obtaining of x-rays of the upper airway and neck. Familiarity with normal radiologic anatomy is helpful here. As Figure 2–15 suggests, when distance from the lower anterior aspect of the second cervical vertebra to the posterior wall of the pharynx (retropharyngeal space) exceeds 7 mm. or the retrotracheal distance from the lower anterior aspect of C6 to the posterior trachea wall exceeds 22 mm, abnormal retropharyngeal swelling should be considered.[52]

2. As noted above, a swollen epiglottis may rarely be visualized below the posterior base of the tongue if adequate tongue depression and patient cooperation are achieved. Rarely, lingual tonsillitis (infection in an anomalously located tonsil at the base of the tongue)[53] may be mistaken for epiglottitis.

3. Bull neck (Fig. 2–16) refers to marked swelling of the submandibular area, often with elevation and posterior displacement of the tongue due to sublingual swelling. This problem is rare, but it is associated with various infectious processes, all of which are potentially fatal. Ludwig's angina[54, 55] is probably most common, but diphtheria, suppurative thyroiditis, and other deep neck and mediastinal infections may also so present.

Ludwig's angina is an infection of the sublingual space that may extend inferiorly to cause upper airway obstruction. A dental abscess is the most

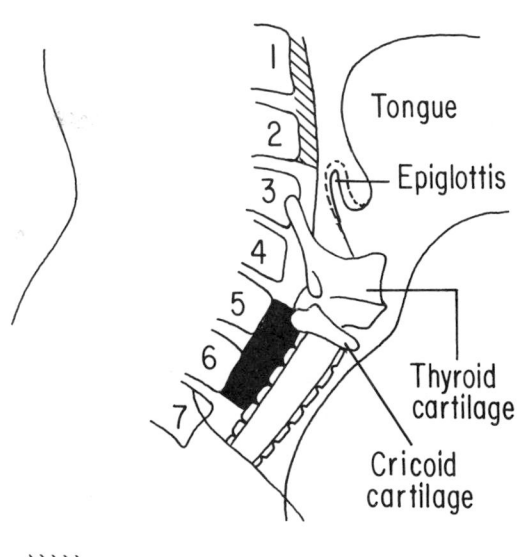

FIGURE 2–15. *A,* Normally, the retropharyngeal space does not exceed 7 mm when measured from the anterior aspect of the C2 verteral body to the posterior pharynx.

B, Normally, the retrotracheal space does not exceed 22 mm when measured from the anterior aspect of C6 to the trachea.

C, Dotted lines depict the "thumbprint" made by a swollen epiglottis.

common precipitating event, while mandibular fractures or oral lacerations may also be complicated by this infection. Streptococcus is the most common organism,[56] but staphylococci and other "mixed" oral pathogens are not rare: Antibiotic treatment usually includes high-dose penicillin (10 million units per day) and an antistaphylococcal drug (nafcillin, for example). Hospitalization and careful airway maintenance are always essential; surgical drainage is sometimes (but not always) necessary. In advanced cases, respiratory failure and death are common because endotracheal intubation is virtually impossible, and only an emergency tracheotomy will be life saving.

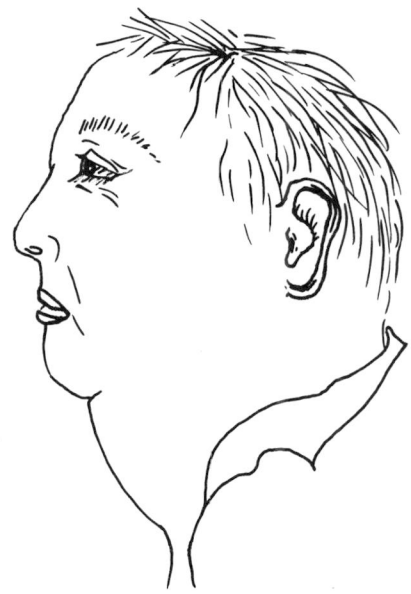

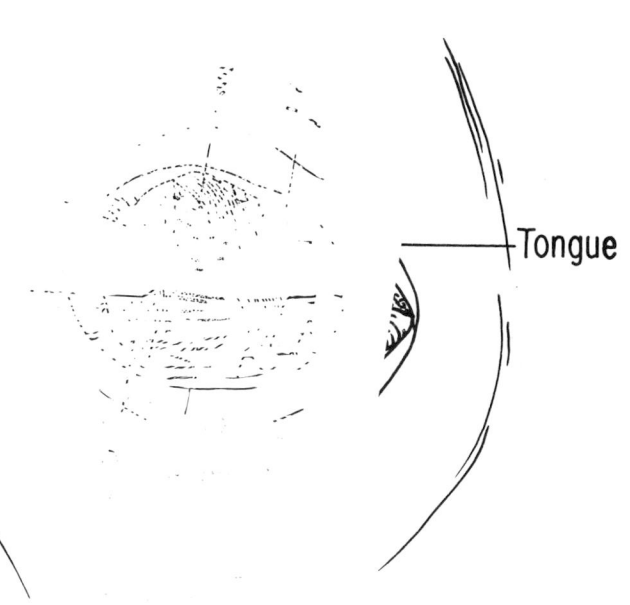

FIGURE 2–16. "Bull neck." The submandibular area is markedly swollen *(above).* There is dramatic elevation of the floor of the mouth by soft tissue swelling, elevating the tongue and displacing it posteriorly *(below).*

Bull neck should not be confused with asymmetric submandibular swelling, usually the result of acute unilateral salivary gland infection (acute sialadenitis) or dental abscesses of the lower jaw. Familiarity with salivary gland and duct location will be helpful here (Fig. 2–1).

Rarely, "complicated sore throat" will be associated with an (apparently) completely normal examination of the head and neck. Especially when respiratory symptoms are prominent, lateral soft tissue neck x-rays or laryngoscopy or both should be performed. Only then will epiglottitis, retropharyngeal abscess, diphtheria, and other serious problems not be missed.

When sore throat is severe or worrisome but all of these examinations are normal, the systemic and referred causes of sore throat (Table 2–1) must be reviewed. Occasionally, such complaints will be psychogenic (page 93), but in patients with confusing, dramatic, or "worrisome" sore throat symptoms (Fig. 2–12), evaluation must be thorough if rare but life-threatening diseases are to be diagnosed promptly.

> Two days later, Quentin Quinsy is remarkably better, but he now admits that he is concerned about VD and asks that he be checked out while in the hospital. Quentin admits that he and his roommate, Phil Pharyngitis, maintain a mostly monogamous homosexual relationship but do have sexual relations with other men on occasion. Cultures from the urethra, rectum, and pharynx are plated on Thayer-Martin medium at the bedside (and all are subsequently negative).

> Phil Pharyngitis, on the other hand, is now entirely well, 6 days after the onset of his sore throat. He reluctantly submits to gonococcal cultures, which, in his case, are positive from the rectum and pharynx. Appropriate therapy is given.*

While it is likely that Quentin's gonococcal cultures were negative because of his intravenous penicillin therapy, it is highly unlikely that his peritonsillar abscess was in any way related. Gonococcal pharyngitis may occasionally be severely symptomatic, but the great majority of patients are completely asymptomatic.[57, 58] (It is unknown whether even Phil's illness was related to his gonococcal infection, since viral or streptococcal pharyngitis will often spontaneously improve in 6 days.) The point here is that occasionally bacterial pharyngitis may not be streptococcal, and other pathogens should be sought in certain circumstances:

1. *Neisseria gonorrhoeae*—Thayer-Martin medium should be plated with a pharyngeal swab when homosexual males (or women who practice fellatio) complain of sore throat (the association with cunnilingus is less clear), or when the patient is suspected of gonorrhea in other sites (urethra, rectum, pelvis).

2. *Corynebacterium diphtheriae*—Diphtheria bacilli can usually be grown on sheep blood agar, but Löffler's slant and tellurite agar may increase the yield.

3. *Neisseria meningitidis* (meningococcus)—Thayer-Martin medium will also identify the meningococcus; such a search is indicated primarily during meningococcal epidemics or following exposure to a patient with documented meningococcal infection (especially meningitis).

---

*See Chapter 8, "Male Genitourinary Infections."

4. Other pathogens may cause infectious pharyngitis, but these are either very rare *(Francisella tularensis* in tularemia; *Hemophilus influenzae; Staphylococcus* or gram-negative rods in neutropenic immunosuppressed patients); are suspected by physical examination *(Fusobacterium* in Vincent's angina; visible syphilitic chancres); or have not been proven to require antibiotic therapy (mycoplasmal or chlamydial infections and *Yersinia enterocolitica).*[85] Attempted isolation of these various organisms is rarely worth the effort and should be considered only in very unusual circumstances.

5. Just as chronic or recurrent sore throat can be caused by a variety of noninfectious processes (see below), it is worth remembering that acute sore throat may also be the result of trauma (sharp objects, endotracheal intubation) "local dehydration" (mouth breathing, oxygen therapy, jogging), inhaled irritants (fumes, fibers, medicinal inhalers) or even foreign bodies (for example, a peanut in the trachea, a caraway seed embedded in a tonsil).

In summary, Figure 2–17 illustrates an overview of the clinical approach to the patient with acute sore throat.

Subsequently, Quentin Quinsy undergoes uncomplicated tonsillectomy and remains well thereafter.

Phil Pharyngitis, however, develops another sore throat 3 weeks later. Physical examination is unremarkable—he is not ill, and there is no adenopathy or pharyngeal exudate. Both streptococcal and gonococcal

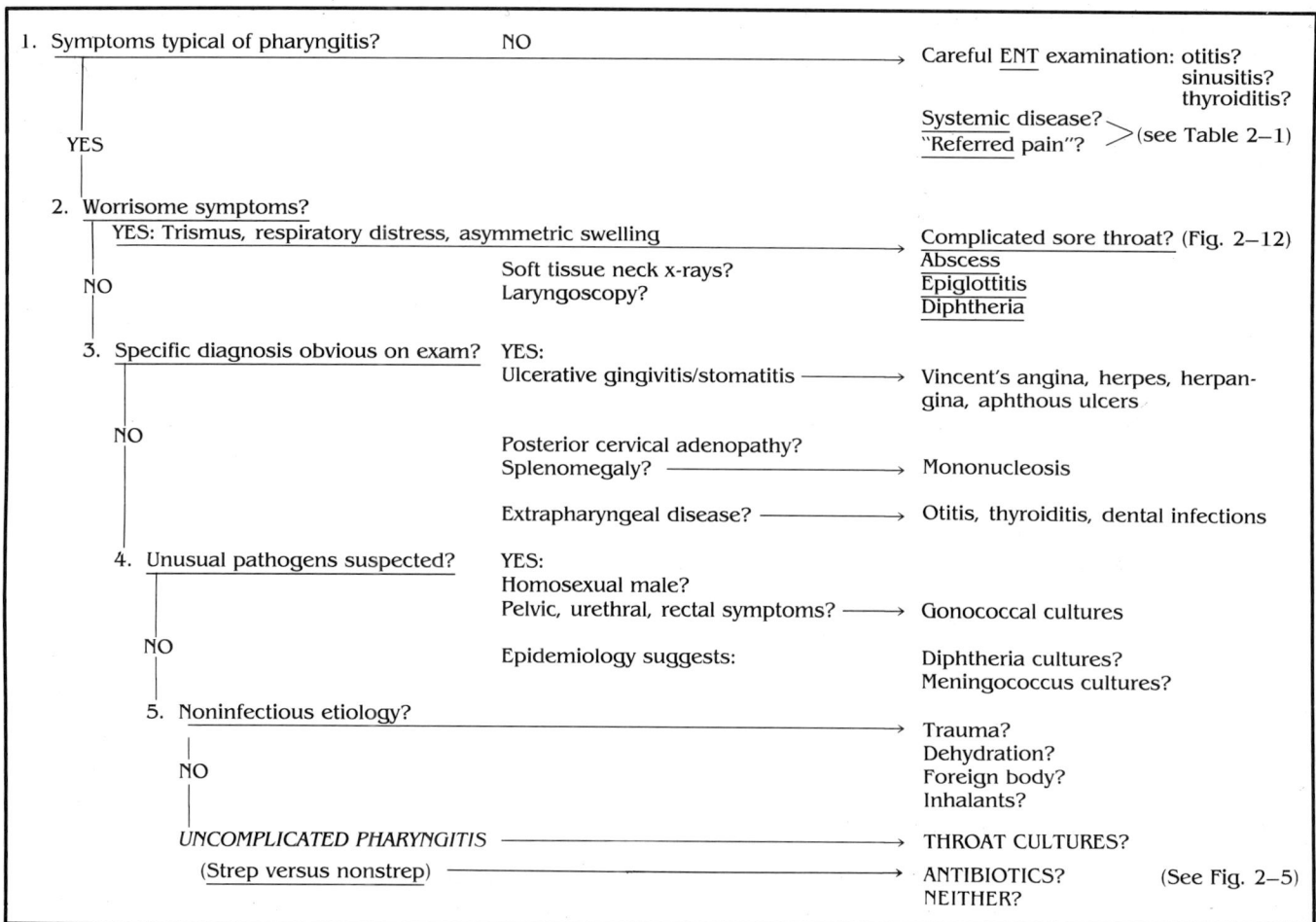

FIGURE 2–17. Acute sore throat.

cultures are negative. There is no tonsillar hyperplasia, and syphilis serologic tests are negative.

Despite reassurance that all is well, Phil continues to complain of mild, chronic sore throat that waxes and wanes over the next several months, and no diagnosis is established despite multiple cultures and examinations; otolaryngologist consultation; repeated culturing of his roommate, Quentin. Empiric antibiotic therapy with three different antibiotics at different times is unsuccessful in relieving Phil's symptoms, as are the usual symptomatic measures.

CHRONIC OR RECURRENT SORE THROAT

This is an uncommon but by no means rare phenomenon—the patient with chronic, recurrent, or relapsing sore throat that eludes specific diagnosis. In such cases, several possibilities should be considered:

1. Chronic tonsillitis. While tonsillectomy is now an unfashionable procedure, there is no question that some patients do develop chronic tonsillitis that requires surgery. Most such patients suffer from recurrent streptococcal tonsillitis—whether streptococci or various other pathogens are more important in this group is unclear.[36, 59] Examination of such patients usually reveals very enlarged tonsils bilaterally with chronic lymphadenopathy. Fever may be absent.

2. Smoking. Heavy tobacco use will cause chronic sore throat in some patients. (Sometimes, stopping smoking will cause throat irritation for a few weeks.) The widespread smoking of marijuana, hashish, and even cocaine has increased the incidence of "hash throat"; here, pharyngeal inflammation and uvular edema often persist for 12 to 24 hours after smoking in susceptible patients, while chronic daily use of these substances may cause persistent, unexplained complaints of sore throat (even with a normal physical examination).

3. Postnasal drip is an extremely common cause of chronic sore throat in adults. Chronic sinusitis and allergic rhinitis are the usual underlying problems—worsening of symptoms in the morning after sleep is common in patients with chronic sinusitis, while atopy, sneezing, asthma, and associated eustachian tube dysfunction with middle ear effusions are often tip-offs to allergic causes.

4. Recurrent subacute thyroiditis[60] may cause puzzling throat and ear pain, but the thyroid is usually tender to palpation, and the sedimentation rate is almost invariably elevated in such patients. Since on occasion the thyroid may not be tender, documentation of this disorder may require a radioiodine scan of the thyroid that will demonstrate marked suppression of iodine uptake during the clinical illness.

5. Infectious mononucleosis may cause relapsing pharyngitis. As noted above, when sore throat persists for more than 1 or 2 weeks, blood counts and monospot tests should be repeated since these may be normal in the first week of illness.

6. Remember that brief episodes of sore throat with a normal examination may represent referred pain—angina pectoris is common, while glossopharyngeal neuralgia is rare.

7. Pharyngeal irritants, especially in smokers or those with chronic rhinitis or sinusitis, should be remembered. The drying effects of home heating systems (especially wood stoves) can be combated with humidification. An occupational history is worth a few minutes' consideration—the textile mill worker, for example, may develop sore throat from wool fiber inhalation. Professional painters, chemical industry workers, asbestos insulation workers, and others may develop puzzling, recurrent throat symptoms.

Each of these possibilities is deemed unlikely after further history and examination in Phil's case. The possibility of psychogenic pharyngitis is raised.

Psychogenic pharyngitis usually occurs in patients who manifest other evidence of anxiety or depression, and very often there is some model in the patient's personal life that implicates the throat as the locale of somatization (a relative with throat cancer, for example). The condition of such patients should, of course, be carefully evaluated, but subsequent management may be difficult, especially if the underlying fear, frustration, or specific psychiatric disorder remains undiscovered.

It is carefully explained to Phil that his gonococcal infection probably did not produce Quentin's illness, that Phil himself is no longer infected, and that, in the future, periodic checks for sexually related illness should be performed on both Phil and Quentin, given their commitment to their chosen life style. Every 3 to 4 months thereafter for the following year, both Phil and Quentin are screened for asymptomatic venereal disease. During that time, Phil's complaints of sore throat gradually diminish, and he remains well.

Throat Cultures, Streptococcal Infections, and the Cost-Benefit Debate

THROAT CULTURES

Throat cultures are usually obtained to diagnose or exclude the presence of group A beta hemolytic streptococci in the pharynx. Under these circumstances, the laboratory will not attempt to isolate any other bacteria and will purposely inhibit the growth of organisms that commonly colonize the oral cavity (pneumococcus, *Hemophilus influenzae*, anaerobes, *Staphylococcus*). Attempts to isolate nonstreptococcal organisms from the pharynx are rarely, if ever, indicated (see page 90).

When streptococcal infection is suspected and culture results will influence treatment (see pages 76 to 79), a sterile swab should be rubbed firmly over the posterior pharynx, tonsils, and any pharyngeal exudate. (The tongue and uvula should be specifically avoided—the tongue depressor helps here.) Gentleness is laudable, but procuring a proper specimen is more important. Because a single swab is associated with a false negative rate of at least 10 percent,[38] some clinicians obtain a second swab (and inoculate it on the same culture plate as the first). The specimen can be plated immediately on sheep blood agar or preserved temporarily in liquid transport medium ("culturette") for further handling by the laboratory technician. Colony growth and beta hemolysis are usually apparent within 12 to 24 hours, but since not all beta hemolytic streptococci are group A, another 12 to 24 hours is often needed to confirm or exclude the presence of group A streptococci (usually by fluorescent antibody techniques or bacitracin disc inhibition). Only group A streptococci deserve treatment,* and even a few colonies are significant. (Attempts have been made to distinguish carrier state from true infection—see below—on the basis of the number of colonies grown on culture, but this is unreliable.)[62, 63]

WHEN IS A STREP THROAT A STREP THROAT?

The principal purpose of treating streptococcal pharyngitis is to prevent subsequent acute rheumatic fever (see below). Only patients with active streptococcal infection, i.e., those with pharyngeal streptococci who also mount a systemic immunologic response to streptococcal antigens, are at risk of developing acute rheumatic fever.[42, 62, 64] Patients who grow group A streptococci on throat culture but who do not develop serial rises in anti-streptococcal antibody titers over time are called strep carriers and are not

---

*A recent report of an epidemic of group G beta hemolytic streptococcal pharyngitis deserves notice,[61] but it is of uncertain significance to the general population.

at risk of acute rheumatic fever. At least half of all patients with strep throat by culture criteria are, in fact, strep carriers who thus do not theoretically require antibiotic therapy to prevent acute rheumatic fever. Unfortunately, there is no current rapid method to differentiate strep carriers from those with active infection, since diagnostic antibody titers rise over the course of several *weeks*. Thus, all current clinical strategies must utilize the operative definition of strep throat—a positive throat culture. A strep throat is always a strep throat.*

WHY IS STREPTOCOCCAL PHARYNGITIS WORTH DIAGNOSING AND TREATING?

1. To alter the natural history of the pharyngitis illness itself?—Probably not.

As noted in the text proper, most studies suggest that streptococcal pharyngitis resolves with or without antibiotic treatment, usually in less than a week, and neither the duration nor severity of clinical symptoms is lessened by antibiotic treatment.[22, 23, 24, 65, 66] These data are far from irrefutable,[67] but more careful studies are unlikely to be undertaken in the future. There are some patients who do appear to subjectively improve more quickly with penicillin treatment but, anecdotal experience aside, this is not the current "scientific" rationale for antibiotic treatment of strep throat.

2. To decrease the spread of infection?—Maybe.

Streptoccocal epidemics can probably be aborted by antibiotic therapy of infected patients, and perhaps further contained by prophylactic treatment within the afflicted community,[68, 69] but the clinical significance of these data in adult endemic infection is unknown. There is some evidence that early treatment of streptococcal pharyngitis in children will reduce subsequent pharyngeal streptococcal colonization among siblings and close household contacts.[70] In general, however, asymptomatic contacts of patients with endemic streptococcal pharyngitis do not require cultures or treatment.

3. To prevent suppurative complications?—Probably.

There is no question that the incidence of parapharyngeal abscess, suppurative cervical adenitis, mastoiditis, and other septic complications of streptococcal pharyngitis is remarkably lower now than during the preantibiotic era. Suffice it to say that such complications are now rare, probably in large part as a result of the widespread use of antibiotics.

4. To prevent "nonsuppurative" complications?—Yes and no.

It is unlikely that poststreptococcal glomerulonephritis can be prevented by treatment of individuals with antecedent streptococcal pharyngitis.[71] Occasionally, guttate psoriasis or erythema nodosum may follow (symptomatic or asymptomatic) streptococcal infection, but there is no evidence that antibiotic therapy will prevent these developments.

Acute rheumatic fever is another matter. Treatment of streptococcal

---

*The one possible exception here is the patient who is treated with appropriate antibiotics and whose follow-up throat culture remains positive for group A streptococci.[32] Since most patients whose post-treatment cultures remain positive are probably carriers, obtaining post-treatment cultures is not usually recommended. When follow-up cultures are obtained, for whatever reason, the patient with a persistently positive culture deserves one repeat course of antibiotics, but no more.

pharyngitis during streptococcal *epidemics* will clearly reduce the incidence of acute rheumatic fever. The attack rate of acute rheumatic fever following an epidemic of streptococcal pharyngitis may be as high as 2 or 3 per cent when the pharyngitis is not treated. Denny et al. found 17 cases of acute rheumatic fever among 804 untreated patients,[72] while Wannamaker et al. diagnosed definite acute rheumatic fever in 28 patients among 996 untreated controls.[73] Antibiotic treatment, even in doses suboptimal by today's standards, will reduce the incidence of acute rheumatic fever tenfold to about 0.2 per cent (2 cases among 798 patients treated by Denny's group,[72] and 2 cases among 978 patients treated in Wannamaker's study.[73]) The impact of antibiotic therapy of *endemic* streptococcal pharyngitis in preventing acute rheumatic fever is less well documented. Siegel et al.[74] diagnosed acute rheumatic fever in 2 children among over 500 patients with positive throat cultures who did not receive antibiotics—an incidence of 0.4 per cent; there were no cases of acute rheumatic fever among a similar number of children who were treated with antibiotics. Endemic streptococcal pharyngitis is, thus, probably associated with a much smaller risk of acute rheumatic fever than is epidemic streptococcal infection. This difference is probably in part due to the greater virulence of streptococcal strains during epidemics (which are rare today) and the higher rate of "active infection" among patients with positive throat cultures during epidemics.[64] There is good reason to believe that even a 0.4 per cent attack rate (4 per 1000 in Siegel's study[74]) is too high an incidence of acute rheumatic fever in current untreated endemic situations.[75, 86] While we can debate the precision of the numbers, the low order of magnitude of acute rheumatic fever risk following streptococcal infection does shed some light on the cost-benefit controversy.

THE COST-BENEFIT DEBATE

If the incidence of acute rheumatic fever in untreated endemic streptococcal pharyngitis is 0.4 per cent (4 per 1000), and if only about 10 per cent of adults with sore throat have positive throat cultures[16, 17] (but only half again of these have active infection, i.e., 5 per cent of the total), then one might expect 20 cases of acute rheumatic fever per 100,000 adult patients (4 per 1000 multiplied by 5 per 100) complaining of sore throat, even if no diagnosis or treatment is pursued. This rough estimate is, in fact, close to some computed estimates of rheumatic fever risks.[76, 77] Since it costs (conservatively) $20 to diagnose and treat the average sore throat, we may be spending $2 million in attempting to prevent 20 cases of acute rheumatic fever, or $100,000 per case.

What happens to the patient who is unlucky enough to develop acute rheumatic fever? Beyond the acute illness (which can be very debilitating), the few available data on this subject suggest that the majority of such patients do not develop serious chronic sequelae.[78] One study group followed 441 patients with acute rheumatic fever an average of 8 years:[78] There were 12 deaths, and 5 other patients had developed Class IV cardiac disability. More than 95 per cent of the total group, however, were asymptomatic or had Class I heart disease at the conclusion of the study. This study does not answer our question, since the latency period between acute rheumatic fever and development of disabling rheumatic valvular disease is often longer than 8 years. For this and other reasons, no one can deny that acute rheumatic fever is a serious disease nor that its reduced incidence in recent years is a major medical success story. Nevertheless, the fact remains that the statistical risk of serious disease in the adult patient with a sore throat is very small, even if we ignore the patient completely.

Many sticky philosophic, scientific, political, and economic issues under-lie the big question—is diagnosing one case of acute rheumatic fever "worth" $100,000 (or whatever)? Such issues may one day form the crux of societal decisions about allocation of health resources, but the individual physician's responsibility is first and always to his or her own patient. The fact is that patients do not consult physicians to assess their statistical risk of danger from a sore throat—they seek comfort, reassurance, and protection. However the statistics read, a $10 throat culture to determine the need for $4 worth of penicillin that can prevent a rare but potentially serious disease represents, to most Americans today, a wise investment.

This does not mean, however, that practical clinical decision making should disregard statistical cost-benefit analysis. In fact, close attention to the clinical details in each individual patient with sore throat can foster cost effectiveness. As noted in the text, in some patients antibiotics should be prescribed without the use of throat cultures (but these are few); in others, neither cultures nor antibiotics are necessary (among adults, these are many). All patients should be educated about the rationale for such decisions. It is, rather, the unthinking "cookbook" approach to the sore throat that limits cost effectiveness (and which may also discourage the careful patient evaluation that will occasionally be critical when sore throat is "complicated").

From another perspective, the individual physician must understand his or her somewhat limited role in helping achieve societal medical goals. The fact that as few as one third of patients who develop acute rheumatic fever consult physicians beforehand because of a sore throat[79] illustrates the impossibility of limiting or abolishing acute rheumatic fever in our society simply by providing adequate "primary care." In fact, very different strategies are needed—development of rapid, inexpensive tests to identify "rheumato-genic" streptococci;[80] improved understanding of host/organism interactions that can be therapeutically disrupted;[37] and formulation of immunogenic but nontoxic vaccines.[81] Such strategies will depend on basic science research advances and are currently only "aspirations which . . . may prove naive."[82] For the time being, though, it is possible to be both thorough and cost conscious.[84] The individual patient need not be shortchanged, while the overall economic impact of limiting "abuse of low-level technologies" can be dramatic indeed.[83]

REFERENCES

1. Bujak, JS, et al.: Juvenile rheumatoid arthritis presenting in the adult as fever of unknown origin. Medicine 52:431, 1973.
2. Volpe, R, Johnston, MW: Subacute thyroiditis: A disease commonly mistaken for pharyngitis. Can Med Assoc J 77:297, 1957.
3. Raskin, NH, Prusiner, S: Carotidynia. Neurology 27:43, 1977.
4. Renson, CE (ed): Oral Diseases. London: Update Books, 1978, pp. 25–30, 40–47, 47–52.
5. Aronson, MD, et al.: Heterophile antibody in adults with sore throat. Frequency and clinical presentation. Ann Intern Med 96:505–508, 1982.
6. Hoagland, RJ: Infectious mononucleosis. Am J Med 13:158, 1952.
7. Lai, PK: Infectious mononucleosis: Recognition and management. Hosp Pract 12:47, 1977.
8. Schleupner, CJ, Overall, JC: Infectious mononucleosis and Epstein-Barr virus. Postgrad Med 65:83, 95, 1979.
9. Chervenick, PA: Infectious mononucleosis. DM December, 1974.
10. Horwitz, CA, et al.: Clinical and laboratory evaluation of elderly patients with heterophile antibody positive infectious mononucleosis. Am J Med 61:333, 1976.
11. Carter, JW, et al.: Infectious mononucleosis in the older patient. Mayo Clinc Proc 53:146, 1978.
12. English, EC, Geyman, JP: The efficiency and cost effectiveness of diagnostic tests for infectious mononucleosis. J Fam Pract 6:977, 1978.
13. Horwitz, CA, et al.: Heterophile negative infectious mononucleosis and mononucleosis-like illness. Laboratory confirmation of 43 cases. Am J Med 63:47, 1977.
14. Klein, E, et al.: The effects of short-term corticosteroid therapy on the symptoms of infectious mononucleosis pharyngotonsillitis. A double blind study. J Am Coll Health Assoc 17:446, 1969.
15. Bender, CE: The value of corticosteroids in the treatment of infectious mononucleosis. JAMA 199:529, 1967.
16. Walsh, T, et al.: Recognition of streptococcal pharyngitis in adults. Arch Intern Med 135:1493, 1975.
17. Glezen, WP, et al.: Group A streptococci, mycoplasmas, and viruses associated with acute pharyngitis JAMA 202:119, 1967.
18. Crawford, G, et al.: Streptococcal pharyngitis: Diagnosis by Gram stain. Ann Intern Med 90:293, 1979.
19. Cantanzaro, FJ, et al.: Symposium on rheumatic fever and rheumatic heart disease: The role of the streptococcus in the pathogenesis of rheumatic fever. Am J Med 17:749, 1954.
20. Spagnuolo, M, et al.: Risk of rheumatic fever recurrences after streptococcal infections. N Engl J Med 285:641, 1971.
21. Taranta, A, et al.: Rheumatic fever in children and adolescents. A long-term epidemiologic study of subsequent prophylaxis, streptococcal infections, and clinical sequelae. V. Relation of the rheumatic fever recurrence rate per streptococcal infection to pre-existing clinical features of the patients. Ann Intern Med 60 (Suppl 5):58, 1964.
22. Denny, FW, et al.: Comparative effects of penicillin, aureomycin, and teramycin on streptococcal tonsillitis and pharyngitis. Pediatrics 11:7, 1953.
23. Brink, WR, et al.: Effect of pencillin and aureomycin on the natural course of streptococcal pharyngitis and tonsillitis. Am J Med 10:300, 1951.
24. Brumfitt, W, Slater, JDH: Treatment of acute sore throat with penicillin: A controlled trial in young soldiers. Lancet 1:8, 1957.
25. Stillerman, M, et al.: Antibiotics in the treatment of beta hemolytic streptococcal pharyngitis: Factors influencing results. Pediatrics 25:27, 1960.
26. Breese, BB, Disney, FA: Penicillin in the treatment of streptococcal infection. A comparison of effectiveness of five different oral and one parenteral form. N Engl J Med 259:57, 1958.
27. Breese, BB, Disney, FA: A comparison of intramuscular and oral benzathine penicillin G in the treatment of streptococcal infection in children. J Pediatr 51:157, 1957.
28. Mohler, DN, et al.: Studies in the home treatment of streptococcal disease. II. A comparison of the efficacy of oral administration of penicillin and intramuscular injection of benzathine penicillin in the treatment of streptococcal pharyngitis. N Engl J Med 254:45, 1956.
29. Green, JL, et al.: Recurrence rate of streptococcal pharyngitis related to oral penicillin. J Pediatr 75:292, 1969.
30. Breese, BB: Treatment of beta hemolytic streptococcic infections in the home: Relative value of available methods. JAMA 152:10, 1953.
31. Colcher, IS, Bass, JW: Penicillin treatment of streptococcal pharyngitis. JAMA 222:657, 1972.
32. Schwartz, RH, et al.: Penicillin V for group A streptococcal pharyngotonsillitis. A randomized trial of seven versus ten days' therapy. JAMA 246:1790–1795, 1981.
33. Cantanzaro, FJ, et al.: Prevention of rheumatic fever by treatment of streptococcal infection. II. Factors responsible for failures. New Engl J Med 259:51–57, 1958.
34. Idsøe, O, et al.: Nature and extent of penicillin side reactions with particular reference to fatalities from anaphylactic shock. Bull WHO 38:159, 1968.
35. Rudolph, AH, Price, EV: Penicillin reactions among patients in venereal disease clinics: A national survey. JAMA 223:499, 1973.
36. Brook, I, et al.: Surface vs. core-tonsillar aerobic and anaerobic flora in recurrent tonsillitis. JAMA 244:1696, 1980.
37. Ferrieri, P: Treatment of group A streptococcal pharyngitis: Reflections on glue and other things. JAMA 246:1813–1814, 1981.
38. Tompkins, RK, et al.: An analysis of cost effectiveness of pharyngitis management and acute rheumatic fever prevention. Ann Intern Med 86:481, 1977.
39. Harner, SG: Peritonsillar, peripharyngeal, and deep neck abscess. Postgrad Med 57:147, 1975.
40. McCurdy, JA: Peritonsillar abscess. A comparison of treatment by immediate tonsillectomy and interval tonsillectomy. Arch Otolaryngol 103:414, 1977.

41. Gorbach, SL, Bartlett, JG: Anaerobic infections. N Engl J Med 290:1177, 1237, 1289, 1974.
42. Brumfitt, W: Benign streptococcal sore throat. Lancet 2:419, 1959.
43. Seidenfeld, SM, et al: Fusobacterium necrophorum septicemia following oropharyngeal infection. JAMA 248:1348–1350, 1982.
44. Ossoff, RH, Wolff, AP: Acute epiglottitis in adults. JAMA 244:2639, 1980.
45. Hawkins, DB, et al.: Acute epiglottitis in adults. Laryngoscope 83:1211–1220, 1973.
46. Bass, JW, et al.: Acute epiglottitis. A surgical emergency. JAMA 229:671, 1974.
47. Gorfinkel, HJ, et al.: Acute infectious epiglottitis in adults. Ann Intern Med 70:289, 1969.
48. Dobie, RA, Tobey, DN: Clinical features of diphtheria in the respiratory tract. JAMA 242:2197, 1979.
49. McCloskey, RV, et al.: The 1970 epidemic of diphtheria in San Antonio. Ann Intern Med 75:495, 1971.
50. Crossley, K, et al.: Tetanus and diphtheria immunity in urban Minnesota adults. JAMA 242:2298, 1979.
51. Bryan, CS, et al.: Retropharyngeal infection in adults. Arch Intern Med 134:127, 1974.
52. Wholey, MH, et al: The lateral roentgenogram of the neck. Radiology 71:350–356, 1958.
53. Case records of Massachusetts General Hospital, #42-1977. N Engl J Med 297:878, 1977.
54. Meyers, BR, et al: Ludwig's angina. Case report, with reviews of bacteriology and current therapy. Am J Med, 53:257, 1971.
55. Finch, RG, et al.: Ludwig's angina. JAMA, 243:1171, 1980.
56. Hough, RT, et al: Ludwig's angina: Report of two cases and review of the literature from 1945 to January 1979. J Oral Surg, 38(11):849–855, 1980.
57. Wiesner, PJ, et al.: Clinical spectrum of pharyngeal gonococcal infection. N Engl J Med 288:181, 1973.
58. Kraus, SJ: Incidence and treatment of gonococcal pharyngitis. Sex Transm Dis 6(Suppl):143, 1979.
59. Davidson, TM, Calloway, CA: Tonsillectomy and adenoidectomy. Its indications and its problems. West J Med 133:451, 1980.
60. Greene, JN: Subacute thyroiditis. Am J Med 51:97–108, 1971.
61. McCue, JD: Group G streptococcal pharyngitis. Analysis of an outbreak at a college. JAMA 248:1333–1335, 1982.
62. Kaplan, EL, et al.: Diagnosis of streptococcal pharyngitis: Differentiation of active infection from carrier state in the symptomatic child. J Infect Dis 123:490, 1971.
63. Breese, BB, et al.: Beta hemolytic streptococcal infection: The clinical and epidemiologic importance of the number of organisms found in cultures. Am J Dis Child 119:18, 1970.
64. Peter, G, Smith, AL: Group A streptococcal infections of the skin and pharynx. N Engl J Med 297:311, 365, 1977.
65. Gould, JR: Streptococcal pharyngitis. JAMA 241:1573, 1979.
66. Evans, AS, Dick, EC: Acute pharyngitis and tonsillitis in University of Wisconsin students. JAMA 190:699, 1964.
67. Weissbluth, M: Streptococcal pharyngitis. (Letter to the Editor) JAMA 242:1735, 1979.
68. Wannamaker, LW, et al.: The effect of penicillin prophylaxis on streptococcal disease rates and the carrier state. N Engl J Med 249:1, 1953.
69. Poskanzer, DC, et al.: Epidemiology of civilian streptococcal outbreaks before and after penicillin prophylaxis. Am J Public Health 46:1513, 1956.
70. Breese, BB, Disney, FA: Factors influencing the spread of beta hemolytic streptococcal infection within the family group. Pediatrics 17:834, 1956.
71. Weinstein, L, LeFrock, J: Does antimicrobial therapy of streptococcal pharyngitis or pyoderma alter the risk of glomerulonephritis? J Infect Dis 124:229, 1971.
72. Denny, FW, et al.: Prevention of rheumatic fever. JAMA 143:151, 1950.
73. Wannamaker, LW, et al.: Prophylaxis of acute rheumatic fever by treatment of the preceding streptococcal infection with various amounts of depot penicillin. Am J Med 10:673, 1951.
74. Siegel, AL, et al: Controlled studies of streptococcal pharyngitis in a pediatric population. I. Factors related to attack rates of rheumatic fever. N Engl J Med, 265:559, 1961.
75. Pantell, RH: Cost effectiveness of pharyngitis management and prevention of rheumatic fever. Ann Intern Med 86:497, 1977.
76. Gordis, L, et al.: Studies in the epidemiology and preventability of rheumatic fever: Demographic factors and the incidence of acute attacks. J Chronic Dis 21:645, 1969.
77. Valkenburg, HA, et al.: Streptococcal pharyngitis in patients not treated with penicillin. II. The attack rate of rheumatic fever and acute glomerulonephritis in patients not treated with penicillin. J Infect Dis 124:348, 1971.
78. Feinstein, AR, et al.: Rheumatic fever in children and adolescents. A long-term epidemiologic study of subsequent prophylaxis, streptococcal infection, and clinical sequelae. VII. Cardiac changes and sequelae. Ann Intern Med 60(Suppl 5):87, 1964.
79. Markowitz, M: Eradication of rheumatic fever. An unfulfilled hope. Circulation 41:1077, 1970.
80. Bisno, AL: The diagnosis of streptococcal pharyngitis. Ann Intern Med 90:426, 1979.
81. Stollerman, GH: Streptococcal vaccines and global strategies for prevention of rheumatic fever. Am J Med 68:636, 1980.
82. Bisno, AL: Worldwide control of rheumatic fever. Ann Intern Med 91:918, 1979.
83. Moloney, TW, Roger, DE: Medical technology—A different view of the contentious debate over costs. N Engl J Med 301:1413, 1979.
84. Komaroff, AL: A management strategy for sore throat. JAMA 239:1249, 1978.
85. Tacket, CO, et al.: Yersinia enterocolitica pharyngitis. Ann Intern Med 99:40, 1983.
86. Land, MA, Bisno, AZ: Acute rheumatic fever. A vanishing disease in suburbia. JAMA 249:895, 1983.
87. Bell GF, Rogers, R: Observation on the diagnosis of recurrent ophthrous stamatitic. Mayo Clin Proc 57:297, 1982.

3

DIARRHEA

ACUTE DIARRHEA 100
    Symptoms and Signs......................... 100
    Tests? 106
    Treatment 108
    Acute Dysentery 111
    When Acute Diarrhea Persists 115
    Lactose Intolerance 119
CHRONIC DIARRHEA............................. 121
    The Initial Approach.......................... 121
    Sequence of Investigation... Figure 3–6, page 128
    Chronic Bloody Diarrhea 129
    Therapeutic Trials 133
    Steatorrhea................................... 138
    Hospitalization 142
APPENDIX I: Acute Proctitis....................... 145
APPENDIX II: Food-Borne Diarrhea................ 148
    Food Poisoning............................... 148
    Food Intolerance 150
    Traveler's Diarrhea ("Turista")................. 151
APPENDIX III: Postoperative Diarrhea............. 152
APPENDIX IV: Diets 155
APPENDIX V: Pancreatic Enzyme Replacement.... 158
REFERENCES...................................... 160

ACUTE DIARRHEA

Symptoms and Signs

> Ernie Enteritis, a 36-year-old traveling salesman, enters the clinic complaining of diarrhea for the previous 36 hours. Two days before, Ernie noted myalgias, malaise, and a low-grade fever. The next day he developed diffuse mild abdominal cramping associated with loose, watery bowel movements and anorexia. Since then he has passed "around 15" bowel movements, each watery liquid without grossly visible blood, pus, or mucus. He has been awakened from sleep several times because of the diarrhea, but he denies tenesmus or fecal incontinence.

Acute diarrhea is usually a brief inconvenience, commonly attributed to viral gastroenteritis or food poisoning, which most often resolves spontaneously after a few days. A precise cause is not usually identified, and specific infectious agents are isolated in only a minority of patients with acute diarrhea.[1-3] Thus, most patients with acute diarrhea treat themselves; among those who seek medical attention, laboratory studies are usually unrevealing (and unnecessary), and only symptomatic treatment is needed in most.

Nevertheless, the differential diagnosis of acute diarrhea is lengthy, as Table 3–1 illustrates. Several of these disorders do require specific therapy;

TABLE 3–1. CAUSES OF ACUTE DIARRHEA

VIRAL	BACTERIAL	IATROGENIC	OTHER
Norwalk agent	*Staphylococcus aureus*	Drug induced	Diverticulitis
Rotavirus	*Clostridium perfringens*	Laxatives	Fecal impaction
Herpes (proctitis)	*Bacillus cereus*	Antibiotics	Ischemic bowel disease
Viral hepatitis (prodrome)	Toxigenic *Escherichia coli*	Antihypertensives	Inflammatory bowel disease
Infectious mononucleosis	*Vibrio cholerae*	Colchicine	Irritable bowel syndrome
(prodrome)	*Salmonella* species	Indomethacin	Malabsorption
Others?	*Shigella* species	Quinidine	Food allergy
	Campylobacter species	Digitalis	Colon carcinoma
PARASITIC	*Yersinia enterocolitica*	Theophylline	Intestinal endometriosis
	Vibrio parahaemolyticus	Caffeine	Appendicitis
Entamoeba histolytica	Invasive *Escherichia coli*	Alcohol	
Giardia lamblia	Gonococcal (proctitis)	Bethanechol chloride	
Strongyloides stercoralis	Syphilis (proctitis)	Antacids	
(See also Table 3–6)	*Chlamydia* (proctitis)		
		Postoperative	
TOXINS		(See App. III)	
Mushrooms			
Heavy metals			
Monosodium glutamate			
Paralytic fish poisoning			
Botulism			
(See App. II)			

a few are serious and even potentially life threatening. How then does one decide whether the "watch-and-wait" approach is appropriate in the individual patient with acute diarrhea? Several considerations help:

1. How "acute" is the diarrhea? Most cases of "benign infectious" diarrhea—usually due to food-borne toxins or viral gastroenteritis—resolve spontaneously within a few days. The patient who presents with diarrhea that has already lasted a few weeks or whose acute diarrhea does not resolve within a week despite symptomatic therapy (see page 109) deserves a different approach. (See "Chronic Diarrhea," page 121.)

> Ernie has had diarrhea for only 2 days. He admits that he has experienced several bouts of diarrhea during the past year, but he had had "normal" bowel movements for at least 1 month before the acute onset of his current symptoms.

2. How "sick" is the patient? Benign infectious diarrhea does not cause high fevers, rigors, bloody stools, or localized abdominal pain and tenderness. Instead, most such patients are only mildly ill and describe rather abrupt onset of lower abdominal cramping, watery diarrhea, nausea and vomiting, or a combination of these. Fever (if present at all) is low grade and brief in duration, bowel sounds are hyperactive, mild generalized abdominal tenderness is common, and the peripheral white blood cell count is usually normal.

"Sick diarrhea" is suggested when the clinical presentation includes dysentery, localized or severe abdominal pain, or orthostatic hypotension.

Dysentery refers to a clinical syndrome that usually results from bacterial invasion of the colonic mucosa. Such "invasive" diarrhea causes fever, toxicity, (occult or grossly) bloody stool, and abdominal pain—illness may be prolonged if left untreated. The most common cause of acute dysentery in the United States is bacterial infection with *Campylobacter, Shigella* or *Salmonella,* but there are other less common and more serious causes as well (see below). Clinical dysentery requires investigation (since specific treatment is often necessary—see page 111).

Localized abdominal pain and tenderness are uncommon in benign infectious diarrhea. Localized right lower quadrant tenderness in the "sick" patient with acute diarrhea should raise the question of acute appendicitis, Crohn's disease, or (rarely) amebic colitis, right-sided diverticulitis, or cecal carcinoma. Localized left lower quadrant tenderness should suggest acute diverticulitis, fecal impaction, colon cancer, and various causes of acute proctocolitis (see below).

Orthostatic hypotension due to dehydration may occur with any diarrheal illness that results in large fluid (or blood) losses. The elderly, the chronically ill, and those who cannot replace fluid losses with oral intake are most susceptible. In the immunosuppressed patient evaluation must be very careful, since even benign infectious gastroenteritis can be serious in such patients.[4]

Ernie denies high fever, rigors or bloody stools.

Ernie appears healthy, if a little tired. Vital signs are normal—he is afebrile and there is no orthostatic fall in blood pressure or rise in pulse. The abdomen is minimally tender, diffusely. Bowel sounds are hyperactive.

3. Do symptoms suggest acute proctocolitis? Rectal pain, frank rectal bleeding, visible anorectal purulent discharge, severe tenesmus, rectal urgency, or fecal incontinence should suggest acute proctocolitis when associated with acute diarrhea. Ulcerative colitis, anorectal venereal disease, bacterial dysentery, amebic dysentery, antibiotic-induced pseudomembranous colitis, and a variety of other disorders must be considered in these circumstances. The clinical setting and results of proctosigmoidoscopy will usually point to the correct diagnosis. In Appendix I the differential diagnosis is briefly discussed.

There is no history of rectal pain or bleeding, and, while Ernie often "has to go quickly," there is no frank tenesmus, rectal urgency, or incontinence.

4. Are there clues that suggest a specific treatable cause? Drug-induced diarrhea includes diarrhea as a side effect of medication—antibiotics, antihypertensives, anti-inflammatory drugs, antacids, and chemotherapeutic drugs are the common offenders here; diarrhea due to specific pharmacologic effect—laxative use (or abuse), most often; and the diarrhea of pseudomembranous colitis, most commonly associated with clindamycin or lincomycin use, but reported with many other drugs, sometimes as long as several weeks after discontinuation of the offending agent. Inquiries about all current prescription and nonprescription medications should be routine in the patient with acute diarrhea.

Sexual habits may be important. Homosexual males (and, much less often, women who practice anal intercourse) are susceptible to a variety of "venereal enteric" infections—especially shigellosis, amebiasis, giardiasis, and infectious hepatitis. Even in the absence of symptoms of acute dysentery or acute proctocolitis, these organisms should be suspected in the homosexual male with acute diarrhea. Thus, laboratory testing (stool cultures, parasite searches) is usually indicated in such patients. This is discussed in Appendix I.

Travel history, particularly recent travel to areas where certain infections are endemic—especially parasitic disease—is always worth noting. Acute diarrhea in this setting is usually due to "turista," most often caused by enterotoxigenic *Escherichia coli* infection, which usually does not require specific therapy (but laboratory testing is often indicated in this situation). Turista is discussed briefly in Appendix II.

Recent surgical procedures—gastrectomy, cholecystectomy, vagotomy, bowel resection, ileocolostomy, "blind loop" formation, or jejunoileal bypass procedures—can result in puzzling diarrhea, by a variety of mechanisms (see Appendix III).

Food poisoning is usually suspected when the patient is one of several others afflicted with acute diarrhea following a common meal. When the patient is the only symptomatic sufferer, clinical symptoms, "incubation period," duration of illness, and suspected food vehicle will usually suggest the correct diagnosis (see Appendix II).

> Ernie travels extensively along the Atlantic Seacoast and throughout the Caribbean. He uses no medications. He denies anal sexual intercourse. There is no history of prior abdominal surgery. Ernie knows of no acquaintances with similar symptoms, but he does "eat in restaurants all of the time" and ate seafood, poultry, and mixed salads while in Florida around the time his symptoms began 2 days before.

5. Does examination of the stool reveal occult blood or fecal leukocytes? Benign infectious diarrhea is usually caused by viruses or enterotoxin-producing bacteria that induce a net fluid loss into the intestinal lumen without "invading" the intestinal mucosa. The pathophysiologic interaction of such "noninvasive" infectious agents with the intestinal mucosal cells is incompletely understood[5, 6] (see also page 109), but the preservation of intestinal mucosal integrity usually precludes bleeding or an outpouring of leukocytes from the afflicted intestine into the intestinal lumen. As a general rule, then, blood or fecal leukocytes are not found among patients with "benign" diarrhea.

Much less often, acute diarrhea results from bacterial (or parasitic) invasion of intestinal mucosa—pathologic mucosal disruption is here often associated with gross or occult blood in the stool or an outpouring of leukocytes into the intestinal lumen. Usually these pathologic events are recognized clinically as dysentery (see above), and the same organisms that commonly cause dysentery (Table 3–5) are the usual causes of invasive diarrhea. Some patients with invasive diarrhea, however, will not be so clinically ill, and examination of the stool for fecal leukocytes and occult blood can help differentiate benign infectious diarrhea from invasive diarrhea in such patients. (In other words, invasive—usually bacterial—diarrhea does not always cause clinical dysentery, but the finding of fecal blood or leukocytes is a clue that invasive pathogens are present.)* This is important since invasive diarrhea often requires further testing and specific therapy, while noninvasive diarrhea usually does not.

Fecal leukocytes (Fig. 3–1) are detected by placing a small fleck of fecal mucus or stool on a microscopic slide, mixing it thoroughly with 2 drops of methylene blue, and then examining the coverslipped slide under high power microscopy (after 2 to 3 minutes to allow adequate "staining" of the cellular nuclei with the blue dye).[7] Fecal leukocytes are commonly found in diarrheal illness due to infection with *Shigella, Campylobacter,* and (some) *Salmonella* and may also be found in infections due to invasive *E. coli* and in inflammatory bowel diseases (especially ulcerative or Crohn's colitis). The absence of fecal leukocytes does not exclude these diagnoses, but their presence is a

---

*This does not mean that all patients with acute diarrhea require stool testing (see page 106). The afebrile mildly ill patient does not.

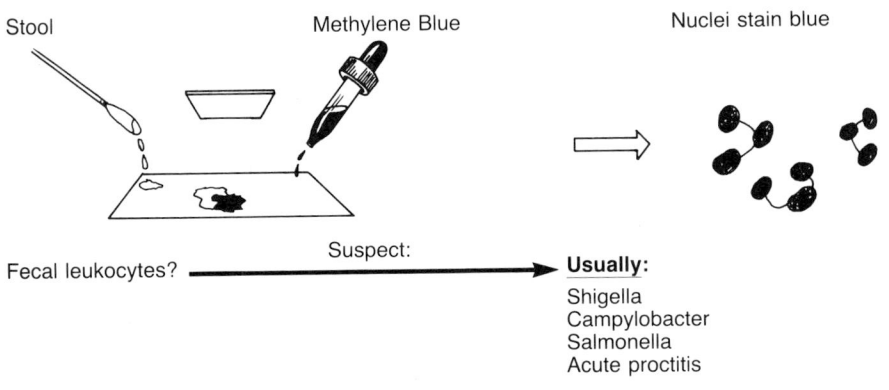

Stool   Methylene Blue   Nuclei stain blue

Fecal leukocytes? ————————— Suspect:

Usually:

Shigella
Campylobacter
Salmonella
Acute proctitis

Less often:

Amebic dysentery
Crohn's disease
Ulcerative colitis
Pseudomembranous colitis
Invasive *E. coli*
Yersinia enterocolitica
Acute diverticulitis
Vibrio parahaemolyticus

FIGURE 3–1. Staining for fecal leukocytes.

valuable diagnostic clue. (Amebiasis—unless associated with severe dysentery—and other parasitic diseases (Table 3–6) usually do not cause fecal leukocytosis.)

Occasionally transient (occult) <u>blood</u> will be found in stools of patients with acute benign diarrhea; more often such a finding indicates mucosal invasion or disruption—usually due to bacterial or amebic dysentery, inflammatory bowel disease, or neoplasms. (Chronic "bloody diarrhea" is briefly discussed on page 129.)

<u>Thus, the presence of fecal leukocytes or (gross or occult) blood in the stool implies an infectious, inflammatory, or neoplastic process that requires investigation.</u> Severe bloody diarrhea (or frank hematochezia) should always suggest acute ulcerative colitis in the young patient, while in the elderly such symptoms are more commonly due to ischemic bowel disease,[8] diverticular bleeding,[9] or intestinal neoplasms. Acute lower gastrointestinal bleeding cannot be adequately discussed here.

Figure 3–2 illustrates the general approach to the patient with acute diarrhea. Note that the clinical history, physical examination, and rapid stool examination for blood and fecal leukocytes will determine whether watchful wating and symptomatic treatment are appropriate or whether more specific diagnostic measures are necessary. <u>The great majority of patients with acute diarrhea are not sick and do not have dysentery or acute proctocolitis, and stool examinations are benign.</u> These patients can be treated simply and inexpensively.

Stool is watery, brown, and heme negative. Microscopic examination for stool leukocytes is negative.

What does this mean?

Ernie's acute diarrhea is probably benign (or "noninvasive")—he is not in a toxic condition, does not have (clinical) dysentery or proctitis, and his stool is negative for both blood and fecal leukocytes. His history and physical examination are compatible with the diagnosis of acute noninvasive gastroenteritis.

Ernie says that he has experienced similar episodes in the past, usually when traveling, but examinations for parasites and bacterial infections have always been normal, and taking diphenoxylate hydrochloride (Lom-

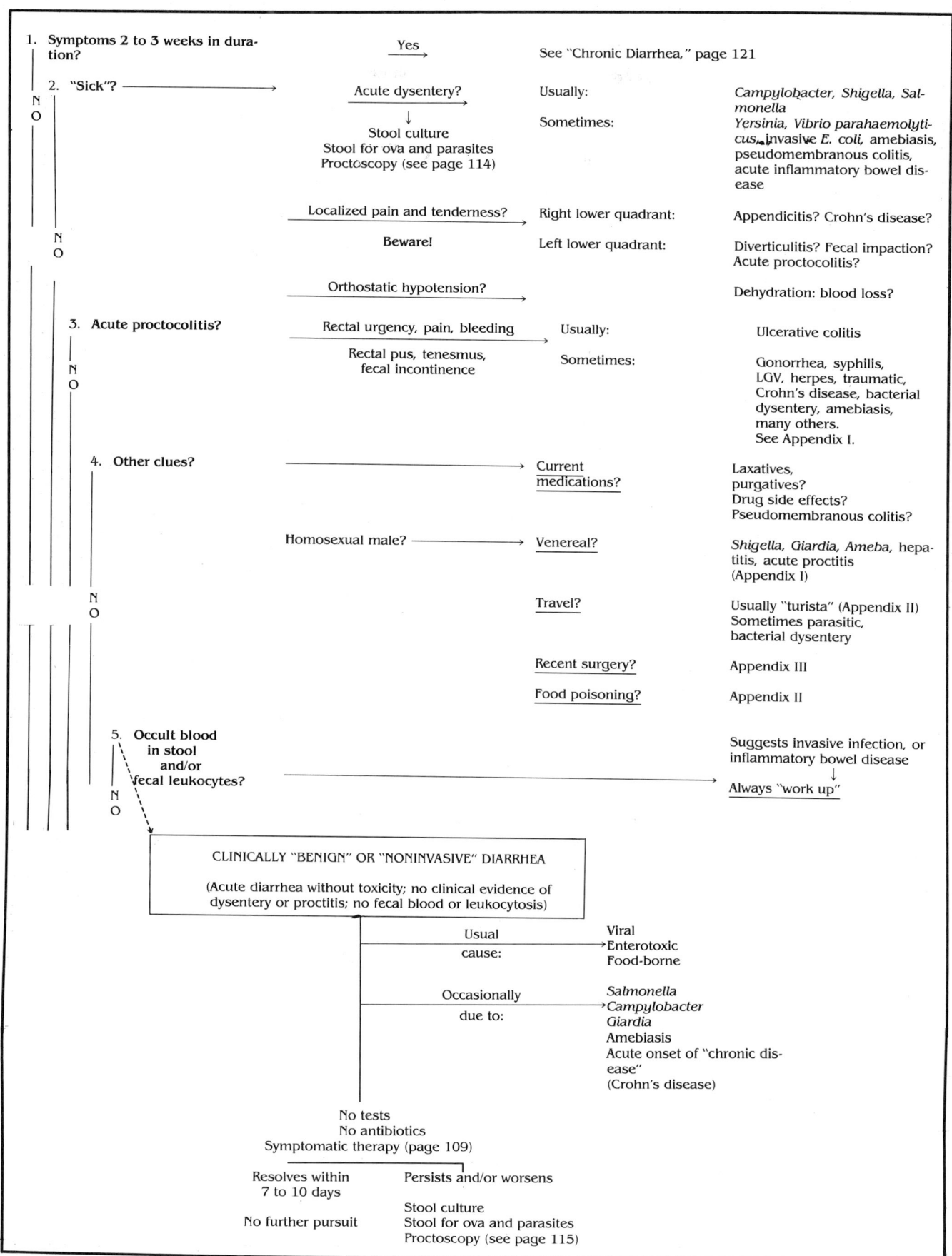

1. **Symptoms 2 to 3 weeks in duration?** — Yes → See "Chronic Diarrhea," page 121

N
O

2. **"Sick"?** →

Acute dysentery? →
↓
Stool culture
Stool for ova and parasites
Proctoscopy (see page 114)

Usually: Campylobacter, Shigella, Salmonella

Sometimes: Yersinia, Vibrio parahaemolyticus, invasive E. coli, amebiasis, pseudomembranous colitis, acute inflammatory bowel disease

N
O

Localized pain and tenderness? →
Beware!

Right lower quadrant: Appendicitis? Crohn's disease?

Left lower quadrant: Diverticulitis? Fecal impaction? Acute proctocolitis?

Orthostatic hypotension? → Dehydration: blood loss?

3. **Acute proctocolitis?**

Rectal urgency, pain, bleeding →

Rectal pus, tenesmus, fecal incontinence

Usually: Ulcerative colitis

Sometimes: Gonorrhea, syphilis, LGV, herpes, traumatic, Crohn's disease, bacterial dysentery, amebiasis, many others. See Appendix I.

N
O

4. **Other clues?** →

Current medications? — Laxatives, purgatives? Drug side effects? Pseudomembranous colitis?

Homosexual male? → Venereal? — Shigella, Giardia, Ameba, hepatitis, acute proctitis (Appendix I)

N
O

Travel? — Usually "turista" (Appendix II) Sometimes parasitic, bacterial dysentery

Recent surgery? — Appendix III

Food poisoning? — Appendix II

5. **Occult blood in stool and/or fecal leukocytes?** →

Suggests invasive infection, or inflammatory bowel disease
↓
Always "work up"

N
O

CLINICALLY "BENIGN" OR "NONINVASIVE" DIARRHEA

(Acute diarrhea without toxicity; no clinical evidence of dysentery or proctitis; no fecal blood or leukocytosis)

Usual cause: → Viral
Enterotoxic
Food-borne

Occasionally due to: → Salmonella
Campylobacter
Giardia
Amebiasis
Acute onset of "chronic disease"
(Crohn's disease)

No tests
No antibiotics
Symptomatic therapy (page 109)

Resolves within 7 to 10 days | Persists and/or worsens

No further pursuit | Stool culture
Stool for ova and parasites
Proctoscopy (see page 115)

FIGURE 3–2. Acute Diarrhea.

otil) for a few days makes him better. He asks for a prescription for Lomotil, since he is due to travel again next week to the Caribbean. He has just returned from the Florida coast (where his current symptoms began).

At the conclusion of the initial clinical evaluation, two decisions must be made:

1. Are tests necessary?
2. Pending the results of tests (if any), what treatment is recommended?

Tests?

Stool cultures are indicated initially when any of the invasive bacterial diseases (see Table 3–5) are suspected. All patients with clinical dysentery, acute proctitis, or fecal blood or leukocytes should therefore have stool cultures. Most clinical laboratories have little difficulty identifying *Salmonella* and *Shigella* species; many now routinely culture stool on a special medium (for example, Campy-BAP) to detect *Campylobacter;* special procedures are needed to identify rarer organisms—e.g., *Yersinia enterocolitica* and *Vibrio parahaemolyticus.* Invasive *E. coli* cannot be identified by simple culture techniques; special tests are required to detect "enteroinvasiveness" of (normally commensal) *E. coli* (see also Table 3–5).

Stool cultures should also be obtained when the acute diarrheal illness is prolonged (more than 1 week), when the patient remains sick or febrile without obvious cause, and when epidemiologic factors are pertinent (when the patient is a food handler or a foreign traveler or a male homosexual, for example). The therapeutic implications of positive and negative stool cultures in these and other settings are discussed below.

Stool examination for ova and parasites is indicated in patients with clinical dysentery or proctitis (primarily to detect amebiasis), prolonged "noninvasive" diarrhea (primarily to detect giardiasis), or when specific parasites are suspected because of foreign travel or endemic parasitic disease.

Proctosigmoidoscopy is indicated when symptoms suggest acute procto-colitis (see above and Appendix I) and sometimes in the patient with clinical dysentery whose stool cultures and smears for parasites are unrevealing (see page 115). Rectal biopsy may or may not be helpful, depending on the gross findings at proctoscopy. Such findings are discussed further below.

Blood counts are not usually helpful. Most patients with acute diarrhea have white blood counts of less than 10,000 (a few with severe dysentery due to *Campylobacter* or *Shigella* may have peripheral leukocytosis). Eosinophilia is usually not associated with amebic or giardia infection but may be seen with strongyloides infection and other rarer parasitic diseases.

Barium x-rays may occasionally be helpful in the diagnosis of acute diarrhea but never before other studies are performed (unless inflammatory bowel diseases are specifically suspected).

"Routine" testing of all patients with acute diarrhea can be very expensive (see Table 3–2).

Most patients with acute diarrhea that is clinically noninvasive do not require any tests. If illness persists or worsens, tests will be necessary at that time.

Stool specimens are obtained for culture and parasite examination.

TABLE 3–2. TESTS IN ACUTE DIARRHEA

Test	Cost	When
Stool cultures (Table 3–5)	$22	Acute dysentery Acute proctitis Fecal blood or leukocytes Prolonged acute diarrhea? Food handler? Homosexual male?
Stool for ova and parasites (× 3) (Table 3–6)	$25	Acute dysentery Acute proctitis Foreign traveler? Homosexual male? Prolonged acute diarrhea?

Proctosigmoidoscopy
  Rigid (25 cm)
  Flexible (60 cm)
  Rectal biopsy
	
	$60
	$140
	$50–100
		
		Acute proctitis
		Dysentery with negative stool studies
		Pseudomembranous colitis?
		Inflammatory bowel disease?
		Rectosigmoid neoplasm?

Barium enema	$130	Rarely: When diarrhea persists and all studies are negative.
Upper GI series (with small bowel follow-through)	$130 ($150)	
Colonoscopy	$450	

NOTE

1. Stool specimens for culture and parasites are obtained here, in spite of the fact that the gastroenteritis is not clinically of the invasive type. Ernie's travel history, the severity of his diarrhea, and his request for antimotility drugs (see page 110) are "soft" findings that suggest that such examinations might be helpful.

For example, Ernie may "carry" various intestinal parasites, even if these organisms are unrelated to his present illness. Foreign travelers and recent immigrants should always be suspected of parasitic infestation.[10]

The severity of Ernie's diarrhea is compatible with benign diarrhea, but, since diarrhea could persist beyond 24 to 48 hours (see below), documentation of negative stool cultures now would be useful information at that time (see page 111). In addition, sometimes invasive diarrhea begins as noninvasive diarrhea—frequent watery diarrhea without blood or fecal leukocytes sometimes progresses to frank dysentery—early stool cultures that document a specific pathogen can be helpful in those cases.

These special considerations in Ernie's case do not alter the fact that most patients with this type of clinical illness require neither stool cultures nor examination for parasites.

2. The microbiology laboratory must be aware of the differential diagnosis when stool cultures and smears for parasites are obtained, since various pathogens will require specific isolation procedures (see Tables 3–5 and 3–6). Similarly, laboratories not expert in parasitology should send specimens to more experienced laboratories when parasitic infestation is clinically likely but pathogens are not identified (see below).

Ernie is told that his diarrhea is probably viral and will likely resolve in the next few days. Oral fluids are prescribed and explained (Table 3–3). Antimotility drugs are not prescribed, with explanations. Ernie is told to call if he worsens over the next 24 to 48 hours.

Treatment

As Figure 3–2 suggests, the initial treatment of acute diarrhea can sometimes be highly specific—when diarrhea is drug-induced, postoperative (see Appendix III), or due to venereal proctitis (see Appendix I), for example. Much more often, treatment must be symptomatic only (see below).

Antibiotic therapy of acute diarrhea is indicated only uncommonly. Why? Because:

1. Clinically "noninvasive" diarrhea—usually a 48- to 72-hour illness, most often caused by enterotoxic viral or food-borne gastroenteritis—does not require antibiotics. Current antiviral agents are ineffective, and a viral etiology is rarely documented anyway (except in clinical studies or frank epidemics).[11] Toxin-mediated diarrhea[5, 6] does not respond to antibiotic therapy directed at the microorganism, probably because it is the toxin itself that is pathogenic.

2. Even invasive bacterial diarrhea may or may not require antibiotic therapy. Both the results of the stool culture and the patient's clinical course determine the need for antibiotics.

For example, consider the following:

a. Salmonella gastroenteritis, in general, does not require antibiotics. Clinical illness is usually mild and brief (fever lasts 24 to 48 hours), and there is evidence that antibiotic treatment may prolong fecal shedding of salmonellae,[12, 13] select resistant strains, or (rarely) precipitate systemic salmonella infection (bacteremia, sepsis).[14] Only the unusual patient who remains clinically ill for more than a week or who may be especially susceptible to salmonella osteomyelitis (the patient with sickle cell disease) or salmonella endocarditis (the patient with valvular heart disease) should be considered for therapy with antibiotics (see Table 3–5).

b. Campylobacter enteritis[15] has a broad spectrum of clinical severity. While erythromycin (or tetracycline) is generally recommended for proven campylobacter enteritis, many patients are clearly improving spontaneously by the time stool cultures identify the organism. It is debatable whether such patients should be treated in these circumstances. Certainly the patient with campylobacter enteritis who is not improving should be treated.

c. Shigella enteritis may also cause mild, self-limited illness, but acute dysentery is more common in adults. In general, antibiotic therapy is recommended for shigellosis, even if illness is mild, since therapy both shortens the clinical illness and decreases the duration of fecal shedding (and infectivity).[13] There remain, however, some controversial issues (see page 113)[16] regarding treatment of shigellosis.

d. Rarer causes of bacterial invasive diarrhea—*Y. enterocolitica*,[17, 18] *V. parahaemolyticus*,[19] invasive *E. coli*—may resolve without antibiotic therapy, but treatment decisions depend on the severity of clinical illness.

Thus, even when a specific pathogenic organism is recovered from the stool of a patient with acute diarrhea, antibiotic therapy is often unnecessary. As Table 3–5 indicates, acute diarrhea due to potentially invasive bacterial pathogens often requires only symptomatic treatment. This is especially true when clinical illness is mild, and the patient has neither acute dysentery nor symptomatic proctocolitis.

Symptomatic treatment of acute diarrhea includes fluid and electrolyte replacement and (sometimes) antimotility drugs.

Intravenous replacement of fluids and electrolytes will be necessary when the patient is severely dehydrated or sick enough to require hospitalization. Usually, however, oral rehydration is sufficient and successful.[20, 21] Two general principles should be remembered:

1. Oral fluids should contain glucose and electrolytes, and the solution should be hypo-osmolar.[22, 23] Noninvasive diarrheal illness is often mediated by the interaction of bacterial toxins with toxin receptors on the epithelial surfaces of small-intestinal mucosal cells.[6] The bacterial toxin activates the intracellular enzyme adenyl cyclase, which produces increased amounts of cAMP, which then mediates both a decrease in active absorption of sodium into the mucosal cell and an increase in active secretion of chloride out of the mucosal cell (into the bowel lumen). The net result is diminished absorption of water and electrolytes from the bowel lumen and a loss of water and electrolytes into the stool. (*Vibrio cholerae* is the classic example of this pathogenic process, but enterotoxigenic *E. coli, Staphylococcus aureus, Clostridium perfringens,* and *Bacillus cereus*—see also Appendix II—are probably pathogenic by related—if not identical—mechanisms.[6]) This impairment of active sodium absorption can be overcome when sodium is administered orally together with glucose.[22, 23] Hence the importance of glucose- and electrolyte-containing fluids for oral rehydration. Table 3–3 illustrates a useful homemade oral fluid and electrolyte replacement.[24]

Fluid should be hypo-osmolar to avoid intraluminal osmotic pressures that would further worsen fluid losses by "sucking" water into the bowel lumen. (Boiled milk, for example, should be avoided.) In addition,

2. Lactose-containing liquids and food should be avoided. Acute gastroenteritis can unmask previously inapparent, mild lactose intolerance (a very common disorder—see page 119). Similarly, transient lactase deficiency may sometimes be induced de novo by acute gastroenteritis. Continued ingestion of lactose during acute gastroenteritis may thus worsen symptoms or prolong an otherwise brief illness. As noted above, some lactose-containing foods are hyperosmolar as well. The problem of lactose intolerance is

TABLE 3–3. HOMEMADE ORAL FLUID REPLACEMENT[24]

Prepare 1 glass of each:

Glass no. 1
Orange, apple, or other fruit juice (potassium)	8 oz
Honey or corn syrup (glucose)	½ tsp
Table salt (sodium chloride)	1 pinch

Glass no. 2
Tap water (boiled or carbonated if water is suspect)	8 oz
Baking soda (sodium bicarbonate)	¼ tsp

Drink alternately from each glass.
Supplement with carbonated beverages, water, tea, coffee, broth.

discussed further on page 119, and in Appendix IV a lactose-free diet is discussed.

Antimotility drugs may be very helpful for symptomatic control of diarrhea, but in general they are unnecessary, and (rarely) they may be dangerous.

Since diarrhea is the "clearance mechanism" whereby intestinal infection is eliminated, pharmacologic reduction of diarrhea can be counterproductive. This is especially true of invasive diarrhea. Clinical worsening or prolongation of disease has been reported in both shigellosis[25] and salmonellosis[12] when antimotility drugs are prescribed. This is primarily a problem when the patient is very ill with dysentery. Mild cases of shigellosis, for example, are probably not worsened by antimotility drugs.[26] In general, antimotility drugs should not be used when invasive diarrhea is clinically suspected (high fever, dysentery) or documented (by culture).

Similarly, these drugs are usually unnecessary in noninvasive disease, since such illness is usually brief and self-limited. Exceptions to this rule may include patients with prolonged bouts of turista (see Appendix II) in whom stool cultures and examinations for ova and parasites are negative and perhaps patients afflicted with epidemic viral diarrhea (i.e., when a community outbreak of noninvasive diarrhea is documented).

However, many patients with acute diarrhea seek medical attention precisely because the nonprescription remedy has not helped.* Table 3–4 lists some of the commonly prescribed antimotility drugs. In general, the prescription drugs are favored because they are more effective, cost differences are small, and (narcotic) abuse potential of (briefly prescribed) prescription antidiarrheals is very small. Associated pain and cramps of acute gastroenteritis will often improve with (especially prescription) antimotility drugs.

Other treatment priorities are sometimes important as well. Epidemic gastroenteritis or suspected food-borne disease often requires further study, for various "public health" reasons (see Appendix II). Prevention of transmission of sporadic gastroenteritis to others usually requires simple hygienic

---

*Many patients with mild diarrhea *will* improve symptomatically with the over-the-counter drugs.

TABLE 3–4. ANTIMOTILITY DRUGS

	DOSAGE	QUANTITY/COST
Nonprescription drugs		
Kaolin and pectin (Kaopectate)	4 tbsp prn q4h	Two 12 oz bottles/$5.80
Kaolin/pectin concentrate (Kaopectate concentrate)	2 tbsp prn q4h	One 12 oz bottle/$3.80
Bismuth subsalicylate (Pepto-Bismol)	2–4 tbsp q4h	Two 8 oz bottles/$4.40
Calcium polycarbophil (Mitrolan)	Chew 2 tables q4–6h (do not exceed 12 tab/day)	36 tabs/$4.75
Prescription drugs*		
Diphenoxylate HCl w/atropine (Lomotil)	2 tablets q4h 2 tsp q4h	25 tabs/$3.60 4 oz/$4.75
Loperamide HCl (Imodium)	4 mg (2 capsules) initially, then 2 mg q4h prn	15 cap/$6.95
Tincture of opium	5–10 drops prn q4h	1 oz/$6.30

*These should be prescribed with no more than one refill.

precautions, while prevention of turista is another matter entirely (see Appendix II). Abdominal cramping associated with diarrhea may be aided by brief fasting (the first 8 to 12 hours of illness) or applying warm packs to the abdomen. Antiemetics (rectal suppositories) will help when nausea and vomiting are severe (most often, with viral, salmonella, and certain food-borne diseases—see Appendix II).

> Two days later, Ernie returns, "worse." He has been febrile—his temperature reaching 102° F each night—abdominal pain persists, and diarrhea continues day and night. Stools are not grossly bloody, there are no symptoms of proctitis, and Ernie is able to ingest fluids.
>
> Examination is unchanged, except for an oral temperature of 101° F. The abdomen is mildly diffusely tender. The stool is now Hematest positive, and abundant leukocytes are visible on methylene blue stain of the stool.
>
> Stool cultures from 2 days previously are growing *Campylobacter jejuni*. Stool examinations for ova and parasites are negative, except for questionable cysts of *Entamoeba histolytica*.

NOTE

1. Most patients presenting with Ernie's initial clinical illness will be better after 48 hours. Ernie's course is not typical of benign gastroenteritis.

2. Ernie's clinical illness is now characteristic of acute dysentery—he has fever, abdominal pain, severe and (occult) bloody diarrhea with fecal leukocytosis. Unlike (presumed) acute, uncomplicated gastroenteritis (above), the syndrome of acute dysentery always requires investigation (Fig. 3–3).

3. Stool cultures from 2 days previously identify *Campylobacter jejuni*, a common cause of bacterial dysentery. Especially since Ernie is not improving spontaneously, treatment with erythromycin (see Table 3–5) is indicated.

4. Identification of *Entamoeba histolytica* cysts does not imply active amebic dysentery but rather a (usually asymptomatic) carrier state. Treatment for active amebiasis is not necessary when only cysts are identified. (It should be remembered that fecal leukocytes and the cysts of *Entamoeba histolytica* can easily be mistaken for each other—the methylene blue stain of nuclear detail will usually distinguish the two.) For these reasons, it makes sense to treat the active, documented infection (*Campylobacter*) and delay consideration of the therapeutic significance of amebic cysts (see also page 116).

> Ernie is informed of the campylobacter infection and is treated with erythromycin, 250 mg qid for 7 days. He is told to remain on a liquid diet for another 2 to 3 days and then to gradually resume a solid, bland diet.

While it is not rare for acute dysentery to begin as a more benign-appearing gastroenteritis (as in Ernie's case), the clinician usually does not have stool culture results at the time the patient initially presents with acute dysentery. Figure 3–3 outlines the general approach to patients with clinical acute dysentery, the treatment of which is discussed further below.

Acute Dysentery

Most patients with acute dysentery suffer from one of the common invasive bacterial infections:[27] *Campylobacter*, *Shigella*, or *Salmonella*. Less

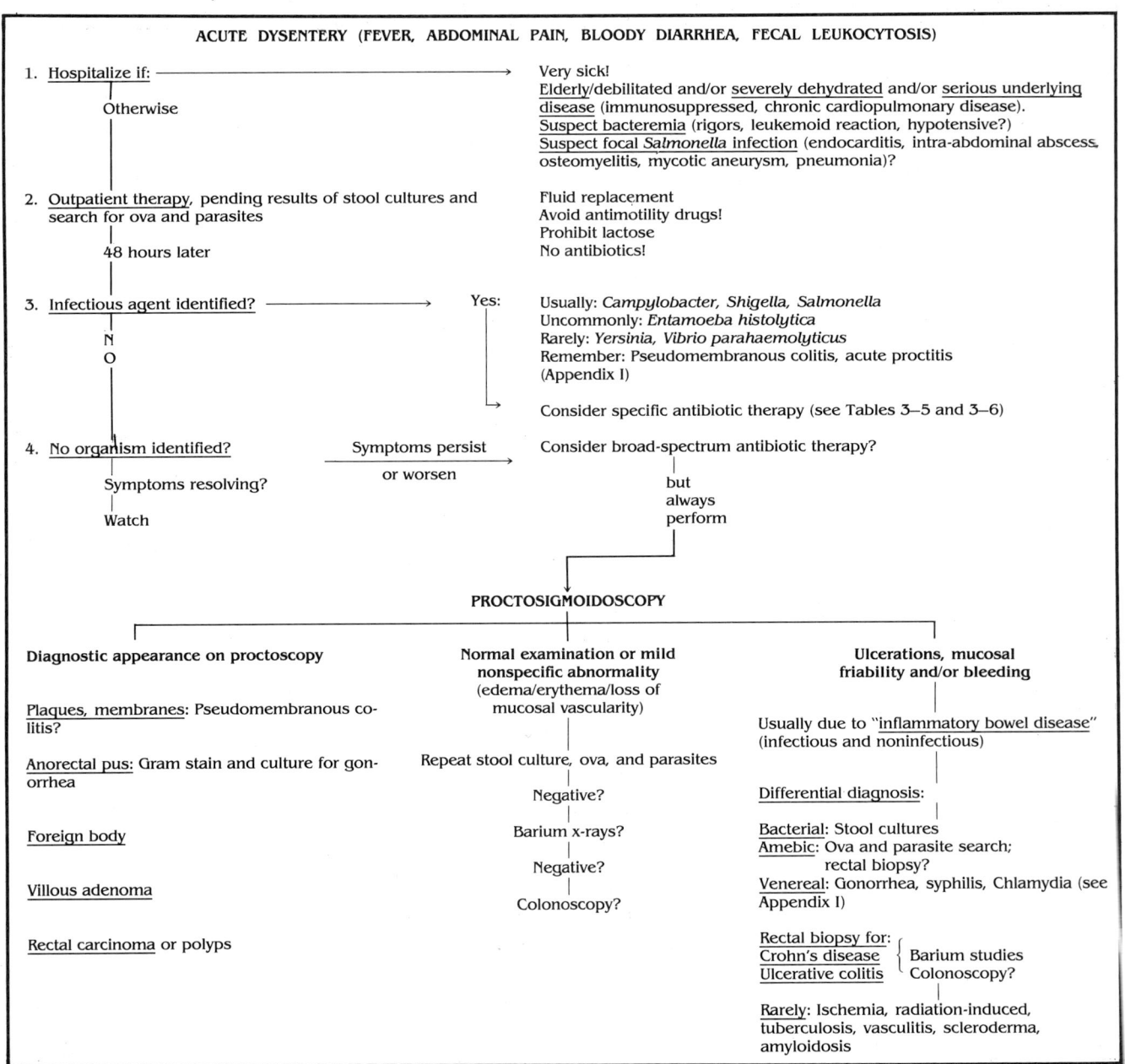

ACUTE DYSENTERY (FEVER, ABDOMINAL PAIN, BLOODY DIARRHEA, FECAL LEUKOCYTOSIS)

1. Hospitalize if: ⟶ Very sick!
Elderly/debilitated and/or severely dehydrated and/or serious underlying disease (immunosuppressed, chronic cardiopulmonary disease).
Suspect bacteremia (rigors, leukemoid reaction, hypotensive?)
Suspect focal Salmonella infection (endocarditis, intra-abdominal abscess, osteomyelitis, mycotic aneurysm, pneumonia)?

Otherwise

2. Outpatient therapy, pending results of stool cultures and search for ova and parasites
Fluid replacement
Avoid antimotility drugs!
Prohibit lactose
No antibiotics!

48 hours later

3. Infectious agent identified? ⟶ Yes:
Usually: Campylobacter, Shigella, Salmonella
Uncommonly: Entamoeba histolytica
Rarely: Yersinia, Vibrio parahaemolyticus
Remember: Pseudomembranous colitis, acute proctitis (Appendix I)

NO

Consider specific antibiotic therapy (see Tables 3–5 and 3–6)

4. No organism identified? — Symptoms persist or worsen — Consider broad-spectrum antibiotic therapy?

Symptoms resolving?

Watch

but always perform

PROCTOSIGMOIDOSCOPY

Diagnostic appearance on proctoscopy

Plaques, membranes: Pseudomembranous colitis?

Anorectal pus: Gram stain and culture for gonorrhea

Foreign body

Villous adenoma

Rectal carcinoma or polyps

Normal examination or mild nonspecific abnormality (edema/erythema/loss of mucosal vascularity)

Repeat stool culture, ova, and parasites

Negative?

Barium x-rays?

Negative?

Colonoscopy?

Ulcerations, mucosal friability and/or bleeding

Usually due to "inflammatory bowel disease" (infectious and noninfectious)

Differential diagnosis:

Bacterial: Stool cultures
Amebic: Ova and parasite search; rectal biopsy?
Venereal: Gonorrhea, syphilis, Chlamydia (see Appendix I)

Rectal biopsy for:
Crohn's disease ⎱ Barium studies
Ulcerative colitis ⎰ Colonoscopy?

Rarely: Ischemia, radiation-induced, tuberculosis, vasculitis, scleroderma, amyloidosis

FIGURE 3–3.

often, uncommon infections (amebiasis, *Yersinia, Vibrio parahaemolyticus*), venereal proctitis, pseudomembranous colitis, acute manifestations of inflammatory bowel disease (Crohn's disease, ulcerative colitis, diverticulitis, ischemic or radiation colitis), neoplasms or very rare disorders (for example, vasculitis) will be responsible for the syndrome of acute dysentery. Figure 3–3 emphasizes several points about the approach to acute dysentery:

1. Most patients do not require hospitalization. Exceptions include elderly or severely dehydrated patients, patients who are less able to tolerate infection (immunosuppressed) or fluid losses (chronic cardiopulmonary disease), and those initially suspected of disease that will require careful observation, parenteral antibiotics, or other intravenous therapy (for example, the patient with suspected acute ulcerative colitis).

2. Initial outpatient therapy is nonspecific.

As noted above, oral fluid replacement (Table 3–3) and avoidance of both lactose and antimotility drugs are usually appropriate for the patient with acute dysentery. Specific therapy depends on the specific cause, however.

While some clinicians initiate broad-spectrum antibiotic therapy when bacterial dysentery is suspected, this is usually inappropriate and may be harmful. As Table 3–5 indicates, no one antibiotic will be helpful for all common causes of bacterial dysentery. As we have seen, salmonella enteritis should not be treated with antibiotics, except rarely.* Antibiotic treatment of campylobacter enteritis depends on the clinical severity of illness. Shigel-

*Remember: Other clinical syndromes due to *Salmonella,* for example, typhoid fever, do require antibiotic therapy (but these illnesses are not usually characterized by diarrhea).[13] When salmonella bacteremia or "metastatic" infection is suspected, e.g., osteomyelitis or endocarditis, hospitalization and antibiotics certainly are indicated (Table 3–5).

TABLE 3–5. "INVASIVE" BACTERIAL DIARRHEA

ORGANISM	CLINICAL SYNDROME	DIAGNOSIS	TREATMENT
Salmonella species Most common: S. typhimurium S. heidelberg S. enteritidis S. newport	Usually headache, fever, watery diarrhea Occasionally acute dysentery Usually acquired from food or water	Stool culture (SS agar)	Symptomatic only No antibiotics unless prolonged; toxic illness?; bacteremia?; suspect focal infection (e.g., endocarditis, osteomyelitis)? Preferred treatment: chloramphenicol Alternatives: ampicillin, trimethoprim-sulfamethoxazole
Shigella species Most common: S. sonnei S. flexneri	Acute dysentery or mild gastroenteritis Children most often afflicted Remember: may be food borne or person-to-person spread (N.B. venereal infection in homosexual male)	Stool cuture Sometimes difficult to grow (Special medium: MacConkey)	Antibiotics not always necessary (mild illness) When necessary: antibiotic sensitivity is crucial (resistant strains common) Usual treatment: trimethoprim-sulfamethoxazole 160/800 mg bid × 5–7 days Alternative: ampicillin 500 mg qid × 5–7 days or tetracycline 2.5 gm (single dose)
Campylobacter species most common: C. jejuni	Mild gastroenteritis or acute dysentery	Stool culture (Special medium: Campy-BAP)	Antibiotics sometimes unnecessary (mild illness) Preferred treatment: erythromycin 250 mg qid × 7 days Alternative: tetracycline 250 mg qid × 7 days
Vibrio parahaemolyticus (rare)	Acute dysentery or mild gastroenteritis Seafood usual source Usually, brief and self-limited	Stool culture (Special media: thiosulfate, citrate, bile salts, sucrose agar [3% sodium chloride])	Symptomatic only Antibiotics rarely necessary: ampicillin, tetracycline, cephalosporins
Yersinia enterocolitica (rare)	Febrile diarrhea (sometimes very sick) Often prolonged (weeks?) May mimic appendicitis, Crohn's disease, ulcerative colitis	Stool culture (Alert the laboratory!)	Usually supportive therapy alone When illness is prolonged or severe trimethoprim-sulfamethoxazole 160/800 mg bid × 7 days Alternatives: ampicillin, tetracycline
Invasive *Escherichia coli* (rare)	Acute dysentery with negative stool cultures	Stool culture to isolate E. coli Serenyi test: guinea pig conjunctival inoculation to determine invasiveness of E. coli	Antibiotics usually unnecessary Sometimes tetracycline 2.5 gm (single dose)
Pseudomembranous colitis due to *Clostridium difficile*	Usually acute proctocolitis, often with characteristic plaques/membranes on proctoscopic visualization Occasionally nonspecific but prolonged diarrhea Usually antibiotic induced	Proctoscopy Identify toxin of C. difficile in stool	Vancomycin 500 mg qid × 10 days Alternative: cholestyramine (Questran), 1 packet q6h × 10 days

losis usually does require antibiotic treatment,[28] but many *Shigella* strains possess transferable R factors that induce resistance to various antibiotics—shotgun broad-spectrum antibiotic therapy may select out resistant strains. Antibiotic therapy of shigellosis should thus always be chosen according to documented antibiotic sensitivities (unless the patient is critically ill and requires hospitalization and "presumptive" antibiotic therapy).

In general, then, consideration of antibiotic therapy should be deferred until the results of stool cultures and sensitivities are available. The presumptive use of oral tetracycline (2.5 gm single dose or 500 mg qid for 7 days) or oral trimethoprim-sulfamethoxazole (160/800 mg bid) cannot be recommended here, but this is a common strategy.

When stool cultures are negative, acute dysentery due to invasive *E. coli* should be considered, since standard stool cultures will not make this diagnosis. In such instances, perhaps tetracycline therapy should be considered (Table 3–5) but so should:

3. Proctosigmoidoscopy.

Direct examination of the anorectal area is frequently a valuable diagnostic aid in the patient with acute dysentery.

Proctoscopy should be performed immediately under certain conditions: When pseudomembranous colitis or venereal proctitis is specifically suspected (see Appendix I), when rectal bleeding is a major symptom/sign, and when symptoms are more suggestive of acute proctitis than of bacterial dysentery (see page 102). In general, proctoscopy should be performed without a "prep," since enemas and cathartics may interfere with identification of some specific pathogens (see below).

Otherwise, proctoscopy can usually be reserved for situations in which acute dysentery is associated with negative stool cultures and parasite examination and when the patient remains ill. As Figure 3–3 notes, sometimes the proctoscopic findings are diagnostic; much more often, the findings are either mildly and nonspecifically abnormal (edema, erythema, loss of mucosal vascularity) or strongly suggest one of several inflammatory bowel diseases. As discussed in Appendix I, a common diagnostic error is to attribute proctoscopic inflammation (ulcerations, bleeding, friability) to idiopathic inflammatory bowel diseases (ulcerative colitis or Crohn's disease). Such proctoscopic findings are highly nonspecific and infectious causes should always be excluded.

When amebic dysentery[29, 30] (or its complications) is suspected clinically, aspirates of mucosal debris or rectal ulcerations should be immediately examined for the trophozoites of *Entamoeba histolytica*. (Cotton swabs should not be used to prepare the microscopic slides, since amebic trophozoites may stick to the cotton, resulting in a false negative microscopic examination.[31]) Rectal biopsy (see below) may be helpful, as may serologic tests for invasive amebiasis (antibodies by indirect hemagglutination are positive in about 80 percent of patients with amebic dysentery).[32] Various "interfering substances"—barium, bismuth, antibiotics, enemas—may all cause false negative examination for amebiasis.

Rectal biopsy may also be helpful in the diagnosis of ulcerative colitis or Crohn's disease,[33, 34] which must occasionally be distinguished from other rare diseases (ischemic proctitis,[35] vasculitis, or amyloidosis[36]). Histologically rectal biopsy may be highly nonspecific,[37] and common treatable infectious causes should always be excluded by obtaining stool cultures and smears for parasites at the time of proctoscopy.

Pseudomembranous colitis (usually antibiotic-induced) may sometimes have a nonspecific proctoscopic appearance—the characteristic plaques and membranes may not be apparent—and thus specimens should be obtained for measurement of *Clostridium difficile* toxin whenever this entity is suspected.[38, 39] Vancomycin treatment must often be begun presumptively.[40, 41]* (Other forms of acute proctocolitis are discussed in Appendix I.)

When Acute Diarrhea Persists

Four days later, Ernie calls to say that he is afebrile and "much better." He now has only three to four bowel movements a day, and there is no tenesmus or abdominal pain. He is told to complete his course of erythromycin. Ernie postpones his trip to the Caribbean.

One week later, Ernie has completed the course of erythromycin and feels "well" but continues to have three to four diarrheal stools per day and occasionally is awakened from sleep by the diarrhea. There is no fever, abdominal pain, or grossly bloody stool.

When acute diarrhea, presumed or proven to be infectious, does not resolve after 7 to 10 days, consideration of three basic concepts will determine whether (and when) further investigations are indicated (see also Fig. 3–4):

I. The expected natural history of diarrheal illness caused by the (suspected or proven) pathogen.

Viral gastroenteritis and "food-borne" diarrhea usually resolve within 3 days. Turista (usually due to enterotoxigenic *E. coli*) lasts an average of 1 week. Bacterial gastroenteritis due to *Salmonella, Shigella, Campylobacter,* or *Yersinia* may (occasionally) last for weeks if untreated, while giardiasis and amebiasis commonly cause prolonged diarrhea if untreated.

Thus, the initial clinical diagnosis—based on the history and stool examination—and the expected response to antibiotic and/or symptomatic therapy will allow a forecast of the expected duration of illness. When presumed viral gastroenteritis or food poisoning persists beyond a week, for example, the diagnosis should be reconsidered (even though, in some such cases, prolonged diarrhea does occur—see below). When the duration of illness exceeds expectations, one must also consider:

II. The accuracy (the sensitivity) of stool microbiology studies. Stool cultures may be false negative for several reasons:

A. Improper handling—fresh specimens should be plated on a specific culture medium as soon as possible, preferably immediately. Swabs obtained directly from the rectum during protoscopy or immediately after passage of stool yield the best results. Specimens exposed to the air and allowed to dry, or those plated after a delay of longer than 2 to 3 hours, will often be falsely negative.

B. The Laboratory must know what to look for!

Salmonella species are usually easy to grow, but *Shigella* may be inhibited even on so-called salmonella-shigella (SS) agar. Multiple specimens should be plated on MacConkey (or other specific) agar when *Shigella* is suspected. *Campylobacter* requires a specific medium

---

*Oral vancomycin is extremely expensive (several hundred dollars for a 10-day course). Cholestyramine (Questran) will help in very mild cases and is less expensive.

(usually, Campty-BAP). *Yersinia enterocolitica* usually grows readily enough, but the laboratory must be alerted to look for it. *Vibrio parahaemolyticus* requires a special medium (TCBS).

C. Prior antibiotic therapy may interfere with stool culture results.

D. Invasive E. coli[42] will not be identified by standard cultures. *E. coli* is commensal in the bowel—specific tests of "enteroinvasiveness" are required to document invasive *E. coli*. These are usually performed only in reference laboratories (and are rarely necessary).

Stool examination for ova and parasites may be falsely negative for other reasons:

A. Experienced parasitologists clearly do better than inexperienced examiners. When the laboratory does not often deal with parasitic problems, specimens should be sent to reference laboratories.

B. Stools must be fresh and warm, devoid of interfering substances (see page 114), and three separate specimens examined before studies are designated negative.

C. Know what to look for. Different parasitic diseases result in shedding of various forms of the organism.[31, 43-45] Amebiasis is diagnosed when trophozoites are observed; cysts of *Entamoeba histolytica* usually reflect an asymptomatic carrier state (as noted above) and may be mistaken for either leukocytes or nonpathogenic amebas—for example, *E. coli* or *E. hartmanni.* Conversely, trophozoites are usually not found in giardiasis—identification of giardia cysts is diagnostic of active infection with *Giardia lamblia.* Experienced examiners will find *Giardia* in 95 per cent of cases when three separate fresh stool specimens are examined,[43] but occasionally duodenal aspiration is needed to demonstrate the organism.

Other parasitic causes of diarrhea are rare in the United States, but as noted in Table 3–6, larvae are identified in the stools of patients infected with *Strongyloides* and *Trichuris trichiura,* while ova are identified in capillariasis. Ascariasis is usually diagnosed when the patient identifies a long worm found in the stool. Pinworm *(Enterobius)* rarely causes diarrhea, but associated pruritus ani should prompt the perianal cellophane tape test* to look for this pathogen.

Thus, the patient in whom acute diarrhea persists, whose initial stool studies are nondiagnostic, should undergo repeat testing, especially if one of these potential false negative factors can be identified. When repeat studies are also negative, one must then also consider:

III. Drugs, diet, and therapeutic trials

Some of the antibiotics used to treat infectious diarrhea may themselves cause diarrhea—erythromycin and ampicillin are common offenders. When diarrhea thus persists in spite of appropriate antibiotic therapy (and especially when subsequent cultures become negative), it makes more sense to stop the antibiotic than to renew it. Similarly, all other drugs taken by the patient should always be reviewed (see Table 3–1).

---

*Cellophane tape is applied to the perianal mucosa before bedtime—in the morning the tape is removed by the patient, taped to a microscopic glass slide, and brought to the laboratory for attempted identification of pinworms trapped under the tape (and usually easily visible under the microscope).

TABLE 3–6. PARASITIC DIARRHEA

Organism	Clinical Syndrome	Diagnosis	Treatment
Entamoeba histolytica (amebiasis)	Acute dysentery or mild diarrhea Remember: travel, sexual contacts Complication: liver abscess! (rare)	Examine fresh, warm stool for trophozoites (or cysts) Rectal biopsy/proctoscopy Serum indirect hemagglutination antibody	Active infection: metronidazole 750 mg tid × 7 days or diiodohydroxyquin 650 mg tid × 20 days Asymptomatic cyst carrier: dilanozide furonate (Furamide) 500 mg tid × 10 days
Giardia lamblia (giardiasis)	Sometimes asymptomatic Usually epigastric discomfort, borborygmi, watery diarrhea, nausea/vomiting	Stool examination for *Giardia* cysts (trophozoites usually not found) Duodenal aspiration occasionally necessary	Quinacrine 100 mg tid × 7 days or metronidazole 250 mg tid × 7 days
Strongyloides stercoralis (strongyloidiasis)	Often asymptomatic Epigastric pain, vomiting, watery diarrhea (beware of life-threatening systemic infection when patient is immunosuppressed!)*	Stool examination for larvae	Thiabendazole 25 mg/kg bid × 2 days
Trichuris trichiura (trichuriasis)	Often asymptomatic Abdominal pain, diarrhea Sometimes rectal prolapse	Stool examination for larvae	Mebendazole 100 mg bid × 3 days
Ascaris lumbricoides (ascariasis)	Diarrhea Sometimes, intestinal obstruction	Identify worm (patient often finds in stool)	Mebendazole 100 mg bid × 3 days or pyrantel pamoate 11 mg/kg, single dose
Necator americanus (hookworm)	Diarrhea, iron deficiency (rarely, asthma or pneumonia)	Stool examination for ova	Mebendazole 100 mg bid × 3 days or pyrantel pamoate 11 mg/kg or pyrvinium pamoate 5 mg/kg, one dose; repeat dose in 2 weeks
Enterobius vermicularis (pinworm)	Pruritus ani Diarrhea, uncommonly	Perianal cellophane tape test × 3 consecutive mornings (ova or worms)	Mebendazole 100 mg bid × 3 days or pyrantel pamoate 11 mg/kg or pyrvinium pamoate 5 mg/kg, one dose; repeat dose in 2 weeks
Capillaria philippinensis (capillariasis)	Watery diarrhea Malabsorption	Stool examination for ova	Thiabendazole 25 mg/kg × 2 to 3 weeks

*Cryptosporidiosis may also be a cause of diarrhea in the immunosuppressed patient.[161]

Some patients develop persistent diarrhea because they continue to ingest only liquids ("what goes in, will come out"). Solid foods should be reinstituted, usually after a few days of the initial liquid diet. Such solids/liquids should not include any lactose-containing products. Simply resuming a lactose-free but otherwise normal diet (see Appendix IV) will often cure persistent "postinfectious" diarrhea.

As Figure 3–4 suggests, occasionally therapeutic trials will be helpful in persistent diarrhea when a specific pathogen has not been documented even after repeated stool examinations for parasites and invasive bacteria:

In travelers, tetracycline or trimethoprim-sulfamethoxazole has been advocated for the treatment of turista. Antibiotics are rarely necessary for this usually self-limited problem, but persistent turista may be worth a therapeutic trial. When *Giardia* is clinically suspected (but unproven), 1 week's treatment with metronidazole or quinacrine is not unreasonable.

Persistent, unexplained dysentery should always be investigated, although a trial of erythromycin (for campylobacter infection) or ampicillin or trimethoprim-sulfamethoxazole (for shigellosis) is often considered before expensive, invasive testing (for example, colonoscopy) in the patient who is not severely ill.

A combination of a lactose-free solid diet, avoidance of nonessential drugs and occasional use of brief therapeutic trials will result in cure of

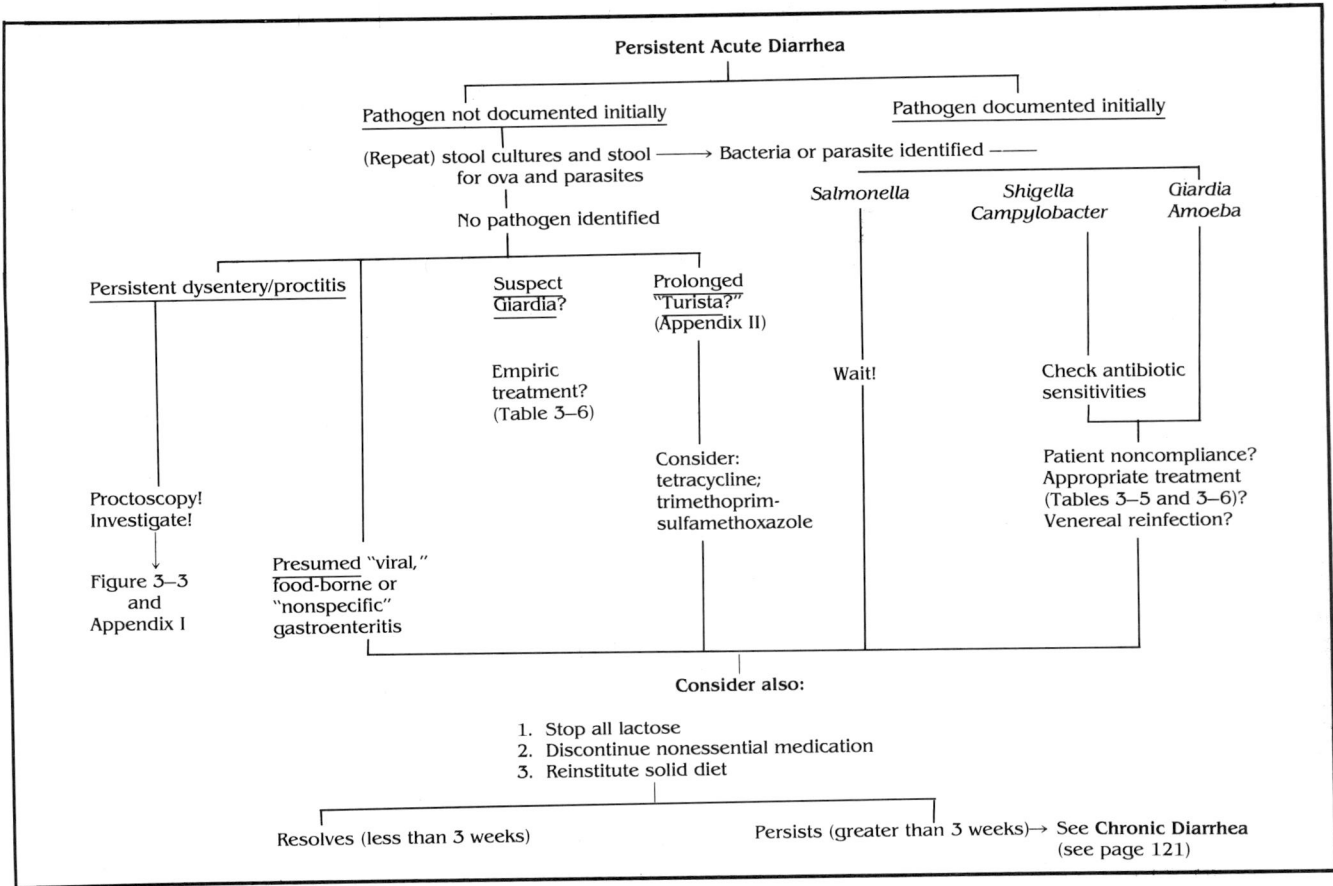

FIGURE 3—4. An approach to persistent acute diarrhea (greater than 7 days).

acute diarrhea in all but a very few patients. Those patients whose diarrhea persists beyond 3 weeks in spite of such measures must be considered to have chronic diarrhea (see page 121). In Ernie's case:

Physical examination is normal. Stool is brown, watery, and heme negative. Fecal leukocytes are absent. Repeat stool culture is obtained, as are two separate stools for ova and parasite examinations. No bacteria or parasites are subsequently identified. No cysts of *Entamoeba histolytica* can be found.

All medications are discontinued. Ernie is instructed to avoid all milk and other lactose-containing foods.

NOTE

1. Repeat stool cultures are usually not necessary in the patient who becomes symptom free following culture-proven bacterial diarrhea. Exceptions here include patients who are an epidemiologic risk to many others, for example, food handlers or day-care workers. Cure of shigellosis especially should be confirmed by subsequent negative stool cultures in such patients.

Since salmonella enteritis is not usually treated with antibiotics, it must be remembered that the organism may still be found on stool culture 1 to 2 months following initial clinical symptoms, but that a chronic carrier state is quite rare if treatment is withheld.

When infection with *Shigella, Campylobacter, Giardia,* or ameba persists or seems to relapse and recur despite appropriate treatment, venereal transmission should be considered, and the patient's sexual habits reviewed. Male homosexuals are commonly so afflicted.

2. Lactose intolerance may cause symptoms when even small amounts of dairy products are consumed. Patients must be specifically instructed about exact dietary restrictions (see Appendix IV). Most (but not all) patients with preexisting lactose intolerance are aware of gaseous indigestion, nausea, bloating, or diarrhea when milk is consumed. Those with transient (postinfectious) lactose intolerance can usually resume lactose ingestion within a week or two after clinical improvement.

Ten days later, Ernie calls to say that he is "cured." Since discontinuing all dairy products, he has had only one or two bowel movements per day, which are soft but "solid." Two days before, he "tested" himself with a glass of milk and soon developed bloating and diarrhea. In retrospect, he believes that much of his intermittent diarrhea of the past several months "could be explained" by ingestion of dairy products.

Ernie is told to avoid dairy products for the next month or so and then to "test himself" again with different lactose-containing foods.

Lactose Intolerance

Lactose intolerance[45-47] is a very common clinical problem. As many as 10 to 15 per cent of adult Caucasian Americans may be afflicted; perhaps 30 million Americans have this problem. (Adult blacks, Orientals, and American Indians are especially susceptible.) Symptoms vary from bloating and "gas" to severe diarrhea, abdominal pain, and vomiting. Because lactose intolerance is often not an all-or-none phenomenon—varied amounts of lactose in different forms may be well tolerated by different patients—the association between ingestion of dairy products and symptoms may be inapparent. Symptoms due to lactose intolerance are very often attributed to the irritable bowel syndrome, "colitis," anxiety, and many other conditions (see **Chronic Diarrhea** below).

The cause of lactose intolerance is usually either a genetic or an "age-related" deficiency of lactase in the small-intestinal mucosa, and, except for the transient lactose intolerance that may complicate infectious gastroenteritis, there is usually no "underlying disease" or anatomic disorder responsible for lactase deficiency. However, lactose intolerance may also result from small-bowel resection, gastrectomy or pyloroplasty (which alter intestinal transit or reduce mucosal surface area or both), or from a more diffuse abnormality of the small-intestinal mucosa wherein lactose intolerance is but one manifestation. Such disorders include celiac sprue, tropical sprue, Whipple's disease, giardiasis, bacterial overgrowth syndromes, Crohn's disease, and intestinal lymphangiectasia (see below).

The diagnosis of lactose intolerance can be made by one of three methods:

1. Intestinal biopsy, with quantitative biochemical assays for lactase content, is the definitive procedure but is rarely necessary. It is usually reserved for research studies or when lactose intolerance is suspected of being due to another process—sprue, for example—in which intestinal biopsy is indicated anyway.

2. The lactose tolerance test is helpful but is usually unnecessary as well. Figure 3–5 illustrates that, when ingestion of lactose causes clinical symptoms and is associated with a rise in blood glucose of less than 20 to 25 mg per 100 ml (blood specimens drawn each half hour for the 2 hours following

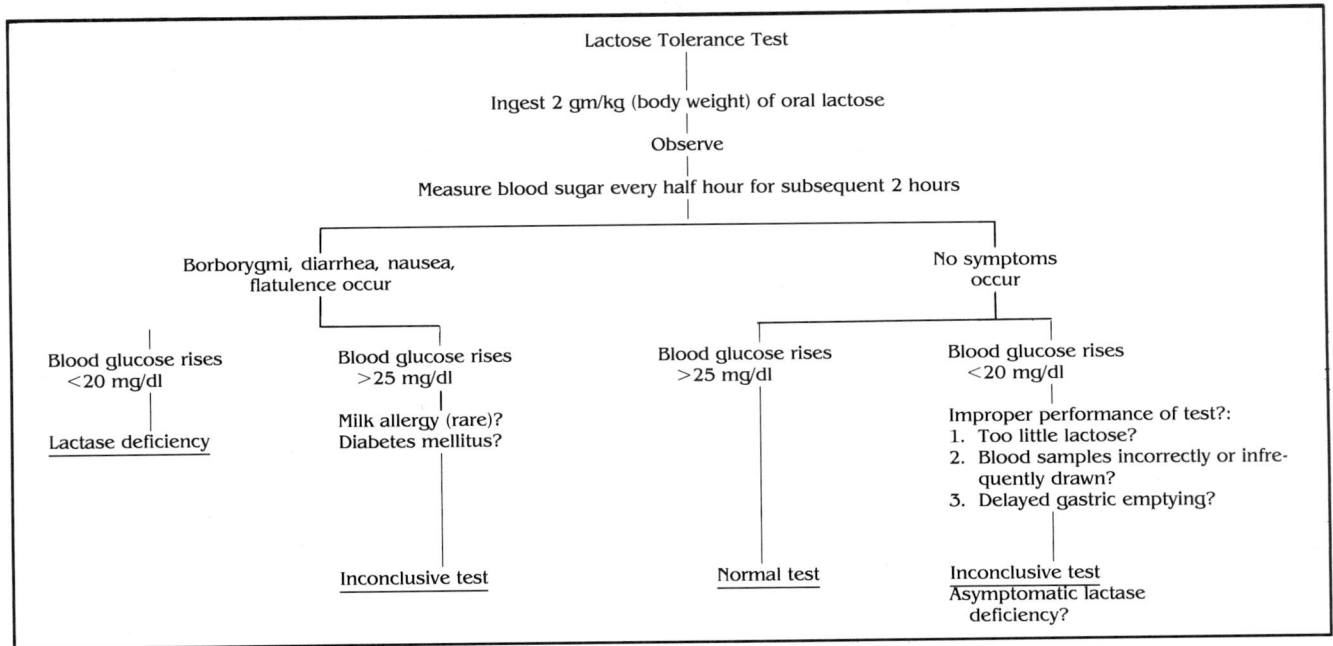

FIGURE 3–5. Lactose tolerance test.

lactose ingestion), the diagnosis of lactase deficiency is usually confirmed. When only one or the other of these criteria is met, the test is inconclusive and other possibilities must be considered.

Thus, while the lactose tolerance test is not difficult to perform, it is usually unnecessary because most often the diagnosis is made more simply by:

3. A clinical trial of a lactose-free diet. The patient is instructed to consume no dairy products for 2 weeks and then to drink two glasses of milk on an empty stomach. Symptoms will develop within 2 hours. Subsequent ingestion of different dairy products can then be "tested" to determine the patient's threshold for symptoms. Appendix IV provides one example of a lactose-free diet.* (Determining the pH of the stool in the patient with diarrhea is sometimes helpful—a stool pH less than 6 is often associated with lactose intolerance.)

> Two months later, Ernie returns complaining, "I guess the diarrhea really never went away."
>
> Two weeks after his last visit, Ernie had been well, having only one or two "slightly loose" bowel movements per day. A test dose of milk at that time caused an episode of abdominal discomfort and diarrhea, but, in spite of discontinuing all lactose-containing foods and liquids, Ernie has continued since then to have daily diarrhea—five to six large malodorous liquid stools per 24 hours—sometimes awakening him from sleep. He feels that this diarrhea is similar to that which has intermittently bothered him during the past several months (but is clearly different from his bout of acute bacterial dysentery). Diarrhea is now daily and is sometimes accompanied by mild periumbilical discomfort. In retrospect, he believes he has had "some" diarrhea for at least 6 months.
>
> Ernie has continued to travel widely along the Atlantic coast and through the Caribbean. He is taking no medications, and denies any laxative use.

---

*An oral lactase (LactAid, Lactozyme) is now commercially available, without prescription. This substance (liquid or powder) is added to milk, which is then shaken and refrigerated for 24 hours. About 70 per cent of the lactose is thus hydrolyzed. This product allows some patients otherwise intolerant to it to ingest lactose.

CHRONIC DIARRHEA[48]

As Table 3–7 illustrates, the possible causes of chronic, persistent, or recurrent diarrhea are legion. The diversity of these disorders presents a difficult problem: Comprehensive evaluation of chronic diarrhea may require an extraordinary array of investigations, ranging from the mundane (stool culture) to the "mega work-up." Table 3–8 illustrates the number and variety of investigations that may be required in the evaluation of chronic diarrhea. Surely, however, not all patients with chronic diarrhea deserve serum measurements of vasoactive intestinal peptide! Clinical judgment and a pragmatic cost-conscious approach usually allow accurate (and much more limited) differential diagnosis, as well as prudent selection of tests and therapeutic trials. Table 3–7, then, can be much less intimidating if we recognize several generalizations about chronic diarrhea.

The Initial Approach

I. Iatrogenic diarrhea is not uncommon, and a careful history alone will make the diagnosis.

A variety of gastrointestinal surgical procedures may be complicated by persistent or recurrent postoperative diarrhea. The pathophysiologic mechanisms and approach to therapy are briefly outlined in Appendix III.

TABLE 3–7. CAUSES OF CHRONIC DIARRHEA

INFLAMMATORY	NEOPLASTIC	MALABSORPTION
Infectious	Colorectal cancer	Chronic pancreatitis
Parasites	Polyposis	Pancreatic carcinoma
Bacteria	Villous adenoma	Biliary obstruction
Viral	Intestinal lymphoma	Bacterial overgrowth syndromes
Tuberculosis	Carcinoid	Disaccharidase deficits
Fungal	Others (rarely)	Celiac sprue
		Tropical sprue
Regional enteritis		Whipple's disease
Ulcerative colitis		Lymphangiectasia
Ischemic bowel disease		Hypogammaglobulinemia
Radiation enteritis		Eosinophilic gastroenteritis
Diverticulitis		Amyloidosis
Proctocolitis (see App. I)		Abetalipoproteinemia
		Nongranulomatous jejunitis

IATROGENIC	METABOLIC/SYSTEMIC	MISCELLANEOUS
Drug induced (see Table 1)	Diabetes mellitus	Irritable bowel syndrome
Poisons/chemicals	Hyperthyroidism	Food allergies
Laxative abuse	Hypoparathyroidism	Zollinger-Ellison syndrome
Postoperative (see App. III)	Adrenal insufficiency	Medullary carcinoma of thyroid
Gastrectomy	Uremia	Vasoactive intestinal peptide
Enteric fistulas	Connective tissue diseases	syndromes
Jejunoileal bypass	(scleroderma, SLE, polyarteritis)	Chronic, severe congestive heart
Cholecystectomy	Dermatitis herpetiformis	failure
Pancreatectomy	Cystic fibrosis	
Short-bowel syndrome	Mastocytosis	
Ileocolostomy	Cystinuria	
Blind loop syndrome	Pellagra	
Billroth II	Porphyria	
Vagotomy	Pheochromocytoma	
Pyloroplasty	Fabry's disease	
Ileal resection		

TABLE 3–8. TESTS SOMETIMES USEFUL IN THE EVALUATION OF CHRONIC DIARRHEA

STOOL
Cultures for enteric pathogens
Ova and parasites ($\times$ 3)
Occult blood
Fecal leukocytes
pH
Alkalinization test
24-hour volume/weight
72-hour fecal fat determination
Osmolality
Quantitative electrolytes/24 hours

BLOOD
Cultures
Amebic serology
CBC
Chemistries
B_{12}, folate
Protein electrophoresis
Quantitative immunoglobulins
Electrolytes
Carotene
Thyroid functions
Cortisols
Lactose tolerance test
Serum gastrin
Vasoactive intestinal peptide
Calcitonin

URINE
Schilling test
D-Xylose test
Urinary 5-HIAA
24-hour urine VMA/
    metanephrines
Urine potassium (diuretic abuse)
Laxative/cathartic assays

INTUBATION/ENDOSCOPY
Proctoscopy, biopsy
Colonoscopy, biopsy
Duodenal aspiration
Gastric acid analysis
Small bowel (jejunal) biopsy
Pancreatic exocrine testing
Intestinal perfusion studies
ERCP

X-RAYS
Plain film of abdomen
Upper GI with small-bowel series
Barium enema
Abdominal CT

MISCELLANEOUS
72-hour fast
Bile acid breath test
Small-intestine cultures
Search for surreptitious drugs/
    laxatives

All medications must be reviewed (Table 3–1). As noted previously, various prescription and nonprescription medications will cause diarrhea. Laxative abuse is common, but patients may not readily admit to it. Persistent surreptitious laxative abuse is rare, but it is a very difficult diagnostic problem (see below).

II. Parasitic infestation—especially with *Giardia lamblia*—is a common cause of persistent diarrhea.

Travel history and familiarity with parasites endemic to various regions of the United States are always important,[49] since brief antibiotic therapy is almost always curative in cases of giardiasis, amebiasis, or (rarely) strongyloidiasis (and other unusual parasites listed in Table 3–6). *Giardia lamblia*, in particular, is now endemic in many parts of the United States. While careful examination of fresh warm stools for the cysts of *Giardia* will usually make the diagnosis, sometimes duodenal intubation and aspiration may be necessary to confirm the diagnosis. When three stool examinations are negative, but giardiasis is still suspected (prolonged watery diarrhea with borborygmi, flatulence, and upper abdominal discomfort in a patient living in or visiting endemic areas), a therapeutic trial of antiparasitic therapy often makes sense.

Bacterial and viral infections rarely cause prolonged (several weeks or longer) diarrhea.

III. Look at the whole patient.

Various systemic diseases may cause chronic diarrhea, but a thorough history and physical examination almost always suggest these diagnoses.

Diabetic enteropathy,[50, 51] for example, usually occurs only when diabetes mellitus is complicated by obvious peripheral and autonomic neuropathy[52]—orthostatic hypotension, stocking-glove sensory loss, sweat disorders, impotence, and other such manifestations will usually be apparent.

Occasionally diarrhea will be the presenting manifestation of thyrotoxicosis, adrenal insufficiency, uremia, cystic fibrosis, or various connective tissue diseases (especially scleroderma or systemic lupus), but a careful history and complete examination will almost always raise

TABLE 3–9. LOOK AT THE WHOLE PATIENT: SYSTEMIC CLUES TO THE CAUSE OF CHRONIC DIARRHEA[48, 53]

SYSTEMIC CLUE	CONSIDER
Vital signs	
Fever	Ulcerative colitis, Crohn's disease, amebiasis, lymphoma, tuberculosis, Whipple's disease, thyrotoxicosis, adrenal insufficiency, yersinia infection
Hypotension, postural	Severe dehydration or hemorrhage
	Drug induced (e.g., antihypertensives)
	Diabetic or other autonomic neuropathy
	Adrenal insufficiency, pheochromocytoma
Severe weight loss, normal appetite	Malabsorption, thyrotoxicosis, pheochromocytoma
Severe weight loss, anorexic	Cancer, inflammatory bowel disease, adrenal insufficiency
Skin	
Hyperpigmentation	Addison's disease, Whipple's disease, celiac sprue, Peutz-Jegher's syndrome
Red-purple flush	Carcinoid, systemic mastocytosis
Sclerodactyly	Scleroderma
Erythema nodosum	Ulcerative colitis
Pyoderma gangrenosum	Ulcerative colitis, Crohn's disease
Dermatitis herpetiformis	Celiac sprue
Ecchymoses	Malabsorption
Rarely: Steven Johnson's syndrome, Fabry's disease, acanthosis nigricans with intestinal cancer, acrodermatitis enteropathica with zinc deficiency, pancreatic tumors (glucagonoma, VIPoma)	
Head and Neck	
Exophthalmos, lid lag	Thyrotoxicosis
Macroglossia, gingival hyperplasia	Amyloidosis
Glossitis	Malabsorption, B_{12} deficiency
Uveitis	Ulcerative colitis, Crohn's disease
Aphthous stomatitis	Ulcerative colitis, malabsorption, connective tissue disease (systemic lupus, Behçet's)
Thyroid enlargement	Hyperthyroidism or medullary carcinoma of thyroid
Lymphadenopathy	Lymphoma, Whipple's disease, bowel carcinoma, tuberculosis
Edema	Hypoalbuminemia due to malabsorption/malnutrition
	Uremia, severe congestive heart failure
Liver disease	Ulcerative colitis, Crohn's disease, metastatic carcinoma or carcinoid, amebic abscess
Surgical scars	Postoperative diarrhea: (App. III)
Pulmonary disease	Cystic fibrosis, connective tissue disease, tuberculosis
Arthritis	Ulcerative colitis, Crohn's disease, Whipple's disease, connective tissue diseases, yersinia enterocolitis, amyloidosis, postjejunoileal bypass
Neuropathy	Diabetic or autonomic neuropathy, amyloidosis, carcinoma, connective tissue diseases, chronic (alcoholic) pancreatitis
Diffuse vascular disease (claudication, bruits, ischemic events)	Mesenteric ischemia
Tetany	Hypocalcemia, hypomagnesemia, hypokalemia secondary to diarrhea
Alcoholic?	Chronic pancreatitis?
Diabetic?	Diabetic enteropathy?

suspicions of systemic disease. Hyperthyroid diarrhea, for example, will rarely occur without some other clue—weight loss, tachycardia, tremor, ocular signs, and the like.

Similarly, various primary gastrointestinal disorders will sometimes be suggested by their secondary systemic manifestations. Fever, polyarthritis, dermatologic conditions, and a variety of other findings will sometimes point to inflammatory bowel disease and other rarer conditions. Table 3–9 illustrates examples of "systemic clues" in the diagnosis of chronic diarrhea.

When the history and physical examination do not strongly suggest iatrogenic, parasitic, or systemic disease, a few clinical determinations will help narrow the differential diagnosis considerably:

IV. Does the history of diarrhea suggest involvement of the distal colon or more proximal intestinal disease?

When stool passes into the rectosigmoid colon, it is normally homogeneous, i.e., the homogenization of stool is normally already complete. Therefore, visible streaks or flecks of blood, mucus, or pus, on or separate from the stool itself, most often come from somewhere in the left side of the colon, usually the sigmoid or rectum.[48] (The presence of undigested food particles is nonspecific, and is often normal.) In addition, normally the left side of the colon serves a reservoir function—otherwise, chronic diarrhea would be normal. When this reservoir function is impaired by disease of the distal colon, stools tend to be small in volume and very frequent in number and may be accompanied by rectal urgency, tenesmus, or even fecal incontinence. When pain accompanies such "distal colon diarrhea," it is usually located in the left lower quadrant, hypogastrium, or sacral area and is often (at least partly) relieved by the bowel movement (or an enema).

Thus, diarrhea due to disease of the distal colon is typically frequent "small-stool diarrhea," which is often nonhomogeneous (mucus, blood, or pus may be visibly distinguishable from stool itself); rectal urgency, tenesmus, and left lower quadrant pain relieved by defecation often coexist. Various types of proctocolitis, colon carcinoma, diverticular disease, or the irritable bowel syndrome are the most common causes of distal colon or small-stool diarrhea.

Conversely, diarrhea due to disease of the small intestine or proximal colon tends to be "large-stool diarrhea," which is less frequent (two to ten times per day), more homogeneous, and usually unassociated with tenesmus and rectal urgency. When pain is present, it is more often located in the periumbilical or right lower quadrant area and is sometimes associated with borborygmi. Such proximal bowel or large-stool diarrhea is most often caused by food intolerance (especially lactose intolerance), infectious or inflammatory diseases of the small bowel and cecum (parasitic disease, Crohn's disease), or by various malabsorptive disorders.*

Tentative localization of the site of disease on the basis of these clinical correlates often helps narrow the differential diagnosis and guide initial diagnostic testing. For example,

---

*Diarrhea due to malabsorption is classically described as consisting of floating, bulky, loose, greasy, and foul smelling stools, but gross appearance is by no means a reliable or predictive clue.

V. When the history suggests disease of the distal colon, is the clinical presentation entirely compatible with the irritable bowel syndrome?

The irritable bowel syndrome may afflict patients of all ages but usually begins between the ages of 20 and 35 years. While symptoms vary among individuals, diarrhea is usually small-stool diarrhea, often admixed with visible mucus. Periods of diarrhea frequently alternate with periods of constipation, or the diarrhea occurs daily after the initial passage of hard pellets or pencil-thin stools upon arising in the morning.[54] Abdominal distention and crampy abdominal pain often coexist, and rectal urgency tends to be partly relieved by defecation. Total 24-hour stool volume is usually normal (less than 300 gm), and thus the diarrhea of the irritable bowel syndrome is more qualitative than quantitative.

Physical examination is usually normal in patients with irritable bowel, except that a tender sigmoid colon is often palpable in the left lower quadrant, but tenderness tends to lessen as the examiner applies gentle but more prolonged manual pressure over the area of tenderness.

While the irritable bowel syndrome is probably the most common cause of chronic diarrhea in the United States today, there are currently no definitive objective criteria that confirm the diagnosis. Various "positive" findings are helpful in making the diagnosis of irritable bowel syndrome—for example, the young adult with intermittent small-stool diarrhea and mucus, alternating with episodes of constipation, and associated with transient lower abdominal distention and discomfort[55, 56]—but such symptoms are highly nonspecific and may be seen with many other disorders (colon carcinoma, lactose intolerance, or Crohn's disease, for example). Because of this the diagnosis of irritable bowel syndrome is often one of exclusion,[57] and extensive (sometimes repeated) testing is commonly undertaken with this purpose in mind. In fact, testing can often be omitted (or least deferred) when symptoms are typical—a therapeutic trial (see page 133 and Table 3–10) is often the best "diagnostic test."

It is therefore crucial to seek out clinical findings that are either very atypical of or frankly incompatible with the diagnosis of irritable bowel syndrome:[58]

1. Diarrhea that awakens the patient from sleep is atypical (but it does occur occasionally).

2. Weight loss does not occur (except as a biologic sign of coexisting depression). Other evidence of systemic disease is always lacking—anemia, elevated sedimentation rate, and fever do not occur.

3. Blood in the stool (gross or occult) does not occur, nor does fecal leukocytosis.

4. The onset of symptoms after middle age is distinctly unusual.

When the clinical history is suggestive of irritable bowel syndrome, and all other clinical findings are compatible with that diagnosis, most tests can be avoided, at least initially, but many authorities recommend at least proctosigmoidoscopy, stool examination for parasites, and perhaps a trial of a lactose-free diet. Especially when tests are not performed, careful follow-up is essential.

Whether extensive testing is performed or not, the treatment of irritable bowel syndrome requires a multifaceted therapeutic approach.[54, 58, 59] High-fiber diets, bulk agents (for example, daily Metamucil), various medications (antidiarrheal agents, anticholinergics, tranquilizers, antidepressants), psychophysiologic manipulations, and patient education must be considered in different patients. (The treatment of irritable bowel syndrome is discussed further in Chapter 11, "Abdominal Pain.")

When distal colon disease is suspected on the basis of the patient's symptoms, but clinical features are not entirely compatible with irritable bowel syndrome (or the patient does not improve with treatment of irritable bowel), then proctosigmoidoscopy, barium enema or (sometimes) colonoscopy will be necessary.

VI. Are there clinical findings that in and of themselves necessitate diagnostic testing?

All patients with chronic diarrhea must be suspected of serious disease when:

A. The stool contains (gross or occult) blood—neoplasms, inflammatory bowel diseases, and a variety of other disorders must be excluded.

Investigation must be carried out in all patients with heme-positive stool.

B. The stool contains fecal leukocytes—the common bacterial diarrheas are rarely the cause of chronic diarrhea, but other inflammatory bowel diseases must be suspected when stool smear with methylene blue reveals leukocytes (Fig. 3–1).

C. Diarrhea "sounds organic," i.e., the diarrhea awakens the patient from sleep, is associated with documented weight loss, fever, or other evidence of systemic illness (Table 3–9), or begins anew in the elderly patient.

How do these generalizations help in the practical approach to the patient with chronic diarrhea? Consider Ernie again in the light of Figure 3–6, which outlines these considerations:

> Again, Ernie denies taking any medications or use of laxatives. He has never undergone surgery of any kind. He now scrupulously avoids all lactose. Ernie again describes his bowel movements as voluminous and smelly, sometimes watery and sometimes soft, without visible blood, mucus, or pus, occurring about six times per day; the bowel movements do awaken him from sleep occasionally. He describes intermittent vague abdominal discomfort (he points to the periumbilical area) associated with the diarrhea. He believes he has lost 5 or 6 pounds in the last 2 months, but his appetite remains good. Review of systems and family history are entirely unremarkable. Ernie does not consume excess alcohol or caffeine. Physical examination is entirely normal. Rectal examination reveals liquid brown feces that are heme negative and contain no white blood cells.

What does this mean?

1. Ernie has chronic diarrhea.

There is wide variation in frequency of bowel movements in a normal population. More than three bowel movements per day is very unusual as a normal pattern[60] and this usually constitutes "diarrhea." Occasionally, however, the frequency of bowel movements does not define diarrhea. Patients with diarrhea due to anxiety, the irritable bowel syndrome, or disorders of the anal sphincter may have frequent movements that are are small in volume—collection of stool volume for a 24-hour period may thus be helpful since diarrhea can be "objectively" defined as stool volume (weight) exceeding 300 gm per 24 hours.[53]

Most patients know what diarrhea means for them, but it is sometimes wise to quantitate stool volume and frequency before embarking on exhaustive diagnostic studies. When routine testing (stool cultures, parasite examinations, barium studies, and proctoscopy) is unremarkable, a 24-hour stool collection may be very informative.

2. Ernie's diarrhea sounds organic.

Diarrhea that is "functional" or related to the irritable bowel syndrome tends not to disturb sleep and is usually not associated with weight loss or any other systemic symptoms or signs. Ernie has nocturnal diarrhea (i.e., it awakens him from sleep*), and he has lost weight—this is considered "organic" diarrhea until proven otherwise.

3. There is no reason to suspect iatrogenic diarrhea or systemic (non-gastrointestinal) disease. There is no history here of drug or laxative use or of prior abdominal surgery; nor are there any systemic clues on physical examination (see Table 3–9).

4. There is very good reason to suspect parasitic infestation or food intolerance or both.

Ernie's travel history speaks for itself. Multiple negative stool examinations for parasites usually exclude consideration of giardiasis, amebiasis, and rarer pathogens (Table 3–6), but not always. A high index of suspicion demands further testing or a therapeutic trial.

Lactose intolerance is subjectively well documented here, and thus strict avoidance of all milk products should be confirmed by a careful diet history (see Appendix IV).

5. The history suggests involvement of the small intestine (or proximal colon), rather than the distal colon. Ernie's diarrhea is (by description) large-stool diarrhea that is homogeneous in appearance and associated with periumbilical abdominal discomfort. There are no symptoms suggesting distal colon disease. As noted above, this diarrhea pattern suggests small-bowel or proximal colon disease—it may be seen with inflammatory bowel disease and various disorders of malabsorption, but lactose intolerance or parasitic infestation will cause this pattern as well.

6. There are no clinical findings that themselves warrant specific investigations. The stool examination demonstrates no blood or fecal leukocytes.

The differential diagnosis of fecal leukocytosis has been discussed previously. In the patient with chronic diarrhea and fecal leukocytosis, proctoscopy and barium enema are always indicated.

Diarrhea with (gross or occult) blood in the stool always demands immediate attention. This subject deserves a brief diversion.

---

*Always review the patient's sleep pattern when diarrhea is nocturnal. More than a few anxious patients with "functional" diarrhea will also have insomnia—nocturnal diarrhea refers not just to the time of day when diarrhea occurs but to the fact that sleep is disturbed by the diarrhea.

1. **Define "diarrhea!"** — Subjectively: Change in normal pattern? ≥3 bowel movements per day?
   Objectively: Stool weight >300 gm/24 hr? — No → Review history! "True" diarrhea? "Small stool" (irritable bowel) diarrhea

NO

2. **Iatrogenic diarrhea?** ——————— Medication? ————→ Discontinue
   Postoperative? ————→ Appendix III
   Laxative (ab)use? ————→ Discontinue

NO

3. **Systemic disease/"systemic clues"** — Thorough physical examination! Table 3–9 ——Evaluate accordingly
   "Organic"? Weight loss? Nocturnal diarrhea?

NO

4. **Travel history/parasites suspected?** ——————— Three stools for ———→ Parasite identified! → Table 3–6
   ova and parasites   None found ———→ Duodenal aspiration? (*Giardia*)
   ↓
   Therapeutic trial? (Table 3–6)   Procto/colonoscopy? and/or Amebic serology? (amebiasis)

NO

5. **Suspect food-related diarrhea?** Lactose intolerance? ———→ Lactose tolerance test? (Appendix IV)
   Therapeutic diet trial?

NO

6. **Stool hemoccult?** ——————— Positive ——————→ | Always investigate! | Inflammatory bowel disease? Neoplasm?

Stool leukocytes? ——————— Fecal white blood cells present ——————→ Inflammatory bowel disease? | Investigate! | Stool cultures!

NO

↓

CHRONIC DIARRHEA, NO OBVIOUS CAUSE BY HISTORY/EXAMINATION

Stool for ova and parasites! ——————————Diagnostic ——————————→ Table 3–6

Negative

Symptoms suggest distal colon?   Small, frequent, inhomogeneous stool? — PROCTOSCOPY ——→ PROCTITIS? (Appendix I)
   Rectal urgency, left lower quadrant pain?   ↓ Normal?

No
or
workup negative

All features suggest irritable bowel?   Any features atypical of irritable bowel?
   ↓   ↓
Treat irritable bowel ——————— No better? ——→ Barium enema Colonoscopy?

Proximal bowel symptoms? ——————— Large, homogeneous stool? ——————————→ Lactose intolerance? → Test? (Fig. 3–5)
   Periumbilical, right lower quadrant pain?   Inflammatory bowel disease?

Barium studies non-diagnostic   Upper GI with small bowel follow through Barium enema CBC, sedimentation rate, electrolytes

or

Symptoms/clues suggest: (Table 3–9) ——————————————→ Metabolic/systemic disease? Thyroid function, glucose, BUN, calcium, cortisols (Tables 3–7 and 3–8)

Malabsorption? ——————→ Large stool diarrhea, weight loss, ——————→ 72-hr fecal fat collection
   abnormal serum vitamin B_{12}, carotene, albumin, protime   See Figure 3–16

↓

FIGURE 3–6. Chronic diarrhea: An approach.

Illustration continued on opposite page

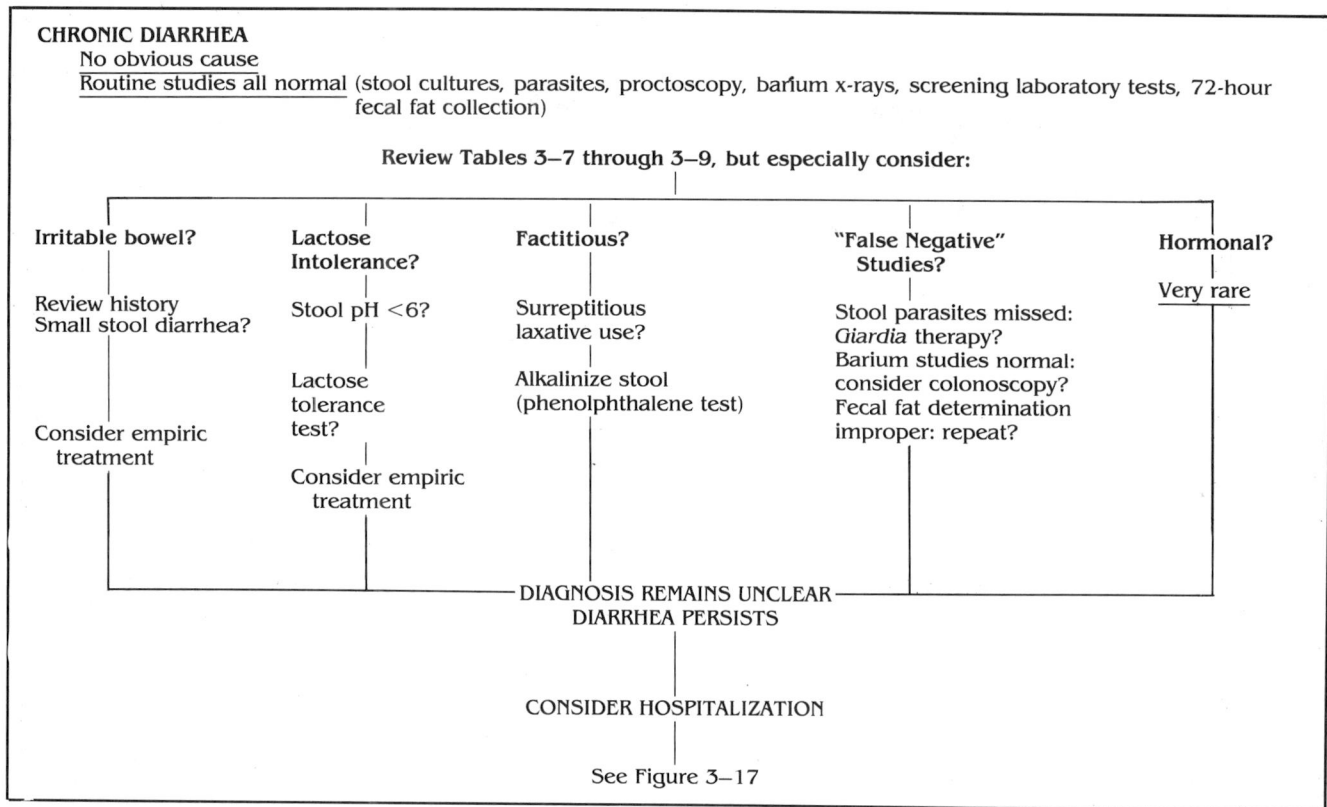

CHRONIC DIARRHEA
No obvious cause
Routine studies all normal (stool cultures, parasites, proctoscopy, barium x-rays, screening laboratory tests, 72-hour fecal fat collection)

Review Tables 3–7 through 3–9, but especially consider:

Irritable bowel?

Review history
Small stool diarrhea?

Consider empiric treatment

Lactose Intolerance?

Stool pH <6?

Lactose tolerance test?

Consider empiric treatment

Factitious?

Surreptitious laxative use?

Alkalinize stool (phenolphthalene test)

"False Negative" Studies?

Stool parasites missed: Giardia therapy?
Barium studies normal: consider colonoscopy?
Fecal fat determination improper: repeat?

Hormonal?

Very rare

DIAGNOSIS REMAINS UNCLEAR
DIARRHEA PERSISTS

CONSIDER HOSPITALIZATION

See Figure 3–17

FIGURE 3–6. *Continued.*

Chronic Bloody Diarrhea

In the young patient, chronic bloody (or heme-positive) diarrhea usually results from ulcerative colitis, although Crohn's disease, amebic colitis, and various forms of proctocolitis (see Appendix I) must always be remembered as well.

Ulcerative colitis typically afflicts patients under the age of 50 years (although 20 to 25 per cent of cases may begin later in life) and usually causes chronic, relapsing bouts of (grossly) bloody diarrhea and abdominal pain, each bout usually lasting a few weeks. The first bout is often the most severe and dangerous,[61, 62] but onset of ulcerative colitis may also be indolent and mild and is not infrequently mistaken for irritable bowel syndrome. Proctoscopy with rectal biopsy will usually establish the diagnosis,[63] since more than 90 per cent of patients with ulcerative colitis will have abnormal proctoscopic and histologic findings (although the gross and microscopic appearance may be mimicked by many other causes of proctocolitis—see Appendix I). The barium enema (Fig. 3–7) usually documents the extent of disease (there is a substantial prognostic difference between "pancolitis" and "limited" ulcerative proctitis[64]) and also excludes other disorders (especially colon cancer).

Acute ulcerative colitis is usually treated with sulfasalazine or corticosteroids.[65, 66] Hospitalization is sometimes required for the acutely ill patient, especially if toxic megacolon (Fig. 3–8), severe abdominal pain, or extensive bleeding occurs. Medical therapy (sulfasalazine or steroids) will help prevent recurrences, but surgical colectomy is the only definitive cure (but fortunately is necessary only uncommonly).

FIGURE 3–7. This 44-year-old man complained of intermittent bloody diarrhea, lower abdominal cramps, and rectal urgency for 3 weeks. Examination was unremarkable except for mild lower abdominal tenderness and (occult) heme-positive stool. Proctoscopy revealed mild, nonspecific inflammation, but this barium enema demonstrates extensive involvement of the transverse, descending, and rectosigmoid colon by (biopsy-proven) ulcerative colitis. Note that there is "thumb printing" in the left colon.

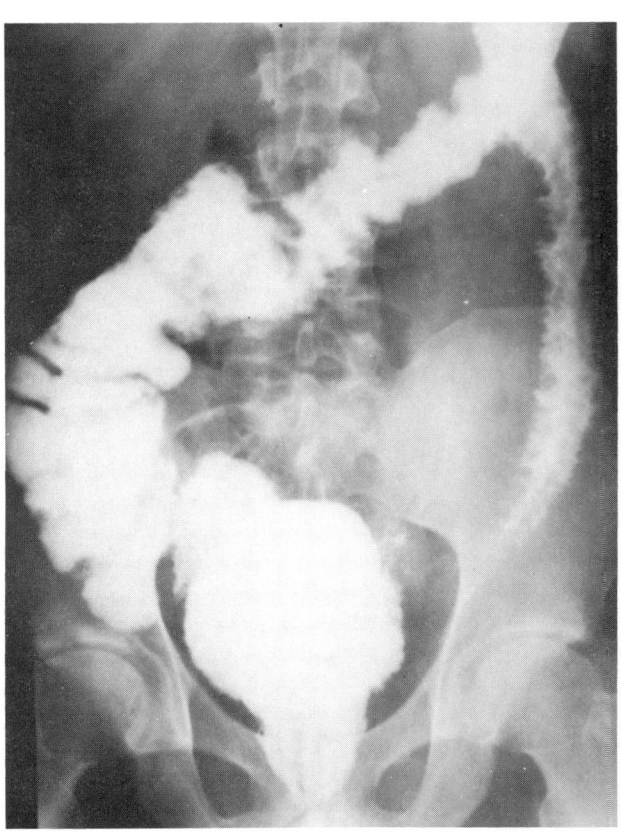

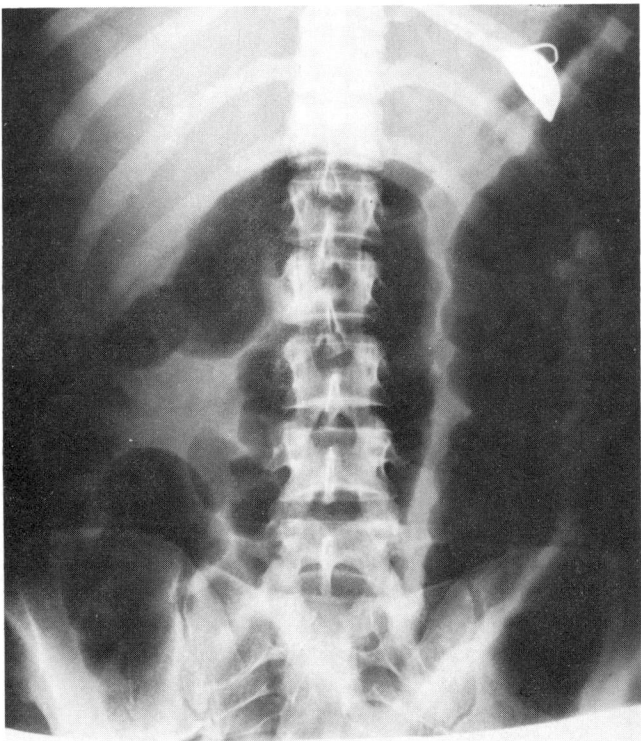

FIGURE 3–8. This 32-year-old woman presented with 2 months of intermittent bloody diarrhea, followed by 3 days of worsening abdominal pain and fever with diminution of diarrhea. She was very ill. X-rays revealed dilatation and edema of the large bowel—"toxic megacolon."

Hospitalization, IV fluids, and corticosteroids did not improve the situation. Total colectomy was required (pathology: severe ulcerative *pancolitis*).

FIGURE 3–9. Crohn's disease. This 33-year-old woman complained of intermittent diarrhea, periumbilical abdominal discomfort, and mild weight loss over the previous 8 months. Prior investigations had revealed no infectious etiology, and a previous barium swallow, proctoscopy, and barium enema had been normal. This small bowel x-ray demonstrates extensive narrowing and inflammation of the distal 25 to 30 cm of the ileum *(arrows)*. Systemic corticosteroids, followed by maintenance sulfasalazine (Azulfidine), resulted in prompt remission.

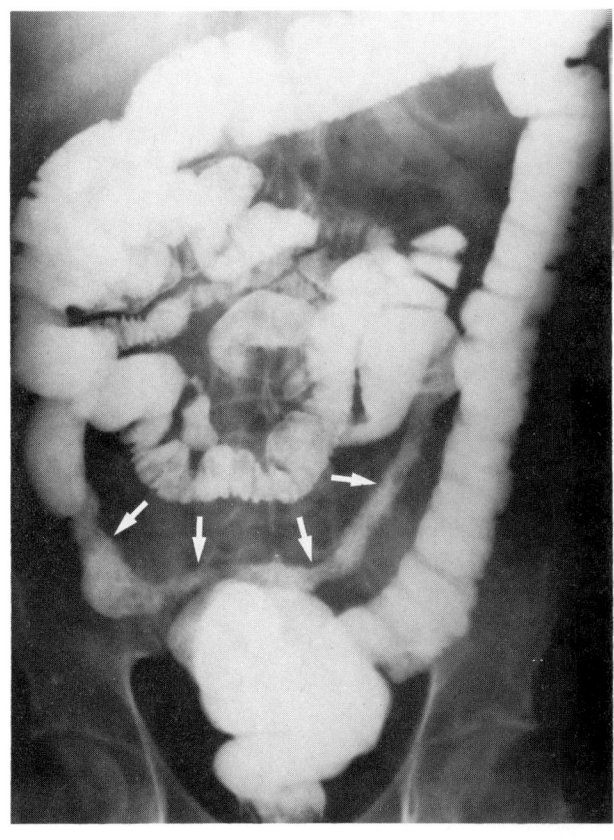

Occasionally, yersinia[18] or amebic enterocolitis[67] will simulate acute ulcerative colitis in all clinical and radiographic respects, just as various infectious types of proctitis can mimic ulcerative proctitis. Stool cultures and parasite searches should always be obtained in the patient with chronic bloody diarrhea (amebic serologic studies or colonoscopic biopsy specimens examined directly for parasites should be obtained when suspicion of amebiasis is high).

Sometimes Crohn's disease limited to the colon (Crohn's—or granulomatous—colitis) is difficult to distinguish from ulcerative colitis. Features that favor Crohn's disease include "sparing" of the rectum, prominent perianal disease (or fistulas), extensive cecal colitis without sigmoid colitis, patchy involvement ("skip lesion") on barium enema, and definite "full-thickness" granulomatous histologic findings on proctoscopic (or colonoscopic) biopsies. Conversely, ulcerative colitis is usually a mucosal (not full-thickness) nongranulomatous inflammatory process involving an anatomically contiguous segment of bowel, most commonly the rectosigmoid colon, without perianal disease or fistula formation.

Disease limited to the colon occurs in only about one quarter of patients with Crohn's disease. In most patients the small intestine, the ileocolic area, or both (Figs. 3–9 and 3–10) are the major sites of disease,[68, 69] but any site in the gastrointestinal tract may be affected. Crohn's disease (regional enteritis) typically afflicts young adults (75 per cent of cases begin before the age of 40 years) and induces recurrent bouts of diarrhea, lower abdominal pain, weight loss, and (sometimes) fever, often remitting and relapsing

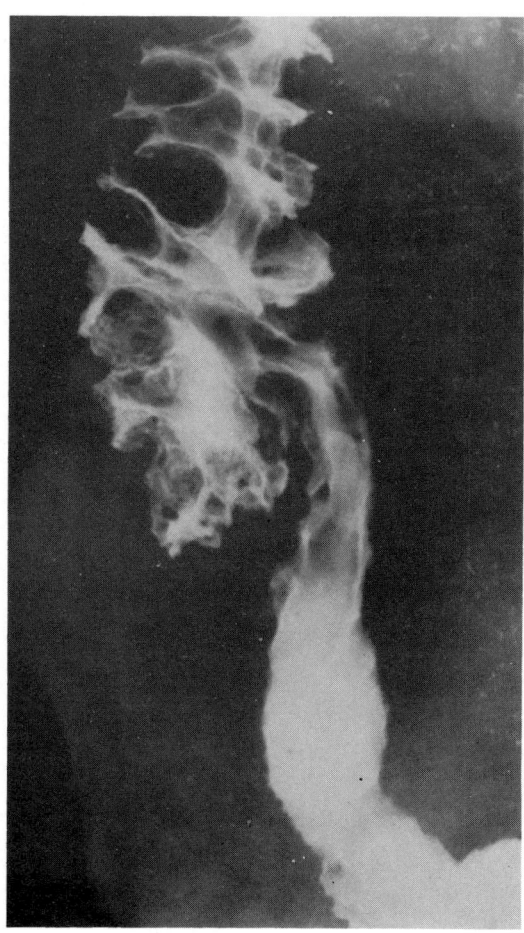

FIGURE 3–10. This 22-year-old man complained of 3 months of right lower quadrant discomfort and intermittent diarrhea. Barium enema demonstrated extensive inflammation and "thumb printing" of the cecum with narrowing and inflammatory changes of the terminal ileum. Despite systemic corticosteroids, resection of this segment of bowel was ultimately necessary. Crohn's disease was proven pathologically.

spontaneously. Crohn's disease may produce acute severe illness, but more often it becomes apparent only after prolonged clinical illness (the delay between onset of symptoms and clinical diagnosis averaged 3 years in the National Cooperative Crohn's Disease Study).[69] Extraintestinal manifestations—arthritis, uveitis, skin lesions (see Table 3–9)—may occasionally antedate gastrointestinal symptoms or overshadow them.[70]

The diagnosis of Crohn's disease usually depends on characteristic radiographic abnormalities on barium x-rays (Figs. 3–9 and 3–10) or the biopsies obtained during proctoscopy or colonoscopy,[72] but such findings must always be correlated with the clinical history and examination. Yersinia enterocolitis, for example can cause a subacute illness (weeks in duration) with radiographic abnormalities suggestive of Crohn's disease, and yet it will resolve completely with appropriate antibiotic treatment. Thus, the recurrent and relapsing natural history of Crohn's disease is often crucial to diagnosis. Treatment[65, 66] usually involves oral corticosteroids (or sulfasalazine 4 to 6 gm a day in mild cases); surgery is avoided whenever possible, since surgical resection does not cure the disease (as it does in ulcerative colitis), but more than half of patients with Crohn's disease ultimately require some surgical resection. Hospitalization is frequently required during acute and recurrent illness.

In the older patient, chronic/subacute bloody diarrhea should also suggest colon cancer or, rarely, ischemic colitis. Ischemic colitis[74] refers to a process that may have an acute onset (frank hematochezia) or progress to frank bowel infarction, but it may sometimes follow a more benign and subacute course. Proctoscopy may be helpful when ischemic proctitis is observed,[35] but barium enemas often reveal characteristic thumbprinting of the (usually distal) colon (Fig. 3–11). As Sullivan's review emphasizes,[8] ischemic proctocolitis is but one of several distinctive intestinal vascular disease syndromes.

Fecal impaction with stercoral ulceration may cause subacute bloody diarrhea, especially in the elderly. Diverticular bleeding[75, 76] may be the most

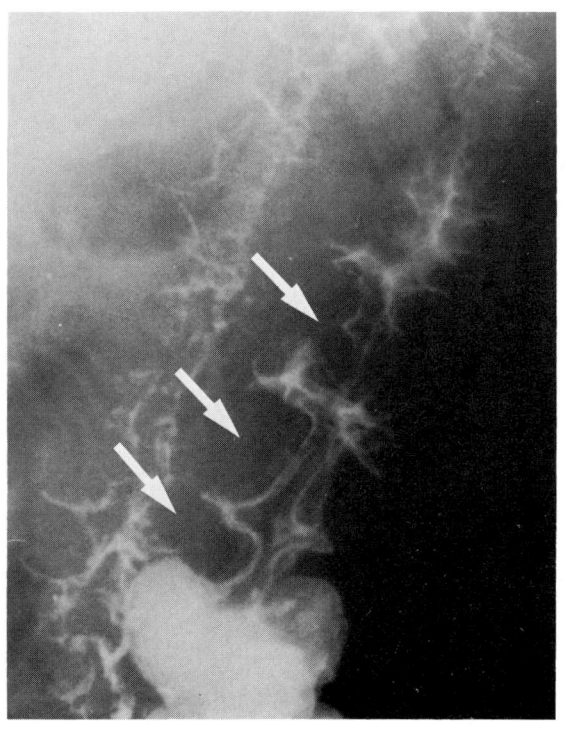

FIGURE 3–11. This 67-year-old man presented with 1 week of bloody diarrhea. Examination was relatively unremarkable, except for mild left upper quadrant discomfort and frank hematochezia. Barium enema demonstrated narrowing and "thumb printing" *(arrows)* of an isolated segment of the splenic flexure of the colon. This is a characteristic appearance of ischemic colitis, but colonoscopy was performed to exclude ulcerative colitis and Crohn's disease. The patient improved spontaneously without further ischemic events.

common cause of rectal bleeding in adults over all (except for hemorrhoids), but diverticulosis usually presents with acute hematochezia rather than with chronic insidious rectal bleeding and diarrhea. Diverticulitis may cause heme-positive diarrhea, but this, too, is usually more acute, and the pain and tenderness usually overshadow any bleeding.

Thus, chronic bloody diarrhea will raise different clinical suspicions, depending upon the patient's age and other clinical clues. Immediate investigation is always required.

As Figure 3–6 illustrates, a careful history and physical examination of the patient with chronic diarrhea usually will suggest a specific diagnosis.

In Ernie's case, parasitic infestation and continuing lactose intolerance both seem a good bet.

> A lactose tolerance test is performed. Abdominal cramping and worsening of diarrhea occur within 1 hour of lactose ingestion, and the blood glucose rises only 10 mg per 100 ml over a 2-hour period. Nevertheless, careful review of Ernie's diet detects few, if any, lactose-containing foods (see appendix IV), and the stool pH is greater than 7.

> Stool cultures are repeated and three separate specimens of fresh stool are collected for ova and parasite examinations. Metronidazole, 750 mg tid, is prescribed for 7 days.

Therapeutic Trials

NOTE

I. Lactose intolerance is documented, but its significance is uncertain.

Lactose intolerance is so common that its objective documentation does not necessarily diagnose the cause of diarrhea, unless a lactose-free diet (see Appendix IV) also eliminates symptoms. Thus, in this case, it is difficult to implicate lactose intolerance alone. (The stool pH greater than 7 is also "soft" evidence that lactose intolerance is not a major culprit at this time.)

II. Despite the negative stool studies, a therapeutic trial of antiparasitic medication is a reasonable option here.

As noted above, giardiasis will cause proximal bowel diarrhea, may induce reversible lactose intolerance, and may be missed, especially if inexperienced parasitologists examine the stool.

The large dose of metronidazole (750 mg tid) is chosen to cover both giardiasis and the very unlikely possibility of amebiasis (Table 3–6). (Ernie's travel history is impressive).

There are several clinical situations in which the therapeutic trial may be worthwhile for the patient with chronic diarrhea: in general, when therapy is benign and when a diagnosis is strongly suspected but difficult (expensive or inconvenient) to prove. Table 3–10 lists some such clinical situations and the indicated therapeutic trial. In general, such strategies should be restricted to the use of short courses of antibiotics or antiparasitic agents, dietary changes, and occasionally other maneuvers (for example, pancreatic enzyme replacement). These treatments should be undertaken only when there is strong presumptive evidence of the disease in question.

TABLE 3–10. THERAPEUTIC TRIALS IN CHRONIC DIARRHEA

TREATMENT	CONSIDER WHEN SUSPECT	"PROOF" OF DIAGNOSIS
Antibiotics		
Tetracycline 2.5 gm, single dose, or	Prolonged turista	*Escherichia coli* toxin studies?
Trimethoprim-sulfamethoxazole 160/800 mg bid		Exclude parasites, bacterial disease
Tetracycline 500 mg qid × 2 weeks	Bacterial overgrowth syndromes (blind loops, stasis, diverticula of small bowel, etc.)	Schilling test Small-bowel cultures Bile acid breath test
Metronidazole 250 mg tid × 7 days, or	Giardiasis	Stool ova and parasites × 3
Quinacrine 100 mg tid × 7 days		Duodenal aspiration
Metronidazole 750 mg tid × 7 days, or	Amebiasis	Stool parasites × 3 Proctoscopy
Diiodohydroxyquin 650 mg tid × 20 days		Colonoscopy Serologies
Tetracycline 250 mg qid × 2 weeks, plus folic acid, 1 mg bid	Tropical sprue*	Small-bowel biopsy
Procaine penicillin 600,000 units IM bid × 10 days, and/or streptomycin	Whipple's disease*	Small-bowel biopsy
Sulfasalazine		
Sulfasalazine 1.0 gm qid	Crohn's disease*/ulcerative colitis*	Barium studies Colonoscopy Clinical course
Diet		
Lactose free	Lactose intolerance	Lactose tolerance test and/or small-bowel biopsy
Gluten free	Celiac sprue*	Small-bowel biopsy
Low fat	Steatorrhea, whatever cause	See Fig. 3–16
High fiber	Irritable bowel, diverticular disease	Clinical findings Barium enema
Elimination diet	Food allergy	Response to diet
Low carbohydrate, frequent feedings	Dumping syndrome	See App. III
Others		
Pancreatic enzyme replacement	Pancreatic exocrine insufficiency	Exocrine pancreatic function tests See App. V
Cholestyramine 4 gm tid or qid	Postcholecystectomy diarrhea Postileal resection	See App. III
Corticosteroid enemas	Limited proctitis (noninfectious)	See App. I
Bulk agents, Metamucil, etc.	Irritable bowel, diverticular disease	

*Proof of diagnosis should always be attempted when these disorders are suspected. Therapeutic trials are only rarely indicated in such patients.

Systemic corticosteroids should never be used in a therapeutic trial (except perhaps in patients hospitalized with severe clinical inflammatory bowel disease, before definitive studies can be performed).

All stool studies are normal. Ten days later, Ernie's diarrhea persists, unchanged. Ernie is eating normally, but now has lost an additional 4 pounds (10 pounds total).

NOTE

III. Diarrhea persists.

As Figure 3–6 suggests, proctoscopy, barium x-rays of the upper and lower bowel, and screening laboratory studies are now indicated in Ernie's case. Several disorders should be excluded:

Inflammatory bowel disease (especially Crohn's disease) must be considered.

Intestinal neoplasms, both rare and common varieties, may present with persistent diarrhea. Colorectal adenocarcinoma, by far the most common colon cancer, will do so in about 10 per cent of cases. Villous adenoma "secretes" water and mucus and often induces major fluid loss with hypokalemia and acid-base disturbances. Intestinal lymphomas[77] are rare and usually do not present as nonspecific chronic diarrhea (abdominal pain, weight loss, constipation, and palpable lymphadenopathy are more common). Carcinoid tumors are very rare[78] but may easily be missed on radiographic examination.

Malabsorption should be strongly considered in Ernie's case. Persistent proximal bowel diarrhea, weight loss in spite of normal food intake, and documented lactose intolerance should suggest the possibility of a primary malabsorptive disease (with secondary lactose intolerance). Proof of malabsorption generally centers around quantitative (72-hour) fecal fat excretion, and subsequent differential diagnosis depends on initial documentation of excessive fecal fat excretion (page 138). Several "screening tests" may be used here, but each is nonspecific and insensitive. These include:

A. Microscopic stool examination for fat (see Fig. 3–12A)

Small specimens of stool (5 mm in diameter) are mixed with water (2 drops) and then 95 per cent ethyl alcohol (2 drops). Several drops of saturated solution of Sudan III in 95 per cent ethyl alcohol are then added, and this preparation is examined under a coverslip at high dry microscopic magnification. Numerous yellow or pale orange refractile fat globules usually correlate reasonably well with subsequent quantitative demonstration of steatorrhea.[79]

B. Blood specimens that reveal macrocytic anemia (due to folate or vitamin B_{12} deficiency), hypoalbuminemia, hypoprothrombinemia, decreased serum cholesterol or carotene all point to malabsorption, but all are both insensitive and nonspecific as screening tests.

Complete blood count, BUN, electrolytes, glucose, cholesterol, liver enzymes, calcium, phosphate, thyroid function tests, protein electrophoresis, and serum carotene are all normal. A stool specimen is alkalinized with sodium hydroxide but is negative for phenolphthalein. Sedimentation rate is 32.

What does this mean?

1. The normal blood tests help in two ways: (1) They exclude a few unlikely systemic causes of chronic diarrhea—hyperthyroidism, hypoparathyroidism, diabetes mellitus, uremia, severe liver disease, and agammaglobulinemia. (2) They indicate that there are no dangerous electrolyte

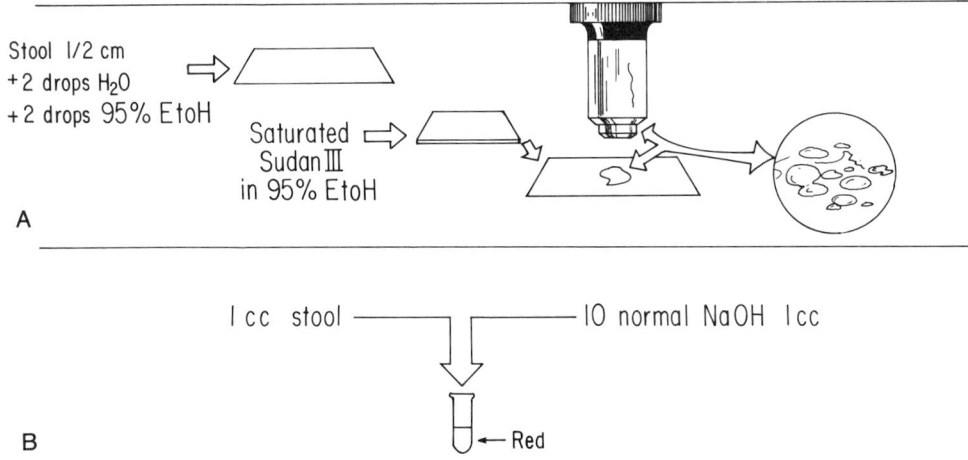

Stool 1/2 cm
+2 drops H₂O
+2 drops 95% EtOH

Saturated Sudan III in 95% EtOH

A

1 cc stool —————————————— 10 normal NaOH 1 cc

← Red

B

FIGURE 3–12. A, Microscopic examination for stool fat (see text, p. 135). B, Addition of 10 normal sodium hydroxide to stool will result in red coloration of the mixture when phenolphthalein laxatives are present.

imbalances induced by the chronic diarrhea. In addition, if malabsorption is present, it is not severe or protracted enough to have caused anemia or hypoproteinemia. These results, however, by no means exclude malabsorption.

2. Alkalinization of the stool (with sodium hydroxide)—Figure 3–12B—will turn stool red if phenolphthalein laxative derivatives are present. (Nonphenolphthalein laxatives will not be detected by simple stool alkalinization, and other tests are needed.) Chronic diarrhea due to surreptitious laxative abuse is not a common problem,[80, 81] but it may be a very difficult diagnosis to make. Sophisticated studies are often required.[80]

Proctoscopy, barium enema, and upper GI series with small-bowel follow-through are completely normal, except for equivocal dilatation of proximal jejunal bowel loops.

NOTE

1. A normal proctoscopic examination excludes the various forms of proctocolitis (see Appendix I), rectal neoplasms, and, usually, ulcerative colitis.[7]

2. The normal barium studies are strong, but by no means absolute, evidence against the diagnosis of an intestinal neoplasm.

As many as 15 to 20 per cent of colon cancers may be missed on routine barium enema[82, 83] (air contrast barium enema is probably more sensitive). Thus, unexplained occult blood in the stool or a family history of colorectal carcinoma (especially in older patients with new symptoms) will occasionally require colonoscopy to exclude colon neoplasms even when barium x-rays are normal.

3. Similarly, the barium studies do not exclude inflammatory bowel disease, but Crohn's disease and ulcerative colitis are much less likely in such a setting. As we shall see, the normal barium studies are also helpful in the differential diagnosis of malabsorption (see below).

A diet of 100 gm of fat per day is begun (lactose free), and stools are collected for 72 hours during the fourth, fifth, and sixth days of that diet. Pending results, an abdominal flat plate from the barium enema is reviewed: No pancreatic calcifications are visible, and there is no evidence of bowel dilatation.

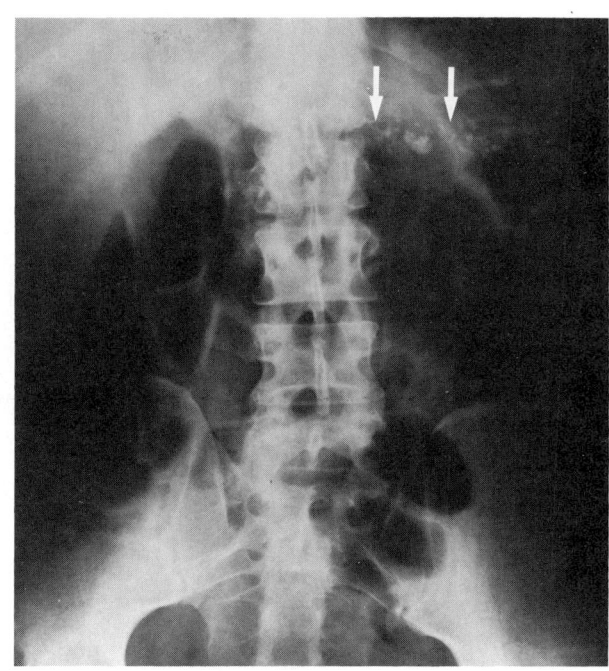

FIGURE 3–13. This 46-year-old alcoholic described chronic, worsening diarrhea over the previous 6 months. He had lost 10 pounds in spite of a normal appetite. Physical examination was completely unremarkable. Tests for infectious pathogens and barium x-rays were unremarkable. Steatorrhea was documented (72-hour fecal fat: 64 gm). Review of the abdominal flat plate at the time of the barium enema demonstrates extensive calcification within the pancreas (left upper quadrant) *(arrows)*. Pancreatic enzyme replacement resulted in marked symptomatic improvement.

NOTE

1. The plain abdominal x-ray is helpful in two ways. (1) It demonstrates no pancreatic calcifications (Fig. 3–13): Such a finding would be most helpful, especially if steatorrhea is documented (see below). (2) Such an x-ray should always be obtained before barium studies in the patient with possible colonic inflammatory bowel disease, to exclude toxic megacolon (Fig. 3–8). (Most patients with toxic megacolon are very ill and require hospitalization and often presumptive therapy without barium studies. Clinically, Ernie does not have toxic megacolon.)

2. In Appendix IV the diet used for the 72-hour fecal fat collection is described. This test can easily be done on an ambulatory basis if patients are instructed properly. Hospitalization is occasionally required to ensure more accurate results. When both fat collections and barium studies are planned, the former should be done first, since barium and the various bowel preparations may interfere with fecal fat collections.

It should be noted, as Figure 3–6 suggests, that when all of these tests are normal in the patient with chronic diarrhea, it is much more likely that we have missed a common problem than that a very rare disorder is the culprit. The history must be carefully reviewed (for example, is diarrhea due to the irritable bowel?), diets reexamined (lactose, for example), embarrassing questions asked (about laxative abuse and sexual habits, for example), and all prior studies reviewed carefully to exclude "false-negative" results of x-rays, fecal fat collections, or stool examination. Only after these considerations (and perhaps a diarrhea check list—see Tables 3–7 to 3–9) are reviewed should hospitalization and more sophisticated studies be considered.

In this case, however, all studies are not normal.

Fecal fat excretion for 72 hours measures 49 gm in a total stool output weighing 2100 gm.

Steatorrhea[84-86]

Steatorrhea is defined as excretion of more than 7 gm of fat per 24 hours while the patient is maintained on a 100 gm-per-day fat diet. Since a 72-hour collection is usually recommended, more than 21 gm of fat excreted in 72 hours (greater than 7 percent of ingested total fat) is considered abnormal. Such results are reliable only if the diet is carefully followed, fat ingestion is quantitated, and the stool collection is complete (see Appendix IV).

When chronic diarrhea is associated with excessive fecal fat excretion, one (or more) of three basic physiologic processes must be abnormal: intraluminal lipolysis, micellar fat solubilization, or mucosal fat uptake and transport. Ingested fat (mainly triglycerides) is hydrolyzed in the proximal small bowel by pancreatic enzymes (especially lipase). The hydrolyzed products—the fatty acids and monoglycerides—are insoluble in water and thus cannot be absorbed unless they are incorporated into "micelles," after which they can passively diffuse into the intestinal mucosal epithelial cell. (These solubilizing micelles are composed of bile acids secreted by the hepatobiliary system into the proximal small bowel after food ingestion.) Once fatty acids and monoglycerides are thus solubilized and diffuse into the intestinal mucosa, they can be reesterified into triglycerides within the intestinal epithelial cell and incorporated into chylomicrons that are then transported via the lymphatics into the systemic circulation. Figure 3–14 illustrates these different stages of fat digestion and absorption.

While the differential diagnosis of steatorrhea is large, the practical diagnostic approach usually centers around analysis of these three basic physiologic processes responsible for fat absorption: intraluminal lipolysis

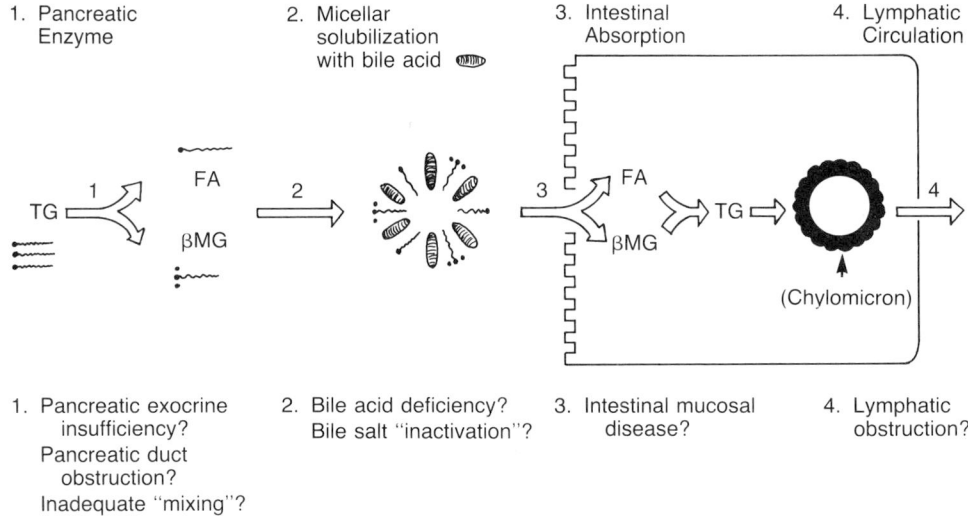

1. Pancreatic Enzyme
2. Micellar solubilization with bile acid
3. Intestinal Absorption
4. Lymphatic Circulation

1. Pancreatic exocrine insufficiency? Pancreatic duct obstruction? Inadequate "mixing"?
2. Bile acid deficiency? Bile salt "inactivation"?
3. Intestinal mucosal disease?
4. Lymphatic obstruction?

FIGURE 3–14. Fat digestion and absorption. The various causes of steatorrhea will interrupt one or more of these four key steps.

1. Pancreatic exocrine insufficiency, pancreatic duct obstruction and/or inadequate "mixing" of pancreatic enzymes with ingested food will impair the initial breakdown of triglycerides.

2. Bile acid deficiencies or bile salt "inactivation" or both will interfere with micelle formation and solubilization of bile acids.

3. A whole variety of diseases that affect the intestinal mucosa will interfere with intestinal absorption.

4. Disorders of lymphatics—lymphatic obstruction, lymphangiectasia—will interfere with the last step.

(Key: TG = triglycerides; FA = fatty acids; BMG = Beta monoglycerides.)

(pancreatic function), micelle formation (bile acid delivery), and intestinal mucosal cell integrity. There are many different tests that can analyze each of these physiologic processes, but usually a careful clinical history and physical examination, together with barium x-rays and the quantitative fecal fat determination, will allow selective testing or suggest a therapeutic trial without extensive testing.

CONSIDER

1. Insufficient pancreatic enzyme activity usually results from exocrine pancreatic insufficiency due to chronic pancreatitis, pancreatic resection, or cystic fibrosis. Chronic pancreatitis is usually recognized after unmistakable painful recurrences of acute pancreatitis documented over the course of many years, usually in the alcoholic patient, at times ultimately resulting in visible pancreatic calcification on abdominal x-rays (Fig. 3–13). Cystic fibrosis may now be seen in adolescents or young adults, but usually there is an obvious associated history of chronic respiratory problems.

Occasionally, pancreatic duct obstruction (by stone or neoplasm) may be responsible, as may a variety of surgical procedures (gastrectomy, vagotomy and pyloroplasty, for example) that impair mixing of ingested food fat with pancreatic enzymes. A history of these surgical procedures will usually be obvious.

Thus, pancreatic causes of steatorrhea often will be strongly suspected purely on the basis of the clinical history (or calcifications on abdominal x-rays). When this is so, pancreatic enzymes can be prescribed as a therapeutic trial (see Appendix V). More sophisticated studies of pancreatic exocrine function[87] often will not be necessary.

2. Bile acid deficiencies may reflect either insufficient delivery of bile acids (due to hepatobiliary disease, surgical biliary diversion, cholecystocolonic fistulas, for example) or cumulative fecal loss of bile acids (usually due to ileal disease or ileal surgical resection). Bile salt inactivation by overgrowth of enteric bacteria in the small intestine is a more common cause of bile acid deficiency.[88] Such bacterial overgrowth syndromes will usually be due to prior surgery (gastrectomy, intestinal resection, blind loop formation), or radiographically visible abnormalities (small bowel diverticula, strictures or fistulas), or specific clinical disorders (diabetic enteropathy, scleroderma, radiation enteritis, or achlorhydria).

Remember, such bile acid deficiencies will usually be strongly suspected on the basis of the clinical and surgical history, as well as examination of the barium x-rays. When this is the problem, broad-spectrum antibiotic therapy (Table 3–10) or reversal of the primary anatomic disorder will be helpful. At times, the Schilling test (with intrinsic factor, before and after broad-spectrum antibiotic therapy),[86] small-bowel cultures,[88] or the bile acid breath test[89] will help—both to document the problem and to objectively follow the response to therapy.

3. Intestinal mucosal disorders are many, and the clinical and radiographic findings (Fig. 3–15) alone are often inadequate to achieve a specific diagnosis. As noted in Table 3–9, certain clues may suggest Whipple's disease, celiac sprue, parasitic infestation, amyloidosis, or mesenteric ischemic disease, but usually a diagnostic peroral small-bowel biopsy is required[86, 90] when these disorders are suspected.

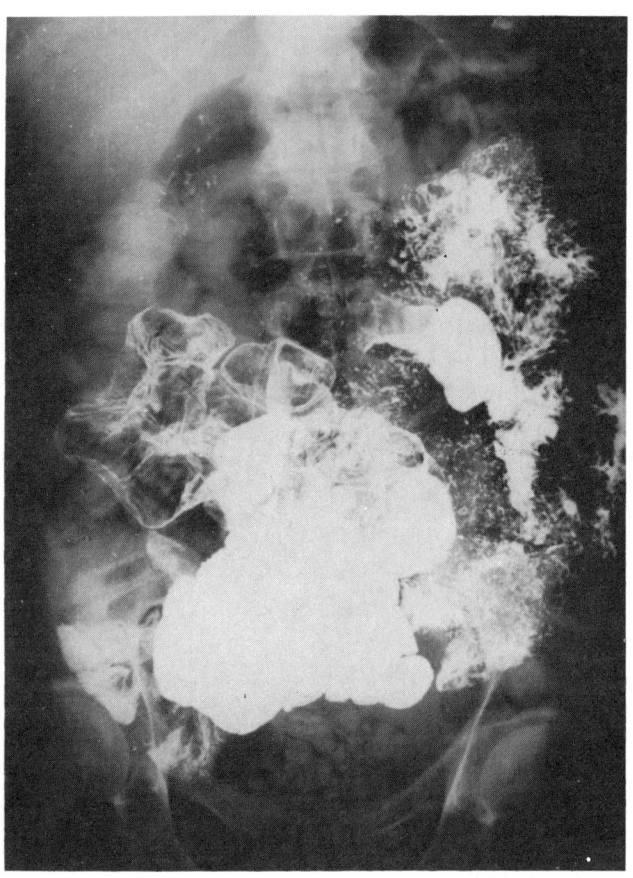

FIGURE 3–15. This 52-year-old chronic alcoholic presented with chronic diarrhea and weight loss. Steatorrhea was documented. This small bowel series was initially interpreted as "compatible with celiac sprue," but pancreatic enzyme replacement alone resulted in amelioration of symptoms and marked reduction of steatorrhea after a small bowel biopsy was normal.

The barium x-ray has a very limited role in the diagnosis of intestinal mucosal disease. Nonspecific abnormalities are common.

In Ernie's case, then, what should be done now? Figure 3–16 illustrates a general approach to the problem of steatorrhea.

1. On the basis of the clinical history, it is very unlikely that pancreatic insufficiency is responsible for Ernie's diarrhea. Some authorities recommend that a D-xylose excretion test be performed at this point[86] to help resolve this issue. This test involves oral administration of 25 gm of xylose (a five-carbon monosaccharide normally absorbed by the proximal small intestine via passive diffusion), followed by a 5-hour urine collection from which is measured quantitative xylose excretion (excretion of more than 4.5 gm implies normal xylose absorption). When xylose excretion is normal in the patient with steatorrhea, pancreatic insufficiency is more likely since such a result usually implies integrity of the small-bowel mucosa (and since bacterial overgrowth syndromes—the most common subtle cause of bile salt deficiency—usually also result in abnormal xylose excretion). When xylose excretion is low, jejunal mucosal disease or bacterial overgrowth syndromes are more likely. Difficulties in interpretations of the D-xylose test have somewhat lessened its diagnostic usefulness: Variations in the patient's age and renal function, as well as various "artifacts" (vomiting, inadequate hydration, delayed gastric emptying) during testing may be responsible for "falsely low" xylose excretion.

2. There is no clinical or radiographic reason to suspect a bacterial overgrowth syndrome or any other bile salt disorder. Such an impression does not exclude these disorders, but as implied in Figure 3–16, it is reasonable in this case to conclude that:

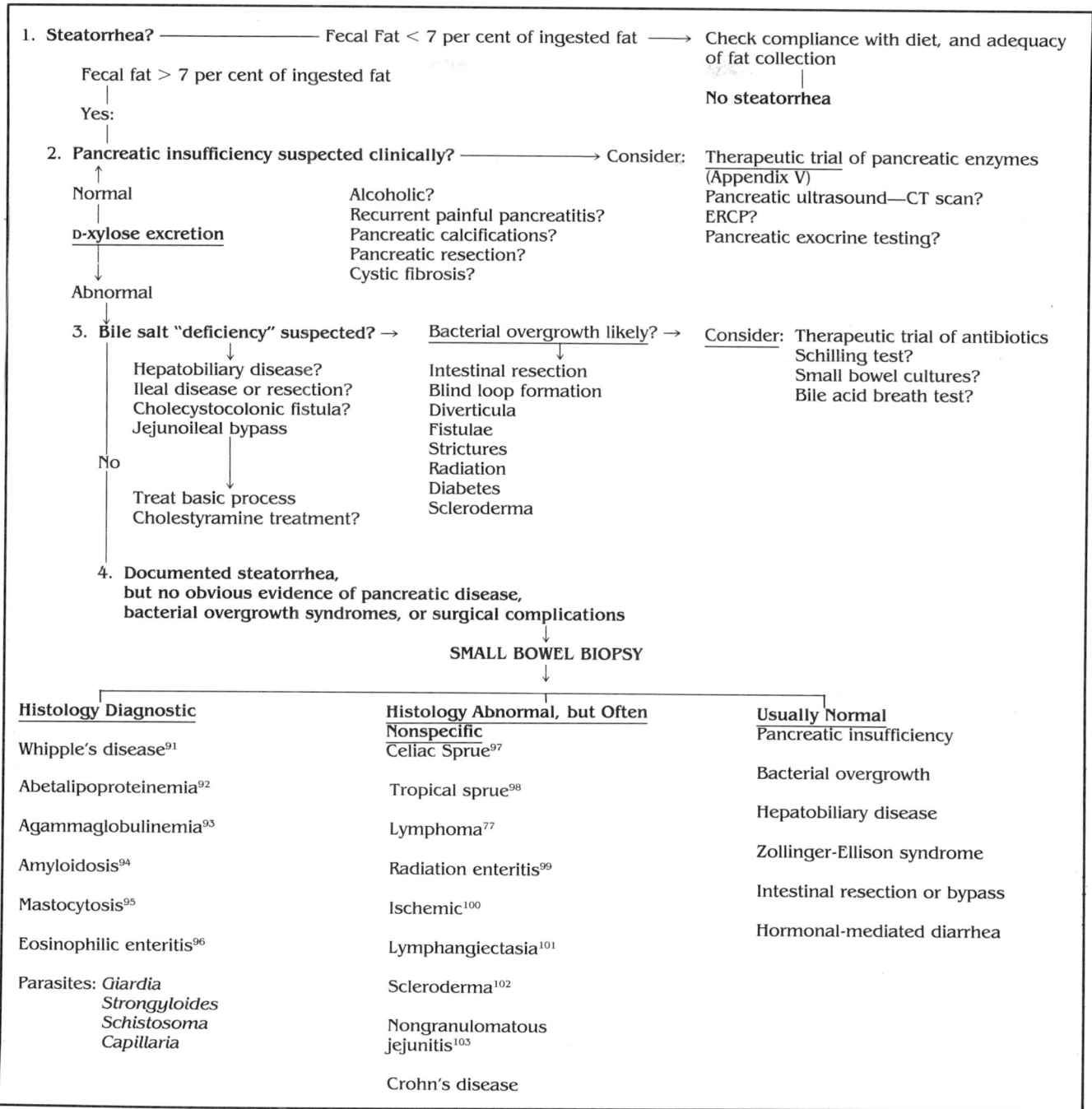

1. Steatorrhea? ——————————— Fecal Fat < 7 per cent of ingested fat ——→ Check compliance with diet, and adequacy of fat collection

    Fecal fat > 7 per cent of ingested fat   No steatorrhea
    Yes:

2. Pancreatic insufficiency suspected clinically? ——————→ Consider: Therapeutic trial of pancreatic enzymes (Appendix V)

Normal   Alcoholic?   Pancreatic ultrasound—CT scan?
                         Recurrent painful pancreatitis?   ERCP?
D-xylose excretion   Pancreatic calcifications?   Pancreatic exocrine testing?
                         Pancreatic resection?
Abnormal   Cystic fibrosis?

3. Bile salt "deficiency" suspected? →   Bacterial overgrowth likely? →   Consider: Therapeutic trial of antibiotics
                                                              Schilling test?
          Hepatobiliary disease?   Intestinal resection   Small bowel cultures?
          Ileal disease or resection?   Blind loop formation   Bile acid breath test?
          Cholecystocolonic fistula?   Diverticula
          Jejunoileal bypass   Fistulae
                               Strictures
No   Radiation
                               Diabetes
          Treat basic process   Scleroderma
          Cholestyramine treatment?

4. Documented steatorrhea, but no obvious evidence of pancreatic disease, bacterial overgrowth syndromes, or surgical complications

SMALL BOWEL BIOPSY

Histology Diagnostic	Histology Abnormal, but Often Nonspecific	Usually Normal
Whipple's disease[91]	Celiac Sprue[97]	Pancreatic insufficiency
Abetalipoproteinemia[92]	Tropical sprue[98]	Bacterial overgrowth
Agammaglobulinemia[93]	Lymphoma[77]	Hepatobiliary disease
Amyloidosis[94]	Radiation enteritis[99]	Zollinger-Ellison syndrome
Mastocytosis[95]	Ischemic[100]	Intestinal resection or bypass
Eosinophilic enteritis[96]	Lymphangiectasia[101]	Hormonal-mediated diarrhea
Parasites: Giardia Strongyloides Schistosoma Capillaria	Scleroderma[102]	
	Nongranulomatous jejunitis[103]	
	Crohn's disease	

FIGURE 3–16. Malabsorption.

3. <u>Small-bowel biopsy is indicated</u>. In Figure 3–16 are enumerated some of the diseases that cause steatorrhea in which small-bowel biopsy may be diagnostically helpful. <u>Except for parasitic infestations, most of the diseases in which small-bowel histology is unequivocally diagnostic are very rare.</u> The more common mucosal diseases—especially celiac sprue and tropical sprue—are often strongly suspected on the basis of the histologic findings on jejunal biopsy, but only subsequent therapeutic trials (and success) will be truly diagnostic, since the histologic picture is not specific.

A gastroenterologist is consulted. The gastroenterologist performs a D-xylose absorption test: Only 2.1 gm are excreted in 5 hours. Thereafter, peroral small-bowel biopsy is performed on an ambulatory basis without complications. Histologic examination reveals mild to moderate villous atrophy, with pleomorphic plasma cells in the lamina propria and pleomorphic lymphoid cell infiltration of the crypts. No parasites are identified. The findings are interpreted as compatible with, but not diagnostic of, tropical sprue, celiac sprue, or, perhaps, nongranulomatous jejunitis. Lymphoma cannot be excluded, but is unlikely.

Because of Ernie's travel history, tropical sprue is deemed most likely. Tetracycline, 500 mg qid, and folic acid, 1.0 mg bid (Table 3–10), as well as continuation of the lactose-free diet, are prescribed.

Three weeks later, Ernie is completely asymptomatic and is having one formed bowel movement per day. He has regained 5 pounds.

Tetracycline, 250 mg qid, and folic acid are continued for another 6 weeks. Ernie remains well. A repeated lactose tolerance test is now normal.

Medications are discontinued, and a normal diet is resumed, without recurrence of any symptoms. Ernie transfers to the West Coast and avoids the Caribbean.

NOTE

The diagnosis of tropical sprue is confirmed as much by a successful therapeutic trial (Table 3–10) as by diagnostic testing and small-bowel histology. Failure to respond to broad-spectrum antibiotics and folic acid would necessitate consideration of the other entities included in the histologic differential diagnosis. Further discussion of small-bowel disease is beyond the scope of this text.

Hospitalization

Very few patients with chronic diarrhea will require hospitalization for diagnostic purposes. Obvious exceptions include the very elderly, those who are systemically or seriously ill, and those whose evaluation requires inpatient procedures—the latter will vary according to local practice, but most of these diagnostic procedures (Fig. 3–6) can now be performed on an ambulatory basis.

Hospitalization usually is necessary, however, when the approach outlined in Figure 3–6 or Figure 3–16 is unrevealing. When a careful history and physical examination, stool studies (cultures, parasite searches, leukocytes, occult blood, pH, alkalinization test), proctoscopy, barium x-rays, screening blood tests, and fecal fat excretion do not suggest a diagnosis and various therapeutic trials (Table 3–10) do not produce clinical improvement, hospitalization is helpful in several ways. Figure 3–17 illustrates very briefly the hospital approach to chronic, mysterious, or unexplained diarrhea.

NOTE

1. The patient and stools can be observed. A 24-hour stool collection containing less than 300 gm of stool or a stool frequency of three or less may simply warrant further observation, since this suggests that the patient does not have true diarrhea. As noted above, the irritable bowel syndrome,

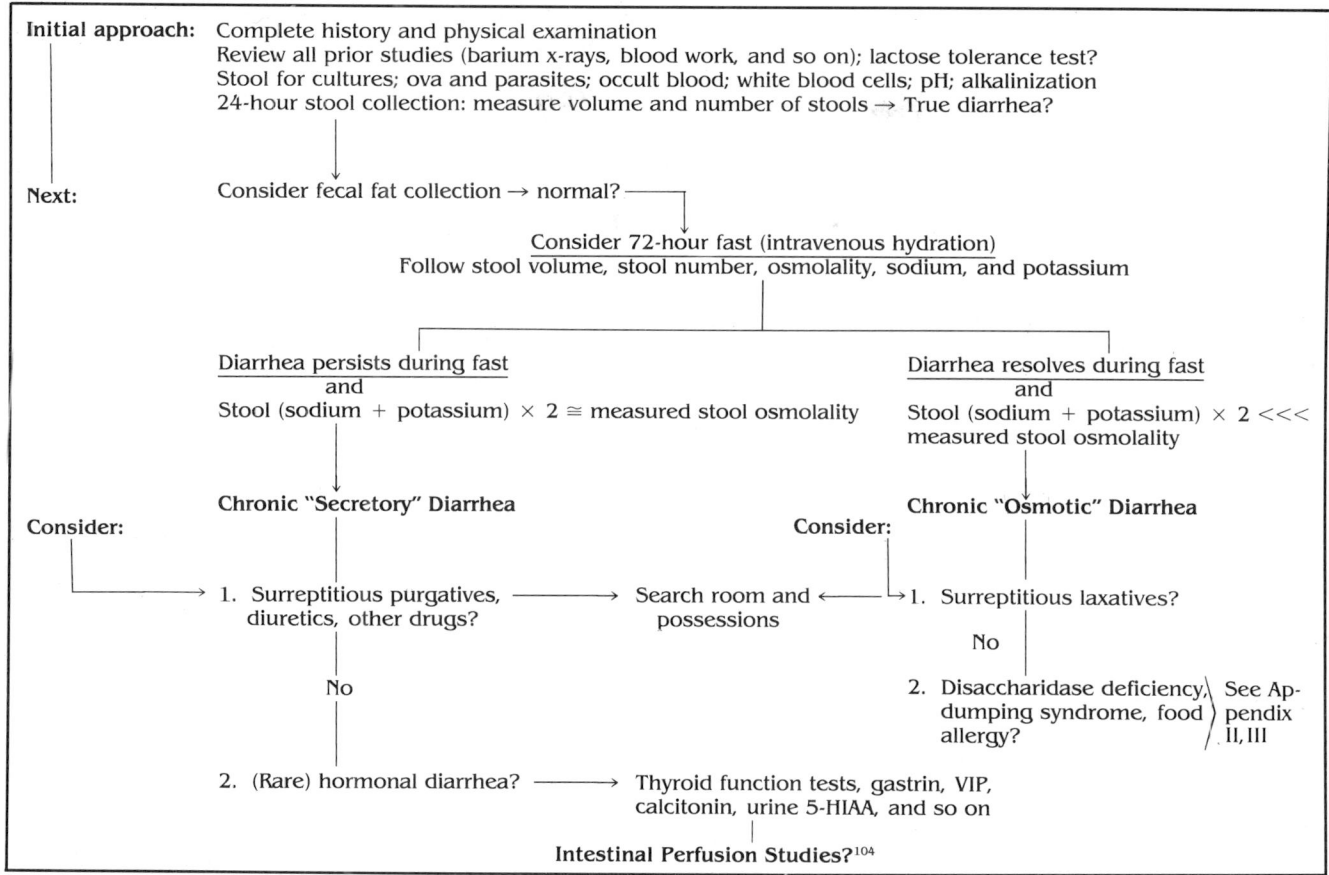

Initial approach: Complete history and physical examination
Review all prior studies (barium x-rays, blood work, and so on); lactose tolerance test?
Stool for cultures; ova and parasites; occult blood; white blood cells; pH; alkalinization
24-hour stool collection: measure volume and number of stools → True diarrhea?

Next: Consider fecal fat collection → normal?

Consider 72-hour fast (intravenous hydration)
Follow stool volume, stool number, osmolality, sodium, and potassium

Diarrhea persists during fast
and
Stool (sodium + potassium) × 2 ≅ measured stool osmolality

Diarrhea resolves during fast
and
Stool (sodium + potassium) × 2 <<< measured stool osmolality

Chronic "Secretory" Diarrhea

Chronic "Osmotic" Diarrhea

Consider:

Consider:

1. Surreptitious purgatives, → Search room and ← 1. Surreptitious laxatives?
diuretics, other drugs? possessions

No

No

2. Disaccharidase deficiency, See Ap-
dumping syndrome, food) pendix
allergy? II, III

2. (Rare) hormonal diarrhea? → Thyroid function tests, gastrin, VIP,
calcitonin, urine 5-HIAA, and so on

Intestinal Perfusion Studies?[104]

FIGURE 3–17. Hospitalization for chronic unexplained diarrhea.

functional diarrhea, anal incompetence, or intermittent diarrhea (e.g., due to food intolerance or drug or laxative ingestion) might then be further suspected.

All prior studies should be reviewed, since it is much more likely that a common disease has been overlooked than that a rare disease has not yet been discovered. Again, a review of Tables 3–7 and 3–8 may be helpful as check lists.

2. If diarrhea is confirmed in the hospital and all prior studies are truly normal, two determinations may help distinguish chronic secretory diarrhea from chronic osmotic diarrhea, each of which has distinctive diagnostic implications. Osmotic diarrhea implies that some osmotically active substance, when ingested, creates diarrhea by (passive) osmosis of water and electrolytes into the bowel lumen. Examples include malabsorption syndrome (fat is the osmotically active substance), lactase deficiency (lactose is the culprit), dumping syndromes (see Appendix III—glucose is the problem), and surreptitious use of osmotic purgatives (magnesium antacids, for example). Osmotic diarrhea thus should stop when the patient has fasted for 48 to 72 hours (i.e., when the ingested osmotic agent is eliminated). Similarly, collection of stool from patients with osmotic diarrhea will demonstrate that the measured osmolality of stool (using an osmometer) will exceed its expected osmolality (stool sodium plus potassium concentrations multiplied by 2). A measured stool osmolality that exceeds this "electrolyte osmolality"

by more than 50 mOsm suggests osmotic diarrhea (i.e., a nonelectrolyte osmolar solute must be present in the stool).

Secretory diarrhea implies that water and electrolytes are secreted into the intestinal lumen by the intestinal mucosal cells in the absence of any osmotically active intraluminal stimulus. Such secretory diarrhea may be the result of neoplasms (villous adenoma or lymphoma, for example) inflammatory bowel disease, or bile salt disorders (for example, when bile salt malabsorption in the ileum causes a secretory colonic diarrhea). These disorders are usually suspected, however, on the basis of the clinical history, the results of barium x-rays, or both. When there are no such clinical or radiographic clues, one must strongly consider the diagnosis of surreptitious laxative abuse or other covert drug ingestion (for example, diuretics*), as well as very rare hormone-secreting tumors (gastrinoma, VIPoma, carcinoid, and so on). These rare problems will thus be clinically suspected when diarrhea persists in spite of a 48- to 72-hour fast and when measured stool osmolality approximates "electrolyte osmolality" (sodium plus potassium concentration multiplied by 2).

Thus, as Figure 3–17 suggests, when hospitalization and observation suggest the presence of chronic osmotic diarrhea, further evaluation should concentrate on surreptitious (osmotic) laxative abuse[80, 81] and various types of malabsorption and food intolerance.[80] When chronic secretory diarrhea is suspected, searches of the patient's room and personal possessions for drugs and (nonosmotic) laxatives is worthwhile, but sophisticated intestinal perfusion studies[104] may ultimately be required to separate such factitious diarrhea from rare hormone-secreting tumors, which may be very difficult to diagnose, even at laparotomy.[78, 105–109]

It cannot be overemphasized that simple clinical observations should always be clarified before sophisticated diagnostic maneuvers are undertaken. Talking to the patient, reviewing the clinical history and prior diagnostic studies, evaluating the patient's diet, medications, and psychologic history, and performing simple bedside observations and stool examinations will almost always be more productive than expansive (expensive) shotgun testing (Table 3–8).

---

*Diuretics may cause both diarrhea and electrolyte imbalance. The latter is due to *urinary* excretion of electrolytes, but sometimes the coexisting electrolyte disturbance will be mistaken as evidence for chronic, severe diarrhea (thus measuring *urine* electrolytes may be helpful in the patient with diarrhea and hypokalemia).

Acute Proctitis[110]

Acute proctitis refers to inflammatory rectal disease that usually presents with symptoms of rectal pain or painful defecation, mucopurulent anal discharge, hematochezia, tenesmus, rectal urgency, or other changes in bowel habits (constipation or diarrhea). When such symptoms arise in the patient with acute diarrhea, proctosigmoidoscopy should be performed immediately. Unfortunately the proctoscopic appearance of different types of acute proctitis may be nonspecific, and this commonly results in a hasty diagnosis of idiopathic ulcerative (procto) colitis. As Table 3–11 illustrates, idiopathic inflammatory bowel disease (especially ulcerative colitis) is a common cause of acute proctitis,[64] but very many other diseases that require distinctive treatment must be considered as well. These various diseases will be recognized and successfully treated if a few generalizations are remembered:

1. Always inquire specifically about prior inflammatory bowel disease, recent radiation or antibiotic therapy, travel history, and sexual habits. Prior history of (proven or suspected) Crohn's disease or ulcerative colitis will usually be evident. Similarly, radiation-induced proctitis is also usually apparent. Recent antibiotic therapy (even as long as several weeks previously) should always raise suspicion of pseudomembranous colitis. Recent travel or epidemiologic exposure to enteric bacterial pathogens or parasites must be noted.

Probably most important is a history of homosexuality in the male, recent anal intercourse, or oral-rectal sexual practices. The venereal transmission of enteric pathogens (especially *Shigella, Campylobacter, Giardia,* and amebas), the growing awareness of anorectal manifestations of venereal diseases (especially gonorrhea, syphilis, herpes simplex, and chlamydial infections), and a variety of other common noninfectious complications of anal intercourse (i.e., foreign bodies, rectal lacerations, "contact" proctitis from anal lubricants, and rectal fissures) emphasize the crucial importance of any history of anorectal sexual activity.[113, 118–120, 159] Because the proctoscopic appearance of many of these disorders is nonspecific, precise diagnosis often requires additional testing, informed by the specific clinical suspicion (Table 3–11).

In the homosexual male with acute proctitis, several studies should be performed, regardless of the proctoscopic appearance. Cultures for gonorrhea are always indicated. This may be done without proctoscopy—an anal swab is passed 1 to 2 cm into the anal canal, rotated back and forth a few times, and then plated on Thayer-Martin medium (unless the swab contains gross fecal matter, in which case the procedure should be repeated). Anorectal gonorrhea is frequently asymptomatic and may thus coexist with other apparent causes of acute proctitis. When anorectal gonorrhea is symptomatic, the patient usually complains of perianal discomfort or itching, mucopurulent anal discharge, or "white matter on the stool"[111] Gram's stain of purulent

TABLE 3–11. ACUTE PROCTITIS

CAUSE	PROCTOSCOPIC FINDINGS	DIAGNOSIS	TREATMENT
Gonorrhea[111]	Mucopurulent anal discharge Mucosal erythema/erosion Not ulcerative	Gram's stain Culture	Procaine penicillin, 4.8 million units IM, 1 gm probenecid orally, or Ampicillin 3.5 gm orally, 1 gm probenecid, repeat dose 12 hours later[112] or Spectinomycin 2 gm IM
Syphilis[113, 114]	Painful, indurated, necrotic ulcerations and/or masses on anterior rectal wall	Dark field exam VDRL, FTA-ABS (see Male Genitourinary Infection, App. 2)	Benzathine penicillin 2.4 million units IM, or Erythromycin 750 mg qid × 10 days (30 gm total) or 250 mg qid × 30 days
Chlamydial[113] Non-LGV[115]	Nonspecific proctitis, usually not ulcerative	Gram stain: polymorphonuclears, no organisms	Tetracycline 500 mg qid × 3 weeks, or
LGV[116]	Often ulcerative (granulomatous histologically)	Gonorrhea cultures negative Chlamydial cultures Chlamydial serology	Erythromycin 500 mg qid × 3 weeks
Herpes simplex[113, 117, 160]	Perianal, anal, or rectal vesicles or confluent erythematous ulcerations	Visual appearance Tzanck smear/vesicles Viral cultures	Nonspecific: analgesics, stool softeners, sitz baths

Enteric pathogens[113, 118–120]
  Shigella
  Salmonella[121]
  Campylobacter[122]
  Yersinia
  Vibrio parahaemolyticus
	Nonspecific, may be ulcerative	Stool culture	See Table 3–5; text

Entamoeba histolytica[123]	Nonspecific or ulcerative (sometimes multiple discrete ulcers)	Aspirate exudate from rectal mucosa Examine slide for trophozoites (do not use cotton swabs)	See Table 3–6
Idiopathic ulcerative (procto)colitis[64]	Nonspecific: ranges from loss of mucosal vascularity to diffuse ulcerations and bleeding Biopsy: nonspecific mucosal inflammation	Exclude infectious, venereal, other causes Establish extent of disease (barium enema)	Corticosteroid enemas (for disease limited to rectum) Sulfasalazine?
Crohn's disease	Perianal disease common Biopsy: granulomatous	Clinical composite: small-bowel and/or colon involvement, too	Oral corticosteroids and/or sulfasalazine
Pseudomembranous colitis[38–41]	Yellow-white plaques and/or membranes May be nonspecific	Proctoscopic appearance Clostridium difficile toxin in stool	Discontinue offending agent Vancomycin 500 mg qid × 7 days, or Cholestyramine
Ischemic proctocolitis[35]	Nonspecific May be nodular or membranous	Usually elderly patient with obvious diffuse vascular disease (or, rarely, vasculitis) Thumbprinting on barium enema	Observe Surgery if proceeds to frank infarction Follow for strictures Corticosteroid enemas?
Radiation-induced proctitis[124]	Nonspecific	History of pelvic, sacral radiation therapy	Observe Follow for strictures Corticosteroid enemas?
Allergic "contact" proctitis[113]	Distal few centimeters of inflammation: abrupt transition to normal mucosa	History of anal intercourse: lubricants, soaps, etc.	Observe Corticosteroid enemas?
Traumatic[113, 120]	Lacerations and/or bleeding	History of anal intercourse and/or foreign bodies	Observe for bleeding, perforation
Foreign bodies[113, 125]	Bottles, vibrators, pencils, etc.	Proctoscopic findings Abdominal x/ray	Remove[125]
Condylomata acuminata[113]	Perianal/rectal warts	Visualization	Topical podophyllin, or Dichloroacetic acid
Rectal ulcers, fissures, fistulas, hemorrhoids[113]	—	Rule out infectious, venereal, neoplastic causes	Expectant, sitz baths, stool softeners, etc.

discharge will then often make a presumptive diagnosis, but cultures (also from the pharynx and urethra) are needed. (When a Gram's stain of mucopurulent anal discharge reveals many leukocytes but no microorganisms, and subsequent cultures are negative for gonorrhea, nongonococcal proctitis due to chlamydial infection[113, 115] should be considered.)

A serologic test for syphilis and stool cultures should also be obtained, and stool should be examined for ova and parasites. Amebiasis causes proctocolitis; giardiasis does not, but both of these parasites can be transmitted venereally. Similarly, blood tests for hepatitis (hepatitis B surface antigen and liver function tests) should also be considered because of the increasing problem of venereal hepatitis transmission, especially in homosexual males.

2. Proctoscopy and rectal biopsy may be nonspecific, but usually help. Sometimes the proctoscopic appearance will be typical of (purulent) anorectal gonorrhea, herpes simplex, pseudomembranous colitis, allergic contact proctitis, lacerations, foreign bodies, rectal warts, or other common anorectal disorders (for example, hemorrhoids and fissures). When this is so, specific diagnostic and therapeutic procedures then follow (Table 3–11).

Tender, necrotic/indurated ulcerations should always raise suspicion of syphilis (perform a darkfield examination and VDRL test), lymphogranuloma venereum (chlamydial cultures and serologic studies are indicated), or herpes proctitis (a Tzanck smear and/or herpes culture should be obtained).

Diffuse inflammatory changes (bleeding, friability, or ulcerations) should prompt culture of the stool for invasive pathogens and aspiration examinations for amebas. (Amebiasis occurs primarily in foreign travelers or homosexuals in the United States, but this is certainly not always the case, and amebiasis should always be considered in cases of acute proctocolitis.) As noted in the text proper, rectal biopsy may be necessary when slide examinations are nondiagnostic for amebiasis.

When there is no history of anal intercourse or other helpful historical clues (see above), and when stool cultures and parasite examinations (especially for amebas) are unremarkable, the differential diagnosis often involves ulcerative colitis and Crohn's disease. Rectal biopsy is usually helpful—granulomatous changes are suggestive of Crohn's disease, but the composite clinical picture must always be considered. Perianal disease, prominent small-bowel involvement, and "cobblestoning" of rectal mucosa on sigmoidoscopy all suggest Crohn's disease. (It must be remembered that granulomatous inflammation on rectal biopsy is nonspecific—syphilis, lymphogranuloma venereum, and other diseases may also produce that histologic picture.)

3. Treatment should be as specific as possible. As Table 3–11 indicates, most of the infectious causes of proctitis require specific treatment. Broad-spectrum antibiotics (tetracycline or erythromycin) may be worth a trial when chlamydial proctitis is suspected in the homosexual male ("nonspecific" proctitis at proctoscopy with negative cultures for gonorrhea and enteric pathogens). Otherwise, in general, antibiotic therapy should be tailored to the specific (proven or suspected) infection.

Corticosteroid enemas once nightly will be helpful in cases of ulcerative colitis limited to the rectum, and perhaps in radiation-induced and allergic proctitis.[64] Routine use of corticosteroid enemas for all patients with proctoscopically nonspecific acute proctitis without consideration of the entities noted in Table 3–11 will often lead to misdiagnoses. The widespread presumptive use of steroid enemas should be avoided, pending studies for venereal and enteric infections. Further examination of the colon and small bowel for the more generalized intestinal involvement in ulcerative colitis, ischemic colitis, or Crohn's disease is usually wise, since systemic steroid or surgical therapy or both may be indicated.

Food-Borne Diarrhea

FOOD POISONING[67]

Most food poisoning in the United States is caused by *Staphylococcus, Clostridium perfringens,* and *Salmonella* species. *Staph. aureus* usually causes a brief, afebrile illness characterized more by "upper intestinal" symptoms—retching and vomiting—than by severe diarrhea. Clostridial and salmonella food poisoning usually cause abdominal cramping or watery diarrhea or both, most often without fever. The diagnosis of these illnesses is usually not systematically confirmed by stool or food cultures because the illness is usually very brief and requires no specific therapy. Most food poisoning outbreaks are thus not reported to health authorities.

Nevertheless, as Table 3–12 illustrates, food-borne gastroenteritis may be caused by a wide variety of chemicals, toxins, or infectious pathogens. Most of these result in brief, self-limited illnesses that do not require treatment. A few, however, may be life threatening (for example, mushroom poisoning, shellfish poisoning, or botulism), and others require antibiotic therapy (for example, shigellosis). Moreover, achieving a specific diagnosis may be important to prevent further spread of disease, to provide the patient with an accurate prognosis, and, when epidemiologic investigation is warranted, to identify factors (usually faulty food handling) that resulted in the outbreak. As such, while it is often difficult to distinguish clinically between nonspecific (or viral) infectious gastroenteritis and food poisoning, a few generalizations will help:

1. Food poisoning is usually suspected when several persons develop a similar illness after eating the same food. When this is the case, the incubation period and the specific clinical symptoms will usually point to a specific diagnosis. As Horwitz teaches us,

> In many cases, the mean incubation period (MIP) can be calculated directly. However, when it cannot be, as when a meal or food has not yet been incriminated, it may be indirectly inferred by noting the span of time over which patients become ill. When most patients become ill within a few minutes, hours, or days of each other, the MIP is usually of comparable duration, i.e., minutes, hours, or days, respectively. An exception to this rule is the continuing common source outbreak, in which the MIP may bear no relationship to the span of time over which cases have onset.[67]

Calculation of the incubation period is an important step in differential diagnosis, as noted in Table 3–12. Food-borne illness with a very brief incubation period (under 2 hours) is usually toxic or chemical in origin, and a specific diagnosis can then almost always be suspected by identifying the food or beverages ingested and considering the specific clinical symptoms (which are often predominantly extraintestinal, but associated with diarrhea). Food-borne illness with longer incubation periods is usually manifested primarily by gastrointestinal symptoms—either "upper" (vomiting) or "lower" (diarrhea) symptoms tend to predominate—but here the duration of illness and the degree of clinical toxicity usually determine what action to take. When diarrhea is the predominant symptom, and especially when clinical dysentery or prolonged diarrhea (more than a few days) develops,

TABLE 3–12. FOOD-BORNE GASTROENTERITIS

Cause	Incubation Period	Clinical Clues	Common Vehicle	Diagnosis
Monosodium glutamate[126]	Minutes to 2 hours	Chinese restaurant syndrome Burning in abdomen, neck, chest, extremities Lightheadedness, chest pain	Chinese food	Large amount of monosodium glutamate found in incriminated food
Heavy metals	Minutes to 2 hours	Metallic taste Vomiting prominent No fever	Carbonated or acidic beverages	Chemical study of incriminated beverage
Mushroom toxin*[127]	Minutes to 2 hours	Altered mental status with visual disturbance (encephalopathy) Hepatitis	Non-commercially obtained mushrooms	Identify mushroom and/or toxic chemical (muscarine, psilocybin, etc.)
Fish/Shellfish*[128] Scombrotoxin[129]	Minutes to 2 hours	Histamine reaction: flushing, headache, dizziness, burning of throat and mouth	Tuna, mackerel, bonito, skipjack, mahi-mahi	Identify fish and/or chemical toxin (ciguatoxin, tetrodotoxin, histamine, etc.)
Shellfish toxin	Minutes to 2 hours	Paresthesias, dizziness Sometimes paralysis "Red tide" in incriminated water	Mussels, clams, oysters, scallops	
Puffer fish toxin	Minutes to 2 hours	Paresthesias	Puffer fish	
Ciguatoxin[130, 131]	2 to 24 hours	Paresthesias Itching, arthralgias, metallic taste, visual disturbances "Loose" painful teeth	Barracuda, red snapper, grouper, amberjack	
Staphylococcus aureus	2 to 8 hours	Prominent vomiting No fever Duration less than 24 hours	Ham, poultry, pastries (cream filled), mixed salads	Isolate 10^5 organisms from food
Bacillus cereus[132, 133] Emetic form	2 to 8 hours	Prominent vomiting No fever Duration less than 48 hours	Fried rice Macaroni/cheese	Isolate 10^5 organisms from food
Diarrhea form	8 to 14 hours	Abdominal cramps Severe diarrhea No fever Duration less than 48 hours	Fried rice Macaroni/cheese	Isolate 10^5 organisms from food
Clostridium perfringens	8 to 14 hours	Abdominal cramps Severe diarrhea No fever Duration less than 48 hours	Meat, poultry	Isolate 10^5 organisms from food and/or stool
Enterotoxigenic *Escherichia coli*[134]	12 hours to several days	Abdominal cramps, watery diarrhea May be prolonged (up to 1 week)	Incomplete data (rarely reported)	Isolate organism and test for enterotoxin production
Vibrio cholerae	12 hours to days	Abdominal cramps, watery diarrhea May be prolonged (up to 1 week)	Incomplete data (very rare in U.S.)	Isolate organism in stool and/or food
Invasive *E. coli*	12 hours to days	Prolonged febrile diarrhea and/or dysentery	Incomplete data	Isolate organism in stool and test for enteroinvasiveness
Shigella	12 hours to days	Prolonged febrile diarrhea and/or dysentery	Fish, mixed salads	Stool culture (or food culture)
Salmonella	12 hours to days	Prolonged febrile diarrhea and/or dysentery	Meat, poultry, dairy products, eggs, various salads	Stool culture (or food culture)
Vibrio parahemolyticus	12 hours to days	Prolonged febrile diarrhea and/or dysentery	Seafood	Stool culture (or food culture)
Campylobacter[135]	12 hours to days	Prolonged febrile diarrhea and/or dysentery	Unpasteurized milk Poultry, meat	Stool culture (or food culture)
Clostridium botulinum[136]	12 hours to days	Diarrhea Cranial nerve palsies, paralysis, ventilatory, failure	Home-canned foods	Botulinum toxin in food, stool, and serum

*Potentially dangerous—observation in hospital often required.

stool cultures are always indicated. Antibiotic therapy is then determined by the results of stool cultures (see text proper).

2. Isolated cases of food poisoning are more difficult to diagnose, because non–food-borne infectious gastroenteritis is usually (hastily) assumed. As Table 3–12 illustrates, analysis of clinical symptoms, duration of illness, and degree of toxicity (fever or dysentery or both) will suggest a more limited differential diagnosis. When extraintestinal symptoms predominate, chemical and toxic causes must be strongly suspected, especially since early diagnosis of botulism,[136] mushroom poisoning,[127] or paralytic shellfish poisoning[128–131] may be lifesaving. When diarrhea predominates, indications for stool cultures and antibiotic therapy are similar to those noted in the text proper.

3. Specific diagnosis and therapy vary widely. Most chemical and toxic causes require identification of the etiologic substance in the incriminated food—this will take time, and thus clinical suspicion often determines immediate presumptive therapy (gastric lavage, cathartics, and careful observation, often in the hospital, when toxic or chemical poisoning is suspected). Early administration of botulinum antitoxin and careful observation for neurologic or ventilatory impairment is necessary when botulism is suspected.

Most bacterial food poisoning does not require specific treatment, but the stool culture and clinical symptoms usually indicate those that do.

FOOD INTOLERANCE[137]

Food intolerance in humans may cause an extraordinary variety of clinical symptoms and metabolic abnormalities, most of which are very rare and only some of which are well understood. Diarrhea due to food intolerance has many different possible causes, but those most commonly observed (or suspected) in adults are:

1. Lactose intolerance is certainly the most common. This is discussed in more detail in the text proper.

2. Milk allergy occurs primarily in atopic infants and usually disappears in early childhood. Most adults who cannot tolerate milk are lactose intolerant—true milk allergy in adults is probably rare, but this entity is poorly understood.

3. Other carbohydrate intolerance diarrhea is very rare (sucrose/starch intolerance) or occurs primarily in young children with various enzyme deficiencies (for example, hereditary fructose intolerance) or is related to a dumping syndrome (see Appendix III). Sometimes sudden administration of large amounts of oral carbohydrates in patients subsisting on low carbohydrate diets will cause temporary diarrhea (probably because of transient inactivation of jejunal glycolytic enzymes).

4. Protein-induced diarrhea is usually related to gluten intolerance (most often associated with celiac sprue or dermatitis herpetiformis, but IgA deficiency and systemic mastocytosis are rare causes of diarrhea that may respond to gluten-free diets).

Protein allergy (for example, eggs, wheat) probably does occur, but true gastrointestinal protein allergy is very difficult to prove. In such circumstances, a more generalized malabsorptive disorder (see text proper) should always be considered.

5. Fat intolerance diarrhea usually implies steatorrhea, as discussed briefly in the text proper.

6. Heavy consumption of sorbitol-containing foods can cause "dietetic food diarrhea."[138] Sugarless gum, candy, and cookies ingested in large amounts for purposes of weight reduction can cause an easily reversible form of diarrhea.

7. A few other forms of diarrhea due to food intolerance are easy to identify if a careful diet history is obtained. Excessive use of prune juice, high bulk/fiber diets, and caffeine are common examples.

TURISTA (TRAVELER'S DIARRHEA)[139-144]

Traveler's diarrhea refers to a clinical syndrome usually characterized by mild to moderate watery diarrhea (three to eight bowel movements per day, usually without fever or clinical dysentery), beginning a few days after arrival in a foreign country, and persisting for an average of 2 to 5 days in most patients. Perhaps 70 per cent of cases are due to infection with enterotoxigenic *Escherichia coli,* usually acquired by ingestion of food or water containing strains of *E. coli* to which the individual is unaccustomed.[139] (The attack rate is between 10 and 50 per cent, varying with many epidemiologic factors.[144]) Occasionally, *Shigella, Salmonella, Giardia,* or other parasites may be implicated. While travelers to underdeveloped countries are most often afflicted (or reported), foreign travelers to the United States may develop turista, too. The ubiquity of the problem is well illustrated by its many local appellations: Montezuma's revenge, Turkey trot, Delhi belly, Aztec two-step, Casablanca crud, the lower Burmas, and many others.

Prevention of turista is uppermost in the minds of many incipient travelers, but no current therapy is both effective and convenient. Pepto-Bismol (bismuth subsalicylate) will reduce the incidence of turista—in one study, from 60 to 20 per cent[143]—but only when large doses (2 ounces qid for 2 to 3 weeks) are used. Ingesting one bottle per day (and transporting many more bottles) of Pepto-Bismol is not considered practical by most travelers. Prophylactic tetracycline (doxycycline 100 mg qid) has also been shown effective (in Peace Corps volunteers in Kenya[142]), but tetracycline-resistant *E. coli* are now common in some parts of the world, side effects (from doxycycline) are not uncommon (photosensitivity, candida vaginitis), and there is the theoretic risk of increased susceptibility to invasive bacterial diseases (shigellosis, for example) due to doxycycline alteration of normal gut flora.

Thus, while Pepto-Bismol or antibiotic prophylaxis can be helpful, the mildness of the usual case of turista in light of the above considerations often weighs in favor of avoiding such treatment. Perhaps the elderly or infirm traveler, or those travelers planning brief visits that demand their persisting good health (spies?) should be especially considered for prophylactic treatment.

In general, the approach to traveler's diarrhea in the patient returning to this country is similar to that described in the text proper. Symptomatic therapy is usually sufficient. The great majority of patients with turista do not require medical attention at all. The occasional case that causes prolonged or more troublesome symptoms may be improved with therapeutic Pepto-Bismol, tetracycline, trimethoprim-sulfamethoxazole, or bicozamycin.*[145] Stool cultures and examinations for parasites should always be performed when diarrhea is persistent.

---

*An antibiotic not currently marketed.

APPENDIX III

Postoperative Diarrhea

Several types of intra-abdominal surgical procedures may be complicated by postoperative diarrhea. Because the onset of diarrhea may be delayed, the association between surgery and symptoms is not always obvious. Since there may be several different pathophysiologic mechanisms responsible for diarrhea after a particular surgical procedure, the precise cause and indicated therapy may be elusive, in some instances. The most common surgical procedures that may be complicated by postoperative diarrhea are:

I. Ulcer operations.[146-148]

Many different operations are advocated for the surgical treatment of peptic ulcer disease. Most common are partial or subtotal gastrectomy; vagotomy and pyloroplasty; vagotomy and antrectomy; and various types of "selective" vagotomy. In general, diarrhea that begins immediately or soon after ulcer operations will be due to:

A. Dumping syndrome.

The loss of reservoir function of the stomach following partial gastrectomy (especially with a Billroth II procedure), or after vagotomy and pyloroplasty, may cause an unaccustomed rush of a hypertonic meal into the proximal small bowel. In a small percentage of such patients, symptoms of diarrhea, sweating, palpitations, nausea, pallor, borborygmi, and dizziness appear within 10 to 20 minutes of eating—such symptoms last up to an hour. (Occasionally, symptoms of reactive hypoglycemia may follow, usually after about 90 minutes.) In a few patients, this dumping syndrome is intractable and incapacitating, but most often the use of small feedings of a diet high in fat and protein but low in carbohydrate, as well as reduced fluid intake during meals, will ameliorate symptoms (see Appendix IV). Occasionally, drug therapy—sedatives, antispasmodics, cyproheptadine, or oral hypoglycemic agents—will be necessary.

B. Postvagotomy diarrhea is a poorly understood phenomenon that is usually postprandial, mild, and transient, sometimes responding to antiperistaltic or anticholinergic agents.

Truncal vagotomy may be responsible more often than newer selective vagotomy operations. Dumping symptoms are absent. Only rarely is this an incapacitating problem, but remedial surgery is occasionally necessary.[149]

C. Inadvertent gastroileostomy or gastrocolostomy, it is hoped, is very rare.

Barium x-rays will be diagnostic, and surgical revision is always necessary.

II. Diarrhea that does not begin until weeks or months after ulcer surgery may be caused by a whole host of problems, and in general the approach outlined in the text proper should be followed, because intercurrent infection, malabsorption, pancreatic insufficiency, and many other problems may be responsible. For example:

A. Steatorrhea may occur for many reasons.

Rapid transit after vagotomy may cause "inadequate mixing" of pancreatic enzymes with ingested food—anticholinergic therapy may help here. Partial gastrectomy with Billroth II anastomosis commonly causes inadequate mixing because the duodenum is bypassed and pancreatic/biliary secretions are inadequately stimulated. Oral pancreatic enzyme replacement with meals may help (see Appendix V). The Billroth II procedure may also lead to bacterial overgrowth in the afferent loop; in this situation, steatorrhea will respond to broad-spectrum antibiotic therapy. Mild pancreatic insufficiency may sometimes develop after gastric resection—hypochlorhydria and rapid intestinal transit probably play a role, but oral pancreatic enzymes may be helpful.

B. Infection with *Salmonella* organisms is theoretically enhanced by a gastric pH greater than 3. Giardiasis may follow gastric surgery as well.

C. Lactose intolerance is so common in the general population that mild subclinical lactose intolerance may become symptomatic when gastric surgery accelerates intestinal transit.

D. The rare Zollinger-Ellison syndrome[150] should be remembered, especially when ulcer disease is refractory to even surgical measures. Diarrhea is a presenting manifestation in about one third of Zollinger-Ellison patients and may antedate ulcer symptoms.

Thus, chronic diarrhea that occurs in the patient who has had recent or remote peptic ulcer surgery may require stool cultures, barium examinations, fecal fat collections, lactose tolerance tests, trials of antibiotics, or pancreatic enzyme replacements, depending on the specific clinical circumstances.

III. Cholecystectomy[151] is not usually complicated by diarrhea, but occasionally a chronic "secretory" diarrhea may be caused by bile acid–mediated mechanisms that can respond dramatically to treatment with oral cholestyramine (which binds bile acids).

IV. Small-intestinal resection.[152]

The management of patients after small-bowel resection is a complicated subject that cannot be adequately covered here. Factors responsible for diarrhea (as well as malnutrition and metabolic complications) include the extent and site of bowel removed, the competence of the ileocecal valve, the absorptive capacity of remaining bowel, and the function of hepatobiliary and pancreatic organs. In general, however, a few mechanisms should be remembered:

A. Ileal resection limited to less than 100 cm often results in bile acid–induced diarrhea (due to malabsorption of bile acids and their irritant effect on the colon), which will respond to cholestyramine therapy (8 to 12 gm a day).

Fecal fat excretion should always be measured, since steatorrhea will occur (and will worsen with cholestyramine therapy) when the bile acid pool is sufficiently reduced to cause inadequate micelle formation and superimposed fat malabsorption. Ileal resections of greater than 100 cm are more often associated with a reduced bile acid pool and subsequent steatorrhea.

B. <u>Bacterial overgrowth</u> is a common problem when the ileocecal valve is resected or when a blind loop is created (as in intestinal jejunoileal bypass for morbid obesity).

The bile acid breath test[89] or Schilling test may help here.[88]

C. Gastric hypersecretion is a common problem after extensive small-bowel resection.

This may cause diarrhea when excessive acid renders pancreatic enzymes relatively inactive, resulting in steatorrhea. Antacids or cimetidine may help.

Otherwise the management of diarrhea after (especially extensive) small-bowel resection will require barium studies (to exclude fistulas, strictures, and the like) and attention to many different details: low-fat diet with or without use of medium-chain triglycerides, avoidance of lactose, judicious use of anticholinergic and antimotility drugs, vitamin and mineral supplements, and other considerations.[152]

Diets[153]

1. <u>Diagnostic 100-gm fat diet.</u> Table 3–13 illustrates specific directions for a 72-hour fecal fat collection. It is crucial that the patient record the total amount of fat ingested each day, and that the diet be continued for 6 days, even though the stool collection will take place only on days 4 through 6. Notice that many fat-containing foods also contain lactose, but the patient with known or suspected lactose intolerance can still achieve 100 gm of fat intake a day (see also Table 3–14).

TABLE 3–13. 100-GRAM FAT DIET

This is a special test diet that will help determine how well your body absorbs fat. You must follow this diet for 3 days, then continue the diet and collect all your stools for a second 3 days. It will be a total of 6 consecutive days that you must follow this diet continuously. A container for stool collection and a laboratory slip will be given to you with the diet. Keep the stools in a cool place until you return the container on the seventh day.

Food	Amount	Fat Content (gm)
Whole milk	1 cup	10
Ice cream	½ cup	10
Cottage cheese	¼ cup	5
Hard cheese	1 ounce	5
Cream cheese	1 tbsp	5
Egg	1	5
Peanut butter	2 tbsp	15
Tunafish, packed in oil	¼ cup	5
Meat, fish, poultry	1 ounce	5
Cold cuts	1 ounce	5
Butter, margarine, mayonnaise	1 tsp	5
Salad dressings	1 tbsp	5
Bacon	1 strip	5
Plain doughnut	1	10
Peanuts	12 whole	5
Olives	5 small	5

While you must keep a record of the above foods to give you a total of 100 gm of fat per day, the following foods may be used AS DESIRED:

Bread, rice, potato, macaroni, spaghetti, noodles, fruits, fruit juices, vegetables, vegetable juices, skim milk and skim milk products, coffee, tea, bouillon, jelly, syrup, sugar, hard candy, soda, jello, angel food cake, puddings made with skim milk, sherbet

DIET TO BE FOLLOWED ON   Day 1 ,   Day 2 ,   Day 3 ; THEN DIET PLUS STOOL COLLECTION ON   Day 4 ,   Day 5 ,   Day 6 .

MEAT _____oz.

MILK _____cups

OTHER FAT _____   _____ gm TOTAL FAT

TABLE 3-14. COMMON LACTOSE-CONTAINING FOODS*

Milk (all types)	Sherbet
Cream	Frankfurters
Ice cream	Bologna
Cheese	Vienna bread
Powdered cream	Party dips
Sour cream	Puddings
Instant potatoes	Pie fillings
Cottage cheese	Frozen desserts
Yogurt	Salad dressings
Butter	Milk chocolate
(Most) margarines†	

*See reference 153 for further details.
†Nucoa margarine contains no lactose.

2. <u>Lactose-free diet.</u> Table 3–14 enumerates common lactose-containing foods and beverages. Floch's book[153] has a more complete list of lactose-free foods.

In general, all lactose is discontinued initially in the patient with known or suspected lactose intolerance, but many patients with documented lactase deficiency can still tolerate small amounts of lactose. Therefore, gradual reinstitution of various lactose-containing foods can be attempted—most patients will tolerate small amounts of many of the foods listed in Table 3–14. Patients with this problem must be instructed to read food labels carefully, since many of the foods in Table 3–14 are not commonly thought of as dairy products.

3. <u>High-fiber diet.</u> Especially for patients with the irritable bowel syndrome (and probably for patients with symptomatic diverticulosis), a diet high in "fiber" is often helpful. While the definition of fiber is somewhat controversial, daily intake of bran cereals, whole wheat bread, and various fruits and vegetables usually is helpful. Table 3–15 includes various common foods that have high fiber content.

4. <u>Gluten-restricted diet.</u> Table 3–16 illustrates various foods that are permitted or restricted in the patient with celiac sprue. Again, the patient must learn to read labels. The food prohibitions here are extensive, and this diet is disliked by most patients. It is always wise to document gluten enteropathy (usually by small-bowel biopsy) before instituting such a diet. Therapeutic trials (see text proper) with a gluten-free diet should only rarely be recommended.

5. <u>Dumping syndrome diet.</u> Postgastrectomy dumping is usually treated with a low-carbohydrate, high-protein, high-fat diet. Usually milk is restricted to small amounts, and liquids are taken only 30 to 45 minutes before or after ingestion of solid food (to avoid increasing osmotic loads and intestinal transit). Frequent small feedings are usually helpful, and the addition of dietary fiber is often useful.

TABLE 3-15. HIGH-FIBER FOODS

Bran cereals	Peas	Peaches
Whole wheat bread	Apples	Coconuts
Wheat bran	Celery	Lentils
Maise	Apricots	Carrots
Walnuts	Blackberries	Lettuce
Red kidney beans	Figs	Prunes

TABLE 3-16. RESTRICTED GLUTEN DIET

REMEMBER: Use only those foods for which the ingredients are completely known. READ LABELS!

BEVERAGES	ALLOWED:	Carbonated beverages, coffee, decaffeinated coffee and instant coffee that does not contain cereal products, milk, buttermilk, skim milk, homemade chocolate milk, tea, vodka, wines, and brandy
	AVOID:	Coffee substitutes, commercial chocolate milk, malted milk, Postum, Ovaltine, ale, beer, and all other alcoholic beverages
BREADS (as desired)	ALLOWED:	Bread products made from arrowroot, corn, gluten-free wheat starch flours, rice, or soybean, and PURE BUCKWHEAT flour
	AVOID:	All bread products made from wheat, rye, oats, or barley. All commercial products and mixes, buckwheat flour mixes, and bread crumbs.
CEREAL (as desired)	ALLOWED:	Hot cereals: corn meals, cream of rice, grits Ready-to-eat cereals: corn and rice products made with allowed ingredients
	AVOID:	All others, including Rice Krispies and Corn flakes
CONDIMENTS (as desired)	ALLOWED:	Salt, pepper, sugar, herbs, and spices
	AVOID:	None
DESSERTS (as desired)	ALLOWED:	Homemade custard, gelatin, cornstarch, or tapioca puddings; ice cream and sherbet without gluten stabilizers; water ice. Desserts prepared with allowed flours and starches
	AVOID:	Desserts prepared from wheat, rye, oats, or barley; all commercial desserts and mixes; ice cream and sherbet with cereal stabilizers
FATS (as desired)	ALLOWED:	Butter, cream, margarine, fats, real mayonnaise; commercial salad dressings without gluten stabilizers, shortenings, vegetable oil, and lard
	AVOID:	Commercial salad dressings with gluten stabilizers
FRUIT AND FRUIT JUICES (as desired, include 1 citrus daily)	ALLOWED:	All
	AVOID:	None
MEATS AND SUBSTITUTES (2 or more servings daily)	ALLOWED:	Beef, fish, lamb, pork, poultry, veal, and liver; pure, ALL MEAT cold cuts, frankfurters, and sausage; cheese, eggs, and peanut butter; all prepared without the addition of wheat, rye, oats, or barley
	AVOID:	Commercially prepared entrees; processed cheese and cheese products containing gluten stabilizers; processed meats with fillers; meat alternatives or protein substitutes that may have gluten stabilizers
POTATO AND SUBSTITUTES (as desired)	ALLOWED:	White and sweet potatoes; grits, hominy, and rice; low-gluten products
	AVOID:	Barley, macaroni, noodles, and spaghetti; any prepared with wheat, rye, or oats
SOUPS (as desired)	ALLOWED:	Clear broth. Homemade cream soups (thickened with allowed flours) and vegetable soups made with allowed ingredients
	AVOID:	Any containing wheat, rye, oats, or barley; canned soups containing prohibited ingredients
SWEETS (as desired)	ALLOWED:	Pure candies, honey, jams, jellies, marshmallows, sugars, syrups, molasses, and corn syrup
	AVOID:	Any containing wheat, rye, oats, or barley
VEGETABLES AND VEGETABLE JUICES (as desired, include dark green or yellow daily)	ALLOWED:	All
	AVOID:	Any prepared with wheat, rye, oats, or barley such as cream sauces and bread crumbs
MISCELLANEOUS (as desired)	ALLOWED:	Baking powder, baking soda, chocolate, cocoa, coconut, gravies (made with allowed flours and starches), nuts, olives, vinegar, mustard, catsup, and pickles
	AVOID:	Any containing wheat, rye, oats, or barley

APPENDIX V

Pancreatic Enzyme Replacement

As noted in the text, steatorrhea due to exocrine pancreatic insufficiency is usually strongly suspected on the basis of the clinical history and the quantitative documentation of steatorrhea. While there are many sophisticated tests available to quantitate exocrine pancreatic function,[87] a therapeutic trial of pancreatic enzyme replacement is often more practical. In the absence of documented steatorrhea, pancreatic enzymes should not be used (for example, the patient with chronic dyspepsia or flatulence is sometimes treated inappropriately with these agents).

There are many different enzyme preparations, but, in general, several facts should be remembered:

1. Lipase activity treats steatorrhea. The variability of in vitro lipase activity among commercially available enzyme preparations is very wide, as Graham has demonstrated.[154] Table 3–17 lists a few enzyme preparations that have acceptably high levels of in vitro lipase activity.

2. In general, in vivo activity (as measured by therapeutic reduction of steatorrhea) correlates with in vitro activity, but large amounts of oral enzyme replacements are usually required. In one study, 28,000 units of lipase were administered with each of four meals consisting of no more than 25 gm of fat per meal, and yet steatorrhea was reduced only 59 per cent.[155] As Table 3–17 illustrates, several tablets or capsules must be given to most patients with each meal to achieve best therapeutic results. Usually, 4 tablets or capsules per meal are used, but as many as 8 or 12 may be required in individual patients.

TABLE 3–17. PANCREATIC ENZYME PREPARATIONS

	LIPASE ACTIVITY PER DOSE (Advertised/Graham Study[154])	USUAL DAILY DOSE*	NUMBER/COST PER MONTH
Ilozyme tablets	9600/3600	4 tablets with each meal (usually, 12 per day)	360/$42
Cotazyme capsules	8000/2000	4 capsules with each meal (12 per day)	360/$32
Viokase tablets	6500/1600	4 tablets with each meal (12 per day)	360/$13
Pancrease (enteric-coated) capsules	4000/not studied	4 capsules with each meal (12 per day)	360/$53
Cimetidine†	—	300 mg q6h	120/$42

*The daily dose required for improvement of steatorrhea varies dramatically in different patients. In some patients, the enteric-coated capsules will be very effective in much smaller numbers per day than will the noncoated tablets. Therefore, these cost differences can be misleading and in some patients the enteric-coated preparations are cost effective.

†May be useful as adjunctive therapy—see text.

3. Enteric-coated tablets may be no more effective and are more expensive than the noncoated preparations[156] (see Table 3–17), but gastric pH does have a major influence on in vivo lipase activity. Maintenance of a gastric pH greater than 4 appears to improve in vivo activity of oral pancreatic enzyme replacements. This does not mean that gastric pH must be monitored in every patient, but failure to respond to apparently adequate amounts of oral lipase should prompt the addition of antacids[157] or cimetidine (300 mg q6h) or a change to enteric-coated capsules.[156]

4. Enzymes can be given with meals.[158] More frequent (hourly) dosage probably is not advantageous for most patients and is certainly less convenient.

5. Documentation of therapeutic benefit by repeat fecal fat collections is usually wise. As noted above, the amounts of enzyme tablets/capsules required for optimal benefit will vary greatly with each patient. It should be remembered that complete eradication of steatorrhea is almost never possible. Nevertheless, improvement in steatorrhea and symptomatic benefit are almost always possible, but attention to detail (as above) is crucial.

REFERENCES

1. Pickering, LK, et al.: Fecal leukocytes in enteric infection. Am J Clin Pediatr 68:562–565, 1977.
2. Blaser, MJ, et al.: Campylobacter enteritis in Denver. West J Med 136:287–290, 1982.
3. Blaser, MJ, et al.: Campylobacter enteritis: Clinical and epidemiological features. Ann Intern Med 91:179–185, 1979.
4. Yolken, RH, et al.: Infectious gastroenteritis in bone marrow transplant recipients. N Engl J Med 306:1009–1012, 1982.
5. Blackow, NR, et al.: Acute infectious nonbacterial gastroenteritis. Etiology and pathogenesis. Ann Intern Med 76:993–1008, 1972.
6. Plotkin, GR, et al.: Gastroenteritis: Etiology, pathophysiology, and clinical manifestations. Medicine 58:95–114, 1979.
7. Harris, JC, et al.: Fecal leukocytes in diarrheal illness. Ann Intern Med 76:697–703, 1972.
8. Sullivan, JF: Vascular disease of the intestines. Med Clin North Am 58:1473–1485, 1974.
9. Renny, A, Snape, WJ: Diverticular disease: A common disorder, a common mimic. Diagnosis (March) 1982, pp. 28–32.
10. Borchardt, KA, et al.: Intestinal parasites in Southeast Asia refugees. West J Med 135:92–95, August 1981.
11. Estes, MK, Graham, DY: Epidemic viral gastroenteritis. A review. Am J Med 66:1001–1007, 1979.
12. Aserkoff, B, Bennett, JV: Effect of antibiotic therapy in acute salmonellosis on the fecal excretion of salmonellae. N Engl J Med 281:636–640, 1969.
13. DuPont, HL: Salmonellosis and shigellosis. Hosp Med (Oct) 1977, pp. 51–80.
14. Rosenthal, SL: Exacerbation of Salmonella enteritis due to ampicillin. N Engl J Med 280:147, 1969.
15. Blaser, MJ, Reller, LB: Campylobacter enteritis. N Engl J Med 305:1444–1452, 1981.
16. Weissman, JB, et al.: Shigellosis: to treat or not to treat? JAMA 229:1215–1216, 1974.
17. Gutman, LT, et al.: An inter-familial outbreak of Yersinia enterocolitica enteritis. N Engl J Med 288:1372–1377, 1973.
18. Vantrappen, G, et al.: Yersinia enteritis and enterocolitis: Gastroenterological aspects. Gastroenterology 77:220–227, 1977.
19. Bolen, JL, et al.: Clinical features in enteritis due to Vibrio parahaemolyticus. Am J Med 57:638–641, 1974.
20. Santosham, M, et al.: Oral rehydration therapy of infantile diarrhea. A controlled study of well-nourished children hospitalized in the United States and Panama. N Engl J Med 306:1070–1076, 1982.
21. Carpenter, C: Oral rehydration. Is it as good as parenteral therapy? N Engl J Med 306:1103–1104, 1982.
22. Hirschhorn, N, et al.: Decrease in net stool output in cholera during intestinal perfusion with glucose-containing solutions. N Engl J Med 279:176–180, 1968.
23. Field, M: New strategies for treating watery diarrhea. N Engl J Med 297:1121–1122, 1977.
24. Gangarosa, EJ: Recent developments in diarrheal diseases. Postgrad Med 62:113–117, 1977.
25. DuPont, HL, Hornick, RB: Adverse effect of Lomotil therapy in shigellosis. JAMA 226:1525–1528, 1973.
26. Dupont, HL: Using OTC drugs for acute diarrhea. Drug Ther 13:138, 1983.
27. Hornick, RB: Acute bacterial diarrheas. Adv Intern Med 21:349–361, 1976.
28. Greenberg RN, Pearson, RD: Clinical approaches in shigellosis. Hosp Pract 17:216–240, 1982.
29. Adams, EB MacLeod, IN: Invasive amebiasis. I. Amebic dysentery and its complications. Medicine 56:315–323, 1977.
30. Adams, EB, MacLeod, IN: Invasive amebiasis. II. Amebic liver abscess and its complications. Medicine 56:325–334, 1977.
31. Krogstad, DJ, et al.: Current concepts in parasitology. Amebiasis. N Engl J Med 298:262–265, 1978.
32. Healy, GR: Laboratory diagnosis of amebiasis. Bull NY Acad Med 47:478–493, 1971.
33. Morson, BC: Rectal biopsy in inflammatory bowel disease. N Engl J Med 287:1337–1339, 1972.
34. Goodman, MJ, et al.: Usefulness of rectal biopsy in inflammatory bowel disease. Gastroenterology 72:952–956, 1977.
35. Kilpatrick, ZM, et al.: Ischemic proctitis. JAMA 205:74–80, 1968.
36. Goldgraber, MB, Kirsner, JB: "Specific" diseases simulating "nonspecific" ulcerative colitis. Ann Intern Med 47:939–955, 1957.
37. Dickinson, RJ, et al.: Rectal biopsy in patients presenting to an infectious disease unit with diarrheal disease. Gut 20:141–148, 1979.
38. Hoberman, LJ, et al.: Colitis associated with oral clindamycin therapy. A clinical study of 16 patients. Dig Dis 21:1–17, 1976.
39. Rifkin, GD, et al.: Neutralization by Clostridium sordellii antitoxin of toxins implicated in clindamycin-induced cecitis in the hamster. Gastroenterology 75:422–424, 1978.
40. Tedesco, F, et al.: Oral vancomycin for antibiotic-associated pseudomembranous colitis. Lancet 2:226–228, 1978.
41. Silva, J, et al.: Treatment of Clostridium difficile colitis and diarrhea with vancomycin. Am J Med 71:815–822, 1981.
42. DuPont, HL, et al.: Pathogenesis of E. coli diarrhea. N Engl J Med 285:1–9, 1971.
43. Wolfe, MS: Current concepts in parasitology. Giardiasis. N Engl J Med 298:319–321, 1978.
44. Blumenthal, DS: Current concepts. Intestinal nematodes in the United States. N Engl J Med 297:1437–1439, 1977.
45. Bayless, TM, et al.: Lactose and milk intolerance: Clinical implications. N Engl J Med 292:1156–1159, 1975.
46. Bayless, TM: Recognition of lactose intolerance. Hosp Pract 11:97–102, 1976.

47. Lipshutz, WH: How to spot the patient who is lactose intolerant. Mod Med (July 15) 1977, pp. 41–44.
48. Almy, TP: Chronic and recurrent diarrhea. In Barondess, J (ed): Diagnostic Approaches to Presenting Syndromes. Baltimore: Williams and Wilkins, 1971, pp. 167–196.
49. Farthing, MJG, Keusch, GT: Giardiasis: The wilderness disease. Drug Ther 115–126 (Jan) 1982.
50. Malins, JM, Mayne, N: Diabetic diarrhea. A study of 13 patients with jejunal biopsy. Diabetes 18:858–866, 1969.
51. Katz, LA, Spiro, HM: Gastrointestinal manifestations of diabetes. N Engl J Med 275:1350–1361, 1966.
52. Hosking DJ, et al.: Diabetic autonomic neuropathy. Diabetes 27:1043–1054, 1978.
53. Krejs, GJ, Fordtran, JS: Diarrhea. In Sleisenger, M, Fordtran, J (eds): Gastrointestinal Disease, 2nd ed. Philadelphia: W. B. Saunders, 1978, pp. 313–335.
54. Drossman, DA, et al.: The irritable bowel syndrome. Gastroenterology 73:811–822, 1977.
55. Prout, BJ: The irritable colon syndrome—very common but often missed. Mod Med 36–40 (July) 1977.
56. Kirsner, JB: The irritable bowel syndrome. Some personal reflections. Practical Gastroenterol III (6):50–55, 1979.
57. Manning, AP, et al.: Towards a positive diagnosis of the irritable bowel. Br Med J 2:653–654, 1978.
58. Shah, SM, Texter, EC: Managing the irritable bowel: Keep it from being an exercise in frustration. Consultant (Jan) 1978, 190–202.
59. Whitehead, WE, Schuster, MM: Psychological management of the irritable bowel syndrome. Practical Gastroenterol III(6):32–36, 1979.
60. Connell, AM, et al.: Variations of bowel habit in two population samples. I. Results in an industrial community. II. Results in general medical practice. Br Med J 2:1095–1099, 1965.
61. Edwards, FC, Truelove, SC: The course and prognosis of ulcerative colitis. Gut 4:299–315, 1963.
62. DeDombal, FT: Ulcerative colitis. Epidemiology and etiology, course and prognosis. Br Med J 1:649–655, 1971.
63. Matts, SF: The value of rectal biopsy in the diagnosis of ulcerative colitis. Q J Med 30:393, 1961.
64. Sparberg, M, et al.: Ulcerative proctitis and mild ulcerative colitis. A study of 220 patients. Medicine 45:391–412, 1966.
65. Kirsner, JB: Observations on the medical treatment of inflammatory bowel disease. JAMA 243:557–564, 1980.
66. Singleton, JW: Current therapy of inflammatory bowel diseases. Drug Ther 12:89–96, 1982.
67. Horwitz, MA: Specific diagnosis of food-borne disease. Gastroenterology 73:375–381, 1977.
68. Farmer, RG et al.: Clinical patterns in Crohn's disease: A statistical study of 615 cases. Gastroenterology 68:627–635, 1975.
69. Mekhjian, HS, et al.: Clinical features and natural history of Crohn's disease. Gastroenterology 77:898–906, 1979.
70. Greenstein, AJ, et al.: The extraintestinal complications of Crohn's disease and ulcerative colitis: A study of 700 patients. Medicine 55:401–412, 1976.
71. Goldberg, HI, et al.: Radiographic findings of the National Cooperative Crohn's Disease Study. Gastroenterology 77:925–927, 1979.
72. Hill, RB, et al.: Clinical usefulness of rectal biopsy in Crohn's disease. Gastroenterology 77:938–944, 1979.
73. Sales, DJ, Kirsner, JB: The prognosis of inflammatory bowel disease. Arch Intern Med 143:294–299, 1983.
74. Whittenberg, J, et al.: Ischemic colitis. Radiology and pathophysiology. Am J Roentgenol 123:287–300, 1975.
75. Almy, TP, Howell, DA: Diverticular disease of the colon. N Engl J Med 302:324–331, 1980.
76. Cello, JP: Diverticular disease of the colon. West J Med 134:515–523, 1981.
77. Lewis, KJ, et al.: Lymphoma of the gastrointestinal tract: A study of 117 cases presenting with gastrointestinal disease. Cancer 42:693–707, 1978.
78. Kowlessar, OD: The carcinoid syndrome. In Sleisenger, M, Fordtran, J (eds): Gastrointestinal Diseases, 2nd ed. Philadelphia: W. B. Saunders, 1978, pp. 1190–1201.
79. Drummey, GD, et al.: Microscopical examination of the stool for steatorrhea. N Engl J Med 264:85–87, 1961.
80. Morris, AI, Turnberg, LA: Surreptitious laxative abuse. Gastroenterology 77:780–786, 1979.
81. Cummings, JH, et al.: Laxative-induced diarrhea: A continuing clinical problem. Br Med J 1:537, 1974.
82. Miller, RE: Detection of colon carcinoma and the barium enema. JAMA 230:1195–1198, 1974.
83. Saunders, CG, MacEwen, DW: Delay in diagnosis of colon cancer. A continuing challenge. Radiology 101:207, 1971.
84. Bliss, CM: Fat absorption and malabsorption. Arch Intern Med 141:1213–1215, 1981.
85. Sleisenger, MH: Malabsorption syndrome. N Engl J Med 281:1111–1117, 1969.
86. Wilson, FA, Dietschy, JM: Differential diagnostic approach to clinical problems of malabsorption. Gastroenterology 61:911–931, 1971.
87. Arvanitakis, C, Cooke, AR: Diagnostic tests of exocrine pancreatic function and disease. Gastroenterology 74:932–948, 1978.
88. Drude, RB, Hines, C: The pathophysiology of intestinal bacterial overgrowth syndromes. Arch Intern Med 140:1349–1352, 1980.
89. Lauterburg, BH, et al.: Clinical value of the bile acid breath test. Evaluation of the Mayo Clinic experience. Mayo Clin Proc 53:227–233, 1978.
90. Rubin, CE, Dobbin, WO: Peroral biopsy of the small intestine. A review of its diagnostic usefulness. Gastroenterology 49:676–690, 1965.
91. Maizel, H, et al.: Whipple's disease: A review of 19 patients from one hospital and a review of the literature since 1950. Medicine 49:175–205, 1970.

92. Isselbacher, KJ, et al.: Congenital beta-lipoprotein and transport of lipids. Medicine 43:347, 1964.
93. Ament, ME, Rubin, CE: Relation of giardiasis to abnormal intestinal structure and function in gastrointestinal immunodeficiency syndromes. Gastroenterology 62:216, 1972.
94. Gilat, T, et al.: Deposition of amyloid in the gastrointestinal tract. Gut 10:98, 1969.
95. Ammann, RW, et al.: Gastrointestinal involvement in systemic mastocytosis. Gut 17:107, 1976.
96. Klein, NC, et al.: Eosinophilic gastroenteritis. Medicine 49:299, 1970.
97. Trier, JS: Celiac sprue disease. In Sleisenger, M, Fordtran, J (eds): Gastrointestinal Diseases, 2nd ed. Philadelphia: W.B. Saunders, 1973, pp. 1029–1051.
98. Klipstein, FA: Tropical sprue. Gastroenterology 54:275–293, 1968.
99. Earnest, DL, Trier, JS: Radiation enteritis and colitis. In Sleisenger, M, Fordtran, J (eds): Gastrointestinal Diseases, 2nd ed. Philadelphia: W. B. Saunders, 1978, pp. 1736–1745.
100. Birchir, J, et al.: Syndrome of intestinal arterial unsufficiency ("abdominal angina"). Arch Intern Med 117:632, 1966.
101. Sleisenger, M, Fordtran, J (eds): Gastrointestinal Diseases, 2nd ed. Philadelphia: W. B. Saunders, 1978, p. 289.
102. Kahn, IJ, et al.: Malabsorption in intestinal scleroderma. Correction by antibiotics. N Engl J Med 274:1339, 1966.
103. Jeffries, GH, et al.: Chronic ulcerative (nongranulomatous) jejunitis. Am J Med 44:47, 1968.
104. Krejs, GJ, et al.: Intractable diarrhea. Intestinal perfusion studies and plasma VIP concentration in patients with pancreatic cholera syndrome and surreptitious ingestion of laxatives and diuretics. Dig Dis 22:280–292, 1977.
105. Schein, PS, et al.: Islet cell tumors: Current concepts and management. Ann Intern Med 79:239–257, 1973.
106. Said, SI, Faloona, GR: Elevated plasma and tissue levels of vasoactive intestinal polypeptide in the watery diarrhea syndrome due to pancreatic, bronchogenic, and other tumors. N Engl J Med 293:155–160, 1975.
107. Larsson, LI, et al.: Pancreatic somatostatinoma. Clinical features and physiological implications. Lancet 1:666–668, 1977.
108. Ebeid, AM, et al.: VIP and the watery diarrhea syndrome. Ann Surg 187:411–416, 1978.
109. Walsh, JH, et al.: Gastrointestinal hormones in clinical disease: Recent developments. Ann Intern Med 90:817–828, 1979.
110. Babb, RR: Evaluation of acute proctitis. JAMA 244:358–359, 1980.
111. Klein, EJ, et al.: Anorectal gonococcal infection. Ann Intern Med 86:340–346, 1977.
112. Sands M, Sellers, T: Therapy of anorectal gonorrhea in men. Efficacy of oral antibiotic regimens. West J Med 133:469–471, 1980.
113. Sohn, N, Robilotti, J: The gay bowel syndrome. A review of colonic and rectal conditions in 200 male homosexuals. Am J Gastroenterol 67:478–484, 1977.
114. Gluckman, JB, et al.: Primary syphilis of the rectum. NY State J Med 74:2210–2211, 1974.
115. Quinn, TC, et al.: Chlamydia trachomatis proctitis. N Engl J Med 305:195–200, 1981.
116. Bolan, RK, et al.: Lymphogranuloma venereum and acute ulcerative proctitis. Am J Med 72:703–706, 1981.
117. Jacobs, E: Anal infection caused by herpes simplex virus. Dis Colon Rectum 19:151–157, 1976.
118. Venereal aspects of gastroenterology. West J Med 130:236–246, 1979.
119. Owen, WF: Sexually transmitted diseases and traumatic problems in homosexual men. Ann Intern Med 92:805–808, 1980.
120. Heller, MB: Special medical problems of hoxosexual men. The gay bowel syndrome. Resident Staff Physician 28:19s–25s, 1982.
121. Saffouri, B, et al.: Colonic involvement in salmonellosis. Dig Dis Sci 24:203–208, 1979.
122. Quinn, TC, et al.: Campylobacter proctitis in a homosexual man. Ann Intern Med 93:458–459, 1980.
123. Giacchino, JL, et al.: The therapeutic dilemma of acute amebic and ulcerative colitis. Surg Gyneco Obstet 146:599–603, 1978.
124. Gelfand, MD, et al.: Acute irradiation proctitis in man. Gastroenterology 54:401–411, 1968.
125. Eftaiha, M, et al.: Principles of management of colorectal foreign bodies. Arch Surg 112:691–695, 1977.
126. Schaumburg, HH, et al.: Monosodium L-glutamate: Its pharmacology and role in the Chinese restaurant syndrome. Science 163:826–828, 1969.
127. Olson, KR, et al.: Amanita phalloides-type mushroom poisoning. West J Med 137:282–289, 1982.
128. Hughes, JM, Merson, MH: Fish and shellfish poisoning. N Engl J Med 295:1117–1120, 1976.
129. Lerke, PA, et al.: Scombroid poisoning. Report of an outbreak. West J Med 129:381–386, 1978.
130. Lawrence, DW, et al.: Ciguatera fish poisoning in Miami. JAMA 244:254–258, 1980.
131. Morris, JG, et al.: Clinical features of ciguatera fish poisoning. A study of the disease in the U.S. Virgin Islands. Arch Intern Med 142:1090–1092, 1982.
132. Terranova, W, Blake, PA: Bacillus cereus food poisoning. N Engl J Med 298:143–144, 1978.
133. Holmes, JR, et al.: Emetic food poisoning caused by Bacillus cereus. Arch Intern Med 141:766–767, 1981.
134. Taylor, WR, et al.: A food-borne and outbreak of enterotoxigenic E. coli diarrhea. N Engl J Med 306:1093–1095, 1982.
135. Robinson, DA, et al.: Campylobacter enteritis associated with consumption of unpasteurized milk. Br J Med 1:1171–1173, 1979.
136. MGH Case Records, 48:1980: N Engl J Med 303:1347–1355, 1980.
137. Herman, RH, Hagler, L: Food intolerance in humans. West J Med 130:95–116, 1979.
138. Ravry, MJR: Dietetic food diarrhea. JAMA 244:270, 1980.
139. Gorback, SL, et al.: Travelers' diarrhea and toxigenic E coli. N Engl J Med 292:933–936, 1975.

140. Merson, MH, et al.: Travelers' diarrhea in Mexico. A prospective study of physicians and family members attending a congress. N Engl J Med 294:1299–1305, 1976.
141. DuPont, HL, et al.: Symptomatic treatment of diarrhea with bismuth subsalicylate among students attending a Mexican university. Gastroenterology 73:715–718, 1977.
142. Sack, DA, et al.: Prophylactic doxycycline for travelers' diarrhea. Results of a prospective double-blind study of Peace Corps volunteers in Kenya. N Engl J Med 298:758–763, 1978.
143. DuPont, HL, et al.: Prevention of travelers' diarrhea (emporiatric enteritis). Prophylactic administration of subsalicylate bismuth. JAMA 243:237–241, 1980.
144. Steffen, R, et al.: Epidemiology of diarrhea in travelers. JAMA 249:1176–1180, 1983.
145. Ericsson, CD, et al.: Bicozamycin, a poorly absorbable antibiotic, effectively treats travelers' diarrhea. Ann Intern Med 98:20–25, 1983.
146. Jordan, PH: Operations for peptic ulcer disease and their early postoperative complications. In Sleisenger, M, Fordtran, J (eds): Gastrointestinal Diseases, 2nd ed. Philadelphia: W. B. Saunders, 1978, pp. 932–946.
147. Meyer, JH: Chronic morbidity after ulcer surgery. In Sleisenger, M, Fordtran, J (eds): Gastrointestinal Diseases, 2nd ed. Philadelphia: W. B. Saunders, 1978, pp. 947–969.
148. Morns, SJ, Rogers, AI: Diarrhea after gastrectomy and vagotomy. Postgrad Med 65:219–230, 1979.
149. Herrington, HL: Remedial operations for postgastrectomy syndromes. Curr Probl Surg 1:63, 1970.
150. Jensen, RT, et al.: Zollinger-Ellison syndrome: Current concepts and management. Ann Intern Med 98:59–75, 1983.
151. Hutcheon, DF, et al.: Postcholecystectomy diarrhea. JAMA 241:823–824, 1979.
152. Weser, E: The management of patients after small bowel resection. Gastroenterology 71:146–150, 1976.
153. Floch, MH: Nutrition and Diet Therapy in Gastrointestinal Disease. New York: Plenum Press, 1981.
154. Graham, DY: Enzyme replacement therapy of exocrine pancreatic insufficiency in man. Relation between in vitro enzyme activities and in vivo potency in commercial pancreatic extracts. N Engl J Med 296:1314–1317, 1977.
155. Malagelada, JR: Enzyme replacement in chronic pancreatitis. Role of H_2 blockers. Drug Ther 12:67–82, 1982.
156. Regan, PT, et al.: Comparative effects of antacids, cimetidine, and enteric coating on the therapeutic response to oral enzymes in severe pancreatic insufficiency. N Engl J Med 297:854–858, 1977.
157. Graham, DY: Pancreatic enzyme replacement: The effect of antacids or cimetidine. Dig Dis Sci 27:485–490, 1982.
158. DiMagno, EP, et al.: Fate of orally-ingested enzymes in pancreatic insufficiency. Comparison of two dosage schedules. N Engl J Med 296:1318–1322, 1977.
159. Quinn, TC, et al.: The polymicrobial origin of intestinal infection in homosexual men. N Engl J Med 309:576–582, 1983.
160. Goodell, SE, et al.: Herpes simplex virus proctitis in homosexual men: clinical, sigmoidoscopic and histopathological features. N Engl J Med 308:868–871, 1983.
161. Current, WL, et al.: Human cryptosporidiosis in immunocompetent and immunodeficient persons. N Engl J Med 308:1252–1257, 1983.

4

HEADACHE

NEW (ACUTE) HEADACHE 165
    Intracranial Hemorrhage 166
    Ocular Headache 169
    Post-traumatic Headache 172
    Headache in the Elderly 173
    Infectious Headache 175
PHYSICAL EXAMINATION OF THE HEADACHE
PATIENT 176
HEADACHE IN SPECIAL CIRCUMSTANCES 181
CHRONIC, RECURRENT HEADACHE 184
    Classic Migraine 186
    Cluster Headache 188
    Trigeminal Neuralgia 189
    Common Migraine versus Tension Headache 191
DIAGNOSTIC TESTS IN HEADACHE 196
ANALGESICS AND HEADACHE 202
TREATMENT OF MIGRAINE 202
    Pharmacologic Therapy 203
        Symptomatic Treatment 203
        Preventive Therapy 205
TREATMENT OF TENSION HEADACHE 209
REFERENCES 213

Headache is so universal a symptom in Western society that it is often not considered a medical problem at all, but rather a common, if unwelcome, reminder of the stress of modern living. So familiar are headaches to most of us that their transience and benignity are usually assumed, and we are almost always right. Mass media advertising for nonprescription headache remedies runs to enormous expense, itself unassailable evidence that headaches are ubiquitous, their treatment empirical, and medical consultation rarely necessary. Even the word has achieved the status of idiom in our society: a headache is a nuisance, a vexing burden to be borne, presumably temporary, but nonetheless a "real headache."

The patient who consults a physician about headache is, then, different in some way. The physician must deal with "selected" patient populations who are, for whatever reason, concerned enough about the headache to seek help. The great majority of such patients suffer from common, benign headaches—due to tension, viral infections, mild trauma or migraine[1]—and the correct diagnosis is usually apparent. But, physician-patient interaction here may be quite complex. Most headache diagnosis is subjective,[2] basic pathogenetic mechanisms are obscure,[3-5] diagnostic labels often are arbitrary,[6] and treatment is frequently nonspecific. While tension and anxiety commonly cause headache,[7] the converse is also true. As more patients demand of physicians "proof" of health, a symptom that is only rarely a harbinger of serious illness results almost routinely now in extensive (expensive) diagnostic testing.[8] While a careful history and physical examination are often sufficiently diagnostic,[9] this time-honored approach now often invites patients' skepticism and demands for technologic "work-up."

Successful treatment of headache then, must address all these interdependent elements—anxiety, fear, misinformation, skepticism, and uncertainty—in the patient whose headache is often difficult to explain or treat "scientifically." No wonder the diagnosis and treatment of headache are such a headache!

It is not wise, then, to be too dogmatic about patients with headache. The need for diagnostic testing, specialist consultation and various treatments must be individualized. Of great importance, however, is the fact that a careful history and physical examination can almost always provide (or strongly suspect) a specific diagnosis.

In general, the history is most important in the patient with chronic or recurring headache (see page 184). Perhaps 90 per cent of such headaches are either vascular (migraine) or tension (muscle contraction) headaches.[10] When headaches have been a problem "for years," one of these syndromes can usually be assumed,[11] unless atypical or worrisome features suggest otherwise (see Fig. 4–9). Familiarity and ongoing clinical experience with the common chronic headache syndromes[12] is far more important than is sophisticated technologic testing in most patients—only rarely will the patient with chronic recurrent headache have serious organic (usually intracranial) disease.[13]

NEW (ACUTE) HEADACHE

"New" headache is a different matter. While chronic/recurrent headache must begin sometime, and more than a few patients with new headache suffer from new tension or migraine headache, a specific disease is more often the cause of new headache.[14-16] Serious disease must always be suspected in the patient with new headache, but attention to a few specific guidelines in the history and physical examination will usually help exclude such problems in favor of the more common and benign causes. Physical examination of the head, neck, eyes, and neurologic systems is crucial.

Various systems of headache nomenclature have been proposed. Table 4–1 illustrates one method of classifying headache. However, such classifications tend to be more helpful in standardizing clinical research than in differential diagnosis per se.

TABLE 4–1. CLASSIFICATION OF HEADACHE[17]

1. Vascular headache of migraine type
   a. Classic migraine
   b. Common migraine
   c. Cluster headache
   d. Hemiplegic and ophthalmoplegic migraine
   e. Lower-half headache
2. Muscle contraction headache
3. Combined headache: vascular and muscle contraction
4. Headache of nasal vasomotor reaction
5. Headache of delusional, conversional, or hypochondriac states
6. Nonmigrainous vascular headaches
7. Traction headache
8. Headache due to overt cranial inflammation
9–13. Headache due to disease of ocular, aural, nasosinusal, dental, or other cranial or neck structures
14. Cranial neuritides
15. Cranial neuralgias

CONSIDER

> Mary Migraine, a 32-year-old housewife, enters the clinic complaining of headache. For the past week she had "just not felt well and figured I had a cold, but, since yesterday, I have had a real bad headache." She describes sore throat, rhinitis, myalgias, dry cough, and a low-grade fever since 1 week ago, but was feeling generally better until 24 hours ago when her headache became very severe, kept her awake last night, and is now associated with nausea. The headache is generalized and "behind my eyes." Her muscle aches have "settled in my lower back" and her eyes "bother" her but nonspecifically. She has taken 12 aspirin in the last 24 hours without much relief.
>
> Mary admits to a long history of "tension headaches," but is adamant that "this headache is different, something new." Mary is worried.

NOTE

1. Mary is a chronic headache sufferer, but this particular headache is considered different. While not always reliable, such an observation by the patient should be taken as seriously as is the complaint that headache is new.

The clinical analysis of headache must then include those elements of the history that pertain to any symptom: severity, location, timing, duration, date and manner of onset, prodromal or associated symptoms, factors that precipitate, relieve, or exacerbate the headache, as well as the course of the headache since its onset (constant, episodic, progressively worsening, and the like). In general, the historical features that tend to be most helpful in the patient with new headache are location, timing, associated symptoms, and exacerbating factors.

2. In Mary's case the headache is severe and (this headache) has been present for only 24 hours.

Often the subjective severity of the headache is not diagnostically helpful. Tension headaches may be described as excruciating, while the patient with a brain tumor may have only mild or occasional headache.

The timing of headache is more often helpful (especially in the diagnosis of chronic headache syndromes—see page 184).

New headache that is constant (day and night), prevents sleep, and progressively worsens over several weeks is worrisome and must be carefully investigated. Brain tumors and other causes of increased intracranial pressure should be suspected.

Similarly, new headache that is very abrupt in onset ("like a hammer coming down on my head") and extremely severe ("the worst headache of my life") must prompt immediate suspicion of serious disease, even (uncommonly) when physical examination is unremarkable. Specifically, intracranial and subarachnoid hemorrhage must be unequivocally excluded in such circumstances.

Intracranial Hemorrhage

As a rule, the patient who suffers intracranial hemorrhage of any kind does not walk into a clinic simply complaining of headache. Such events are usually catastrophic, resulting in obvious neurologic compromise. Subdural or epidural hematomas usually occur after some type of trauma (see page 172), and impaired mental status is the rule in such cases. Intracerebral

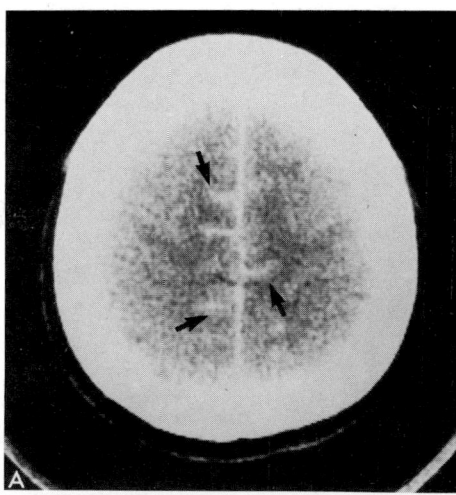

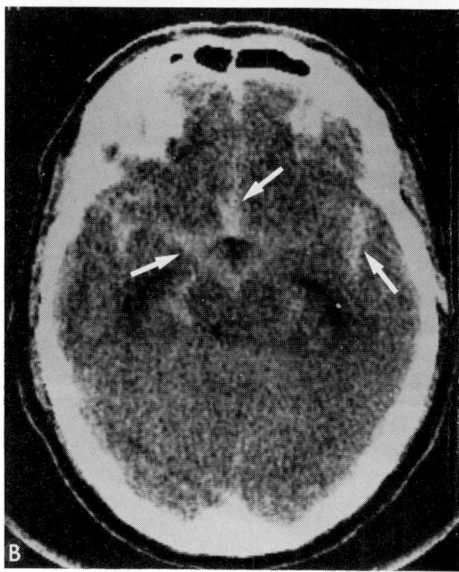

FIGURE 4–1. *A* and *B*, This unfortunate 33-year-old man complained of abrupt onset of severe headache, followed within the next hour by progressive unresponsiveness. Examination revealed low-grade fever, meningismus, and deep coma. CT scan demonstrated extensive subarachnoid bleeding. (Contrast is visible in the basal cisterns and cortical sulci—see *arrows.*) The patient died 2 days later.

Regrettably, this patient had suffered a similar event 3 weeks previously—sudden onset of severe headache and stiff neck but without impairment of mental functioning. The headache and stiff neck gradually resolved, and the patient did not seek medical attention at that time. Had he done so, surgical clipping of the aneurysm found at autopsy might have prevented his death.

hemorrhage presents as stroke or sudden coma, with associated neurologic findings defined by the site of the bleeding (most frequently the putamen, thalamus, and pons). The clinical picture and the CT scan[18] are virtually always diagnostic.

Two types of intracranial bleeding—subarachnoid hemorrhage and cerebellar hemorrhage—deserve special emphasis here because occasionally neurologic abnormalities may be subtle or even absent in such patients, and only the history of sudden severe headache will suggest the correct diagnosis.

Subarachnoid hemorrhage[19-23] produces sudden severe headache, usually reaching peak intensity within a minute or two of onset. Sometimes strenuous physical exertion precipitates the event (by raising intracranial pressure), and the headache is often associated with vomiting, transient loss of consciousness, or subsequent meningismus. (Rarely, headache will be mild, insidious, or altogether absent.) The headache usually lasts one to several days in patients who remain conscious long enough to complain of it. A reduced level of consciousness, nuchal rigidity, preretinal hemorrhages, and obvious neurologic impairment (Fig. 4–1*A* and *B*) are the rule, however, either immediately (in 50 per cent of patients) or within 24 hours (in more than 75 per cent of patients), but some patients remain alert and manifest no abnormal neurologic findings.[24, 25] Since these (alert) patients have a good

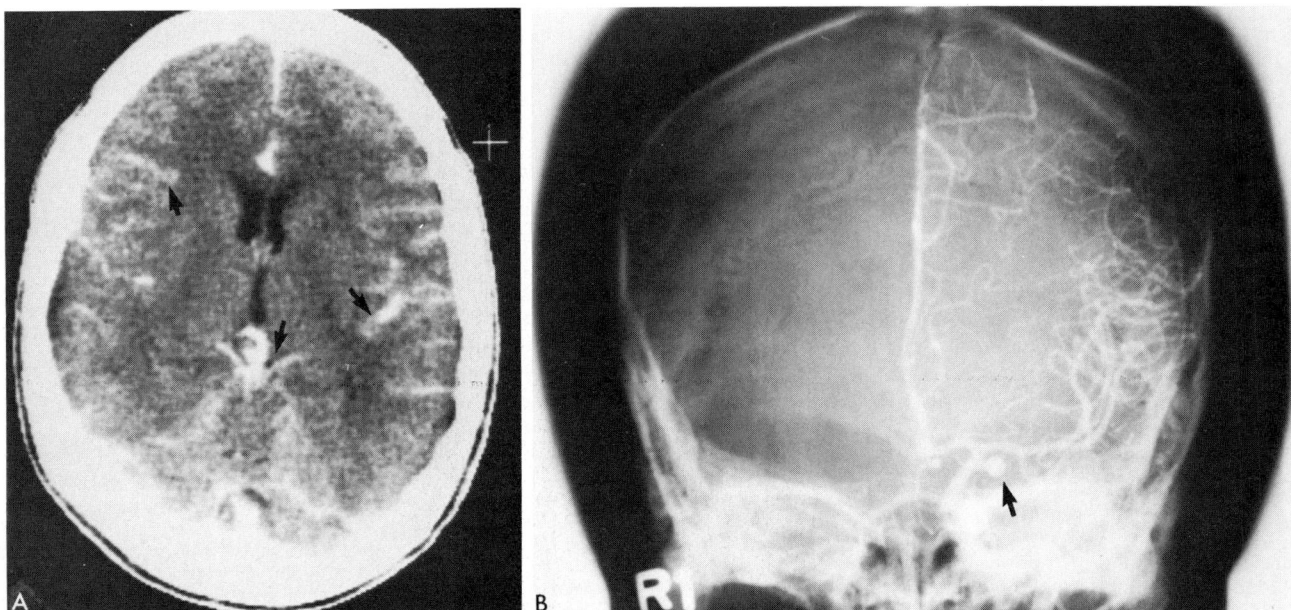

FIGURE 4–2. This 22-year-old man described 8 hours of severe occipital headache that had begun quite abruptly. He sought attention when he became nauseated and the headache did not improve. Examination was unremarkable except for mild meningismus and lethargy.

CT scan *(A)* reveals extensive subarachnoid hemorrhage (contrast in subarachnoid space—*arrows*). Surgical resection of the aneurysm demonstrated on arteriography *(B)* was successful, and the patient is well today.

prognosis when diagnosis is made early and the condition is managed correctly, a high index of suspicion of subarachnoid hemorrhage is crucial in patients with sudden severe headache (Fig. 4–2). Computerized tomography (CT scan) will be diagnostic in more than half of patients and is the initial procedure of choice, when available.[20] When the CT scan is normal or unavailable, but the diagnosis is strongly suspected, lumbar puncture will confirm acute (bloody CSF) or recent (xanthochromic CSF) bleeding. Arteriography usually localizes the source of the bleeding—an aneurysm much more commonly than an arteriovenous malformation, but there are occasionally other rare causes.

Untreated subarachnoid hemorrhage is often fatal. Rebleeding is common among survivors of an initial (unrecognized) hemorrhage. Hence the importance of early diagnosis (Figs. 4–1 and 4–2).

Cerebellar hemorrhage[26] is a life-threatening event that usually presents with sudden (often occipital) headache, vomiting, dizziness, and ataxia. While many patients are drowsy or frankly comatose, and exhibit both cranial nerve dysfunction and ataxia on neurologic examination (Fig. 4–3), some such patients are fully alert and demonstrate neurologic findings that may be quite subtle (Fig. 4–4), especially if the patient is examined "laconically."[26] Most (carefully examined) patients show some combination of appendicular or truncal ataxia, ipsilateral gaze palsy, and (peripheral) facial nerve paresis. Such a clinical picture in the typical patient (hypertensive, anticoagulated, or traumatized) should prompt emergency CT,[27] which is usually diagnostic. Skull x-rays, electroencephalograms, and isotope brain scans are usually not helpful here. Lumbar puncture is potentially dangerous in these circumstances but should be considered when CT or arteriography is not available, since the cerebrospinal fluid is usually bloody and a neurosurgeon must then be consulted immediately.

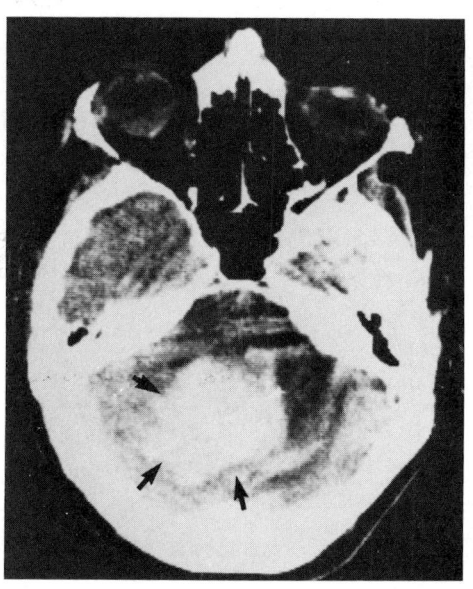

FIGURE 4–3. This 73-year-old man taking oral anticoagulants developed mild but persistent occipital headache. His family brought him to the emergency room when he appeared unable to walk.

Examination revealed marked truncal ataxia and a distracted, inattentive affect. CT scan demonstrated a huge cerebellar hemorrhage (*arrows*). Neurosurgical evacuation was successful, but the patient remains neurologically impaired.

The mortality from cerebellar hemorrhage is high, even under ideal circumstances. Neurosurgical evacuation of the hematoma is probably more successful when the diagnosis is made very early.

3. Mary's headache is generalized, but there are complaints referable to the eyes. Some patients with local disorders of eyes, ears, nose, sinuses, throat, temporomandibular joint, or neck will complain of headache when, in fact, pain is more localized to the face, orbit, jaw, or neck. Always ask the patient where the headache hurts and whether it involves or "spreads" to any specific anatomic structure.

Ocular Headache

Headache in the orbital or periorbital area should suggest several possibilities. Usually the history and a careful examination of the external orbit, pupil reactivity and size, extraocular movements, visual acuity, and funduscopic detail will differentiate among these possibilities.[28, 29] Table 4–2

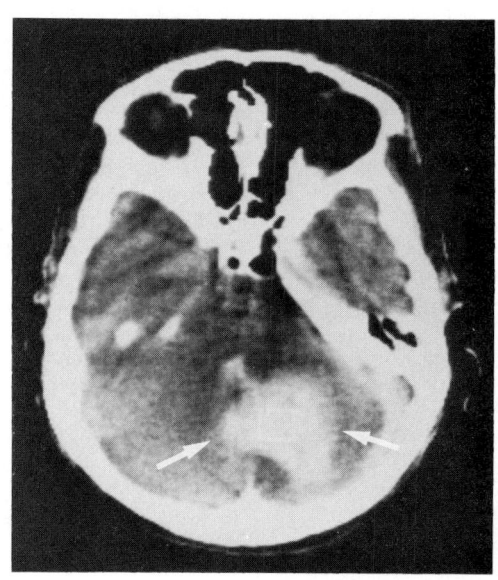

FIGURE 4–4. This 62-year-old woman presented with the sudden onset of severe occipital headache. Examination was remarkably normal, except for marked dysmetria of the left hand and a (peripheral) facial nerve palsy. CT scan demonstrates extensive cerebellar hemorrhage (*arrows*). Neurosurgical evacuation of the hematoma was undertaken 8 hours later, when the patient began to deteriorate. The patient recovered fully.

lists a few salient diagnostic points about headache around the eye that is of ocular origin.

Acute glaucoma[32] (angle closure glaucoma) induces pain in the eye or orbit and is almost always associated with an abnormal eye examination. The patient is usually quite sick, often vomiting repeatedly. The globe is tender or hard, the pupil dilated, the cornea "steamy," and the conjunctiva injected. (Rarely, patients will experience intermittent brief eye pain precipitated by episodic pupillary dilatation—e.g., walking into a dark movie theater or after using medication with anticholinergic properties. Symptoms may resolve completely before examination, and tonometry may be normal at this time, but this history alone is usually suggestive.)

Iritis (uveitis) is associated with eye pain, conjunctival injection ("red eye"), decreased visual acuity, and a unilaterally small pupil, often with extreme photophobia.

Optic neuritis is not a common cause of headache or eye pain but should be suspected when orbital pain and headache are associated with a decreased pupillary light reflex, blurring of the disc, and hyperemia of the retina (which may mimic papilledema), or painful extraocular movements. Visual acuity is diminished (and the patient may complain of "looking through a steamed-up window").

Occlusion of the central retinal artery (due to cardiac emboli, vasculitis, carotid disease, and the like) causes sudden complete unilateral visual loss with a "gray" fundus, constricted arterioles, and retinal edema.[31] Central retinal vein thrombosis[31] causes less severe but acute diminution of vision with retinal hemorrhages, engorged veins, and retinal edema. Both of these conditions (especially the latter) may be mistaken for papilledema.

Eye strain is a much overdiagnosed cause of headache, but some patients will experience orbital or retro-orbital headache after prolonged reading or close work, relieved by refractive or other correction. Presbyopia, strabismus, or astigmatism is much more often the underlying problem than is myopia.[30]

TABLE 4–2. COMMON OCULAR CAUSES OF HEADACHE[28, 30, 31]

DISEASE	SYMPTOMS AND SIGNS	TREATMENT RECOMMENDATIONS
Acute glaucoma	Severe unilateral eye pain; sick, vomiting; pupil dilated; "red eye," "steamy" cornea; diminished vision	Pupillary constriction; acetazolamide; urgent ophthalmology consultation
Iritis	Eye pain; "red eye"; small pupil; photophobia; diminished vision	Find cause! Corticosteroids; pupillary dilatation; consult ophthalmologist
Optic neuritis	Diminished vision; pupillary light reflex decreased; hyperemia of fundus and disc; painful extraocular movements	Consult ophthalmologist Toxins, infections? Young patient: multiple sclerosis? Elderly patient: temporal arteritis?
Vascular occlusion (retinal artery or retinal vein)	Sudden eye pain and loss of vision; "gray" avascular fundus (arterial occlusion); retinal hemorrhages and edema (venous occlusion)	Consult ophthalmologist immediately; acetazolamide?; analgesics
Eye strain	Presbyopia? Strabismus? Astigmatism	Consult ophthalmologist

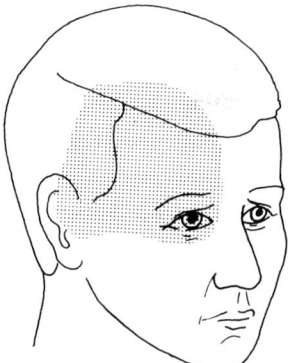
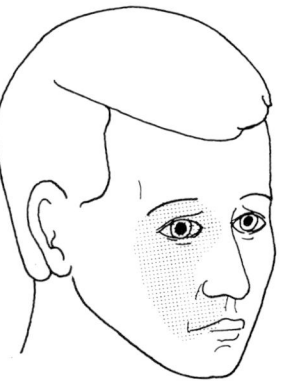

FIGURE 4–5. Periorbital headache.

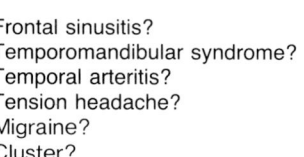

Frontal sinusitis?
Temporomandibular syndrome?
Temporal arteritis?
Tension headache?
Migraine?
Cluster?

Maxillary sinusitis?
Dental infection?
Allergic/vasomotor rhinitis?
Nasopharyngeal tumor?
Trigeminal neuralgia?
Migraine?
Cluster?

As is noted in Table 4–2, an ophthalmologist should be consulted (sometimes urgently) when these conditions are suspected. In many other circumstances, however, pain around the eye or headache associated with various visual complaints may not fall within the province of the eye specialist. For example, headache associated with photophobia is very common in migraine; systemic viral infection, aseptic meningitis, subarachnoid hemorrhage, and pituitary tumors may also cause photophobia.[30] In these circumstances, examination of the eye itself is often normal.

When headache is associated with demonstrable visual loss, pupillary dilatation (or constriction), or cranial nerve palsies (ophthalmoplegia), many other conditions must be considered (see Table 4–7).

Orbital or periorbital pain with a normal eye examination should suggest migraine, cluster headache, trigeminal or postherpetic neuralgia—here, the history alone is often diagnostic (see page 185). Other causes of periorbital headache are enumerated in Figure 4–5. Sinus disease is especially common.

Frontal sinusitis causes pain above the eyes; maxillary sinusitis causes pain below the eye, in the upper teeth, or both; ethmoid sinusitis causes pain along the medial orbit, straddling the nose. Rarely, isolated sphenoid sinusitis[33] causes pain at the vertex of the skull and "behind the eyes." Thus, while the headache of sinusitis may be generalized,[34, 35] other clues are usually helpful: the precise location, coexistent nasal congestion or postnasal drip, symptomatic variations with seasonal or barometric changes, prominence of symptoms on awakening or bending over. Sometimes the basic process is allergic or vasomotor rhinitis without frank sinus infection. (Conversely, nasal symptoms in association with headache may have many other causes— nasal congestion or rhinorrhea is common with cluster and migraine headache, for example.)

4. In Mary's case, there is no history of trauma.[36, 37] Major head trauma that results in intracranial hemorrhage, cerebral contusion, major skull fractures, or prolonged coma is far beyond the scope of this text.[148] Such patients are usually seriously impaired. The patient with reduced mental status, focal neurologic findings, CSF rhinorrhea or otorrhea, bloody CSF, or an abnormal CT scan following head trauma always requires neurosurgical observation or intervention.

Post-traumatic Headache

Epidural hematoma is rare but deserves brief mention here. The classic picture is that of brief loss of consciousness (usually in the setting of severe head trauma with a skull fracture through the ipsilateral middle meningeal artery), thereafter followed by a lucid interval of minutes to days during which the patient may appear well. Subsequent relapse into coma with focal neurologic compromise (hemiparesis, dilated pupil, etc.) then announces the seriousness of the problem. Neurologic deterioration may be preceded by worsening headache and vomiting during this lucid interval. CT scan is usually diagnostic; surgical decompression is required.

A much more common problem for the generalist physician is the patient with headache following minor head trauma. Usually this is a self-limited headache that resolves gradually over several days. "Whiplash" injuries, scalp hematomas, and uncomplicated skull fractures are usually treated conservatively and expectantly. While such patients must be carefully examined and followed (sometimes in the hospital for the first 1 to 2 days), most of these headaches are uncomplicated. A few such cases are more difficult:

Postconcussion* (or post-traumatic) syndrome refers to persistent headache and associated nonspecific symptoms—insomnia, emotional instability, fatigue, vertigo, impaired concentration, antisocial behavior—usually beginning hours to days after minor head trauma. These headaches are usually generalized; may worsen with cough, exertion, or changes in head position; often improve with rest or sleep; but may gradually intensify for days or weeks, only to slowly abate over the ensuing several weeks. Usually these post-traumatic headaches mimic either tension or vascular headache (see page 191). In the former subset, headache tends to be constant, generalized or occipital, and nonpulsatile—persistent anxiety following the traumatic event may contribute. Other headaches seem clearly "vascular"—visual auras and nausea and vomiting may occur, and these headaches may be more localized and throbbing. Some such patients develop a "vascular" headache repeatedly precipitated by "mild" trauma (the football player who develops a "migraine" after each practice session, for example).

Two points must be emphasized about the post-traumatic syndrome. (1) While poorly understood, this may be a debilitating affliction, all the more so when clinicians' misunderstanding allows many such patients to be labeled neurotic or actual malingerers. Emotional and analgesic support are important. The long-term prognosis is generally good. (2) It must be

---

*Concussion traditionally refers to loss of consciousness, however brief, at the time of trauma, but this syndrome may also occur without "true" concussion.

TABLE 4–3. POST-TRAUMATIC HEADACHE

CONSIDER
Epidural hematoma
Subdural hematoma
Cerebral contusion
Skull fracture
Cervical spine fracture

USUALLY DUE TO
Postconcussion syndrome
Whiplash injury
Scalp contusion/hematoma

TABLE 4–4. NEW HEADACHE IN THE OLDER PATIENT

CONSIDER
Giant cell arteritis
Occlusive cerebrovascular disease
Accelerated hypertension
Neoplasm (primary or metastatic)
Trigeminal neuralgia
Postherpetic neuralgia
Cluster headache
Acute glaucoma
Subdural hematoma

remembered that even trivial trauma may cause intracranial hemorrhage, especially in the elderly, alcoholic, or anticoagulated patient. Obvious focal neurologic deficits are sometimes inapparent in the patient with subdural hematoma. Subtle personality changes, mild inattention, intermittent drowsiness, or slowed mentation in association with a steady, generalized, progressively worsening (but not always severe) headache may be the only clues to the diagnosis of subdural hematoma. CT scan is virtually always diagnostic in patients with subdural hematoma[38] (Fig. 4–6).

5. Mary is young. Patients of any age may develop headaches of any kind. However, new headache in the older patient (beyond 50 years of age) is always cause for concern. Several "special considerations" should be remembered:

Headache in the Elderly

Temporal arteritis,[39–43] better termed giant cell arteritis, is a serious, not at all rare, and eminently treatable condition that almost always afflicts patients over the age of 50. Sharply localized pain over a tender, nodular, superficial temporal artery in the elderly patient should never be a diagnostic dilemma, but the diagnosis of this disorder is often not so obligingly obvious. Headache does not occur in all patients; when it does occur, it is often nonspecific in quality and generalized in location. Most patients do have other subtle systemic symptoms (fever, malaise, depression, anorexia, or weight loss) or clinical polymyalgia rheumatica. Almost all have (Westergren) sedimentation rates above 50. Jaw claudication (ischemic jaw and face pain with repetitive chewing) occurs in only a minority but is highly suggestive of the diagnosis when present.

Most patients with this disease will have headaches and other systemic symptoms for weeks before the onset of visual loss—the major danger of giant cell arteritis (due to ischemic optic neuritis or retinal artery occlusion)—but blindness may also occur suddenly (and is usually irreversible). The older patient with new headache and an elevated sedimentation rate should be treated promptly with daily high-dose corticosteroids (prednisone 60 mg a day) even before more specific diagnostic studies are undertaken (temporal artery biopsies*). This is especially critical when visual symptoms (amaurosis fugax, diplopia, or ptosis) are already present or when the patient has already sustained unilateral visual loss—irreversible involvement of the contralateral eye often follows soon thereafter if the patient is not treated promptly.

---

*Because an elevated ESR is not rare in elderly patients without temporal arteritis, the biopsy is essential.

Arteriosclerotic headache[44-46] is a poorly understood, but probably real, phenomenon. Completed infarctions (stroke) or transient ischemia involving carotid or vertebrobasilar vascular territory may be associated with headache in 25 percent of cases, but the associated neurologic symptoms and signs usually dominate these clinical presentations. (Such syndromes may be confused, rarely, with classic migraine—see page 186.) Some elderly patients with carotid or vertebrobasilar stenosis (or frank occlusion) may experience headache without symptoms of neurologic ischemia, however. Sometimes these headaches "sound vascular"—pulsatile and "throbbing"—and may be appropriately localized: occipital when vertebrobasilar disease is the problem, or hemicranial when unilateral carotid disease is the problem. More often the headache is nonspecific in quality and location. Whether such headaches are due to vasodilatation of extracranial collateral vessels is unknown. Nevertheless, new headache in the elderly patient should prompt at least a noninvasive search for treatable extracranial vascular disease—e.g., a careful history for symptoms of transient ischemia, careful neck auscultation for carotid or posterior vascular bruits, or noninvasive carotid vascular studies (ultrasound and plethysmography).

Hypertension is mentioned here only because so many elderly patients have systolic or diastolic hypertension or both, and it is thus often tempting to attribute recent headache in hypertensive patients to transient blood pressure elevations. With few exceptions, this temptation should be resisted. While a few patients "can tell when my blood pressure is up" because of (usually mild) headache, this is not the rule. Various studies[47, 48] support the notion that, in general, hypertension causes headache only in unusual circumstances: malignant hypertension, eclampsia, pheochromocytoma, and when diastolic pressures exceed 130 mm of mercury.

Neoplasms,[36] whether primary or metastatic to the brain, cause headache that is usually very nonspecific. Such tumors are by no means restricted to the older population. In fact, primary intracranial neoplasms are more common in children and adolescents (glioma, craniopharyngioma, hemangioma) or in early middle age (meningioma, fibroma, glioma, and pituitary tumor). Metastatic neoplasms are, however, more common than are primary tumors, and metastatic carcinomatosis does occur much more often in the older patient population. New headache in an older patient always should

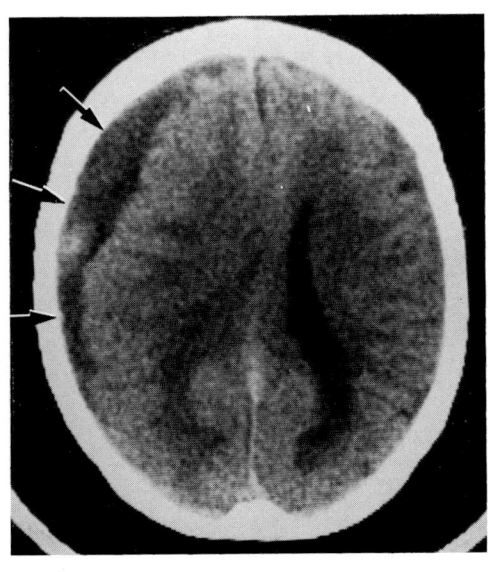

FIGURE 4–6. This 72-year-old gentleman fell and hit his head while climbing out of the bathtub. He did not lose consciousness, but for the next 3 days, he complained of mild headache. His wife brought him to medical attention when he appeared to her to be slightly confused. Examination was entirely unremarkable, except for mild impairment of mental status (short-term recall, calculations, and orientation to time). CT scan demonstrates a subdural hematoma on the right (arrows). Surgical evacuation resulted in prompt improvement.

prompt a complete physical and neurologic examination, chest x-ray, urinalysis, stool examination for occult blood, and a chemistry profile. Headache that is constant, progressive, related to head position, or that awakens the patient from sleep is worrisome.

Various other headache disorders are also more common in the older patient (Table 4–4). Cluster headache (see page 188) usually occurs in middle age. Trigeminal neuralgia and postherpetic neuralgia (see page 189) are usually diseases of the elderly. Acute glaucoma, nasopharyngeal carcinoma, subdural hematoma, and temporomandibular joint dysfunction are more often seen in the older patient as well.

6. In Mary's case the clinical setting suggests infection.

Infectious Headache

Most headache in the setting of fever and other evidence of systemic infection is only mild or moderate in severity and probably results from the cranial vasodilatation that accompanies fever. The headache usually resolves with subsidence of fever.

Table 4–5 lists a variety of common and uncommon infectious diseases in which headache may be a prominent symptom. Most often, associated symptoms point to a specific diagnosis.

A stiff neck (meningismus) may suggest meningitis, but subarachnoid hemorrhage, deep neck abscesses, cervical osteomyelitis, brain abscess, juvenile rheumatoid arthritis, or other cervical spondylitides may also present with fever and stiff neck. Bacterial meningitis or brain abscess is usually accompanied by severe systemic toxicity and mental status impairment. Aseptic meningitis—usually caused by enteroviruses or mumps virus—is another matter: Such patients are sometimes only mildly ill and may even be afebrile (see below). Photophobia and painful eye movements are frequent clues to the diagnosis of aseptic meningitis in the patient with minimal or no meningismus who is not in a toxic state. Encephalitis is almost always accompanied by impaired mental status.

Most patients with headache and fever have an obvious viral infection or another common infectious disease (Table 4–5).

TABLE 4–5. SYSTEMIC INFECTION IN WHICH HEADACHE MAY BE A PROMINENT SYMPTOM

COMMON ILLNESS	UNCOMMON ILLNESS	UNCOMMON, BUT MOST SERIOUS
Viremia	Typhoid fever	Meningitis
Influenza	Tularemia	Brain abscess
Pharyngitis	Toxoplasmosis	Retropharyngeal abscess
Otitis media	Cytomegalovirus infection	Cervical osteomyelitis
Sinusitis	Mumps	Suppurative intracranial
Mononucleosis	Measles	thrombophlebitis
Pneumonococcal	Poliomyelitis	Subdural empyema
pneumonia	Psittacosis	Encephalitis
Mycoplasma pneumonia	Dengue	Septicemia
	Trichinosis	Endocarditis
	Q fever	Rocky Mountain spotted fever
	Legionnaires' disease	Malaria
	Leptospirosis	
	Typhus	

Mary says that her headache, while severe, did <u>not</u> begin abruptly with sudden immediate severity but has gradually progressed over the course of the day. There is no history of head trauma, hypertension, or anticoagulation.

Mary believes that her "cold" had been improving at the time her headache began and that she had been afebrile for several days. The nausea is new, as is the discomfort in the eyes—"the light hurts my eyes today." Mary denies a stiff neck.

PHYSICAL EXAMINATION OF THE HEADACHE PATIENT

Physical examination reveals normal vital signs, but the temperature is 38°C orally. Examination of the ears, nose, and throat is normal. Funduscopic examination reveals normal findings, with visible venous pulsations, but the light hurts Mary's eyes. The pupils are equal in size and react to light normally. There is no corneal or conjunctival injection. Extraocular movements, visual fields, and visual acuity are normal, but the extraocular movements cause discomfort. The neck is supple, and there are no definite meningeal signs, but the lower back feels "tight" with neck and hip flexion.

There are no focal neurologic abnormalities. Mary is fully alert, and formal mental status testing—orientation to place, person, and time; remote and recent memory; and attention span—is completely normal.

What does this mean?

1. <u>The patient is fully alert. This is the most critical determination in patients with new headache.</u> Any suggestion of even mildly impaired mental status in the patient with acute headache warrants investigation (usually in the hospital). Formal mental status testing should be performed—a "screening" mental status examination can be briefly accomplished in tandem with the history and examination (Table 4–6).

2. <u>There are no focal neurologic abnormalities.</u> Such findings—hemiparesis, cranial nerve or cerebellar dysfunction, asymmetric reflexes, or upgoing toes (Babinski's)—would raise many important diagnostic considerations, depending upon the clinical setting and particular neurologic deficit. Ischemic or hemorrhagic disease of the cerebral cortex, cerebellum, or brain

TABLE 4–6. "SCREENING" MENTAL STATUS TESTING

INSIGHT
What is your problem? How are you sick? Why are you here?

ORIENTATION
Person: What is your name? Where do you live? What is your occupation?
Place: How did you get here today? Where are we now?
Time: What is the date and day of the week today? What time is it?

MEMORY
Remote: What jobs have you held in the past?
Recent: What did you have for breakfast today?
Short term: Repeat these numbers: 7–5–1–4–9.
            Now, repeat these numbers backwards: 8–4–2–7–3.

CALCULATION
Subtract 7 from 100, serially ("serial 7's").

LEARNING
Name three objects and ask patient to remember those objects.
Ask patient to recall these three objects 5 minutes later.

stem is far beyond the scope of this text, as is a detailed discussion of intracranial mass lesions.

Focal neurologic findings in the patient with fever must raise the question of brain abscess,[49, 50] bacterial endocarditis with septic cerebral emboli, mycotic intracranial aneurysms, meningitis, and subdural empyema.

3. Mary has a low-grade fever. In general, the absence of fever excludes most of the problems listed in Table 4–5. Exceptions include head and neck infections, which may themselves induce local headache without fever. Hence the importance of the fact that:

Examination of the ears, nose, throat, and neck is normal.

Otologic causes of headache[34] include otitis media, otitis externa, and mastoiditis—pain is almost invariably unilateral, and examination is usually diagnostic.

Sinusitis will occasionally cause generalized headache, but usually other symptoms (see page 171) and the location of pain and tenderness are highly suggestive. Figure 4–5 illustrates the usual location of pain and tenderness referred from the frontal and maxillary sinuses.

Allergic rhinitis or vasomotor rhinitis without sinusitis may also cause headache—pale, watery, engorged nasal mucosa is usually visible on examination of the "allergic nose" (and eosinophils will be present on Wright's stain of the nasal secretions). The nasal mucosa of vasomotor rhinitis is often a purple blue.

Nasopharyngeal neoplasms[51] may cause generalized headache, at times with "secondary" cranial neuralgias (when advanced tumor infiltrates the base of the skull).

Pharyngotonsillitis is usually obvious, as are dental infections. Subacute thyroiditis, carotidynia,[52] deep neck abscesses,[53] and temporomandibular disorders may be less obvious. Cervical spine disease[54] is a common cause of (usually occipital) headache (see page 210).

4. The absence of frank meningismus usually, but not always, excludes meningitis. In the first few hours of bacterial meningitis, the neck may be supple. Usually there is resistance to passive flexion of the neck or Brudzinski's or Kernig's signs will be apparent (Fig. 4–7A and B) Especially in

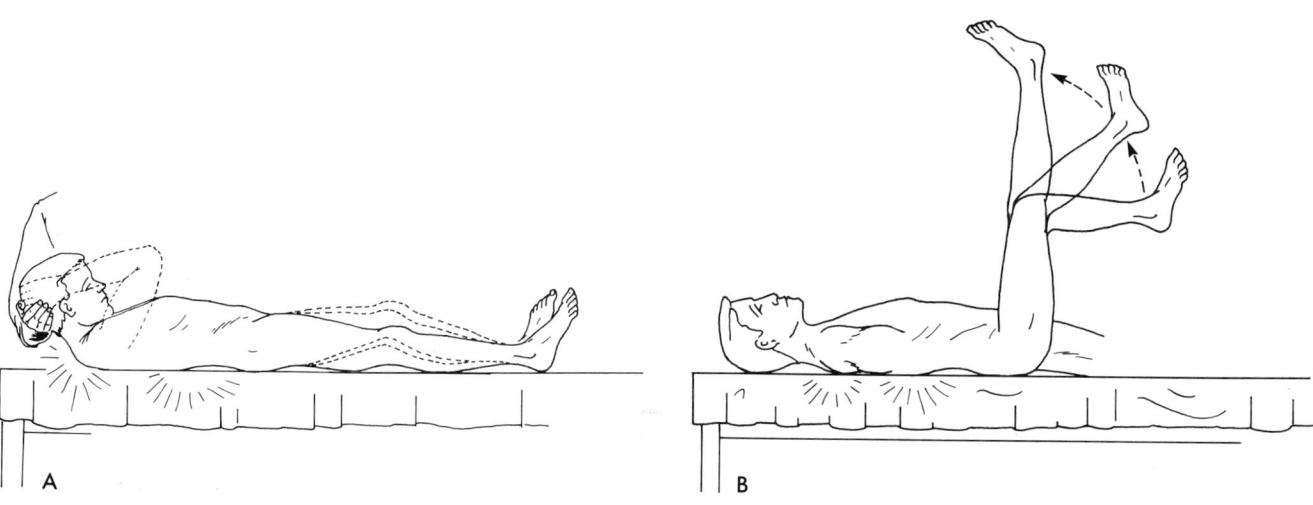

FIGURE 4–7. A, Brudzinski's sign. The patient lies supine—the head is passively elevated from the table by the examiner. The patient complains of neck and low back discomfort and attempts to relieve the meningeal irritation by involuntary flexion of the knees and hips. B, Kernig's sign. The patient lies supine with the hip and knee flexed. The knee is then gradually extended—complaints of pain in the lower back, neck and/or head are suggestive of meningeal irritation.

aseptic meningitis, however, meningismus may be absent or very subtle. Unimpressive complaints of mild "tightness" of the cervical or lumbar spine on "meningeal testing" (Fig. 4–7) are noted in some cases of proven viral meningitis. In rarer types of meningitis—for example, tuberculous, fungal, or neoplastic—the neck may be supple.

5. Mary's eye symptoms—primarily photophobia and painful extraocular movements—are not accompanied by any obvious abnormality of vision or eye anatomy, and there is no ophthalmoplegia. Common ocular causes of headache are usually apparent on physical examination (Table 4–2 above). Confirmation examination by an ophthalmologist is required when these are suspected. Tonometry, slit lamp examination, full field funduscopy, and other procedures may be necessary.

When new headache is associated with new visual impairment or ophthalmoplegia, many possibilities must be considered.[30] A specific diagnosis can often be at least strongly suspected on the basis of the pattern of visual loss (e.g., monocular, binocular, homonymous hemianopia), the history, and physical examination.[29, 31, 32, 55, 56] Table 4–7 lists some of the distinguishing

TABLE 4–7. CONDITIONS THAT MAY CAUSE NEW HEADACHE AND EYE SIGNS

DIAGNOSIS	DISTINGUISHING FEATURES
Headaches with Visual Loss	
Headache with Monocular Visual Loss	
Optic neuropathies[56]	
Temporal arteritis	Elderly patient, elevated sedimentation rate, accompanying systemic symptoms
Nonarteritic optic neuropathy	Sudden visual loss; funduscopy may be normal
Optic neuritis	Usually decreased pupillary light reflex, disc blurring with hyperemia of the fundus, sometimes with painful extraocular movements
Infiltrative neuropathies	Progressive, more gradual visual loss—pituitary tumors, intracranial aneurysms, increased intracranial pressure common cause
Ophthalmic transient ischemic attack[28] (amaurosis fugax)	Typically brief (3–5 min), sudden visual loss, with associated diffuse atherosclerosis; carotid bruits common
Ophthalmic migraine	More gradual onset of visual loss than amaurosis fugax, lasts longer (25–30 min), and often followed by typical headache
Iritis (uveitis)	Conjunctival infection, miosis, photophobia (see Table 4–2)
Meningovascular syphilis	May mimic temporal arteritis; positive VDRL in CSF (and pleocytosis)
Acute glaucoma	Sick, nausea and vomiting, tender or hard globe, pupil dilated, cornea "steamy," "red eye."
Headache with Binocular Visual Loss	
Temporal arteritis	Usually sequential eye involvement
Iritis (bilateral)	Gradual visual loss, abnormal eye examination (see Table 4–2)
Basilar migraine[57]	Usually young female with other vertebrobasilar neurologic symptoms—ataxia, vertigo, weakness, loss of consciousness (see page 187)
Vertebrobasilar transient ischemia	Older patient, diffuse atherosclerosis, other vertebrobasilar symptoms—vertigo, dysarthria, leg weakness
Chiasmal tumor	Often bitemporal hemianopia, enlarged sella turcica on tomograms of skull (Fig. 4–16)
Increased intracranial pressure: benign intracranial hypertension[58]	Fluctuating headache, papilledema
Episodic hypoglycemia	*Transient* episode in which visual symptoms may (occasionally) predominate, often followed by headache
Presyncope (usually cardiac)	*Transient* episode sometimes followed by headache

Table continues on opposite page.

features of various conditions that may cause new headache associated with visual loss, ophthalmoplegia, or pupillary abnormalities.

6. Mary's headache is compatible with acute migraine, but there are atypical features. When there are no symptoms and signs that clearly point to a specific diagnosis, the decision to investigate further with laboratory or radiologic testing or both (see Fig. 4–8) often depends on whether the new headache can be confidently diagnosed as tension headache or migraine or, more rarely, as cluster headache or cranial neuralgia (see page 185).

In this case, generalized headache associated with nausea, photophobia, and painful extraocular movements is compatible with common migraine headache (see page 193). On the other hand, such a headache occurring in the setting of a recent "viral" illness, that is associated with low-grade fever and symptoms suggestive of subtle meningeal irritation must raise the question of aseptic meningitis.

Lumbar puncture, performed in the clinic, reveals clear, colorless cerebrospinal fluid with an opening pressure of 220 cm of water. There are 90 white blood cells, 90 percent of which are lymphocytes. Spinal fluid glucose, Gram's stain, and protein are normal.

TABLE 4–7. CONDITIONS THAT MAY CAUSE NEW HEADACHE AND EYE SIGNS (Continued)

DIAGNOSIS	DISTINGUISHING FEATURES
Headache with Homonymous Hemianopia	
Classic migraine	Typical history (see page 186).
Posterior cerebral transient ischemia	Carotid or basilar atherosclerosis, with other neurologic symptoms
Occipital lobe disease (neoplasm, hemorrhage)	Visual loss and headache occasionally may be only manifestation
Headache with Ophthalmoplegia	
Intracranial aneurysm (especially posterior communicating artery)	Third cranial nerve paresis, pupil dilated
Diabetic neuritis	Third cranial nerve paresis, pupil normal; eye usually very painful
Ophthalmoplegic migraine[59]	Typical history (see page 187)—usually third cranial nerve
Temporal arteritis	Mild ptosis occasionally observed without other visual symptoms
Basilar meningitis[60]	Usually chronic symptoms with abnormal spinal fluid
Cavernous sinus disease or parasellar disease[30]	Paresis of third through sixth cranial nerves
Brain tumor or other causes of hydrocephalus	Bilateral sixth cranial nerve paresis—often a "false localizing" sign
Exophthalmos of any cause	Proptosis
Syphilis	CSF VDRL
Nasopharyngeal carcinoma[51]	Usually when cancer advanced and involving base of skull
Multiple sclerosis	Episodic neurologic deficits of different types, occurring widely spaced over time; optic atrophy sometimes a clue
Idiopathic (Tolosa-Hunt syndrome)[61]	May be responsive to corticosteroid therapy
Headaches with Pupillary Asymmetry	
Headache with Unilateral Dilated Pupil	
Transtentorial herniation due to mass effect	Decreased mental status with usually obvious neurologic compromise
Intracranial aneurysm	Other cranial nerve findings (third)
Optic neuritis	Table 4–2
Acute glaucoma	Table 4–2
Headaches with Unilateral Constricted Pupil	
Cluster headache (with partial Horner's syndrome)	Typical history (see page 188)
	Ptosis, miosis during headache
Mediastinal neoplasm with intracranial metastases or superior vena cava obstruction (with Horner's syndrome)	Chest x-ray diagnostic
	Unilateral ptosis, miosis, anhydrosis

NOTE

1. While these CSF findings are not absolutely diagnostic of viral meningitis, the clinical setting combined with this "CSF profile" makes that diagnosis virtually certain. Other causes of mild lymphocytic (30 to 300 cells) pleocytosis with normal glucose and protein in the CSF may include partially treated bacterial meningitis, tuberculous or fungal meningitis, cerebral abscess or neoplasm, cerebral infarction or neoplastic meningeal infiltration. Usually other clinical and CSF findings suggest these much more serious diagnoses.[36, 62]

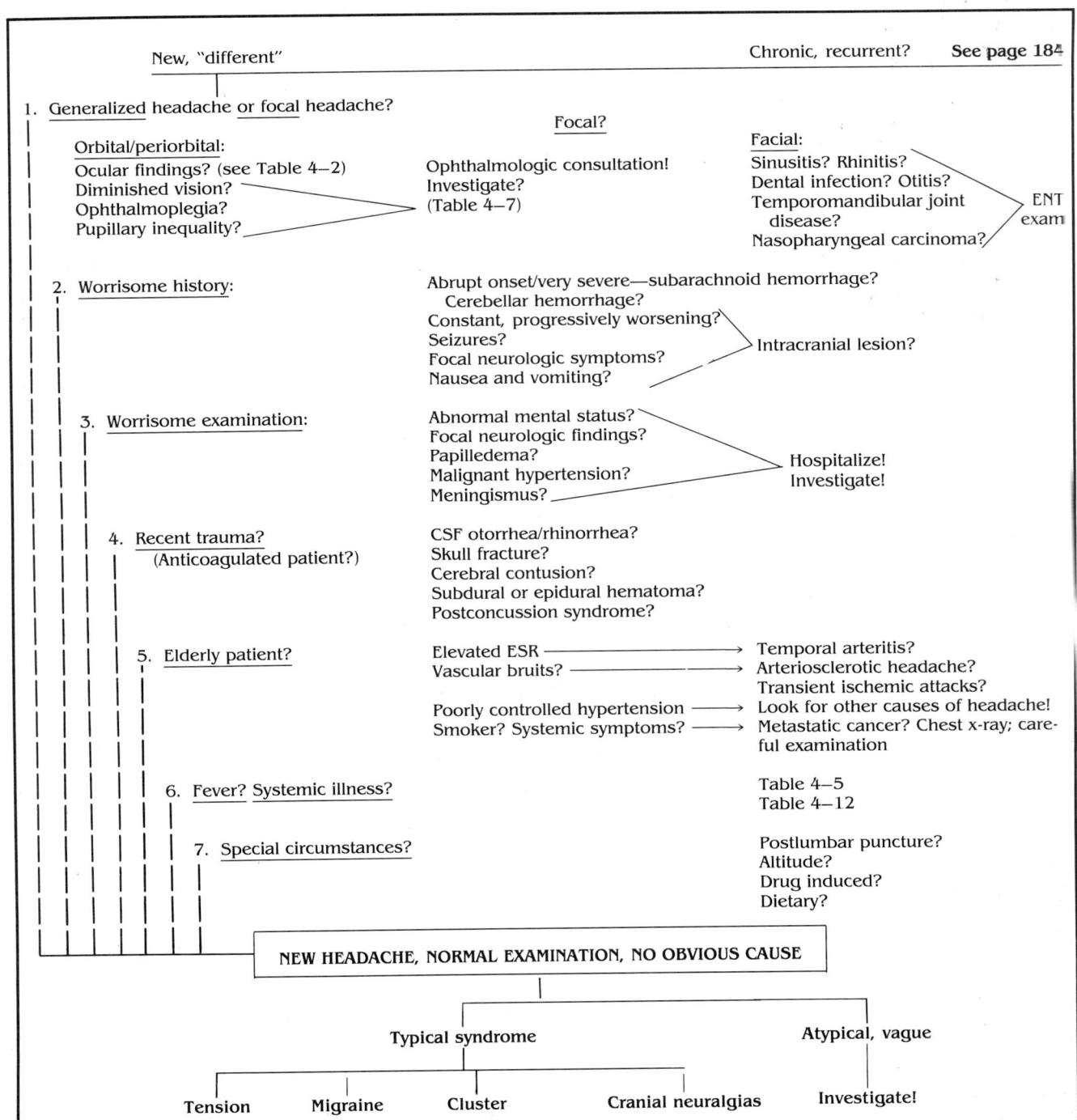

FIGURE 4–8. Headache.

2. The decision to perform lumbar puncture[63] in this case can be criticized since viral meningitis does not require specific therapy—it is usually a self-limited process that resolves spontaneously in 1 to 2 weeks, often without the need for hospitalization. (Occasionally, headache will recur for several weeks thereafter.) In this case, however, the presence of low-grade fever and subtle meningeal findings in a patient who is ill (nauseated) with acute headache should warrant some concern about (early) bacterial meningitis or even (more rarely) subarachnoid hemorrhage. These CSF findings virtually exclude both diagnoses. Of equal importance is the fact that we are now able to identify a "specific" diagnosis* in Mary's case.

3. Some cases of new headache are not so easily diagnosed. Since most new headaches are benign (especially in the young patient), careful follow-up is sometimes as useful as extensive laboratory investigations. Figure 4–8 attempts to emphasize clinical findings that are worrisome enough to warrant thorough evaluation (often in the hospital), clues that may point the clinician in specific diagnostic dirrections, and the final "bottom line": new headaches that are otherwise unexplained and that are not typical of any of the common headache syndromes deserve careful continuing attention. Whether that attention involves clinical follow-up or extensive testing (see pages 196 to 201) must be individualized.

> Mary returns home, given a presumptive diagnosis of viral meningitis. Two days later, CSF cultures are normal, but Mary calls to say that she is "much worse." Closer questioning reveals that her headache has changed: The headache is quite mild when Mary is supine, but any attempt to sit up or stand produces a severe bifrontal throbbing headache that quickly resolves with resumption of the supine position. There are no neurologic symptoms. Mary feels well when lying down.

This "lumbar puncture headache" (see below) is one example of several headache syndromes that can be recognized immediately, simply on the basis of the special circumstances in which they occur.

HEADACHE IN SPECIAL CIRCUMSTANCES

Lumbar puncture headache[64–66] is typically a severe, generalized headache precipitated by sitting or standing but completely relieved by lying supine. The headache begins 12 to 72 hours after the lumbar puncture, usually persists for hours to a few days, but (rarely) can last for weeks. This complication will occur much less often when small-bore needles are used for the procedure, when the CSF is obtained with a single, atraumatic "pass," and when the patient is instructed to lie prone for 3 hours immediately after the procedure. These measures all address the likely pathogenetic mechanism of LP headache: leak of CSF from the site of puncture, resulting in low CSF pressures and postural symptoms. At times, an epidural patch[66] may be necessary to "seal the leak": Here, 10 cc of the patient's own blood is injected into the site of lumbar puncture to coagulate around the puncture site.

Headache that occurs only on standing (or which is clearly posturally exacerbated) may also be seen with serious neurologic disease—especially

---

*Serologic studies over time would be needed to identify a specific viral cause—this is usually not necessary.

posterior fossa masses. The absence of neurologic findings and the clinical setting usually clearly distinguish LP headache. Nevertheless, radiographic examination (especially CT scan) should be performed before lumbar puncture if there is any suspicion of an intracranial mass or increased intracranial pressure.

Altitude headache is a typical feature of mountain sickness, usually occurring after climbs to altitudes above 8000 feet and almost universally occurring at altitudes above 12,000 feet.[67] The clinical setting alone is usually sufficiently diagnostic, extensive work-up is usually unnecessary, and furosemide or acetazolamide may help in treatment or prophylaxis.[67]

Post-traumatic headaches are discussed briefly above.

Effort headache (exertional headache)[68, 69] refers to abrupt onset of headache that originates during some type of strenuous physical exertion (running, weight lifting) or Valsalva maneuver (cough,[68] sneeze, strain). This headache is brief in duration (seconds to minutes) and may be recurrent. (This syndrome must be carefully distinguished from headaches that transiently worsen during exertion—this is a nonspecific finding common to many types of headache. Similarly the headache of subarachnoid hemorrhage may be precipitated by exertion—this headache usually persists beyond just a few minutes, usually then worsens, and is associated with other clinical findings—see page 167.) Effort headache has been associated with potentially serious organic disease in perhaps 10 per cent of cases—craniovertebral anomalies are most common, but brain tumors or subdural hematomas are occasionally responsible. Conversely, most such patients have "benign exertional headache."[69] Nevertheless, brain tumors are common; benign exertional headache is not. Cervical spine films and CT scans should be considered in patients with exertional headache.*

Paroxysmal headache[70] refers to a sudden, very brief jolt of a headache that occurs for no apparent reason at all, lasts minutes to an hour, and vanishes as quickly as it arrives. This is a very unusual headache and is probably most often benign. On occasion, such headaches may be associated with intracranial masses or abnormalities of the intracranial ventricular system. Especially when such a headache is associated with leg weakness, frank "drop attacks," vomiting, or loss of consciousness, investigation should be vigorously pursued. Cystic masses of the third ventricle are perhaps most commonly found in this setting.

Orgasmic (or coital) headache[71] is an uncommon disorder wherein severe (usually "vascular") headache occurs during sexual arousal or at the time of sexual orgasm. While an obviously frightening and frustrating phenomenon, most patients do not have serious disease as the cause of the headache. Nevertheless, it is difficult not to be concerned about an intracranial neoplasm or aneurysm when the patient first presents with such a history. Investigation, while usually unrevealing, is often pursued.

Drug-induced headache may take several forms:

1. Headache due to pharmacologic properties of specific drugs—nitrates, nitrites, and other vasodilators (hydralazine, for example)—is common and usually obvious.

2. Conversely, headache may occur as a side effect of drug treatment. Many drugs may produce headache as a side effect, but indomethacin, theophylline, terbutaline, reserpine, and oral hypoglycemic agents are espe-

---

*Rarely, exertional headache will be caused by an *unruptured* intracranial aneurysm—here, even the CT scan may be normal and arteriography is needed (see also Table 4–13).

cially common offenders. Of special note are patients with vascular headache treated with ergotamine preparations (see page 205) who develop "ergot tolerance" and gradually escalating headache, relieved only transiently by further increasing the ergotamine dose.[72]

3. Certain drugs will precipitate organic causes of headache. Typical examples are monoamine oxidase inhibitors, which may induce hypertensive crises, and anticholinergic drugs, which may precipitate acute glaucoma. Vitamin A intoxication is an uncommon cause of generalized headache, but the popularity of "vitamin cults" in recent years deserves notice.

4. The literature on the relationship between estrogens and patients with headache is most confusing. Headache may occur following the use of estrogens, following the withdrawal of estrogens, or sometimes in association with various endogenous hormonal fluctuations.[73-76] The most common association is that of migraine headaches with the oral contraceptive pill. It is prudent to discontinue oral contraceptives in this setting (or at least to reduce the estrogen dose component of the combination pill).

5. Certain drugs may not be considered "drugs" at all. Alcohol will, of course, induce headache "the morning after," but in some patients will also cause a vascular headache during consumption. Caffeine may produce a puzzling syndrome in heavy caffeine users (coffee, tea, cola drinks), who experience "withdrawal" headaches following abstinence from caffeine for several hours (especially in the morning, after sleep). This usually occurs only in patients who use very large amounts of caffeine (for example, 10 to 20 cups of coffee per day), but moderate consumers may be susceptible too.

A whole variety of foods may precipitate headache, and this has been best studied in migraine sufferers. However, even in nonmigraine patients, ice cream, hot dogs, and monosodium glutamate may induce headache reproducibly. Foods most commonly incriminated among migraineurs include alcohol beverages (especially beer), chocolate, cheese, citrus fruit, tyramine-containing foods, and cured meat. Analysis of diet will sometimes play an important role in the overall management of the patient with migraine headache.[77]

Sleep (nocturnal) headache is, in general, nonspecific. Many of the chronic, common headache syndromes, especially migraine and tension headache, may awaken the patient during the night. Nevertheless, patients whose headache commonly awakens them from sleep deserve especially careful attention. Brain tumors, cluster headache, pheochromocytoma, and glaucoma may be associated with prominent nocturnal headache, and nocturnal headache is thus one of several "soft" worrisome findings which warrants attention. As noted above, headache that is positional, exertional, or paroxysmal must also be analyzed carefully—see also Figure 4–9.

Mary Migraine recovers from her viral meningitis over the next 2 weeks. Three months later, Mary returns to the clinic asking for help with her chronic problem, which seems "worse than ever." She feels she has completely recovered from her meningitis headache, but her "old headaches" are bothering her more.

Mary has been troubled with chronic recurring headaches for the past 10 years. Beginning in her senior year in college, the headaches were initially infrequent, but quite severe. Occurring perhaps every month or two, the headaches were generalized bilateral throbbing pains that would last for 1 or 2 days, would often be associated with nausea and vomiting, and would not allow her to work or study. Mary was told by her physician that these were tension headaches, probably induced by her impending graduation and engagement to be married, and were at least partly relieved with

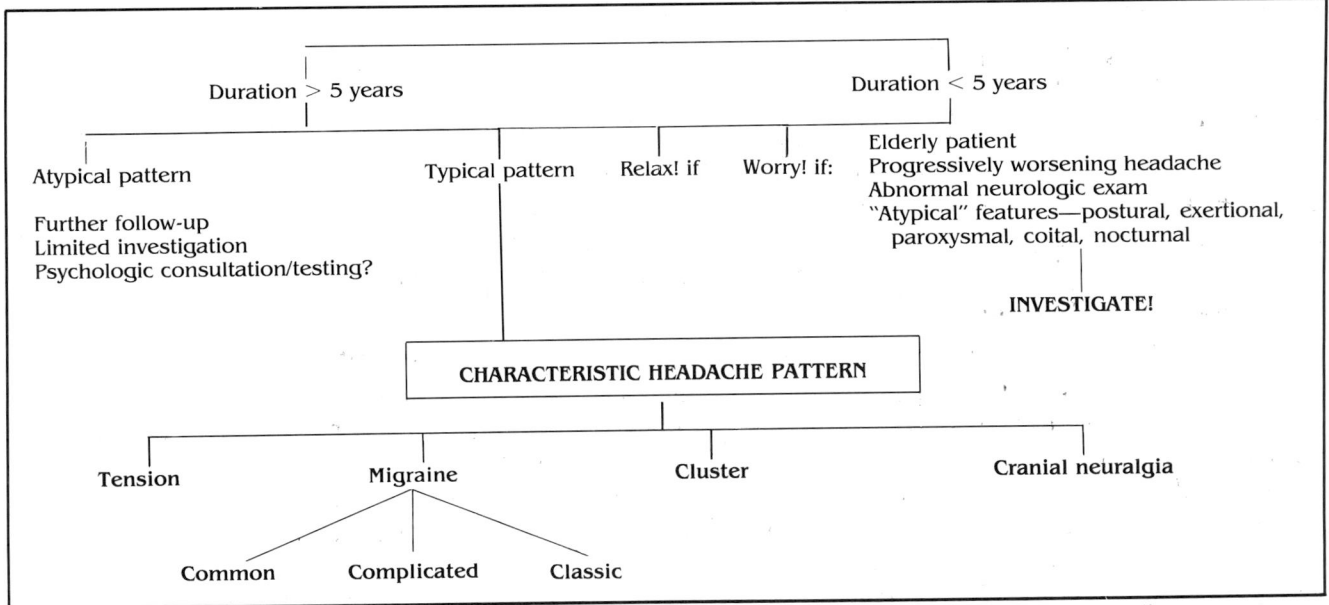

FIGURE 4—9. Chronic, recurrent headache.

various analgesics. On a few occasions, Mary had to go to her physician for parenteral pain medications. There was never any warning of the headache, and there were never any visual symptoms or associated neurologic abnormalities. There was no family history of headache or migraine. Mary thought that her headaches might be associated with her periods, but she could not be sure. She agreed with her physician at that time that she was under a lot of pressure and, over the next few years, the headaches became less frequent, and became virtually nonexistent during each of her three pregnancies "when I was most contented and satisfied."

Over the past 5 years, however, Mary's headaches have become more frequent and less stereotyped. Sometimes, perhaps once or twice a month, she develops an "old sick tension headache that puts me to bed, bangs on my head, and hurts all over for a whole day or more." More often, though, she notes a different headache, which seems to come and go, but may occur daily for weeks at a time, and is often quite severe. "I go on with my work; what choice do I have?" The headache feels like "pressure or tightness all around my head from front to back." Mary has tried various analgesics, tranquilizers, and "some migraine medicines," none of which has helped appreciably.

Recently, over the past 3 weeks, Mary has been having "almost daily" headaches. Some are severe, others mild. They are almost always generalized, but sometimes on only one side or the other. While she feels "generally lousy" during the headaches (but rarely vomits), there is no prodrome nor are there visual or neurologic symptoms.

Mary is especially concerned because, "while I guess I get tension headaches, I do not feel any tension or worry in my life right now, and yet my headaches seem worse than ever. Besides, I have been on the "pill" for 5 years now, and I read that they might cause a stroke. Could I have a brain tumor?"

CHRONIC, RECURRENT HEADACHE

Most patients with chronic recurring headache are diagnosed as having tension (muscle contraction) or migraine (vascular) headaches.[10] Such diagnoses are often highly subjective and the differential diagnosis, at times, seems semantic, since there are no specific diagnostic tests that clearly separate tension from migraine headache, and there is much clinical overlap between the two. In fact, some authorities wonder whether basic pathogenetic mechanisms in these disorders define a common continuum, rather than sharp differences.[78] Clinical diagnosis usually depends on the recognition of a characteristic headache pattern that is typical of a particular disorder.

Figure 4–9 illustrates a general, if simplified, approach to the patient with chronic or recurrent headache.

Consider Mary's headache history:

1. Headaches have been present for 10 years. This, in itself, is very reassuring, since the likelihood of serious systemic or neurologic disease thus becomes minutely small. Usually a careful history will place such patients' headaches into one of the several characteristic chronic headache patterns that are briefly summarized in Table 4–8. Each of these is discussed in greater

TABLE 4–8. TYPICAL CHARACTERISTICS OF COMMON CHRONIC HEADACHE DISORDERS[9, 10, 79–85]

	CLASSIC MIGRAINE (see page 186)	COMPLICATED MIGRAINE (see page 187)	COMMON MIGRAINE (see Table 4–9)
	Migraine usually begins in adolescence or young adulthood.		
Age at Onset			
Prodrome (aura)	Stereotyped; usually visual (scotomata); lasts 10–30 min; disappears with onset of headache	Neurologic symptoms and signs overshadow and outlast headache	Often absent entirely; prodrome may be vague—irritability, fluid retention, insomnia; headache often related to menstruation, psychologic stress, depression, diet
Headache	Episodic; unilateral (usually); throbbing (usually); "sick"—nausea/vomiting, prostration; gradual increase in severity; lasts 1–6 hours; several headaches per year	May be mild or inapparent; duration unpredictable	Unilateral or bilateral; throbbing, usually; usually "sick"; may last 1–3 days; frequency very variable
Examination	"Sick"; hibernating; photophobia	Neurologic deficit: aphasia, hemiplegia, ophthalmoplegia, confusion, "brain stem" symptoms	"Sick"; no neurologic findings; hibernating; photophobia
Differential diagnosis	Depends on nature of aura (See p. 186)	Depends on neurologic deficit: Intracranial aneurysm "Stroke" Transient ischemic attack Intracranial neoplasm Multiple sclerosis	Tension headache Sinusitis

	CLUSTER HEADACHE (see page 188)	TENSION HEADACHE (see Table 4–9)	TRIGEMINAL NEURALGIA (see page 189)
Age at Onset	Usually middle age (30–50)	Usually begins in young adulthood	Usually occurs in elderly
Prodrome (aura)	None	None	None
Headache	Excruciating; periorbital; unilateral (always same side); nonpulsatile; occurs in "clusters" of 1–3 months; lasts about 1 hour; often precipitated by alcohol; often nocturnal	Often mild/moderate; waxes and wanes; often every day, or constant; less episodic than migraine; generalized headache often "tight," "pressure," band-like	Severe, lancinating, sudden "electric"; very brief—10 to 45 sec but recurrent—may appear to last 15 to 45 min; intermittent
Examination	Photophobia; tearing; nasal stuffiness; ?Horner's syndrome; agitated, even violent, behavior	Normal; occasional muscle spasm and tenderness of occipital and trapezius muscles; ?depression; ?anxiety	Trigger points; pain limited to trigeminal nerve; (usually II or III division); normal neurologic examination
Differential diagnosis	Trigeminal neuralgia Pheochromocytoma Temporal arteritis Glaucoma Sinusitis	Common migraine Cervical spine disease or whiplash Depression Psychiatric disease Tumor Sinusitis	Depends on neurologic examination[86, 87]

detail below. Note that the patient's age, the presence or absence of prodromal symptoms before onset of headache, the timing, quality, and location of the headache, and the physical examination (which attempts to exclude other diseases that may mimic each headache type) form the basis for clinical diagnosis.

As illustrated in Figure 4–9, when headaches are more recent, the clinician must be especially concerned about the elderly patient, the patient with progressively worsening symptoms, and the patient with an abnormal neurologic examination. Recurrent headaches that are exertional, paroxysmal, coital, nocturnal, or positional also warrant caution, as noted above. Diagnostic studies (see below) must be individualized according to specific circumstances.

2. There is some suggestion of another new headache. Obviously, patients with typical tension or migraine headache may also develop intercurrent disease, as we have seen in Mary's case. The evaluation of new or different headache must follow the guidelines outlined in Figure 4–8.

> On further questioning, Mary says that she does not believe her recent headaches are any different from her longstanding headaches, but only that they are more of a daily problem than previously. There is no recent history of fever, head trauma, or dietary or medication changes.
>
> Physical and neurologic examinations are completely normal.

3. There are no worrisome features that, in and of themselves, should prompt extensive diagnostic testing. The patient is young, has a normal examination, and, while headaches are frequent and chronic, they are not truly progressive. (Progressive headache refers to daily or constant headache that progressively and ineluctably worsens over time—usually over weeks to months.)

4. The history alone can exclude classic migraine, cluster headache, and cranial neuralgias.

Classic Migraine

Classic migraine[79–85] usually begins abruptly as a vivid, stereotyped visual or neurologic prodrome without headache. This prodrome (or aura) usually lasts 10 to 30 minutes before gradually receding as the headache begins. The headache itself is usually pulsatile, unilateral (often contralateral to the prodromal symptoms), and accompanied by nausea, vomiting, anorexia, and photophobia/phonophobia. The headache usually lasts for 1 to 6 hours, during which time the patient is often incapacitated by pain and the need to seek shelter in a quiet, dark environment. This "hibernation behavior," and digital compression of throbbing superficial scalp vessels, provide some relief, but the patient often gratefully succumbs to the sleep that finally brings comfort.

Prodromal symptoms are most often visual. These may include flashes of color, wavy lines, shimmering spots or stars, scintillations, visual distortions or frank hallucinations, and all varieties of transient visual loss (total blindness rarely, but monocular or hemianopic deficits most often). These visual symptoms are nonspecific—intraocular or embolic vascular disease may cause similar symptoms. Fortification spectra[88] (Fig. 4–10), however, are virtually pathognomonic of migraine: Vision blurs, and there appears a slowly ex-

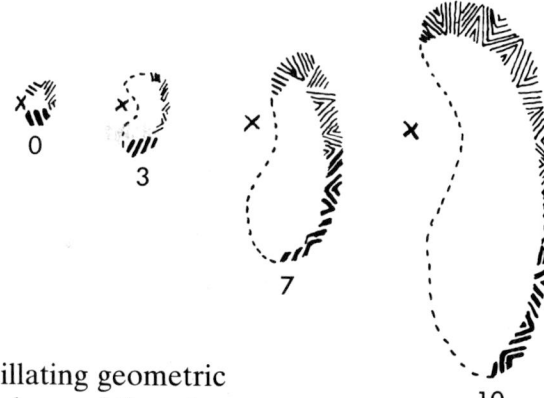

FIGURE 4–10. Fortification spectra—the classic visual prodrome to migraine. These four figures are depictions of Lashley's (1941) own visual prodrome, signaling the onset of his own migraine attack. The "X" represents the visual fixation point; each picture represents the progression of the visual image after the designated number of minutes has passed (see numbers below figures). The area of visual loss gradually expands and proceeds laterally. (From Lashley, KS: Arch Neurol Psychiatry 46:331–339, 1941. Copyright 1941, American Medical Association; reproduced with permission.)

panding paracentral scotoma, surrounded by luminous scintillating geometric forms, which enlarges and moves laterally until it disappears beyond the edge of peripheral vision—the entire sequence usually occupying 10 to 30 minutes.

Neurologic prodromes of migraine vary with the cerebrovascular territory involved by the vasospastic phenomenon of migraine. Hemisensory paresthesias, hemiparesis, or dysphasia may occur contralateral to subsequent headache. Vertebrobasilar symptoms—vertigo, diplopia, dysarthria, weakness— are not rare. Often, a mix of vascular territory syndromes will occur, since several segments of the cerebral circulation may be afflicted simultaneously. When such neurologic symptoms resolve (usually in 10 to 30 minutes) and then elide into the classic headache, the diagnosis is rarely in doubt. Two circumstances are more difficult:

1. Complicated migraine is characterized by persistence of the neurologic prodrome long after the headache has resolved—sometimes, for several days or more. At times, the headache is very mild and is completely overshadowed by the neurologic problem. Hemiplegic migraine is a (usually familial) disorder in which the complication is persistent hemiparesis (always on the same side), often associated with dysarthria, aphasia, or both. Ophthalmoplegic migraine[59] causes ptosis, usually ipsilateral to the headache, followed by development of complete third nerve palsy over the next several hours, which then gradually resolves over several days. Basilar migraine[57] may be complicated by persistent (days) vertebrobasilar insufficiency—usually vertigo, ataxia, or cranial nerve paresis, but including, at times, coma and seizures.

Especially when the headache is unimpressive or a history of recurrent episodes cannot be obtained, it is easy to understand how complicated migraine may be confused with more serious events—stroke, intracranial aneurysms, and even cerebral or cerebellar hemorrhage. Fortunately, such attacks are usually few and far between, tend to occur in young patients (adolescents and young adults), and resolve uneventfully.

2. Occasionally only the migraine prodrome occurs, without headache. This is not a rare phenomenon, and such symptoms are usually mistaken for more ominous problems—transient ischemic attacks usually—when the middle-aged or elderly are afflicted. Multiple sclerosis is often suspected in the younger patient.

The timing of the migraine prodrome is often helpful here—the slow march of the migraine neurologic prodrome (for example, thumb to hand to face over 20 to 30 minutes) is unusual in other types of transient ischemic attacks or focal seizures; the duration of the visual prodrome in migraine (20 to 30 minutes) is longer than the typical episode of atheroembolic monocular visual loss (amaurosis fugax), which usually lasts only 3 to 5 minutes.

(Treatment of migraine is discussed on pages 202 to 209.)

Cluster Headache

Cluster headache[89-94] is probably a type of vascular headache, about one-tenth as common as migraine (in referral clinics), whose diagnosis is usually apparent from the clinical history alone. Kudrow presents a first-person account of a cluster headache, which is dramatic and informative.[89] These headaches (Fig. 4–11) are usually unilateral (frontotemporal or oculofrontal), extremely severe, and stereotyped; they begin suddenly, last for 30 to 60 minutes with gradually increasing intensity, are usually nonthrobbing, and are often associated with unilateral nose and eye symptoms—tearing, running nose, and (occasionally) a mild Horner's syndrome. While one single cluster headache may be confused with various other disorders—migraine, sinusitis, glaucoma, for example—it is the recurrent periodicity—the "clustering"—of the headaches that is so often diagnostic.

"Clusters" last an average of 1 to 3 months. During this time, headache occurs once or several times each day, often at the same time each day, not infrequently awakening the patient from sleep or other restful relaxation. During such clusters, patients await in dread the onset of headache and may be thrown into a state of panic, agitation, or frank terror by the severity of the recurrent pain. The pacing, frantic, and sometimes violent raging behavior that may be prompted by the pain is considered by some experts almost diagnostic of this disorder. (Note the difference here from the migraineur, who usually seeks "hibernation" during headache.) Most cluster headache sufferers then enter periodic remissions during which they are totally free of headache for months or years (average 12 months) until another cluster recurs. Family history of headache is usually unimpressive, unlike that of many patients with migraine.

Most patients with cluster headache are middle-aged males, and not uncommonly they have a characteristic (but unexplained) facies that has been described as alcoholic or acromegalic.[90] Alcohol (and other vasodilators) often precipitates attacks, such that many cluster sufferers (but not all) become teetotalers, at least during their cluster.

The differential diagnosis of recurrent cluster headache is very limited. The periodicity and timing of the headache (episodic, 45-minute duration) may be mimicked by pheochromocytoma, but those patients usually have other symptoms and signs (sweating, tachycardia, hypertension, pallor) during their headache, which is itself usually generalized and more often throbbing (unlike cluster headache). The location, severity, and type of pain may be mimicked by temporal arteritis, but those patients usually have more persistent headache and an elevated sedimentation rate. Trigeminal neuralgia may superficially resemble cluster, especially when repetitive bursts of neuralgic pain add up to a 30- to 60-minute duration, but the timing and quality of trigeminal neuralgic pain are usually distinctive (see page 189). Sphenopalatine neuralgia is probably another name for cluster headache, but some such pains may last for several hours and be relieved with cocaine instillation into the sphenopalatine ganglion by an otolaryngologist. Migraine usually occurs much less frequently than daily, lasts hours to days, and is more often throbbing in nature. Chronic paroxysmal hemicrania is a very rare disorder in which repeated attacks of hemifacial pain occur during the course of each day. (Indomethacin may be dramatically effective.)[91] Recurrent sinusitis may also mimic cluster.

The pharmacologic therapy of cluster headache is quite similar to that of migraine, with these important differences:

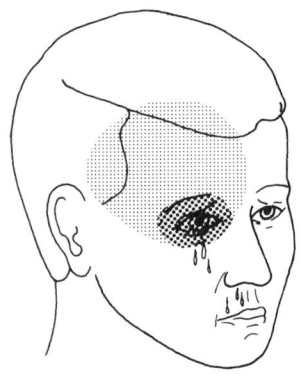

Periorbital or frontotemporal location is usual

Tears and nasal stuffiness, often unilateral, accompany the headache

Duration is usually brief (1 hour)

FIGURE 4–11. Cluster headache (see text).

1. Since there is no aura and the headache is quite brief, immediate ergotamine therapy to abort the headache is often unsuccessful because the nonparenteral ergotamine preparations often take full effect only after about 1 hour. (Ergotamine by sublingual or aerosol administration—see page 203—may occasionally be helpful.) In some cluster patients, inhalation of 100 per cent oxygen may help, but it is cumbersome and expensive.

2. Prophylactic therapy is then most reasonable. Ergotamines (several times daily or 1 or 2 hours before an expected attack) and methysergide are probably most effective. These are especially attractive since ergotism and fibrotic complications of methysergide therapy (page 202 ff.) are much less a problem in the treatment of cluster when therapy is continued only for a few weeks or months until clusters disperse. Similarly, prednisone[92] (40 mg a day with a slow "taper" over 1 month) and lithium carbonate[93] (300 mg bid to qid) may be especially effective in cluster headache. These drugs are probably more effective as prophylaxis than propranolol, tricyclic antidepressants, cyproheptadine, phenothiazines, or indomethacin (see Table 4–16).

3. Some ill-fated patients with cluster headache have chronic cluster in which remissions do not occur (or last only a few weeks out of the year); here, prophylactic therapy with ergotamine, methysergide, and prednisone is less attractive. Lithium[93] is probably the drug of choice for these (rare) patients.

4. Nonpharmacologic methods—biofeedback, acupuncture, exercise, dietary manipulation, psychotherapy, relaxation techniques—are usually ineffective, and most experts do not advise the time and expense involved.

Trigeminal Neuralgia

Trigeminal neuralgia[87, 95] (tic douloureux) is a relatively rare disorder, primarily afflicting the elderly, which usually presents as facial pain rather than headache. Usually an extremely severe electric or lancinating (nonthrobbing) pain that involves unilaterally the second or third division of the trigeminal nerve (rarely the first) (Fig. 4–12), this neuralgia sometimes occurs

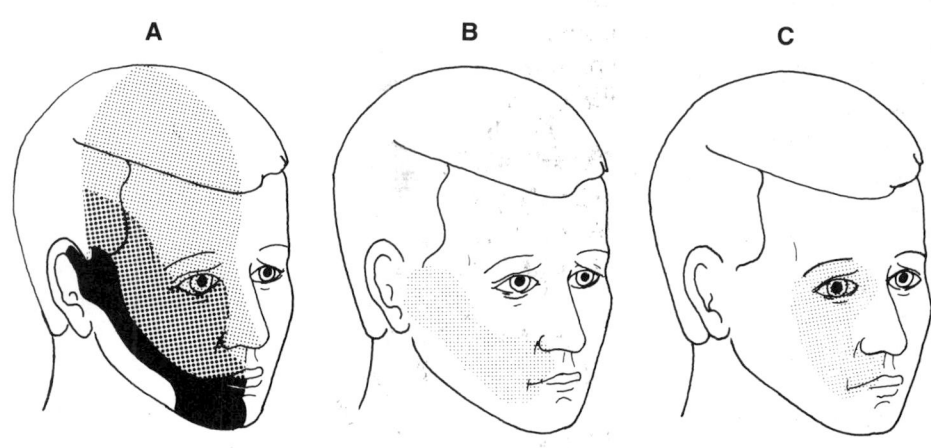

FIGURE 4–12. Trigeminal neuralgia.

The three divisions of the trigeminal nerve:
I. Ophthalmic
II. Maxillary
III. Mandibular

The most common locations of the pain of trigeminal neuralgia many times per day, each "burst" lasting only seconds to a few minutes, but sometimes repeating in such staccato fashion that the patient may describe a duration of attack up to an hour in length. (A careful history, however, will usually reveal that the hour is punctuated by repetitive interrupted salvos.) As Amols has described,

> Few disorders are as striking or distinctive in appearance. The patient, previously composed if not relaxed, suddenly freezes in whatever position he may be holding when the attack strikes. His hand rises involuntarily to his face, but he rarely touches it. His faces contorts and draws to one side. His eyes become narrow slits or close tightly. If his nature is stoical, he remains in the position until the attack subsides. If of a more volatile temperament, he may cry out piteously and dash frantically about the room. Fortunately, each acute episode is usually short-lived and the sufferer's relief upon its conclusion is matched only by his apprehension of the next attack. When witnessed, the episode is unmistakable as tic douloureux.[87]

In addition to the typical quality, timing, and location of the pain, many patients have learned to prevent triggering an attack by avoidance of various sensitive areas of the face or gums that may induce an attack when stimulated during routine daily activities—for example, brushing the teeth, washing the face, shaving, or chewing on one side. These "trigger points" may be purposefully stimulated to provoke an attack as a diagnostic maneuver, but the patient is rarely enthusiastic about that approach.

Carbamazepine[96, 97] (Tegretol) is helpful in managing tic, in doses of 400 to 800 mg per day. Many patients note excellent relief within the first few days of beginning this drug. There are, however, serious side effects, especially bone marrow suppression, that require monitoring blood and platelet counts on a weekly basis at least for the first few months of therapy. Other side effects (dermatitis, abnormal liver function tests, diarrhea, and dizziness) will perhaps be rendered less frequent if the drug is begun at 200 mg per day and gradually increased. If Tegretol is ineffective or cannot be tolerated, diphenylhydantoin may be helpful. When all drug therapies are unsuccessful, an experienced neurosurgeon should be consulted about the possibility of performing one of the various available surgical procedures.[98]

Several disorders may be mistaken for trigeminal neuralgia:

Cluster headache also usually involves the periorbital area and is paroxysmal, but this pain usually lasts up to an hour, builds to intensity, and fades more gradually than does tic; cluster often occurs at night (tic almost never does) and is not usually lancinating or electric in quality. As noted above, sphenopalatine neuralgia may be confused occasionally with it as well, but, again, this pain usually lasts a few hours, and is relieved with topical measures.

Postherpetic neuralgia may involve the same facial distribution within the trigeminal nerve (but is more often in the first division of the trigeminal nerve). There is almost always a history of the typical herpes zoster rash, there is usually not a trigger point, and postherpetic pain is much more constant (or waxing and waning) than is the truly paroxysmal tic.

Glossopharyngeal neuralgia is of the same quality and timing as trigeminal neuralgia but is usually deep in the throat (tonsillar) or on one side, and often seems to involve the ear. Tegretol may also be helpful here.

Occipital neuralgia is commonly overdiagnosed as an explanation for unilateral occipital or occipitoparietal head pain. (Most such headaches are tension or vascular in origin.) True occipital neuralgia is a brief, lancinating "neuralgic" pain that "shoots" from the occiput over a C2 distribution on the scalp. It may be associated with various craniovertebral or cervical spine anomalies.[99]

Atypical facial pain is probably a "wastebasket" diagnosis for a variety of facial pain syndromes (usually involving the lower part of the face) in which pain is often deep, constant, non-neuralgic, in unusual anatomic distributions (for example, face, neck, and shoulder on one or both sides), and which often prompts constant massaging. (There are no trigger points). While anatomic causes are sometimes found (temporomandibular joint disease or dental problems, for example), many such patients have no known explanation for their symptoms and are very difficult to treat. Depression, either primary or secondary, is extremely common among these (usually middle-aged female) patients.

Finally, a whole host of central nervous system (posterior fossa tumors, demyelinating diseases) and ear, nose, and throat disorders (parotid tumors, nasopharyngeal carcinoma) may masquerade as trigeminal neuralgia. Neurologic examination with careful attention to cranial nerve testing (especially corneal reflexes and facial sensation) is critical, since the patient with primary trigeminal neuralgia invariably has a normal physical and neurologic examination.[86] When this is not the case, testing and consultation are mandatory.

Thus, familiarity with the typical clinical picture of classic migraine, cluster headache, and cranial neuralgias usually permits suspicion of these (unusual) diagnoses quite readily. On the other hand, Mary's history is most compatible with common migraine or tension headache.

Common migraine is "common" in two ways: (1) It comprises probably 90 percent of all "vascular" headache in the general population,[79] and, (2) its typical characteristics are much less dramatic and memorable than are those of classic migraine. The clinical quandary is that common migraine has much in common with tension headache, from which it must be distinguished if therapy is to be optimal.

Common Migraine versus Tension Headache

Table 4–9 indicates some of the clinical features that may be useful in distinguishing common migraine from tension headache. Note that many of the clinical features that allow differentiation among the other types of chronic headache (Table 4–8)—the patient's age, the nature of the headache prodrome, and the timing, quality, and location of pain—are less helpful here.[79-81] Both tension and common migraine headaches tend to begin before the age of 30 years, neither is associated with a dramatic prodrome, each may be unilateral or bilateral, pulsatile or nonpulsatile, and the duration of headache is quite variable for each.

Tension headache is typically described as tightness or pressure that is nonpulsatile and generalized. Two locations are most common: the occipital location, where the patient describes headache in the upper cervical and craniovertebral junction area, often involving the occipital and occipitotemporal cranium bilaterally; and the "hatband" location, where discomfort encircles the head, the patient often describing with gestures a bifrontal "band" extending around the head. There is no prodrome, precipitating factors are nonspecific, and physical examination is usually normal except sometimes for tenderness of the trapezius and upper cervical neck muscles. Tension headaches are extremely variable in timing and duration—often, the patient describes them as coming and going every day, or, sometimes, as constant. Tension headaches rarely interfere with sleep, and aspirin is often

TABLE 4–9. DISTINGUISHING CHARACTERISTICS OF TENSION HEADACHE AND COMMON MIGRAINE HEADACHE

	COMMON MIGRAINE HEADACHE	TENSION HEADACHE
Age at onset	About 70% under age 30	60% under age 30
Quality	Often throbbing	Tight, constricting pressure, but may "throb"
Location (see Figure 4–13)	More often unilateral than bilateral	Usually generalized, hatband or occipital
*Timing**	Usually sporadic episodes (with headache-free intervals)	Less episodic—often daily
*Duration**	Each episode lasts several hours to (2–3) days	Extremely variable—brief to "all of the time"
Severity	Often disabling (cannot continue with daily activities)	Patient usually remains functional in spite of headache
Prodrome (aura/warning)	Vague, if present at all: irritability, fluid retention, e.g.	None
*Associated symptoms**	Sometimes nausea/vomiting, anorexia, photophobia, polyuria, abdominal distention, diarrhea	General unhappiness
Family history	Positive for migraine 65%	Positive for tension 40%
*Precipitating factors**	Menses, stress, visual glare, fatigue, hunger, foods, drugs, excess or lack of sleep	Nonspecific
Aspirin therapy	Usually does not help	Often helps
*Ergot therapy**	Predictably helps in 50–80%	Variable response; (placebo response to ergotamine may be as high as 50%)

*Most helpful differential features.

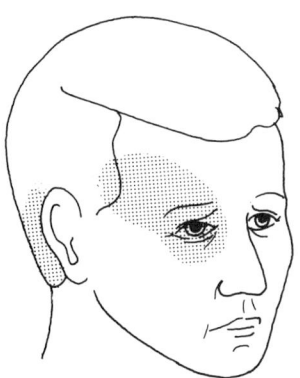

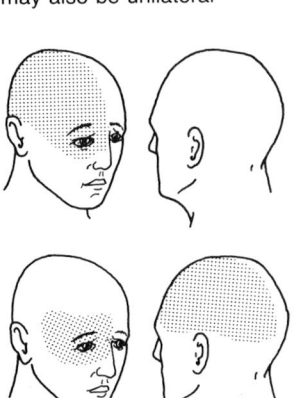

Common locations of migraine headache—tension headache may also be unilateral

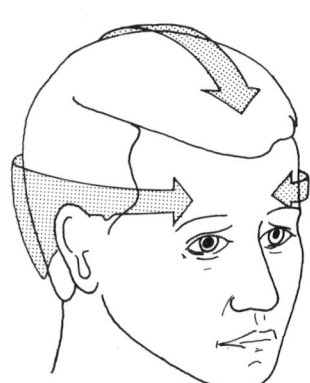

Common locations of tension headache—migraine may occur in the same location

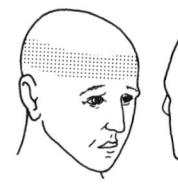
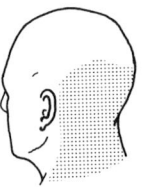

"Hatband" distribution   Occipital distribution

A   **B**

FIGURE 4–13. Common location of migraine *(A)* and tension *(B)* headaches.

an effective analgesic. The patient is usually able to continue daily activities, and, while the pain may be severe, it is rarely incapacitating.

Common migraine usually occurs in clearly delineated episodes of pulsatile unilateral headache, which often are associated with nausea, vomiting, and anorexia, and which usually last for several hours to a few days, often preventing the patient from continuing usual daily activities. Some patients "can tell a headache is coming" a few hours or days before (especially women whose migraine correlates with menstruation), but vague irritability, bloating, fluid retention, and anorexia may antedate the headache in others. In many patients there is no prodrome at all. Aspirin is often ineffective* even in large doses. Ergotamine therapy is predictably helpful in many, but not all (see below).

These typical features are most helpful in recognizing a clinical "gestalt" about headache patterns. No one clinical characteristic is diagnostic. Probably the most helpful diagnostic features are the truly episodic nature of migraine and its tendency to make the patient "sick" (nausea/vomiting), and the "tight, tense" constant pressure of the generalized tension headache.

Any clinician who carefully listens to patients' descriptions of chronic recurrent headaches will be impressed by "overlap" problems—that is, clinical features suggesting both common migraine and tension headache. Such mixed tension/vascular headache is more than just a semantic classification. Some patients with common migraine, occurring in typical episodic attacks, also experience mild or generalized "pressure" headaches that may appear daily or frequently and yet respond well to "migraine pharmacology" (see below).[10, 100] Are these tension headaches responding to ergotamine or are they atypical common migraine? Since psychologic tension states may induce migraine and vice versa, and since the response to ergotamine is not specific for migraine, unambiguous clinical definitions are sometimes impossible in the patient with "mixed" headache.

In Mary's case (pages 183 to 184) the infrequent, clearly episodic, often incapitating "sick" headaches, which are prolonged, which may be related to hormonal events (menstruation, pregnancy, contraception), and which began in adolescence, strongly suggest common migraine (despite the previous physician's clinical diagnosis). Other headaches—the constant, daily, nonpulsatile, generalized "tightness" that is manageable but annoying—suggest tension headache despite the denial of "any tension or worry in my life." (See also page 211.)

What should we do now?

Mary is told that she may have two different types of headache, common migraine and muscle contraction headache. The problem of overlap is briefly explained, and we suggest that we need to discover which type of headache is currently the major problem, since treatment depends on this understanding. A brief explanation of the pathogenesis of migraine (the vascular model) and of tension headache (the muscle contraction model) is offered. Mary is told that there is no reason to be concerned about any serious illness like a brain tumor.

We recommend that Mary stop the birth control pill for the next few months. We ask that Mary keep a "headache calendar" for the next 4 to 6 weeks and to return at that time to review her symptoms. Mary is told to use aspirin or acetaminophen (Tylenol) when needed, but is given a prescription for propoxyphene (Darvon)—see page 203—to be used when aspirin is ineffective. A rectal ergotamine preparation is prescribed (see Table 4–15—Cafergot (ergotamine 2 mg, caffeine 100 mg)—and Mary is

---

*Migraine headaches vary greatly in severity—certainly, "mild migraine" may be relieved with aspirin.

TABLE 4–10. TYPICAL MIGRAINE HEADACHE CALENDAR

DATE	TIME	SEVERITY OF HEADACHE	TREATMENT USED	DOSE	RELIEF
2-4-83					
2-5					
2-6					
2-7					
2-8					
2-9	6 AM	Severe	Cafergot	2 mg, 2 doses	Almost complete
2-10					
2-11					
2-12					
2-13	12 noon	Moderate	Cafergot	2 mg, 1 dose	Complete
2-14					
2-15					
2-16					
2-17					
2-18					
2-19					
2-20					
2-21					
2-22					
2-23					
2-24	8 PM	Severe	Cafergot	2 mg, 2 doses	Moderate
2-25					
2-26	4 PM	Mild	Cafergot	2 mg, 1 dose	Complete
2-27					
2-28					
3-1-82					
3-2					
3-3					

instructed in its use. Mary is told to try the Cafergot at the first sign of one of her sick headaches, and also to see whether the Cafergot has any effect on her more recent daily headaches.

A complete blood count and chemistry profile are obtained (and are normal).

NOTE

I. Every patient with headache deserves education and reassurance about the nature of the problem.

Unexpressed fears of serious disease are the rule, rather than the exception, among headache patients. The patient should be told early and emphatically that he or she does not have a brain tumor, aneurysm, or other malicious illness. A brief explanation of the pathogenesis of the specific headache disorder is always helpful—the vasoconstriction/vaso-dilatation phenomenon in migraine, the muscle contraction/muscle spasm mechanism in tension headache.[82] Vasoconstrictive therapy for migraine

TABLE 4–11. TYPICAL TENSION HEADACHE CALENDAR

DATE	TIME	SEVERITY OF HEADACHE	TREATMENT USED	DOSE ×	RELIEF
4-10-83	All day	Severe	Empirin #3	4	Moderate
4-11	Evening & night	Severe	Darvon	4	Slight
4-12	All day	Severe	Darvon	4	Complete
4-13	Off & on all day	Mild	Aspirin	1	Slight
4-14	Evening	Severe	Empirin #3	4	None
4-15	Morning	Moderate	Fiorinal	2	Moderate
4-16	Night	Severe	Darvon	3	Moderate
4-17	All day	Moderate	Darvon	3	Slight
4-18	Morning	Moderate	Tylenol	4	Slight
4-19	All day	Severe	Empirin #3	4	None
4-20	Off & on all day	Mild	Tylenol	1	Complete
4-21	Night	Severe	Fiorinal	4	Moderate
4-22	Morning	Moderate	Aspirin	4	None
4-23	Morning	Severe	Empirin #3	3	Moderate
4-24	Evening & night	Severe	Empirin #3	4	Moderate
4-25	All day	Mild	Aspirin	3	Slight
4-26	Off & on all day	Moderate	Fiorinal	2	Moderate
4-27	Off & on all day	Moderate	Darvon	2	None
4-28	Evening	Severe	Darvon	4	Slight
4-29	All day	Moderate	Tylenol	2	Slight
4-30	All day	Moderate	Fiorinal	1	Moderate
5-1-82	Evening	Severe	Fiorinal	4	Moderate
5-2	Morning	Mild	Aspirin	4	Slight
5-3	Morning	Mild	Aspirin	2	Complete
5-4	All day	Moderate	Fiorinal	1	None
5-5	Evening & night	Severe	Empirin #3	4	Slight
5-6	Morning	Mild	Tylenol	4	Moderate
5-7	All day	Moderate	Darvon	2	Slight

(see page 203) and the "holistic" approach to the treatment of tension headache (see page 209) are more likely to be effective and followed when the rationale for treatment is made clear to the patient.

(It is true that the pathogenesis of tension headache and common migraine remains controversial. It is impossible, however, to convey to the patient a sense of diagnostic certainty and yet simultaneously admit total ignorance of the precise pathogenesis of migraine and tension headache.)

II. There is no specific reason to incriminate the oral contraceptive as the cause of Mary's headaches, but, in general, all drugs that can produce headache as a side effect should be discontinued before additional drugs are prescribed to treat the headache.

Commonly prescribed drugs that cause headache are discussed briefly on page 182.

III. Several strategies can be useful to better identify the nature and dominant mechanism of recurrent headache.

These include:

1. Repeated careful history taking over a period of weeks or months is always helpful.

   A specific diagnosis can usually be strongly suspected after one attentive interview, but getting to know the patient, assessing response to various treatments, and reevaluating the initial hypothesis is crucial.

2. A headache calendar may help, in some patients.

   Tables 4–10 and 4–11 illustrate calendars that are quite typical of migraine headache and tension headache, respectively. Diamond and Dalessio have used this technique to good advantage.[82] It is true that the vague or forgetful historian may also be an unreliable record keeper. A patient like Mary, however, whose various symptoms are so entangled and unfocused may be better understood after reviewing a month or two of such a calendar (see page 208). The timing and severity of headache and the effect of various medications/treatments can thus be better assessed in certain patients.

3. The response to ergotamine therapy must be carefully determined. When even part of the headache complex is suspected to be vascular, a trial period of ergotamine therapy is often helpful diagnostically, but only when precise instructions about dose and administration are provided to the patient (see page 204).

IV. When is diagnostic testing indicated?

DIAGNOSTIC TESTS IN HEADACHE

Most patients with chronic recurrent headache require no testing at all. As noted above, exceptions always include the patient with more recent onset of unexplained headache, especially when the patient is elderly, the headache is atypical, or the neurologic examination is abnormal.

Nevertheless, it often makes sense (to the physician and the patient) to "noninvasively exclude" unlikely but potentially serious and treatable diseases.

Blood counts and blood chemical determinations are occasionally helpful, since a number of common and uncommon systemic or metabolic disorders may occasionally present with recurrent headache (see Table 4–12). Most of these disorders are usually suspected because of other accompanying symptoms and signs.

Lumbar puncture will occasionally help uncover the patient with (very rare) infectious or noninfectious chronic meningitis,[60] but there are almost always other clues to these diagnoses. Lumbar puncture is rarely worthwhile in the patient with chronic headache and a normal neurological examination.

More often the patient and physician need to be reassured that one of several intracranial processes is not responsible for headache. While "testing for reassurance" is worthwhile in some circumstances, specific tests should be chosen for specific purposes.

When a specific disorder is suspected (or "worried about"), the sensitivity of the test is most important, i.e., how often will the test be abnormal in patients suffering from that specific disease? For example, the elderly patient with new headache whose sedimentation rate is normal can usually be reassured that temporal arteritis is not the problem since the sedimentation rate is a very sensitive "screening" test for this disease. (Conversely, since

TABLE 4–12. HEADACHE: SYSTEMIC AND METABOLIC CAUSES

COMMON	UNCOMMON
Hyperthyroidism	Carbon monoxide poisoning
Hypothyroidism	Toxic hemoglobinopathies
Anemia	Pheochromocytoma
Polycythemia	Parathyroid disease
Hypoxemia	Cushing's disease
Hypercarbia	Addison's disease
Hypoglycemia	Vitamin A intoxication
Hypertension	Paget's disease (cranial)
Uremia	Cranial neoplasm
Hyponatremia	Chronic leukemia

the sedimentation rate is also a very nonspecific test, an elevated sedimentation rate in such a patient is by no means diagnostic of temporal arteritis.)

When testing is done for reassurance purposes, however, one is looking for a negative test result and is hoping to derive from such a negative test the assurance that disease is not present. The reassurance value of a test, then, relates to the likelihood of falsely negative tests among all negative tests: The lower the ratio of a false negative test, the more reassuring is that test when it is normal. When one is concerned about a brain tumor, for example, a normal skull x-ray and electroencephalogram (EEG) are not reassuring at all; a normal CT scan is very reassuring. Table 4–13 compares costs, sensitivity, and reassurance values of various tests in the diagnosis of commonly "worried about" intracranial diseases.*

NOTE

Skull x-rays are always helpful in patients with acute traumatic headache, but only rarely otherwise.[101] A normal skull x-ray has a poor reassurance value in the chronic headache patient, since most serious diseases resulting in chronic headache will not be apparent on plain radiography. When disease of the cranial vault is considered, x-rays are helpful (Figs. 4–14 and 4–15). In addition, pituitary tumors may present with nonspecific headache and a normal neurologic examination—here the lateral skull film (especially with tomograms of the sella turcica)[102] (Fig. 4–16) will be a "sensitive" (and usually reassuring) test.

The EEG[103] is usually a waste of time and money in the patient with chronic headache. Patients with migraine may have nonspecifically abnormal EEGs, just as the patient with a brain tumor or aneurysm may have a normal EEG.

Radionuclide brain scan will detect most patients with chronic subdural hematomas, metastatic intracranial malignant disease, and cerebral abscesses.[104] While the CT scan has rendered this test obsolete in many medical centers, the patient with a normal neurologic examination and a normal radionuclide brain scan is most unlikely to have one of these disorders (which are among the most commonly "worried about" problems in the patient with chronic headache). On the other hand, pituitary tumors, intracranial aneurysms and arteriovenous malformations, posterior fossa tumors, and slow-growing primary CNS neoplasms will often be missed on the radionuclide scan.

The CT scan[8] must be considered the single most reassuring test and is

*Table 4–13 is included here, with apologies. "Sensitivity" and "reassurance value" are statistical terms and should be presented as quantitative, not qualitative, values. Adequate quantitative data are not available, however.

TABLE 4–13. HEADACHE TESTS

DISEASE	SENSITIVITY/REASSURANCE VALUE*			
	Skull X-Ray ($90)	EEG ($100)	Radionuclide Brain Scan ($200)	CT Scan ($400)
Primary CNS neoplasm				
Cerebral cortex	Poor/poor	Poor/poor	Poor/poor	Very good/very good
Cerebellum/brain stem	Poor/poor	Poor/poor	Poor/poor	Very good/very good
Pituitary	Good/good†	Poor/poor	Poor/poor	Very good/very good
Metastatic CNS neoplasm				
Skull	Good/poor‡	Poor/poor	Poor/poor	Very good/very good
Cerebral cortex	Poor/poor	Poor/poor	Good/good	Very good/very good
Cerebellum	Poor/poor	Poor/poor	Poor/poor	Very good/very good
Cerebral abscess	Poor/poor	Poor/poor	Very good/very good	Very good/very good
Subdural hematoma				
Acute	Poor/poor	Poor/poor	Poor/poor	Very good/very good
Chronic	Poor/poor	Poor/poor	Good/good	Very good/very good
Hydrocephalus	Poor/poor	Poor/poor	Poor/poor	Very good/very good
Intracranial aneurysm§				
Unruptured	Poor/poor	Poor/poor	Poor/poor	Poor/poor
Ruptured	Poor/poor	Poor/poor	Poor/poor	Good/good

*Definitions:

Sensitivity $= \dfrac{\text{No. patients with positive test}}{\text{No. patients with disease}}$ (The higher this value, the more sensitive the test.)

Reassurance value $= \dfrac{\text{No. false negative tests}}{\text{No. false negative tests} + \text{No. true negative tests}}$ (The lower this value, the more reassuring the test.)

†Tomogram of the sella turcica (additional $90) is better than the simple skull x-ray in evaluating enlargement of the sella.

‡A radionuclide bone scan will greatly improve the diagnostic sensitivity/reassurance value in looking for metastases to the cranium.

§Arteriography is the diagnostic procedure of choice for intracranial aneurysms.

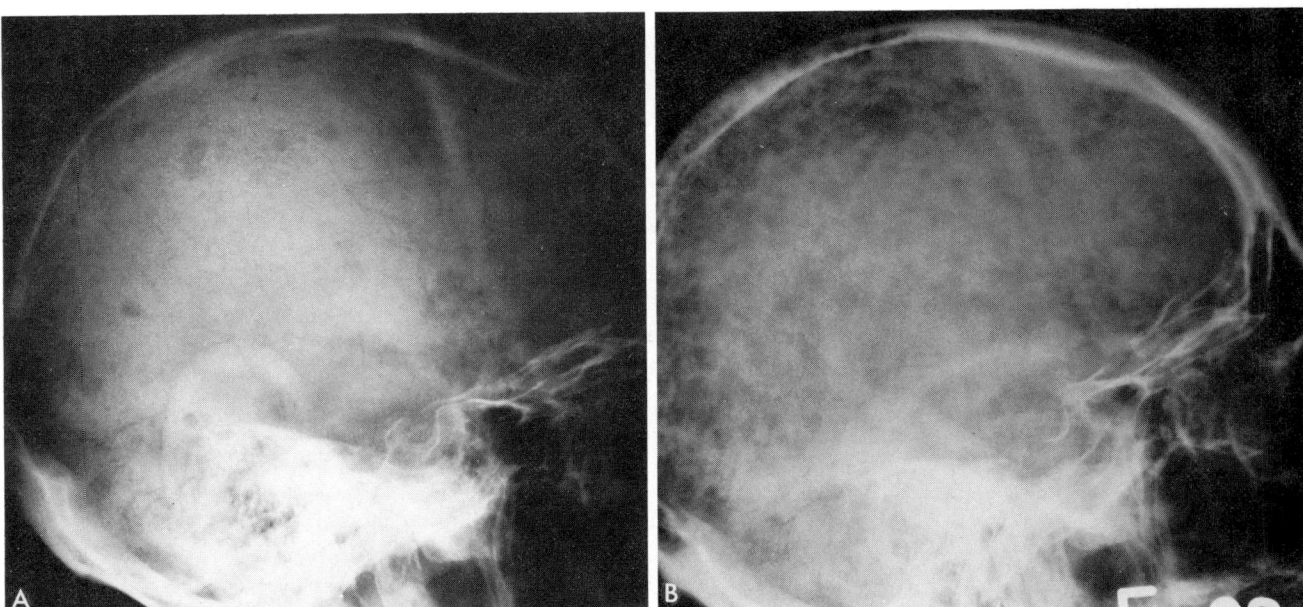

FIGURE 4–14. This 77-year-old man complained of weakness and a progressively worsening diffuse headache for the previous 2 months. Examination was unremarkable, except for marked pallor and diffuse bony tenderness of the cranium. The x-ray (A) reveals multiple lytic defects in the skull. Bone marrow examination and serum protein electrophoresis confirmed the diagnosis of multiple myeloma. Despite therapy, disease progressed (B).

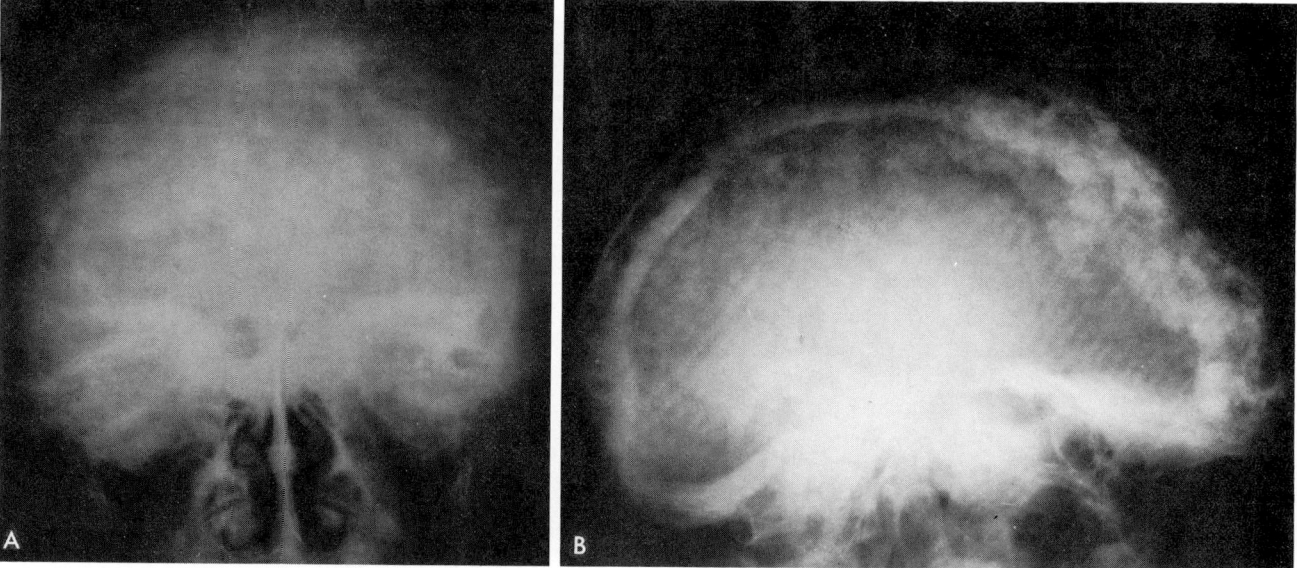

FIGURE 4–15. *A, B,* This 66-year-old man complained of progressively worsening headache for the previous year. He had also developed marked bilateral deafness, for which he had not sought medical attention. Examination revealed marked bony enlargement of the skull. Paget's disease was found in many bones, but the skull was dramatically involved.

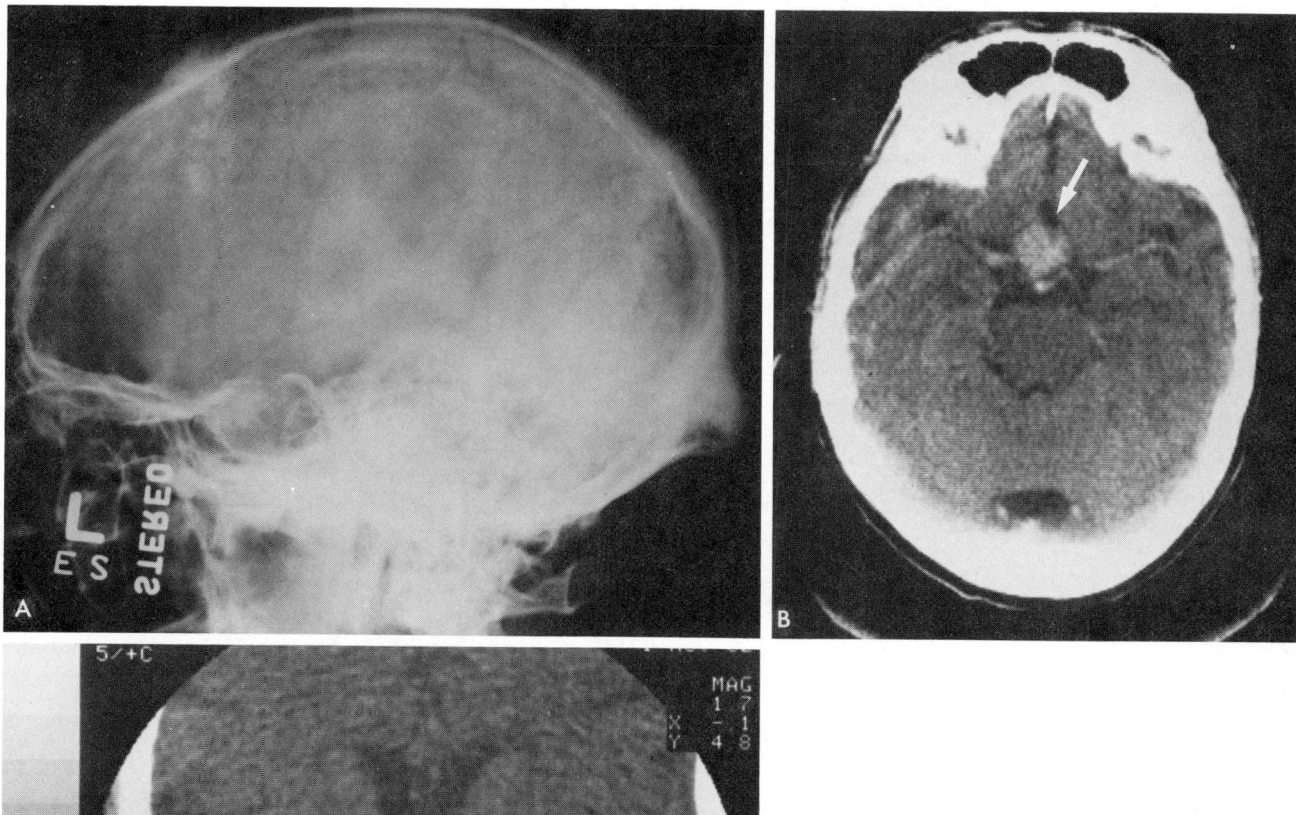

FIGURE 4–16. *A–C,* This 33-year-old woman complained of worsening diffuse headaches over the previous 3 weeks. Examination suggested a bitemporal visual field defect. The skull x-ray (*A*) revealed marked enlargement of the sella turcica, ultimately proven the result of a chromophobe adenoma. CT scan demonstrates a large sellar mass *(arrows)* (*B, C*).

199

TABLE 4–14. FINAL DIAGNOSIS AMONG 161 SELECTED PATIENTS WITH HEADACHE

FINAL DIAGNOSIS	BEFORE CT AVAILABLE No. (%)	AFTER CT AVAILABLE No. (%)
Migraine	15 (27)	25 (24)
Tension	18 (32)	35 (34)
Cluster	2 (4)	0
Cervical spondylosis	2 (4)	9 (8)
Post-traumatic	0	4 (4)
Tumor	1 (2)	1 (1)
Seizure disorder	2 (4)	3 (3)
Psychiatric disease	7 (12)	11 (11)
Unknown	7 (12)	12 (12)
Other*	2 (4)	5 (5)
Total	56 (100)	105 (100)

*Uremia, bacterial endocarditis, drug toxicity, Meniere's disease, transverse myelitis, carpal tunnel syndrome.
Adapted from Reference 8.

certainly more sensitive in detecting posterior fossa masses, primary CNS neoplasms, acute subdural hematomas, and vascular anomalies than is the radionuclide scan.[105] Even the CT scan may miss pituitary tumors, aneurysms, and other (especially small) intracerebral lesions,[106] but the "newer generation" CT scans are increasingly more accurate, even in these areas. The CT scan, however, is very expensive (Table 4–13) and the value of performing CT scans in (even highly selected) headache patients who have a normal neurologic examination is vanishingly small.[8, 107] Table 4–14 indicates the range of final diagnoses established among 161 highly selected patients referred for headache evaluation, some before and others after the availability of CT. Thus, while the CT scan has revolutionized neurologic diagnosis, the physical examination and history are the best "test" in most patients with headaches (Fig. 4–17).

Cerebral arteriography and pneumoencephalography should be reserved for specific diagnostic dilemmas, usually only after consultation with a neurologist or neurosurgeon.

Thus, again, specific tests should be chosen for specific purposes. Careful

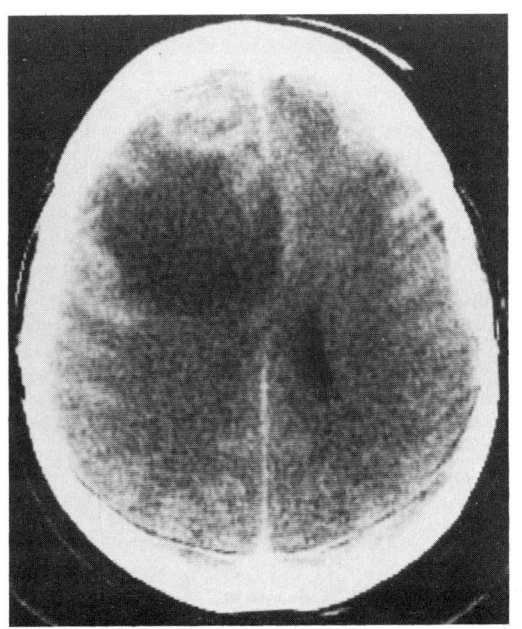

FIGURE 4–17. This 52-year-old accountant complained of mild, intermittent headache for two months, which was not severe enough to prompt him to seek medical attention. When he began to experience difficulties in concentration and in performing complicated mathematical computations, he sought medical examination. Physical examination was unremarkable except for mental status testing, which revealed mild inattention, extreme passivity, and some apraxia of gait. The CT scan demonstrated a huge neoplasm (an unresectable glioblastoma) in the right frontal lobe.

clinical evaluation is always more important than any one test. "Shotgun testing" should be avoided.

Mary asks many questions and seems skeptical. How can we be sure about her headaches without x-rays and other tests? How can she be having tension headaches when she denies any stress or worry in her life?

Even in the patient who is not skeptical, when common migraine or tension headache are clinically most likely the stage should be set for further discussion of psychosocial factors. Both vascular and tension headaches are so often related to, exacerbated by, or symptomatic of emotional conflicts, pressured life styles, unresolved ambivalence, anxiety, or depression that these issues must at least be reviewed if treatment is to be successful. Each clinician will, of course, approach this in his or her own way; the following is just one way to begin to talk about such issues:

> Headaches may be caused by specific troubles like an illness in the family or trouble paying the bills, and you've probably gotten headache at times like that, just as I have. Very often, though, the cause of headaches is more hidden and harder to see and admit. Tension and stress build up inside all of us and come out or show themselves in different ways in different people. Some of us scream and yell and "let off steam," but some of us don't do that, and sometimes we are not even aware of the stress we feel until it shows itself in some physical way. This happens to all of us, and while some of us develop headaches, others develop other physical symptoms, which you yourself may also have experienced at one time or another—trouble sleeping, bowel troubles, chest pains, dizziness, or whatever. I don't know why some of us get headaches at times like this and others get diarrhea, but I do know that some feeling of frustration or helplessness or "being stuck" in a situation we don't know how to resolve plays a big part in causing the headache. Most of us, at one time or another, want something (or someone) we can't have, have some ambition we can't fulfill, are mad at someone but can't say so—we get "caught in the middle" of something that is very important to us deep down. Often, though, we tend to push it all "under the rug," and we don't deal with it straight out because, although it is important to us, we can't see any easy way out. Each of us can only take this for so long before it begins to affect us in a physical way. In a sense, the headache is like a safety valve—it helps release a little of this pressure before it gets unbearable. At the same time, though, it is a warning—it means that we must do something to resolve our problem, it means that we can't keep on this way. We must try to recognize and deal with the underlying problem—otherwise, the headaches won't go away.

This does not mean that psychoanalysis or psychiatric consultation is needed—these interventions are only rarely productive in the patient with chronic headache. Rather, the physician must get to know the patient and must treat the whole person, not just the headache. Patients must be made aware of the kinds of covert conflicts or anxiety that may contribute to chronic headache (see also page 209).

Mary remains skeptical but agrees to be "open-minded about it."

Eight days later, Mary calls to say that she has a severe headache that has now lasted over 12 hours and is no better despite 6 mg of ergotamine and several aspirins and Darvons. She has vomited several times. Examination in the clinic at this time is entirely normal, but Mary is obviously uncomfortable, holding her right temple and preferring to sit quietly and not be disturbed. The headache is unilateral over the right temple, was not associated with any prodrome or other symptoms except nausea and vomiting, and is now throbbing and quite severe. Mary says this headache is similar to her sick headaches of the past. Rectal antiemetic suppositories and intramuscular meperidine improve her greatly within an hour. She is given a few codeine tablets and sent home.

This is the typical picture of common migraine headache. Usually migraine will respond to ergotamine and mild analgesics, but not always (see below). Acute migraine unresponsive to ergotamine should be treated with potent analgesics, sedatives, and antiemetics, in a quiet environment.

ANALGESICS AND HEADACHE[108]

Most patients with chronic headache have received many different pain medications, and more than a few are addicted to various analgesics. Over-the-counter remedies—aspirin or acetaminophen, for example—have invariably been found unsatisfactory by such patients, and this, in part, prompts the visit to the physician—"better pain medicine" is needed. While analgesics are an important element in the treatment of all chronic headache, pain relief is only one of many goals of the headache sufferer, and analgesics must be prescribed as but one part of a broader approach.[109]

Some clinicians categorically refuse narcotics to chronic headache patients. This is, at times, cruel and therapeutically counterproductive. No headache treatment program is completely effective. All chronic headache sufferers will develop painful headaches intermittently. The patient with acute, severe migraine is a good example (see above)—refusal to relieve such distress because of dogmatic opposition to narcotic administration will engender hostility (and even shame) in otherwise well-intentioned patients, such that the ongoing therapeutic venture is subverted. The importance of developing a trusting physician-patient relationship cannot be overemphasized here—such relationships allow the judicious use of potentially abusive medication.

Patients who "use" headache to obtain narcotics, often with sporadic visits to doctors' offices or emergency rooms, are clearly a different problem. Frustrating encounters with these patients should not distort therapeutic relationships with all headache patients, however. Most well-intentioned patients respond to the notion that analgesics are adjunctive therapy, to be used wisely and sparingly. Fiorinal (butalbital 50 mg, aspirin 200 mg, phenacetin 130 mg, caffeine 40 mg), propoxyphene (Darvon), and Norgesic (orphenadrine citrate) are among the many remedies that are found to be helpful by some patients, and that have lesser addiction potential than commonly prescribed narcotics (codeine, pentazocine [Talwin], oxycodone [Percodan, Tylox], meperidine [Demerol]). The potential hazards of all analgesics should be explained. Even the non-narcotic analgesics may induce serious illness—analgesic nephropathy with (especially) phenacetin-containing drugs, and hepatotoxicity and gastrointestinal toxicity with salicylates are among the better known such hazards.

It is rare for patients with correctly diagnosed chronic headache syndromes to be completely refractory to all preventive or symptomatic therapy and thus to require daily use of potentially addictive drugs. In such instances the specific diagnosis should be questioned, a second opinion from a physician more experienced with headache problems should be recommended, and the patient's motivation should be scrutinized—usually in that order.

TREATMENT OF MIGRAINE

In general, the mainstay of migraine therapy is pharmacologic (see below), but several nonpharmacologic measures must be remembered:

1. Exogenous and endogenous triggers. The precise pathogenesis of migraine is poorly understood. It is clear, however, that in many migraineurs, headache may be triggered by a wide variety of often inapparent influences: diet,[110-112] drugs, lighting and glare, hormonal fluctuations,[73-76] psychologic stress, disordered sleep patterns, and many others.[113] Of great importance is the fact that specific precipitants of migraine may be only intermittently a problem—for example, the migraineur whose headache is often induced by drinking red wine does not always get a headache in that situation. Migraineurs must understand this. It is not possible for all migraine sufferers to consistently avoid all potentially precipitating factors, but the migraineur should be encouraged to "keep track" of the circumstances in which migraine occurs—its relation to menstrual cycles, food and beverage intake over the prior 24 hours, medications, stressful situations, for example. When connections are made, temporary modification of suspected precipitants makes sense. It is remarkable how timidly some patients act on their own diagnostic and therapeutic hunches—the patient must be told to observe and to experiment with possible "triggers." An elimination diet has been advocated to establish the dietary precipitants of migraine,[77] but this is rarely necessary.

2. Many nonspecific health measures are helpful. A balanced diet, maintenance of ideal body weight, adequate sleep (and predictable sleep habits), relaxing avocational interests, and regular strenuous physical exercise are often neglected by the headache patient (and the physician). Simple life adjustments may be crucial in individual patients. Measures that engender a sense of physical well-being—jogging is a classic example—may be of more psychologic than physiologic benefit, but they are beneficial nonetheless.

3. Various behavioral modification techniques—biofeedback, relaxation training, meditation, yoga—may be remarkably helpful in selected patients.[114-117] Such techniques require that the patient be highly motivated, cooperative, and enthusiastic—disappointment with these techniques is the rule rather than the exception unless patients are so selected.

Pharmacologic Therapy[118-121]

Drug therapy of migraine may be symptomatic (to abort or modify an acute attack) or prophylactic (to prevent the attack before it occurs).

Symptomatic Treatment. Many patients with acute migraine headache will improve if able to rest in a darkened environment, take mild analgesics, and perhaps apply ice locally to the area of head pain. Aspirin, acetaminophen, propoxyphene, or codeine may be helpful, especially in mild or moderate cases. Midrin, a combination of isometheptene (a vasoconstrictor), dichloralphenazone (a sedative), and acetaminophen, in doses of 2 to 3 capsules immediately and repeated once 45 minutes later, is helpful to some. Inhalation of 100 per cent oxygen may be dramatically effective in some patients, but is impractical for most. When ergotamines cannot be taken or tolerated (see below), nonsteroidal anti-inflammatory agents (for example, ibuprofen [Motrin] or indomethacin [Indocin]) may be useful.

Ergotamine preparations are the drugs of choice for symptomatic therapy.[80, 122] Most migraines (common, classic, and complicated) will respond to ergotamines, but success depends upon individualizing treatment for different patients.[123] Most "ergotamine failures" are the result of too little taken too late by inappropriate routes of administration, or relate to ergotamine side

TABLE 4–15. ERGOTAMINE PREPARATIONS

BRAND/GENERIC NAME	ROUTE	ERGOTAMINE DOSE	"ADDITIVES"
Ergotamine	Subcutaneous/ intramuscular	0.25 mg/0.5 ml	
Bellergal	Oral	0.3 mg	Belladonna 0.2 mg, phenobarbital 20 mg
Ergotamine (Medihaler)	Aerosol	0.36 mg/puff	
Bellergal-S	Oral	0.6 mg	Belladonna 0.2 mg, phenobarbital 40 mg
Cafergot	Oral	1.0 mg	Caffeine 100 mg
Cafergot P-B	Oral	1.0 mg	Caffeine 100 mg, belladonna 0.125 mg, phenobarbital 30 mg
Gynergen	Oral	1.0 mg	
Migral	Oral	1.0 mg	Caffeine 50 mg, cyclizine 25 mg
Wigraine	Oral	1.0 mg	Caffeine 100 mg, belladonna 0.1 mg, phenacetin 130 mg
Wigraine	Rectal suppository	1.0 mg	Caffeine 100 mg, belladonna 0.1 mg, phenacetin 130 mg
Cafergot	Rectal suppository	2.0 mg	Caffeine 100 mg
Cafergot P-B	Rectal suppository	2.0 mg	Caffeine 100 mg, belladonna 0.25 mg, phenobarbital 60 mg
Ergostat	Sublingual	2.0 mg	
Ergomar	Sublingual	2.0 mg	

effects (primarily nausea), which can often be circumvented by careful choice of dose and specific preparations. Table 4–15 lists many of the ergotamine-containing drugs commonly used today. Several points deserve emphasis:

1. While many of these preparations contain other drugs, ergotamine is the primary active agent.[122] The key to successful therapy lies in establishing for each individual patient the dose of ergotamine that is necessary to control headache and that is also well tolerated. Note that different oral, rectal, sublingual, aerosol, and parenteral preparations contain different doses of ergotamine, ranging from 0.25 mg to 2 mg per dose—an eightfold difference. Failure of one preparation or intolerable side effects from another should prompt trials with different dosages and routes of administration. Authorities with large clinical experience note that oral preparations are generally less satisfactory[118] than rectal, sublingual, or aerosol preparations in the treatment of acute attacks. (Slowed drug absorption from the upper intestinal tract during acute migraine may be partly responsible for this. The addition of caffeine to some preparations—Table 4–15—may improve drug absorption, but this is controversial.) Parenteral preparations are more rapid acting but are usually impractical for outpatients. Aerosol and sublingual preparations may be more rapid acting than the suppositories, but this varies with individual patients. Rectal suppositories are especially useful when nausea is a prominent part of the headache syndrome (often).

Sedatives or belladonna preparations are added to erogtamine for general comfort or when the gastrointestinal effects of migraine are troublesome.

2. As such, when one is initiating therapy, test doses of ergotamine should be administered on headache-free days. Nausea is the most common

side effect. Therefore, increasing amounts of a specific preparation should be administered as a test trial until the full recommended dose is reached or side effects occur. For example, a 2-mg ergotamine rectal suppository (Cafergot PB or Cafergot) can be cut in halves or thirds, each partial dose being inserted rectally at 60-minute intervals. If the full 2 mg is well tolerated, this should be the initial dose used for acute migraine; if only 1 mg is tolerated before nausea occurs, then one half of the Cafergot suppository or 1 Wigraine suppository (containing only 1.0 mg ergotamine—Table 4–15) should be used when migraine strikes. It is unusual for a patient to be unable to tolerate any dose of ergotamine. The drug should be taken at the first sign of headache, and repeated hourly, up to a (usual) maximum dose of 4 mg rectally or 8 mg orally.

Aerosol preparations should be shaken thoroughly and deeply inhaled following a forced expiration.

Sublingual tablets should perhaps be chewed but not swallowed to speed absorption.

Shelf life of ergotamine may be short (several months); failure to respond to previously effective doses should prompt a new prescription refill.

3. Side effects of ergotamine,[118] beside nausea and vomiting, include myalgias, abdominal pain, diarrhea, vertigo and dizziness, paresthesias, and mouth dryness. Rarer side effects include angina pectoris, vascular claudication, syncope, and dyspnea.

Ergotism is a rare but dramatic complication of erogotamine use. In this condition, severe vasoconstriction afflicts (usually) the lower limbs bilaterally and symmetrically, but it is almost always heralded by preceding symptoms of distal paresthesias, coldness of the digits, and symptoms of exertional claudication. Gangrene has been reported, but only when patients continue to use ergotamine in spite of these premonitory symptoms.[118] As such, all patients should be warned of this uncommon but serious side effect.

Ergot dependence is a separate phenomenon in which daily use of ergotamine leads to apparent tolerance, increasingly refractory headache, and need for progressively larger doses, with only transient benefit.[72] In general, patients should be instructed to take no more than 10 mg of ergotamine per week. The need for larger weekly doses should prompt reevaluation—preventive therapy is almost always indicated in such circumstances (see below).

4. Contraindications to ergotamine therapy include pregnancy, sepsis, angina, peripheral vascular disease, and hepatic or renal disease. Hypertension is probably not a contraindication.[118] Thrombophlebitis has been reported[124] but is rare.

5. Note that side effects or contraindications may relate as much to other drugs (in combination preparations) as to ergotamine. Common "additives" (Table 4–15) include caffeine, anticholinergics, and barbiturates; hence, tachycardia, glaucoma, urinary retention, or drowsiness may develop, but usually not from ergotamine per se.

Preventive Therapy. Preventive therapy should be considered when migraine occurs frequently (several times per month) or is especially incapacitating or when ergotamine or analgesics are contraindicated, ineffective, or abused. Nonpharmacologic measures must always be remembered as well (see page 203).

Table 4–16 lists several drugs that have been studied and found effective

TABLE 4–16. DRUGS IN MIGRAINE PROPHYLAXIS

Drugs	Daily Dose (Initial) (Average) (Maximum)	Efficacy (Definite Improvement)	Side Effects	Contraindications	Cost/Month
Amitriptyline[125, 126] (trial, 6–8 weeks)	10–25 mg qhs 50–75 mg qhs 300 mg qhs	50–60%	Dry mouth, sedation, drowsiness, weight gain	Arrhythmias, urinary retention, glaucoma	50 mg, #30, $6
Propranolol[127–131] (4–6 weeks)	10–20 mg tid 40 mg tid 320 mg qd	50%	Drowsiness, flatulence; beware sudden withdrawal!	Congestive heart failure, asthma, brittle diabetes	40 mg, #60, $12
Cyproheptadine[10, 132] (4–6 weeks)	4 mg bid 6–12 mg bid 16 mg bid	40%	Drowsiness, weight gain		4 mg, #90, $10
Ergonovine[100, 122] (4–6 weeks)	0.2 mg bid 0.4 mg bid 1.0 mg bid	*	Nausea, abdominal pain	Prinzmetal's angina, venous disease, pregnancy	0.2 mg, #120, $23
Papaverine[133, 134] (4–6 weeks)	300 mg qd 5 mg/kg qd 900 mg qd	*	Constipation, nausea, facial flushing, sweating, sedation, tachycardia		150 mg, #60, $8
Methysergide[10, 132, 135, 136] (4–6 weeks)	1–2 mg bid 3–4 mg bid 4–6 mg tid	60–80%	Myalgias, dizziness, drowsiness, nausea, vomiting, weight gain, fibrotic disorders[137]	Angina, ?hypertension, ?venous thrombosis, liver/kidney disease, valvular heart disease	2 mg, #120, $60
Ergotamine	1.0 mg qd/bid no more than 10 mg per week	60% (?)	See page 205; tolerance; ergotism	See page 205	1 mg, #30, $10

Others*
  Chlorpromazine
  Bromocriptine
  Prednisone
  Dilantin
  Phenelzine
  Indomethacin
  Other nonsteroidal anti-inflammatory drugs
  Clonidine
  Calcium channel blockers

*Data available on relatively few patients.

in migraine prophylaxis. While unifying hypotheses explaining modes of drug action have been offered,[118] precise understanding of these drugs is controversial. Note that no drug is 100 per cent effective, and sequential trials of different drugs are often necessary to find the drug that is both well tolerated and effective for the individual patient.

Drug trials reported in the literature are often difficult to interpret because of differences in diagnostic definitions, the high rate of placebo response (20 to 50 per cent), patient selection biases, variable control of simultaneous medications, and variable grading systems for headache measurements. Several generalizations, however, are valid:

1. Likely efficacy must be balanced against frequency and severity of side effects. For this reason, drugs that produce uncommon or mild side effects are preferred, at least initially. Methysergide is probably the most effective drug, but it is also the least well tolerated and is associated with both common minor side effects and uncommon serious side effects. (It is also expensive.) Table 4–16 lists prophylactic drugs in the order in which they might be sequentially tried. Amitriptyline is recommended initially since it is usually well tolerated, is effective at low doses (and probably independently of its antidepressant effects), and is often completely effective when it is effective at all[125] (unlike other drugs that are often helpful, but are less commonly completely effective). Sequential trials of amitriptyline, propranolol, cyproheptadine, ergonovine, or papaverine—each drug slowly increased in dosage over a trial period of at least 4 to 6 weeks—will result in benefit

in the great majority of patients; one of these drugs will usually be both effective and well tolerated. Methysergide (and various other drugs—Table 4–16) should generally be reserved for patients who fail these trials. (Note that other beta blockers, tricyclic antidepressants, and antihistamines may not be as effective as are propranolol, amitriptyline, and cyproheptadine.[118])

Ergotamine is not a drug of choice as a prophylactic agent, unless small doses (1 mg per day) are both successful and well tolerated. This is unusual. However, migraine that occurs primarily before or during menstruation can sometimes be suppressed with daily ergotamine dosages for several menstrual days.

2. Each prophylactic drug takes time to work. During the trial of these preventive drugs, symptomatic and ergotamine treatment should be continued. (Ergotamine may be even more effective when taken simultaneously with ergonovine or methysergide.)

Even "effective" prophylactic drugs will not be 100 per cent effective. The quantitative weekly use of ergotamine for symptomatic treatment will be one useful measure of the efficacy of prophylactic drugs (and the need for increasing dosages of the latter).

3. Each drug should be given at low doses initially and increased at periodic intervals until failure or efficacy is established or until a maximum dose is reached. Average daily doses that are effective vary considerably (especially for propranolol), but rough guidelines are given in Table 4–16. Most drugs will be effective when taken only once or twice per day, but propranolol and methysergide *may* require thrice daily dosage.

4. Drugs found to be effective should be tapered slowly every 4 to 6 months to assess ongoing needs. It is often possible to take "drug holidays" after several months of effective prophylaxis. When methysergide is used, discontinuation of the drug for 1 month every 4 to 6 months probably helps avoid fibrotic complications[137] and is very strongly recommended.

Intractable migraine may require hospitalization. Status migraine is a rare event that refers to a single, prolonged (days to weeks) vascular headache that is unresponsive to vigorous therapy of acute migraine, or migraine that recurs at such frequent intervals that the patient is incapacitated. Such patients usually require withdrawal of all vasoactive drugs, heavy sedation (barbiturates or chlorpromazine up to 1000 mg per 24 hours), narcotics, or high-dose corticosteroid therapy (60 mg of prednisone per day). Convalescence may be prolonged (weeks).

Four weeks later, Mary returns for her appointment and says she is no better. She has had two more "sick headaches," and the ergotamine suppositories clearly helped these. Nevertheless, she continues to have almost daily headaches that require both aspirin and Darvon, and ergotamine does not help these headaches at all. (Table 4–17 is Mary's headache calender.)

Again the common covert psychodynamic tension headache relationships are discussed. Mary admits that she is not entirely free of such conflicts, "but then who is?" She is a college-educated woman who has devoted her adult life to her husband and children. She admits that she is no longer personally fulfilled by her housewife role and yet continues to infuse all of her considerable energy into her family—she rarely leaves the children with baby-sitters; she has become obsessed with decorating and cleaning the house. Mary seems somewhat resentful of her husband's long work hours and obvious personal satisfaction with his own career. When asked, "Are you happy with your life as it is?" she briefly breaks down and cries. She admits that she awakens in the middle of the night for no apparent

TABLE 4–17. MARY'S HEADACHE CALENDAR

DATE	TIME OF DAY	SEVERITY	MEDICATION	RELIEF
9/16/83	4:00 PM	Moderate	Aspirin, Darvon	Moderate
9/17	10:00 AM	Mild	Aspirin, Darvon	Moderate
9/18	All day	Mild	Aspirin, Darvon	Moderate
9/19	10:00 AM	Moderate	Aspirin, Darvon	Moderate
9/20	All day	Severe	Cafergot, aspirin	None
9/21*	5:00 AM	Very severe, vomited	Cafergot × 3 Aspirin, Darvon	No relief Clinic visit (parenteral Demerol) Eventual relief
9/22	No headache			
9/23	6:00 PM	Mild	Aspirin, Darvon	Complete
9/24	2:00 PM	Mild	Aspirin, Darvon	Moderate
9/25	No headache			
9/26	All day	Severe	Cafergot, aspirin, Darvon	Moderate
9/27	6:00 PM	Mild	Aspirin	Complete
9/28	10:00 AM	Moderate	Aspirin, Cafergot	None
9/29	All day	Mild	Aspirin	Moderate
9/30	9:00 AM	Mild	Aspirin, Darvon	Complete
10/1*	11:00 PM	Very severe, vomited	Cafergot × 1	Complete in 1 hour
10/2	11:00 AM	Mild	Aspirin	Complete
10/3	No headache			
10/4	6:00 PM	Mild	Aspirin	Complete
10/5	7:00 PM	Mild	Aspirin, Darvon	None
10/6	9:00 AM	Mild	Aspirin	Moderate
10/7	6:00 PM	Moderate	Aspirin	Moderate
10/8	4:00 PM	Severe	Cafergot	None
10/9	5:00 PM	Mild	Aspirin	Complete
10/10	No headache			
10/11*	6:00 AM	Very severe, vomited	Cafergot × 4	Moderate in 4 hours
10/12	No headache			
10/13	6:00 PM	Mild	Aspirin, Darvon	Complete
10/14	7:00 PM	Mild	Aspirin, Darvon	None

*Probably migraine.

reason and has some difficulty falling asleep again. She denies any change in libido or appetite for food.

It is suggested that tension headaches are Mary's major problem now and that these may well be making her migraine headaches more of a problem. Mary is encouraged to discuss her feelings with her husband and to think more about how she might deal with the conflicts in her life.

Mary admits that some of these conflicts could have something to do with her headaches, but she remains skeptical, and again asks whether she does not need some "tests and x-rays." "If I have a brain tumor, I want you to tell me."

Neurologic examination is repeated and is normal. At Mary's insistence, a CT scan is performed and is normal. Amitriptyline, 25 mg at bedtime, is prescribed, and ergotamine suppositories are continued. Mary is encouraged to stay off the oral contraceptive and to consider other methods of birth control, to begin a regular exercise program, and to return again in 6 weeks.

TREATMENT OF TENSION HEADACHE

There is no single best approach to the treatment of chronic tension headache. Drug therapy of some kind is almost always necessary, but the goal of treatment is helping the patient to find some means of coping with a complex, usually multifactorial problem. Therapeutic success demands patience and insight—qualities that are difficult for physicians to sustain in a busy clinical practice (and are inadequately reimbursed by third-party payors) and that few chronic headache sufferers themselves have in abundance.

Flexibility of approach is crucial—different patients respond to different methods. Patients whose headache is a psychophysiologic symptom of some recognizable and remediable emotional conflict often do well with simple reassurance and explanation. When such conflicts are recognizable but insoluble, reassurance combined with ongoing opportunities for the patient to ventilate his or her frustrations is helpful. When psychodynamic stresses are apparent but serious psychiatric disease (psychosis, severe depression) is also suspected (uncommonly), psychiatric consultation is certainly worthwhile.

Much more often, though, chronic headache patients either do not possess the insight required to recognize subtle covert psychodynamic conflicts or openly refute the suggestion that such conflicts are present or, if present that they are avoidable. These patients generally do not respond to the "psychophysiologic approach"—i.e., achieving insight into the "meaning" of tension headache as a symptom. Excessive emphasis on avoiding stress or modulating anxiety in such patients can be a mistake. Many such patients are best served by emphasis on the physical model—e.g., explaining the pathogenesis and treatment of muscle spasm in "muscle contraction" headache. Most patients can at least understand the notion that muscle spasm can cause pain and that emotional or psychologic stress can cause the muscle spasm. Whether tension headache is always synonymous with muscle contraction headache (an interesting pathophysiologic controversy) may not be so important practically as long as the patient responds to one or the other explanation.

NOTE ALSO

1. The patient and the physician must be convinced that organic diseases have been ruled out. This step is crucial, since primary treatment involves educating these patients (see below). As long as the possibility of a "hidden" physical disease remains, the patient will not be receptive to such efforts.

While some patients will persist in their insistence that "something has been missed" and will "shop around" for different opinions (and usually will find someone who will tell them what they want to hear), this can be avoided in many patients. A careful, detailed history and physical examination (with thorough neurologic examination) usually will detect those organic disorders that commonly masquerade as tension headache.

The occipital pattern of tension headache may be mimicked by cervical spine disease, craniovertebral anomalies, and post-traumatic (whiplash) syndromes.[54] (Rarely, intracranial—especially posterior fossa—tumors, vertebrobasilar vascular disease, or polymyalgia rheumatica may be confused with occipital tension headache.) Cervical spondylosis is an especially common cause of occipital headache, especially in the middle-aged and elderly. Abnormal x-rays of the cervical spine are not themselves diagnostic of the cause of headache, however, given the high prevalence of *asymptomatic* cervical spondylosis.[138] Unilateral neck and shoulder pain, limitation of motion of the neck, radicular neurologic symptoms, and abnormal postures of the head and neck are much more helpful. Relief of headache with aspirin, local heat, and physical therapy (especially home traction) usually confirms the diagnosis of cervical spondylosis.

The bifrontal or hat band pattern of tension headache is easily confused with sinus or ocular disease, and, more rarely, with temporal arteritis or intracranial (or pituitary) mass lesions.

Even in patients with classic tension headache—chronic, recurrent, typical headache in a younger patient with a normal physical and neurologic examination—evaluation with noninvasive testing may be reassuring (see page 197). A common pitfall here is allowing the patient to think that tension headache is a diagnosis of exclusion—"all the tests are normal, so it must be a tension headache." While this approach is temporarily effective for some, it is often valuable to impress upon the patient immediately after the history and physical examination that the headaches are clinically typical of tension headache. Subsequent negative diagnostic tests can then be used (if at all) to support the initial clinical diagnosis, thereby reinforcing the certainty of that diagnosis in the patient's mind. Most patients are aware of the fallibility of tests—a "positive" diagnosis of tension headache will often not be accepted by patients with chronic headaches simply because tests for other disorders are negative at one point in time. The physician must look elsewhere when the clinical picture is atypical but should convincingly communicate to the patient his or her own "certainty" when the clinical picture is typical, even before (or without) diagnostic testing. It must be repeated that thoroughness of the history and physical examination is the crucial first step here.

2. Significant underlying psychiatric disorders are uncommon but must be remembered. Headache certainly occurs as the presenting manifestation of psychosis, hysteria, conversion reactions, or serious affective disorders[139] but is uncommon.

Bizarre descriptions ("My head is crawling with snakes") must prompt a careful evaluation of mental status—the psychotic patient may well have organic headache, but a psychiatrist's help is usually necessary. Depression is very common among chronic headache sufferers—whether primary or reactive is often a moot point,[140, 141] given the effectiveness of amitriptyline in such patients.[142, 143] Coincident emotional life events (childbirth, parental death, divorce) should always be explored, as should the presence of any biologic signs of depression—anorexia, insomnia, decreased libido—or any suicidal intent. A prior history of conversion reactions or hysterical disease is helpful information in some—inappropriate indifference to pain or overly supportive relatives who dignify the patient's "invalid role" occasionally raise such suspicions.

Some patients without serious psychiatric illness may benefit from psychiatric consultation—especially the highly motivated, insightful patient who is unable to unravel or confront psychodynamic conflicts—but most patients with tension headache do not require, or benefit from, psychiatric attention.

3. Patients must be educated about tension headache. One must avoid a common mistake—failing to explain that tension headache is often not associated temporally with any specific recognizable stress or tension. Patients who experience headache during obviously stressful situations—arguments, following a particularly harrowing day, during school examination periods, for example—rarely need help in making such connections. However, pointing out the obvious association between headache and these overt stresses may help set the stage for the more elusive recognition of a relationship between covert stress and headache. It is almost axiomatic that the patient with chronic tension headache who consults a physician has failed to appreciate the types of subliminal psychodynamic stresses that are the prevalent triggers of headache. Generally these stresses include ongoing (and not acute) interpersonal conflicts, anxiety, frustration, ambivalence, or helplessness revolving around issues of dependency, sexuality, or suppressed hostility. Such experiences are universal and are usually recognizable when introduced to patients in simple nonmedical terms—see page 201.

It must also be made clear to the patient that the physician is not implying that the headache is "made up" or imaginary. The physician who admits that he or she, too, has had similar experiences—"I, like you, have had headaches like this, and I know how real they are, believe me!"—goes a long way toward reassuring the patient that the patient is not alone, unique, or "crazy."

4. Ongoing longitudinal care is crucial. Accessible, continuing physician interest is just as important for the patient with chronic headache as it is for the patient with chronic cardiac or renal disease. Follow-up is essential.

5. Analgesic therapy is usually necessary, at least intermittently, but narcotics should be strictly (if not absolutely) discouraged in treatment of chronic tension headache. Combinations of sedative–analgesic–muscle relaxant drugs (for example, Fiorinal) are often helpful, but long-term daily use of these too should be discouraged.

6. Preventive pharmacologic therapy may be helpful, in some, but is generally less effective than is drug therapy of migraine. Amitriptyline, even in low doses (25 mg nightly) may be very useful, and its effect may not be simply the result of its antidepressant efficacy. Incremental doses to 300 mg a day should be tried before the drug is discontinued.

For some patients, tranquilizers[10, 144]—diazepam, chlordiazepoxide, thioridazine (Mellaril), meprobamate or barbiturates—are effective. Such drugs should always be tapered after several months of treatment.

7. Many nonspecific therapies should be adjunctively used, as noted

above.[145] Heat, massage, and stretching exercises (especially for occipital headache patterns) are active participatory treatments, while behavioral modification techniques may also be helpful in selected patients.[116, 117] While biofeedback may be more promising than other behavioral treatments for migraine, various relaxation techniques are probably more useful in tension headache.[3] Nevertheless, the value of meditation, hypnosis, yoga, and the "relaxation response" for treatment of chronic tension headache remains controversial. Promoting relaxation in the patient with tension headache certainly will not hurt!

> **Six weeks later, Mary is smiling. She says that she has had only two migraines, and the ergotamine helped both times. She continues to have occasional tension headaches, but these are much less frequent and she goes for several days without any headache at all. When asked how she "cured herself," she says that she and her husband have agreed on several changes in their life style. Mary has decided to look for a part-time job, has begun to go out on her own more often, and is jogging during the day. Her husband has agreed to have a vasectomy, and Mary now wants "to get on with the rest of my life."**

Recognition of covert tension headache conflicts rarely happens with sudden self-awakening. Ongoing discussion, ventilation of feelings, and emphasis on development of patient insight take time. The whole patient must be treated. Advice about birth control, encouragement of physical exercise, and responsiveness to Mary's anxiety about the need for tests may be just as helpful as drugs and ongoing pursuit of psychodynamic insight.

To illustrate some approaches that help some patients, the happy ending to this story, of course, ignores the many similar patients who do not do so well. A few patients do not want to improve. The "manipulative help rejector"[146] will move on to another symptom complex that sanctions read-mission to the physician's care if the headache is "explained away." Many such patients benefit from regular "ventilation visits" with a nonthreatening physician who takes them seriously. Such patients often say, "No, my headache isn't better but I feel better just talking to you." Success here is measured more by the patient's gratitude than by "headache grading systems."

The most difficult patients are those who are refractory to all nonanalgesic treatment. Some of these become "hateful patients."[46] Others are best considered chronic pain problems.[147] Even when the multidisciplinary approach at "headache clinics" is available, such patients manipulate physicians, abuse analgesics, and remain major "headaches." Depression is often a component of such illness. Tricyclic antidepressants can potentiate analgesic effects, and thus these drugs are commonly helpful, both in limiting analgesic requirements and in ameliorating common biologic accompaniments of depression (for example, anorexia and insomnia), which may themselves be nonspecific "triggers" or "fellow travelers" in the vicious holistic cycle of chronic tension headache.

> **Six months later, Mary continues to do well, and the amitriptyline is withdrawn. Ergotamines are needed once or twice a month, and while tension headaches still occur with some regularity, Mary "can cope with those all right."**

Most patients with chronic headache can be helped. Relatively few are cured. Realistic expectations must be emphasized.

REFERENCES

1. Dhopesh, V, et al.: A retrospective assessment of emergency department patients with complaints of headache. Headache 19:37–42, 1979.
2. Ryan, RE, Ryan, RE, Jr.: Headache and Head Pain: Diagnosis and Treatment. St. Louis: C. V. Mosby, 1978.
3. Lance, JW: Mechanisms and Management of Headache, 3rd ed. Boston: Butterworth, 1978.
4. Raskin, NH, Appenzeller, O: Headache. In Smith, LH (ed): Major Problems in Internal Medicine. Philadelphia: W.B. Saunders, 1980, vol. 19, pp. 84–110.
5. Dalessio, DJ: Classification and mechanisms of migraine. Headache 19:114–121, 1979.
6. Olesen, J: Some clinical features of the acute migraine attack. An analysis of 750 patients. Headache 18:268–271, 1978.
7. Friedman, AT, von Storch, T: Tension headache. JAMA 151:174–177, 1953.
8. Larson, EB, et al.: Diagnostic evaluation of headache. Impact of computerized tomography and cost effectiveness. JAMA 243:359–362, 1980.
9. Kunkel, RS: Evaluating the headache patient: History and workup. Headache 19:122–126, 1979.
10. Lance, JW, et al.: Investigations into the mechanism and treatment of chronic headache. Med J Aust 2:909–914, 1965.
11. Friedman, AP: Clinical approach to the patient with headache. Med Clin North Am 62:433–450, 1978.
12. Caviness, VS, O'Brien, P: Current concepts: Headache. N Engl J Med 302:446–450, 1980.
13. Friedman, AP: Recurring headache. Diagnosis and differential diagnosis. Primary Care 1:275–292, 1974.
14. Kudrow, L: Systemic causes of headache. Postgrad Med 56:105–111, 1974.
15. Hatfield, WB: Headache associated with metabolic and systemic disorders. Med Clin North Am 62:451–458, 1978.
16. Raskin, N.: Headaches associated with organic diseases of the nervous system. Med Clin North Am 62:459–466, 1978.
17. Ad Hoc Committee of the National Institute of Neurological Diseases and Blindness: Classification of Headache. JAMA 179:717–718, 1962.
18. Walshe, T, et al.: The diagnosis of hypertensive intracerebral hemorrhage: The contribution of computerized tomography. Comput Tomogr 1:63–69, 1977.
19. Walton, JN: Subarachnoid Hemorrhage. London: Livingstone, 1976.
20. Scotti, G, et al.: Computed tomography in the evaluation of intracranial aneurysm and subarachnoid hemorrhage. Radiology 123:85–90, 1977.
21. McKissock, W, et al.: An analysis of the results of treatment of ruptured intracranial aneurysms. J Neurosurg 17:762–776, 1960.
22. Winn, HR, et al.: The long-term prognosis in untreated cerebral aneurysms. I. The incidence of late hemorrhage in cerebral aneurysm: A 10-year evaluation of 364 patients. Ann Neurol 1:358–370, 1977.
23. Graf, CJ, Nibbelink, DW: Cooperative study of intracranial aneurysms and subarachnoid hemorrhage. Report on a randomized treatment study. Stroke 5:559–601, 1974.
24. Brust, J: Subarachnoid hemorhage: Early detection and diagnosis Hosp Pract 17:73–80, 1982.
25. Dhopesh, VP, Bouzarth, WF: The subtle subarachnoid hemorrhage. Emergency Med 14:203–217, 1982.
26. Ott, K, et al.: Cerebellar hemorrhage: Diagnosis and treatment. Arch Neurol 31:160–167, 1974.
27. Turner, DA, Howe, JF: Cerebellar hemorrhage as evaluated by computerized tomography. West J Med 136:198–202, 1982.
28. Hedges, TR: An ophthalmologist's view of headache. Headache 19:151–155, 1979.
29. Sanders, MD: Sudden visual loss. Practitioner 219:43–52, 1977.
30. Behrens, M: Headaches associated with disorders of the eye. Med Clin North Am 62:507–521, 1978.
31. Pau, H: Differential Diagnosis of Eye Diseases. Philadelphia: W.B. Saunders, 1978.
32. Schwartz, B: The glaucomas. N Engl J Med 299:182–184, 1978.
33. Wyllie, JW, et al.: Isolated sphenoid sinus lesions. Laryngoscope 83:1252, 1973.
34. Birt, D: Headaches and head pain associated with diseases of the ear, nose, and throat. Med Clin North Am 62:523–531, 1978.
35. Ryan, RE, Ryan, RE, Jr.: Headache of nasal origin. Headache 19:173–179, 1979.
36. Adams, RD, Victor, M: Principles of Neurology. New York: McGraw-Hill, 1977, Chap. 29.
37. Raskin, N, Appenzeller, O: Headache. In Smith, LH (ed): Major Problems in Internal Medicine Vol. 19. Philadelphia: W.B. Saunders, 1980, pp. 199–209.
38. Forbes, GS, et al.: Computed tomography in the evaluation of subdural hematoma. Radiology, 126–143–148, 1978.
39. Raskin, N, Appenzellar, O: Headache. In Smith, LH (ed): Major Problems in Internal Medicine Vol. 19. Philadelphia: W.B. Saunders, 1980, pp. 220–234.
40. Hamilton, CR, et al.: Giant cell arteritis: Including temporal arteritis and polymyalgia rheumatica. Medicine 50:1–27, 1971.
41. Sandok, BA: Temporal arteritis. JAMA 222:1405–1406, 1972.
42. Hollenhorst, RW, et al.: Neurologic aspects of temporal arteritis. Neurology 10:490–498, 1960.
43. Goodman, BW: Temporal arteritis. Am J Med 67:839–852, 1979.
44. Dinsdale, HB: Headache in vascular disease and hypertension. Headache 13:85–90, 1973.
45. Medina, JL, et al.: Headache in patients with transient ischemic attacks. Headache 15:194–197, 1975.
46. Edmeads, J: The headaches of ischemic cerebrovascular disease. Headache 19:345–349, 1979.
47. Waters, WE: Headache and blood pressure in the community. Br Med J 1:142–143, 1971.
48. Badran, R, et al.: Hypertension and headache. Scott Med J 15:48, 1970.

49. Crocker, EF, et al.: Technetium brain scanning in the diagnosis and management of cerebral abscess. Am J Med 56:192–201, 1974.
50. Samson, DS, Clark, K: A current review of brain abscess. Am J Med 54:201–210, 1973.
51. Jackson, RT, et al.: Malignant neoplasms of the nasal cavities and paranasal sinuses. A retrospective study. Laryngoscope 87:726–736, 1977.
52. Raskin, N, Prusiner, S: Carotidynia. Neurology 27:43–46, 1977.
53. Harner, SG: Peritonsillar, peripharyngeal and deep neck abscesses. Postgrad Med 57:147, 1975.
54. Edmeads, J: Headaches and head pains associated with diseases of the cervical spine. Med Clin North Am 62:533–544, 1978.
55. Chisholm, IA: Gradual visual loss. Practitioner 219:64–71, 1977.
56. Lessell, S: Optic neuropathies. N Engl J Med 299:533–536, 1978.
57. Bickerstaff, ER: Basilar artery migraine. Lancet 1:15, 1961.
58. Weisberg, LA: Benign intracranial hypertension. Medicine 54:197–207, 1975.
59. Friedman, AP, et al.: Ophthalmoplegic migraine. Arch Neurol 7:320–327, 1962.
60. Ellner, JJ, Bennett, JE: Chronic meningitis. Medicine 55:341–369, 1976.
61. Mathew, NT, Chandy, J: Painful ophthalmoplegia. J Neurol Sci 11:243, 1970.
62. Hyslop, NE, Swartz, MN: Bacterial meningitis. Postgrad Med 58:120, 1975.
63. Petito, F, Plum, F: The lumbar puncture. N Engl J Med 290:225–226, 1974.
64. Tourtellotte, W, et al.: A randomized double-blind clinical trial comparing the 22 vs. the 26 gauge needle in the production of post LP syndrome in normal individuals. Headache 12:73–78, 1972
65. Brocker, RJ: A technique to avoid spinal tap headache. JAMA 168:261–263, 1958.
66. Glass, PM, Kennedy, WF, Jr.: Headache following subarachnoid puncture: Treatment with epidural blood patch. JAMA 219:203–204, 1972.
67. Appenzeller, O: Altitude headache. Headache 12:126–129, 1972.
68. Symonds, C: Cough headache. Brain 79:557–568, 1956.
69. Rooke, ED: Benign exertional headache. Med Clin North Am 52:801–808, 1968.
70. Harris, W: Paroxysmal and postural headaches from intraventricular cysts and tumors. Lancet 2:654–655, 1944.
71. Paulson, GW, Klawans, HL: Benign orgasmic cephalgia. Headache 13:181–187, 1974.
72. Rowsell, AR, et al.: Ergotamine-induced headaches in migrainous patients. Headache 13:65–67, 1973.
73. Kudrow, L: The relationship of headache frequency to hormone use in migraine. Headache 15:36–40, 1975.
74. Somerville, BW: The role of estradiol withdrawal in the etiology of menstrual migraine. Neurology 22:355–365, 1972.
75. Chaudhuri, TK, Chaudhuri, ST: Estrogen therapy for migraine. Headache 15:139, 1975.
76. Esptein, MT, et al.: Migraine and reproductive hormones throughout the menstrual cycle. Lancet 1:543–548, 1975.
77. Grant, ECG: Food allergies and migraine. Lancet 1:966–969, 1979.
78. Raskin, NH, Appenzeller, O: Headache. In Smith, LH (ed): Major Problems in Internal Medicine Vol. 19. Philadelphia: W.B. Saunders, 1980, pp. 182–183.
79. Friedman, AP: Migraine. Med Clin North Am 62:481–494, 1978.
80. Selby, G, Lance, JW: Observations on 500 cases of migraine and allied vascular headaches. J Neurol Neurosurg Psychiatry 23:23–32, 1960.
81. Friedman, AP, et al.: Migraine and tension headaches. A clinical study of 2000 cases. Neurology 4:773–788, 1954.
82. Diamond, S, Dalessio, D: The Practicing Physician's Approach to Headache. New York: Medcom Press, 1973.
83. Lance, JW, Anthony, M: Some clinical aspects of migraine. Arch Neurol 15:356–361, 1966.
84. Friedman, AP: The migraine syndrome. Bull NY Acad Med 44:45–62, 1968.
85. Raskin, N, Appenzeller, O: Headache. In Smith, LH (ed): Major Problems in Internal Medicine Vol. 19. Philadelphia: W.B. Saunders, 1980, pp. 172–184.
86. Needham, CW: Major cranial neuralgias and the surgical treatment of headache. Med Clin North Am 62:545–557, 1978.
87. Amols, W: Differential diagnosis of trigeminal neuralgia and treatment. Headache 8:50–53, 1969.
88. Raskin, N, Appenzeller, O: Headache. In Smith, LH (ed): Major Problems in Internal Medicine Vol. 19. Philadelphia: W.B. Saunders, 1980, pp. 28–83.
89. Kudrow, L: Cluster headache: Diagnosis and management. Headache 19:142–150, 1979.
90. Graham, JR: Cluster headache. Headache 10:175–185, 1972.
91. Price, RW, Posner, JB: Chronic paroxysmal hemicrania: A disabling headache syndrome responding to idomethacin. Ann Neurol 3:183–184, 1978.
92. Jammes, JJ: The treatment of cluster headache with prednisone. Dis Nerv Syst 36:375–376, 1975.
93. Kudrow, L: Lithium prophylaxis for chronic headache. Headache 17:15–18, 1977.
94. Duvoisin, RC: The cluster headache. JAMA 222:1403–1404, 1972.
95. Wepsic, JG: Tic douloureux: Etiology, refined treatment. N Engl J Med 288:680, 1973.
96. Mancall, EL: Guidelines for managing the cranial neuralgias. Drug Ther 5:125, 1980.
97. Crill, WE: Carbamazepine. Ann Intern Med 79:844, 1975.
98. Voorhies, R, Patterson, RH: Management of trigeminal neuralgia (tic douloureux). JAMA 245:2521–2523, 1981.
99. Dugan, MC, et al.: Occipital neuralgia in adolescents and young adults. N Engl J Med 267:1166–1172, 1962.
100. Barrie, MA, et al.: Analysis of symptoms of patients with headaches and their response to treatment with ergot derivatives. Q J Med 37:319–336, 1968.
101. Komar, N: Radiological techniques in the examination of patients with headache. Med Clin North Am 62:585–620, 1978.

102. Kricheff, I: The radiologic diagnosis of pituitary adenoma. Radiology 131:263–265, 1979.
103. Masland, W: Electroencephalography and electromyography in the diagnosis of headache. Med Clin North Am 62:571–584, 1978.
104. Evens, RG, Jost, RG: The clinical efficacy and cost analysis of cranial computed tomography and the radionuclide brain scan. Semin Nucl Med 7(2):129–136, 1977.
105. Abrams, HL, McNeil, BJ: Medical implications of computed tomography ("CAT scanning"). N Engl J Med 298:255–261, 1978.
106. Messina, AV: Cranial computerized tomography. Arch Neurol 34:602–607, 1977.
107. Carrera, GJ, et al.: Computerized tomography of the brain in patients with headache or temporal lobe epilepsy: Findings and cost effectiveness. J Comput Asst Tomogr 1:200–203, 1977.
108. Diamond, S, et al.: The use of analgesics in headache. Headache 19:185–190, 1979.
109. Packard, RC: What does the headache patient want? Headache 19:370–374, 1979.
110. Raskin, N, et al.: Migraine. West J Med 123:211–217, 1975.
111. Dalton, K: Food intake prior to a migraine attack—study of 2,313 spontaneous attacks. Headache 15:188–193, 1975.
112. Medina, JL, Diamond, S: The role of diet in migraine. Headache 18:31–34, 1978.
113. Raskin, N, Appenzeller, O: Headache. In Smith, LH (ed): Major Problems in Internal Medicine Vol. 19. Philadelphia: W.B. Saunders, 1980, pp. 42–53.
114. Turin, A, Johnson, W: Biofeedback therapy for migraine headaches. Arch Gen Psychiatry 33:517–519, 1976.
115. Medina, J, et al.: Biofeedback therapy for migraine. Headache 16:115–118, 1976.
116. Diamond, S, et al.: The value of biofeedback in the treatment of chronic headache: A five-year retrospective study. Headache 19:90–96, 1979.
117. Diamond, S: Biofeedback and headache. Headache 19:180–184, 1979.
118. Raskin, N, Appenzeller, O.: Headache. In Smith, LH (ed): Major Problems in Internal Medicine Vol. 19. Philadelphia: W.B. Saunders, 1980, pp. 111–171.
119. Friedman, AP: Migraine headache. JAMA 222:1399–1402, 1972.
120. Graham, JR: Migraine headache: Diagnosis and management. Headache 19:133–141, 1979.
121. Friedman, AP: Medicine for migraine: What to use when. Mod Med 48:36–49, 1980.
122. Lennox, WG: Ergonovine versus ergotamine as a terminator of migraine headaches. Am J Med Sci 195:458–468, 1938.
123. Waters, WE: Controlled clinical trial of ergotamine tartrate. Br Med J 2:325–327, 1970.
124. Carter, ER: Bilateral thrombophlebitis after a single dose of ergotamine tartrate for migraine. Br Med J 2:1452–1453, 1958.
125. Couch, J, et al.: Amitriptyline in the prophylaxis of migraine. Neurology 26:121–127, 1976.
126. Gomersall, J, Stuart, A: Amitriptyline in migraine prophylaxis. J Neurol Neurosurg Psychiatry 36:684–690, 1976.
127. Diamond, S, Medina, J: Double-blind study of propranolol for migraine prophylaxis. Headache 16:24–27, 1976.
128. Forssman, B, et al.: Propranolol for migraine prophylaxis. Headache 16:238–245, 1976.
129. Widerøe, T, Vigander, T: Propranolol in the treatment of migraine. Br Med J 2:699–701, 1974.
130. Malvea, BP, et al.: Propranolol prophylaxis of migraine. Headache 12:163–167, 1973.
131. Weber, R, Reinmuth, O: The treatment of migraine with propranolol. Neurology 22:366–369, 1972.
132. Lance JW, et al.: Comparative trial of serotonin antagonists in the management of migraine. Br Med J 2:327–330, 1970.
133. Poser, C: Papaverine in prophylactic treatment of migraine (Letter). Lancet 1:1290, 1974.
134. Sillanpaan, M, Koponen, M: Papaverine in the prophylaxis of migraine and other vascular headache in children. Acta Paediatr Scand 67:209–212, 1978.
135. Curran, DA, Lance, JL: Clinical trial of methylsergide and other preparations in the management of migraine. J Neurol Neurosurg Psychiatry, 27:463–469, 1964.
136. Friedman, AP, Elkind, AH: Appraisal of methylsergide in the treatment of vascular headaches of the migraine type. JAMA 184:125, 1963.
137. Graham, JR, et al.: Fibrotic disorders associated with methylsergide therapy for headache. N Engl J Med 274:359–368, 1966.
138. Elias, F: Roentgen findings in the asymptomatic cervical spine. NY State J Med 58:3300–3303, 1958.
139. Packard, RC: Psychiatric aspects of headache. Headache 19:168–172, 1979.
140. Dalessio, DJ: Some reflections on the etiologic role of depression in head pain. Headache 8:28, 1968.
141. Davis, RA, et al.: Personality, depression, and headache. Headache 16:246, 1976.
142. Lance, JW, Curran, DA: Treatment of chronic tension headache. Lancet 1:1236–1239, 1964.
143. Diamond, S, Baltes, BJ: Chronic tension headache—treated with amitriptyline—a double-blind study. Headache 10:110–116, 1971.
144. Weber, MB: The treatment of muscle contraction headache with diazepam. Curr Ther Res 15:210–216, 1973.
145. Raskin, N, Appenseller, O: Headache. In Smith, LH (ed): Major Problems in Internal Medicine Vol. 19. Philadelphia: W.B. Saunders, 1980, pp. 172–184.
146. Groves, JE: Taking care of the hateful patient. N Engl J Med 298:883–887, 1978.
147. Janowsky, DS, Sternbach, RA: The patient with pain. In Abram, HS (ed): Basic Psychiatry for the Primary Care Physician. Boston: Little, Brown, 1976, pp. 99–116.
148. Friedman, W: Head injuries. CIBA Clin Symp 35(4):1–32, 1983.

5
KNEE PAIN

HISTORY 216

PHYSICAL EXAMINATION OF THE KNEE 221

LOCALIZED SWELLINGS AND TENDERNESS 229

PATELLOFEMORAL SYNDROMES 233

    Treatment of Patellofemoral Syndromes 239

TRAUMATIC KNEE PAIN 241

THE SWOLLEN KNEE 255

    Arthrocentesis and Synovial Fluid Analysis 256

MONARTHRITIS OF THE KNEE 258

APPENDIX: FUNCTIONAL KNEE ANATOMY 265

REFERENCES 271

HISTORY

> Mike Meniscus, a college sophomore, enters the clinic complaining of right knee pain. Mike has always been healthy and has never had any problem with his knees until 3 weeks ago when he began to note vague, poorly localized discomfort in the right knee. Initially his discomfort occurred only after heavy exercise—running several miles over hilly terrain; brief rest or an icepack relieved the pain. More recently Mike's knee has begun to hurt during exercise, and he is now unable to run more than a few hundred yards before pain stops him.
>
> Mike insists that he has never injured his knee. He has not fallen, twisted his knee, or experienced pain during sports activities previously. He has never noticed swelling of the knee—remotely or recently.

Knee pain occasionally presents a difficult diagnostic problem, and an experienced orthopedist must be consulted on such occasions. The great majority of ambulatory patients with knee pain can be managed at least initially by the generalist physician, however. As with all medical symptoms, a careful clinical history very often makes the diagnosis. Consider the key points in Mike's case:

1. There is no history of direct trauma or knee injury. Traumatic knee pain requires a specific diagnostic approach, as briefly outlined on page 241. Precise mechanisms of injury, functional internal knee anatomy, and careful physical examination of ligaments, menisci, and bony structures must be understood and reviewed in such circumstances. While some sedentary pundits will declare that running several miles up and down hills is traumatic, there is a major clinical difference between actual knee trauma (for example, a fall or blow) and the case in which:

2. Knee pain is directly related to mechanical use of the knee. Most disorders to be discussed cause pain that is clearly associated with movement of the knee and related structures. Thus, bending the knee, walking, climbing,

jumping, or running exacerbate or precipitate the pain. Such a history suggests a "mechanical" knee problem.

Occasionally pain in the knee is not mechanical or is referred from another site. When pain cannot be attributed to the use of the knee (and especially when knee examination is normal—see below), several other problems should be remembered (Fig. 5–1). Disorders of the hip—trochanteric bursitis and degenerative arthritis, for example—can cause pain referred to the knee. Lumbosacral radiculopathy often causes pain in the posterior portion of the knee along the "sciatic" distribution, and occasionally the only site of pain will be the back of the knee. Less commonly, lesions of the L3 or L4 nerve root (or the femoral nerve) will cause anterior knee pain (see Chapter 1, Low Back Pain). Entrapment of the saphenous nerve[1] in the subsartorial canal can cause puzzling knee pain—here, manual pressure over the saphenous opening (four fingers above the medial femoral condyle—see Figure 5–22 and Low Back Pain, Chapter 1) will elicit pain and often dysesthetic radiation down into the lower leg. Arterial claudication will cause exertional pain and "tightness" in the knee when the femoral system is occluded—rest relieves the pain. Popliteal thrombophlebitis will frequently cause posterior knee pain (Fig. 5–2).

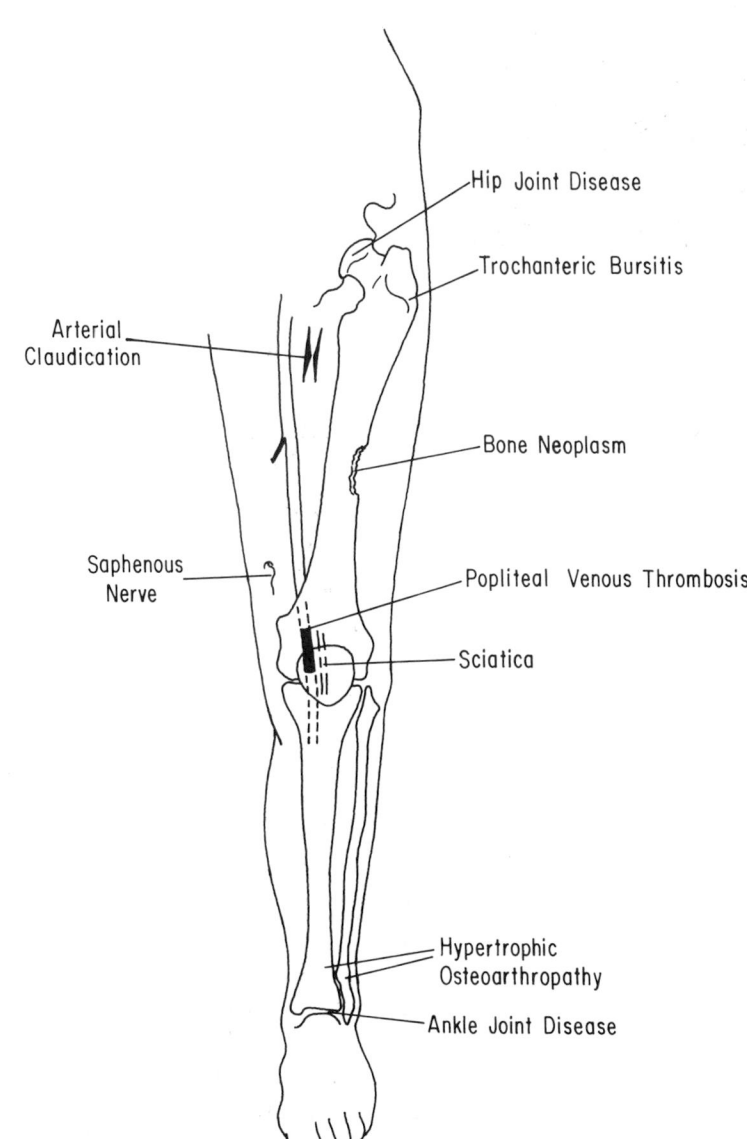

FIGURE 5–1. "Nonmechanical" knee pain.

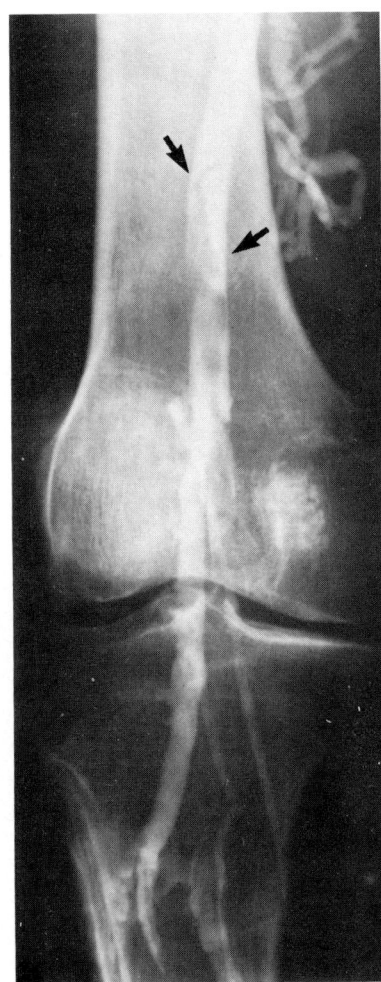

FIGURE 5–2. This 72-year-old man complained of 10 days of increasing knee pain. Examination of the knee was normal, but there was slight edema of the lower leg on that side. The venogram demonstrates a clot in the popliteal vein (*arrows*).

Thus, when knee pain is atypical of "mechanical pain," and especially when examination of the knee joint itself appears normal, remember to examine the hips, low back (and straight leg raising), pulses, venous system, and the neurologic system.

3. There is no history of a knee effusion. This must be verified on physical examination (see below), but the presence of a knee effusion raises many specific questions, which are discussed briefly later (page 255).

4. Specific associated symptoms should be reviewed. Locking of the knee refers to sudden fixation of the knee in one position, usually at about 20 degrees of flexion, with inability to further flex or extend the knee. Acute knee trauma that results in a locked knee may have many causes: fractures, dislocations, severe hemarthrosis, torn meniscus, or major ligament damage. Recurrent locking, on the other hand, that the patient learns to "unlock," is usually due to a torn meniscus (but may also occur with degenerative arthritis or osteochondritis dissecans[2] in which a bony fragment is "trapped" within the joint (Fig. 5–3). Incomplete tears of the anterior cruciate ligament (see also page 248) may also cause locking.[3]

Clicking of the knee is very common and usually does not imply any disease. Clicking refers to an audible sound that occurs during knee flexion or extension—for example, during deep knee bends. Occasionally a symptom of meniscus tears, degenerative arthritis, osteochondritis dissecans, or chondromalacia patellae (see below), clicking usually results from benign snapping of the hamstring tendon over the femoral condyle or from mild patellofemoral friction.

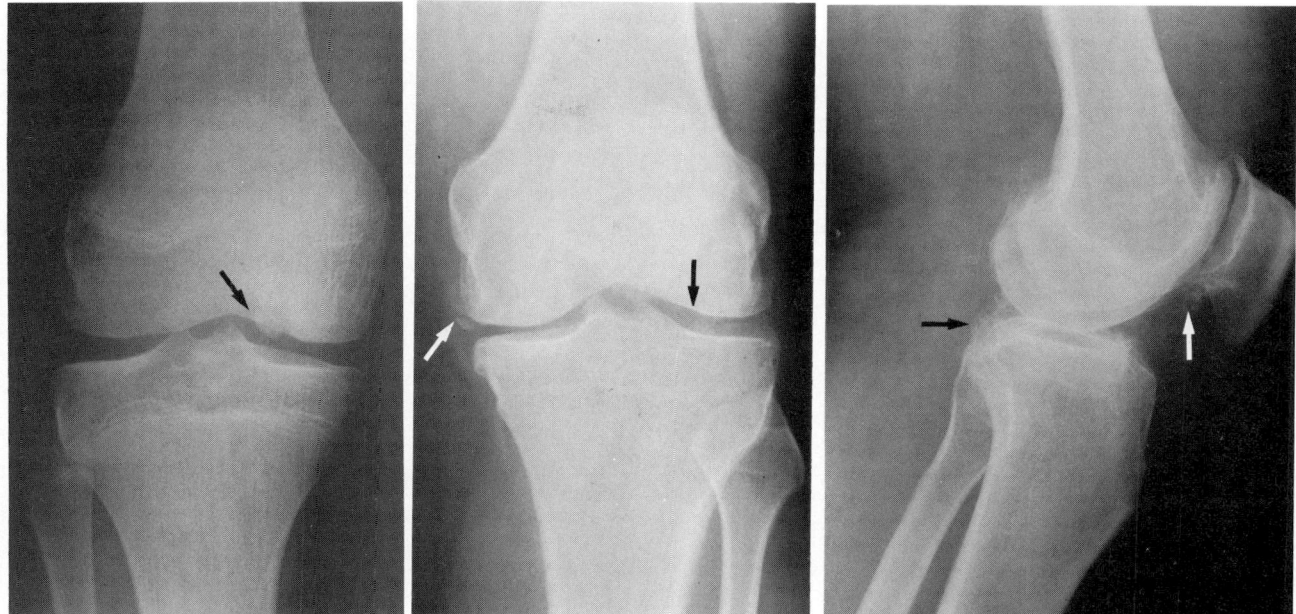

FIGURE 5–3. Locking. *A,* Osteochondritis dissecans. This patient complained of recurrent locking of the knee. There was no history of trauma. X-ray demonstrates a loose body beneath the medial femoral condyle (*arrows*). Arthroscopic removal of the loose body relieved all symptoms.

B, This patient with longstanding degenerative arthritis developed intermittent "locking" of the left knee. There are several loose bony fragments within the joint—small fractures of osteophytes (*arrows*).

Buckling of the knee refers to giving way of the knee—for example, during walking, climbing, or arising from a sitting position. Several disorders cause "true buckling"—ligamentous instability (especially cruciate ligament problems), meniscus tears, patellar dislocation, or tibiofibular disarticulation can cause sudden mechanical instability of the knee—here the leg will not bear weight, and the patient often falls. Much more common and benign is "pseudobuckling"—this refers to transient, incomplete giving way of the knee, usually without a fall, most often because of pain from various extensor mechanism disorders (patellofemoral syndromes—see page 233) or simple weakness of the quadriceps muscles (especially in the sedentary or elderly).

5. The patient is young, healthy, and active, and has no prior history of knee problems. While the physical examination will be all-important in diagnosis, Sutton's law ("go where the money is") dictates that subacute knee pain in the young athletic patient (without trauma or effusion) is most often due to one of the patellofemoral syndromes (see page 233). The more sedentary or middle-aged adult is more apt to develop one of the overuse syndromes—jogging syndromes, bursitis, or tendinitis (see below). The elderly patient is much more likely to suffer from degenerative joint disease.

6. A precise history of the factors that precipitate, exacerbate, or relieve the knee pain is essential. As noted above, it must first be established that pain is related to mechanical use of the knee. When this is so, certain specific complaints can sometimes be helpful. When pain is clearly related to stress of the extensor mechanism (see page 233 and Appendix), various patellofemoral syndromes should be suspected. Repetitive flexion and extension of the knee during weight bearing—climbing and descending stairs or hills, for example—causes symptoms in these cases.

When complaints are related to pivoting or "cutting," i.e., sudden changes in direction during walking or running, disorders of the meniscus or patella should be remembered.

When the knee appears to "gel," i.e., stiffen up during rest but then gradually "warm up" during subsequent exercise, inflammatory conditions (arthritis, tendinitis, bursitis) or (early) patellofemoral syndromes should be suspected. In contrast, when knee pain becomes progressively worse throughout the day or with more prolonged use, degenerative conditions (arthritis or later stages of patellofemoral syndromes) may be more likely.

When nontraumatic knee pain is constant, unrelenting, nocturnal, and unrelieved by rest of the leg, advanced arthritis, local neoplasms, osteomyelitis, or osteonecrosis of the femur should be suspected, since this is always a worrisome history.

Figure 5–4 summarizes important historical clues in patients with knee pain.

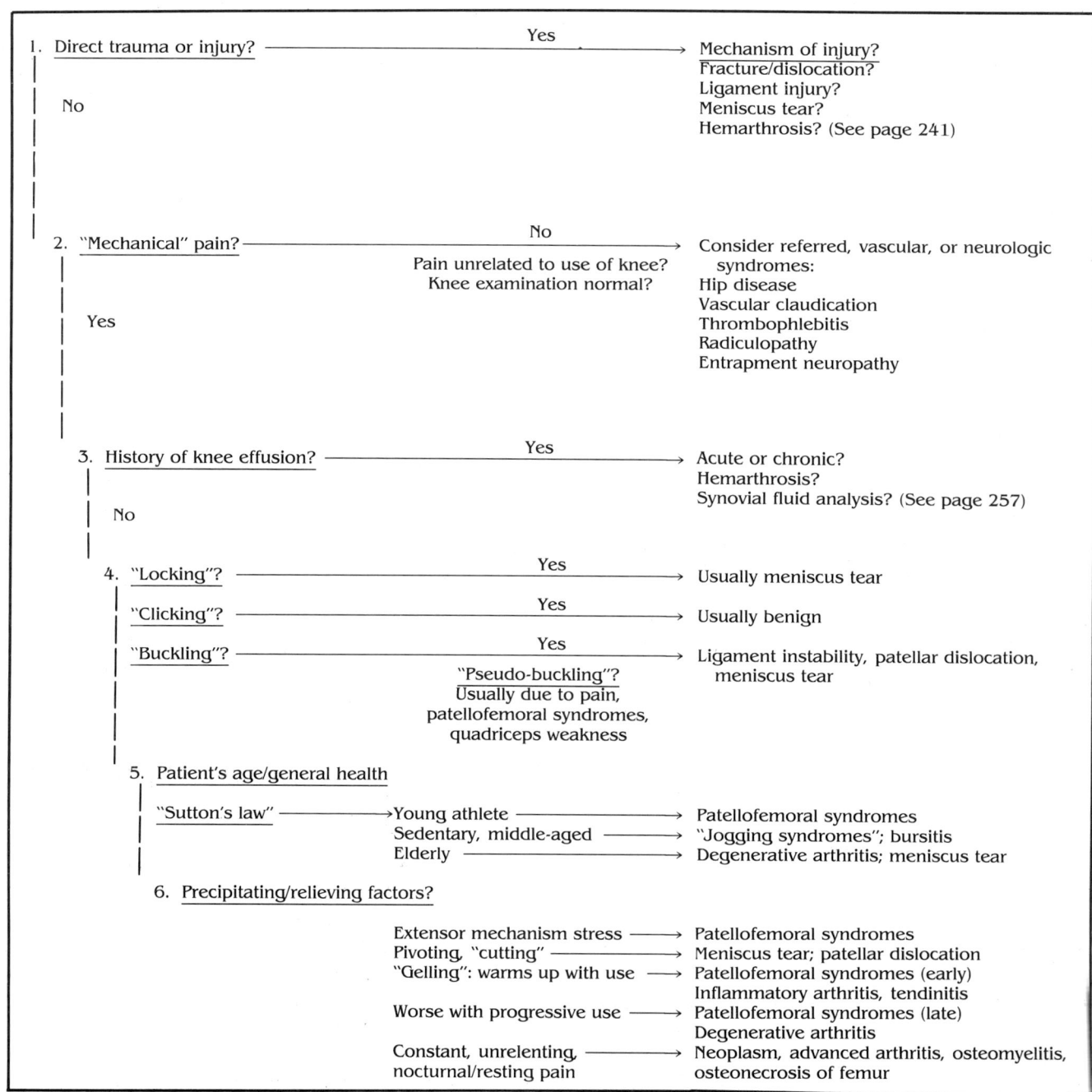

FIGURE 5–4. Knee pain: history.

One month ago, Mike's knees felt normal. At this time, he began an exercise program to "get into shape" for an upcoming intramural soccer program at school. He had never engaged in any daily training program before and began by gradually increasing jogging distances up to several miles per day, often up and down hills. After about 1 week, Mike noticed vague, mild discomfort in the right knee after running about 1 mile, but this would subside as he continued to run and the knee "warmed up." By the next week, the knee pain persisted for the latter half of each workout and has since progressively worsened to the point that he is unable to run at all without pain. Recently even routine daily activities, like climbing stairs, produce pain in the knee, and the pain often persists for a few hours after stopping all climbing or running. An ice pack and aspirin help.

Mike is most comfortable with his right leg bearing no weight, with the knee fully extended and relaxed. For the last week, Mike has avoided all running and climbing, and his knee has improved, but yesterday he tried to run again and immediately developed recurrent pain.

Mike notes clicking of the knee occasionally when bending, but denies any history of locking or buckling.

What does this mean?

1. Mike describes the subacute onset of unilateral knee pain, unrelated to any known direct trauma, without a history of swelling, buckling, or locking of the knee, and that appears clearly related to mechanical use of the knee. In the absence of trauma, serious internal derangements are unlikely. The intermittent timing and the mechanical nature of the pain make both serious bone/joint disease and referred pain, respectively, less likely.

2. The most likely diagnosis in a young, healthy, physically active person with such a history is one of the patellofemoral syndromes, while bursitis or one of the causes of "jogger's knees" should also be suspected. The differential diagnosis of these disorders is usually easy, when the history is accurate, but:

3. Careful physical examination of the knee must confirm the diagnosis suspected by the history. As noted above, an intra-articular effusion must be carefully sought or excluded—its presence raises other questions (see page 255). Similarly, thorough examination of the ligaments and menisci of the knee is especially important in the patient with traumatic knee pain (see p. 247). In this particular case, however, manual palpation of various structures and an understanding of the patellofemoral mechanism are more likely to be helpful. Consider, then:

PHYSICAL EXAMINATION OF THE KNEE[4-7]

The patient should be undressed below the waist. The hips, lower extremity pulses, and lower back should be quickly examined. A few common types of knee deformity will be obvious on simple inspection (Fig. 5–5).

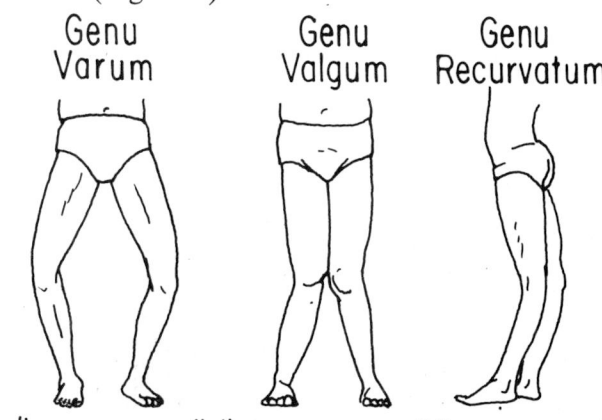

FIGURE 5–5. Common knee deformities.

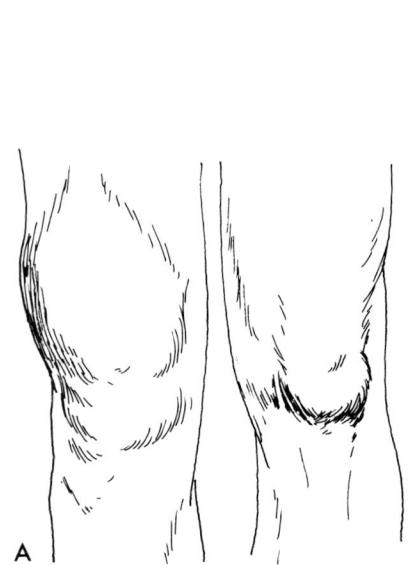

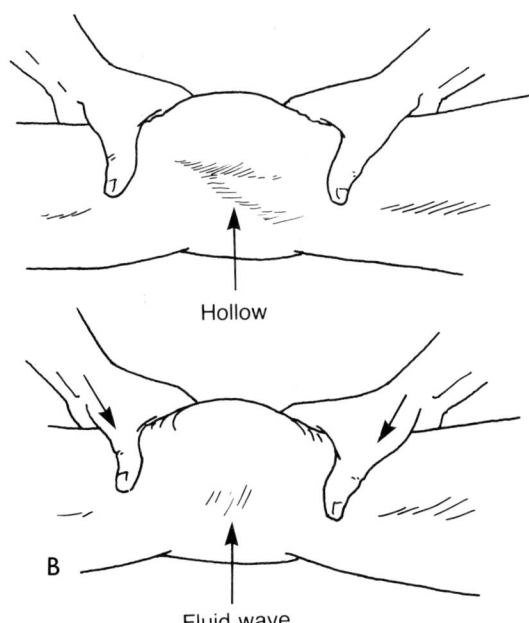

Hollow

Fluid wave

FIGURE 5–6. Knee effusion. A, Obvious right knee effusion. B, Subtle "fluid wave" sign.

The patient should be asked to point where the pain is felt. Sometimes the patient will point to a circumscribed area—here an appreciation of visible and palpable knee anatomy will often allow rapid, precise diagnosis (see page 229). When the pain is poorly localized to the "whole knee," several steps must be reviewed:

1. Inspect the knee and leg with the patient lying supine on the examining table, knee fully extended and relaxed. Compare the painful knee with the contralateral knee.

Intra-articular knee effusions are usually obvious on visual inspection but may be subtle. The normal knee appears slightly "hollow" on either side of the patella, and (less so) in the "space" just superior to the patella. Small accumulations of fluid within the synovial cavity fill in these hollows or spaces. A large effusion will produce obvious bulging that is often especially prominent superior to the patella where the joint cavity is most spacious (Fig. 5–6A). Very small effusions may be detected by "milking" the synovial fluid into the medial hollow—here, both of the examiner's hands compress the superior, inferior, and lateral peripatellar pouches and the medial hollow is seen to fill with a visible "fluid wave" (Fig. 5–6B). Knee effusions must always be distinguished from extra-articular (usually bursal) fluid collections—see page 229. The approach to unexplained intra-articular effusions is discussed on page 257.

Full extension of the knee is the first step in assessment of knee range of motion (Fig. 5–7). The normal knee extends to at least 0 degrees (the posterior aspect of the knee is flush to the table). Most patients can flex the knee beyond 135 degrees, and some can reach almost 180 degrees (sitting on their heels). Limitation of motion of the knee may be caused by a joint effusion, a mechanical internal derangement of the joint, menisci, or ligaments, or pain.

The most subtle limitation of motion is usually incomplete extension. One way to evaluate this is to support the patient's leg, one examining hand supporting the back of the thigh, the other holding the lower leg. The patient is then asked to completely relax the leg, and the knee is allowed to "drop" or fully extend itself passively. Pain, or limitation of motion, with this attempt

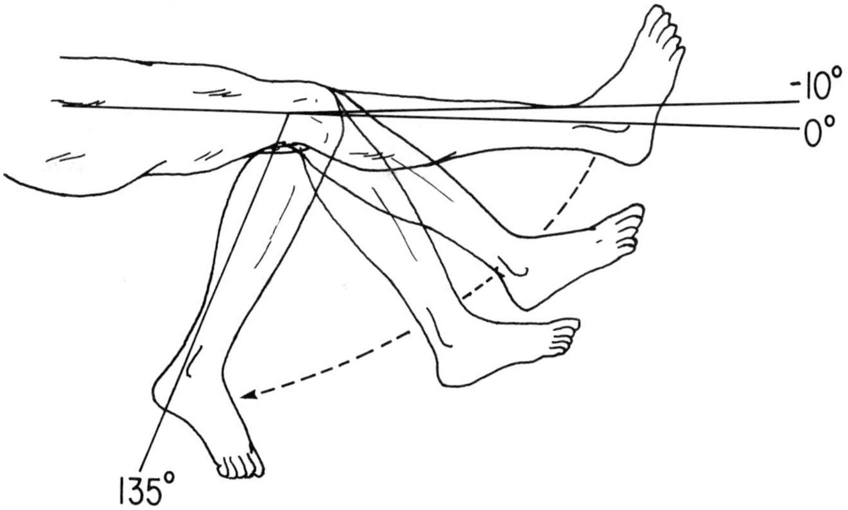

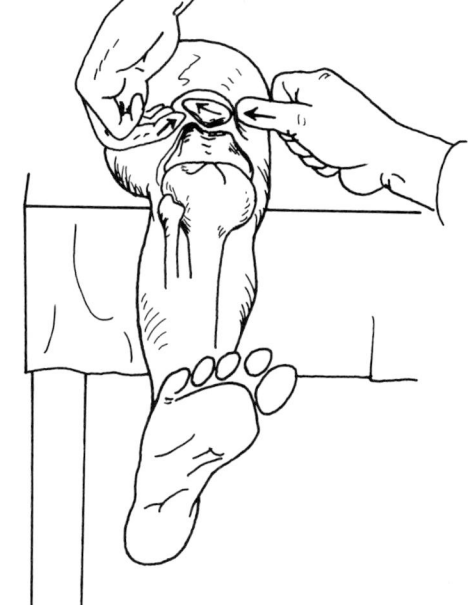

FIGURE 5–7. Normal range of motion of the knee.

-10°
0°
135°

at passive <u>hyperextension</u> should suggest an internal derangement. (See also page 241 and Appendix.)

2. With the patient's knee fully extended and relaxed, <u>manipulate the patella</u> (Fig. 5–8).

With the knee flexed, the patella is difficult to palpate and is immobile. With the quadriceps apparatus fully relaxed, the patella "floats" above the femoral condyles and is more mobile medially than laterally. Palpation and manipulation of the patella are helpful in diagnosing chondromalacia patellae, patellar dislocation, and other patellofemoral syndromes (see pages 233).

3. <u>Test the integrity of the collateral and cruciate ligaments.</u> Ligament damage is usually suspected on the basis of the history (see page 243), but all patients with knee pain should be briefly examined for ligamentous laxity, rupture, or tenderness as is illustrated in Figure 5–33. The painful knee must always be compared with the normal knee. The performance and interpretation of these maneuvers are discussed in more detail on page 247.

4. Perform tibiofemoral rotatory testing to <u>examine the menisci.</u> As with ligament injuries, meniscal tears are usually suspected for specific reasons

FIGURE 5–8. The patella is mobile only with the knee extended and relaxed.

(see page 244). Nevertheless, gently rotating the tibia internally and externally with the knee flexed will often elicit localized pain, tenderness, or clicking when meniscus problems are the source of knee pain. The McMurray test is nonspecific, but both this maneuver and Apley's compression test exemplify the desired manipulation: manual torsion of the tibia on the femoral articulating surface (see page 250).

5. With the patient's knee flexed to 90 degrees, examine the external knee surface for palpable tenderness or swelling. An appreciation of palpable knee anatomy is essential here. Figure 5–9 illustrates initial points of orientation for palpation of the knee. The patellotibial tendon extends from the inferior pole of the patella across the tibiofemoral joint line to insert into the tibial tubercle. If the examiner's thumbs straddle the patellotibial tendon while the fingers of each hand surround the medial and lateral circumference of the leg, important palpable structures are easy to find:

The patella will be situated just above the examiner's thumbs. The superior border of the patella forms the insertion for the quadriceps tendon—this broad, firm tendon will be palpable when the patient actively extends the knee against resistance. The inferior border of the patella forms the attachment of the patellotibial tendon, which can be palpated for an inch or two below the patella until it inserts into the tibial tubercle. Many of the patellofemoral syndromes (see below) and various types of patellar bursitis will be diagnosed by examination of this patellofemoral (or extensor mechanism) complex.

Palpating medially, the examiner's thumb now feels the medial joint space that separates the medial tibial plateau inferiorly from the medial femoral condyle superiorly, until these structures seem to fuse (the space disappears) as the thumb moves further medially (away from the patellar tendon—Figure 5–10). The medial meniscus (an internal structure) can sometimes be palpated within the medial joint space as the lower leg is internally and externally rotated—during external rotation the joint space is deep and hollow, but internal rotation then fills the hollow as the medial meniscus slides anteriorly (see Appendix). Tenderness along this medial joint line is common in disorders of the medial meniscus. The medial femoral epicondyle is the bony promontory just above the fusion of the medial joint space—the medial collateral ligament originates here, then crosses the medial joint space to insert into the medial tibial plateau below. Normally the medial

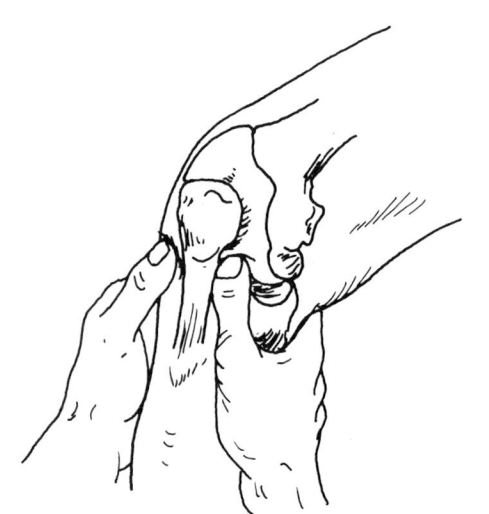

FIGURE 5–9. Points of orientation for palpating the knee.

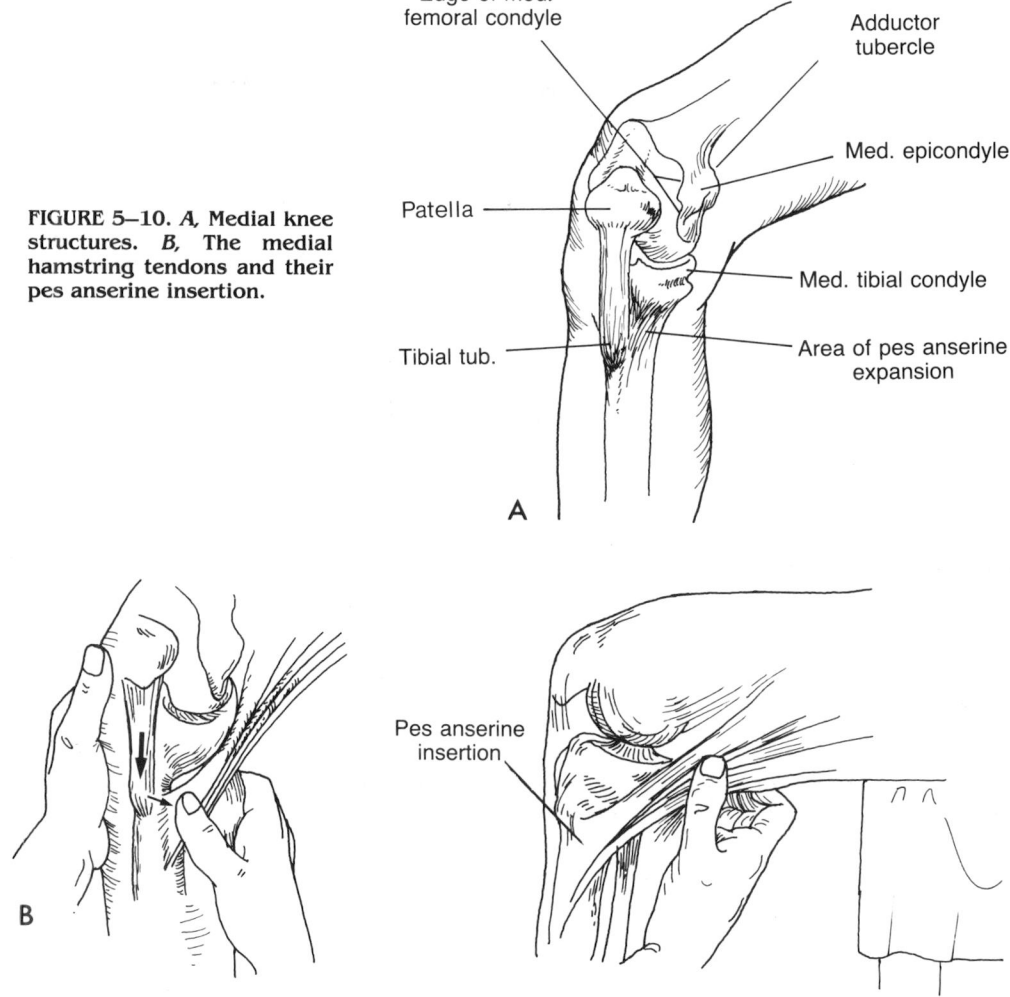

FIGURE 5–10. *A,* Medial knee structures. *B,* The medial hamstring tendons and their pes anserine insertion.

Edge of med. femoral condyle

Adductor tubercle

Med. epicondyle

Patella

Med. tibial condyle

Area of pes anserine expansion

Tibial tub.

A

Pes anserine insertion

B

collateral ligament is difficult to palpate since the tendons of the medial hamstring muscles obscure it as they cross the medial joint space to insert into the medial tibia (Fig. 5–10*B*). These tendons are more prominently palpable when the patient forcefully flexes the knee against resistance, and this common insertion of the sartorius, gracilis, and semitendinosus muscles— the pes anserine tendon—is a common site of bursitis (see page 229). This pes anserine insertion is located medial to the tibial tubercle. These structures are illustrated in Figure 5–10*B*.

Palpating laterally, the examiner's thumb now feels the lateral joint space that separates the lateral femoral condyle superiorly from the lateral tibial plateau inferiorly, until palpation further laterally senses "joining" of the femur and tibia (the space disappears—Figure 5–11). Superior to this junction is the lateral femoral epicondyle, the bony promontory from which the lateral collateral ligament originates before it crosses the lateral joint space to insert into the head of the fibula (which is just lateral and inferior to the more prominent lateral tibial condyle). Analogous to the medial structures, the lateral ligament is partially obscured by the lateral hamstring tendons (the biceps femoris—Figure 5–12), which stand out more during resisted knee flexion and which insert into the fibula. The lateral collateral ligament is more easily palpable than the medial ligament, especially when the patient crosses his legs—Figure 5–12*B*. The popliteus tendon (Fig. 5–13) —which inserts on the lateral femoral condyle after crossing the posterior

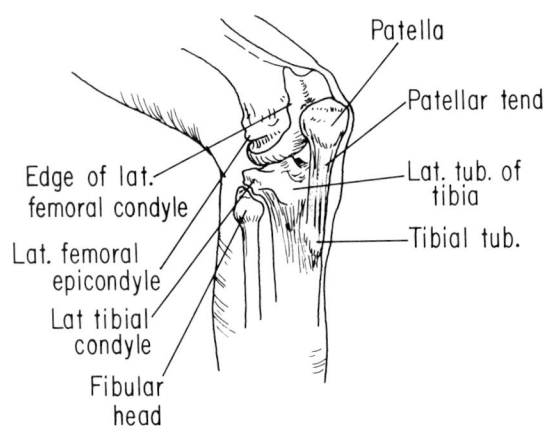

Patella

Patellar tendon

Edge of lat.
femoral condyle

Lat. tub. of
tibia

Lat. femoral
epicondyle

Tibial tub.

Lat tibial
condyle

Fibular
head

FIGURE 5–11. Lateral knee structures.

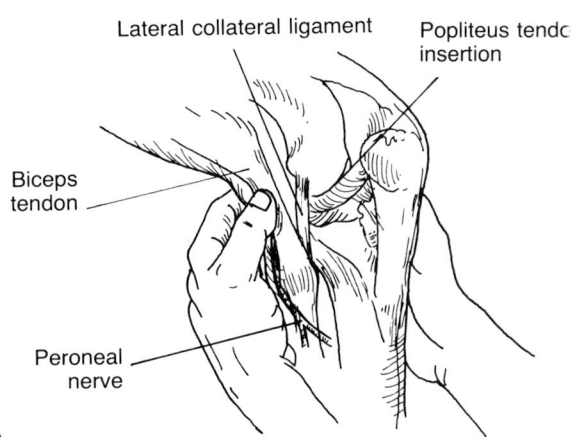

Lateral collateral ligament

Popliteus tendon
insertion

Biceps
tendon

Peroneal
nerve

A

FIGURE 5–12. *A,* The examiner's thumb palpates the biceps tendon. *B,* The lateral collateral ligament is deep but can be palpated when the patient "crosses his legs."

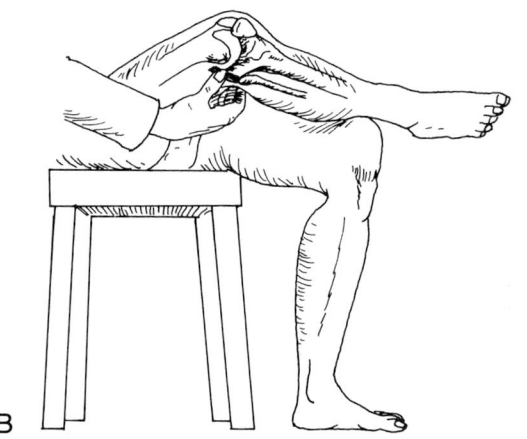

B

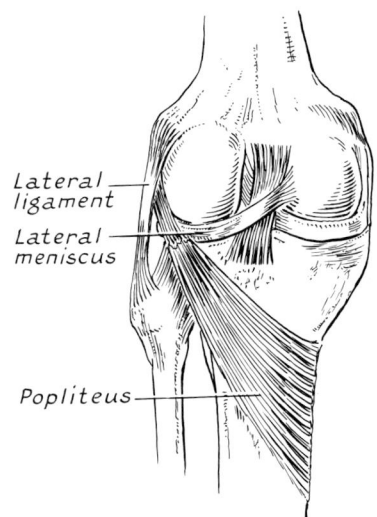

Lateral
ligament

Lateral
meniscus

Popliteus

FIGURE 5–13. The popliteus muscle is <u>posterior</u>, as illustrated by this <u>posterior</u> view of the knee. The insertion of the popliteus tendon, however, occurs just <u>anterior</u> to the lateral collateral ligament (Fig. 5–12*A*). Popliteus tendinitis may cause pain in the posterior knee, but tenderness is usually most easily elicited over the insertion of the tendon (anteriorly). (Reproduced with permission from Helfet, AJ: Disorders of the Knee. Philadelphia: J.B. Lippincott Co., 1982, p. 13.)

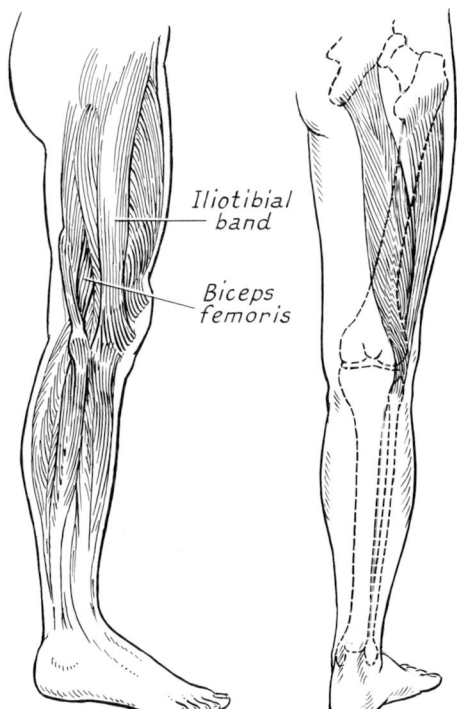

FIGURE 5–14. The iliotibial band. (Reproduced with permission from Helfet, AJ: Disorders of the Knee. Philadelphia: J.B. Lippincott Co., 1982, p. 6.)

aspect on the knee from the posterior portion of the tibia—can be felt just anterior to the upper insertion of the lateral collateral ligament. (Popliteus tendinitis causes localized tenderness here—see page 232). The peroneal nerve (Fig. 5–12) can be palpated just below the fibular head—it feels like a mobile cord—as it coils around the fibular neck. (Peroneal nerve trauma or entrapment[8] is a common cause of pain and dysesthesias in the lower leg— see Chapter 1, Low Back Pain.) The iliotibial band (Fig. 5–14)—a thick band of fascia extending along the entire lateral thigh that inserts into the lateral tibial condyle—is easily palpable just lateral to the patella but only when the knee is fully extended and the entire leg raised. Tenderness of this band is a common problem in joggers (see page 232).

Finally the examiner's hands palpate the posterior surface of the knee. The medial and lateral borders of this popliteal space are bounded by the medial and lateral hamstrings respectively. As Figure 5–15 illustrates, the hamstrings, the primary flexors of the knee, originate from the ischial tuberosity of the pelvis, run down the posterior thigh, separate into medial and lateral groups, and insert into tibia and fibula respectively after crossing the posterior joint line. The medial muscle group includes the semimembranosus and semitendinosus—the latter join with the thigh adductors, the gracilis and sartorius, to form the pes anserine insertion (Fig. 5–10); the semimembranosus attaches to the posterior tibia just above the popliteus muscle. The biceps femoris muscle (Figs. 5–12 and 5–14) forms the lateral "group."

The superior border of the popliteal space is thus formed by the "branching" of the hamstrings into medial and lateral groups; the inferior border is formed by the origin of the calf muscles—the gastrocnemius, soleus, and plantaris. Normally the only palpable structure within this popliteal space is the popliteal artery, since the popliteal vein, posterior tibial nerve, and popliteus muscle are usually not palpable. However, popliteal artery aneurysms, popliteal thrombophlebitis, and Baker's cysts (page 230) may cause swelling or tenderness in this popliteal "fossa."

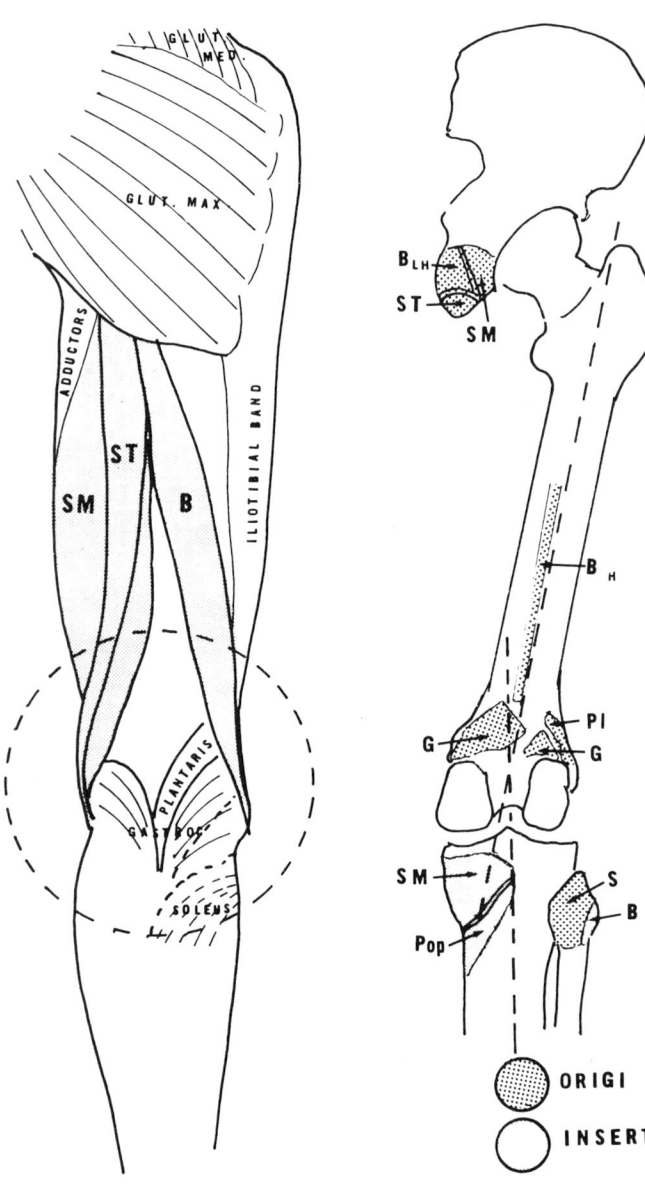

FIGURE 5–15. Posterior thigh muscles: flexors. *Left,* Semimembranosus (SM); semitendinosus, (ST); and biceps muscles of thigh (B). The other muscles are labeled. *Right,* The origin and insertion of the posterior muscle groups.

B$_{LH}$—Biceps long head
B$_{SH}$—Biceps short head
B—Biceps
S—Soleus
Pl—Plantar
Pop—Popliteus
G—Heads of gastrocnemius

(Reproduced with permission from Cailliet, R: Soft Tissue Pain and Disability. Philadelphia: F.A. Davis Co., 1977, p. 226.)

With a little practice, this full examination can be completed in just a few minutes. How does this help? Consider Mike's examination:

> Mike appears generally healthy, and is afebrile. Mike walks easily and without a limp, but step climbing on and (especially) off the examining table causes knee pain. There is no obvious bony deformity. Hips, thighs, ankles, and lower extremity pulses are normal. There is no swelling of the leg, nor is there any apparent knee effusion. Range of motion of the knee is entirely normal. All ligaments are stable, and rotatory testing elicits no pain or palpable clicks.*
>
> With the knee flexed 90 degrees, all superficial palpable structures are identified—none is tender, and there is no visible swelling. Specifically, the medial and lateral joint spaces, patellar tendon, tibial tubercle, pes anserine tendons and insertion, medial femoral epicondyle, fibular head, lateral collateral ligament, popliteus tendon, and iliotibial band are normal. The popliteal space is unremarkable.
>
> With the knee passively extended, however, manipulation of the patella causes moderate discomfort, similar to Mike's complaint.

What does this mean?

---

*See pages 247–250.

I. There is no evidence of an internal knee derangement.

Neither the history nor the physical examination suggests a disorder of ligaments, menisci, or intra-articular structures: the ligaments are stable (page 247); "meniscus testing" is normal (page 250); there is no history of injury; range of motion of the knee is normal; and there is no intra-articular effusion.

II. There is no localized swelling or discrete palpable tenderness of external knee structures.

LOCALIZED SWELLINGS AND TENDERNESS

Bursal effusions are the usual cause of localized swellings around the knee. Figure 5–16 illustrates those knee bursae that most commonly are associated with clinical bursitis—the infrapatellar, prepatellar, pes anserine, and popliteal bursae (in approximate order of frequency). Infrapatellar and prepatellar bursitis are usually related to direct trauma—a direct blow to the knee—in which case the bursal effusion is usually bloody; or they may be due to repetitive friction and pressure, as with prolonged kneeling (housemaid's knee, surfer's knobs, and canoer's knees are common eponyms)—here, bursal effusion is usually subacute and serous. Pes anserine bursitis may also be either traumatic or due to repetitive medial hamstring stress (for example, in cyclists or rowers) with inflammation of those tendons and the adjacent bursa. These types of bursitis may thus be either acutely traumatic or subacute in onset.

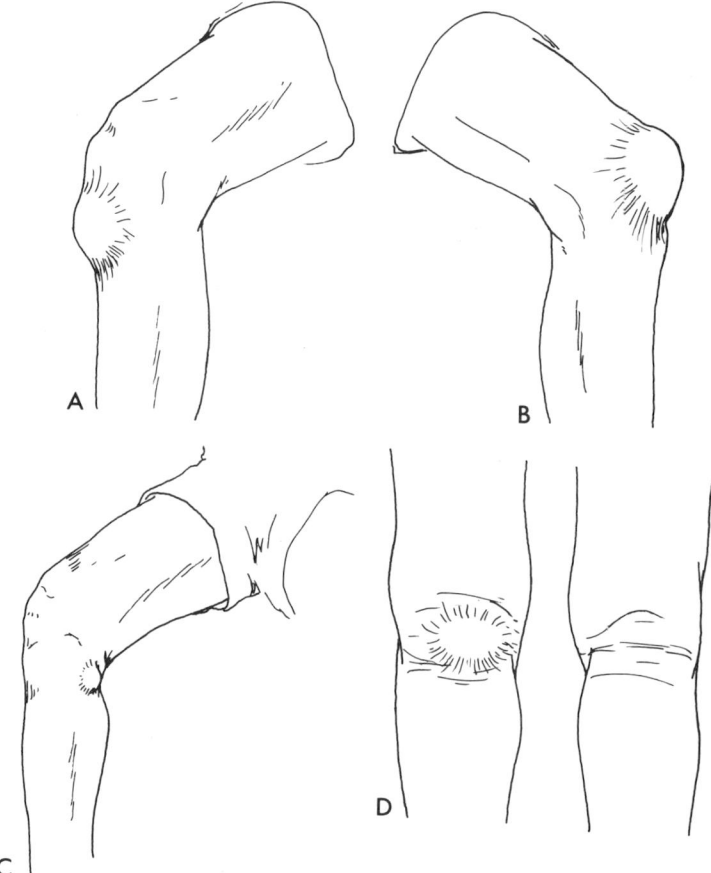

FIGURE 5–16. *A,* Swelling of the infrapatellar bursa. *B,* Swelling of the prepatellar bursa. *C,* Swelling of the pes anserine bursa. Note that this swelling is below the joint line (unlike a cyst of the medial meniscus, as in Figure 5–18*A*). *D,* A Popliteal (Baker's) cyst.

At times, there is no palpable fluid collection, and only local tenderness, thickening, or crepitus precisely localized to the bursal area will be found. When a bursal effusion is present, however, great care must be taken to exclude septic bursitis.[9-11] Fever is often inapparent in septic bursitis, although pain, bursal tenderness, and visible erythema or frank overlying cellulitis is usually prominent. Often there is a prior history of a skin abrasion or overlying skin infection that serves as the portal of entry for *Staphylococcus aureus*—the etiologic organism in over 90 per cent of cases of septic bursitis.

Only bursal fluid aspiration will diagnose or exclude septic bursitis. Aspiration is very simple to perform, since the fluid accumulation is so superficial. Aseptic technique is crucial. Most sterile effusions contain fewer than 1000 white blood cells per milliliter, mostly mononuclear; septic effusion should be assumed when the white blood count is over 10,000 and predominantly polymorphonuclear. Most septic effusions contain fluid that is grossly cloudy or purulent (with more than 50,000 polymorphonuclears). The Gram's stain very often does not reveal microorganisms even when the staphylococcus is subsequently grown on culture. Thus the initial diagnosis of septic bursitis often depends on the clinical examination and the bursal fluid cell count alone. When the patient is febrile, diabetic, or has an overlying cellulitis, hospitalization and parenteral antibiotics are indicated. When the patient is afebrile and the infection appears confined to the bursa alone, i.e., there is no cellulitis, oral antibiotic therapy (dicloxacillin 500 mg qid, pending cultures) for 2 to 3 weeks is often successful, and outpatient treatment can be attempted. Frequent follow-up is necessary.

When bursitis is known to be noninfectious, oral anti-inflammatory drugs[12] (see Table 1–4) often suffice. Persistent (especially traumatic) effusions can be aspirated and injected with intrabursal corticosteroids (20 to 40 mg triamcinolone hexacetonide [Aristospan], for example)—sometimes, repeat injections (once or twice) are necessary. Surgery is only rarely needed.

Other localized swellings of the knee may include:

A. Popliteal cysts (Baker's cysts)[13-16] are distended gastrocnemiosemi-membranosus bursae (Fig. 5–16), usually presenting as painless, palpable swellings in the popliteal fossa.

   Popliteal aneurysms, which are pulsatile, are usually easily differentiated. Popliteal cysts are actually bursal effusions, which communicate with the intra-articular knee joint, and are thus usually associated with an intra-articular effusion as well. Thus, in adults, popliteal cysts are usually secondary to some primary intra-articular process (most often, rheumatoid arthritis), and treatment often requires aspiration of the knee joint or medical therapy of the "primary process."

   Popliteal cysts usually become symptomatic when they enlarge (painlessly) or, less often, if they rupture—usually into the popliteal and calf tissues. Cyst rupture is usually announced by the very sudden onset of calf pain and swelling, often after arising or after "stretching" the popliteal space. The very abrupt onset usually distinguishes this problem from that of popliteal thrombophlebitis (Fig. 5–2), with which it is frequently confused. Careful distinction between a ruptured popliteal cyst and popliteal thrombophlebitis is crucial, since anticoag-

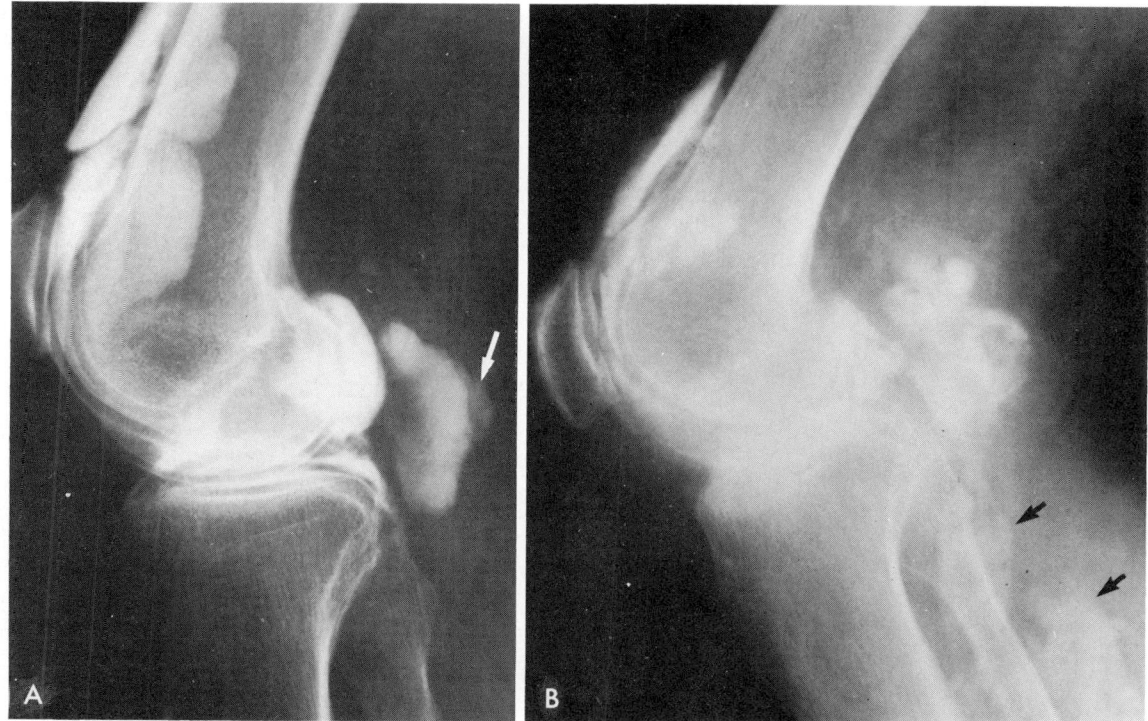

FIGURE 5–17. Popliteal (Baker's) cyst. This 74-year-old man presented with the acute onset of calf pain and swelling, without knee pain. The initial suspected diagnosis was popliteal thrombosis. A venogram was normal.

A, An arthrogram reveals a collection of dye posterior to the joint space—this is the popliteal (Baker's) cyst *(arrow).*

B, Subsequent x-ray demonstrates extravasation of dye from the popliteal cyst down into the calf—this is a ruptured popliteal (Baker's) cyst *(arrows).*

ulation of a ruptured popliteal cyst can be disastrous. (Rarely, the two diagnoses may coexist,[14] when rupture of the popliteal cyst leads to venous stasis and secondary thrombophlebitis.) The precise diagnosis requires arthrography that demonstrates extravasation of intra-articular dye into the calf tissues (Fig. 5–17).

B. Meniscal cysts[4, 7] are not common but may be confusing (Fig. 5–18).

Cysts of the medial meniscus usually present as relatively painless localized swellings along the medial joint line. (When swelling is considerable and localized posteromedially—behind the medial ligament—these may be mistaken for popliteal cysts.)

Cysts of the lateral meniscus are more common and usually

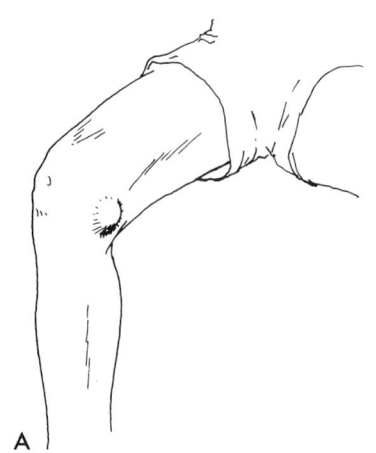
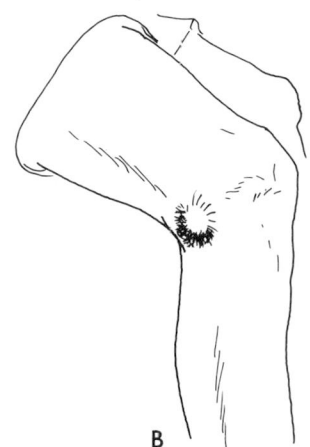

FIGURE 5–18. *A,* A cyst of the medial meniscus. *B,* A cyst of the lateral meniscus. These swellings are best appreciated with the knee slightly flexed—swelling usually occurs along the joint line.

A

B

present with pain and tenderness along the lateral or posterolateral joint line.

    Meniscal cyst swelling is most prominent with the knee in 45 degrees of flexion, and these cysts <u>may disappear</u> when the knee is fully flexed or extended. (This is not true of bursal swellings.)

C. <u>Painful fat pads</u>[4, 7] are common causes of (often bilateral) knee pain and swelling in young females and usually present with symptoms of recurrent pain, tenderness, and swelling on either side of the patellar tendon (Figs. 5–9 to 5–11).

    Symptoms and palpable swelling are more prominent with the patient standing and the knees fully extended. Cyclic edema of the fat pads sometimes related to the menstrual cycle may be the cause in some. Pain is usually worse during physical activity and forced knee extension (going down stairs, for example) and better with rest and knee flexion. Heeled shoes may help (slight knee flexion decompresses the fat pads). Reassurance, quadriceps strengthening (see page 239), or restoration of hormonal/fluid balance usually helps. Surgery is rarely indicated.

D. <u>Other swellings</u> may include lipomas and areas of localized muscle contusion, trauma, or hematomas.

    Localized swelling of various components of the patellofemoral mechanism are also often diagnostic (see pages 233 to 238).

III. While <u>Mike's knee problem seems related to jogging</u>, there is no evidence of either <u>popliteus tendinitis</u> or the <u>iliotibial band syndrome</u> (see pages 228 and 229).

    The jogging craze has resulted in legions of sore-kneed runners. While internal derangements may occur, and many orthopedists are concerned about the development of premature osteoarthritis in the dedicated long distance runner, two more benign syndromes are more common,[17] especially in the novice runner like Mike:

    <u>Popliteus tendinitis</u>[17] usually results from running downhill or on banked surfaces (for example, the beach or the edge of the road), since the popliteus muscle (Fig. 5–13) and tendon are strained by repetitive forward thrust of the femur on the tibia or by hyperpronation of the foot, respectively. <u>Point tenderness</u> is found just anterior to the lateral collateral ligament where the popliteus tendon inserts into the lateral femoral condyle (Fig. 5–12). Rest, local ice or anti-inflammatory drugs, running on flat surfaces, or use of orthotic devices in running shoes (to prevent excessive pronation)—or combinations of these—is helpful.

    <u>The iliotibial band syndrome</u>[17] refers to inflammation and tenderness over the lateral femoral epicondyle due to repetitive friction of the overlying iliotibial band (Fig. 5–14) as this fascial tract glides backward and forward with flexion and extension of the knee during running. Tenderness may be localized precisely at the insertion of the fascial band into the lateral tibia, but it is more often diffuse or associated with <u>point tenderness of the band when palpated with the knee forcefully extended.</u> Treatment is similar to that for popliteus tendinitis, but iliotibial stretch exercises (hip abduction) before running are helpful as well. Local steroid injections may be necessary in the competitive runner, but certainly repetitive injections should be avoided.

IV. <u>In Mike's case, physical examination (page 228) supports the initial suspicion of a patellofemoral syndrome, especially chondromalacia patellae.</u>

PATELLOFEMORAL SYNDROMES

Patellofemoral syndromes[4, 6, 18] refer to a variety of disorders in which the patella itself or its musculotendinous connections or both are abnormal. (The Appendix briefly discusses the extensor mechanism of the knee, which includes the quadriceps muscles and tendons, the patella and the patellofemoral articulation, and the patellotibial tendon). All these disorders (Table 5–1) are characterized by knee pain (with or without localized tenderness) that is symptomatically related to repetitive use of the extensor mechanism, i.e., activities that repetitively flex/extend the knee while weight bearing. Thus, running, jumping, climbing, and descending inclines are common inciting factors.

The most common patellofemoral syndrome is chondromalacia patellae.[18] This is an incompletely understood degenerative condition of the cartilage-lined posterior patella, which dynamically articulates with the femoral condyles during knee flexion and extension (see Appendix). Various anatomic or mechanical factors create repetitive frictional "drag" of the posterior patella against the femoral condyle, gradually resulting in progressive cartilaginous inflammation, fragmentation, and erosion of the posterior patellar surface, if uncorrected (Fig. 5–19). Sometimes preexisting disorders of patellar biomechanics are the underlying cause (see Appendix), but often exertional overuse of an inadequately conditioned quadriceps apparatus will be the major problem.

The typical clinical history is that of an individual (usually young female) who experiences pain around or "under" the kneecap, initiated or aggravated by excessive or unaccustomed knee extensor stress—running up and down hills, climbing and descending stairs or inclines, i.e., repetitive weight bearing, quadriceps contraction. (Descending an incline is often most painful—feel the palpable stress on your own lower quadriceps as you step downstairs!) Symptoms are usually mild initially and often improve with continued activity (warming up), but symptoms

TABLE 5–1. PATELLOFEMORAL SYNDROMES

PROBLEM	WHEN TO SUSPECT	FINDINGS: LOCATION OF PAIN AND TENDERNESS (REFER TO FIG. 5–22)	X-RAY
Chondromalacia patellae	Any age—usually young	Pain with patellar compression and manipulation: 1	Usually normal (unless advanced)
Jumper's knee	Young athlete	Tender inferior pole of patella: 2	Normal
Sinding-Larsen-Johansson's disease	Adolescent	Tender inferior pole of patella: 2	Osteochondritis of patella
Osgood-Schlatter's disease	Adolescent	Tender tibial tubercle: 4	Traction epiphysitis tibial tubercle (Fig. 5–20)
Patellar tendinitis	Any age	Tender ± swollen patellotibial tendon: 3	Normal
Recurrent patellar dislocation	Young female	+ Patellar apprehension test: 1 (Fig. 5–21)	Usually normal
Patellofemoral osteoarthritis	Older patient; prior chondromalacia?	Usually, tibiofemoral degenerative joint disease too: 1, 7, 8	Degenerative joint disease (Figs. 5–3, 5–41)
Quadriceps disorders	Elderly (often)	Quads weakness: 11	Normal

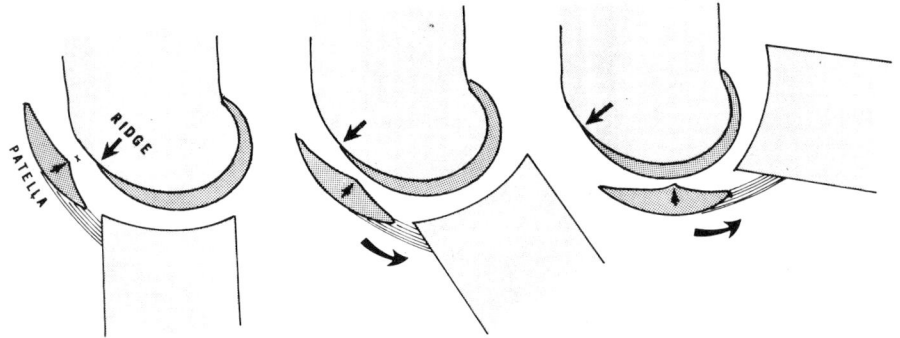

FIGURE 5–19. Mechanism of chondromalacia caused by the femoral condylar ridge. As the knee flexes, the patella is dragged across the ridge and irritates the patellar cartilage. The irritation occurs between 15 and 30 degrees of flexion. (Reproduced with permission from Cailliet, R: Knee Pain and Disability. Philadelphia: F.A. Davis Co., 1973, p. 79.)

can progress until even mild extensor stress (rising from a chair) is painful, and the knee may feel stiff after prolonged rest. Some patients describe clicking due to crepitus of the patellofemoral articulation as well as buckling (which is in fact usually "pseudobuckling"—see page 219). Chondromalacia is frequently bilateral.

Often the history alone must make the diagnosis, since physical examination may be remarkably normal, especially when compared to the degree of symptomatic discomfort. Sometimes manual pressure on the patella during resisted extension of the knee will elicit pain or palpable crepitus. Joint effusions or ligament instability must always suggest another diagnosis, although small joint effusions may occasionally occur. X-rays are usually normal, although "skyline" views (see Fig. 5–28D) of the patellofemoral surfaces may reveal asymmetry or loss of joint space (or, rarely, subchondral bone sclerosis when the lesion is advanced). Arthroscopy is occasionally necessary to confirm the diagnosis and exclude other disorders that may mimic it, but this is unusual.

Differential diagnosis of chondromalacia includes other patellofemoral syndromes, in which physical examination is often more helpful and specific (see below and Table 5–1). Occasionally chondromalacia must be distinguished from painful fat pads, meniscal cysts, and patellar bursitis. Treatment is discussed below.

As Table 5–1 suggests, other patellofemoral syndromes are usually suspected by certain physical findings in patients of varied ages:

Jumper's knee[19] refers to inflammation, and usually palpable tenderness, at the attachment of the patellotibial tendon to the inferior pole of the patella. Usually a problem in young adult athletes (high jumpers, basketball players), there may be localized swelling over the lower patellar tendon insertion (coexisting infrapatellar bursitis may occur as well). Kneeling may be painful, but knee extension exercise is the major problem; relaxed extension of the knee is most comfortable.

Sinding-Larsen-Johansson disease (osteochondritis of the inferior pole of the patella) is clinically very similar, but it occurs in adolescents and is associated with radiographic fragmentation of the inferior pole of the patella (unlike jumper's knee in which x-rays of the fully mature patella are usually normal).

Osgood-Schlatter's disease is an analogous condition in the adolescent (the Little League catcher is a common victim), in which pain, tenderness, and swelling involve the distal patellar tendon insertion into the tibial tubercle. The tibial tubercle is very tender, and x-rays may reveal "traction epiphysitis" of the tubercle (Fig. 5–20).

Patellar tendinitis is a nonspecific term for tenderness or swelling

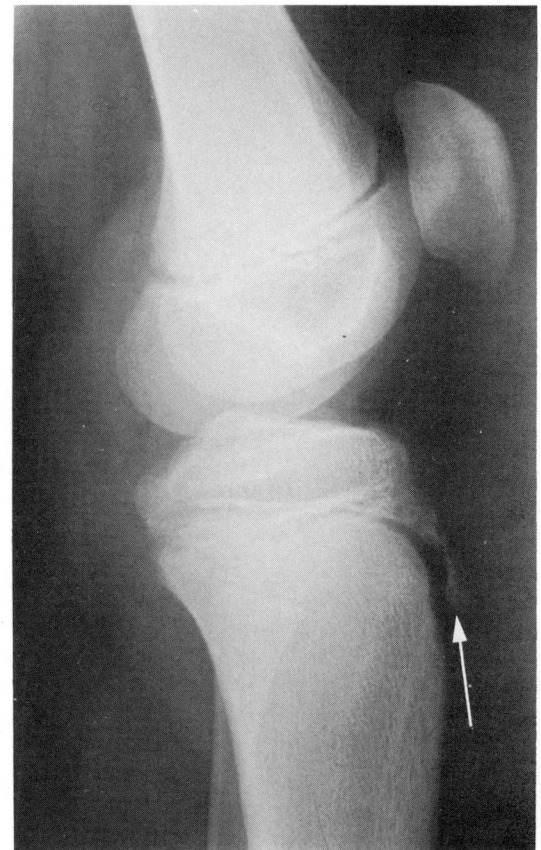

FIGURE 5–20. Osgood-Schlatter's disease. This 14-year-old boy complained of bilateral knee pain with prominent tenderness over the tibial tubercles bilaterally. X-ray demonstrates "traction epiphysitis" of the tibial tubercle (arrow).

along the patellotibial tendon itself, with or without associated infrapatellar bursitis. Local trauma or overuse syndromes are the usual cause.

Recurrent patellar dislocation is an uncommon cause of intermittent knee pain, often associated with buckling of the knee. The (usually young female) patient develops pain and "giving way" of the knee with forced knee extension, often when turning away (pivoting) from the affected side. Manipulation of the patella in such patients is usually painful, and the patellar apprehension test (Fig. 5–21) may be pathognomonic.

(Remember that the patella is most mobile and most easily tested with the knee fully extended and relaxed. In this position, displacement of the patella laterally will cause obvious apprehension as the patient recognizes the unpleasant sensation that precedes frank subluxation of the patella. Treatment is often surgical.)

Patellofemoral osteoarthrosis usually coexists with more generalized tibiofemoral osteoarthrosis (Fig. 5–3B) in the older patient. Severe degenerative changes limited to the patellofemoral joint may be the end result of longstanding chondromalacia patellae, however. A common complaint is stiffness of the knee when driving a car and an intermittent urge to get out and stretch the knee, since continued contraction of the quadriceps muscle for operation of the car pedals causes repetitive patellofemoral apposition and grinding. The middle-aged or elderly female may worsen the condition by wearing high-heeled shoes, which cause slight but continuous knee flexion while walking.

Disorders of the quadriceps muscles themselves may cause knee pain. Quadriceps rupture presents with sudden anterior knee and lower

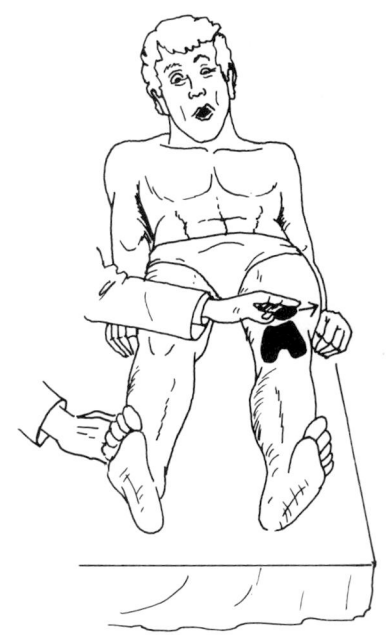

FIGURE 5–21. Patellar apprehension test. Attempted manipulation of the patella caused "anticipatory pain" in the patient with patellar dislocation.

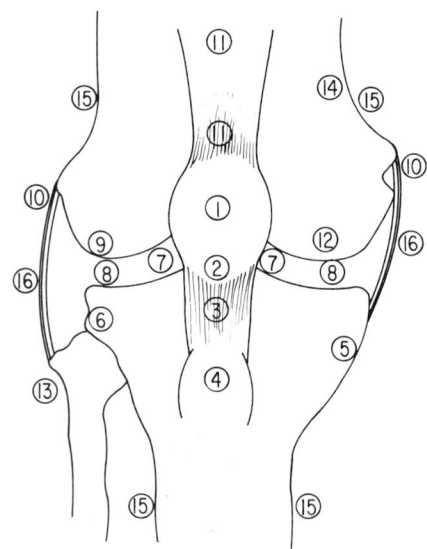

FIGURE 5–22. Localization of swelling and/or tenderness in various painful knee syndromes (see also Tables 5–1 and 5–2).

Key:

1. Patella: dislocation; chondromalacia; prepatellar bursitis or neuralgia
2. Jumper's knee; Sinding-Larsen-Johanssen's disease
3. Patellar tendinitis; infrapatellar bursitis
4. Osgood-Schlatter's disease
5. Pes anserine bursitis
6. Iliotibial band insertion
7. Fat pads; degenerative arthritis
8. Meniscal tears or cysts; intra-articular foreign bodies; degenerative arthritis
9. Popliteus tendinitis
10. Pellegrini-Stieda syndrome; collateral ligament syndromes
11. Quadriceps tendinitis strain or rupture; suprapatellar bursitis
12. Aseptic necrosis femoral condyle (medial)
13. Peroneal nerve
14. Saphenous nerve
15. Osteoarthropathy
16. Collateral ligament strains, tears, ruptures

thigh pain immediately after sudden extensor stress (jumping downward, for example), usually in the middle-aged or elderly. With complete rupture (which may occur at any of multiple sites along the musculotendinous apparatus, but usually just above the patella), the patient falls and is unable to maintain active knee extension. Surgery is usually necessary in these circumstances. Incomplete tears may result only in swelling and local tenderness, without complete quadriceps motor loss. Conservative treatment often suffices here. Any disorder that results in quadriceps weakness (old age, disuse, steroid myopathy, diabetic amy-

TABLE 5–2. LOCAL SWELLINGS OR TENDERNESS

PROBLEM	WHERE SWOLLEN/TENDER: (REFER TO FIG. 5–22)	REMEMBER
Bursitis		
Prepatellar	Superficial to patella: 1	? Intra-articular effusion too?
Infrapatellar	Deep to patellotibial tendon: 3	
Pes anserine	Tibial attachment of medial hamstrings and adductor: 5	Aspirate fluid
Popliteal (Baker's)	Popliteal space (Fig. 5–16D)	Thrombophlebitis? Popliteal aneurysm?
Popliteus tendinitis	Lateral femoral condyle (just anterior to lateral ligament): 9	Runners and joggers
Pellegrini-Stieda	Medial (or lateral) femoral epicondyle: 10	X-ray usually diagnostic (Fig. 5–23)
Iliotibial band	Distal lateral femur or tibial insertion: 6	Runners and joggers
Meniscus cysts	Medial or lateral joint line: 8	May disappear in full flexion/extension
Painful fat pads	Soft tissue straddling patellotibial tendon: 7	Young females
Osteonecrosis, femoral condyle	Medial femoral condyle; usually older patients: 12	X-rays often normal (but see Fig. 5–25); bone scan if x-ray normal
Osteoarthropathy	Distal femur or along tibia: 15	Finger clubbing; (usually) pulmonary disease (Fig. 5–24)
Traumatic prepatellar neuralgia	Anterior patella: 1	History of recent trauma
Meniscus tears	Medial or lateral joint line: 8	Mechanism of injury? Rotatory testing! (see p. 250)
Saphenous nerve entrapment	Above and medial to medial femoral epicondyle: 14	May cause paresthesias—down medial foreleg
Degenerative arthritis	Bony proliferation: 7, 8, 9, 12	X-ray diagnostic (Figs. 5–3, 5–41)
Peroneal nerve entrapment	Neck of fibula: 13	Common cause of knee and lower leg/foot pain
Collateral ligament strains	Lateral or medial ligament: 16	Strain versus rupture (pp. 241 ff.)

otrophy, myositis ossificans, suprapatellar bursitis, femoral neuropathy) may predispose to quadriceps tears or will disrupt the extensor mechanism and predispose the patient to superimposed patellofemoral disorders.

Figure 5–22 and Tables 5–1 and 5–2 provide an overview of disorders causing knee pain in which examination often reveals tenderness or localized swelling of involved structures. In addition to patellofemoral syndromes (Table 5–1), bursitis (Fig. 5–16), popliteus tendinitis and iliotibial band syndromes, meniscal cysts (Fig. 5–18), painful fat pads, popliteal cysts, and recurrent patellar dislocation, careful palpation of external structures may help diagnose other much more unusual problems. These include:

Pellegrini-Stieda syndrome refers to calcification of either the medial or lateral collateral ligament attachment to the femoral epicondyle, usually appearing 3 to 4 weeks after a knee "strain" in a patient with progressive difficulty flexing and using the knee at a time when simple knee strains should be improving (see also page 241). Pain gradually disappears but may be very prolonged (months). X-rays will often demonstrate calcification adjacent to the femoral epicondyle (Fig. 5–23).

Hypertrophic osteoarthropathy[20] (Fig. 5–24) may cause pain and tenderness of the distal femur or along the lower leg, usually in association with finger clubbing and one of various pulmonary (or systemic) diseases. Treatment of the underlying condition is essential here.

Traumatic prepatellar neuralgia[21] refers to exquisite (superficial) tenderness of the anterior patella beginning a few weeks after direct trauma to the patella. Local injections with steriod/anesthestic combinations usually help.

Osteonecrosis of the femoral condyle[22] may cause sudden, severe, and persistent pain in (usually) older patients, in which pain and tenderness are localized to the femoral condyle. X-rays are often normal,

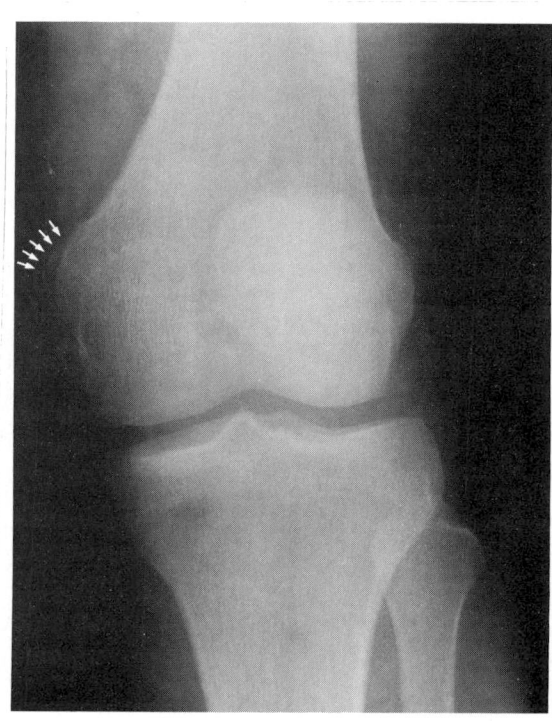

FIGURE 5–23. Pellegrini-Stieda syndrome. This 42-year-old man complained of persistent knee pain for several months. Examination revealed marked tenderness of the medial femoral epicondyle, without laxity of the medial ligament. X-ray demonstrates calcification of the insertion of the medial collateral ligament on the epicondyle (arrow). Anti-inflammatory medicines alone were successful in treatment.

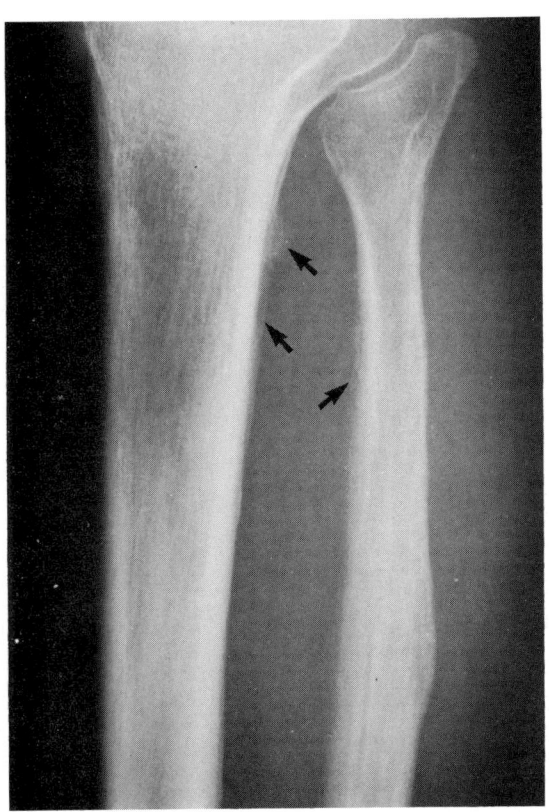

FIGURE 5–24. This 63-year-old woman complained of bilateral aching in both lower legs, most prominent around the knees. Examination was unremarkable except for tenderness along the entire length of both tibias. X-ray demonstrates remarkable periosteal elevation along the shaft of both the tibia and fibula *(arrows)*. Treatment of the primary process, diffuse interstitial pneumonitis, resulted in improvement of leg pain.

but a bone scan will be diagnostic (Fig. 5–25). Pain usually resolves spontaneously but may be prolonged (weeks or months).

> Mike is told that his knee pain is caused by chondromalacia patellae. The nature of the problem is briefly explained. On examination there is no evidence of patella alta, patella baja, or genu valgum. The "Q angle" is measured and appears normal (see Appendix).
>
> Mike is told to temporarily discontinue his training program and to perform only normal daily activities, but to avoid specific movements that cause pain—climbing stairs, for example. He is instructed in the mechanics of isometric quadriceps exercises and told to progress gradually through weighted isometric exercise. Aspirin, 2 tablets four times a day, is suggested for the next 1 to 2 weeks.
>
> Mike is told to return in 4 weeks. X-rays are not obtained.

NOTE

1. X-rays are unnecessary at this time. Most patellofemoral syndromes are associated with nondiagnostic x-rays (Table 5–1). If symptoms were to persist in spite of appropriate treatment, x-rays would be indicated.

X-rays are always necessary when knee pain is traumatic (see below).

2. When chondromalacia patellae is diagnosed, recognition of anatomic patellar abnormalities may be important. Patella alta, patella baja, and abnormal Q angles are example of these (see Appendix).

Most patients with patellofemoral syndromes do not require orthopedic consultations. When, however, anatomic or biomechanical disorders of the patellofemoral mechanism are present, specialist consultation is often worthwhile (see Appendix).

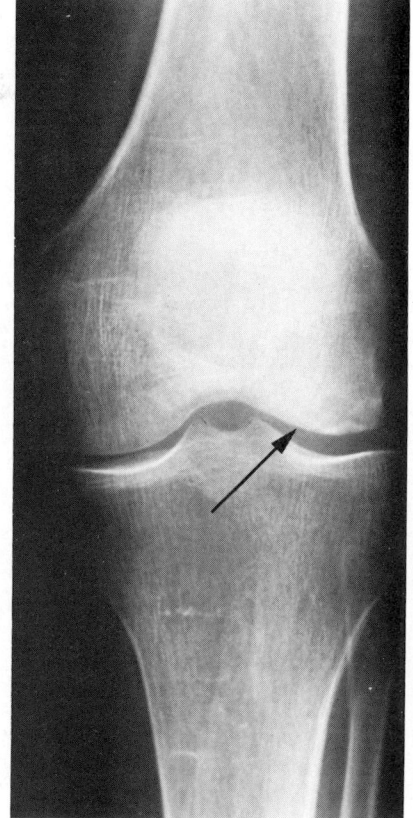

FIGURE 5–25. Osteonecrosis of the femoral condyle. This 59-year-old woman presented with the acute onset of severe pain in the left knee. Examination revealed exquisite tenderness over the lateral femoral condyle. The x-ray reveals some flattening and sclerosis of the inferior border of the lateral femoral condyle (arrow). A bone scan obtained on the same day was markedly "positive" in the same area. Conservative therapy with anti-inflammatory medication and physical therapy ultimately resulted in marked improvement. Surgery was not required.

Treatment of Patellofemoral Syndromes

Fundamental to the treatment of all patellofemoral syndromes are (temporary) avoidance of precipitating activities, isometric quadriceps exercises, anti-inflammatory measures, and reassurance.

Immobilization in a cast is rarely required but is sometimes needed in advanced cases of chondromalacia or Osgood-Schlatter's disease. A week or two in an immobilizing splint sometimes helps (Fig. 5–36). While rehabilitation is proceeding, however, running, jumping, climbing, and the various other pain precipitants must be avoided.

Even when acute pain and tenderness require (analgesics or) anti-inflammatory drugs (see Chapter 1, Table 1–4), isometric quadriceps exercises should be begun. These "isometric" exercises (Fig. 5–26) are not, strictly speaking, isometric, since both the patella and quadriceps muscle do move during their performance, but these exercises strengthen the extensor apparatus without movement of the knee joint itself. Figure 5–26 illustrates three different maneuvers, each of which is a successive stage in a quadriceps strengthening program:

1. Quadriceps muscle "setting." With the knee fully extended and relaxed, the quadriceps muscles are actively contracted ("set"), without either lifting the leg or moving the tibiofemoral joint through any flexion or extension. The patella will visibly ride slightly upward on the femur as the quads contract—this position is maintained for several seconds, relaxed, and repeated over and over. This initial stage can be begun even when pain has not completely resolved, since it usually does not cause worsening of symptoms, and can be done repeatedly during the day.

2. Straight leg raising, unresisted. The patient sits in a chair, the knee

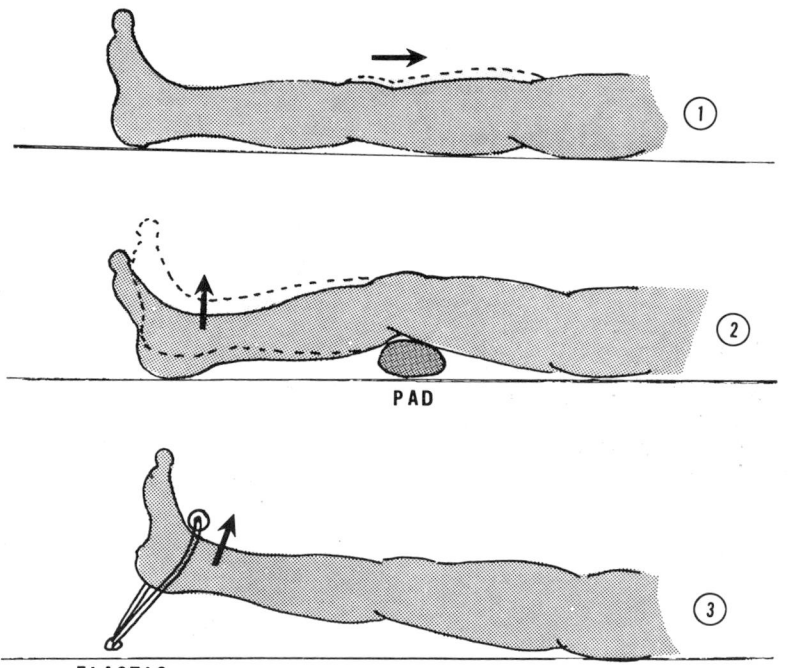

PAD

ELASTIC

FIGURE 5–26. <u>Types of quadriceps exercises.</u> <i>1,</i> Quad setting. Knee is fully extended, muscle shortens with no joint motion, and patella ascends. <i>2,</i> With a 3-inch pad under the knee, the quadriceps function is enhanced and joint motion is minimal. <i>3,</i> Straight leg raising against resistance (isometric exercises) further strengthens quadriceps without joint motion. (Reproduced with permission from Cailliet, R: Soft Tissue Pain and Disability. Philadelphia: F.A. Davis Co., 1977, p. 243.)

relaxed and fully extended, with the foot resting comfortably on another chair (or another, slightly lower, support). The patient's hands support the thigh (helping to lift the femur and relieving any stress on the hip flexors) as the patient lifts the outstretched foot and lower leg a few inches above its support and holds it, usually for 10 seconds or longer. Here the quadriceps muscles support the weight of the extended lower leg, but <u>without any movement of the knee joint itself</u> (and without any downward patellar "drag," Figure 5–19). These exercises are repeated, 10 seconds up, 10 seconds down, for 5 or 10 minutes <u>with each leg</u>.

3. When <u>unresisted straight leg raising is performed repeatedly, easily and without pain, resisted straight leg raising</u> is begun. Small weights (1 or 2 pounds to start) are suspended from the outstretched foot (an old handbag is a useful weight container), and straight leg raising is repeated, as above. Over time, additional weight is added—the ultimate goal must be individualized since the competitive athlete may lift 50 pounds, the sedentary older person only 5 pounds. Again the quads lift the weighted lower leg <u>without knee flexion and extension</u> (the converse are <u>isotonic</u> exercises, which can be used for further conditioning at a later date—see Figure 5–27).

In patients with chondromalacia, progressive isometric exercises are pursued for 6 to 8 weeks, with gradual increase of weight resistance. Pain during exercise implies improper performance of the maneuver, excessive weight, or need for reexamination of the knee. Muscular exercise of the <u>hamstrings</u> is also wise, especially during the latter phase of recovery, to <u>insure a "balance"</u> of strength between the flexors and extensors of the knee.[23]

Anti-inflammatory measures may or may not be necessary. Aspirin four times a day is usually sufficient in chondromalacia and is much less expensive than other nonsteroidal anti-inflammatory drugs (see Table 1–4). Local steroid injections may be helpful when swelling and tenderness of the patellar tendon or bursa are present, but this is rarely helpful in uncomplicated chondromalacia patellae.

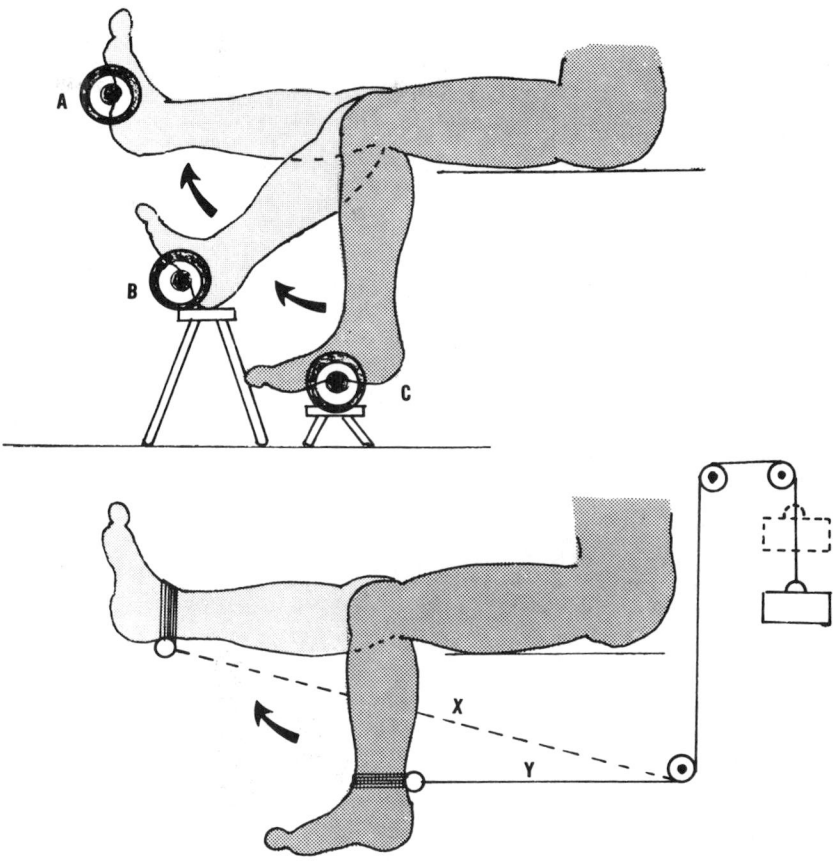

FIGURE 5–27. Progressive resistive exercises (isotonic). *Above, A,* Full extension is attempted. *B,* With stool to support weighted foot, only the last degrees of extension are exercises. This is most desired and strengthens the vastus medialis. *C,* Resistance is minimal, and there is ligamentous strain on the knee when the leg is fully dependent. *Below,* Pulley exercises. Maximum resistance occurs in the first 45 degrees of extension and none at full extension. (Reproduced with permission from Cailliet, R: Soft Tissue Pain and Disability. Philadelphia: F.A. Davis Co., 1977, p. 206.)

> Four weeks later, Mike is lifting 20 pounds with each leg during resisted isometric quadriceps maneuvers, and is symptom free, even when climbing stairs.
>
> Examination at this time is entirely normal, and quadriceps strength is excellent bilaterally. Mike is told to continue his exercise, but to avoid isotonic weight lifting, at least for the present. Running up and down hills is discouraged, but Mike is told he may resume his prior training program, but gradually.

Chondromalacia patellae in the absence of underlying anatomic abnormalities usually improves gradually with this program. Isotonic exercises can be performed when isometric exercises are painlessly managed, but "isotonics" do recreate the repetitive flexion-extension stress and are usually discouraged, at least until all symptoms have completely resolved. Isotonic exercises are more useful in progressive rehabilitation following knee trauma, when the extensor mechanism is not the major problem (see below).

> Three months later, Mike returns, complaining of right knee pain. Mike had been playing competitive soccer since his last visit and had not experienced any difficulty until yesterday when he injured his knee during a soccer match.
>
> This morning there is much pain and swelling of the injured knee. Mike walks into the office but is limping badly.

TRAUMATIC KNEE PAIN[5, 24-29]

The diagnosis and treatment of major knee injuries are far beyond the scope of this book. Nevertheless, most knee injuries are minor and respond well to simple conservative measures. Distinguishing these less serious injuries

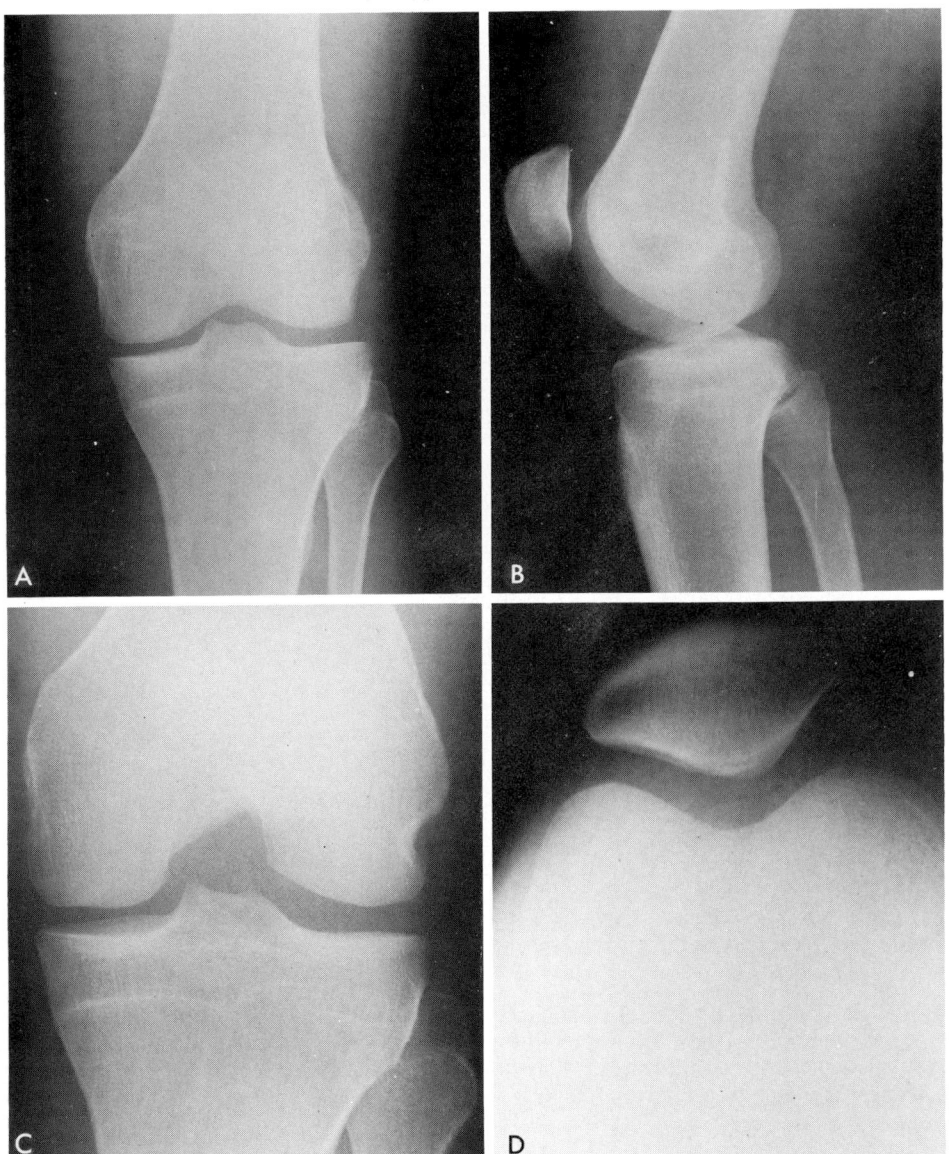

FIGURE 5–28. The knee x-ray. The anteroposterior *(A)*, lateral *(B)*, "tunnel" *(C)*, and "skyline" *(D)* views of the knee. These x-rays are normal.

from significant internal knee derangements is a common problem in adult ambulatory medicine. When should the orthopedist be consulted?

All fractures and dislocations require immediate orthopedic attention. These problems cannot be reviewed here; however, x-rays should always be obtained when knee pain follows an acute injury (Fig. 5–28). Four x-ray views should be obtained: anteroposterior, lateral, "tunnel" view, and a "30-degree sunrise" view. When x-rays reveal no fracture or dislocation, the major initial concerns must include:

1. Is there serious ligament damage? Surgical repair of serious (or third-degree) ligament tears is probably optimal within the first 7 to 10 days of injury. Early recognition of this problem is thus important to the patient's eventual full recovery (see below). Most ligament injuries, however, are simple "strains" (or first-degree tears) that improve with rest and conservative therapy.

2. Is a meniscus torn? Most meniscal injuries do not require immediate orthopedic consultation, and very few require immediate surgery. Nevertheless, early diagnosis facilitates appropriate treatment (see below).

3. Is the extensor apparatus disrupted? Patellar fractures and dislocations will usually be obvious on x-ray. However, tears or disruptions of the quadriceps muscles, quadriceps tendon, or patellar tendon may also require immediate orthopedic consultation (and will not be demonstrated by x-rays).

4. Is hemarthrosis present? Even when x-rays are normal, acute traumatic hemarthrosis warrants orthopedic referral. Inapparent (especially osteochondral) fractures, synovial contusion with hemorrhage, tears of the joint capsule, major (especially cruciate) ligament tears, patellar dislocations, and (occasionally) peripheral meniscal tears are among the causes of acute traumatic hemarthrosis (Table 5–3, page 245). Some of these problems are managed by aspiration of the hemarthrosis and conservative therapy, but an orthopedist should usually make those decisions.

These questions can usually be answered by obtaining a detailed history of the precise mechanism of injury and by performing a careful examination of the knee. Correlation of these findings with some understanding of functional internal knee anatomy is essential (see Appendix).

CONSIDER

> Mike recalls the circumstances of his injury quite vividly: While running at top speed and about to kick the ball with his right foot, Mike was bumped by an opposing player coming from his (Mike's) left side. The toe of Mike's shoe jammed into the turf as he swung it forward to kick the ball, and he experienced sudden, severe pain on the inside of his right knee. Mike fell to the ground and had some difficulty getting up again, but he was ultimately able to walk off the field without assistance. He was unable to continue playing, however, and his knee felt weak. Over the next 8 hours, Mike noted increased stiffness of the knee. The knee is worse this morning and is now swollen, but Mike is able to bear weight, albeit painfully.

NOTE

1. Mike is able to walk. Major fractures, (especially cruciate) ligament injuries, or locked meniscal tears will often render weight bearing impossible, but the ability to walk should not exclude suspicion of serious internal knee derangement. Every patient is different.

2. The mechanism of injury is primarily indirect and of a rotational nature, rather than a direct blow to the knee. Most serious ligament injuries occur from a direct blow to the knee. Figure 5–29 illustrates typical mecha-

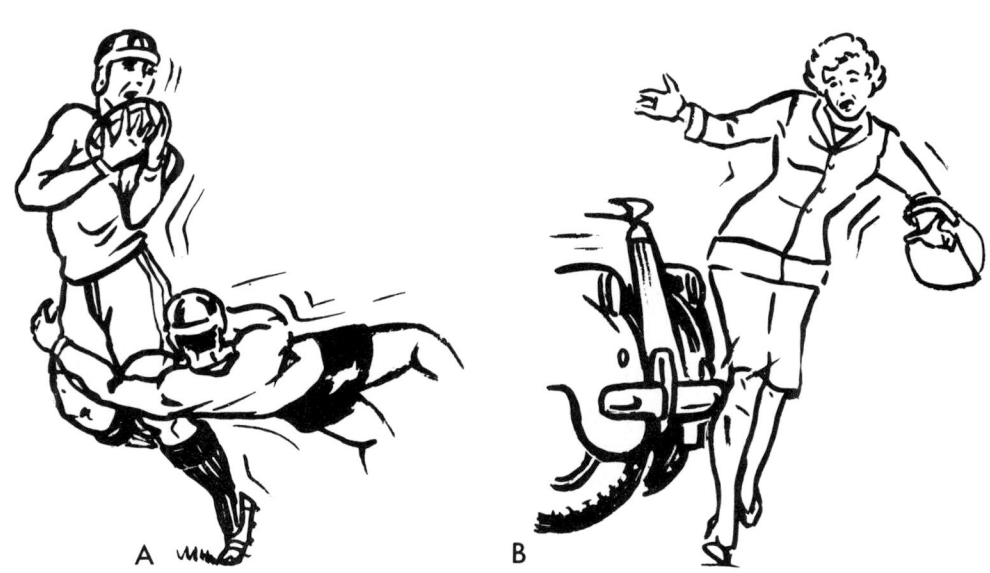

FIGURE 5–29. Typical mechanisms of ligamentous injury. Note that the knee is weight-bearing and is subjected to forceful valgus stress. In both of these circumstances, injury to the medial collateral ligament, cruciate ligaments, and/or medial meniscus would be likely. A, Violent abduction or adduction injuries with the leg straight produce ruptures of the medial or the lateral ligaments. B, The foot is caught, and the rest of the body is thrown violently. This accident caused rupture of the medial and the cruciate ligaments. (Reproduced with permission from Helfet, AJ: Disorders of the Knee. Philadelphia: J.B. Lippincott Co., 1982, pp. 102 and 103.)

A   B

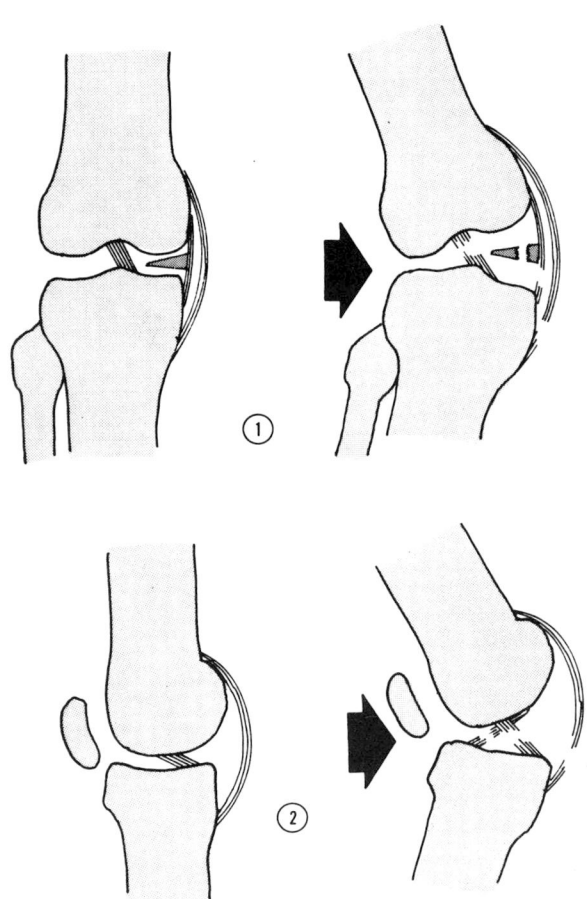

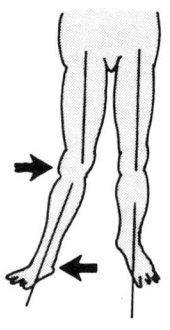

FIGURE 5–30. Severe ligamentous sprain (the unhappy triad). *1*, Lateral (valgus) stress causing disruption of the medial collateral ligament, the medial meniscus, and the anterior cruciate ligament (the unhappy triad). *2*, Lateral view of a severe anterior stress causing hyperextension of the joint and disrupting both anterior and posterior cruciate ligaments and the posterior capsule. Clinically, it has a positive drawer sign (Fig. 5–33*B*). (Reproduced with permission from Cailliet, R: Knee Pain and Disability. Philadelphia: F.A. Davis Co., 1973, p. 66.)

nisms of abduction (valgus) injury to the knee—usually a direct blow to the outer aspect of the weight-bearing knee with resultant stretching or actual rupture of the medial knee compartment. Under these circumstances the medial collateral ligament, medial meniscus, anterior cruciate ligament, and joint capsule may (all) be damaged (Fig. 5–30). An audible "pop" at the time of injury is suspicious of ligament injury.

Varus stress produces analogous injury to the lateral knee compartment—the lateral collateral ligament or deep capsular ligaments or both are at risk in these less common circumstances. Hyperextension stress damages the posterior joint capsule and may tear either or both cruciate ligaments (see Fig. 5–30 and Appendix). Note that "stress vectors" are not always unidirectional—combined valgus stress and hyperextension may damage the knee's entire ligamentous support, resulting in very serious injury.

Most isolated meniscus injuries are the result of indirect, rotational stress on the weight-bearing knee. (As noted above, the meniscus may be torn together with ligaments in direct blow injuries.) The precise mechanism of meniscal tears remains controversial, but a shearing of different arcs of the meniscal circumference usually results from some combination of tibiofemoral compression (weight bearing) and nonphysiologic tibiofemoral rotation. Figures 5–31 and 5–32 illustrate a few examples, the first of which is similar to Mike's injury. Note that, in addition to weight bearing and rotation, some component of sudden extension/flexion or adduction of the upper leg is often involved. In Mike's case, external rotation of the tibia is maintained (because, as in Figure 5–31*A*, the player catches his toe in the turf) in spite of forced tibiofemoral extension (the kick) and resisted thigh adduction.

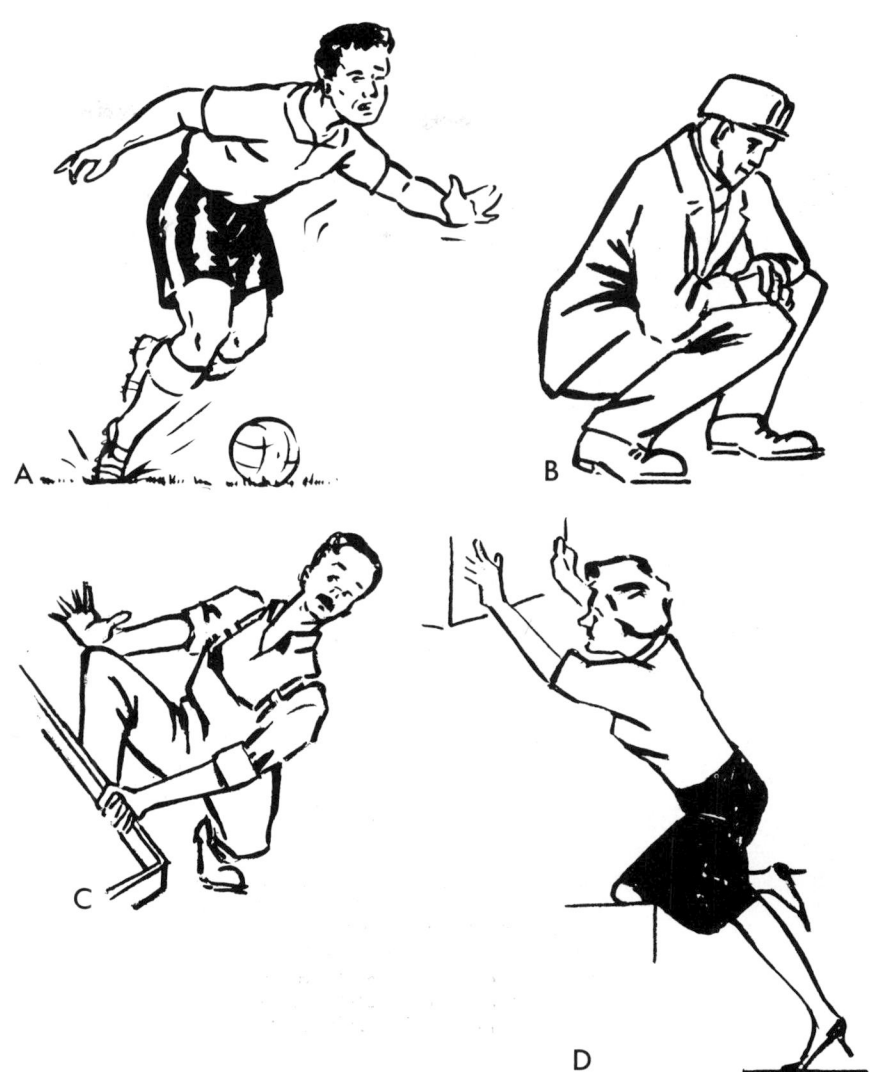

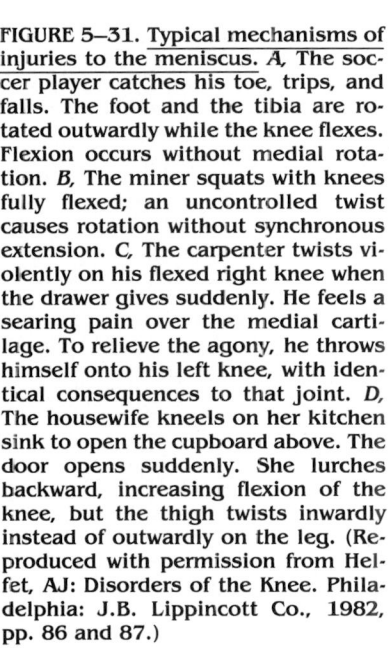

FIGURE 5–31. Typical mechanisms of injuries to the meniscus. *A*, The soccer player catches his toe, trips, and falls. The foot and the tibia are rotated outwardly while the knee flexes. Flexion occurs without medial rotation. *B*, The miner squats with knees fully flexed; an uncontrolled twist causes rotation without synchronous extension. *C*, The carpenter twists violently on his flexed right knee when the drawer gives suddenly. He feels a searing pain over the medial cartilage. To relieve the agony, he throws himself onto his left knee, with identical consequences to that joint. *D*, The housewife kneels on her kitchen sink to open the cupboard above. The door opens suddenly. She lurches backward, increasing flexion of the knee, but the thigh twists inwardly instead of outwardly on the leg. (Reproduced with permission from Helfet, AJ: Disorders of the Knee. Philadelphia: J.B. Lippincott Co., 1982, pp. 86 and 87.)

In the older patient, meniscal tears may occur with little or no apparent injury since the menisci degenerate with age. In such patients, mild twisting—as when getting out of a car—may induce a painful tear. Some meniscal tears are painless and remain unrecognized in older patients.

3. The time lapse between injury and the onset of swelling suggests that a reactive effusion, not hemarthrosis, is present. Bleeding into the joint is usually immediate and is apparent within the first few hours after the injury. Later onset of effusion usually speaks against hemarthrosis and suggests a "reactive" serous effusion instead. Table 5–3 lists some causes of hemarthrosis.

TABLE 5–3. HEMARTHROSIS

TRAUMATIC CAUSES (X-RAY MAY BE NORMAL)	NONTRAUMATIC CAUSES
Fracture (osteochondral)	Hemophilia
Synovial contusion with hemorrhage	Other bleeding disorders
Tears of joint capsule	Scurvy
Ligament tears	Villonodular synovitis
Patellar dislocation	Neoplasm
Meniscus tears (peripheral)	Hemangioma
Traumatic arthrocentesis	

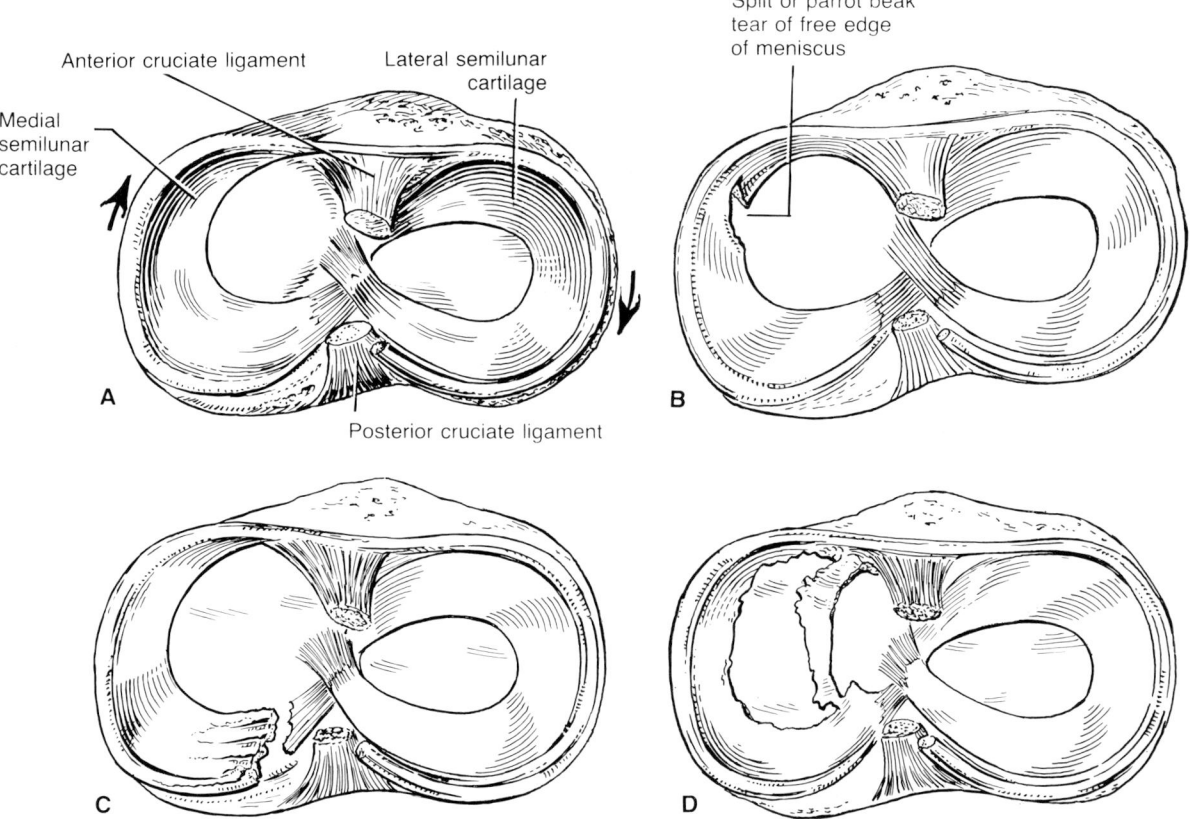

FIGURE 5–32. The anatomy of the semilunar cartilages (menisci) and examples of common types of meniscal tears. A, Normal. B, This minor "split" is most common. C, Rupture of its firm attachments to the cruciate ligament and the posterior capsule produces the ragged retracted posterior horn. D, The "bowstring," or bucket-handle, results from splitting of the cartilage longitudinally to allow the free border to bowstring across the joint. The separation is roughly equivalent to the distance the tibia normally rotates. (Reproduced with permission from Helfet, AJ: Disorders of the Knee. Philadelphia: J.B. Lippincott Co., 1982, pp. 9, 87, 88, and 89.)

REMEMBER

The absence of a joint effusion does not exclude serious internal damage. In fact, among the more severe injuries are those that rupture the joint capsule as well as the ligaments, such that blood dissects out of the joint space into the soft tissues; in these cases, an effusion or hemarthrosis may not be present.

Physical examination reveals a healthy young male whose only abnormality involves his right knee. There is an obvious intra-articular knee effusion (Fig. 5–6A). Knee range of motion is limited by tightness and generalized discomfort at 90 degrees of flexion; full extension of the knee cannot be achieved because of pain in the posteromedial knee at 15 degrees of flexion. Mike is able to elevate his leg; the extensor mechanism and patella appear intact.

There is moderate tenderness over the medial joint line and peripherally around the posteromedial joint line, and it is difficult to tell whether the medial ligament is tender or not. The collateral ligaments do not appear lax during varus and valgus stress, and both anterior and posterior drawer signs are negative, but Mike is unable to fully relax his hamstring muscles during testing and complains of discomfort during all these maneuvers. Rotatory testing is not performed at this time.

X-rays of the knee are normal except for obvious knee effusion.

What does this mean?

I. A fracture is unlikely when x-rays are normal. An inapparent (osteochondral) fracture must still be suspected if hemarthrosis is present, even if x-rays are normal.

II. Serious ligament damage[27, 30] is unlikely, but the examination is inconclusive.

While ligament laxity cannot be demonstrated in Mike's case, testing for ligamentous laxity must be interpreted with caution in the setting of an acute injury in which muscular (usually hamstring) spasm may "falsely stabilize" the knee. When a large joint effusion is present, palpable landmarks are obscured, and ligament testing may be even more difficult.

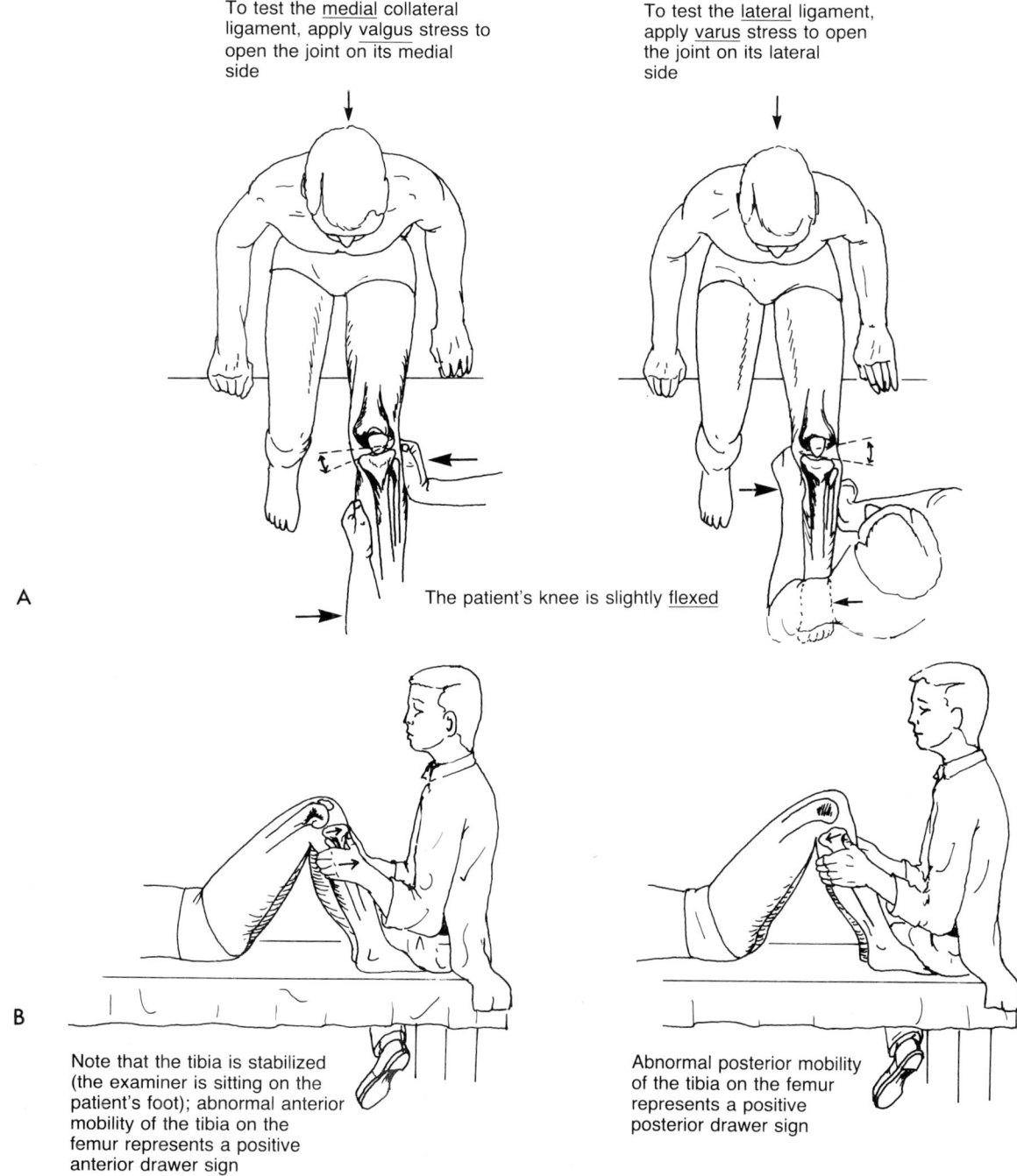

To test the medial collateral ligament, apply valgus stress to open the joint on its medial side

To test the lateral ligament, apply varus stress to open the joint on its lateral side

A

The patient's knee is slightly flexed

B

Note that the tibia is stabilized (the examiner is sitting on the patient's foot); abnormal anterior mobility of the tibia on the femur represents a positive anterior drawer sign

Abnormal posterior mobility of the tibia on the femur represents a positive posterior drawer sign

FIGURE 5–33. A, Collateral ligament testing. B, The "drawer" signs for cruciate ligament testing.

When the patient is relaxed (feel the hamstring tendons!) and an effusion is small, absent, or has been aspirated (see below), ligament testing may still be confusing, even for the specialist, but Figure 5–33 illustrates the essentials. Note:

A. The injured knee must always be compared with the normal knee, since asymmetric instability is the critical finding.

For example, the patient with congenitally lax (or even absent) lateral collateral ligaments will reveal bilateral laxity on varus testing (Fig. 5–33A) that is of no clinical importance. Such a finding could be confused with acute ligament rupture. Pain or tenderness during ligamentous testing may reflect a strain, but, in general, ligament injuries that require immediate orthopedic referral are those that cause the joint to "open up" on stress testing (Fig. 5–33).

B. Collateral ligament testing should be performed with the knee in full extension and again with the knee flexed 30 degrees.

As described in the Appendix, the bony contours of the tibiofemoral joint "lock" in full extension, and all ligamentous support is taut in this position. When medial or lateral laxity can be appreciated with the knee fully extended, very extensive internal derangement is present. Such straight medial instability (medial laxity with valgus stress on the fully extended knee) indicates damage to medial collateral, deep capsular, and cruciate ligaments, and often the posterior capsule as well. Straight lateral instability on varus testing implies analogous injury to lateral collateral and cruciate ligaments, as well as deep capsular structures.

Since isolated collateral ligament instability cannot be detected with the knee fully extended, "unlocking" the knee and slackening its ligamentous support by flexing the knee 20 degrees allows more sensitive testing of the collateral ligament alone.

C. The drawer tests for cruciate ligament instability must be carefully interpreted.

As Figure 5–33B illustrates, these tests are designed to elicit anterior or posterior displacement of the stabilized tibia (the examiner should sit on the patient's foot) on the flexed femur, such that anterior "draw" implies anterior cruciate laxity and posterior draw, posterior cruciate laxity.

First, remember that effusions and muscle spasm may render these tests insensitive, (i.e., ligament injury may be inapparent).

Second, examine both knees for any visible anterior or posterior subluxation before testing. Why? If the posterior drawer test is initiated with the tibia already anteriorly displaced following anterior cruciate injury, the tibia may move posteriorly "back to neutral" during the drawer test, simulating posterior cruciate injury.

Third, remember that disruption of other internal structures may produce positive drawer signs when the cruciates are in fact intact. For example, medial or lateral compartment injuries that damage collateral ligaments or the joint capsule may result in rotational laxity when drawer tests are being performed. Anteromedial rotatory instability refers to a positive anterior drawer sign due to medial compartment injuries when only the medial tibia draws anteriorly, simulating anterior cruciate laxity. (Conversely, straight anterior instability refers to forward displacement of the entire tibia during the anterior drawer test; this is due to cruciate laxity.) Posterolateral rotatory instability (due to lateral compartment injury) may analogously be confused with straight posterior laxity (due to posterior cruciate ligament injury).

Even the experienced orthopedist may have difficulty interpreting these findings. Arthroscopy may be needed[31] to answer the question definitively.

III. Range of motion of the knee is markedly impaired, but this may be due to the joint effusion.

Inability to fully flex or extend the knee often indicates an internal knee derangement. Meniscus tears (or rarer intra-articular foreign bodies, Fig. 5–3) are common examples. As is indicated in the Appendix, full extension requires a tight "fit" between opposing tibial and femoral articular surfaces.

The presence of a large joint effusion allows no conclusion to be drawn about the cause of limited range of motion. Only by removing the joint fluid can range of motion be adequately tested.

IV. Rotatory testing is not performed in Mike's case because these maneuvers are often very painful in the patient with an acute meniscus tear. Usually the mechanism of injury, tenderness along the medial joint line, and the absence of definite ligament injury suffice, at least initially, to heighten suspicion of meniscus injury (as in this case).

Figure 5–34 illustrates two types of rotatory testing. Both involve rotation of the tibia on the femur with the knee in flexion or extension. These maneuvers allow indirect assessment of the integrity of the menisci, which rotate together with the tibia and move posteriorly and anteriorly during flexion and extension of the knee, respectively (see Appendix). The McMurray test involves palpation of the medial and lateral joint lines with one hand while the other hand rotates the tibia, thus allowing the palpating hand to appreciate any clicking (sometimes audible) or pain during the rotational maneuver. This test is nonspecific in that it was originally described in the diagnosis of posterior longitudinal meniscus tears, which comprise only a minority of all meniscus tears. Nevertheless, this test and the Apley compression test are useful in that each attempts to elicit pain, grating, tenderness, or click/crepitus along the joint line during tibiofemoral rotation—such findings often indicate a torn meniscus, especially when the mechanism of injury is appropriate (Fig. 5–31).

Tables 5–4 and 5–5 (page 251) summarize clinical features of ligament and meniscus injuries.

Arthrocentesis reveals 40 cc of serous fluid with a white blood count of 80 and a red blood count of 950. Following the tap, the right knee is able to flex beyond 135 degrees, but there is still discomfort and limitation of motion on extension of the knee, with a 5-degree flexion "contracture." Hamstring spasm persists, but ligament testing appears stable.

NOTE

1. Arthrocentesis is helpful diagnostically and therapeutically in this situation (see also page 255). The serous effusion is reassuring, since acute hemarthrosis should prompt orthopedic referral (even when x-rays are normal). When visible fat globules are present within the syringe after

A

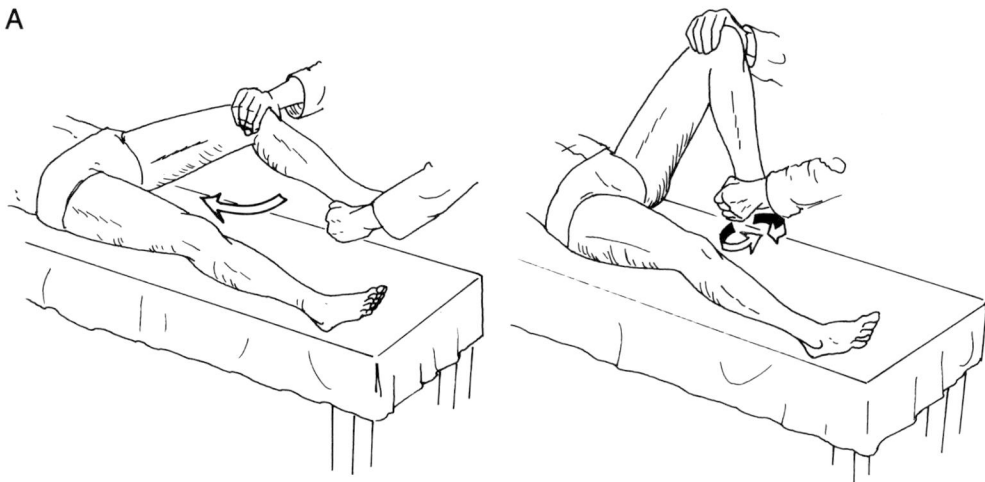

The knee is flexed, and the tibia is rotated internally and externally on the femur

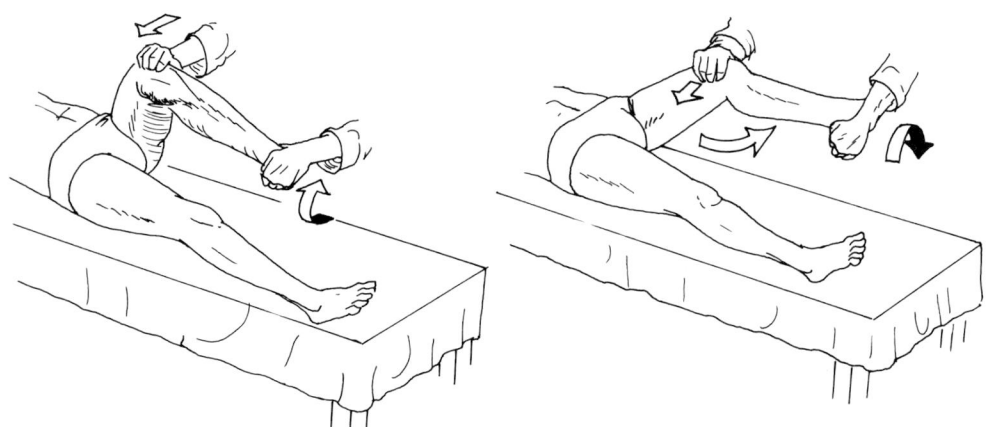

With the tibia externally rotated, exert valgus stress on the knee and then slowly extend the knee; a palpable or audible "click" during this maneuver is "positive"

FIGURE 5–34. Rotatory testing of the knee. A, The McMurray test. B, The Apley test.

B

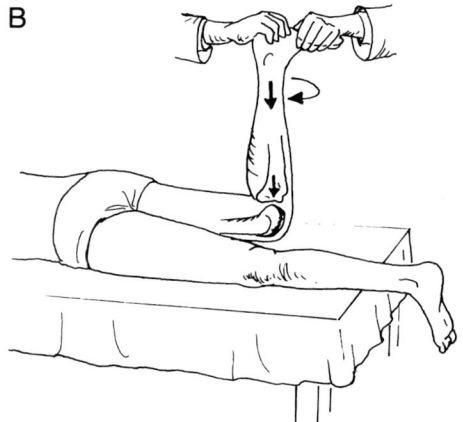

The compression test rotates the tibia while applying downward pressure on the tibiofemoral joint (the patient prone); this "grinds" a torn meniscus

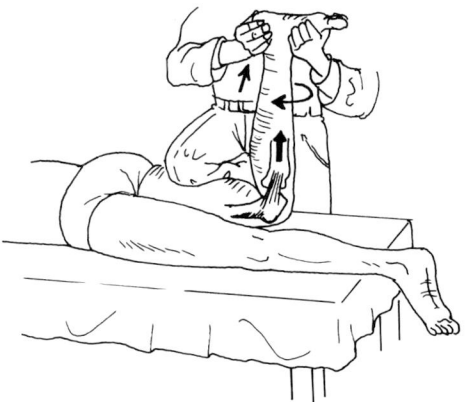

Rotation of the tibia during upward traction on the tibiofemoral joint stresses ligaments, not menisci

TABLE 5–4. LIGAMENT INJURIES

HISTORY
Sudden onset localized knee pain; "pop"?
Usually direct blow, fall, or other extreme valgus, varus, and/or hyperextension stress
   to the knee.

EXAMINATION
Effusion common
Tenderness over involved ligaments
Range of motion often restricted by pain/effusion
Ligamentous instability?
      Varus/valgus laxity in full extension: —————————→ severe injury
      Varus laxity at 30° flexion: ————————————→ lateral collateral ligament
      Valgus laxity at 30° flexion: ———————————→ medial collateral ligament
      Anterior drawer: ——————————————————→ anterior cruciate
      Posterior drawer: —————————————————→ posterior cruciate
Remember: Combined injuries common!

X-RAYS
Usually normal

ARTHROCENTESIS
Hemarthrosis common

DEFINITIVE DIAGNOSIS
Arthroscopy
Examination under anesthesia
Surgery?

aspiration of the hemarthrosis, an unsuspected fracture should be especially considered.

In addition, joint aspiration allows more accurate testing of range of motion and will make the patient more comfortable more quickly. This does not mean that all traumatic joint effusions must be aspirated. Small effusions that do not impair range of motion and that clearly developed many hours (or days) after the traumatic event (and thus are unlikely to be hemarthroses) need not be tapped. The risk of introducing infection by arthrocentesis is very small, but real.

TABLE 5–5. MENISCUS INJURIES[26]

HISTORY
Sudden onset localized knee pain
Usually rotatory mechanism of injury without direct blow
Knee may lock, buckle, or click
Often recurrent with subacute exacerbations

EXAMINATION
Effusion common
Tenderness over joint line (medial most common)
Range of motion often limited; especially extension
Rotatory testing reproduces pain, produces click/crepitus

X-RAYS
Usually normal

ARTHROCENTESIS
Effusion usually serous, noninflammatory
Hemarthrosis unusual, except with peripheral tear

DEFINITIVE DIAGNOSIS
Arthroscopy
Arthrogram

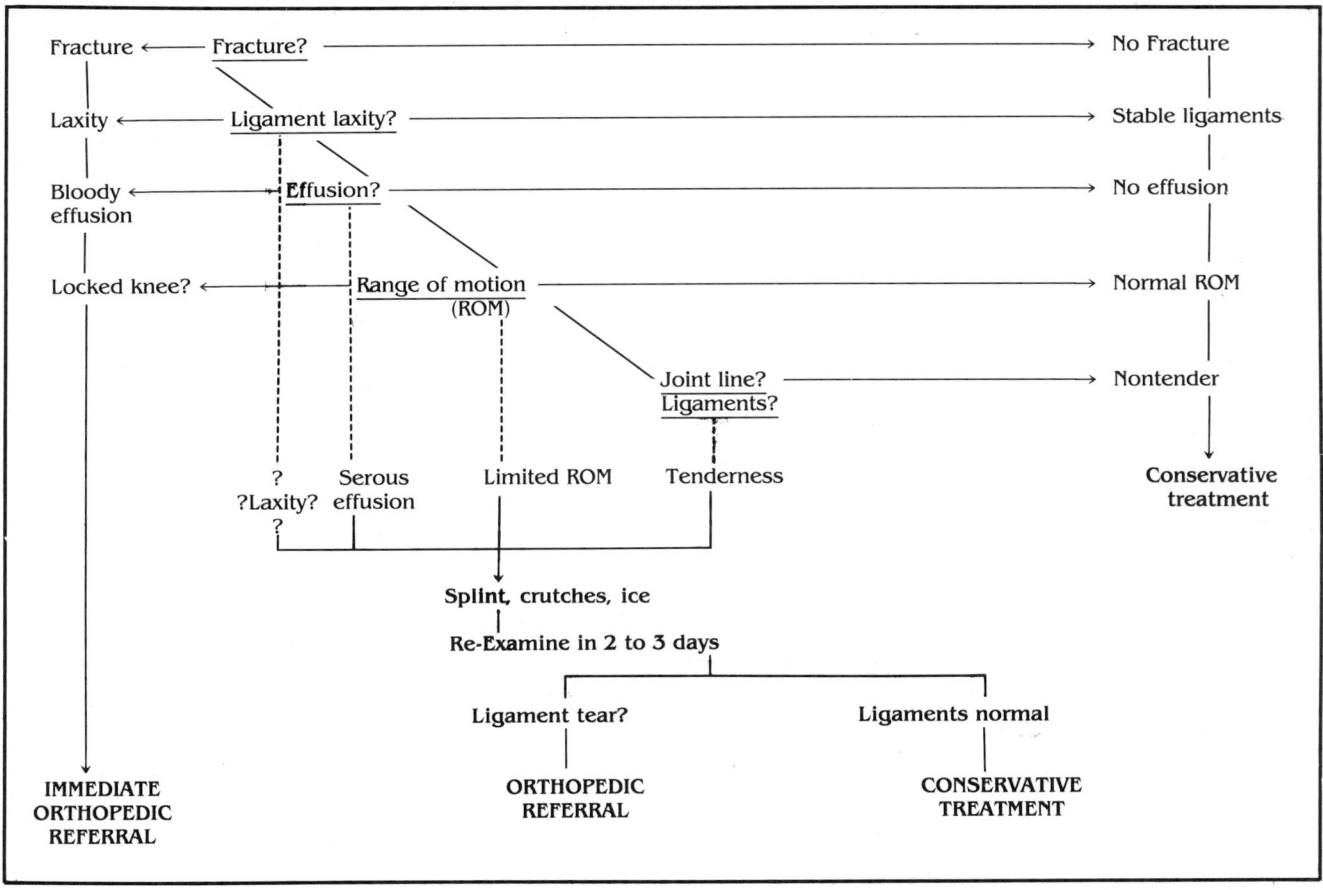

FIGURE 5–35. Acute knee injury.

2. There is no need to consult an orthopedist immediately. The most likely diagnosis here is a meniscus injury—the mechanism of injury is typical, there is tenderness along the medial joint line, a serous effusion is present, and there is no evidence of fracture, major ligament instability, or hemarthrosis.

Figure 5–35 illustrates the general approach to the initial management of the acute knee injury.

What should be done now?

Mike is told that he has a torn cartilage that will likely repair itself over the next several weeks.

A posterior splint is applied to the knee; Mike is instructed in the use of crutches and told not to bear weight on the injured knee. Local ice and elevation of the leg for the next day or two are recommended. Mike is told to begin daily quadriceps setting (see page 240) exercises to preserve muscle tone but to avoid any other knee exercise for the time being.

Mike is told to return 3 days hence for a repeat examination.

NOTE

1. Unless there is obvious major internal derangement on examination, most acutely injured knees should be splinted (weight bearing forbidden), ice and aspirin recommended, and the patient should be reexamined in 2 to 3 days when, it is hoped, both swelling and muscle spasm will have lessened to allow more sensitive physical examination of ligamentous structures.

The posterior knee splint illustrated in Figure 5–36 is most helpful and convenient and should be worn 24 hours a day.

2. Quadriceps atrophy can be documented as early as 1 week following immobilization. More rapid functional recovery will result when measures are undertaken early to prevent even mild muscular weakness. Isometric exercises (especially simple quad setting) are always desirable. Isotonic exercises should be avoided initially.

3. Proof of a meniscus tear requires arthrography (Fig. 5–37), arthroscopy, surgical exploration or a combination of these. Indications for such procedures vary according to different authorities and different clinical circumstances. Since most acute meniscus injuries do not require surgery, and since conservative therapy usually suffices, the initial diagnosis is often based on the clinical history and examination without resorting to invasive procedures. (Exceptions include the competitive or professional athlete who cannot await the results of the conservative approach. Similarly, an acute knee injury, presumably a meniscus tear, in a patient whose knee will not "unlock" with simple manipulation—see Figure 5–38—is an orthopedic emergency who must be referred immediately.)

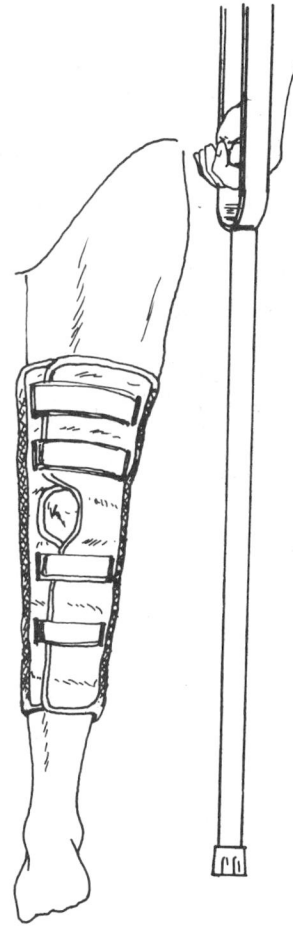

FIGURE 5–36. The posterior knee splint. The knee splint simply prevents flexion of the knee. Prevention of weight-bearing will, of course, be possible only if the patient also uses crutches.

Three days later, Mike returns for reexamination. There is now only a minimal knee effusion. Range of motion of the injured knee is normal except for mild discomfort and limitation at full extension. Muscle spasm has greatly diminished, and there is no ligamentous laxity of collateral or cruciate ligaments, although valgus stress elicits mild discomfort over the medial collateral ligament. There is persistent tenderness of the medial and posteromedial joint line. Rotational torque of the tibia on the femur elicits pain in the medial knee, especially on external tibial rotation, but rotatory testing otherwise reveals no click, crepitus, or palpable mass on palpation of the medial joint space during tibial rotation and full knee extension.

What does this mean?

1. Reexamination within a few days of the acute injury is essential if ligamentous tears are to be diagnosed or suspected early enough to allow an orthopedist to achieve optimal surgical repair. If doubt remains after several days about the integrity of the ligaments, an orthopedist must be consulted.

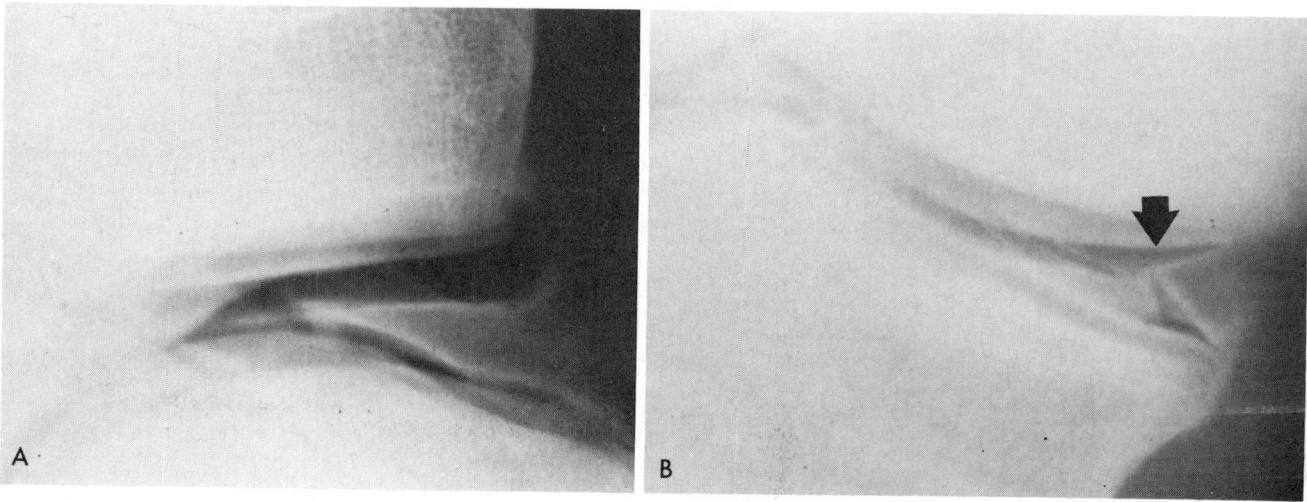

FIGURE 5–37. Arthrogram demonstrating torn meniscus. The normal meniscus on the lateral side (A) is compared here with the easily demonstrated tear in the medial meniscus in the same patient (B) (arrow).

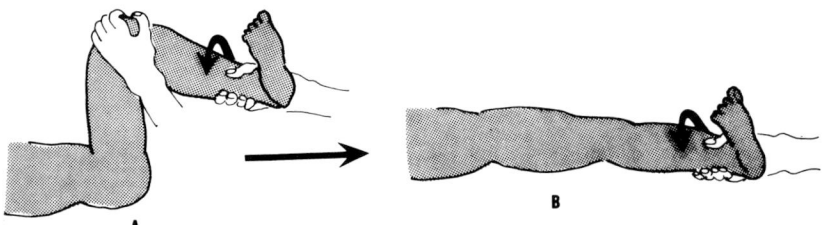

FIGURE 5–38. Manipulation of "locked knee." The purpose of manipulation to unlock the meniscus is to relieve pain and prevent further damage to the meniscus. A, In lateral meniscus the knee is fully flexed and some pressure is exerted to cause varus of the leg. B, The leg is externally rotated. Then the physician suddenly (but not forcefully) extends the leg A to B. For lesions of the medial meniscus, the opposite motion (internal rotation varus) is used. (Reproduced with permission from Cailliet, R: Knee and Pain Disability. Philadelphia: F.A. Davis Co., 1973, p. 53.)

2. In this case there is good evidence for a torn medial meniscus, perhaps with a strain of the medial collateral ligament. Tenderness along the collateral ligament in the setting of an acute injury may indicate either minor or serious ligament damage. In the absence, however, of any demonstrable ligamentous laxity, tenderness in this location probably indicates a strain which usually resolves uneventfully with conservative therapy.

3. Because there is clinical evidence for a medial meniscus injury and perhaps a strain of the medial collateral ligament, the anterior cruciate ligament must be carefully assessed. As the Appendix and Figure 5–30 indicate, injuries to the medial compartment commonly damage all three of these structures.

> Mike is told to continue the same treatment program. Reexamination 4 days later (now 1 week after injury) again reveals no pain, tenderness, or laxity on ligament testing. The effusion has completely resolved, but there remains mild tenderness of the medial joint space, especially with rotatory testing.
>
> Mike is kept in a splint and on crutches for the next 3 weeks. Resisted isometric straight leg raising exercises are begun, and 3 weeks later Mike is lifting 20 pounds without discomfort. Examination at this time reveals no quadriceps atrophy and a totally normal knee. The splint is removed, and Mike is told he can walk without crutches, but that he should continue with isotonic leg lifts up to 30 pounds for the next 3 weeks before resuming athletic activities.
>
> Three weeks later (a total of 6 weeks after injury), Mike is pronounced fit for further training and exercise.

Disability from meniscus injuries will usually resolve within several weeks if immobilization, isometric exercises, and isotonic exercises are undertaken in appropriate stages. Not infrequently, however, recurrent problems ensue.

> Six weeks later, Mike returns to the clinic, again with a swollen knee. Mike has resumed his usual activities and denies any specific injury or stress but has been playing competitive soccer daily for the past 2 weeks. Yesterday Mike noticed that his knee felt weak during a particularly arduous soccer practice, and last night he noted swelling of the knee. Mike says this is the first trouble he has had since his previous injury.
>
> Examination reveals a moderate intra-articular effusion in the right knee but otherwise normal findings except for mild discomfort medially with rotatory testing.

THE SWOLLEN KNEE

Swelling of the knee[4, 32, 33] usually implies an intra-articular effusion, and careful examination (see above) will distinguish this from extra-articular (usually bursal) fluid collections, bony protuberance (degenerative arthritis, Charcot's joints), or soft-tissue swellings (synovial proliferation, bursae, meniscal cysts, hypertrophied fat pads, for example). Recognition of these other types of swellings is discussed above.

The clinical approach to an unexplained knee effusion should involve several caveats:

1. The entire patient must be examined. As is suggested from Table 5–6, the differential diagnosis of polyarthritis involving the knee is different from that of the isolated knee effusion. All other joints must be examined for range of motion and effusions.

Similarly, arthritis of the knee is often a result of systemic disease—the patient should be carefully questioned about other symptoms (fever, venereal disease symptoms, inflammatory bowel disease, jaundice, for example), medications (diuretics induce gout, for example), and prior joint disease. The patient's temperature should always be recorded.

2. Is the effusion acute, or is it chronic and recurrent? Most acute monoarticular knee effusions are traumatic (due to meniscal tears, ligament strains, traumatic synovitis, and the like). Trauma may, however, be trivial

TABLE 5–6. DIFFERENTIAL DIAGNOSIS OF POLYARTHRITIS INVOLVING THE KNEE AND MONARTHRITIS OF THE KNEE

MONARTHRITIS OF THE KNEE

Acute	*Chronic*
Septic arthritis*	Rheumatoid arthritis
Gonococcal arthritis*	Osteoarthritis
Osteomyelitis	Internal derangement
Gout	Osteochondritis dissecans
Pseudogout	Chronic infection (TB, fungal)
Trauma	Sarcoid
Internal derangement	Pigmented villonodular synovitis
Hemorrhage	Synovial chondromatosis
Rheumatoid arthritis	Synovial sarcoma
Palindromic rheumatism	
Intermittent hydrarthrosis	

POLYARTHRITIS INVOLVING THE KNEE

Acute	*Chronic*
Rheumatic fever	Rheumatoid arthritis
Rheumatoid arthritis	SLE
SLE	Other connective tissue diseases
Gonococcal arthritis	Osteoarthritis
Reiter's syndrome	Psoriatic arthritis
Sarcoidosis	Reiter's syndrome
Erythema nodosum	Inflammatory bowel disease
Serum sickness	Gout
Sickle cell disease	Pseudogout
Rubella	Sarcoidosis
Hepatitis	Neoplasia
Inflammatory bowel disease	
Endocarditis	
Gout	

*Gonococcal arthritis is, of course, one subset of septic arthritis.
Adapted from Reference 34.

or remote. Remember also that trauma may occasionally precipitate non-traumatic monarthritis, especially the crystalline diseases (gout and pseudogout).

When trauma cannot be implicated, the differential diagnosis of acute monarticular knee arthritis is very different from that of chronic monarticular arthritis (Table 5–6).

3. The synovial fluid should be aspirated[35] for diagnostic testing.

Arthrocentesis and Synovial Fluid Analysis

The knee is the easiest joint to tap. Strict aseptic technique is crucial. The skin at the site of the needle entrance is usually anesthetized with local anesthesia, but some clinicians do not do so since "one needle is better than two." As Figure 5–39 illustrates, the joint is entered between the posterior surface of the patella and the articular surface of the femoral condyles, with the knee relaxed and extended. Lateral entry is most often recommended, but medial entry is easy as well. Manual compression of the contralateral side of the joint may bring dependent joint fluid toward the aspirating needle and result in greater success.

Gross inspection of synovial fluid is only sometimes helpful. As noted above, hemarthrosis raises specific questions (Table 5–3). Cloudy, turbid fluid is common in septic arthritis, but other inflammatory disorders may result in a similar gross appearance.

Synovial fluid analysis[36–39] should always include total cell count with differential count, Gram's stain, bacterial cultures, and a search for crystals. Many other determinations may occasionally be helpful (LE preparation, glucose, complement, TB cultures, for instance), but these are expensive and only rarely useful.

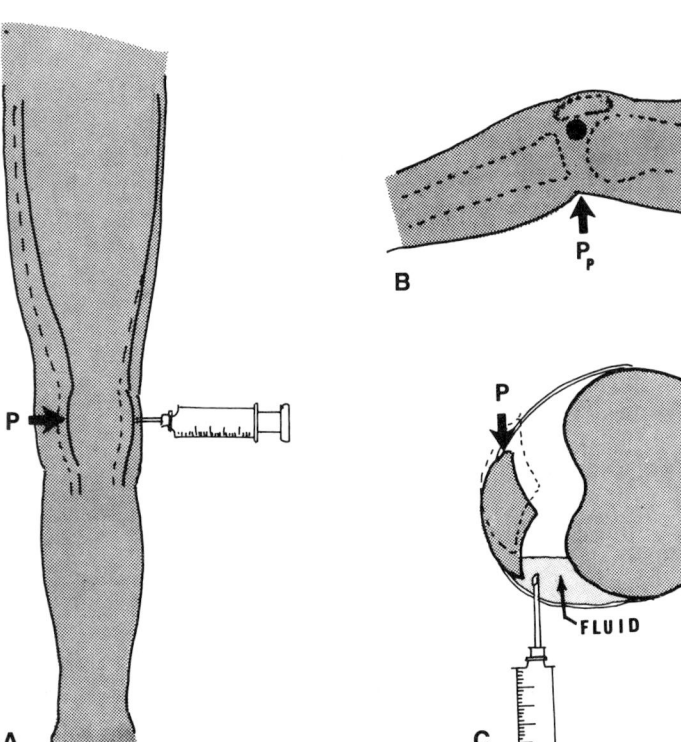

FIGURE 5–39. Knee aspiration technique. *A,* Patella (P) is moved laterally. *B,* Lateral view of site of injection (black dot). Pressure upon popliteal space (P$_p$) brings fluid toward needle tip. *C,* In lateral position, gravity localizes fluid to permit easier withdrawal. Knee aspiration from the medial side is just as easy. (Reproduced with permission from Cailliet, R: Soft Tissue Pain and Disability. Philadelphia: F.A. Davis Co., 1977, p. 245.)

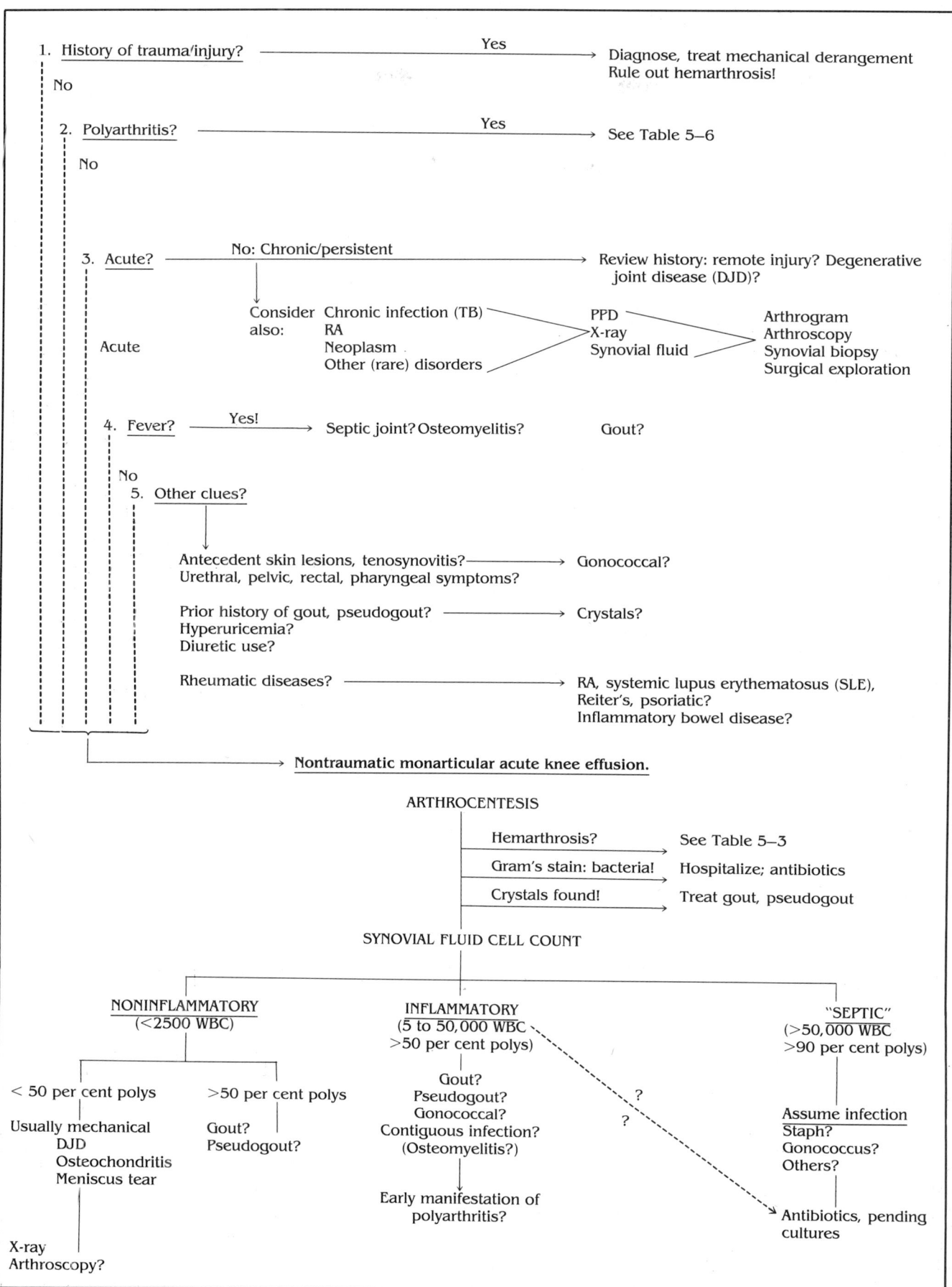

1. History of trauma/injury? ——————————— Yes ——→ Diagnose, treat mechanical derangement
   No   Rule out hemarthrosis!

2. Polyarthritis? ——————————————— Yes ——→ See Table 5—6
   No

3. Acute? ——————— No: Chronic/persistent ————————————→ Review history: remote injury? Degenerative
                                                                            joint disease (DJD)?

          Consider   Chronic infection (TB)   PPD   Arthrogram
          also: RA   X-ray   Arthroscopy
   Acute   Neoplasm   Synovial fluid   Synovial biopsy
                      Other (rare) disorders   Surgical exploration

4. Fever? —— Yes! ——→ Septic joint? Osteomyelitis?   Gout?
   No
   5. Other clues?

      Antecedent skin lesions, tenosynovitis? ————————→ Gonococcal?
      Urethral, pelvic, rectal, pharyngeal symptoms?

      Prior history of gout, pseudogout? ——————→ Crystals?
      Hyperuricemia?
      Diuretic use?

      Rheumatic diseases? ————————————————→ RA, systemic lupus erythematosus (SLE),
                                                            Reiter's, psoriatic?
                                                            Inflammatory bowel disease?

   ——→ **Nontraumatic monarticular acute knee effusion.**

                    ARTHROCENTESIS

                    Hemarthrosis? ————————→ See Table 5—3
                    Gram's stain: bacteria! ——→ Hospitalize; antibiotics
                    Crystals found! ——————→ Treat gout, pseudogout

                 SYNOVIAL FLUID CELL COUNT

   NONINFLAMMATORY   INFLAMMATORY   "SEPTIC"
   (<2500 WBC)   (5 to 50,000 WBC   (>50,000 WBC
                                >50 per cent polys)   >90 per cent polys)

   < 50 per cent polys   >50 per cent polys   Gout?
                                              Pseudogout?   ?
   Usually mechanical   Gout?   Gonococcal?   ?   Assume infection
   DJD   Pseudogout?   Contiguous infection?   Staph?
   Osteochondritis   (Osteomyelitis?)   Gonococcus?
   Meniscus tear   Others?

                                              Early manifestation of
                                              polyarthritis?   Antibiotics, pending
   X-ray   cultures
   Arthroscopy?

FIGURE 5—40. Knee effusion: an approach.

Normal joint fluid contains 200 to 300 (usually mononuclear or synovial) cells.

Mechanical (traumatic) and degenerative disorders (degenerative arthritis, osteochondritis dissecans, for example) usually are associated with "noninflammatory" effusions: fewer than 2500 white blood cells (less than 50 per cent polymorphonuclear).

Some patients with gout and pseudogout may have "noninflammatory" total cell counts, but usually there is a predominance of polymorphonuclear cells in such fluid. The importance of searches for crystals under polarized microscopy as a routine procedure must be emphasized.

Noninfectious inflammatory diseases (rheumatoid arthritis, systemic lupus, gout, pseudogout) usually produce fluid with cell counts in the "inflammatory" category: 5000 to 50,000 white blood cells (greater than 60 per cent polymorphonuclear). Usually the clinical setting and other findings help distinguish among these disorders (Table 5–7).

Septic (bacterial) arthritis[40–42] usually is associated with a "septic fluid profile"—greater than 50,000 white blood cells, 90 per cent or more polymorphonuclear. A significant minority of patients with septic arthritis (perhaps 30 per cent) may have initial cell counts under 50,000, but a repeat tap within 1 to 2 days will often then reveal "transition" to the higher cell count (greater than 50,000). (The most common cause of septic arthritis is gonococcal arthritis. Since Gram's stain and even subsequent cultures may sometimes be nondiagnostic in patients with gonococcal arthritis, this diagnosis must often be *presumed* because of concomitant venereal symptoms, antecedent tenosynovitis, or characteristic skin findings (see Chapter 8, "Male Genitourinary Infections").

There is, then, considerable overlap in synovial fluid profiles among noninflammatory, inflammatory, and septic disorders. Nevertheless, the clinical setting, the distinction between monoarticular and polyarticular disease, and the synovial fluid analysis will usually point to the correct diagnosis, as outlined in Figure 5–40. More than half of all cases of acute, nontraumatic monoarthritis of the knee can be diagnosed immediately by clinical examination and synovial fluid analysis (and sometimes x-rays)—Table 5–7.

> **Mike is afebrile. There is no history of other systemic symptoms, exposure to venereal disease, or use of medications recently.**
>
> **Arthrocentesis of Mike's right knee demonstrates 30 cc of clear yellow fluid with 700 white blood cells, 70 per cent mononuclear or synovial. Gram's stain and crystal searches are negative. A repeat knee x-ray is normal.**

What does this mean?

MONARTHRITIS OF THE KNEE

Mike has a noninflammatory monoarticular knee effusion that has arisen soon after a traumatic knee injury (the presumed meniscal tear 6 weeks before). While a specific diagnosis cannot be proven without further testing (arthroscopy, for example), it is most likely that the knee effusion is due to the former mechanical injury to the knee. Recurrent knee effusion and disability are among several reasons to consider definitive testing and surgical repair of a torn meniscus. Others include repetitive locking, buckling, or recurrent pain.

TABLE 5–7. ACUTE MONARTHRITIS OF THE KNEE

Disease	Consider When	Synovial Fluid	X-Rays	Diagnosis
Mechanical disorders (meniscus, ligament, osteochondritis, etc.)	Trauma history; known internal derangement; suggestive exam	Noninflammatory	May be diagnostic: fracture? osteochondritis: (Fig. 5–3A) loose bodies?	Exam; x-ray; arthroscopy?; arthrogram?
Degenerative arthritis	Older patient, or history of remote trauma; exam: crepitus, bony proliferation	Noninflammatory	Usually diagnostic (Figs. 5–3B and 5–41)	X-ray and exam

Remember: Look for crystals: superimposed gout or pseudogout? Charcot's joint?

Infection

Gonococcal[44, 45]	Young, sexually active; venereal symptoms (urethral discharge, pelvic pain); and/or characteristic skin lesions; and/or antecedent polyarthritis, tenosynovitis, fever; painful joint motion	Inflammatory (usually septic profile); Gram's stain often negative; culture immediately on Thayer-Martin medium	Not helpful	Synovial fluid cultures and Gram's stain; blood culture; culture from other sites

Remember: Culture on specific media specimens from pharynx, rectum, cervix, urethra! (Joint and blood cultures may be negative.)

Staph aureus[40–42] (and some others)	Fever; very painful joint motion; diabetes; antecedent joint disease (rheumatoid arthritis); recent arthrocentesis; immunosuppressed	Inflammatory (usually septic profile); low glucose; Gram's stain may be negative	Not helpful acutely; serial x-rays and/or bone scan may help	Positive culture

Remember: Rule out concomitant osteomyelitis

Osteomyelitis[46] with "sympathetic effusion"	"Clinically septic"; bony tenderness; bacteremia	Inflammatory (>50,000); normal glucose; Gram's stain and culture negative	Bone scan may be positive in 3–7 days; x-rays negative for weeks (Fig. 5–42)	Positive blood culture; positive biopsy (bone) culture

Crystalline disorders

Gout[47]	Adult male (rare in females); prior podagra; increased blood uric acid; diuretics?	Inflammatory, usually; linear, needle-shaped, strongly birefringent crystals (monosodium urate)	Not helpful	Crystals identified!

Remember: Trauma may initiate! May have fever!

Pseudogout[48]	Sudden onset; either sex; often middle aged/elderly; knee most common	Inflammatory (usually); linear or rhomboid, weakly or negatively birefringent (calcium pyrophosphate) crystals	Calcified cartilage identified occasionally (Fig. 5–43)	Crystals identified!

Remember: Usually idiopathic, but may be secondary to hyperparathyroidism, Wilson's disease, hemochromatosis, renal disease

Systemic diseases with monarticular presentations	Suspect: SLE, rheumatoid arthritis, Reiter's, inflammatory bowel disease, ankylosing spondylitis, sarcoidosis, vasculitis, hepatitis, Behçet's syndrome, Henoch-Schonlein disease, Whipple's disease, familial Mediterranean fever	Inflammatory (5000–50,000)	Usually not helpful	Specific tests: ANA, rheumatoid factor, biopsies; other clinical findings

Miscellaneous
Intermittent[4, 34] hydrarthrosis

Hypermobile joints[4] (genu recurvatum)

Mike is told that we do not know the cause of his knee problem, but we suggest an orthopedic consultation since it seems likely that a meniscal tear is responsible for his knee effusion. A posterior splint, crutches, and quadriceps setting exercises are resumed.

An orthopedic consultation 1 week later reveals a persistent synovial effusion, which on repeat synovial fluid analysis is unchanged. Previous fluid cultures are sterile, as is a tuberculin skin test. Arthroscopy is recommended by the orthopedist, but Mike refuses. Conservative therapy is again initiated and, 1 month later, Mike is exercising again.

Over the next 3 months, however, Mike develops intermittent knee pains, occasionally associated with temporary locking of the knee and associated with recurrent knee effusions. Mike is convinced to undergo arthroscopy and subsequent surgical repair. A torn medial meniscus is repaired uneventfully, and ultimately there is full functional recovery.

While Mike's problem is fairly straightforward, given his recurrent mechanical knee problems and the prior history of injury, sometimes monarthritis of the knee[43] remains unexplained. As Table 5–7 illustrates, the clinical findings, synovial fluid analysis, and x-rays (Figs. 5–41 through 5–47) usually point to a specific diagnosis. When this is not the case, it is often necessary to treat the patient symptomatically (rest and anti-inflammatory drugs) and to follow the subsequent course of events. When symptoms persist, repeat arthrocentesis, with careful fluid analysis for crystalline disease, and a review of cell counts and cultures will sometimes provide a diagnosis initally missed.[43] Most such confusing cases will resolve spontaneously even if a specific diagnosis is not made.

However, when monarthritis persists without explanation for 4 to 6 weeks, an orthopedist or rheumatologist or both should be consulted. In such patients, further evaluation may require an arthrogram or arthroscopy if an internal derangement is suspected, while synovial biopsy or even surgical

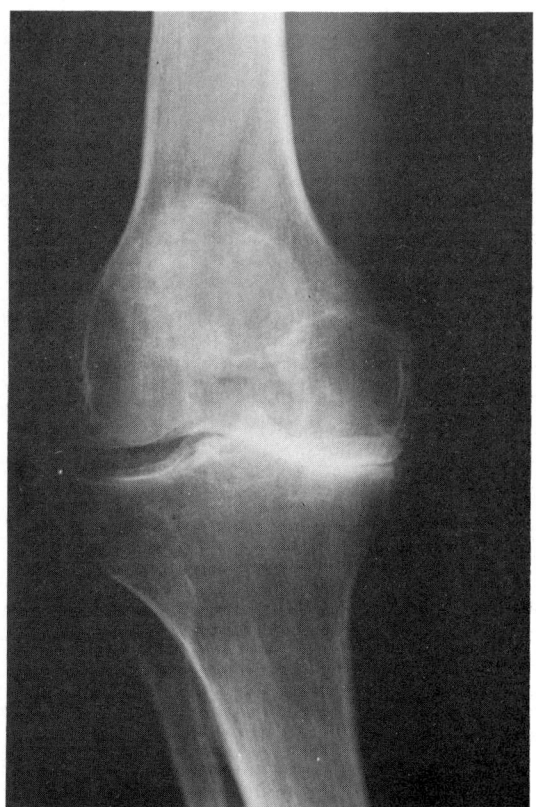

FIGURE 5–41. Degenerative arthritis of the knee. This 63-year-old man complained of chronic pain, stiffness, and swelling of both knees. X-ray of the knee demonstrates extensive degenerative arthritis with marked narrowing of the medial joint space and hypertrophic bony changes throughout the joint. Joint fluid contained 45 white blood cells. There is a valgus deformity of the knee due to the osteoarthritis. This patient ultimately required a total knee replacement for amelioration of symptoms.

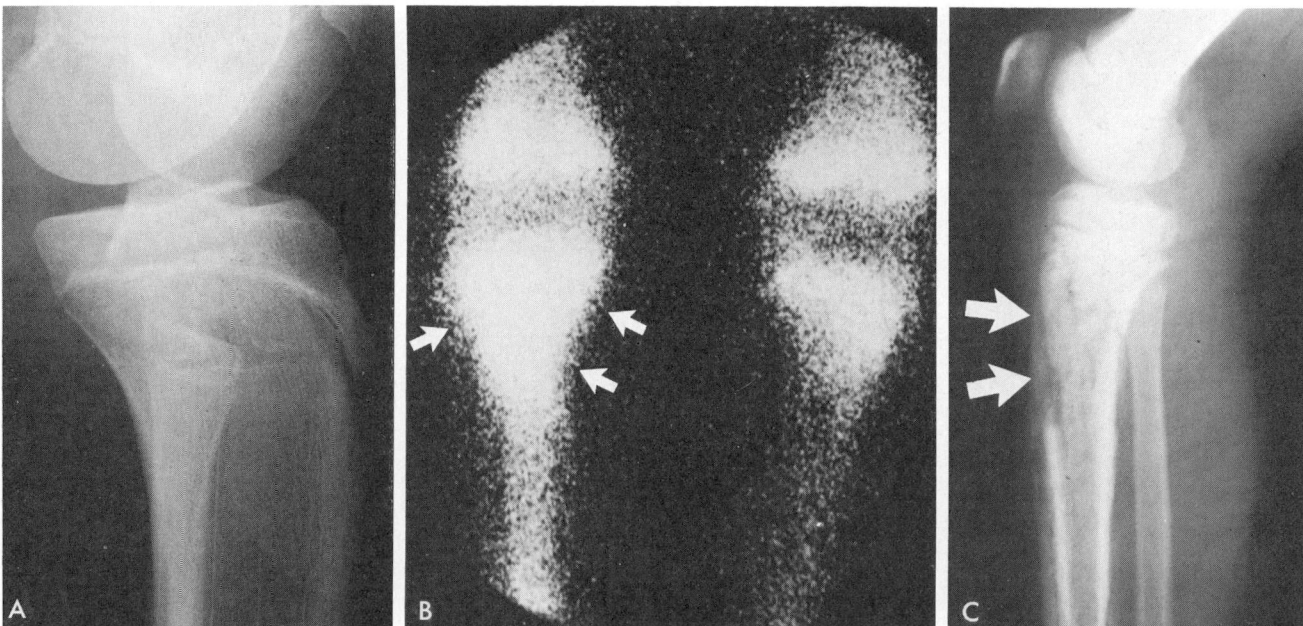

FIGURE 5–42. Osteomyelitis of the tibia. This 14-year-old girl complained of 6 weeks of right knee pain. Examination revealed a low-grade fever (37.7°C.), moderate tenderness of the proximal tibia, and a moderate knee effusion. Arthrocentesis demonstrated inflammatory cells (20,000; 75 per cent polys) without microorganisms. The initial x-ray is unimpressive (A). Bone scan (B) performed on the same day is dramatically "hot." X-rays performed 4 weeks hence (during parenteral antibiotic therapy for *Staphylococcus aureus* osteomyelitis, proven on open biopsy) reveal more "classic" changes of osteomyelitis (C).

Remember that the x-ray may be unimpressive early in osteomyelitis!

FIGURE 5–43. Pseudogout. This 79-year-old man developed an acutely painful and swollen left knee. X-ray demonstrates calcification of the knee cartilage bilaterally (arrow). Arthrocentesis demonstrated inflammatory synovial fluid with visible calcium pyrophosphate crystals on polarized microscopy.

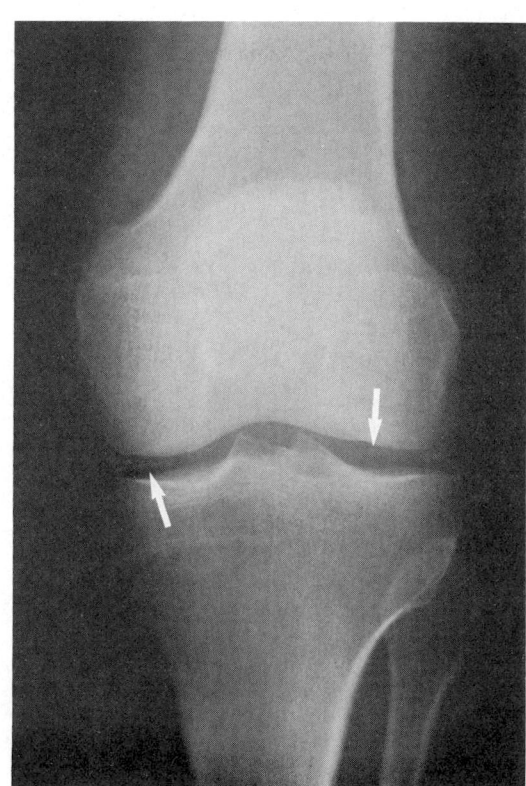

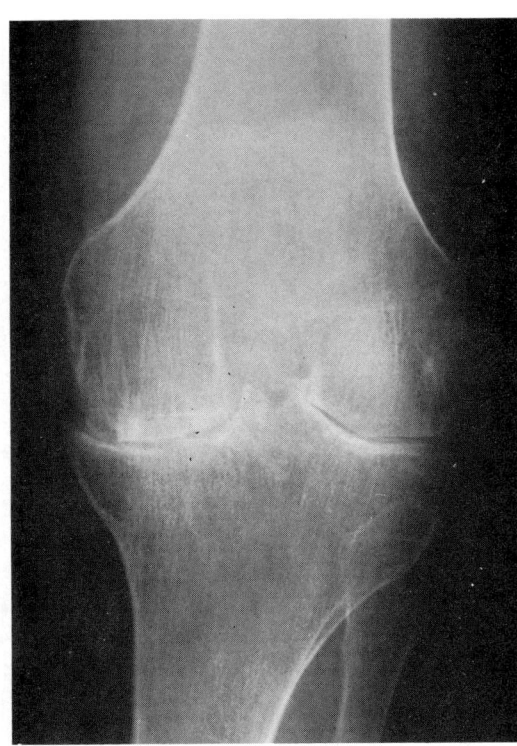

FIGURE 5–44. Severe rheumatoid arthritis of the knee. There is marked osteopenia around the knee joint, diffuse joint space narrowing, and cystic bone reabsorption on both sides of the knee joint. There is also marked soft tissue (synovial) swelling.

exploration may be needed to exclude chronic infection or other rare diseases. Some causes of this unusual problem (unexplained, persistent monarthritis of the knee) include:

Rheumatoid arthritis, especially the juvenile variety, may produce an indolent, inflammatory monarthritis of the knee. The diagnosis may be difficult, since many "specific" tests—rheumatoid factors, synovial biopsies—may be nondiagnostic. Usually, over time, polyarthritis becomes obvious (Fig. 5–44).

Chronic infection, especially tuberculosis,[49] should be considered. While synovial fluid findings are variable in tuberculosis, there is usually inflammatory fluid (10,000 to 20,000 cells with 50 to 70 per cent polymorphonuclear); the purified protein derivative (PPD) skin test is almost always positive; and cultures of the fluid (80 per cent) or synovial biopsy (90 per cent) are usually positive after incubation for several weeks. Acid-fast stains of the synovial fluid are usually negative (80 per cent), however, and a presumptive diagnosis must often be made to initiate specific therapy before culture results are available. Nontuberculous mycobacteria and fungi may also produce chronic monarthritis.

Pigmented villonodular synovitis[50] is a rare disorder, usually considered a benign neoplasm, that produces nodular villous growth throughout the involved synovium. Hemarthrosis or xanthochromic synovial fluid is a clue to the diagnosis, but synovial biopsy or exploration is required to clinch the diagnosis (Fig. 5–45).

Synovial chondromatosis[51] is a benign metaplasia of synovium that induces a nodular cartilaginous proliferation within the synovium. Recurrent pain, joint effusion, and limitation of motion are common, and surgery (synovectomy) may be needed when symptoms persist. When the cartilage calcifies, a typical radiographic appearance may be highly suggestive (Fig. 5–46).

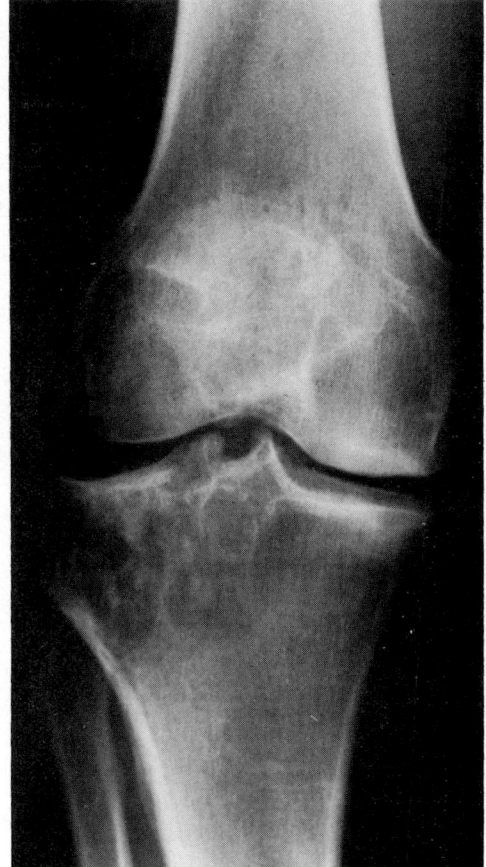

FIGURE 5–45. Pigmented villonodular synovitis. This 47-year-old woman presented with a history of recurrent knee pain and undiagnosed knee effusion. Arthrocentesis on two occasions revealed dark bloody fluid. The x-ray demonstrates destructive changes in the lateral tibia, compatible with some "invasive" process in the bone or joint or both. Total synovectomy resulted in cure.

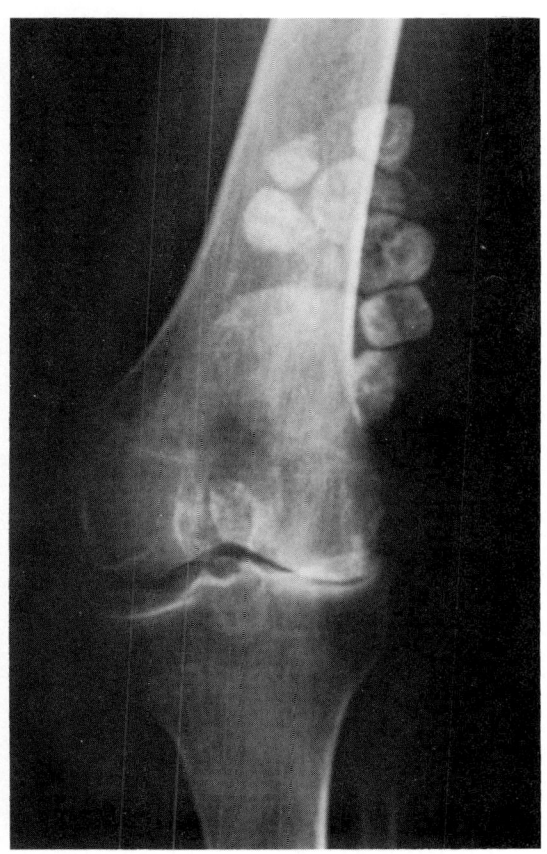

FIGURE 5–46. Synovial chondromatosis. This 50-year-old woman presented with recurrent pain, limitation of motion, and an unexplained knee effusion. There are multiple "popcorn" calcifications overlying the distal femur. Synovectomy abolished most symptoms, but there is degenerative disease here as well.

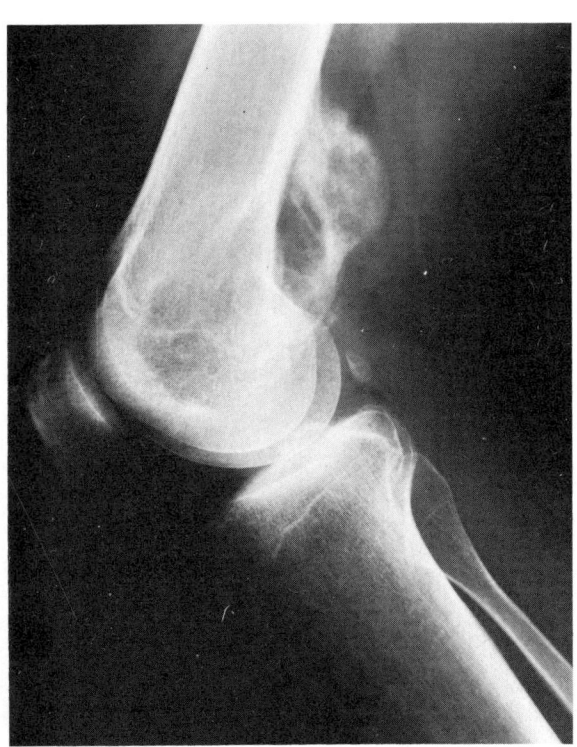

FIGURE 5–47. Osteogenic sarcoma. There is a large, expanding bony lesion of the posterior distal femur.

Synovial sarcoma[52] is a malignant synovial neoplasm that often presents as a soft-tissue mass, with or without calcification or contiguous osteolytic bony defects on x-ray.

Metastatic neoplasms are rare around the knee and usually occur only with advanced and obvious metastatic disease. Osteogenic sarcoma (Fig. 5–47) and other primary malignant tumors of bone usually are demonstrated on x-ray.

Mechanical derangements are probably the most common cause of chronic knee effusions. Examination, arthrography, arthroscopy, and/or exploration may be needed to make the diagnosis.

Osteochondritis dissecans, gout, pseudogout, and inadequately treated bacterial infection (especially monarticular gonococcal infection) may also cause chronic or persistent effusions, but x-rays and synovial fluid analysis will usually be diagnostic in these cases.

Functional Knee Anatomy[4-7, 53, 54]

The knee comprises two separate but interdependent joints—the tibiofemoral and the patellofemoral. The weight-bearing function of the knee involves primarily the tibiofemoral joint: apposing osteochondral surfaces of the femur and tibia, interposed fibrocartilaginous menisci that distribute pressures between those bony surfaces during weight bearing, and ligaments that stabilize this articulation and limit its mobility within physiologic, functional ranges of motion. Tibiofemoral motion is largely one-dimensional—flexion/extension is the primary plane of movement (some tibiofemoral rotation also occurs—see below). Knee flexion is powered primarily by the hamstring muscles. Knee extension is a complex biomechanical action that is powered by the quadriceps muscles but is given leverage by the patellofemoral—or extensor—mechanism.

The extensor mechanism includes the quadriceps muscles, the patella, the articular surface between patella and femur, and the tendinous attachments among these structures (Fig. 5–48).

The quadriceps muscles (Fig. 5–49) include the rectus femoris (which originates from the anterior inferior iliac spine) and the three vasti—vastus medialis, vastus lateralis, and vastus intermedius (all of which originate from the proximal femoral shaft). These four powerful muscles run downward and inward to converge into a common palpable tendon above the patella, part of which then crosses the tibiofemoral joint and inserts into the tibial tubercle. Contraction of these muscles thus extends the tibia on the femur. Other components of the quadriceps tendon insert directly into the patella: the vastus medialis especially centralizes and stabilizes the patella by exerting medial, as well as cephalad, pull (Fig. 5–50). (The vastus lateralis pulls

FIGURE 5–48. The exterior mechanism. The quadriceps extends over the anterior knee joint with three ligamentous extensions: 1, the epicondylopatellar portion attaches to the epicondyle eminence of the femur and guides rotation of the patella; 2, the meniscopatellar attaches to and pulls the meniscus forward during knee extension; and 3, the infrapatellar tendon, which attaches to the tibial tubercle and extends the tibia upon the femur. (Reproduced with permission from Cailliet, R.: Soft Tissue Pain and Disability. Philadelphia: F.A. Davis Co., 1977, p. 225.)

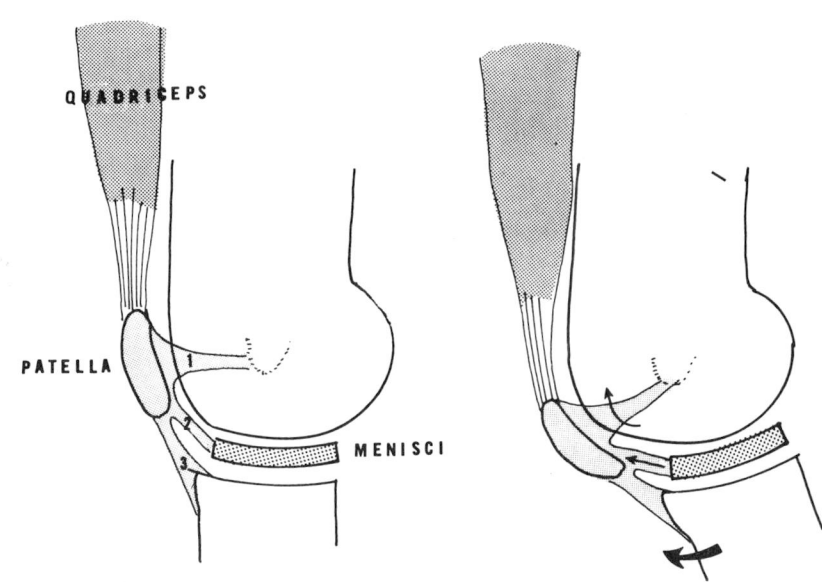

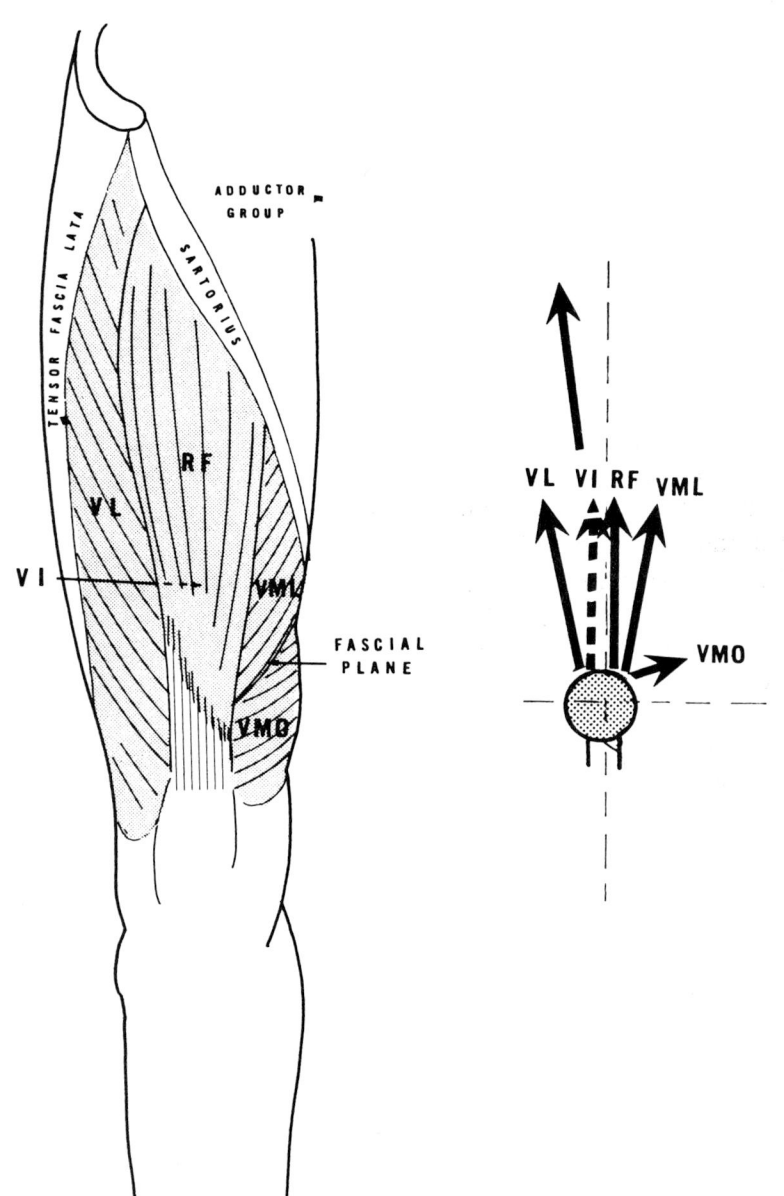

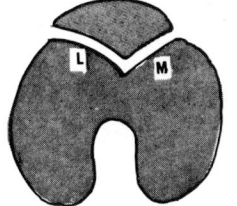

FIGURE 5–49. The quadriceps muscles. Quadriceps femoris: function of quadriceps mechanism. Each long component of the quadriceps group (RF, rectus femoris; VL, vastus lateralis; VI, vastus intermedius; VM, vastus medialis) can extend the knee fully. The vastus medialis oblique fibers, VMO, cannot extend the knee but apparently pull the patella medially *(right)* and keep it centered against lateral pull of the quadriceps *(arrows)*. All long components pull equally throughout extension range, with VMO exerting twice the force of contraction. (Reproduced with permission from Cailliet, R: Knee Pain and Disability. Philadelphia: F.A. Davis Co., 1973, p. 17.)

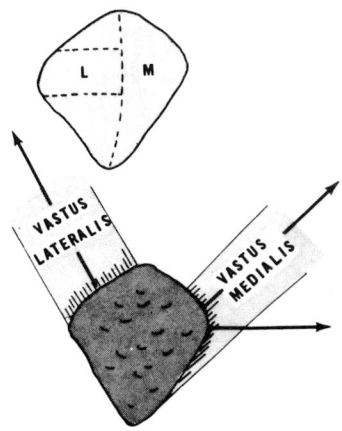

FIGURE 5–50. Patella. *Above,* Patellofemoral articulation. The lateral condyles are broader and more concave than the medial. *Center,* Facet planes of the patella on the articular surface: three planes on the lateral half and one plane on the medial. *Below,* Muscle pull upon the patella, with the vastus lateralis muscle pulling cephalad. The vastus medialis muscle, by attaching lower and more laterally, exerts medial pull, thus centralizing and stabilizing the patella. (Reproduced with permission from Cailliet, R: Soft Tissue Pain and Disability. Philadelphia: F.A. Davis Co., 1977, p. 233.)

primarily cephalad.) Quadriceps contraction thus moves the patella cephalad during extension. Still other fibers of the quadriceps tendon attach the patella to the femoral epidondyles and to the meniscus of the tibiofemoral joint. Quadriceps contraction thus moves the meniscus anteriorly as the knee extends. Figures 5–48 through 5–50 illustrate some of these relationships.

The patella—an asymmetric sesamoid bone—is "contained within" the quadriceps tendon, and its posterior surface articulates with the concave intercondylar groove between the femoral epicondyles. The patella moves within that groove cephalad and caudad as the knee extends and flexes respectively. In full knee extension, the patella lies above the femoral condyles in contact with a suprapatellar fat pad; progressive knee flexion produces increasing contact between patella and the femoral groove (see also Fig. 5–19).

This patellofemoral arrangement confers certain mechanical advantages on the tibiofemoral joint as the latter flexes and extends. These mechanical advantages are lost, however, if the patella is unstable (Fig. 5–21) within the intercondylar groove, if the geometry of the patellotibial tendon is askew, or if the composite "direction of pull" (the Q angle) of the quadriceps apparatus is abnormal (Fig. 5–51). Such abnormal patellofemoral mechanics will create one or more of the patellofemoral syndromes discussed in the text. When the patella is a peculiar shape; or is anomalously located (for example, "high riding" or patella alta; "low riding" or patella baja); or is powered by

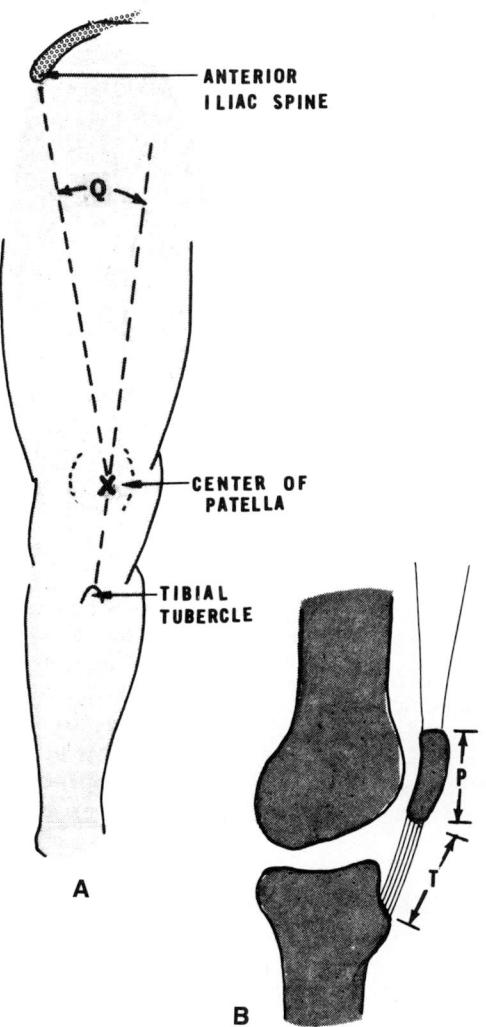

FIGURE 5–51. Q angle A, The Q angle is drawn from a line originating at the anterior iliac spine to the center of the patella (essentially the direction of pull of the quadriceps) and a line from the center of the tibial tubercle to the center of the patella. Normal is considered to be 20 degrees or less.
B, Patella-tendon ratio. Roentgenographic measurement of the length of the patella (P) compared with the length of infrapatellar ligament (T) determines the height the patella rides. T should equal P. If T is longer, it indicates a high-riding patella (patella alta). (Reproduced with permission from Cailliet, R: Soft Tissue Pain and Disability. Philadelphia: F.A. Davis Co., 1977, p. 234.)

discordant quadriceps muscles (for example, when the vastus medialis is weak and the Q angle is wide), patellofemoral articulation may be abnormal (resulting in chondromalacia patellae), or the quadriceps apparatus may be subjected to unusual stresses (resulting in patellar tendinitis, for example). Since the full and normal function of the tibiofemoral joint depends on coordinated, painless extensor mechanics, both weight bearing and walking will be impaired by extensor mechanism disorders (see page 233).

INTERNAL KNEE ANATOMY

A few simple observations of the normal knee during sitting and weight bearing and during flexion and extension illustrate important facts about the internal mechanics of the knee (Fig. 5–52).

While the primary plane of motion of the tibiofemoral joint is flexion/extension, tibiofemoral rotation also occurs, especially at the completion of knee extension. As Figure 5–53 illustrates, the tibia rotates laterally (externally) as the knee moves from flexion into extension. The bony contour of the apposing (convex) femoral condyles and (concave) tibial plateau dictates that full knee extension is characterized by a locking of the femoral condyle into the tibia. This "screw-home" motion results from the longer anteroposterior diameter of the medial compared with the lateral femoral condyle (Fig. 5–53). Because the knee is locked in full extension, rotation (or any other joint motion) is impossible with the knee fully extended. The knee ligaments (see below) are also taut with the knee fully extended—capsular and collateral ligaments thus prevent tibiofemoral motion in the coronal plane; cruciate ligaments check any anteroposterior glide of the femur on the tibia.* <u>Try this for yourself:</u> Stand with the knee fully extended and try to pivot on that

---

*Note that descriptions of tibiofemoral motion depend on whether the leg is weight bearing—when it is, the femur moves "on" the tibia; when not, the tibia moves "on" the femur.

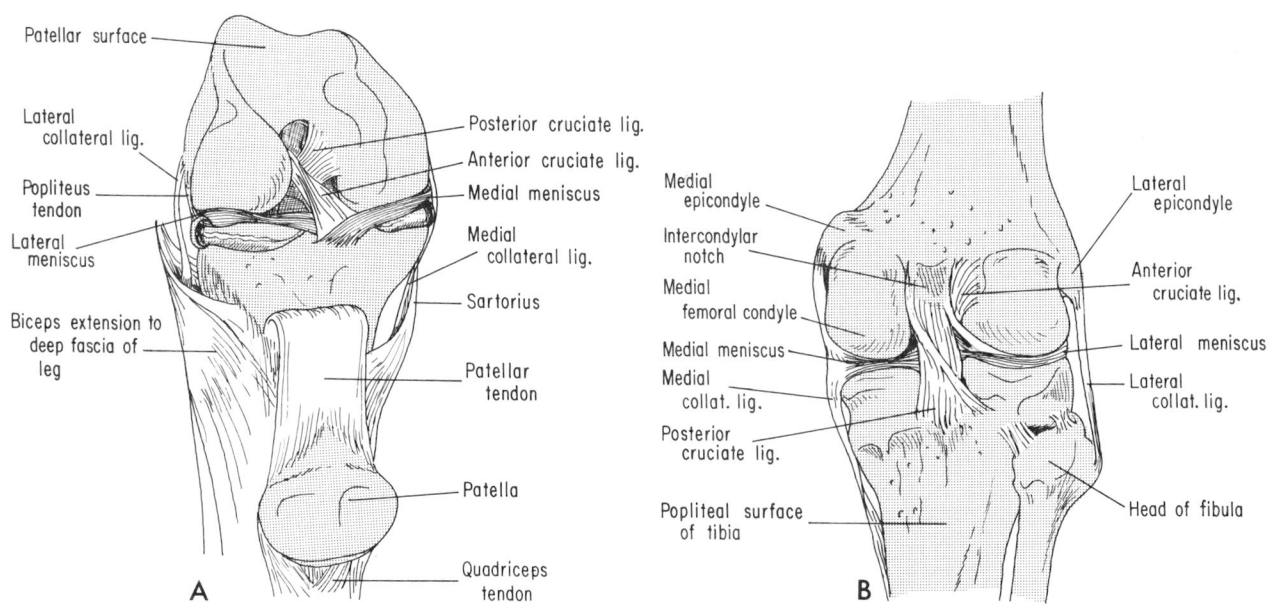

FIGURE 5–52. "Internal anatomy" of the knee. *A,* Anterior view. The knee is flexed, and the patella is "stripped" downward to better illustrate "internal" structure. *B,* Posterior view.

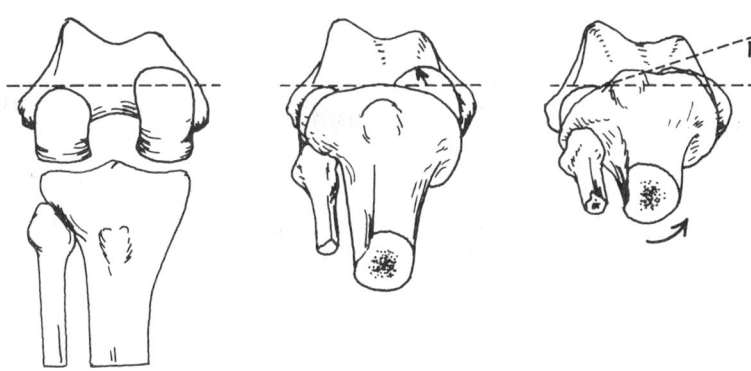

FIGURE 5-53. In the non–weight-bearing position, full extension of the knee involves external rotation of the tibia—the "screw home" motion.

foot in either direction—the knee is locked, and rotation cannot occur at the knee (and will be possible only at the hip and ankle). The pivot (or the "cut" in sports jargon) is crucial to coordinated walking and directional change; rotation at the knee allows the pivot—flexion of the knee allows rotation.

Knee flexion thus begins with unlocking the bony contours of the tibiofemoral articulation. The tibia rotates medially (internally) as the screw-home motion is reversed. The ligaments slacken to allow further mobility. Further flexion then allows fuller tibiofemoral rotation that is passively permitted by slackened ligaments and actively guided by an elaborate figure-of-eight mechanism, as described by Helfet.[7] As Figure 5–54 illustrates, tibiofemoral rotation is "tracked" by the menisci and "checked" by the cruciate ligaments.

The menisci are fibrocartilaginous, semilunar "discs" that move in association with tibiofemoral joint movement—in flexion, extension, and rotation. The medial meniscus is a C-shaped wedge that attaches around its entire periphery to the medial joint capsule and also adheres to the tibial tubercle, anterior cruciate ligament, and lateral meniscus (see also Fig. 5–32). The lateral meniscus, a more oval-shaped structure, attaches its anterior and posterior horns to the medial meniscus and posterior cruciate respectively, but its periphery normally has few capsular attachments (this relative "freedom" of the lateral meniscus is one reason the medial meniscus is more commonly damaged).

That the menisci form the track for tibiofemoral movement can be appreciated by examining yourself. Try this: Sit with your knee flexed and foot dangling. Palpate the medial joint line of that knee while internally and externally rotating the non–weight-bearing tibia, i.e., turn the foot and lower leg in and out. In external rotation the medial joint space feels empty, while internal rotation then "fills in" the empty space as the medial meniscus moves anteriorly. Similarly, extension of the knee will also displace the medial meniscus anteriorly—the hollow is palpable with the knee flexed but is "filled in" in extension. Appreciating that the menisci move during tibiofemoral movement can help in understanding how menisci are injured. Figure 5–31 illustrates various sudden movements that result in combinations of tibiofemoral rotation and flexion, extension, or thigh adduction that might trap the meniscus and "shear" its substance during nonphysiologic rotatory stresses. Figure 5–31A, for example, shows the soccer player with the knee flexed and the tibia externally rotated in preparation for a kick. Sudden forceful extension of the knee with the foot trapped in external rotation could then tear the meniscus.

The "checking action" of the cruciate ligaments is illustrated in Figure

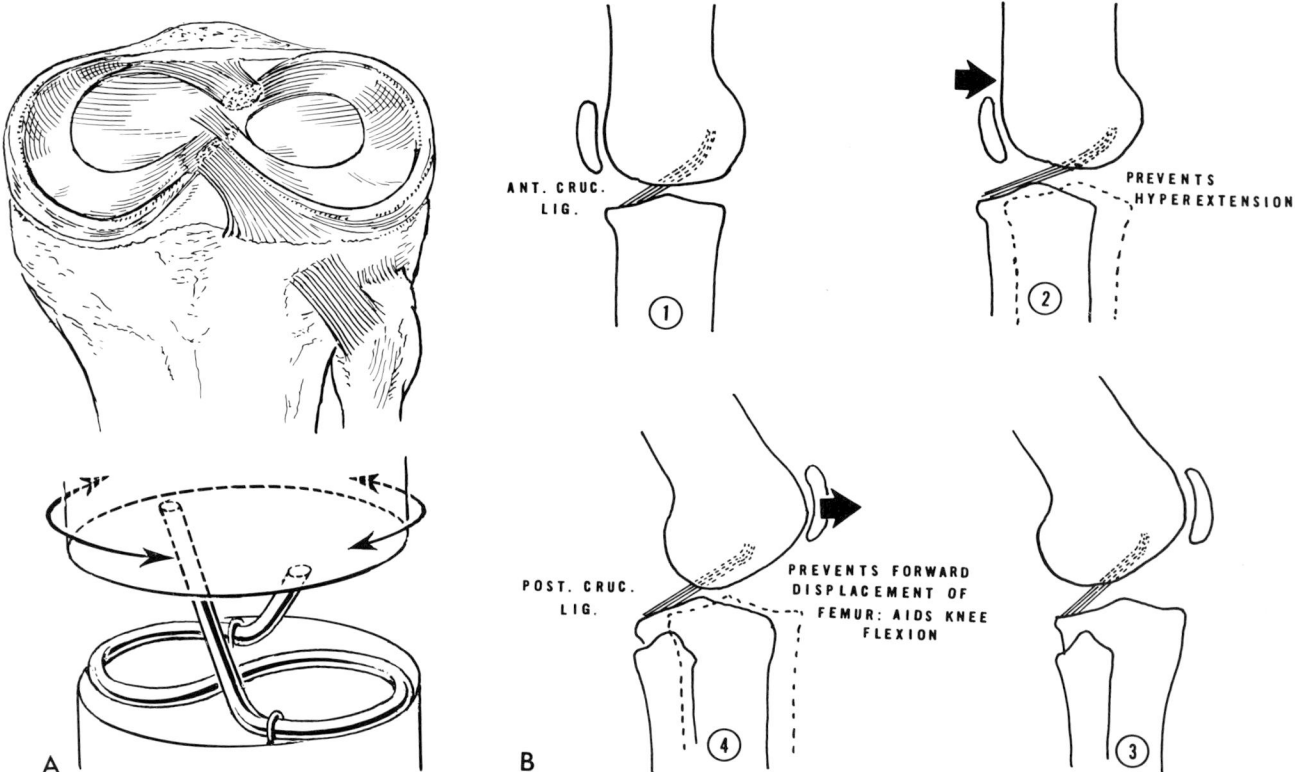

FIGURE 5–54. *A*, The anatomic arrangement and continuity of the cruciates with the semilunar cartilages (menisci) suggest that the function of guiding rotation is shared in this figure eight manner. *B*, Cruciate ligament function. *1* and *2*, Lateral view showing anterior cruciate as it prevents hyperextension. *3* and *4*, Posterior cruciate ligament function, which prevents forward displacement of the femur upon the tibia and aids in normal knee flexion. (*A* reproduced with permission from Helfet, AJ: Disorders of the Knee. Philadelphia: J.B. Lippincott Co., 1982; *B* reproduced with permission from Cailliet, R: Soft Tissue Pain and Disability. Philadelphia: F.A. Davis Co., 1977, p. 221.)

5–54*B*. Cruciate ligaments are named according to their tibial attachments. Each runs diagonally and superiorly from tibia to femoral condyle, crossing the tibiofemoral joint. The anterior cruciate thus originates from the anterior tibia and inserts into the medial face of the lateral femoral condyle, while the posterior cruciate arises from the posterior tibia and attaches to the medial femoral condyle. It can be seen that the anteroposterior orientation of the cruciates limits hyperextension of the femur on the tibia (via the anterior cruciate) and prevents forward displacement of the femur on the tibia during knee flexion (via the posterior cruciate). These ligaments thus stabilize the tibiofemoral joint in its primary plane of motion. The drawer tests during examination are designed to test this stability (Fig. 5–33). The inverse crisscrossing of the cruciates also then guides and limits rotational motion (Fig. 5–54). Severe rotation or hyperextension injuries may then tear the cruciates.

Figure 5–52 illustrates some of the ligamentous knee support. Medial collateral ligaments have varied connections with associated structures (meniscus, joint capsule, quadriceps tendon) while the lateral collateral is less intimately connected with other structures. Not shown in this figure is the joint capsule that surrounds the entire joint as a fibrous envelope that attaches to the femur—just proximal to the epicondylar articular cartilage, and to the tibia below—just distal to the tibial cartilage and attachment of collateral ligaments. Many "capsular ligaments" are not shown in Figure 5–52.

REFERENCES

1. Kopell, HP, Thompson, WAL: Peripheral Entrapment Neuropathies. Baltimore: Williams and Wilkins, 1963, pp. 48–52.
2. Aichroth, P: Osteochrondritis dissecans of the knee. J. Bone Joint Surg 53B:440, 1971.
3. Monaco, BR, et al.: Incomplete tears of the anterior cruciate ligament and knee locking. JAMA 247:1582–1584, 1982.
4. Smillie, IS: Diseases of the Knee Joint. Edinburgh: Churchill Livingstone, 1980, Chaps. 1, 2, 12.
5. Smillie, IS: Injuries of the Knee Joint. Edinburgh: E. & S. Livingstone, 1970, Chaps. 1, 8, 12.
6. Hoppenfield, S: Physical Examination of the Spine and Extremities. Appleton-Century-Crofts, 1976, Chap. 7.
7. Helfet, AJ: Disorders of the Knee. Philadelphia: J. B. Lippincott, 1974.
8. Kopell, HP, Thompson, WAL: Peripheral Entrapment Neuropathies. Baltimore: Williams and Wilkins, 1963, pp. 42–47.
9. Ho, G, et al.: Septic bursitis in the prepatellar and olecranon bursae. Ann Intern Med 89:21, 1978.
10. Engelbrecht, J, Mueller, M: Septic bursitis (Letter). Ann Intern Med 89:1011, 1978.
11. Ho, G, Tice, AD: Comparison of nonseptic and septic bursitis. Arch Intern Med 139:1269, 1979.
12. Simon, LS, Mills, JA: Nonsteroidal anti-inflammatory drugs. N Engl J Med 302:1179–1237, 1980.
13. Kilcoyne, RF, et al.: Ruptured Baker's cyst simulating acute thrombophlebitis. JAMA 240:1517, 1978.
14. Gordon, GV, et al.: Baker's cysts and true thrombophlebitis. Arch Intern Med 139:40, 1979.
15. Burt, TB, et al.: Clinical manifestations of synovial cysts. West J Med 133:99, 1980.
16. Jayson, M, et al.: Popliteal and calf cysts in rheumatoid arthritis. Ann Rheum Dis 31:9, 1972.
17. Brody, DM: Running injuries. Ciba Clin Symp 32(4):1–36, 1980.
18. Bentley, G: Chondromalacia patellae. J Bone Joint Surg 52A:221, 1970.
19. Blazina, ME, et al.: Jumper's knee. Orthop Clin North Am 4:665, 1973.
20. Altman RD, Tenenbaum, J: Hypertrophic osteoarthropathy. In Kelley, WN, et al. (eds.): Textbook of Rheumatology. Philadelphia: W. B. Saunders, 1981, pp. 1647–1657.
21. Gordon, GO: Traumatic prepatellar neuralgia. J Bone Joint Surg 34B:41–44, 1952.
22. Lotke, PA, et al.: Painful knees in older patients. J Bone Joint Surg 59A:617–621, 1977.
23. Levy, IM, Warren, RF: Knee rehabilitation. Essentials of a postinjury exercise program. Consultant (May) 1982, 148–154.
24. Ellison, AE: Skiing injuries. Ciba Clin Symp 29(1):2–40, 1977.
25. O'Donaghue, DH: Treatment of acute ligamentous injuries of the knee. Orthop Clin North Am 4:617, 1973.
26. Nicholas, JA: Injuries to menisci of the knee. Orthop Clin North Am 4:647, 1973.
27. Eriksson, E: Sports injuries of knee ligaments. Their diagnosis, treatment, rehabilitation, and prevention. Med Sci Sports 8:133–144, 1976.
28. Ivey, FM: Evaluating acute knee injuries. Am Fam Physician 25:122–129, 1982.
29. Testa, NN: The disruptions of the knee and ankle. Emergency Med 14:123–132, 1982.
30. Hughston, JC, et al.: Classification of knee ligament instabilities. I. The medial compartment and cruciate ligaments. II. The lateral compartment. Am J Bone Joint Surg 58A:159–172; 173–179, 1976.
31. Ivey, FM, et al.: Arthroscopy of the knee under general anesthesia: An aid to the determination of ligamentous instability. Am J Sports Med 8:235–238, 1980.
32. Kalenak, A: The swollen knee: Noninfectious causes. Consultant, 1979 pp. 108–114.
33. Norden, CW: The swollen knee: Infectious causes. Consultant, 1979, pp. 181–185.
34. Moskowitz, RW: Clinical Rheumatology. Philadelphia: Lea & Febiger, 1975, Chaps. 3, 4–7, 20.
35. Miller, JA: Joint paracentesis from an anatomic point of view. II. Hip, knee, ankle, foot. Surgery 41:999–1011, 1957.
36. Schumacher, HR: Analyzing synovial fluid—A useful diagnostic aid for practitioners. Mod Med 1977, pp. 58–63.
37. Currey, H, Vernon-Roberts, B: Examination of synovial fluid. Clin Rheum Dis 2:149–177, 1976.
38. Krey, PR, Bailen, DA: Synovial fluid leukocytosis. A study of extremes. Am J Med 67:436, 1979.
39. Podell, TE, et al.: Synovial fluid eosinophilia. Arthritis Rheum 23:1060, 1980.
40. Ward, JR, Atcheson, SG: Infectious Arthritis. Med Clin North Am 61:313, 1977.
41. Sharp, JT, et al.: Infectious arthritis. Arch Intern Med 139:1125, 1979.
42. Goldenberg, DL, Cohen, AS: Acute infectious arthritis. Am J Med 60:369, 1976.
43. Freed, JF: Acute monoarticular arthritis. A diagnostic approach. JAMA 243:2314, 1980.
44. Handsfield, HH, et al.: Treatment of the gonococcal arthritis–dermatitis syndrome. Ann Intern Med 84:661–667, 1976.
45. Holmes, KK, et al.: Disseminated gonococcal infection. Ann Intern Med 74:979–993, 1971.
46. Waldvogel, FA, Vasey, H: Osteomyelitis: The past decade. N Engl J Med 303:360, 1980.
47. Kelley, WN: Gout and related disorders of purine metabolism. In Kelley, WN, et al. (eds.): Textbook of Rheumatology. Philadelphia: W. B. Saunders, 1981, pp. 1397–1437.
48. Howell, DS: Diseases due to the deposition of calcium pyrophosphate and hydroxyapatite. In Kelley, WN, et al. (eds.): Textbook of Rheumatology. Philadelphia: W. B. Saunders, 1981, pp. 1438–1454.
49. Wallace, R, Cohen, AS: Tuberculous arthritis. Am J Med 61:277, 1976.
50. Byers, PD, et al.: The diagnosis and treatment of pigmented villonodular synovitis. J Bone Joint Surg 50B:290, 1968.
51. Schiller, AL: Tumors and tumor-like lesions involving joints. In Kelley, WN, et al. (eds.): Textbook of Rheumatology. Philadelphia: W. B. Saunders, 1981, pp. 1787–1790.
52. Schiller, AL: Tumors and tumor-like lesions involving joints. In Kelley, WN, et al. (eds.): Textbook of Rheumatology. Philadelphia: W. B. Saunders, 1981, pp. 1798–1802.
53. Cailliet, R: Knee Pain and Disability. Philadelphia: F. A. Davis, 1973, Chaps. 1, 2, 5.
54. Cailliet, R: Soft Tissue Pain and Disability. Philadelphia: F. A. Davis, 1977, Chaps. 1, 10.

6

FEMALE URINARY TRACT INFECTIONS

THE TRADITIONAL APPROACH..................... 272

COMMON UTI SYNDROMES........................ 275

THE EMPIRIC APPROACH.......................... 280

THE INDIVIDUALIZED APPROACH................. 282

INITIAL TREATMENT OF SUSPECTED UTI.......... 285

    Urine Cultures................................. 288
    When the Patient with Acute UTI Does Not
      Improve..................................... 290
    Follow-up after Treatment..................... 293

RECURRENT UTI 293

    Prophylactic Antibiotics in Recurrent UTI 293

APPENDIX I: ACUTE PYELONEPHRITIS 300

    II: LOCALIZING THE SITE OF
        INFECTION........................... 303

    III: ECONOMICS OF UTI................. 305

REFERENCES...................................... 306

THE TRADITIONAL APPROACH

> Cynthia Cystitis, a 24-year-old woman, enters the clinic requesting "a urine culture and some sulfa pills." When asked to explain, she says she has a "bladder infection and sulfa usually cures it." Cynthia says she has had many "bladder infections" over the past 3 years. Her previous physician (she has just moved to the area) evaluated her problem extensively—she has undergone intravenous pyelography, cystoscopy and urethral dilatation—but the studies "found nothing wrong."
>
> Cynthia has been well for the previous 2 months but describes 2 days of dysuria and urinary urgency, without fever, chills, or flank pain.

While this patient is probably correct about her own diagnosis and need for treatment, urinary symptoms in females are nonspecific—identical symptoms may be caused by genitourinary problems as diverse as vaginitis and acute pyelonephritis. Even when careful evaluation ferrets out those patients with associated vaginal symptoms (due to vaginitis) or those with high fever and flank pain (pyelonephritis), female dysuria and urinary frequency may be due to any of several distinctive syndromes of urinary tract infection (UTI).[1] While most such women will be found to have bacterial cystitis or various forms of urethritis, it is clear that suspecting UTI is only the first step in identifying which specific UTI syndrome is present in an individual patient. Table 6–1 enumerates some of these varied conditions, each of which may require a distinctive therapeutic approach.

Traditionally, efforts to diagnose and treat female UTIs have emphasized the urine culture as the pivotal diagnostic test. There are several reasons for this. (1) Most women with UTI symptoms were thought to have bacterial

272

TABLE 6–1. UTI SYNDROMES

URETHRITIS	CYSTITIS	UPPER TRACT INFECTION
Bacterial	Bacterial	Acute bacterial pyelonephritis
Chlamydial	*E. coli*	Upper tract bacteriuria
Gonococcal	*Enterococcus*	Perinephric abscess
Mycoplasmal (?)	*S. saprophyticus*	Xanthogranulomatous
Traumatic	*Klebsiella*	pyelonephritis
Irritative	Other gram-negative	Tuberculosis
Pelvic disease	organisms	Fungal infection
	Chlamydial	
	Tuberculous	
	Fungal	
	Interstitial	
	Neoplastic	

VAGINITIS	COMPLICATED SITUATIONS
Candida	Recurrent bacterial infection
Trichomonas	Relapsing bacterial infection
Gardnerella	Chronic renal failure
Atrophic	Obstructive uropathy
Herpes	Urolithiasis
Traumatic	Indwelling urinary catheter
Dermatitis	Urologic anomalies: diverticula
(See also vaginitis,	strictures
Chapter 7)	

infection of the bladder or kidney(s), and the urine culture identified these. (2) Those women with similar symptoms who had negative urine cultures either soon became asymptomatic without treatment (the so-called urethral syndrome) or subsequently developed symptoms and signs of some pelvic or vaginal disorder that could then be treated accordingly. (3) Perhaps most important was the traditional dogma that documentation and eradication of bacteriuria per se were as important as the relief of urinary symptoms. Thirty years ago a substantial subset of (then often fatal) chronic renal failure was due to "chronic pyelonephritis," at that time widely believed to be the result of chronic or recurrent bacterial infection of the kidneys. On the assumption that prevention or treatment of bacteriuria, symptomatic or not, might have a beneficial impact on that problem, screening programs for bacteriuria (especially in children) flourished, as did compulsive attempts to eradicate even asymptomatic bacteriuria with (often repeated) antibiotic therapy.[2–6] This traditional paradigm viewed urinary symptoms and urinary bacteriology, in a sense, as related but independent variables. The relief of symptoms was always desirable, but so was bacteriologic sterilization of the urine, even if symptoms were absent.

Figure 6–1 illustrates various outcomes of cases approached in this traditional manner. Positive and negative urine cultures are distinguished by the traditional criterion of greater than or equal to 10^5 bacteria per ml of urine, as developed by Kass and co-workers.[2, 5, 6] When the urine culture is positive, appropriate antibiotic therapy usually results in symptomatic and bacteriologic cure (1A in Figure 6–1). When either symptoms or bacteriuria persist after treatment, the infection is "complicated," (1B, 1C, 1D) and various diagnostic investigations (cystoscopy and intravenous pyelography, for example) are considered; repeated courses of antibiotics are then often prescribed to cure the patient (and the urine culture). On the other hand, when the initial urine culture is negative, we worry less about infection of the kidney and symptoms usually resolve spontaneously anyway (2B).

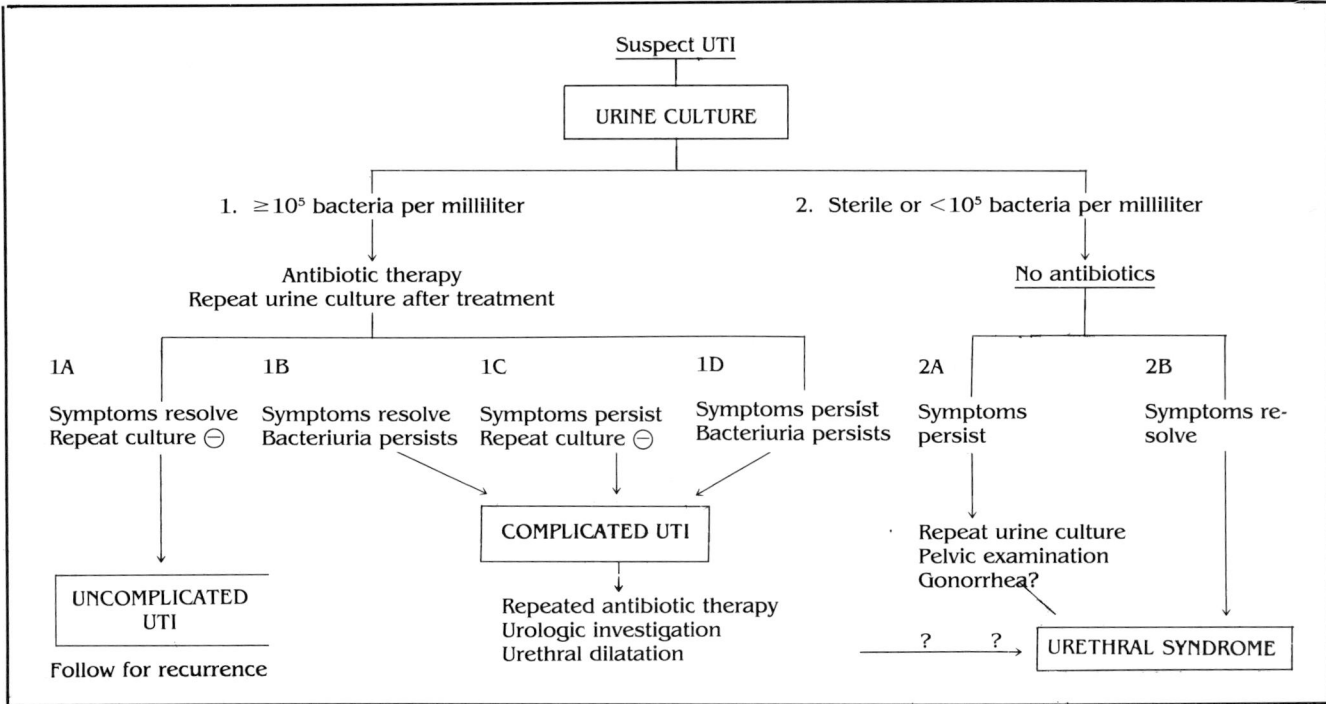

FIGURE 6–1. Traditional approach to UTI.

While this traditional approach still has much merit, it has several theoretic and practical flaws that have come to light in the past decade:

1. There is little evidence that bacteriuria per se causes renal disease. We now know that bacterial infection is rarely, if ever, the sole cause of chronic pyelonephritis,[7–14] a pathologic entity with diverse causes now usually termed chronic (tubulo) interstitial nephritis.[15] Thus the traditional rationale for the widespread detection and compulsive eradication of *asymptomatic* bacteriuria has been shaken.[16–26]

2. The definition of a positive urine culture is unclear. The traditional criterion of greater than or equal to 10^5 bacteria per ml of "clean-catch" urine was derived from studies of asymptomatic women and women with acute pyelonephritis with gram-negative bacteriuria: Greater than or equal to 10^5 bacteria per ml correlated with "true bacteriuria" (defined by bladder aspiration cultures) 80 per cent of the time, and a repeat culture confirming the initial result raised this corrrelation to 95 per cent. These studies have been widely *misinterpreted* to mean that urine cultures that grow fewer bacteria are negative or insignificant. When one notes that any bacterial growth in urine obtained by percutaneous sterile suprapubic aspiration is abnormal,[27] one must look askance at the magic number of 10^5. [28–30] In fact, while low-level bacteriuria may represent urinary contamination, it is frequently of clinical importance, especially in the symptomatic patient.[31, 32] (See also "Urine Cultures," page 288.)

3. Some women with sterile urine cultures do have infections of the bladder or urethra that require antibiotic therapy. We now know that the urethral syndrome comprises a heterogeneous group of infectious and non-infectious disorders.[31, 33, 34] Some of these women clearly benefit from anti-

biotic therapy, especially those with chlamydial infection[31] (which cannot be diagnosed on routine urine culture).

4. Only a very small minority of women with urinary infection have anatomic or functional urorenal disease. Traditionally, the woman with recurrent urinary infection and the woman whose symptoms and bacteriuria did not resolve with appropriate antibiotic therapy have been routinely subjected to urologic investigation: cystoscopy, intravenous pyelography, cystometrography, or a combination. The rationale is that urorenal disease (especially obstructive uropathy) sometimes does cause recurrent or persistent infection; in addition, if bacteriuria ever does cause renal damage, it does so when urorenal abnormalities coexist. We now know that the great majority of women with recurrent UTI are urologically normal;[35, 36] various nonanatomic factors are usually responsible for repeated reinfection (see page 293). Similarly, relapsing infection—when symptoms and bacteriuria do not resolve with antibiotic treatment—usually results from upper tract bacteriuria (see below), which requires more prolonged treatment than simple cystitis, but which is usually also unassociated with any urorenal disease. Urologic investigation of women with UTI is thus sometimes important, but not very often.

To recapitulate, bacteriuria per se is important only sometimes. In addition, the microbiologic definition of significant bacteriuria is problematic—the quantitative urine culture is not always easy to interpret. In fact, even when one can interpret the culture as unequivocally negative (sterile), antibiotics may still be indicated in the woman with symptoms of UTI. Finally, complicated UTI's—when bacteriuria or symptoms persist or recur—are not rare, but the traditional urologic approach to this problem is only occasionally helpful.

How, then, do we reconcile these uncertainties in a practical, cost-conscious approach to the woman with symptoms of UTI?*

COMMON UTI SYNDROMES

CONSIDER

Cynthia describes a "burning" discomfort during and immediately after urination. This feeling is "inside." There is also a sense of urinary urgency and frequency—"I seem to go every half hour"—and there is mild suprapubic discomfort partly relieved by urination.

Cynthia denies any vaginal symptoms—discharge, itching, irritation, or odor. She is married, has sexual relations only with her husband, and says she "could not" be pregnant. There is no history of diabetes or renal disease.

Brief physical examination is normal. Cynthia is afebrile, looks healthy, and has no flank or suprapubic tenderness.

What does this mean? (See also Fig. 6–5, p. 283.)

1. The patient is afebrile and only mildly ill. Acute urinary symptoms in the sick, febrile patient who is in a toxic condition raise several distinctive

---

*For a brief discussion of the economics of UTI, see Appendix III.

questions, and the approach to suspected acute pyelonephritis is outlined in Appendix I. It is important to remember, however, that traditional clinical distinctions between acute pyelonephritis and cystitis are helpful but are far from perfect.[1] Some patients with bladder infection may complain of flank pain or low-grade fever. Some patients with acute pyelonephritis will be only mildly ill (see Table 6–2, page 278).

High fever, chills, nausea and vomiting, severe flank pain and tenderness, tachycardia, and clinical toxicity should always suggest acute pyelonephritis.

2. There are no vaginal symptoms. Vaginitis is a very common cause of urinary symptoms in females. In fact, when dysuria is the "index symptom" in a clinical study, more women will be found to have vaginitis than UTI.[37] When both urinary symptoms (dysuria) and vaginal symptoms (odor, itch, discharge) coexist, vaginitis is six times more likely than UTI.[38, 39] Closer questioning of the woman whose dysuria is caused by vaginitis often reveals that vaginal dysuria is perceived as "external," due to irritation of inflamed labia by the passage of urine.

When "internal" dysuria and urinary frequency are noted by a woman who specifically denies symptoms of vaginitis, a pelvic examination can usually be omitted, since vaginitis is very unlikely. (The approach to suspected vaginitis is discussed in Chapter 7.)

In addition, in this case,

3. There is no specific reason to suspect gonorrhea. Gonorrhea is an uncommon but well-described cause of the urethral syndrome (see below).[40] Young, sexually active women with multiple sexual partners or recent change in sexual partners should undergo a pelvic examination with cervical and urethral cultures for gonorrhea.

4. Symptoms are typical of urinary infection, but the site of infection may be the kidney, bladder, or urethra. Some women with UTI will describe atypical presenting symptoms—vague suprapubic discomfort, malodorous urine, flank pain, or urinary hesitancy without dysuria or urinary frequency. Such symptoms require a broader differential diagnosis—examination of the abdomen and pelvis will be necessary, and urinalysis will help localize the problem to the urinary system when pyuria or hematuria is documented.

On the other hand, when symptoms are typical of UTI—urinary frequency and dysuria without vaginal symptoms—infection of the urethra, bladder, or kidney(s) can usually be presumed, especially when urinalysis reveals pyuria.

Figure 6–2 represents a theoretic group of 100 adult women with typical UTI symptoms and no clinical suspicion of vaginitis or acute pyelonephritis. About 60 per cent of such women will have proven UTI according to the traditional definition of greater than or equal to 10^5 bacteria per ml on urine culture. If these 60 women were subjected to careful study (see Appendix II), two thirds (40) would have infection of the bladder, but one third (20) would be found to have upper tract bacteriuria*—infection localized to the kidney(s).[41, 42] The remaining 40 women with "negative" urine cultures will include those with diagnostic entities traditionally grouped as the urethral syndrome:[31] those with low-level bacteriuria, i.e., less than 10^5 bacteria per ml; those with sterile bacterial urine cultures but proven infection with

*Note that upper tract bacteriuria is not synonymous with acute pyelonephritis. The latter is one subset of upper tract infection—which is distinguished from other UTIs purely on clinical grounds—see Appendix I.

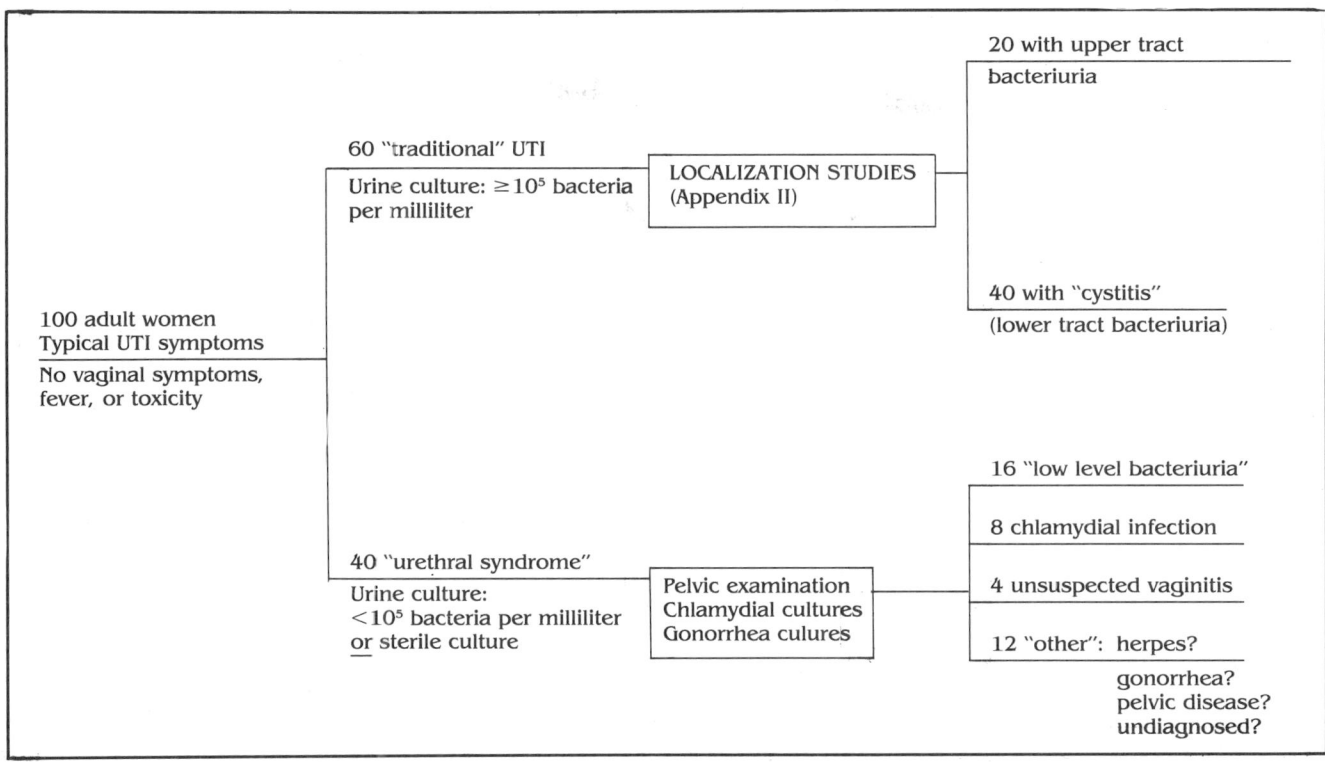

FIGURE 6–2. Common UTI syndromes.

Chlamydia trachomatis; those with unsuspected vaginitis; and those with various other problems—herpes simplex infection, gonorrhea, other pelvic disease (uterine myomas, traumatic urethritis, for example). In a few, no conclusive diagnosis will be reached.

Table 6–2 illustrates clinical characteristics of the common UTI syndromes. While each of these syndromes may require a specific therapeutic approach, symptomatic differences are unreliable in differential diagnosis. In the absence of clinical acute pyelonephritis (see Appendix I), upper tract bacteriuria is clinically indistinguishable from cystitis. Each usually presents with rather abrupt onset (1 to 2 days) of dysuria, frequency, suprapubic pain, or gross hematuria, or combinations of these, without (as a rule) fever or systemic toxicity. Only various localization procedures (see Appendix II) will distinguish upper tract from lower tract bacteriuria, and such studies are not routinely available. Urethral syndrome due to low-level bacteriuria—which "may represent an early phase of cystourethritis or a balance in the interaction between invading microorganisms and host defense mechanisms"[31]—will produce symptoms identical to those of cystitis or upper tract bacteriuria. Urethritis due to chlamydial infection is often more gradual in onset (1 to 2 weeks), usually unassociated with suprapubic pain or hematuria (although pyuria is common), and afflicts primarily young, sexually active women.[31]

Thus, precise definition of a specific UTI syndrome may require elaborate testing—bacterial localization studies, pelvic examination, and cervical and urethral cultures for chlamydiae, gonorrhea, or herpes simplex, among others. While such studies are important in clinical research on UTI, many are impractical in most clinical situations. As we shall see, the practical clinical approach to these problems rarely requires such elaborate testing.

5. Cynthia is a low-risk patient. "Low risk" here refers to the potential acute danger or long-term deleterious effects of bacteriuria per se. High-risk

TABLE 6–2. CLINICAL CHARACTERISTICS OF COMMON UTI SYNDROMES

	SYMPTOMS AND SIGNS	URINALYSIS	URINE CULTURE	RECOMMENDED THERAPY	PROGNOSIS
Urethritis					
Bacterial	Abrupt-onset dysuria, frequency, suprapubic pain; previous UTI?; no recent change in sex partner	Pyuria; bacteriuria	$<10^5$ bacteria/ml (commonly 10^2–10^4); usually *E. coli, S. saprophyticus, Enterococcus, Klebsiella*	Short course antibiotics	Rapid recovery (24–48 hours)
Chlamydial	Gradual-onset dysuria; no hematuria or suprapubic pain; recent change in sex partner	Pyuria; no bacteriuria	Sterile	Tetracycline 500 mg qid × 7 days	Rapid recovery
Gonococcal	Pelvic pain; ± dysuria; cervical discharge; recent VD exposure	May be normal	Usually sterile	Tetracycline 500 mg qid × 5 days, or ampicillin 3.5 gm po (see also Chapters 7 and 8)	Recovery in several days
Cystitis	Identical to bacterial urethritis	Pyuria, bacteriuria	$\geq10^5$ bacteria/ml; *E. coli, S. saprophyticus, Enterococcus, Klebsiella*	Short course antibiotics	Rapid recovery
Upper tract bacteriuria	Identical to bacterial cystourethritis	Pyuria, bacteriuria	$\geq10^5$ bacteria/ml; *E. coli, S. saprophyticus, Enterococcus, Klebsiella*	3 to 12 weeks of oral antibiotics	Commonly relapses after short course antibiotic therapy
Acute pyelonephritis	Fever, flank pain, chills, nausea toxicity	Pyuria, WBC casts? bacteriuria	$\geq10^5$ bacteria/ml (usually gram-negative bacilli or enterococci)	2 to 3 weeks (often parenteral) antibiotics	Gradual improvement (48–72 hours)

patients primarily include women who are pregnant or diabetic or who have underlying renal or urologic disease (Table 6–3).

A significant minority of pregnant women[43–45] with bacteriuria will develop acute pyelonephritis. There may also be other potential risks to maternal and fetal health if (even asymptomatic) bacteriuria is untreated. For these reasons, pregnant women should be screened periodically for asymptomatic bacteriuria during gestation.

Some authorities worry that bacteriuria in association with underlying renal failure or structural/functional urologic disease (Fig. 6–3) may accelerate morbidity or mortality. While we have noted that chronic renal failure is rarely, if ever, caused by bacteriuria per se, those bacteriuric women who do develop chronic renal failure are usually those with associated (especially obstructive) urorenal disorders. Thus the patient with known renal failure or an obstructive urologic disorder should be considered a high-risk patient, even though the natural history of the urorenal disease is probably more responsible for ultimate morbidity than is the bacteriuria per se.

Given their well-known propensity to develop renal and bladder disease, their faulty antibacterial defense mechanisms, and their greater likelihood of

TABLE 6–3. HIGH-RISK PATIENTS

Pregnant	Renal failure
Diabetic	Recurrent acute pyelonephritis
Known urologic disease	Known upper tract bacteriuria (?)

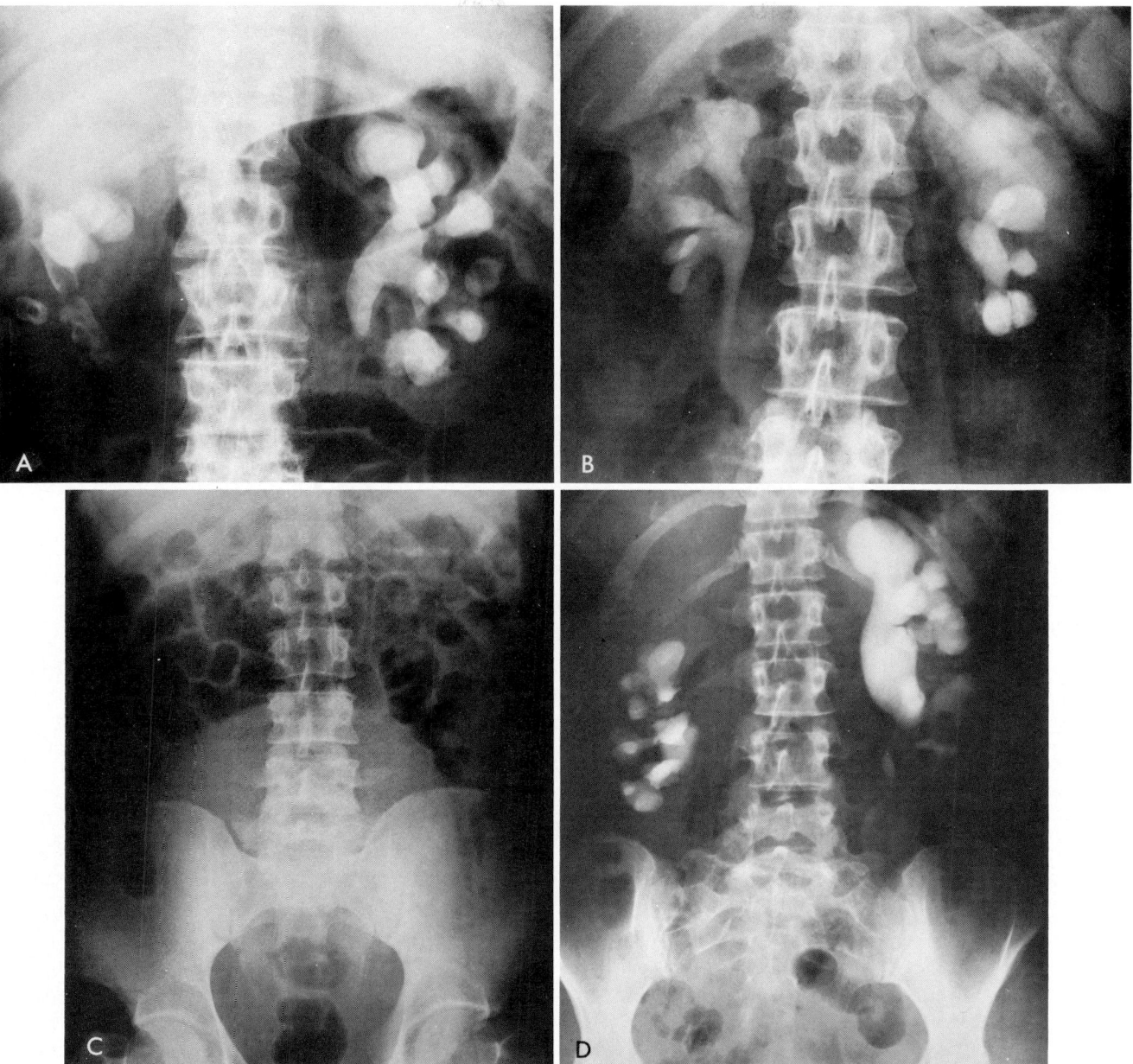

FIGURE 6–3. *A, B,* This 46-year-old woman suffered from recurrent urolithiasis with mild azotemia. X-ray *A* was taken before IVP dye (*B*) was administered. There are giant bilateral staghorn calculi. Recurrent infection in such a patient is difficult to prevent or treat, but aggressive treatment and surveillance are indicated, since recurrent infection may accelerate renal dysfunction.

C, This 30-year-old woman has had insulin-dependent diabetes since age 5. This x-ray demonstrates a huge soft tissue mass filling the entire lower abdomen—this is a distended, neurogenic bladder. Impaired bladder function in diabetics is an important predisposition to urinary tract infection.

D, This 30-year-old woman had suffered recurrent urinary tract infections since adolescence. An IVP demonstrates bilateral hydronephrosis, much more marked on the left. Subsequent study demonstrated this to be the result of vesicoureteral reflux. Such a patient should be considered a "high risk" patient—eradication of bacteriuria is not always possible but is always desirable.

upper tract infection,[46] women with diabetes mellitus should be considered high-risk patients.

6. Cynthia does have a history of recurrent UTIs. This fact is important for three reasons. (1) Some women with allegedly recurrent UTIs have, in fact, suffered from varying, unrelated episodes of vaginitis, urethritis, or true bacterial urinary infection. Thus, bacteriologic documentation of recurrent UTI is important. (2) The diagnostic and therapeutic approach to such women is distinctive—recurrent UTI is discussed on page 293. (3) Women with documented recurrent UTI usually know when they are infected again—Cynthia's self-diagnosis and request for treatment are probably correct.

In summary, Cynthia is a low-risk patient with prior recurrent bladder infection who probably has another one.

What should be done now?

> Urinalysis demonstrates more than 25 leukocytes and "moderate bacilli" per high-power field on a centrifuged urine specimen. Pelvic examination is not performed. A clean-catch urine specimen is collected for bacterial culture. Three tablets of trimethoprim-sulfamethoxazole, each 160/800 mg (total dose 480/2400 mg), are prescribed to be taken immediately in a single dose.
>
> Cynthia is asked to call for the results of her urine culture in 2 days.

Why are both urinalysis and urine culture performed? Does every such patient need a urine culture?

How can we so confidently forgo the pelvic examination?

When is single dose therapy appropriate? When is it contraindicated?

THE EMPIRIC APPROACH

Table 6–4 illustrates typical results of urinalysis and urine cultures among our theoretic group of 100 adult women with symptoms of UTI described in Figure 6–2, as well as their expected response to treatment after short courses (7 to 10 days) of broad-spectrum antibiotics (e.g., tetracycline, sulfonamides, or trimethoprim-sulfamethoxazole). These 100 women are broken down into the several subsets that could be identified if extensive testing were undertaken, i.e., bacterial localization studies (see Appendix II), chlamydial cultures, and the like. In fact, the only information usually available to the clinician during the initial visit is the urinalysis (or Gram stain of the urine) and, 2 days later, the urine culture and sensitivities.

Notice that a brief course of broad-spectrum antibiotics will usually cure at least 80 per cent of women subsequently found to have a "positive" urine culture.* (The exact figure will vary in different populations, depending on how many women with upper tract bacteriuria are included, since this subset will respond to treatment only 50 per cent of the time. The number of cultures that grow organisms resistant to broad-spectrum antibiotics will also influence these figures.)

Among women with "urethral syndrome" (defined by "negative" urine cultures*), the great majority will also be "cured" after 7 to 10 days of antibiotics. Some of these women will improve spontaneously, others as a direct result of the antibiotic therapy. The precise numbers here will also vary, depending upon the population studied—how many have vaginitis or

---

*"Positive" refers to $\geq 10^5$ bacteria per ml.

TABLE 6–4. TYPICAL RESULTS OF URINALYSIS AND URINE CULTURE IN THEORETIC GROUP OF 100 WOMEN WITH UTI SYMPTOMS*

DIAGNOSIS†	NO. PATIENTS	PYURIA?	URINE CULTURE POSITIVE (≥10^5/ml)‡	RESPONSE TO SHORT-COURSE ANTIBIOTICS§ CURE (No. %)	RESPONSE TO SHORT-COURSE ANTIBIOTICS§ NO CURE (No. %)
Upper tract bacteriuria	20	19	20	10 (50)	10 (50)
Cystitis	40	38	40	38 (95)	2 (5)
Urethral syndrome	(40)	(23)	0	(32) (80)	8 (20)
Low level bacteriuria	16	14	0	16 (100)	0
Chlamydial	8	7	0	8 (100)	0
Vaginitis	4	1	0	1 (25)	3 (75)
Other (herpes, gonorrhea, undiagnosed)	12	1	0	7 (58)	5 (42)
Total	100	80	60	80	20

*Dysuria, urinary frequency, no fever or vaginal symptoms.
†If precise diagnosis was achieved by localization studies, chlamydial cultures, and the like. (See also Fig. 6–2.)
‡By definition.
§The number of patients "cured" following 7 to 10 days of antibiotics. This does not necessarily imply that the antibiotics caused the improvement, e.g., among women with herpes or vaginitis.

gonorrhea?—as well as the antibiotics prescribed—broad-spectrum drugs like tetracycline will do best because of their effect on chlamydiae.

The point here is that as many as 80 per cent of a cross section of adult women with UTI symptoms will be cured by short courses of antibiotics, without any tests at all. Note that the urine culture is an unreliable predictor of success—the majority who do not improve have positive cultures (12/20), but many who do improve have negative cultures (32/80). Pyuria on urinalysis is a more accurate prognosticator—of the 80 patients with pyuria, at least 70 will respond. This "dysuria-pyuria" syndrome (whatever its specific diagnostic composition) has been shown to respond well to antibiotic therapy.[47]

This theoretic set of patients (Figure 6–2; Table 6–4) illustrates a few important practical points about women with suspected UTI that have long been apparent to the busy medical practitioner. First, urinary symptoms are extremely common among women and very often resolve spontaneously—many such women do not seek medical attention at all. Second, among those who do seek help, most are symptomatically cured after a short course of broad-spectrum antibiotics, whatever the results of tests and cultures (if any). Some physicians do not therefore perform any tests initially—in fact, the problem is frequently managed by telephone. Finally, those (few) patients who do not improve with antibiotics are those who require a more careful evaluation—urine cultures, pelvic examination, etc.

If our 100 theoretic women with UTI symptoms (Figure 6–2) were managed empirically—no tests, "presumptive" broad-spectrum antibiotics, further evaluation only for those who remain symptomatic after several days—several outcomes would ensue (Fig. 6–4). In the majority (80), symptoms would resolve. A few of these—among those with upper tract bacteriuria (10) and those with simple cystitis (38) due to a resistant organism—might have persistent, albeit now asymptomatic, bacteriuria. In such women, recurrence of symptomatic infection is likely, and there is at least the theoretic risk of acute pyelonephritis. A few others—among them those with various types of urethral syndrome (32)—might have inadequately treated pelvic infections. Finally, among the minority whose symptoms persist in spite of antibiotic therapy (20), urine culture (12) or pelvic examination (8) will often then identify the reason for treatment failure.

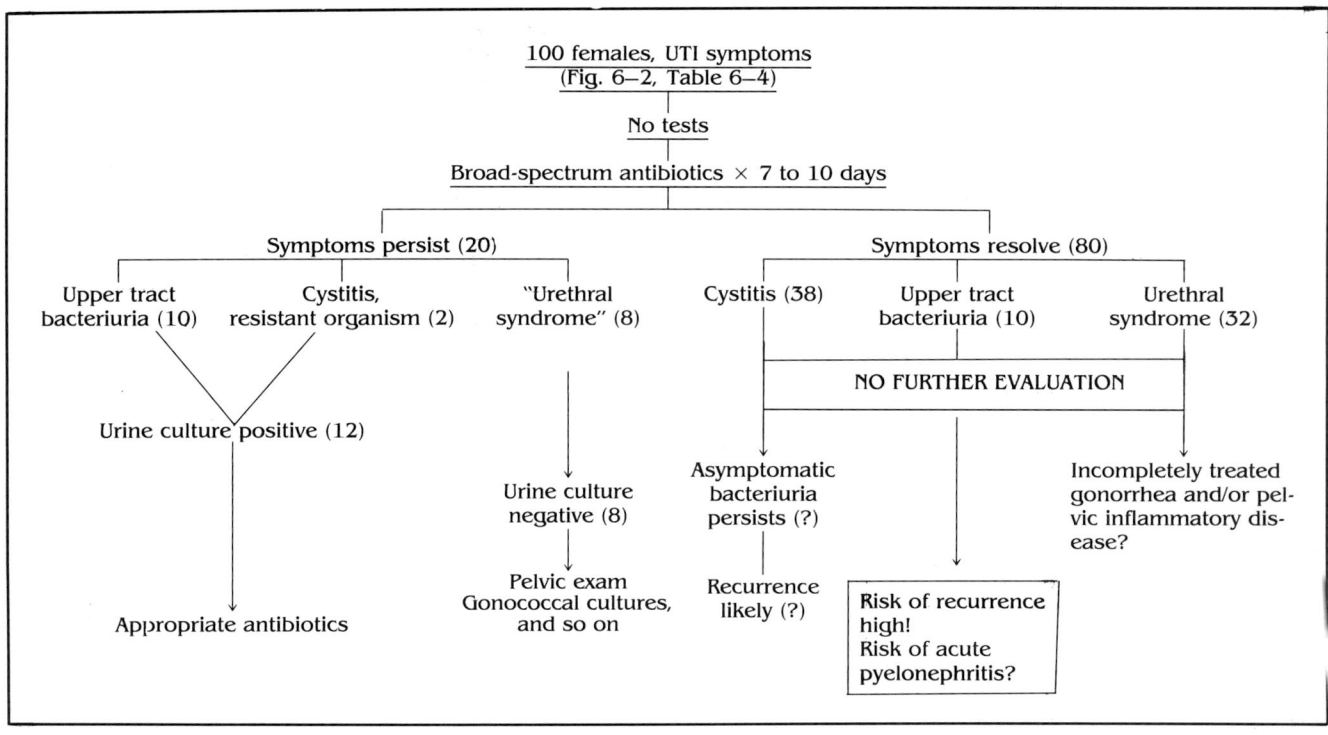

FIGURE 6–4. The empiric approach to UTI.

Thus the "empiric approach" to UTI (Fig. 6–4) will usually be effective, but its disadvantages include:

1. Antibiotics will sometimes be prescribed unnecessarily. For example, some patients with various urethral syndromes do not require antibiotics.[48]

2. Diagnostic precision will be sacrificed. As we have seen, many different UTI syndromes may present with identical symptoms. Specific diagnosis and therapy are always desirable, when possible.

3. Bacteriuria per se sometimes is important. As we have seen, even asymptomatic bacteriuria may be important in the "high-risk" patient (Table 6–3). In addition, persistent asymptomatic bacteriuria following short courses of antibiotics is often a hint that upper tract infection is present (see pages 285 and 304), and more prolonged antibiotic therapy is needed in this situation. Hence, urine cultures sometimes are important (see Table 6–5, page 285).

THE INDIVIDUALIZED APPROACH

Both the traditional approach (Fig. 6–1) and the empiric approach (Fig. 6–4) have certain practical and theoretic shortcomings. Figure 6–5 illustrates an alternative approach that attempts to individualize diagnostic and therapeutic strategies in women with suspected UTI. Here, emphasis is placed on recognizing potentially serious illness (acute pyelonephritis), suspecting other benign disorders that require an entirely different approach (for example, vaginitis—see Chapter 7), and obtaining tests that are either practically useful immediately (the urinalysis) or that will yield information that must itself be acted upon (the urine culture in the high-risk patient, for example).

This approach depends entirely on two simple procedures: the clinical history and the detection of pyuria. The standard urinalysis is the most

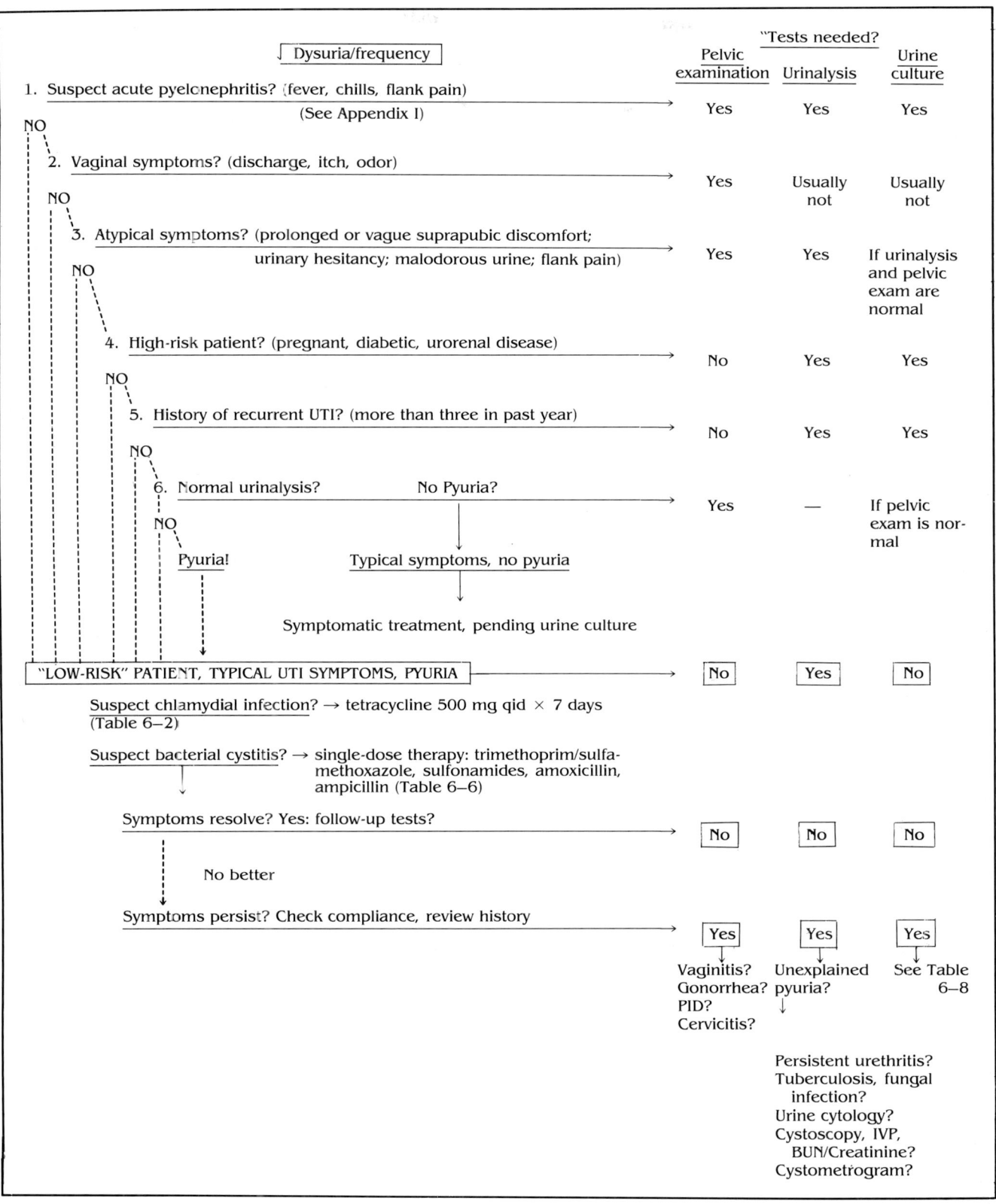

FIGURE 6–5. Suspected UTI: An individualized approach.

common test for pyuria. An aliquot of urine is centrifuged for 5 minutes—the supernatant is discarded and the sediment is mixed with a pipette. One drop of sediment is placed on a slide, covered with a cover glass, and examined under high power (400 to 450) for leukocytes. More than five leukocytes per high power field (10 fields usually counted) is usually designated pyuria. Another method for quantitation of pyuria involves filling a hemocytometer chamber with *uncentrifuged* urine: 10 leukocytes per cu mm is designated pyuria in this counting chamber method (Fig. 6–6). Recently a simple dipstick test for leukocyte·esterase activity in urine was shown to correlate well with pyuria as defined by both urinalysis and counting chamber criteria; this rapid, easy test requires further study.[49]

While centrifugation before standard urinalysis is slightly time consuming, the advantages of the standard urinalysis include the ability to detect bacteriuria as well as pyuria—and occasionally white blood cell casts in acute pyelonephritis (see also Table 6–2).

Occasionally the detection of pyuria may be superfluous. When urine cultures are to be obtained anyway—in the high-risk female or the patient with recurrent infection, for example—the results of urinalysis will often not influence clinical strategies. Even in such circumstances, however, detection of pyuria is helpful in the initial approach to the patient. While the absence of pyuria does not exclude bacterial urinary infection,[50, 51] this finding should at least prompt a pelvic examination, even if vaginal and pelvic symptoms are inapparent.

Most women with typical UTI symptoms will have no fever or vaginal symptoms, and will be low-risk patients without recurrent UTIs. Such women will usually demonstrate pyuria on urinalysis—the dysuria-pyuria syndrome[47]—and should be treated immediately with short courses of broad-spectrum antibiotics. (The precise antibiotic chosen will depend on whether chlamydial urethritis is clinically likely or not—see below.) Urine cultures can usually be omitted in this situation. The great majority of such women become asymptomatic a few days hence. The value of pretreatment or post-treatment urine cultures in the woman with such uncomplicated UTI who becomes asymptomatic after a brief course of antibiotics is highly debatable and is certainly expensive (see Appendix III).

On the other hand, there are several situations in which the urine culture definitely is indicated (Table 6–5). Most often, this is determined by the

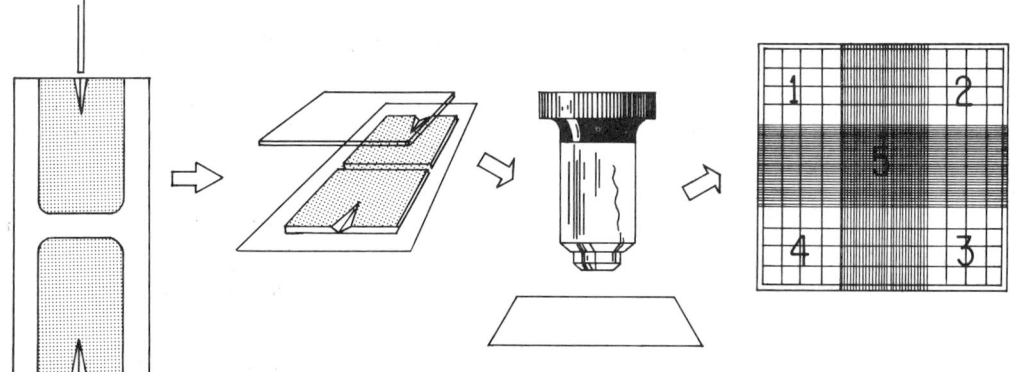

FIGURE 6–6. Quantitation of pyuria by counting chamber method. A microhematocrit tube is used to fill both sides of the hemocytometer chamber with undiluted urine. White blood cells are counted in all five "counting areas" on each side of the chamber. Each of these counting areas represents 1 sq mm. Total cell number is then expressed as cells per cubic millimeter. More than 10 white blood cells per cubic millimeter is considered "pyuria." When significant hematuria is also present, diluting the urine 1:4 in 2 per cent acetic acid will lyse red blood cells. Total white blood cells counted must then be multiplied by 4 to factor in dilution.

TABLE 6–5. INDICATIONS FOR URINE CULTURES

BEFORE TREATMENT

When acute pyelonephritis is the clinical diagnosis—to document the pathogen and guide antibiotic therapy. (see Appendix I)

When upper tract infection is suspected, and the urinary bacterial antibody-coated test (see Appendix II) is to be performed

When "recurrent urinary infection" has not been well documented in the past, and specific documentation of infection is desired in the present

When quantitating bacteriuria and establishing antibiotic sensitivities are important at the outset—for example, in the "high-risk" patient (pregnant, diabetic, urorenal disease, immunosuppressed) or the patient (pregnant, anxious, distrustful, or cantankerous) who will not accept antibiotics without "proof" of infection

When symptoms are typical, but both the urinalysis and pelvic examination are normal

AFTER TREATMENT

When symptoms do not resolve

When documentation of bacteriologic cure is deemed important: by the physician in the "high-risk" patient, or by the patient "who needs to know"

In the patient treated for acute pyelonephritis or for (documented or suspected) upper tract bacteriuria

In the patient with recurrent UTI when attempting to distinguish relapse from reinfection (see page 293)

DURING TREATMENT

During treatment of acute pyelonephritis

When treating presumed upper tract bacteriuria with prolonged courses of antibiotics

---

clinical setting—the patient with acute pyelonephritis, recurrent urinary tract infections, or high-risk conditions. Occasionally the urine culture may be worthwhile when symptoms are typical of urinary tract infection but the urinalysis is normal.

INITIAL TREATMENT OF SUSPECTED UTI

Most women with acute UTI are uncomfortable, and it is the relief of symptoms that they most desire. Antibiotic therapy will relieve symptoms within 24 to 48 hours in most such patients. Whether urine cultures are obtained or not, treatment should be initiated immediately. The choice of antibiotic, dose, and duration of therapy is determined by the specific clinical circumstances:

1. In the low-risk female with typical UTI symptoms and pyuria, either a conventional (7 to 10 days) course of antibiotics or a single-dose regimen will be effective.[39, 42, 52] The great majority of such women quickly respond both symptomatically and bacteriologically to single-dose therapy with any of the agents listed at the top of Table 6–6.[31, 42, 55–59] Single-dose therapy is often less expensive, improves compliance, induces fewer side effects, and "exerts less intense selective pressure for emergence of resistant organisms in gut, urinary, or perineal flora."[55] In addition, women with apparently uncomplicated UTI (Figure 6–5) who do not respond to single-dose therapy are much more likely to have (otherwise unsuspected) "complicated UTI," especially upper tract bacteriuria—failure to respond quickly to single-dose therapy is, in a sense, a diagnostic marker. For all these reasons, single-dose therapy is advocated here.

2. When chlamydial urethritis is clinically suspected (see Table 6–2),

TABLE 6–6. ANTIBIOTIC TREATMENT OF UTI

| | | | RECOMMENDED USE IN | |
DRUG	DOSE	COST*	PREGNANCY	RENAL FAILURE†
Single dose				
Amoxicillin	3 gm	$ 5.50	Not well studied	
Ampicillin	3 gm	3.00	Not well studied	
Sulfisoxazole	3 gm‡	2.00	Not well studied	
Trimethoprim-sulfamethoxazole	0.48/2.4 gm‡	3.00	Not well studied	
Conventional (10 days)				
Tetracycline	250 mg qid	4.00	Avoid	Avoid§
Sulfisoxazole	500 mg qid	3.50	Avoid	Avoid
Ampicillin	250 mg qid	6.75	Acceptable	Acceptable
Trimethoprim-sulfamethoxazole	80/400 mg bid	6.60	Avoid	Avoid
Nitrofurantoin	50 mg qid	3.60	Acceptable	Avoid
Macrodantin	100 mg qid	22.00	Acceptable	Avoid
Nalidixic acid	500 mg qid	14.00	Probably acceptable	Avoid
Keflex	250 mg qid	20.00	Acceptable	Acceptable
Mandelamine and ascorbic acid	1 gm qid + 500 mg qid	9.50	Probably acceptable	Avoid

*Average costs, 1983, in several nonhospital pharmacies.

†These dogmatic recommendations refer to the patient with advanced renal failure (creatinine clearance ≤ 10).

‡Smaller single doses have also been found to be effective—1 gm of sulfisoxazole, 2 gm of sulfisoxazole; 160 mg/800 mg of trimethoprim-sulfamethoxazole or 320 mg/1600 mg of trimethoprim-sulfamethoxazole.[53]

§Doxycycline is probably acceptable in renal failure.

tetracycline 500 mg qid for 7 days should be the initial treatment. A typical example is the young, sexually active female with dysuria and pyuria without bacteria visualized on urinalysis. Of note is the fact that this regimen will also cure gonococcal infection and most cases of bacterial cystitis[54] (bacteriologic sensitivity testing may indicate otherwise, but this can be misleading—see page 289). Erythromycin 500 mg qid for 7 days is preferred in the pregnant woman with suspected chlamydial infection. Currently, chlamydial cultures are neither widely available nor practically useful in most settings.

3. When symptoms are typical of cystourethritis but urinalysis does not reveal pyuria (and pelvic examination is normal, as in Fig. 6–5), symptomatic therapy with phenazopyridine hydrochloride (Pyridium) 200 mg tid, pending urine culture results, may be desirable. In a few such women bacteriuria will be demonstrated on urine culture, and specific treatment is then indicated. In many women, a urethral syndrome of unknown cause[31, 48] is often implicated when cultures and urinalysis are negative, but such patients usually improve without treatment. (Tetracycline may be worth a trial when symptoms persist, but chlamydial urethritis is usually associated with pyuria.) The cause of nonchlamydial urethral syndromes remains debatable—whether fastidious or anaerobic microorganisms are responsible is unclear.[60–66]

The patient with "complicated UTI" (Table 6–7) requires a different approach:

4. Acute pyelonephritis usually (but not always) requires hospitalization and prolonged antibiotic therapy, with or without various diagnostic procedures (see Appendix I).

5. The high-risk patient (Table 6–3) should be treated initially with

conventional (7 to 10 days) doses of antibiotics, which can be adjusted according to results of the urine culture and sensitivities available 48 hours later. Single-dose therapy has not been carefully studied in pregnant women or those with chronic renal failure. Single-dose therapy is not indicated in the patient with known urologic disease or in the patient otherwise suspected of upper tract bacteriuria—diabetics, especially.[46]

Antibiotics must, of course, be chosen carefully in the pregnant patient (Table 6–6).

When severe renal failure is present, several drugs should be avoided.[67] These include tetracycline (but perhaps not doxycycline[54]), which can further impair renal function, as well as nitrofurantoin,[68] sulfonamides,[69] and carbenicillin,[70] which may not achieve therapeutic urinary concentrations in this setting.

When obstructive uropathy, chronic urolithiasis, or other urologic abnormalities (diverticula, strictures, hydronephrosis) are known to be present, antibiotics should be prescribed, but correction of the underlying problem (when possible) should be a higher priority, especially when infections are recurrent.

6. The patient with a permanent indwelling urinary catheter will almost always develop bacteriuria, often asymptomatically. Only when symptomatic infection develops in such patients—fever, chills, bacteremia, severe symptoms—should antibiotics be prescribed, since repeated courses of treatment to eradicate asymptomatic bacteriuria in these patients will rarely be successful[71] and will ultimately result in antibiotic-resistant infection. Careful attention to catheter care and drainage systems are most important.[72, 73] The catheter should, of course, be removed whenever possible; catheter-acquired UTI is a major problem today.[74]

TABLE 6–7. COMPLICATED UTI

ACUTE PYELONEPHRITIS	HIGH-RISK PATIENT*	RECURRENT UTI	INDWELLING URINARY CATHETER
Usually hospitalize			
Blood culture; urine culture before, during, and after treatment	Urine culture; 10 days of antibiotics; post-treatment culture	Urine culture; single dose or 10 days of antibiotics; post-treatment culture	Urine culture; treat only if symptomatic and sick
2–3 weeks of antibiotics	Carefully select antibiotics in pregnancy and renal failure (see Table 6–6)	Distinguish relapse from reinfection (see text)	Avoid multiple course of antibiotics
See Appendix I	Correct obstructive uropathy when possible	See Fig. 6–10	Remove catheter, when possible

*Pregnant, diabetic, renal failure, urologic disease

7. The patient with recurrent UTI deserves a distinctive approach (see page 293). Most such women suffer from recurrent reinfections that respond rapidly to either single-dose or conventional doses of antibiotics. Some, however, experience repeated relapses of a persistent upper tract infection that will be only temporarily suppressed by short courses of antibiotics. When the latter is a possibility (see below), single-dose therapy should be avoided.

In Cynthia's case, then, the clinical symptoms and urinalysis suggest bacterial cystitis or urethritis (Table 6–2). The urine culture is obtained primarily to document bacterial infection, given the (as yet) undocumented history of recurrent infection (see Fig. 6–5 and Table 6–7). In this setting, single-dose therapy is an acceptable option, but documentation of cure with post-treatment cultures will be necessary (see below), again because of the history of recurrent infection. Had there been no such history, single-dose therapy without any urine cultures could be recommended (although many "traditionalists" will object to such a strategy).

> Two days later, Cynthia is completely asymptomatic. Urine culture has grown 50,000 *Escherichia coli* sensitive to trimethoprim-sulfamethoxazole.
>
> Cynthia remains well, and a repeat urine culture 1 week later is sterile.

This happy result raises several important issues:

1. How should we interpret urine cultures?

2. What should we do when the patient does not improve?

3. When are post-treatment cultures and follow-up indicated?

Urine Cultures

Normal urine is sterile. The most specific and sensitive test for urinary infection is the percutaneous needle aspiration of urine directly through the bladder wall under sterile conditions. While this test is primarily useful as a research tool[27] (and sometimes, clinically, in very young children), it is the "gold standard" against which other culture techniques are measured. Suprapubic bladder aspiration that reveals any bacteria indicates infection.

Unfortunately the more practical methods of obtaining urine for culture are subject to contamination by the various microorganisms that heavily colonize the vaginal and periurethral areas. (1) Specimens collected by the patient at home (in a "clean" jar) should always be discarded. (2) Clean-catch urine specimens are the most commonly procured and are usually reliable when all instructions are carefully followed. (The specimens are collected in commercially prepared kits with easy-to-understand instructions.) The clinical value of the clean-catch urine culture is directly proportional to the care with which it is obtained. (3) Urine specimens obtained by passing a sterile catheter through the urethra into the bladder after carefully cleansing the periurethral area ("in-and-out" catheterization) are less often contaminated than are specimens obtained by collecting passed urine, but catheterization is cumbersome, time consuming, and may itself introduce infection.

As noted previously, the traditional definition of "significant bacteriuria" has been primarily quantitative (greater than or equal to 10^5 bacteria per ml), but unwavering adherence to this criterion will be misleading, especially in the symptomatic patient. For example, low-level bacteriuria may be a treatable cause of the urethral syndrome. Between 10^2 and 10^4 organisms per ml may thus represent either contamination or "true" low-level bacteriuria, but this culture result should be considered significant in the woman with typical UTI symptoms[31, 32] especially when the organism is a typical urinary pathogen—see below. (Low-level bacteriuria may also be "falsely low" due to prior antibacterial therapy, urine pH variables, and other metabolic factors that inhibit bacterial growth in the laboratory.)

Usually the organisms responsible for female UTI originate in the patient's own enteric flora that colonize the perineum. *E. coli* is by far the most common organism, but *Enterococcus, Staphylococcus saprophyticus*[75–78] and *Klebsiella* are not uncommon. (The laboratory must be instructed not to disregard *S. saprophyticus* as contaminating micrococci, a common error.) Other gram-negative infections (due to *Proteus, Pseudomonas,* or *Serratia* species) are much less common but occur especially when associated with chronic urorenal disease, when infection is acquired in hospital, following urologic instrumentation, or as a final sequel to repeated infections and antibiotic therapy. *Proteus* infections are not infrequently associated with underlying urinary calculus disease (Fig. 6–7). Mixed bacterial growth (two or more organisms isolated simultaneously) usually represents contamination, but, if confirmed on repeated cultures and in large numbers, may rarely point to significant underlying genitourinary disease (bladder stones, bladder diverticula, enterovesical or vesicovaginal fistulas) and should not be resolutely dismissed as invariably unimportant (Fig. 6–8).

Sensitivity testing for antibiotic susceptibility can be misleading. *Urinary* concentrations of antimicrobial agents correlate best with response of urinary infection to treatment,[27, 79] but antibiotic sensitivity testing in the laboratory

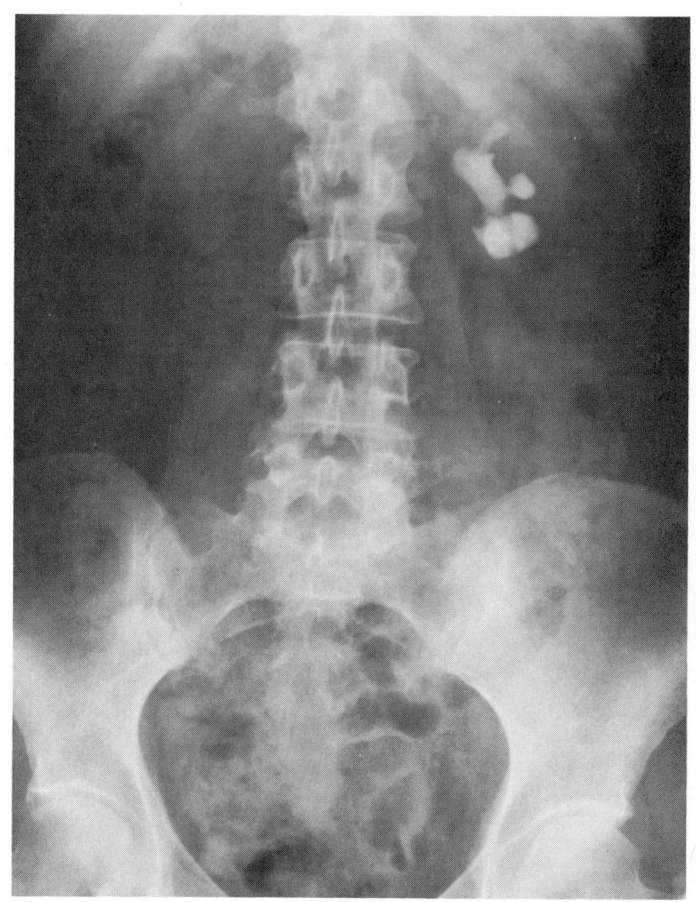

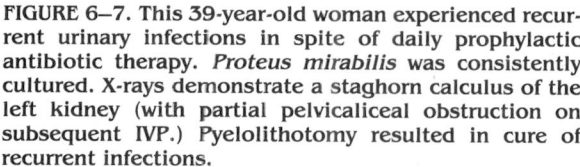

FIGURE 6–7. This 39-year-old woman experienced recurrent urinary infections in spite of daily prophylactic antibiotic therapy. *Proteus mirabilis* was consistently cultured. X-rays demonstrate a staghorn calculus of the left kidney (with partial pelvicaliceal obstruction on subsequent IVP.) Pyelolithotomy resulted in cure of recurrent infections.

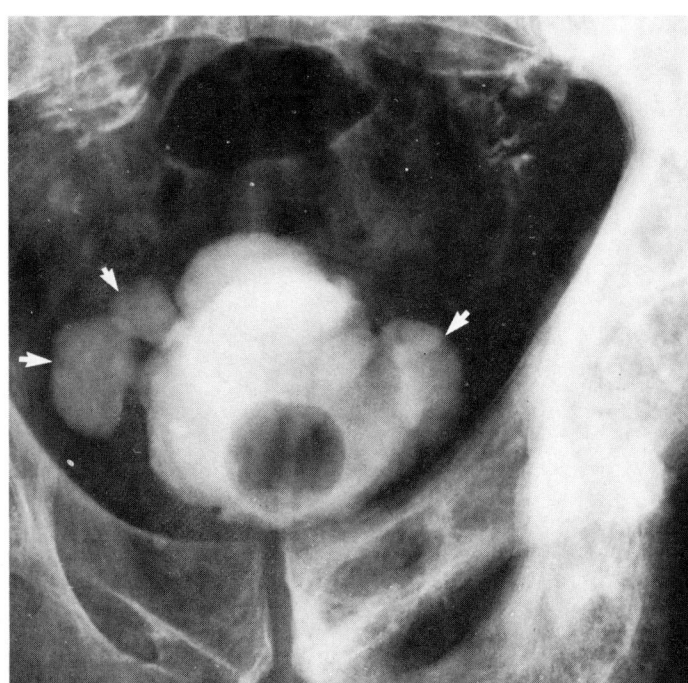

FIGURE 6–8. Recurrent urinary infections, unresponsive to antibiotic therapy, persisted in this 72-year-old woman with Paget's disease. (Note osteoblastic lesions in the left pelvis.) Surgical resection of these bladder diverticula (*arrows*) was considered: operation was refused. Recurrent infections continue. Multiple (mixed) organisms are repeatedly cultured in large numbers ($> 10^5$ per milliliter).

is often performed with concentrations of antibiotics achieved in the *serum*, not in the urine. Thus some organisms are described as resistant to various drugs on in vitro sensitivity testing, but infection may nonetheless be eradicated by these same drugs that are excreted and concentrated in urine. For this reason, prospective sensitivity testing may not always correlate with subsequent clinical results. The patient with symptomatic UTI who is completely free of symptoms after 2 days of therapy with an antibiotic to which the cultured organism is "resistant" need not necessarily be changed to another drug. In general, if one takes the trouble to document bacteriuria by urine culture (see above), it makes sense to tailor antibiotics to sensitivities. However, when (usually in a "complicated" patient [Table 6–7]) an organism is grown that is resistant to all but expensive, toxic, or difficult-to-administer antibiotics (i.e., aminoglycosides), an antibiotic predicted to be ineffective by sensitivity testing may well be worth a try. (Such an approach, of course, is never indicated in sick patients with acute pyelonephritis.)

When the Patient with Acute UTI Does Not Improve

All patients whose apparently uncomplicated UTI does not symptomatically improve within a few days of treatment require urine cultures (whether obtained initially or not), a urinalysis, and sometimes a pelvic examination. Table 6–8 summarizes why:

I. If the woman remains symptomatic after treatment and has a positive urine culture at that time several questions should be raised:

    A. Is the cultured organism sensitive to the (previously) prescribed antibiotic?

        If not, change antibiotics. (When a urine culture is obtained before treatment is initiated, the change in antibiotics can be done confidently and immediately, according to sensitivities. When the

TABLE 6–8. WHAT URINE CULTURES MAY INDICATE IN THE PATIENT WHO DOES NOT IMPROVE AFTER TREATMENT

Urine Culture Positive	Urine Culture Negative
Resistant organisms?	Chlamydial infection
Noncompliance?	Gonorrhea
Upper tract bacteriuria?	Vaginitis or pelvic disease
Renal failure?	Unusual infection—tuberculosis, fungal
Underlying urologic disorder?	Traumatic urethritis
	Irritant urethritis
	Urologic disease
	Interstitial cystitis
	Psychogenic dysuria
	Intrinsic renal disease

urine culture is not obtained initially, final decisions will be based on the culture result 2 more days hence.)

B. Is the patient taking the prescribed antibiotic as directed?

   Patient noncompliance is not a common cause of therapeutic failure of UTI (especially when single-dose therapy is employed), but it certainly does occur.

C. If the persistently symptomatic patient was initially treated with single-dose therapy and the organism grown on culture is sensitive to that drug, assume that the patient has upper tract bacteriuria and treat for 2 to 3 weeks.

   Perhaps half of women with upper tract bacteriuria will require prolonged therapy. Since documentation of upper tract bacteriuria by localization testing (see Appendix II) is not widely available, often it is wise to simply assume upper tract bacteriuria in this setting.

D. Does the patient have renal failure or known urologic disease?

   A serum creatinine determination will be helpful, since certain antibiotics will not be effective in the presence of (usually far-advanced and obvious) renal failure (see page 287). While various other "complicating" problems may prevent cure of symptomatic bacteriuria, urologic investigation should usually be delayed* (until several weeks' antibiotic therapy is attempted) unless there are specific reasons to suspect obstructive uropathy, stones, or other pathoanatomic urorenal abnormalities (see also page 296).

II. In the woman who remains symptomatic but has sterile urine cultures, consider:

A. Is chlamydial (or gonococcal) urethritis likely, i.e., is the patient sexually active with a compatible clinical profile (Table 6–2)? If so, specimens from the cervix and urethra should be cultured for gonococcus and the patient treated with tetracycline 500 mg for 7 days (thus "covering" both gonococcal and chlamydial infection).†

B. If not, does the patient have otherwise unexplained pyuria?

   Tetracycline therapy is probably still worth a trial here, but urinary fungal infection,[80–82] tuberculosis[83, 84] (Fig. 6–9), various interstitial renal diseases (urinary calculi, papillary necrosis, polycystic disease, analgesic nephropathy[85]) must also be considered.

---

*As is noted in Appendix I, the patient with acute pyelonephritis who does not improve rapidly always needs urologic investigation.

†Chlamydial cultures of urine can be obtained, usually in reference laboratories. This is rarely necessary.

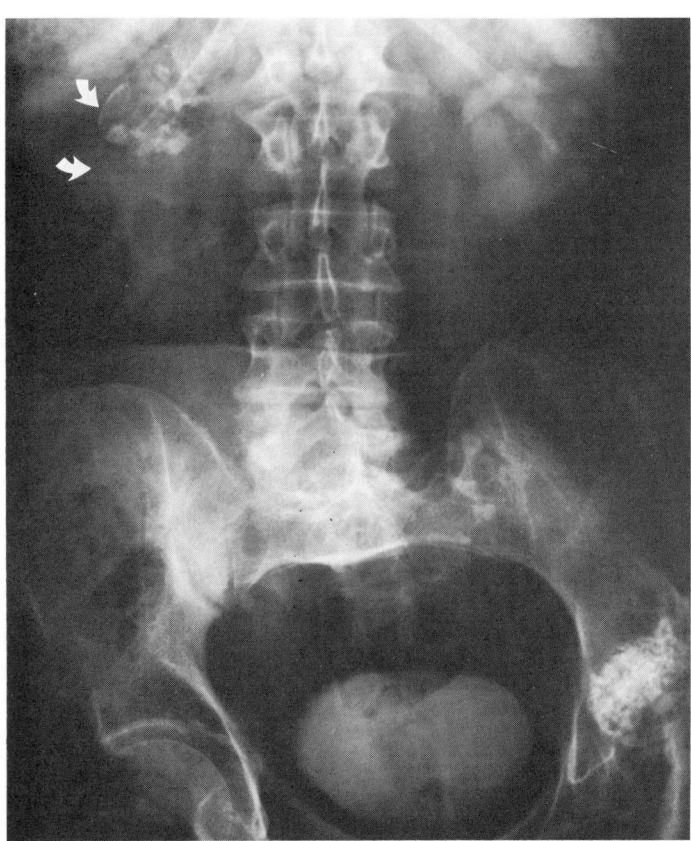

FIGURE 6–9. Sterile pyuria was the clue to the diagnosis of tuberculosis in this 75-year-old woman with vague urinary symptoms. The right kidney is shrunken, and the upper pole is markedly calcified and scarred (*arrows*). Of note is destructive arthritis of the left hip, which is also due to *Mycobacterium tuberculosis*.

C. Pelvic examination must be performed.

Vaginitis, gonorrhea, pelvic inflammatory disease, uterine myomas, urethral prolapse (in older women), urethral caruncle, and pelvic masses are among the many pelvic disorders that may cause unexplained urinary symptoms. Atrophic vaginitis is a common cause of dysuria in postmemopausal women.

D. When symptoms persist beyond a week or two without explanation, urologic consultation is usually worthwhile.

Most instances of acute, "unexplained" dysuria in females resolve spontaneously. Traumatic urethritis (due to sexual intercourse), irritative urethritis (due to douches, deodorants, tampons, etc.), pharmacologic side effects (cyclophosphamide, for example) and nonbacterial causes of the urethral syndrome (see above) are often implicated in such patients.

Persistent, unexplained dysuria, however, usually requires cystoscopy—urethral strictures, bladder stones, or neoplasia may be discovered. Interstitial cystitis[86] is believed to be a specific clinical entity in a few women with unexplained chronic dysuria in whom submucosal hemorrhages or ulcerations of the bladder mucosa are demonstrated on cystocopy. Histology is nonspecific. Topical intravesical instillation of 0.4 per cent oxychlorosene sodium, once or repeatedly, is sometimes effective.

Psychogenic dysuria does occur, usually in patients with obvious psychiatric problems, but this is always a diagnosis of exclusion.

Follow-up after Treatment

Most women with single (or rare) episodes of uncomplicated UTI require no follow-up after therapy. Some authorities still believe that urine cultures should always be obtained after treatment to document "cure," but, when the patient has become asymptomatic, the value of demonstrating persistent (now asymptomatic) bacteriuria in this setting is unknown. It is certainly expensive (see Appendix III).

A critical unanswered question is whether patients with asymptomatic upper tract bacteriuria are "at risk" in any way. If a few such untreated patients do subsequently develop renal failure (an unknown), does this mean that cultures should be obtained after treatment from all women with acute UTI? Probably not. This is the subset of patients (i.e., those with upper tract infection) in whom persistent post-treatment bacteriuria is most common, but most such patients probably subsequently develop recurrent symptomatic infections that thus come to medical attention and then require a specific approach—see below. (This area requires further prospective studies.)

As noted in Table 6–5, post-treatment urine cultures should always be obtained from patients with acute pyelonephritis and those with "high-risk" profiles.

> **Three weeks later, Cynthia develops another infection documented by urine culture that grows 10^5 E. coli with identical antibiotic sensitivities as previously. Her symptoms again resolve within 24 hours of initiation of antibiotic therapy—this time, 10 days of sulfisoxazole 500 mg qid. Follow-up urine culture is sterile, but Cynthia is unhappy. Before further evaluation is undertaken, Cynthia's prior medical records are requisitioned.**

RECURRENT UTI

Most recurrent urinary infections in adult women are *reinfections*—urinary colonization by different organisms at different times, each usually "cured" (or spontaneously resolving) before the next infection supervenes.[87-93] Most reinfections involve only the lower urinary tract (bladder or urethra). In such women, repeated colonization occurs (sequentially) in the periurethral area, urethra, and bladder urine with enteric or vaginal organisms, bacteriuria being without symptoms for varying intervals of time before the unpredictable emergence of symptomatic episodes.*[94] Bacteriuria can be eradicated successfully with antibodies each time, but recurrences nevertheless ensue episodically. There is probably no single etiologic factor in this population, but immunologic,[95] epidemiologic,[35, 96] microbiologic,[97, 98] physiologic,[91, 99] and other factors[96, 100-103] play variably important roles in different women. Very few such "susceptible" women have anatomic or functional urorenal abnormalities detectable by conventional investigative methods (serum creatinine, cystoscopy, intravenous pyelography).[35, 36] The key to the treatment of urinary reinfection is prevention, as discussed below.

Other (and fewer) recurrent urinary infections are, in fact, not recurrent

---

*This well-established sequence of events raises an interesting and unanswered question: What exactly causes urinary symptoms?[1]

at all but represent repeated *relapses* of the same initial infection.[88, 91, 92] This is a very different problem, because here bacteriuria persists in spite of appropriate antibiotic therapy. Most often, relapsing infection is localized in the upper urinary tract (without underlying urorenal disease) and may be either symptomatic or asymptomatic. Such women will either remain symptomatic and bacteriuric during antibiotic therapy of symptomatic UTI, or will appear to be "cured" temporarily (symptomatically, bacteriologically or both) when infection has been suppressed, only to relapse soon thereafter. Six to 12 weeks of therapy may be necessary in this setting, but three weeks is often sufficient. An analogy between relapsing upper tract infection and subacute bacterial endocarditis has been suggested—a persistent "nidus" of infection requires prolonged therapy (the precise pathophysiology is obscure).

The practical problem here is that it is often difficult to distinguish reinfection from relapse in an individual patient. This is an important distinction since the treatment of the former is largely prophylactic, while treatment of the latter requires a single prolonged course of antibiotics. Figure 6–10 illustrates some clues.

When recurrent infections are infrequent or widely spaced over time (months apart), when different species of organisms are recovered during different episodes (for example, *E. coli* now, *Staphylococcus saprophyticus* previously), when post-treatment urine cultures remain negative a few weeks after the initial infection has been treated—these are usually indications that reinfection, not relapse, is the problem.

Documentation of true relapse requires serotyping or other biochemical determinations that establish unequivocally *bacteriologic identity* of the original and the persistent or recurrent microorganism. There are more than 100 different serotypes of *E. coli*, for example—repeated recurrence of *E. coli* bacteriuria in no way distinguishes relapse from reinfection.

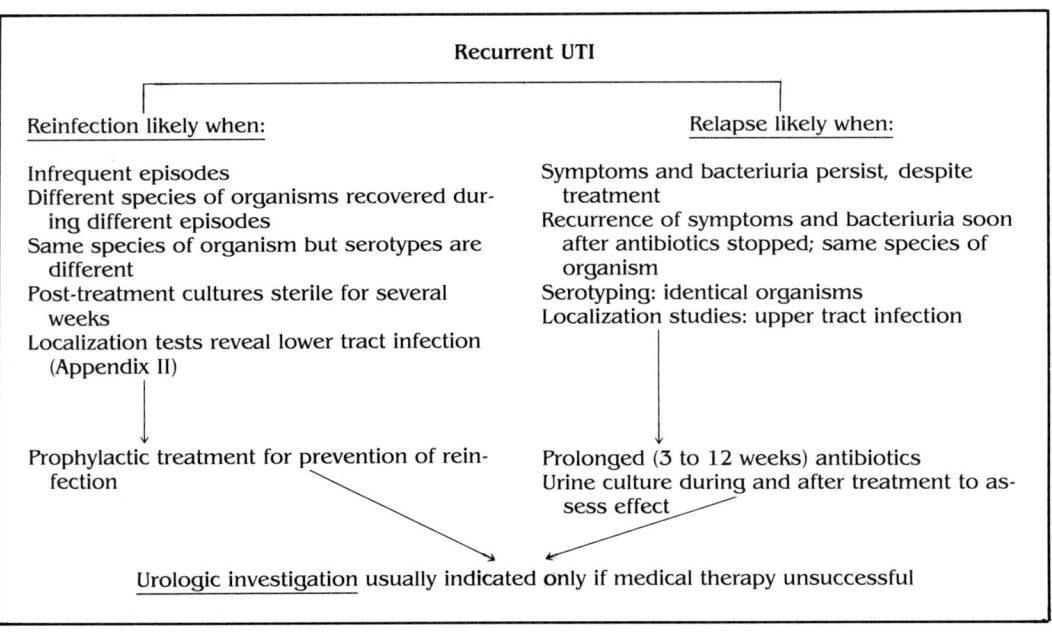

Recurrent UTI

Reinfection likely when:

Infrequent episodes
Different species of organisms recovered during different episodes
Same species of organism but serotypes are different
Post-treatment cultures sterile for several weeks
Localization tests reveal lower tract infection (Appendix II)

Prophylactic treatment for prevention of reinfection

Relapse likely when:

Symptoms and bacteriuria persist, despite treatment
Recurrence of symptoms and bacteriuria soon after antibiotics stopped; same species of organism
Serotyping: identical organisms
Localization studies: upper tract infection

Prolonged (3 to 12 weeks) antibiotics
Urine culture during and after treatment to assess effect

Urologic investigation usually indicated only if medical therapy unsuccessful

FIGURE 6–10. Recurrent UTI.

Similarly, it is not easy to distinguish upper tract from lower tract bacteriuria.* As noted previously, symptoms are usually indistinguishable. If a simple, reliable test were available as a "marker" for upper tract infection, some relapsing infections could probably be prevented by initial treatment with prolonged courses of antibiotics. Recent research offers some hope here. The antibody-coated bacteria test (ACB test)[104-107] is one such development, but this and other localization procedures are far from perfect (see Appendix II).

> Cynthia's previous medical records are now available. She had visited her previous physician 12 times in the previous 30 months because of acute urinary symptoms. The first eight episodes were associated with more than 10^5 bacteria per ml each time, *E. coli* on six occasions, and enterococci on two others. Sulfonamide therapy achieved rapid symptomatic and bacteriologic cure on all occasions but one, when enterococci were resistant to sulfonamides and ampicillin was substituted with quick success. All follow-up cultures (performed between 4 days and 2 weeks after treatment) were sterile.

> Urologic investigation revealed a normal IVP, cystoscopy, and cystometrogram, but urethral dilatation was performed anyway. BUN and creatinine were normal. Following a symptom-free interval of 3 months, symptomatic infection recurred on four more occasions, each treated successfully with sulfonamides or ampicillin as prescribed by telephone, without any urine cultures before or after treatment.

> The most recent infection is Cynthia's fifth in the past year.

These records make several important points:

1. <u>Recurrent bacterial infection is well documented.</u> This is always important before one embarks on any therapeutic course.

Many "definitions" of recurrent infection have been proposed—three per year, ten per 5 years, and so on—but these are useful only in defining a patient population (in clinical studies, for example) and not in any practical way. There is no evidence that quantitating recurrence has any bearing on pathogenesis, treatment, or prognosis. What is important is that recurrent infection is well documented, that the patient senses ongoing disability (for example, anxiety over future morbidity or marital disharmony), and that the recurrences are frequent enough to justify the specific preventive or therapeutic approach employed (see below).

2. <u>It is reasonable to assume that Cynthia's problem is that of repeated reinfections of the lower urinary tract.</u> First, reinfection is much more common than relapse, and lower tract infection is more common than upper tract infection. Second, different species of bacteria have been recovered during different symptomatic episodes. Third, post-treatment urine cultures are always sterile in Cynthia's case, up to 2 weeks after the stopping of antibiotics. As Figure 6–10 illustrates, these factors suggest that reinfection is more likely than relapse. Only sophisticated microbiologic or localization studies will answer this question definitively in some patients, but usually we can make a good guess.

---

*Remember that the distinction between relapse and reinfection is not necessarily identical to the respective distinction between lower tract and upper tract infection. Not all <u>relapses</u> involve the upper tract. A few persistent, relapsing infections may flourish in vaginal or periurethral flora or be associated with structural or functional disorders of the <u>bladder</u>—neurogenic bladder, bladder stones, or diverticula; or <u>urethra</u>—strictures, diverticula, for example. Similarly, some <u>reinfections</u> may repeatedly colonize the upper tract. <u>In general, however, relapse is more often associated with upper tract bacteriuria, reinfection with lower tract bacteriuria.</u>[91, 92]

3. Urologic investigation is usually normal in such women, whether relapse or reinfection is the problem.

The traditional rationale for urologic investigation of patients with recurrent UTI is twofold. First, as noted previously, chronic bacteriuria in association with structural (especially obstructive) urologic disease is more likely to result in long-term complications, while chronic bacteriuria per se is usually benign. Second, anatomic abnormalities—ureteral or urethral obstruction (Fig. 6–11), bladder or kidney calculi or (Fig. 6–12) diverticula—or other disorders—neurogenic bladder (Fig. 6–3C) or vesicoureteral (Fig 6–3D) reflux, for example—may render conventional antibiotic therapy ineffective. Correction of a urologic disorder may then have an impact on long-term prognosis as well as on the "stubbornness" of recurrent infections. For example, an otherwise inapparent giant staghorn calculus may render antibiotic therapy ineffective (Fig. 6–7).[88] Struvite stones, or "infection stones" (composed of magnesium, ammonium, and phosphate), may (at least partly) *result from* chronic infection[108, 109]—urea-splitting organisms like *Proteus mirabilis* may be sequestered within the stone, inaccessible to antibiotics.

In males and children, this traditional rationale for urologic investigation makes sense. In adult women, this is not the case. It is true that most practitioners have encountered women with recurrent infection whose urologic investigation revealed some unexpected abnormality or in whom urologic intervention (urethral dilatation, for example) has resulted in apparent benefit. Such procedures are difficult to justify routinely, however. One primary care physician evaluated recurrent symptomatic infection (more than three per year or more than nine per 5 years) in 40 women—none had urologic abnormalities.[35] A referral urology center evaluated recurrent infection[36] in 102 women—in 5 patients the investigators demonstrated mild abnormalities (e.g., renal cortical scars, ureteritis cystica), the discovery of

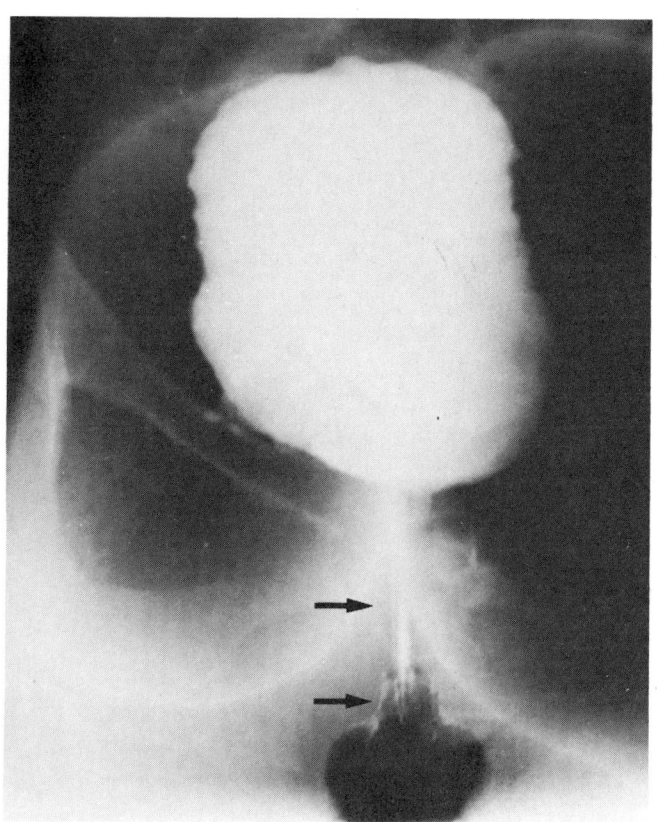

FIGURE 6–11. This voiding cystourethrogram in a 20-year-old woman with recurrent urinary infection demonstrates urethral stenosis *(arrows)* and impaired bladder emptying (this is the "postvoid" film). After urethral dilatation, the patient experienced no further infections.

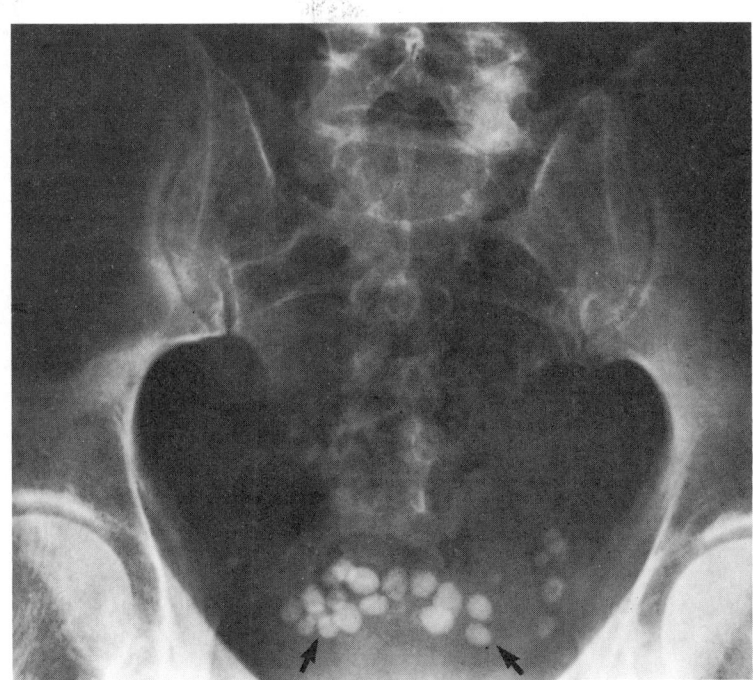

FIGURE 6–12. Multiple bladder (*arrows*) stones were the only urologic abnormality found in this middle-aged female with recurrent urinary infections. (There are several "phleboliths" lateral to the bladder also demonstrated here.) Removal of bladder stones cystoscopically resulted in a marked decrease in the frequency of urinary infections.

which did not alter therapy; 3 urethral diverticula were found, 2 of which were repaired (with uncertain benefit to the patients involved.)

In general, urologic investigation should be reserved for those women who do not respond to prolonged courses of antibiotics for presumed upper tract infection or who fail to improve despite prophylaxis against recurrent infection (see below). Urologic investigation should, however, be considered always in women with: unexplained impaired renal function and recurrent infection; known or suspected urologic disorders (prior stones, hydronephrosis, the diabetic patient, or the neurologically compromised patient with suspected neurogenic bladder); signs or symptoms of urorenal dysfunction (incontinence, hesitancy, hematuria) even when infection is not present. Urologic investigation is always indicated in the woman who has suffered more than one bout of acute pyelonephritis (see Appendix I).

4. Urethral dilatation may have helped Cynthia, transiently. Urethral dilatation is an almost mystical procedure, since it does seem to help some women with recurrent infection even when no abnormality of the urethra is found. Whether these successes result from the dilatation itself, the simultaneous bladder washout procedure (see Appendix II) sometimes performed at the time of instrumentation, or the postprocedure antibiotic therapy is difficult to say.

> Following successful treatment and a sterile urine culture 10 days later, Cynthia is instructed briefly about perineal hygiene—the need to wipe front to back after urination or defecation, urination soon after sexual intercourse, maintenance of high urine volumes during the day following intercourse, substitution of showers for baths, and avoiding nonessential antimicrobial therapy for other illnesses. These instructions are not at all novel to Cynthia, and she says that this has not helped her in the past. She does believe that at least some of her infections have begun soon after sexual intercourse.

NOTE

1. In general, prophylactic antibiotic therapy is the cornerstone of the treatment of recurrent urinary reinfection.[110-118] Such treatment should never

be begun until the prior infection has definitely been eradicated, i.e., urine cultures are sterile for 1 to 2 weeks following antibiotic therapy of the symptomatic infection. Since some women with apparent reinfection do, in fact, suffer from relapses and upper tract bacteriuria, localization studies (see Appendix II) may be helpful, when available. A minority of women with recurrent UTI are permanently cured by weeks or months of daily antibiotic therapy—it seems likely (but is unproven) that many of these women have undocumented upper tract infection. When in doubt, treat the patient for 6 weeks and only thereafter consider ongoing chronic prophylaxis (see below).

2. Antibiotics are not the only way to prevent bacteriuria. While the pathogenesis of recurrent infection is obscure, nonpharmacologic maneuvers relating to personal hygiene, sexual intercourse, and other behavioral factors will sometimes be helpful. Some such measures are folklore and have not been carefully investigated. All, however, are simple, safe, and free of cost (see case above). Occasionally, a sexually active or hygienically unsophisticated woman will benefit from these instructions, without the need for prophylactic antibiotics thereafter.

3. The role of sexual intercourse in initiating female UTI is controversial.[100] Nevertheless, in the sexually active woman a single dose of antibiotics following sexual intercourse is often a reasonable way to begin antibiotic prophylaxis[96] and will be successful in some.

> **Sulfisoxazole 500 mg is prescribed for the evening or morning following sexual intercourse.**
>
> **This appears to be helpful initially, but Cynthia develops two infections in the next 3 months (the second with *E. coli* resistant to sulfisoxazole). Following eradication of symptomatic infection, trimethoprim-sulfamethoxazole 40 mg/200 mg is begun once nightly.**
>
> **For the next 6 months, Cynthia remains completely asymptomatic, and a repeat urine culture is sterile.**

Prophylactic Antibiotics in Recurrent UTI

Several studies have documented the efficacy of prolonged courses of daily (or thrice weekly) antibiotic therapy in diminishing the number of recurrent symptomatic infections.[110-118] There is, however, no evidence that any long-term benefit accrues to the patient following the period of treatment. In other words, the discomfort and inconvenience of recurrent symptomatic infection can be predictably prevented in most cases, but only for as long as antibiotic prophylaxis is continued. Following cessation of prophylaxis, infections commonly reappear. Patients should understand this, just as the clinician must address this problem with several factors in mind:

1. The extent of the patient's disability. One or two brief symptomatic infections per year are not worth the effort or expense of daily prophylaxis. One study suggested that, in most practice settings, daily prophylaxis will be cost effective only in women with more than two symptomatic infections per year.[114] Other strategies should be considered (and studied) in women with infrequent recurrent infections. Diagnosis and treatment by telephone are often possible in the woman with known recurrent reinfections, since the history provides most of the important clinical information (see Figure 6–5).

The strategy employed by Cynthia's physician—allowing the patient to administer her own courses of antibiotics at the onset of recurrent symptoms—should also be studied, especially since various single-dose regimens have proven so effective.

2. Theoretic concerns. Prolonged antibiotic theapy often alters enteric flora—the usual reservoir of recurrent urinary reinfection—by conferring R-factor resistance, thereby selecting the emergence of subsequently more resistant bacteria.[102, 119] Some R factors confer resistance to only a single antibiotic, but others promulgate resistance to several drugs simultaneously. While, in general, daily prophylactic antibiotics have not caused clinically apparent problems with resistant bacterial infections in women studied thus far, the theoretic concern is worth note. For this, and more pragmatic reasons—a few women will be permanently "cured" after several months of daily prophylaxis—attempts should always be made to withdraw antibiotics after 6 to 8 months. Reinstitution of antibiotics is commonly necessary, since in many women reinfections again recur.

3. Varied approaches may help. As noted above, a single dose of antibiotics following sexual intercourse is occasionally sufficient. More often, daily or thrice-weekly prophylaxis is necessary. Prospective studies have shown that excellent results are obtained with trimethoprim-sulfamethoxazole 40 mg/200 mg per day or nitrofurantoin 50 mg per day. Each of these drugs is usually well tolerated and relatively inexpensive (Table 6–6). The (relatively rare) potential dangers of long-term administration of nitrofurantoin[120] tips the balance in favor of trimethoprim-sulfamethoxazole—the current drug of choice. It should be remembered that most studies of antimicrobial prophylaxis have employed newer antibiotics—other drugs, like sulfisoxazole or ampicillin, are also effective in some women. (Whatever antibiotic is used, some patient intolerance will be unavoidable. Warning the patient about common side effects is always important, but providing only a small quantity of pills with the initial prescription is also appreciated by those few patients who do develop drug reactions or side effects and who would otherwise be left with a cache of expensive, intolerable pills.)

Two months later, prophylactic antibiotics are discontinued (after 8 months' prophylaxis). Following a hiatus of 3 months, symptomatic cystitis recurs twice in 2 months. Prophylaxis is resumed.

Most women with recurrent UTI can be helped, but many different approaches should be entertained. Flexibility and practicality should override any one dogmatic bias. Every patient is different.

APPENDIX I

Acute Pyelonephritis

Acute pyelonephritis[121, 122] is a clinical syndrome usually characterized by high fever, rigors, nausea, vomiting, and flank pain in the setting of a urinary infection. The kidney itself is infected (this is one type of upper tract infection), tissue invasion and often bacteremia occur, both local and systemic immunologic responses are recruited, and there may be subtle transient functional kidney impairment (diminished renal concentrating mechanism, for example[123]). Azotemia, however, does not occur in uncomplicated unilateral acute pyelonephritis.

Not all cases of acute pyelonephritis are so dramatically obvious. Low-grade fever, nausea, and mild flank discomfort may occasionally occur even with lower tract infection, but such symptoms should alert one to the possibility of "mild" pyelonephritis, especially in the elderly or immunosuppressed patient.

When one considers that a substantial minority of women with UTI have upper tract infection in the absence of any signs of clinical acute pyelonephritis (Table 6–2; Fig. 6–2)—so–called upper tract bacteriuria (see also Appendix II)—the incidence of acute pyelonephritis is relatively infrequent. The pathophysiologic relationship between such "noninvasive" upper tract bacteriuria and clinical acute pyelonephritis is poorly understood and requires further study. A major advance would be the development of some marker that could predict which patient with UTI is likely to develop acute pyelonephritis.

The patient with classic acute pyelonephritis usually requires hospitalization and parenteral antibiotic therapy since the patient is usually in a toxic state, and may be unable to tolerate oral intake (due to nausea or paralytic ileus); in some, frank sepsis is present. The decision to hospitalize, then, is usually determined by how ill the patient looks, rather than by the suspected site of infection alone. Patients with suspected acute pyelonephritis who are not so sick often can be treated as outpatients. Careful follow-up is crucial in such circumstances.

The approach to the patient with suspected pyelonephritis must be strictly defined (whether the clinical picture is urgent or not), and much less latitude is acceptable here than in the healthy female with simple cystitis. Urinalysis, Gram's stain of the urine, and urine and blood cultures are all helpful and should be performed routinely. Urinalysis will almost always document pyuria and may further suggest the pathologic diagnosis by demonstrating white cell casts in the urinary sediment. The Gram's stain of the urine will usually demonstrate gram-negative bacilli but may reveal gram-positive cocci (enterococci or staphylococci), and initial antibiotic therapy may be more selectively chosen with this information at hand. Urine culture is mandatory initially to document the specific organism and antibiotic sensitivities and to help distinguish acute pyelonephritis from other conditions that may mimic it (for example, papillary necrosis, ureterolithiasis, or renal infarction). Bacteremia is, of course, a serious event per se, but it may also rarely suggest another diagnosis (for example, bacterial endocarditis with secondary "seeding" of the urinary tract in the patient with enterococcal or staphylococcal infection), and thus should be sought with blood cultures.

Antibiotic therapy must be individualized. The hospitalized patient with sepsis and gram-negative infection will usually be treated with parenteral ampicillin and aminoglycosides, while carbenicillin, ticarcillin, piperacillin, amikacin, and various cephalosporins may be added initially in the patient who is immunosuppressed or otherwise suspected of infection with more resistant organisms (*Pseudomonas, Proteus, Serratia*) before urine culture results are available. The patient in a less toxic state treated on an outpatient basis will usually do well initially with oral ampicillin or an oral cephalosporin, but antibiotic sensitivities of the organism cultured must then be addressed. A total of 2 to 3 weeks of antibiotic therapy is usually recommended in acute pyelonephritis, but there are no good data on optimal duration of therapy. Parenteral antibiotics are usually discontinued after the patient has been afebrile for several days, and oral antibiotics are substituted at this time. The urine culture should be repeated during treatment to document efficacy of treatment. A follow-up urine culture several days after completion of therapy is always important to document cure.

The great majority of adult women with acute pyelonephritis have normal urinary tracts. While most clinicians have encountered patients with unexpected functional or anatomic disease of the genitourinary system underlying the development of acute pyelonephritis (Fig. 6–13), routine intravenous pyelography in the acute disease is highly unlikely to add useful information and may (rarely) be dangerous.[124] However, unremitting fever or toxicity after 48 to 72 hours of appropriate antibiotic therapy must suggest some complicating (especially obstructive) urorenal disease. Ultrasound ex-

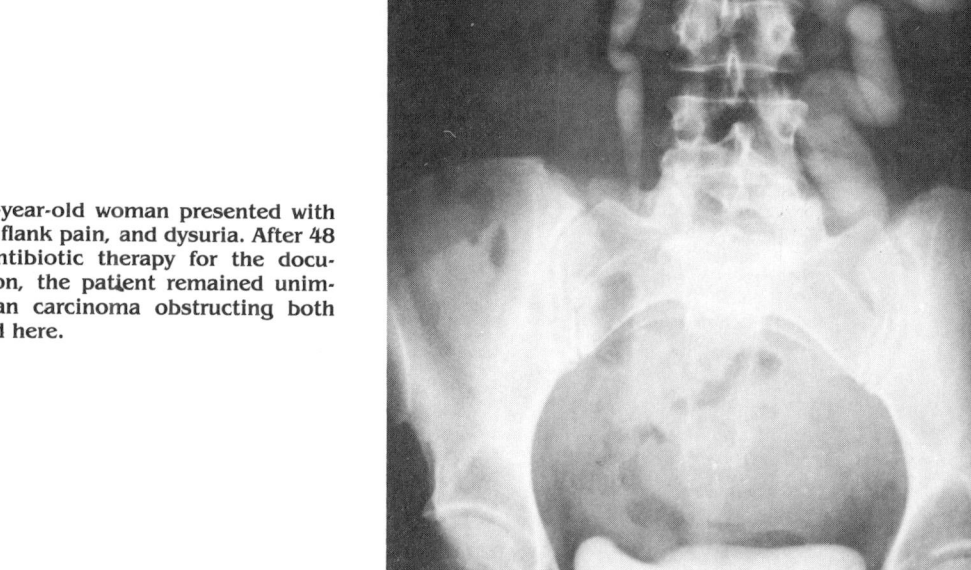

FIGURE 6–13. This 35-year-old woman presented with high fever, chills, right flank pain, and dysuria. After 48 hours of parenteral antibiotic therapy for the documented *E. coli* infection, the patient remained unimproved. A large ovarian carcinoma obstructing both ureters is demonstrated here.

amination of the kidneys, when available, may be especially helpful in detecting obstruction when intravenous pyelography should be avoided (for example, in the dehydrated diabetic with sepsis).[124] Many clinicians obtain IVPs (to exclude underlying disease) after the patient is clinically improved and well hydrated, but the "yield" is very low in the adult woman with her first bout of pyelonephritis. Recurrent acute pyelonephritis always mandates urologic investigation.

When obstructive uropathy cannot be demonstrated (by ultrasound, for example) in the patient with presumed acute pyelonephritis who does not respond rapidly to appropriate parenteral antibiotics, several other conditions should be remembered:

Perinephric abscess[125, 126] usually occurs "behind" some obstructing process in the ureter or pelvicaliceal system, but not always. The patient with diabetes mellitus, polycystic kidneys, or a history of parenteral drug abuse, chronic steroid treatment, or other immunosuppression is at risk for perinephric abscess, as is the patient with bacteremia or some other serious focal infection (such as lung abscess, osteomyelitis, endocarditis). Intravenous pyelography will often suggest the diagnosis, but renal arteriography, CT scan or gallium scan may be necessary. Surgical drainage is the usual treatment of choice.

Intranephric (renal parenchymal) abscess[126] is usually acquired after hematogenous seeding from other sites of primary infection (see above). Parenteral antibiotic treatment of the systemic infection may result in cure, without surgical drainage, in some such patients.

Xanthogranulomatous pyelonephritis[127] is a rare form of renal suppuration that is usually indolent in presentation and is only sometimes associated with fever, flank pain, and bacteriuria. Urine culture is often sterile. Surgery (nephrectomy) is usually required for diagnosis (and treatment).

Tuberculous or fungal infection should also be suspected in the patient with clinical acute pyelonephritis in whom urine culture for bacteria is sterile.

Localizing the Site of Urinary Infection

As noted in the text proper, bacterial urinary infection may involve the lower urinary system (bladder, urethra) or the upper urinary system (kidneys, renal pelvis, ureters), or both. Except for the clinical syndrome of classic toxic acute pyelonephritis (see Appendix I), clinical signs and symptoms are unreliable predictors of the site of infection.[1] Since upper tract infection is more difficult to treat, commonly relapses, and has an uncertain effect on long-term morbidity, its detection is worthwhile. (Certainly, clinical research studies on the treatment of urinary infection must correlate response to treatment with the site of infection, whatever other variables are also analyzed.)

There are several ways to localize the site of infection.

DIRECT TECHNIQUES

Renal biopsy might demonstrate upper tract infection by histologic and bacteriologic study of the biopsy specimen. This procedure is never indicated for this purpose.

Ureteral catheterization[64] is the "gold standard." Under direct cystoscopic observation, quantitative urine cultures are obtained through sterile catheters threaded into each ureter—this clearly distinguishes bladder from renal bacteriuria and localizes infection to one or both upper tracts. The disadvantages of this technique are obvious—it is expensive, logistically cumbersome, and potentially dangerous. While it should remain the standard with which to compare other localization techniques in clinical research, it is rarely recommended in practical patient management.

The bladder washout procedure[128, 129] involves catheterizing the bladder, culturing bladder urine, and subsequently collecting several more serial urine cultures after the bladder is "washed" with saline, a debriding agent (streptokinase), and an (usually aminoglycoside) antibiotic. The results of the "postwashout" urine cultures correlate well with ureteral catheterization studies in localizing the infection. Bladder infection typically demonstrates

TABLE 6–9. BLADDER WASHOUT

SITE OF INFECTION	1 (BLADDER)	2 (IMMEDIATE POST-WASHOUT)	3 (10 MIN)	4 (20 MIN)	5 (30 MIN)	6 (40 MIN)	7 (50 MIN)
Bladder	$>10^5$	0	0	0	0	0	0
Renal	$>10^5$	$\geq 10^2$	10^4	10^4	5×10^4	5×10^4	5×10^4
Not sure	$>10^5$	10^1-10^2	10^3	4×10^3	2×10^3	10^3	10^3

sterile postwashout cultures (the procedure itself will often eradicate the infection). Upper tract infection is diagnosed when bacteriuria persists after washout, and quantitative bacterial counts increase in serial samples over time. Table 6–9 demonstrates typical findings on bladder washout when infections are localized to the bladder or to the kidneys (or when results are equivocal). Morbidity of the bladder washout procedure is minimal, but it is clearly too invasive and cumbersome for routine practical use.

INDIRECT TECHNIQUES

Many different procedures have been advocated for this purpose. X-ray studies (IVP, voiding cystourethrogram), urinalysis, tests of renal physiology (concentrating capacity, response to water loading),[130, 131] white cell excretion studies,[132, 133] gallium scanning,[134, 135] and urinary enzyme determinations[136] are among the many. None of these is useful.

The antibody-coated bacteria test (ACB test)[104-107] is quite reliable in adult women as a predictor of the site of infection. This method visualizes, by direct immunofluorescence, bacteria in the urine (from the urine culture) that have formed a complex with antibodies (presumably produced in the renal parenchyma). A positive antibody test correlates well with upper tract infection, while a negative test correlates well with lower tract infection. This test, however, is far from infallible (it may even be negative in women with classic acute pyelonephritis). Moreover, the ACB test is not widely available, it is not useful in all patients (it is useless in males, for example), and it requires ongoing technical expertise with its performance and standardization.

When the ACB test is available in a laboratory expert in its implementation, it may be very helpful. It has proven very useful in clinical research studies of urinary tract infection. The routine performance of this test in all women with UTI cannot be recommended here, however. Most women with UTI have lower tract infections, and of the minority with upper tract infection, many are cured with short-term antibiotics anyway (Table 6–4). The ACB test should probably be reserved for women with recurrent or persistent bacteriuria in whom one wishes to exclude upper tract infection.

DOCUMENTATION OF RELAPSE: PRESUMPTIVE LOCALIZATION

As noted in the text proper, most relapsing infections reside in the upper tract; most reinfections, in the lower tract. This is by no means invariable, but documentation of relapse is sometimes a helpful clue to the presence of upper tract infection. As we have seen (page 294), only identical serotyping of the original and post-treatment organism is definitive evidence of relapse in the patient with persistent bacteriuria. Reference laboratories will perform serotyping on demand.

Of great practical interest is the fact that failure to respond to single-dose antibiotic therapy often correlates well with the presence of upper tract infection. Identification of the same species of organism with identical antibiotic sensitivities before and after antibiotic therapy is only "soft" evidence favoring a relapsing upper tract infection, but this observation is further recommendation for single-dose therapy of apparently uncomplicated UTI—as a therapeutic diagnostic test.

The Economics of Urinary Tract Infection

Table 6–10 illustrates total direct costs incurred during the evaluation and treatment of single episodes of urinary infection in 117 adult women in a teaching hospital outpatient clinic.[114] Complicated cases—patients with stones, urologic abnormalities, catheters, for example—were *excluded* from the study. While these figures may not accurately reflect costs in some clinical practices, they do underline the striking expense that may result from the routine or "traditional" management of urinary infection. This traditional approach—pretreatment urine cultures, antibiotic therapy, post-treatment urine cultures (see Fig. 6–1)—can be remarkably costly. When one considers that these particular costs involve only patients with uncomplicated urinary tract infection, and that perhaps 5 million such women visit American physicians every year,[137] the economics of urinary infection achieves a relevance sometimes ignored by the individual patient (and the physician). Can we be spending over a billion dollars per year on female urinary tract infections alone?

Most of the financial expense involves physician fees and urine cultures. Antibiotics, when carefully chosen, are relatively inexpensive (see Table 6–6). It seems very likely that selective clinical strategies for individual patients can dramatically reduce the cost of managing UTIs. As discussed in the text proper, the value of pretreatment and post-treatment urine cultures deserves skepticism in many patients. (Note that most of the patients in Table 6–10 are each billed for two urinalyses, two urine cultures, and two clinic visits.) Usually second physician visits are unnecessary. While the physicians in this study employed admirable restraint in the use of high-level technology (cystoscopy, intravenous pyelography), it is common knowledge that such restraint is not universal.

The approach to female urinary tract infection must be individualized. As noted elsewhere in this book, the abuse of "low-level technology" contributes greatly to soaring medical costs.

TABLE 6–10. COSTS OF EVALUATION AND TREATMENT OF SINGLE EPISODES OF UTI IN 117 PATIENTS*

	Cystitis (N = 61)		Urethral Syndrome (N = 48)		Pyelonephritis (N = 8)	
	N	$	N	$	N	$
Urinalysis	127	685.80	80	432.00	18	97.20
Urine culture	133	1276.80	77	739.20	18	172.80
Clinic visit	144	5472.00	87	2784.00	19	722.00
Gonorrhea culture	6	24.00	16	64.00	0	0.
Abdominal film	1	25.00	3	75.00	0	0.
Intravenous pyelography	5	250.00	3	150.00	2	100.00
Cystoscopy	4	400.00	4	400.00	0	0.
Vaginal wet prep	—	—	5	15.00	—	—
Antibiotics	68	303.71	31	229.61	9	67.36
Average cost per episode		139.02		103.46		166.67

*Adapted from reference 114.

REFERENCES

1. Sanford, JP: Urinary tract symptoms and infections. Annu Rev Med 26:485–498, 1975.
2. Kass, EH, Zinner, SH: Bacteriuria and renal disease. J Infect Dis 120:27–46, 1969.
3. Kunin, CM, et al.: Epidemiology of urinary tract infections. N Engl J Med 263:817–823, 1960
4. Kunin, CM, et al.: Urinary tract infection in school children. N Engl J Med 266:1289–1296, 1962.
5. Kass, EH: Asymptomatic infections of the urinary tract. Trans Assoc Am Physicians 69:56–64, 1956.
6. Kass, EH: Bacteriuria and the pathogenesis of pyelonephritis. Lab Invest 9:110–116, 1960.
7. Gower, PE: A long-term study of renal function in patients with radiological pyelonephritis and other allied radiological lesions. In Brumfitt, W., Asscher, AW (eds.): Urinary Tract Infections. London: Oxford University Press, 1973.
8. Freedman, LR: Chronic pyelonephritis at autopsy. Ann Intern Med 66:697, 1967.
9. Burray, AF: A profile of renal disease in Queensland: Results of an autopsy survey. Med J Aust 1:826, 1966.
10. Stewart, JH, et al.: Diseases causing end-stage renal failure in New South Wales. Br J Med 1:440, 1975.
11. Freedman, LR, Andriole, V: The long-term followup of women with urinary tract infections. In Proceedings of the 5th International Congress of Nephrology, Mexico City, 1972, 3:230.
12. Freedman, LR: Natural history of urinary infection in adults. Kidney Int 8(Suppl):96–100, 1975.
13. Freeman, RB: Does bacteriuria lead to renal failure? Clin Nephrol 1:61, 1973.
14. Schechter, H, et al.: Chronic pyelonephritis as a cause of renal failure in dialysis candidates. JAMA 216:514, 1971.
15. Murray, T, Goldberg, M: Chronic interstitial nephritis: Etiologic factors. Ann Intern Med 82:453–459, 1975.
16. Gleckman, R: The controversy of treatment of asymptomatic bacteriuria in nonpregnant women—resolved. J Urol 116:776, 1976.
17. Meares, EM: Asymptomatic bacteriuria: Current concepts in management. Postgrad Med 62:106, 1977.
18. Kunin, CM: Should bacteriuria, whether symptomatic or not, be treated vigorously? In Ingelfinger, FJ, Relman, AS, Finland, M (eds.): Controversies in Internal Medicine. Philadelphia: W. B. Saunders, 1966, pp. 289–301.
19. Petersdorf, RG: Asymptomatic bacteriuria: A therapeutic enigma. In Ingelfinger, FJ, Relman, AS, Finland, M (eds.): Controversies in Internal Medicine. Philadelphia: W. B. Saunders, 1966, pp. 302–312.
20. Kimmelstel P: Asymptomatic bacteriuria, a hypothetical concept, should be treated with caution. In Ingelfinger, FJ, Relman, AS, Finland, M (eds.): Controversies in Internal Medicine. Philadelphia: W. B. Saunders, 1966, pp. 313–327.
21. Relman A: Comment. In Ingelfinger, FJ, Relman, AS, Finland, M (eds.): Controversies in Internal Medicine. Philadelphia: W. B. Saunders, 1966, pp. 328–329.
22. Sussman, M, et al.: Asymptomatic significant bacteriuria in the nonpregnant woman. I. Description of a population. Br J Med 1:799–803, 1969.
23. Asscher, AW, et al.: Asymptomatic significant bacteriuria in the nonpregnant woman. II. Response to treatment and followup. Br J Med 1:804–806, 1969.
24. Asscher, AW, et al.: The clinical significance of asymptomatic bacteriuria in the nonpregnant woman. J Infect Dis 120:17–26, 1969.
25. Summary of invited discussion on bacteriuria. Kidney Int 8(Suppl.):120–121, 1975.
26. Turck, M: Therapeutic guidelines in the management of urinary tract infection and pyelonephritis. Urol Clin North Am 2:443–450, 1975.
27. Stamey, TA, et al.: The localization and treatment of urinary tract infections: The role of bacteriocidal urine levels as opposed to serum levels. Medicine 44:1–36, 1965.
28. Kass, EH: Chemotherapeutic and antibiotic drugs in the management of infections of the urinary tract. Am J Med 18:764–781, 1955.
29. Kass, EH: Bacteriuria and the diagnosis of infection of the urinary tract: Without observations on the use of methionine as a urinary antiseptic. Arch Intern Med 100:709–714, 1957.
30. Sanford, JP, et al.: Evaluation of the "positive" urine culture: An approach to the differentiation of significant bacteria from contaminants. Am J Med 20:88–93, 1956.
31. Stamm, WE, et al.: Causes of the acute urethral syndrome in women. N Engl J Med 303:409–415, 1980.
32. Stamm, WE, et al.: Diagnosis of coliform infection in acutely dysuric women. N Engl J Med 307:463–468, 1982.
33. Gallagher, DJA, et al.: Acute infections of the urinary tract and the urethral syndrome in general practice. Br J Med 1:622–626, 1965.
34. Brooks, D, Maudar, A: Pathogenesis of the urethral syndrome in women and its diagnosis in general practice. Lancet 2:893–898, 1972.
35. Rubinoff, H: Urinary tract infection. Primary Care 4:617–628, 1977.
36. Fowler, JE, Pulaski, ET: Excretory urography, cystography, and cystoscopy in the evaluation of women with urinary tract infections. N Engl J Med 304:462, 1981.
37. Komaroff, AL, et al.: Management strategies of urinary and vaginal infection. Arch Intern Med 138:1069–1073, 1978.
38. Conte, JE: Urinary tract infection/vaginitis protocol. West J Med 129:181–187, 1978.
39. Mabeck, CE: Treatment of uncomplicated urinary tract infection in nonpregnant women. Postgrad Med J 48:69–75, 1972.
40. Curran, JW: Gonorrhea and the urethral syndrome: Sex Transm Dis 4:119–121 (July–Sept), 1977.
41. Fang, LST, et al.: Efficacy of single dose and conventional amoxicillin therapy in urinary tract infection localized by antibody coated bacteria technique. N Engl J Med 298:413–416, 1978.

42. Rubin, RH, et al.: Single dose amoxicillin therapy for urinary tract infection. JAMA 244:561–564, 1980.
43. Andriole, VT: Urinary tract infection in pregnancy: Urol Clin North Am 2:485–498, 1975.
44. Savage, WE, et al.: Demographic and prognostic characteristics of bacteriuria of pregnancy. Medicine 46:385–407, 1967.
45. Brumfitt, W: The effects of bacteriuria in pregnancy on maternal and fetal health. Kidney Int 8(Suppl):113–119, 1975.
46. Forland, M, et al.: Urinary tract infections in patients with diabetes mellitus. JAMA 238:1924–1926, 1977.
47. Komaroff, AL, Friedland, G: The dysuria-pyuria syndrome. N Engl J Med 303:452–454, 1980.
48. Stamm, WE, et al.: Treatment of the acute urethral syndrome. N Engl J Med 304:956–957, 1981.
49. Kusumi, RK, et al.: Rapid detection of pyuria by leukocyte esterase activity. JAMA 245:1653–1655, 1981.
50. Cattell, WR, et al.: Approach to the frequency and dysuria syndrome. Kidney Int 8(Suppl):138–143, 1975.
51. Brumfitt, W, Percival A: Pathogenesis and laboratory diagnosis of nontuberculous urinary tract infection: A review. J Clin Pathol 17:482–491, 1964.
52. Charlton, CAC, et al.: Three-day and ten-day chemotherapy for urinary tract infection in general practice. Br J Med 1:124–126, 1976.
53. Sabath, LD: Tetracycline in the treatment of genitourinary tract infection. Bull NY Acad Med 54:205–215, 1978.
54. Buckwold, FJ, et al.: Therapy for acute cystitis in adult women. Randomized comparison of single-dose sulfisoxazole versus trimethoprim-sulfamethoxazole. JAMA 247:1839–1842, 1982.
55. Stamm, WE: Single-dose treatment of cystitis. JAMA 244:591–592, 1980.
56. Ronald, AR, et al.: Bacteriuria localization and response to single-dose therapy in women. JAMA 235:1854–1856, 1976.
57. Gruneberg, RN, Brumfitt, W: Single-dose treatment of acute urinary tract infection: A controlled trial. Br J Med 3:649–651, 1967.
58. Kabovitz, E, et al.: Single-dose gentamicin therapy for urinary tract infection. Antimicrob Agents Chemother 6:465, 1974.
59. Bailey, RR, Abbott, GD: Treatment of urinary tract infection with a single dose of trimethoprim-sulfamethoxazole. Can Med Assoc J 118:551–552, 1978.
60. O'Donnell, RP: Acute urethral syndrome in women (letter). N Engl J Med 303:1531, 1980.
61. Maskell, R: Acute urethral syndrome in women (letter). N Engl J Med 303:1531–1532, 1980.
62. Maskell, R, Pead, L: Anaerobes and slow growers in urine cultures. Lancet 1:368, 1980.
63. Aarnoudse, JG, et al.: Do anaerobes cause urinary tract infection? Lancet 1:368–369, 1980.
64. Gargan, RA, et al.: Do anaerobes cause urinary infection? Lancet 1:37, 1980.
65. Drabu, YJ, Sanderson, PJ: Urine cultures in urethral syndrome. Lancet 1:37–38, 1980.
66. Maskell, R, et al.: The puzzle of "urethral syndrome": A possible answer? Lancet 1:1058–1059, 1978.
67. Phillips, MF, et al.: Tetracycline poisoning in renal failure. Br J Med 2:419, 1974.
68. Schlegel, JU, et al.: Bacteriuria and chronic renal disease. Trans Am Assoc Genitourin Surg 59:32, 1967.
69. Adam, WR, Dawborn, JK: Urinary excretion and plasma levels of sulfonamides in patients with renal impairment. Aust Ann Med 19:250, 1970.
70. Cox, CE: Pharmacology of carbenicillin indanyl sodium in renal insufficiency. J Infect Dis 127(Suppl):157, 1973.
71. Britt, MR, et al.: Antimicrobial prophylaxis for catheter-associated bacteriuria. Antimicrob Agents Chemother 11:240, 1977.
72. Stamm, WE: Guidelines for prevention of catheter-associated urinary tract infection. Ann Intern Med 82:386–389, 1975.
73. Warren, JW, et al.: Antibiotic irrigation and catheter-associated urinary tract infections. N Engl J Med 299:570–573, 1978.
74. Platt, R, et al.: Mortality associated with nosocomial urinary tract infection. N Engl J Med 307:637–642, 1982.
75. Namavar, R, et al.: Novobiocin resistance and virulence of strains of *Staphylococcus saprophyticus* isolated from urine and skin. Med Microbiol Immunol 11:243–247, 1978.
76. Shrestha, TL, Darrell, JH: Urinary infection with coagulase-negative staphylococci in a teaching hospital. J Clin Pathol 32:299–302, 1979.
77. Jordan, PA, et al.: Urinary tract infection caused by *Staphylococcus saprophyticus*. J Infect Dis 142:510–515, 1980.
78. Anderson, JD, et al.: Urinary tract infection due to *Staphylococcus saprophyticus*, bio type 3. Can Med Assoc J 124:415–418, 1981.
79. Stamey, TA, et al.: Serum vs. urinary antimicrobial concentrations in cure of urinary tract infections. N Engl J Med 291:1159–1163, 1974.
80. Randall, RE, et al.: Cryptococcal pyelonephritis. N Engl J Med 279:60, 1968.
81. Petersen, EA, et al.: Coccidiodiduria: Clinical significance. Ann Intern Med 85:34, 1975.
82. Michigan, S: Genitourinary fungal infections. J Urol 116:390, 1976.
83. Christensen, WE: Genitourinary tuberculosis: Review of 102 cases. Medicine 53:337, 1974.
84. Simon, HB, et al.: Genitourinary tuberculosis: Clinical features in a general hospital population. Am J Med 63:410, 1977.
85. Murray, T, Goldberg, M: Analgesic abuse and renal disease. Ann Rev Med 26:537, 1975.
86. Messing, EM, Stamey, TA: Interstitial cystitis: Early diagnosis, pathology and treatment. Urology 12:381–392, 1978.
87. Kraft, JK, Stamey, TA: The natural history of symptomatic recurrent bacteriuria in women. Medicine 56:55–60, 1977.

88. Stamey, TA: A clinical classification of urinary tract infection based upon origin. South Med J 68:934–939, 1975.
89. Santoro, J, Kaye, D: Recurrent urinary tract infection: Pathogenesis and management. Med Clin North Am 62:1005–1020, 1978.
90. McGeachie, J: Recurrent infections of the urinary tract: Reinfection or recrudescence? Br J Med 1:952–954, 1966.
91. Turck, M, et al.: Relapse and reinfection in chronic bacteriuria. N Engl J Med 275:70–73, 1966.
92. Turck, M, et al.: Relapse and reinfection in chronic bacteriuria. II. The correlation between site of infection and pattern of recurrence in chronic bacteriuria. N Engl J Med 278:422–427, 1968.
93. Gillenwater, JY: Recurrent urinary infection. Postgrad Med 53:124–128, 1973.
94. Stamey, TA, et al.: Recurrent urinary infection in adult women. The role of introital enterobacteria. West J Med 115:1–19, 1971.
95. Stamey, TA, et al.: The immunologic basis of recurrent bacteriuria: Role of cervicovaginal antibody in anterobacterial colonization of the introital mucosa. Medicine 57:47–56, 1978.
96. Vosti, KL: Recurrent urinary tract infection: Prevention by prophylactic antibiotics after sexual intercourse. JAMA 239:934–940, 1975.
97. Brumfitt, W, et al.: Antibiotic resistant E. coli causing urinary tract infection: Relation of fecal flora. Lancet 1:315, 1971.
98. Datta, M, et al.: R-factors in E. coli in feces after oral chemotherapy. Lancet 1:312, 1971.
99. Kaye, D: Host defense mechanisms in the urinary tract. Urol Clin North Am 2:407–422, 1975.
100. Buckley, RM: Urine bacterial counts after sexual intercourse. N Engl J Med 298:321–324, 1978.
101. Addatto, K, et al.: Behavioral factors and urinary tract infection. JAMA 241:2525–2526, 1979
102. Harkness, JL, et al.: R-factors in urinary tract infection. Kidney Int 8(Suppl):130–133, 1975.
103. Schaeffer, AJ, et al.: Association of in vitro E. coli adherence to vaginal and buccal epithelial cells with susceptibility of women to recurrent urinary tract infection. N Engl J Med 304:1062–1066, 1981.
104. Thomas, V, et al.: Antibody coated bacteria in the urine and the site of urinary tract infection. N Engl J Med 290:588–590, 1974.
105. Jones, SR, et al.: Localization of urinary tract infection by detection of antibody-coated bacteria in urine sediment. N Engl J Med 290:591–593, 1974.
106. Mundt, KA, Polk, BF: Identification of site of urinary tract infection by antibody-coated bacteria assay. Lancet 2:1172–1175, 1979.
107. Hawthorne, NJ, et al.: Accuracy of antibody-coated bacteria test in recurrent urinary tract infection. Mayo Clin Proc 53:651–654, 1978.
108. Griffith, DP: Struvite stones. Kidney Int 13:372–382, 1978.
109. Nemoy, NJ, Stamey, TA: Surgical, bacterological and nonchemical management of "infection stone." JAMA 215:1470–1476, 1971.
110. Stamey, TA, et al.: Prophylactic efficacy of nitrofurantoin macrocrystals and trimethoprim-sulfamethoxazole in urinary infection. N Engl J Med 296:780–783, 1977.
111. Harding, GKM, Ronald, AR: A controlled study of antimicrobial prophylaxis of recurrent urinary infection in women. N Engl J Med 291:597–601, 1974.
112. Harding, GKM, et al.: Prophylaxis of recurrent urinary tract infection in female patients. Efficacy of low-dose, thrice-weekly therapy with trimethoprim-sulfamethoxazole. JAMA 242:1975–1977, 1979.
113. Stamm, WE, et al.: Antimicrobial prophylaxis of recurrent urinary tract infection. A double-blind placebo-controlled trial. Ann Intern Med 92:770–775, 1980.
114. Stamm, WE, et al.: Is antimicrobial prophylaxis of urinary tract infection cost effective? Ann Intern Med 94:251–255, 1981.
115. Ronald, AR, Harding, GKM: Urinary infection prophylaxis in women. Ann Intern Med 94:268–270, 1981.
116. O'Grady, F, et al.: Long-term treatment of persistent or recurrent urinary tract infection with trimethoprim-sulfamethoxazole. J Infect Dis 128(Suppl):652–656, 1973.
117. Smellie, JM, et al.: Long-term low-dose cotrimoxazole in prophylaxis of childhood urinary tract infection: Clinical aspects. Br J Med 2:203–206, 1976.
118. Ronald, AR, et al.: Prophylaxis of recurrent urinary tract infection in females: Comparison of nitrofurantoin with trimethoprim-sulfamethoxazole. Can Med Assoc J 112(Suppl):13–16, 1979.
119. Gruneberg, RN, et al.: Changes in antibiotic sensitivities of fecal organisms in response to treatment in children with urinary tract infection. In Brumfitt, W, Asscher, AW (eds.): Urinary Tract Infection. London: Oxford University Press, 1973, pp. 131–136.
120. Holmberg, L, et al.: Adverse reactions to nitrofurantoin: Analysis of 921 reports. Am J Med 69:733–738, 1980.
121. Riff, LJM: Evaluation and treatment of urinary infection. Med Clin North Am 62:1183–1200, 1978.
122. Braude, AI: Current concepts of pyelonephritis. Medicine 52:257–264, 1978.
123. Ronald, AR, et al.: Effect of bacteriuria on renal concentrating mechanism. Ann Intern Med 70:723, 1969.
124. Byrd, L, et al.: Radiocontrast-induced acute renal failure. Medicine 58:270–279, 1979.
125. Thorley, JD, et al.: Perinephric abscess. Medicine 53:441, 1974.
126. Saiki, J, et al.: Perinephric and intranephric abscesses: A review of the literature. West J Med 136:95–102, 1982.
127. Goodman, M, et al.: Xanthogranulomatous pyelonephritis (XGP): A local disease with systemic manifestations. Report of 23 patients and a review of the literature. Medicine 58:171–181, 1979.
128. Fairley, KF, et al.: Simple test to determine site of urinary tract infection. Lancet 2:427–428, 1967.
129. Fairley, KF, et al.: Site of infection in acute urinary tract infection in general practice. Lancet 2:615–618, 1971.

130. Norden, CW, et al.: Predictive effect of urinary concentrating ability and hemagglutinating antibody titer upon response to antimicrobial therapy in bacteriuria of pregnancy. J Infect Dis 121:588–596, 1970.

131. Clark, H, et al.: Correlation between site of infection and maximal concentrating ability in bacteriuria. J Infect Dis 120:47–51, 1969.

132. Little, PJ, deWardener, HE: The use of prednisolone phosphate in the diagnosis of pyelonephritis in man. Lancet 1:1145, 1962.

133. Pears, MA, Houghton, BJ: Response of infected urinary tract to bacterial pyrogen. Lancet 2:1167, 1959.

134. Kersler,WO, et al.: Gallium-67 scan in the diagnosis of pyelonephritis. West J Med 121:91, 1974.

135. Hurwitz, SR, et al.: Gallium-67 citrate to diagnose pyelonephritis. J Nucl Med 15:503, 1974.

136. Ronald, AR, et al.: Failure of urinary beta-glucuronidase activity to localize the site of urinary tract infection. Appl Microbiol 21:990, 1971.

137. National Center for Health Statistics. Ambulatory medical care rendered in physicians' offices: United States, 1975. Adv Data 12:1–2, 1977.

7

VULVO-VAGINAL DISORDERS

SYMPTOMS AND SIGNS........................... 310
THE INITIAL APPROACH......................... 311
DIFFERENTIAL DIAGNOSIS 313
INFECTIOUS VAGINITIS......................... 318
    Treatment of Trichomoniasis 324
    Treatment of Vaginal Candidiasis............ 327
    Recurrent Vaginal Candidiasis 329
ATROPHIC VAGINITIS........................... 333
VULVAR PRURITUS 334
APPENDIX: NONSPECIFIC VAGINITIS............. 337
REFERENCES................................... 339

> Trixi T., a 56-year-old widow, enters the clinic complaining of "a personal problem." Questioning reveals that the patient has noted an increased vaginal discharge over the past 3 weeks, associated with mild itching of the vulvar and perineal area. While for many years she has noted intermittent, light vaginal discharge ("normal for me, I guess"), this is a different problem. There is no history of abdominal or pelvic pain, fever, or previous known vaginal or venereal infections.
>
> This is a new problem.

There are many possible causes of vaginal discharge and itching, but while differential diagnosis may be lengthy, a brief, careful history and examination will reveal the correct diagnosis in most instances.[1–6] If a simple systematic approach is followed in all such patients, the common disorders will be easily recognized and the less common more quickly suspected.

SYMPTOMS AND SIGNS

Abnormal vaginal discharge refers to unaccustomed or excessive flow of secretions from the vagina. The vagina itself normally contains no glandular elements, unlike the vulva, cervix, endometrium, and fallopian tubes, all of which may secrete or "discharge" in response to normal physiologic events. Cervical secretions are prominent during ovulation, vulvar secretions during coitus, endometrial and tubal secretions during the latter phase of the menstrual cycle.[5, 7] The vagina contributes to the normal vaginal discharge by shedding its desquamated nonkeratinized squamous epithelial cells under hormonal influences. Glycogen liberated from these cells is converted to lactic acid by normal vaginal bacterial flora. These physiologic events underscore the facts that vaginal discharge may be either normal or abnormal and

TABLE 7–1. CAUSES OF VAGINAL DISCHARGE

PHYSIOLOGIC	INFECTIOUS	NONINFECTIOUS
Ovulation	Vaginal	Atrophic (senile) vaginitis
Coitus	Candida	Vaginal foreign body
Oral contraceptive	Trichomonas	Vaginal adenosis[8, 9]
use	Gardnerella	Allergic/irritant vulvovaginitis
Pregnancy	Toxic shock syndrome	Vulvar, vaginal carcinoma
Premenstrual		Cervical polyps
Premenarchal	Vulvar	Cervical carcinoma
Intrauterine device	Herpes	Cervical erosion/ulcer
	Condylomata acuminata	Uterine carcinoma
	Syphilis	Endometrial (submucous)
	Bartholinitis	myoma
	Lymphogranuloma venereum	Vesicovaginal fistula
	Chancroid	Enterovaginal fistula
	Granuloma inguinale	
	Urethritis	
	Pyoderma	
	Cervical	
	Gonorrhea	
	Chlamydial or bacterial cervicitis	
	Chronic cervicitis	
	Pelvic inflammatory disease	

that abnormal vaginal discharge may reflect abnormalities in any one of several genital organs.

On the other hand, vulvovaginal itching is never normal. When pruritus is associated with vaginal discharge, infectious vulvovaginitis is the usual cause, but many other conditions are possible (Table 7–1). Similarly, vulvovaginal pruritus alone may be due to a host of disorders—primary dermatologic diseases, infestations, neoplasms, and dystrophic disorders comprise most of these (see pages 334).

THE INITIAL APPROACH

With these facts in mind, our approach to the patient with vaginal discharge or itching should focus on three broad questions:

1. What is the anatomic site of organ involvement? Is the disorder vulvar, vaginal, or cervical? Is there evidence for uterine or tubo-ovarian involvement?

2. Is the problem infectious or noninfectious? Most women with vulvovaginal discharge or itching suffer from one or more types of infectious vulvovaginitis. Simple office examination can confirm specific diagnoses most of the time (see below).

3. Are there complicating factors? There are many potentially complicating factors that may influence our approach, depending upon the site and nature of the problem. Examples include the presence of underlying systemic diseases (for example, diabetes), a history of repeated or refractory vaginal infections, unusual sexual practices, and various psychologic issues surrounding sexual function. Some of these will be discussed below.

How do we answer these questions?

Physical examination provides most of the answers (see below), but the history is also essential. Consider our patient (see also Fig. 7–8):

1. Does the patient complain of pelvic or abdominal pain? Is there a history of fever or systemic illness?

Pelvic inflammatory disease may produce vaginal discharge, but the patient is usually ill and complains of abdominal pain. Low-grade fever, pelvic or low abdominal pain, bilateral tubo-ovarian tenderness and swelling, and exacerbation of pain by manual manipulation of the cervix during pelvic examination ("chandelier sign") are typical findings in the woman with pelvic inflammatory disease (PID). Gonococcal infection is the cause in one third to one half of such women, while various anaerobic bacteria and chlamydiae have been implicated in nongonococcal PID.[10-12] Laparoscopy is sometimes necessary to confirm the diagnosis,[13] but usually the clinical findings are sufficient to presume the diagnosis, obtain gonococcal cultures, and begin broad-spectrum antibiotic therapy. Coverage for gonorrhea should always be provided—tetracycline 500 mg qid for 10 days, or ampicillin 3.5 gm immediately followed by 500 mg qid for 10 days.[14] (In Chapter 11, "Abdominal Pain," other aspects of PID are discussed, since the presenting symptom is only rarely just vaginal discharge; PID is usually considered in the differential diagnosis of abdominal pain.)

Toxic shock syndrome is an acute febrile illness involving multiple organ systems, usually associated with hypotension and a characteristic exfoliative erythroderma, ultimately resulting in desquamation of the skin of the palms and soles.[15-17] It is probably due to various toxins of *Staphylococcus aureus* and was initially associated with the use of certain vaginal tampons. Parenteral antistaphylococcal antibiotics and hemodynamic support are the mainstays of treatment. This disease is rare but potentially fatal. Vaginal discharge is commonly present, but the severity of multisystem illness always overshadows the vaginal symptoms.

Trixi denies abdominal or pelvic pain, feels generally well, and has noted no fever, chills, or rash.

2. Are symptoms most suggestive of vaginitis? The presence of both pruritus and discharge is a helpful clue, since infectious vaginitis is the usual cause when these symptoms coexist. Vaginal discharge without pruritus may or may not be abnormal, but in general requires the same diagnostic approach (see Fig. 7–8). Pruritus without discharge may be caused by vaginitis, but many other infectious and noninfectious disorders are also possible (see Table 7–6).

When urinary symptoms coexist, it is helpful to distinguish between "vaginal" or "external" dysuria (caused by urine flow through inflamed external genitalia) and internal dysuria ("it burns inside"), which more often implies urinary infection (see Chapter 6, "Female Urinary Tract Infections").

Trixi describes both vaginal discharge and itching but denies any urinary symptoms.

3. Is the patient postmenopausal? Virtually all types of infectious and noninfectious disorders are possible in all age groups, but atrophic (senile) vaginitis must be remembered as either a primary or associated cause of vulvovaginal symptoms in the postmenopausal female, since this is such a common problem.

Trixi is 8 years postmenopausal. She uses no hormonal medications.

4. Is the patient sexually active? Various infectious and noninfectious vulvovaginal disorders are either sexually transmitted or related in other ways to sexual activity.[18] Trichomoniasis and *Gardnerella* vaginitis are usually sexually transmitted, while noninfectious irritation due to contraceptive devices, douching apparatus, or other foreign substances may also occur.

Gonorrhea is an uncommon finding among women with symptoms of vaginitis,[1, 2] but occasionally gonorrhea will present with nonspecific vaginal discharge.[19] Other venereal diseases will usually manifest visible vulvovaginal lesions (see Fig. 7–2) and only rarely cause vaginal discharge alone.

The patient's sexual habits are also worth noting because of the rising incidence of asymptomatic cervical gonorrhea in females. Traditional strategies for detecting asymptomatic female gonorrhea have centered around case finding of the female consorts of men with proven gonorrhea, but, since asymptomatic male gonorrhea is now known not to be a rarity,[20] routine cultures from sexually active females can be an important public health measure.[21] The indications for gonococcal cultures are discussed below.

Thus the patient with vulvovaginal symptoms should always be asked whether her sexual partner(s) has had a documented venereal disease or recent genitourinary symptoms.

> A widow for 5 years, Trixi reluctantly admits to a new sexual relationship (her first since her husband's death) over the last 3 months. Her partner has no known genitourinary symptoms.

5. In Trixi's case there is a long history of intermittent vaginal discharge (without pruritus), but have there been documented recurrent vaginal infections? When recurrent vaginal infections are well documented, proper therapeutic strategies will depend on the specific type of infection. Refractory vaginitis raises distinctive questions and deserves a different approach (see page 329).

> Trixi denies any prior history of known vaginal or venereal infections.

DIFFERENTIAL DIAGNOSIS

Once we have this historical information, pelvic examination of the patient with vaginal complaints will answer our initial question: Which anatomic site is the source of symptoms?

Figure 7–1 illustrates normal external female genitalia. Characteristic gross physical findings will often be suggestive of a specific diagnosis in the patient with infectious vaginitis (see page 318) or in the patient with vulvar pruritus without vaginitis (see page 334). In addition, several other common vulvovaginal infectious processes (or local "bulges") can be diagnosed pri-

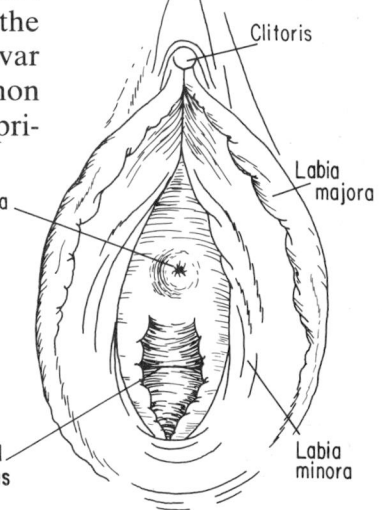

FIGURE 7–1. Normal female external genitalia.

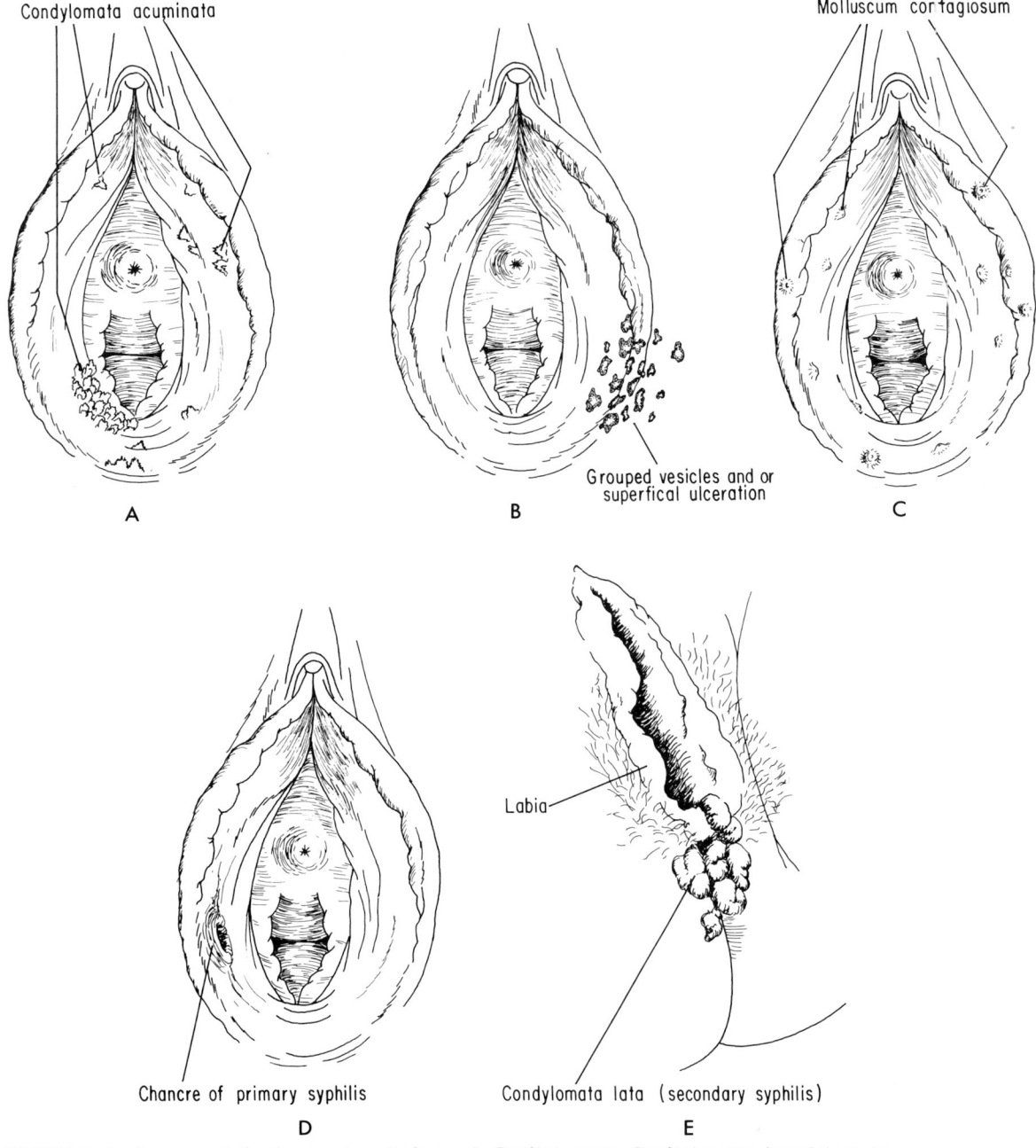

FIGURE 7–2. Common infectious vulvar lesions. A, Genital warts. Genital warts (condylomata acuminata) are usually frondlike excrescences that may appear on the labia or the external or internal vaginal/perineal area (but rarely on the contiguous thighs). They are usually asymptomatic. Treatment of condylomata acuminata involves topical application (weekly, in the office) of podophyllin in 10 to 25 per cent benzoin, liquid nitrogen, or trichloroacetic acid. The normal skin surrounding the warts is usually treated with petroleum jelly before the application of these substances because they are irritating to normal skin. In general, warts that are intravaginal are not treated with podophyllin, and trichloroacetic acid is favored.

Condylomata acuminata are usually easy to distinguish from syphilitic condylomata lata (which are broad-topped and few in number)—these are lesions of secondary syphilis (E).

Condylomatous vulvar carcinoma (which is more indurated, asymmetric and/or ulcerated) is usually distinctive in appearance, but biopsy is necessary to confirm this diagnosis. Infections that are rare in this country—schistosomiasis, amebiasis, chancroid, lymphogranuloma venereum, and granuloma inguinale—may be mistaken for genital warts on occasion.

B, Herpes simplex infection. Genital herpes infections (usually Type II herpes simplex, occasionally Type I) usually are obvious after careful examination of external and internal genitalia. Primary (first time) infections most often present as painful, superficial ulcerations widely distributed over the vulva, but any area of the vagina, cervix, or perineum may be involved. Inguinal adenopathy and dysuria are common; urinary retention and sacral radiculopathy are rare but occasionally necessitate hospitalization. Systemic symptoms (headache, fever) are

Legend continues on opposite page.

marily by their gross physical appearance. These include genital warts (condylomata acuminata), herpes simplex infection, syphilitic chancres, molluscum contagiosum, and condylomata lata (Fig. 7–2). Common "bulges" (which are usually asymptomatic) include Bartholin's cysts, Gartner's duct cysts, uterine prolapse, cystocele, rectocele, and urethral caruncle (Fig. 7–3).

Figure 7–4 illustrates normal appearance of the cervix on speculum examination. Familiarity with normal variations and common pathologic conditions of the cervix is very important, since a variety of cervical disorders can cause vaginal discharge (Table 7–1), and the treatment of these entities is very different from the treatment of infectious vaginitis. Acute cervicitis (see Fig. 7–7) is especially important, since cultures and treatment for gonorrhea are most often the procedure of choice, although other organisms may also be responsible for acute cervicitis. Chronic cervicitis, cervical polyps, cervical erosions, or cervical carcinoma may also cause vaginal discharge and may at times be difficult to distinguish from one another. These latter disorders often require gynecologic consultation, but early recognition by the generalist physician is most important.

Finally, bimanual palpation of cervix, uterus, ovaries, and rectum is performed to detect tenderness, masses, or abnormal position of these organs.

Physical examination reveals a pleasant, afebrile woman who is obviously embarrassed by her predicament. The findings of a brief abdominal examination are normal.

The external genitalia are examined with the patient in the lithotomy position. There is perhaps mild vulvar atrophy and slight erythema of the labia minora. Speculum examination demonstrates a liquid, yellow discharge that pools in the posterior vagina, as well as a few punctate hemorrhagic lesions of the vaginal wall and cervix. The cervical os contains a small amount of similar yellow discharge. Bimanual examination reveals a normal-sized uterus, nonpalpable ovaries, and no cervical or adnexal tenderness; rectal examination is normal.

FIGURE 7–2 *Continued*
surprisingly common. The painful ulcerations persist for an average of 2 to 3 weeks, during which time new lesions commonly develop. Topical acyclovir (5 per cent ointment in polyethylene glycol, four to six times a day for 7 to 14 days) is the treatment of choice.[26]

Recurrent genital herpes more often presents as grouped painful vesicles (which then often erode into superficial ulcerations). There is often a prodrome of itching or tingling for hours to days before eruption of vesicles. Recurrent infections (average, three to four recurrences per year) tend to cause shorter duration of pain and more rapid healing, but there is no known effective treatment for recurrent herpes. Acyclovir is not recommended in this setting, but further studies are needed.

C, Molluscum contagiosum[27] is a pox virus infection that appears as firm, pearly hemispherical papules, usually multiple and of varying sizes (a few millimeters to 1 cm in diameter). Sometimes cheesy material can be expressed from the often umbilicated center of each lesion. Treatment may include curettage, podophyllin and/or liquid nitrogen, but simple expectant therapy is more often used.

D, The chancre of primary syphilis is usually a single, painless, ulcerating papule with indurated, "heaped-up" edges (see also Fig. 8–1B). Darkfield examination of the primary chancre is usually diagnostic.

E, Condylomata lata are usually flat-topped, eroded exudative papules that appear on vulva or perineum most often. Occasionally, these are difficult to distinguish from condylomata acuminata. The VDRL is "always" positive in secondary syphilis (See Chapter 8, Appendix II).

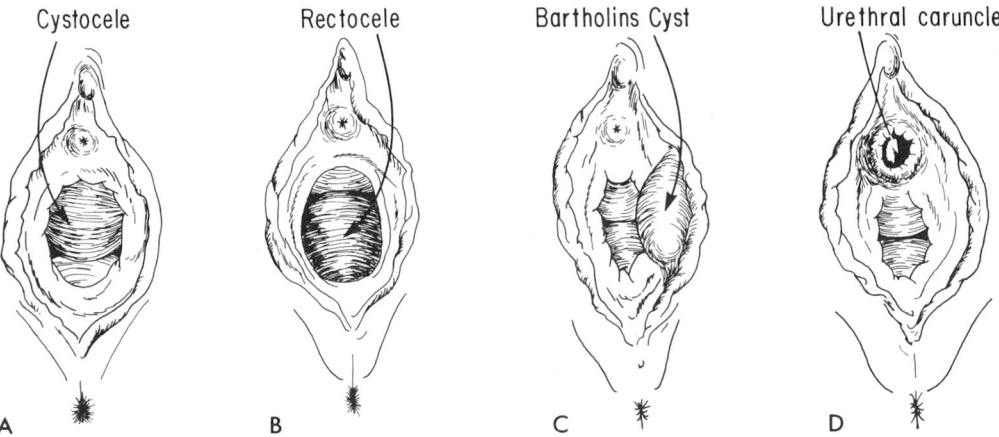

FIGURE 7–3. Visible "bulges." A, B, Cystoceles and rectoceles commonly occur in middle-aged or elderly multiparous or posthysterectomy females. These usually represent disorders of "pelvic relaxation." Not shown in the figure is uterine prolapse, which may coexist with cystoceles or rectoceles. In first-degree prolapse, the cervix "herniates" to, but not through, the vaginal introitus. In second-degree prolapse, the cervix protrudes through the introitus. Third-degree prolapse is rare—the entire uterus herniates through the introitus.

C, Bartholin's glands are located on either side of the inner aspect of the lower vaginal vestibule and may become obstructed (cyst formation) or infected (abscess formation—many different organisms are possible) or, rarely, develop a malignancy. Bartholin's cysts are usually easy to distinguish from Gartner's duct cysts (not shown here), which are often multiple and line the interior vaginal wall.

D, Urethral caruncle is a prolapse of the urethral mucosa that appears as an erythematous enlargement of the urethral meatus. Usually asymptomatic, these may be associated with dysuria and are especially common in women with atrophic vaginitis.

TABLE 7–2. VAGINITIS

CAUSE	TYPICAL SYMPTOMS	GROSS APPEARANCE	PRESUMPTIVE DIAGNOSIS	DEFINITIVE DIAGNOSIS
Candida (yeast)	Vulvar and vaginal itching	White "curds" of vulvovaginal discharge, loosely adherent to vaginal mucosa Vulvar erythema/edema common	Candida hyphae on KOH preparation	KOH prep Rarely, fungal cultures Response to topical therapy (Table 7–4)
Trichomonas ("trich")	Pruritic vaginal discharge	"Strawberry" appearance of vagina and cervix Copious yellow/white liquid discharge	Motile trichomonads identified on wet mount	Wet mount Rarely, *Trichomonas* culture Response to metronidazole therapy (Table 7–4)
Gardnerella (formerly nonspecific or Hemophilus); (see Appendix)	Pruritic or malodorous vaginal discharge	Copious gray, liquid vaginal discharge	Wet mount: clue cells KOH: fishy odor Vaginal pH >5 No candida, trichomonads identified	Culture Response to metronidazole (Table 7–4)
Atrophic (senile)	Vaginal irritation, burning dyspareunia	Atrophic, dry external genitalia and vaginal mucosa	Gross appearance in postmenopausal female	Exclude infectious vaginitis Response to topical estrogens (page 333)

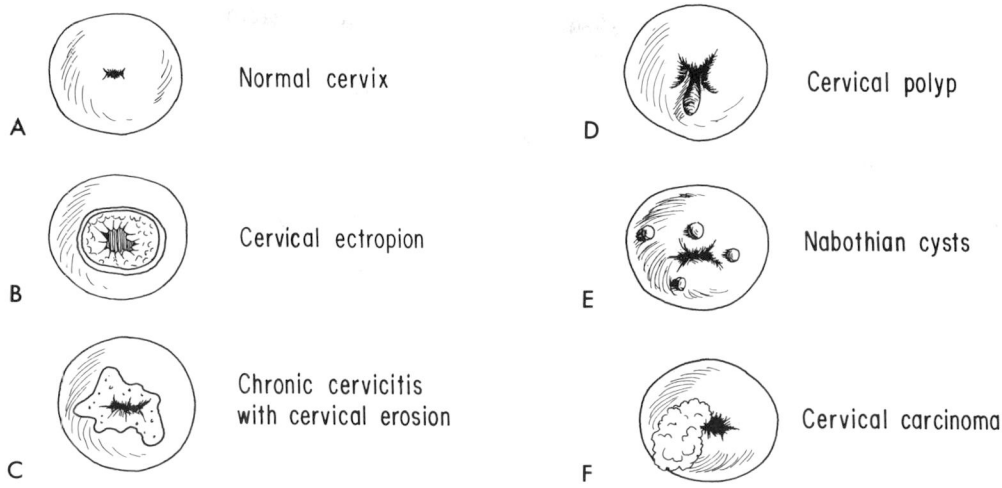

A   Normal cervix

D   Cervical polyp

B   Cervical ectropion

E   Nabothian cysts

C   Chronic cervicitis with cervical erosion

F   Cervical carcinoma

FIGURE 7–4. *A,* The exocervix—the portion visible on speculum examination—is usually a pale, bluish-pink, smooth, mushroom-like structure umbilicated at its center by the external os of the endocervical canal. This homogeneous appearance results from the integrity of squamous epithelium that lines the exocervix before it elides into the columnar epithelium of the endocervix at the squamocolumnar junction.

B, Cervical ectropion (misnamed congenital cervical erosion) refers to prominent visibility of columnar endocervical epithelium, which, in many young women (perhaps 15 to 20 per cent), extends beyond the limits of the endocervical canal. This appears as a discrete, bright-red circumferential band of varying width[70] around the cervical os. This may be mistaken for a cervical erosion (*C*). Mild mucoid discharge may be seen. No therapy is necessary.

C, Chronic cervicitis is a much misunderstood phenomenon. Many (most?) parous women will demonstrate microscopic inflammation of the cervix (leukocytic infiltration on biopsy). Sometimes, this is extensive and severe enough to cause swelling and gross erythema of the cervix or the appearance of an "erosion." Occasionally, subacute pelvic cellulitis will result in back pain and dyspareunia. More often, the patient is asymptomatic, but the gross appearance of this cervix sometimes raises the question of cervical carcinoma. Careful cytologic diagnosis and/or biopsies are often necessary in such cases—a gynecologist should treat such patients.

D, Cervical polyps may be exocervical or endocervical and are occasional causes of vaginal discharge or bleeding. Otherwise, polyps are rarely a cause for concern.

E, Nabothian cysts not infrequently coexist with chronic cervicitis. They are of no specific clinical importance, except that mild mucoid cervical discharge may be seen in their presence.

F, Cervical carcinoma may at times be difficult to distinguish from cervicitis or cervical erosion—often, however, an indurated infiltrating mass will be obvious.

What does this mean?

1. The major anatomic site of abnormality is the vagina. There is slight vulvar abnormality (atrophy and erythema), but this is mild in comparison with the vaginal findings. There may be a cervical discharge, however, and this deserves attention (see below).

There is no evidence of uterine or tubo-ovarian involvement.

2. Infectious vaginitis is most likely.

Most (90 per cent) cases of infectious vaginitis are caused by one or more of three different organisms: *Candida albicans, Trichomonas vaginalis,* or *Gardnerella vaginalis* (Table 7–2 and Fig. 7–5).

Candidal vaginitis usually presents with prominent pruritus and vulvar irritation—heavy liquid discharge is unusual since candidal discharge is usually thick and adheres to the cervical, vaginal, and vulvar mucosa in patches of white, like cottage cheese or curd.

Patients with *Trichomonas* infection more often complain of both pruritus and a discharge, which may be copious, yellow, malodorous, and frothy (bubbly). Vulvar inflammation is usually less severe than with candida infection, but punctate cervical and vaginal mucosal hemorrhages may be

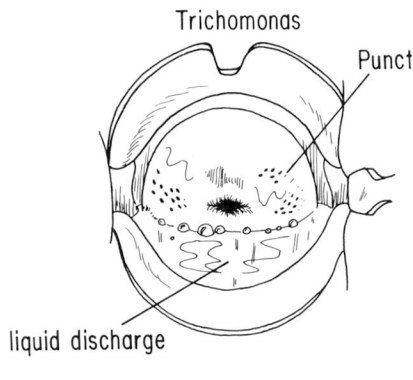

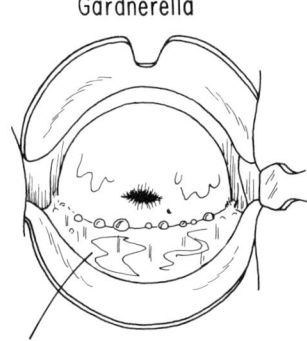

FIGURE 7–5. Common gross appearances of the three common causes of infectious vaginitis.

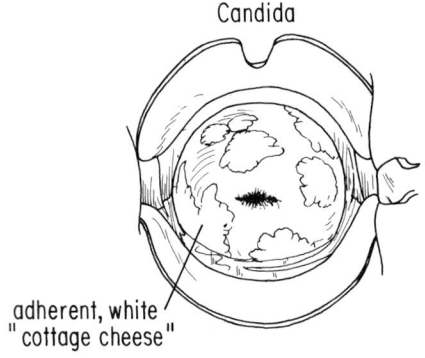

seen (strawberry appearance), and these are quite characteristic of *Tricho-monas* infection when present.

Gardnerella vaginitis (formerly termed nonspecific or *Hemophilus vagi-nalis* vaginitis—see Appendix) is less often pruritic and usually produces a gray liquid discharge that may also be malodorous.

While some other vulvovaginal disorders may be confidently diagnosed simply on the basis of gross appearance (see above), precise diagnosis of infectious vaginitis can be achieved reliably only by integrating historical and physical findings with a few simple "bedside" laboratory procedures (see below). Gross appearance (Fig. 7–5) is nonspecific. Some women with candidiasis may have a thin, liquid discharge, while *Trichomonas* or *Gard-nerella* infection may produce no obvious discharge at all. In addition, mixed infections are not at all uncommon.[28–30]

3. There are a few complicating factors in Trixi's case.

The patient is postmenopausal—atrophic vaginitis should be suspected in addition to the different infectious (and noninfectious) vaginal conditions.

The patient has recently resumed sexual relations and may well have a sexually transmitted infection.

Finally, the patient is distraught and will need careful explanation about the nature of her problem, its relation to her current life situation, and implications for treatment (see below).

What should we do now?

INFECTIOUS VAGINITIS

When vaginitis is suspected, obtain three specimens during the pelvic examination:

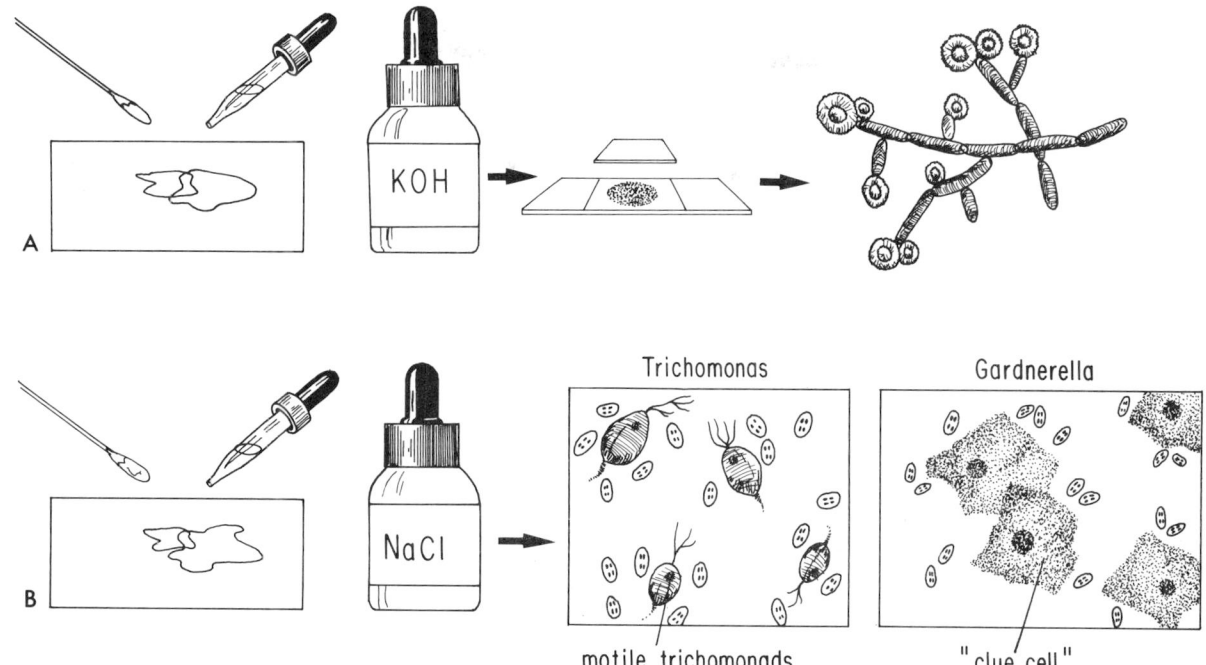

FIGURE 7–6. The KOH preparation for *Candida (A)* and the wet mount for *Trichomonas* and "clue cells" *(B)*.

I. The wet mount (Fig. 7–6*B*).

A swab or drop of vaginal discharge should be placed in a test tube containing 2 cc of saline (or immediately mixed on a microscopic slide with a few drops of saline). A slide containing the liquid mixture is examined (before drying) under the microscope with the low (and then high dry) objective. Motile trichomonads (Fig. 7–6*B*) are usually easy to see under low power. The wet mount is the diagnostic procedure of choice for *Trichomonas vaginalis* infection but may also detect "clue cells," the hallmark of *Gardnerella* infection (see also pages 323 and 337).

II. The KOH preparation (Fig. 7–6*A*).

A second swab (or drop) of vaginal discharge is smeared on a microscopic slide, and 1 drop of 10 per cent potassium hydroxide solution is added to the smear. A coverslip is added, and the slide is examined under the microscope (at low power) after it is flame or air heated until barely dry.

KOH lyses many of the cellular elements that may obscure the hyphal forms of *Candida* fungal species in vaginal discharge. As such, the KOH preparation is a more sensitive examination for *Candida* hyphae than is the routine wet mount. (In some hands, Gram's stain of the vaginal discharge is the preferred method for detection of *Candida* hyphae. The Gram's stain is much more laborious to prepare than is the KOH preparation, however, and the latter is highly sensitive when carefully prepared and examined.)

III. Culture specimens.

A third specimen of vaginal discharge should be obtained with a sterile swab and placed in a transport medium (for example, Culturette). Usually such culture specimens are unnecessary (see below) and can be immediately discarded after examination of the wet mount and KOH

TABLE 7–3. VAGINAL AND CERVICAL CULTURES

ORGANISM	CULTURE MEDIUM	WHEN TO CULTURE	COST
Candida (vaginal swab)	Nickerson's	Almost never; rarely in patients with recurrent/refractory/unexplained vaginitis	$25
Trichomonas (vaginal swab)	Kupferberg's trypticase serum	Almost never; rarely, in patients with unexplained vaginitis or contraindications to metronidazole therapy (for example, during pregnancy)	$10
Gardnerella vaginalis (vaginal swab)	Thioglycolate, chocolate agar, or Casman broth in candle jar at 37° C	When there is no evidence for *Candida* or *Trichomonas* vaginitis and there are no "indirect clues" to diagnosis, i.e., clue cells, amine odor, vaginal pH >5	$22
Neisseria gonorrhoeae (cervical swab)	Thayer-Martin or other specific for gonorrhea	Cervical discharge PID Definite gonorrhea exposure Other venereal disease	$ 9

preparation which will make the diagnosis in perhaps 80 per cent of cases. Occasionally, specific cultures for *Gardnerella* will be needed, but usually indirect clues (Table 7–2 and p. 323) are sufficient to make a presumptive diagnosis of this type of vaginitis. Cultures for *Trichomonas* and *Candida* are only rarely necessary. Table 7–3 illustrates a few salient points about vaginal and cervical cultures.

The incidence of asymptomatic gonorrhea varies widely, ranging from 20 per cent among newly incarcerated young prisoners to much less than 1 per cent among affluent elderly women.[21] Thus, routine gonorrhea cultures will have a high yield in VD clinics and inner city obstetric clinics; suburban geriatric populations are a different matter.

Cultures for gonorrhea should be obtained in several circumstances:

A. When "vaginal" discharge in fact emanates from the cervix (Fig. 7–7).
   The cervical Gram's stain is helpful here but is not a definitive test. False positive smears are common because nonpathogenic *Neisseria* species are vaginal commensals; false negative smears are not rare in culture-proven cervical gonorrhea.[35]

B. When there is any suspicion of PID (see also Chapter 11, "Abdominal Pain").

C. When there is a definite or likely history of exposure to gonorrhea. When the patient's male partner has proven gonorrhea, the woman should be treated immediately after appropriate cultures are ob-

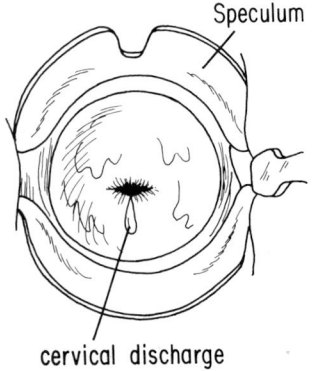

Speculum

cervical discharge

FIGURE 7–7. Acute cervicitis. Acute cervicitis may result from common causes of coexistent vaginitis (especially *Trichomonas*), but "vaginal" discharge emanating from the cervix must suggest venereal cervicitis—gonococcal or chlamydial infection most often, but acute cervicitis is occasionally the result of herpes, syphilis, or rarer venereal diseases. (*Hemophilus influenzae* or streptococcal infections may rarely cause acute cervicitis.) Endocervical Gram's stain will reveal typical intracellular gram-negative diplococci in most patients with gonococcal cervicitis, but cultures are necessary to prove the diagnosis. Chlamydial cultures are currently impractical for routine use.

tained. When the history is less definite, treatment is usually postponed until positive culture results are available.

D. When the patient has evidence of sexually acquired vaginitis, i.e., *Gardnerella* or *Trichomonas*, or other venereal disease—for example, pubic lice, syphilis, herpes, and scabies are infections that are usually sexually acquired.

Mixed infections are not rare, and asymptomatic gonorrhea is probably more prevalent among women with other venereal infections.

Gonococcal cultures should be obtained by first cleaning the exocervix of any mucus or debris and then inserting a sterile swab (1 to 2 cm deep) into the endocervical canal and twirling it for 5 to 10 seconds before removing it and inoculating on selective culture media.[35] (Both rectal and pharyngeal cultures should also be obtained. The rectal swab should be inserted with care not to contaminate the swab with feces—insertion of the swab 1 to 2 cm into the anus is usually sufficient.) Urethral cultures should be obtained if gonorrhea is suspected in the woman without a cervix (posthysterectomy).[36]

A careful history, pelvic examination, and performance of the wet mount and KOH preparation examinations will usually provide at least a presumptive diagnosis. Figure 7–8 summarizes the general approach to the woman with vaginal discharge or irritation.

In this case:

Examination of the wet mount reveals microscopic fields streaming with cellular debris, vaginal epithelial cells, and some polymorphonuclear leukocytes. There are no clue cells. In every field can be seen motile organisms—about twice the size of a polymorphonuclear leukocyte and smaller than a vaginal epithelial cell—that undulate in a cork-screwing motion through the field. At high power, a flagellum can be seen on some of these trichomonads (Fig. 7–6).

The KOH preparation is unremarkable. Fungal hyphae are not seen, and addition of the KOH to the discharge does not produce an unpleasant odor.

Gram's stain of the cervix reveals few polymorphonuclear leukocytes but no gram-negative diplococci.

What does this mean?

I. *Trichomonas vaginalis* infection is documented.

Observation of motile trichomonads on the wet mount is sufficient proof of infection. Cultures for *Trichomonas* are not necessary. A few points should be emphasized here:

A. Trichomonads are not always so obvious.

Often careful scanning of several microscopic fields will be necessary before the organism will be found. The organism is motile only when the wet mount is wet. Drying of the slide will obscure the organisms.

B. The material for wet-mount examination should be obtained from the vagina, not the cervix.

While *Trichomonas* infection involves multiple genitourinary sites (and cervical discharge may be seen with *Trichomonas* infection, as in this case), Grys obtained cultures in 387 women with symptomatic trichomoniasis and demonstrated *Trichomonas* organisms in the vagina in 98.4 per cent, in the urethra in 82.5 per cent, and in

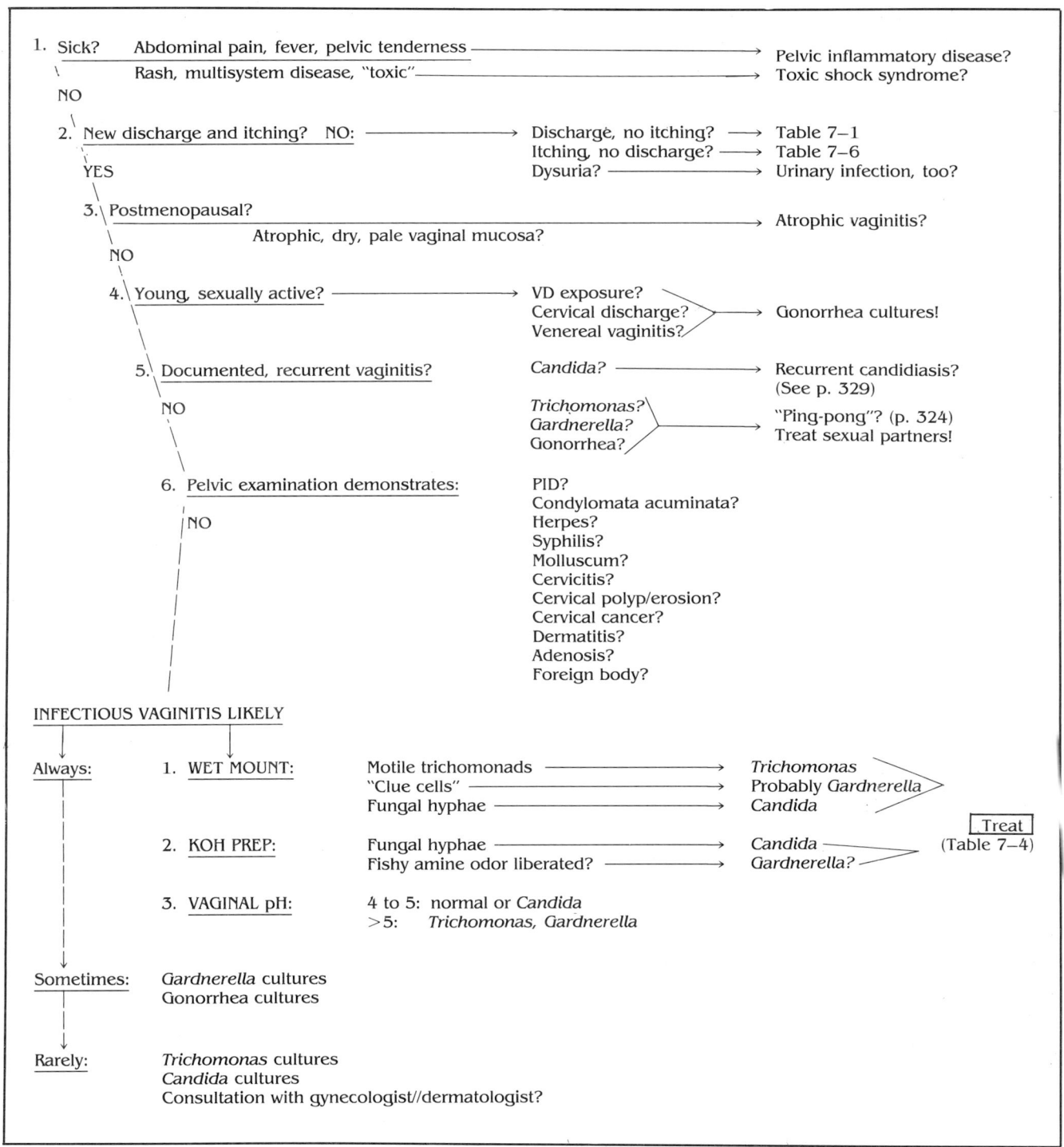

FIGURE 7—8. Vaginal discharge and/or irritation.

the endocervix in only 13 per cent.[37] (When vaginal smears are negative, the likelihood of finding organisms in the urethra is very small (1.7 per cent).

C. Cultures for *Trichomonas* are not usually helpful.

McLennan and associates studied over 200 patients in assessing the diagnostic reliability of wet mounts, cultures, and Papanicolaou smears (where trichomonads may be seen with surprising frequency, even when the patient is asymptomatic).[30] When wet mounts are prepared and examined carefully by a competent observer experienced in its use, the diagnostic yield increases only minimally when cultures for *Trichomonas* are also performed. Occasionally, cultures on Kupferberg's Trypticase medium will help in problem cases (Table 7–3).

    D. *Trichomonas* infection not uncommonly coexists with other types of vaginitis.

        Hence, the important facts that:

II. Candidal infection is unlikely.

As with *Trichomonas* infections, fungal cultures may improve the yield of diagnostic testing for candidal infection by about 10 per cent if a careful KOH preparation reveals no fungal forms.[30] Cultures for *Candida* are not routinely recommended when the KOH preparation is negative, however, since many women will harbor small numbers of *Candida* in the vagina even when asymptomatic, and thus a positive culture (especially for small numbers of *Candida*) may be unrelated to the actual cause of the patient's symptoms. The diagnosis of candidal vaginitis usually rests on the gross appearance and KOH preparation.

III. *Gardnerella* (formerly Hemophilus) vaginitis is also unlikely.

Specific culture methods *are* needed to definitively document this third common type of vaginitis,[38] but such cultures are usually reasonable only when clinical suspicion is high and the wet mount and KOH preparation fail to reveal trichomonads or Candidal organisms (see also Appendix). Even in these circumstances, cultures for *Gardnerella* are often superfluous since three "indirect" findings commonly suggest *Gardnerella* infection:

    A. Clue cells are vaginal epithelial cells covered with short *Gardnerella* bacilli, commonly found on wet mount (or Gram's stain) of discharge in *Gardnerella vaginalis* infection (See Fig. 7–6).

    B. A characteristic amine (fishy) odor is often apparent when KOH is added to vaginal discharge infected with *Gardnerella vaginalis*.[39]

    C. Vaginal pH above 5 in a young woman with vaginitis but no evidence of yeast or *Trichomonas* infection on smears should suggest *Gardnerella* infection.[40]

        Normal vaginal pH is 4, and most vaginal pathogens do not grow in such an acid environment. (This is the rationale for various nonspecific acidification treatments of vaginitis). Vaginal pH during candidal infections is usually normal (4 to 5); during *Trichomonas* infection the pH is usually greater than 5.

        (Table 7–2 illustrates some of the typical symptoms, gross appearance, and methods of presumptive diagnosis for the common causes of vaginitis. In the great majority of cases, presumptive diagnosis is sufficient, and only rarely are specific cultures important.)

IV. Gonorrhea is unlikely, but cultures should be obtained.

The unimpressive cervical Gram's stain makes gonorrhea unlikely, but since the patient's trichomoniasis is likely to have been sexually acquired, since cervical discharge is present (although the *Trichomonas* infection may be a cause of cervical discharge), and since asymptomatic gonorrhea is a major public health problem today, specific gonococcal cultures should be obtained.

What should be done now?

Treatment of Trichomoniasis

Metronidazole (Flagyl) is the drug of choice for vaginal trichomoniasis. The organism is extremely sensitive to this drug, and treatment failure is almost never due to antibiotic resistance. (Keighley achieved a cure rate of 98 per cent when women in prison were treated with metronidazole, thus presumably avoiding patient noncompliance and reducing the likelihood of reinfection during treatment.)[41] Several treatment regimens have been found equally effective:

1. Metronidazole, 250 mg, tid for 7 days.

2. Metronidazole, 500 mg, bid for 5 days.

3. Metronidazole, 2.0 gm, one dose.

Several points should be emphasized:

I. *Trichomonas* vaginitis is almost always acquired via sexual intercourse.[18, 42]

While the organism may be found alive in formites, urine, and even toilets or swimming pools, the patient's sexual partner is the usual source of infection. Since the male is often asymptomatic, failure to treat the female patient and her sexual partner simultaneously may result in repeated reinfections (the ping-pong effect).

II. The most common reason for treatment failure is noncompliance.

Noncompliance refers to failure of the patient or her sexual partner to complete the course of therapy. There are several possible causes of this, which should be anticipated:

A. Abstinence from alcohol intake is recommended during metronidazole therapy.

Abdominal cramping, flushing, nausea and vomiting (Antabuse reaction) occasionally occur when alcohol and metronidazole interact (Metronidazole has even been used to treat alcoholism.[43]) Some women are unwilling to accept this restriction or to impose it upon their sexual partners.

B. When the woman has more than one sex partner, simultaneous treatment of patient and partner may be difficult or impossible.

C. Misinformation about resuming sexual relations.

Abstinence from sexual intercourse (or use of a condom) is not necessary when the patient and her partner are treated simultaneously.

D. Drug side effects are uncommon, but furry tongue and a metallic taste in the mouth are not rare,[44] and the patient should be warned that these are not reasons for alarm.

Nausea, skin rash, and abdominal discomfort may also occur, rarely. Single-dose therapy (2 gm in one dose) probably does not reduce the incidence of these side effects, but has the advantage that treatment is completed (and is usually successful) when (if) side effects do occur.[45, 46]

E. Some patients may be afraid to take the drug.

Popular magazines and health guides may overly emphasize the dangers of metronidazole. Reports of carcinogenesis in rodents[47] and mutagenesis in bacteria[48] after exposure to metronidazole have suggested to some that metronidazole should be used with caution, if at all.[49] There are no studies that implicate this drug as a carcinogen in humans,[50] but it is sometimes wise to briefly inform certain patients about some of the controversies surrounding use of this drug. Metronidazole is clearly the drug of choice for *Trichomonas* infection.

III. Leukopenia has been reported after metronidazole therapy.

While the manufacturer recommends that a blood count be obtained before and after treatment, this is probably necessary only if repeated treatment courses are prescribed for the same patient (see below).

IV. During pregnancy, metronidazole should be avoided.

While some authors argue that *Trichomonas* infection during pregnancy may be dangerous and should therefore be eradicated before delivery,[51] most agree that metronidazole is contraindicated during the first trimester and should be avoided throughout pregnancy when possible. Alternative treatments during pregnancy include:

A. Topical (vaginal inserts) metronidazole—500 mg per day for 10 days—may be effective, but the drug is (partly) systemically absorbed, and caution is also advised here, especially during the first trimester.

This (and other—see below) topical treatment may be symptomatically effective but is generally less successful than oral (systemic) therapy, since *Trichomonas* infection so often also involves paravaginal tissues. Systemic (oral) therapy is therefore usually necessary to permanently eradicate the organism from the vagina, cervix, urethra, and periurethral glands, but symptomatic relief may also be obtained with:

B. Clotrimazole (Gyne-Lotrimin) suppositories (Table 7–4)—this treatment has been effective[6] in relieving vaginitis in some women with *Trichomonas* infection (but probably does not eradicate paravaginal infection).

It is safe during pregnancy.

C. Nonspecific douches (4 teaspoons of baking soda in 1 to 2 quarts of warm water) may be symptomatically effective, but, in general, douches (especially those containing iodine)[52] should probably be avoided during pregnancy.

D. Aci-Jel vaginal jelly.

One instillation twice a day for 2 weeks may lower the vaginal pH and provide symptomatic relief temporarily.

Trixi is told that she has *Trichomonas* vaginitis. She is informed that this infection is usually sexually acquired and that her partner may well be infected too, but that he may not be aware of this because men are so often asymptomatic. Trixi is told that this is not a serious infection, but the treatment will be most effective if both she and her partner take the medication.

Trixi is given a prescription for 250-mg metronidazole tablets, no. 16, and told to take 8 pills herself in one dose, and to ask her partner to do the same. She is told to avoid alcohol on the day of therapy and for 2 to 3 days thereafter.

Vaginal culture specimens for *Gardnerella vaginalis* are discarded, but the cervical gonococcal culture is sent to the laboratory. A Papanicolaou smear is not obtained, but Trixi is told to return in a few weeks since she has not had a Pap smear in 4 years. She is told to call before then should problems or questions arise.

Trixi is uncomfortable throughout this discussion and is clearly embarrassed when sexual matters are mentioned. She agrees with the treatment recommendations but is subdued and asks few questions.

NOTE

1. While different types of vaginitis often coexist simultaneously,[28, 30, 46] it is not necessary to exhaustively study every patient for every cause of vaginitis, especially when a source of the patient's symptoms has already been found. In this setting, cultures for *Gardnerella* are unnecessary (and expensive—Table 7–3), because trichomoniasis has been documented and can easily explain the patient's symptoms and findings. (In addition, metronidazole is the drug of choice for both of these types of infection—see Appendix—although single-dose therapy has not been well studied in *Gardnerella* infections.)

While the culture for *Gardnerella vaginalis* can be discarded, then, cultures for gonorrhea do make sense. The patient does have another venereally acquired infection *(Trichomonas)* and a recent change of sex partner. Metronidazole is not adequate therapy for gonorrhea.

2. Obtaining Pap smears should be delayed until *Trichomonas* infection is eradicated. *Trichomonas* infection commonly induces an inflammatory response or even frank atypia in the cervical Pap smear. These cytologic changes are always reversible after effective treatment of infection. Since Pap smears must often be repeated when inflammatory or atypical smears are found, it makes sense to delay the smear until after treatment.

3. The patient appears troubled. Despite the so-called sexual revolution, there remains much ambivalence among some women about openly discussing sexual matters. In Trixi's case, her life situation should raise a "red flag"—a recently widowed, formerly monogamous woman who has just resumed sexual relations and is now told she has a venereal disease. A return visit may thus be worthwhile here, even though uncomplicated nongonococcal vaginitis that is cured symptomatically does not ordinarily require any follow-up examinations.

Gonococcal cultures are negative.

Two days later, Trixi calls to say she is "a little better" but still has some discharge. She is told that this may be normal and that as long as she is better and has followed the instructions, she can wait to see what happens. She is reassured about gonococcal infection but seems worried.

Ten days later, Trixi calls to say that she is "right back where I started" and is itching even more.

Examination now reveals more prominent vulvar erythema and a white curd-like vulvovaginal patchy eruption but minimal liquid discharge. The cervix is normal in appearance. The KOH preparation reveals abundant fungal hyphae, and the wet mount shows a few motile trichomonads. There are no clue cells.

Trixi says that she took the metronidazole as prescribed but admits that she did not ask her sexual partner to also take the medication. She denies sexual activity since her last visit.

What does this mean and what should be done now?

1. The patient now has vaginal candidiasis. It is possible that candidiasis and trichomoniasis coexisted at the time of the initial visit and that the *Candida* was missed, but vaginal candidiasis commonly develops anew following the use of metronidazole[46] (or any other broad-spectrum antibiotic).

Multiple simultaneous infections are common in vaginitis. This should always be remembered at the initial visit or when symptoms persist or recur. Thus our initial approach (p. 319) to suspected vaginitis should be followed in all patients whenever they are examined, even when a known cause of vaginitis has been recently identified in that same patient. In other words, while the initial suspicion might be that Trixi's *Trichomonas* infection had not responded to treatment (see below), at least three specimens should still be obtained during the repeat pelvic examination—for KOH preparation, wet mount, and (possibly) a culture for *Gardnerella vaginalis* (if smears are negative).

2. Live trichomonads can still be identified. Since we know that metronidazole is highly effective in the treatment of trichomoniasis,[41] we should assume either that Trixi did not take her medication or that she has been reinfected by sexual intercourse with her partner (who may carry the organism asymptomatically and who has not been treated).

A repeat course of metronidazole is thus indicated for both Trixi and her consort.

Treatment of Vaginal Candidiasis

Candidal vaginitis can be successfully treated with a number of different topical preparations:

I. Clotrimazole (Gyne-Lotrimin, Mycelex-G) tablets (inserted intravaginally)* have been found effective in two dosage schedules:

   A. One 100 mg tablet each night for 7 nights.
      Occasional cases are not thoroughly eradicated after 1 week; an additional 7 days is then recommended in those few.
   B. One 100 mg tablet bid for 3 days.†
      This schedule has been less extensively studied, but it is effective (and more convenient) for many.[53]

II. Clotrimazole (Gyne-Lotrimin, Mycelex-G) intravaginal cream nightly for 7 nights.[54]

III. Miconazole nitrate (Monistat) intravaginal cream nightly for 14 nights.[54] (In some, only 1 week's therapy is sufficient.) Miconazole tablets are also available.

IV. Nystatin (Mycostatin) vaginal tablets, 1 tablet (100,000 units) bid for 2 weeks.[55] (In some, only 1 week's therapy may be sufficient.)

These different preparations are all highly effective and of approximately equal cost (Table 7–4). Creams are often more practical than tablets since vulvar involvement is so common in candidiasis and the creams may be applied both externally and internally. Patients should be instructed in the use of the vaginal cream applicators and advised to use the medication after retiring at night to insure adequate deposition of the drug. Thus, 1 week's therapy with clotrimazole cream is favored here. As noted above, however, micronazole cream may also be effective when used for only 7 days. As Table 7–4 indicates, the major cost differences relate to the duration of therapy.† Clotrimazole is not more cost effective for women who require 14

---

*When tablets are used, the patient is instructed to insert the tablet into the vagina at a time when the tablet is not likely to be dislodged from the vagina for an hour or more. Dosage at bedtime is often desirable for this reason.
†Studies of single-dose therapy are pending at this time.

TABLE 7–4. TREATMENT FOR INFECTIOUS VAGINITIS

TREATMENT	DOSE	COST/AMT
Candida		
Clotrimazole vaginal cream		
Gyne-Lotrimin, Mycelex-G	1 applicator nightly × 7	$9.50/45 gm
	1 applicator nightly × 14	$16.50/90 gm
Clotrimazole vaginal tablets		
(100 mg)		
Gyne-Lotrimin, Mycelex-G	100 mg each night × 7	$10.00/7
	100 mg bid × 3 nights or	$10.00/6
	100 mg nightly × 14	$20.00/14
Miconazole nitrate		
Monistat vaginal cream	1 applicator nightly × 7 or	$10.00/47 gm
	1 applicator nightly × 14	$20.00/94 gm
Monistat vaginal tablets	1 tablet nightly × 7	$10.00/7
	1 tablet nightly × 14	$20.00/14
Nystatin*		
Nystatin vaginal tablets	1 tablet bid × 14	$ 7.00/28
(100,000 units)		
Mycostatin vaginal tablets	1 tablet bid × 14	$14.00/28
(100,000 units)		
Mycostatin oral tablets	2 tablets bid × 14	$20.00/56
(500,000)†		
Trichomonas		
Metronidazole‡ tablets (oral)	8 tablets, single dose	$ 6.00/8
(250 mg)	1 tablet tid × 7 days	$13.00/21
	2 tablets bid × 5 days	$13.00/20
Flagyl tablets (250 mg,	2 gm, single dose	$ 9.00
500 mg)	250 mg tid × 7 days	$20.00/21
	500 mg bid × 5 days	$17.00
Gardnerella		
Metronidazole (250 mg)	500 mg bid × 7 days	$15.00/28
Flagyl (500 mg)	500 mg bid × 7 days	$25.00/14
Ampicillin (250 mg)	250 mg qid × 7 days	$ 5.00/28
	(plus anticandidal agent?)[40]	(plus $10.00 or more?)
Cephradine (Velosef)§	500 mg qid × 7 days	$32.00/28

*Nystatin is the generic form of Hycostatin (the trade name) and is thus less expensive.
†Useful as adjunctive therapy for recurrent candidiasis.
‡Metronidazole is the generic name for Flagyl, but Flagyl is marketed in two different dosages.
§Not yet FDA approved for treatment of *Gardnerella*.

days of treatment (but 7 days is usually sufficient.) Many other treatments have been advocated in the past, but none is as effective or tolerable as those discussed above:

Boric acid has been shown to be effective in clinical studies, but there is no reason to prefer this treatment to the fungal antibiotics listed above.[56]

Topical gentian violet (1 per cent) is very effective but usually requires office treatment, may produce severe skin reactions, and often stains clothing (stains can be removed with equal amounts of cold water, vinegar, and alcohol).[6]

Mycolog cream (nystatin-neomycin-gramicidin-triamcinolone combination) is often successful, especially when vulvar pruritus is extreme, but local allergic reactions to the various drugs are common enough to warrant some reluctance to use this preparation, especially since the other single-drug preparations are so effective. (Rarely a few days of topical steroid treatment of the vulva may be indicated when vulvar involvement is severe and an appropriate antifungal agent is used simultaneously, but, in general, steroids should be avoided.)

Commonly used nonspecific treatments, such as AVC cream (sulfanilamide-aminacrine-allantoin) or Sultrin (different sulfonamide preparations), should probably be left on the shelf with the history textbooks.

Douches with sodium lavryl sulfate combinations (Trichotine), povidone-iodine (Betadine), or vinegar may be symptomatically helpful, but are no substitute for specific antifungal therapy.

Other considerations in the treatment of candidiasis include:

1. In general, the male partner does not require treatment. Asymptomatic male infection is not rare,[57] especially in the uncircumcised male, but unless the male is symptomatic (usually a pruritic balanitis) or the female patient suffers from recurrent candidal infections (see below), treatment of the male is not necessary. (Treatment is, however, very simple in the male—application of the vaginal cream to the head of the penis daily for 5 to 7 days is almost always curative.)

2. Abstinence from sexual intercourse during treatment is not mandatory. There is no good evidence that sexual intercourse interferes with antifungal therapy.

3. Candidal vaginitis probably occurs more commonly in patients with predisposing causes. It is generally assumed that diabetes, pregnancy, and the use of oral contraceptives, corticosteroids, and antibiotics predispose women to the development of vaginal candidiasis.[58] This is difficult to prove conclusively, but it is worth remembering. Nevertheless, candidal vaginitis is extremely common in normal, healthy women, and a single bout of candidal vaginitis usually does not warrant extensive investigation for "predisposing causes."

Random bouts of vaginal candidiasis are thus usually easy to treat successfully. The approach to women with frequent or recurrent vaginal candidiasis, however, may be a very difficult and frustrating therapeutic problem.

Recurrent Vaginal Candidiasis

Candida is a fungus that may infect various external and internal bodily areas[59]—nail beds, skin (especially intertriginous areas of breasts, axillae, and groin), mouth, intestinal tract—as well as the vagina. The organism thrives in environments that are warm, moist, and glycogen-rich. Often, minor alterations in hormonal or metabolic factors in the host or transient changes in the normal (commensal) microbial flora will allow these ubiquitous *Candida* organisms to flourish and produce symptomatic infection. Thus several factors should be considered in the woman with recurrent vaginal candidiasis:

1. As noted above, diabetes mellitus, systemic glucocorticoid treatment (or Cushing's syndrome), pregnancy, and oral contraceptive agents may all predispose the patient to symptomatic candidal vaginitis, perhaps because of metabolic/hormonal influences on vaginal glycogen. Elimination or alleviation of the predisposing condition is always desirable but is not always possible. Prophylactic intermittent vaginal antifungal treatment is sometimes necessary in such women.

2. Antibiotic therapy commonly alters host-enteric flora symbiosis and causes recrudescence of symptomatic candidiasis. Long-term antibiotic therapy (for acne, for example) or frequent intermittent antibiotic therapy (for

recurrent urinary infections, for example) will often predispose susceptible women to vaginal candidiasis. Such women often benefit from prophylactic antifungal therapy administered during the (brief) course of antibiotics. Long-term (daily) antibiotic therapy should be avoided whenever possible.

3. Venereal transmission[57] is an uncommon source of vaginal candidiasis, but the sexual partner(s) of women with recurrent candidiasis should always be examined, and, if necessary, treated for penile (or oral) fungal infection.

When the woman with recurrent candidiasis is not diabetic, takes no medications, and when venereal transmission has been excluded (or the sexual partner has been treated "just in case"), two general approaches are worthwhile:

I. Eradication of a persistent focus of infection.

The most common such focus is intestinal "carriage" of *Candida*—probably the source of infection in most women with recurrent candidiasis.[60, 61] One study documented 100 per cent correlation between vulvovaginal infection and simultaneous (usually asymptomatic) anorectal (and enteric) candidiasis.[51] Topical vaginal treatment will not eradicate the intestinal reservoir, but 2 to 3 weeks of oral (swallowed) nystatin (Mycostatin) tablets (500,000 units qid) taken simultaneously with topical vaginal treatment of the symptomatic vaginitis will help some such patients. (The patient should always be reminded to wipe front to back after defecation because of the risk of enteric-vaginal inoculation.)

Very rare sources of recurrent infection may include diaphragms, components of douche apparatus, or other foreign bodies that are repeatedly inserted into the vaginal canal. These devices should be disinfected or replaced when recurrent infection defies other treatment or explanation.

II. Various nonspecific measures may help.

There is an abundance of folklore on this subject, but in some women simple advice is helpful:

A. Weight reduction.

The obese woman is more likely to harbor candidal infection since intertriginal moisture and chafing, especially in the groin area, is common in such women.

B. Clothing changes.

Excessive perspiration or decreased ventilation of the perineal area may predispose to candidal colonization. Clothing changes in summer, avoidance of multiple layers of clothing (especially nylon undergarments—cotton should be used), and sleeping without underwear have been recommended.

C. Diet changes.

Minimizing fruit and carbohydrate intake and increasing protein intake is said to be of benefit to some. Yogurt may acidify enteric and perineal pH, rendering the vagina less hospitable to the fungus.

D. Avoidance of other irritants.

Mild soap, daily perineal cleaning (gentle bath), and application of nonirritating baby cream to the vulva may help. Deodorants, dyed toilet paper, contraceptive foams, and irritating douches should be avoided. (Baking soda douches are probably least irritating of all.)

Trixi is told that she has a yeast infection and that this is probably related to her use of the metronidazole. She is informed that there are still some signs of persistent *Trichomonas* infection, and that this is usually caused by reinfection from her sexual partner. Trixi sheepishly admits that she "might have" had sexual intercourse during her treatment, confirms that her male partner was not treated (and is her only sexual partner), and admits that she does not know if he has had any itching or penile symptoms himself. The ping-pong effect (p. 324) is explained again.

Trixi is given prescriptions for metronidazole, 250 mg tid for 7 days, for both herself and her partner. Clotrimazole vaginal cream is also prescribed, one application (externally and internally) nightly for 7 nights, to be used concurrently with her own and her partner's metronidazole therapy. The symptoms of candidal balanitis and urethritis are explained to Trixi, and it is suggested that the vaginal cream also be used by her friend if he has any such penile symptoms. Instructions about side effects and alcohol abstinence during metronidazole therapy are reemphasized.

Trixi quietly agrees but asks if these are the only treatments for these conditions. Various options for candidiasis are mentioned, but metronidazole is said to be the only truly effective treatment for *Trichomonas* infection. Trixi accepts this, but, when asked to explain her questions, she demurs. Gentle probing about her current sexual relationship is quietly rebuffed. Trixi agrees to call after 10 days, whatever the results of treatment.

Again: Follow-up visits, examinations, and cultures are usually unnecessary when the patient with nongonococcal vaginitis is cured symptomatically.

Two weeks later, Trixi calls to say she is "much better." When questioned, she admits to a slight discharge but says it "is much less and may be normal for me." There is "very little" itching. She says she is pleased with the results of the treatment, and agrees to return in the near future for a Pap smear or to call if she has a recurrence of her symptoms.

Symptomatic cure is the goal of treatment (except in gonococcal infection, in which follow-up cultures are also necessary). Following successful treatment of the common infectious vaginitides, most women are asymptomatic, but discharge or pruritus may persist in some. A cause for persistent pruritus can usually be identified (see page 334); sometimes, mild nonpruritic vaginal discharge will persist in spite of all appropriate efforts, and a "cause" may never be identified.[41, 46] Again—vaginal pruritus is never normal; vaginal discharge may be.

Three months later, Trixi returns for a Pap smear. She says she has felt well, admits to intermittent, mild vulvovaginal pruritus, but is not concerned about this. She also admits that she occasionally notes a slightly malodorous yellow discharge but says the symptoms are "nothing like they were before, and are probably just normal for me."

Physical examination is normal, except for the pelvic examination, which reveals moderate atrophy of the vulvar skin, thinning and pallor of the vaginal mucosa, and a small amount of viscous, yellow-brown discharge. The cervix, uterus, and ovaries are normal.

KOH and wet-mount examinations of the discharge are normal. A Pap smear is obtained. When asked about her current sexual activity, Trixi admits to a relationship (only) with the same man as previously.

Cultures for *Gardnerella* are obtained (and subsequently are negative). A Pap smear reveals moderate inflammation, rare atypical cells, and many trichomonads.

What does this mean?

I. There is clinical evidence of atrophic vaginitis.

In a postmenopausal woman the physical findings described are typical of vaginal atrophy due to estrogen deficiency.[62] This condition alone may cause both vaginal discharge and (occasionally) pruritus. At more advanced stages, "dryness" and pain during sexual intercourse, dysuria (due to concomitant atrophic urethritis), or frank bleeding may result if atrophy is not treated. Therapy involves vaginal estrogen suppositories (see below). Oral estrogens may be used but are usually indicated only when other perimenopausal or postmenopausal problems (hot flashes, osteoporosis) coexist.

II. While routine examination (KOH preparation, wet mount, and *Gardnerella* cultures) does not demonstrate any infectious vaginitis, trichomonads are visible on the Pap smear.

While Pap smears are not a highly sensitive technique for diagnosing trichomoniasis,[18] an experienced cytologist has no difficulty identifying the organisms, and this finding should be taken seriously, for at least three reasons:

A. As noted previously, reversible cervical dysplasia is common in *Trichomonas* infection.[63]

The Pap smear should simply be repeated after antibiotic therapy cures the infection.

B. There is anecdotal experience that hormonal treatment of atrophic vaginitis may render infectious vaginitis more refractory to therapy, especially *Trichomonas* and candidal infection.[44]

There is also some anecdotal experience that atrophic vaginitis predisposes to other bacterial infections. While infectious vaginitis can certainly coexist with atrophic vaginitis, as in Trixi's case, vaginal cultures that demonstrate staphylococci, enterobacteria, or organisms other than those discussed above should be disregarded, except in unusual circumstances—when pelvic inflammatory disease or acute cervicitis is present, when vulvar furunculosis is apparent, when a Bartholin's abscess appears, for example. Streptococcal vulvovaginitis has been reported as a distinct entity,[64] but this must be rare.

C. Again, persistence of *Trichomonas* infection implies noncompliance with therapy or ongoing venereal reinfection.

Trixi is told the results of the Pap smear. She is upset, asks if she has cancer, and is angry that her infection persists.

Trixi is told that most of her symptoms are likely due to atrophy, which can be easily treated, that there is no evidence of cancer, but that the *Trichomonas* infection must be cured before we can repeat the Pap test to be absolutely certain of this. She is again told that persistence of the *Trichomonas* infection means that the metronidazole was not taken correctly or that she has been reinfected by sexual intercourse. She is asked whether she and her sexual partner took the drug, whether she (or he) might have other sexual partners, or if she can think of any other reason the medication might not have worked.

Reluctantly, Trixi now admits that, while she has taken the metronidazole faithfully and has only one sexual partner herself, she cannot say the same for her friend. She suspects that "he sees other women," and, while she asked him to take the metronidazole, she doubts that he did so. The importance of simultaneous treatment is reemphasized, and metronidazole is prescribed again (a peripheral white blood count is normal). Trixi is told that repeated courses of metronidazole are best avoided and that she should do all she can to rid herself of the infection once and for all. She

is told that the vaginal atrophy (and most of her symptoms) can be treated once the *Trichomonas* infection resolves.

ATROPHIC VAGINITIS

Vulvovaginal atrophy that results from estrogen deficiency must be distinguished from the primary atrophic (or dystrophic) vulvar disorders that may be premalignant and require more careful evaluation (see page 335). "Senile" atrophic vaginitis is usually well treated with oral estrogen preparations or intravaginal estrogen creams (Table 7–5). (Conjugated estrogen [Premarin] vaginal cream—1.25 mg per 2 gm of cream— is highly effective.) It should be emphasized that topical vaginal estrogen is absorbed into the circulation[65] and probably exerts its effect systemically as well as topically. Caution is thus advised in women with estrogen-dependent neoplasms (breast, uterus) and (perhaps) other contraindications to estrogen therapy (extensive vascular disease, hypertension, for example).

Vaginal estrogens are best applied once daily for several weeks, then every other day, and ultimately only occasionally (perhaps once a week), according to symptomatic needs. This program is highly successful and acceptable for most women.

Vulvar atrophy (of the senile variety) may occasionally worsen with topical estrogens, since hormonal responsiveness of vaginal mucosa and the vulva differs. Testosterone propionate 2 per cent in petroleum jelly may be more helpful for symptomatic vulvar atrophy (and can be used simultaneously with the intravaginal estrogens for vaginal atrophy).

One month later, Trixi returns for a repeat Pap smear. She continues to have mild vulvovaginal pruritus and a slight discharge but "feels better." When asked to elaborate, Trixi begins to cry and explains that she is sure that her *Trichomonas* infection is now cured. She says that she has not had sexual relations since her last visit and is no longer seeing her friend. Her former sexual partner has repeatedly refused to take the metronidazole since "he drinks very heavily; I know now that he is a real alcoholic, and he is really saying that his whiskey is more important to him than I am. I won't see him again." Trixi seems genuinely relieved but depressed nonetheless.

Pelvic examination is unchanged. The Pap smear is now entirely normal. Daily topical vaginal estrogen is begun, with instructions to taper the dose over the next few months. Trixi is asked if she needs any other help, or if she would like to talk more about her personal situation, but says "I'll be all right."

Three months later, Trixi calls to say she is "still itching on the outside." Repeat, careful examination is normal, except that the vulvar tissue appears pale, thin, and wrinkled. There is no vaginal discharge or inflammation, the vaginal mucosa now appears more normal, and the cervix, uterus, and ovaries are normal.

TABLE 7–5. TREATMENT OF ATROPHIC VAGINITIS

Conjugated estrogen (Premarin) vaginal cream	1.25 mg/2 gm of cream (once daily, topical application for several weeks; less often thereafter)
Oral estrogens	0.625, 1.25 mg qd
2% testosterone propionate in petroleum jelly for associated vulvar atrophy	

TABLE 7–6. SOME CAUSES OF VULVAR ITCHING

COMMON	UNCOMMON	RARE
Candida vaginitis	*Gardnerella* vaginitis	Benign familial pemphigus
Trichomonas vaginitis	Lichen planus	(Hailey-Hailey disease)
Atrophic vaginitis	B_{12} deficiency	Keratosis follicularis
Pediculosis pubis	Diabetic vulvitis	(Darier's disease)
Scabies	Local drug reactions	Fox-Fordyce disease
Insect bites	Lichen sclerosus et atrophicus	Behçet's disease
Tinea cruris	Vulvar dystrophy	
Erythrasma	Leukoplakia	
Intertrigo	Vulvar carcinoma	
Allergic dermatitis	Psychogenic	
Seborrheic dermatitis		
Psoriasis		
Urinary/fecal incontinence		

VULVAR PRURITUS

Vulvar pruritus is a symptom, not a disease. While vaginitis is a frequent cause of vulvar itching, many other common and uncommon disorders (Table 7–6) may be responsible for this symptom.[66] Careful examination (often with a magnifying glass) of the external genitalia is the most important diagnostic aid. Physical findings may be quite subtle when potentially important disease entities are present, hence the value of careful external examination. Comprehensive discussion is beyond the scope of this text,* but several categories of disorders should be remembered:

1. Infection. In addition to the three common infectious vaginitides, a few entities should be remembered. Isolated vulvar candidiasis, often with contiguous perineal skin involvement, is usually obvious and occurs most often in diabetic, obese, or pregnant women. The vulvar tissues are red; infection often involves the mons pubis and inner thighs; and small pustules are commonly noted at the border of the erythematous rash ("satellite" pustules—see Fig. 8–3). KOH preparation for examination of the vulvar erythema is usually diagnostic, and topical treatment is similar to that for candidal vaginitis.

Phthirus pubis (pubic louse) infestation results in a normal-appearing vulva, but careful inspection will reveal tiny nits that adhere to (usually the base of) the pubic hairs (Fig. 8–4). Pruritus is intense; low-power microscopic examination of the nit will demonstrate the pathogenic louse (or egg); and gamma benzene hexachloride (Kwell) 1 per cent treatment is always effective.[71] Kwell is applied topically to the pubic area, rinsed off after 5 to 10 minutes, and nits are combed out with a fine comb. Repeated treatment 24 hours later is sometimes helpful.

Scabies (Fig. 8–4) more often produces visible vulvar perineal inflammation, either as papular linear erythematous areas or as pseudofolliculitis with infestation at the base of hair shafts. Unroofing of the lesion will often reveal the mite, *Sarcoptes scabiei*. Kwell is the treatment of choice.[71]

Tinea cruris or erythrasma may also involve the vulva but almost always is associated with involvement of the perineum and inner thigh as well, and each is usually easily diagnosed (Fig. 8–3). KOH preparation of the rash will usually reveal the small fungal forms in tinea infections, and topical antifungal therapy for 2 to 3 weeks is usually very effective. Tolnaftate (Tinactin),

*See references 67–70.

clotrimazole (Lotrimin), haloprogin (Halotex), and miconazole nitrate (Monistat), applied tid, are all effective. Wood's lamp illumination of erythrasma (a bacterial infection due to *Corynebacterium minutissimum*) will fluoresce the rash a bright coral red, and oral erythromycin is the treatment of choice here.

2. Vulvar dystrophy. Lichen sclerosus et atrophicus refers to atrophy of the vulvar tissue, sometimes indistinguishable from senile atrophy, except that this condition may also involve other areas of the skin (thighs and submammary and periumbilical areas). Gross appearance varies from that of nonspecific atrophy—pale, thinned vulvar skin—to the occurrence of small, flat polygonal lesions in multiple sites on the vulva, which often require biopsy to distinguish them from leukoplakia or carcinoma (see below). This entity may be a premalignant condition.[72] Topical testosterone propionate, 2 per cent in petroleum jelly, is probably the treatment of choice. Other regimens have met with varied success.[73-75] Some authorities suggest a combination of 2 per cent testosterone combined with 1 per cent hydrocortisone.

Leukoplakia[76] of the vulva usually presents as thickened, white patches, which may be excoriated or inflamed. Pruritus, vulvar discomfort, dysuria, and vaginal discharge are prominent symptoms. The perimenopausal or postmenopausal woman is most often afflicted. Leukoplakia itself is not a malignant condition, but the biopsy specimen often demonstrates atypical epithelial cells in the epidermis, and this is definitely considered a premalignant disorder—vulvar carcinoma may occur in more than half of such cases if untreated.

Hyperplastic dystrophy[77] refers to a visible change in the vulvar skin (thickened and white or erythematous and scaly) with nonspecific histologic findings on biopsy that may be similar to those found with irritant vulvitis (see below). As such, topical corticosteroid preparations (perhaps with crotamiton added in a 1:3 proportion) and avoidance of any irritants (sprays, detergents) are usually successful. However, biopsy of these lesions should be done, since hyperplastic lesions that demonstrate cellular atypia on biopsy may (rarely) progress to development of:

3. Vulvar carcinoma. Epidermoid vulvar carcinoma (greater than 90 per cent of all vulvar malignant disease) is not rare but can be diagnosed early (often in situ) if persistent pruritus (the most common symptom) is carefully evaluated, and if biopsy of unexplained vulvar skin lesions is done routinely.[66, 68, 78] This disorder occurs in all age groups. The size and appearance of the lesions of in situ carcinoma are extremely variable and are often unimpressive. The labia are most often involved. Most commonly the gross lesions are white, thickened, and elevated, varying from 1 to 3 cm in size, and may be multiple, separated by normal vulvar skin. Some are flat and erythematous; others, warty and irregularly pigmented. Early biopsy diagnosis is crucial since extensive surgery may not be necessary in many patients when the diagnosis is made at an early stage.

Any vulvar lesion that might represent vulvar dystrophy or that otherwise remains unexplained may require biopsy to exclude carcinoma in situ or frank vulvar carcinoma. A gynecologist or dermatologist must be consulted.

4. Primary dermatologic conditions.[68, 69, 79] Many dermatologic conditions affect the vulva, but relatively few will affect only the vulva. Common disorders that uncommonly so present include seborrheic dermatitis, pso-

riasis, eczema, and lichen planus. The possibility of irritant dermatitis (due to deodorant sprays or douches, for example), or allergic contact dermatitis (due to lubricants, condoms, cosmetics, local anesthetics, or antibiotics, and the like) should always be remembered and offending agents removed or discontinued. Intertrigo is common in the obese or unhygienic and may also be seen when chronic urinary incontinence or diarrhea is the primary problem. Much less common are:

Benign familial pemphigus (Hailey-Hailey disease) usually appears as sore, itchy, hyperpigmented, moist plaques on the vulva; remissions and relapses are common in spite of treatment.

Keratosis follicularis (Darier's disease) appears as red or flesh-colored papular lesions that may become confluent plaques. Histology is distinctive. This most often occurs in adolescents.

Fox-Fordyce disease results in small, dome-shaped, flesh-colored papules that are intensely pruritic but may be difficult to see (like multiple syringomas, which do not itch). Similar lesions may be found in the axillae and areolar areas of the breast.

Many other vulvar dermatoses may itch. These may be primary skin conditions with generalized involvement or skin disorders associated with systemic disease. Ridley's monograph[68] is instructive.

5. Psychogenic. Vulvar pruritus is only rarely a functional or psychiatric symptom (unlike vaginal discharge, which is often physiologic and yet is sometimes allowed to assume inordinate importance for the anxious or disturbed woman). When vulvar pruritus persists without obvious cause, consultation with a gynecologist or dermatologist should be strongly considered before the diagnosis of psychogenic pruritus (a diagnosis of exclusion) can be made.

> Trixi is treated with topical testosterone (and vaginal estrogens are continued), and she is told that improvement will be slow, but that the symptoms will lessen over the next 3 to 6 months.
>
> Several phone calls over the next 6 weeks indicate that pruritus persists, and Trixi is worried (about persistent infections or cancer). Gynecology consultation is obtained. Atrophic vulvitis is documented (vulvar biopsy is performed), and vulvar testosterone and vaginal estrogen are continued.
>
> Over the next 6 months, Trixi becomes asymptomatic, but her depression and loneliness worsen. Ongoing psychologic counseling is begun. Trixi remains physically well, however.

Some women will continue to complain of vaginal discharge or itching even when careful, repeated examinations are nondiagnostic, and after different empiric treatment regimens are attempted. Consultation with a gynecologist is warranted in all such situations, since a wide variety of cervical and uterine disorders (see Tables 7-1 and 7-6) may occasionally present in this way.

Not infrequently, however, the interplay of normal vaginal discharge with various personality types, psychiatric disorders, or covert patient anxieties will be the major problem. Frequently, specific anxieties implicate the vaginal area as the locale for somatization: ambivalence about becoming pregnant, fear of cancer, fear of venereal disease, or psychodynamic stresses surrounding the patient's marriage, sexual attitudes, or sexual identity. While some authorities suggest that it "rarely helps to explain these psychosomatic aspects of vaginitis,"[6] a thoughtful approach toward functional illness[80] may, at times, be dramatically effective.

Nonspecific Vaginitis[81]

The term "nonspecific vaginitis" has long been applied to those instances of vaginitis in which infection with *Candida, Trichomonas,* or the gonococcus could not be documented. This is a very common clinical situation and, depending on the patient population studied, may be the most common situation of all.[6] While our understanding of nonspecific vaginitis is incomplete, and controversy abounds among clinical and microbiology authorities, we can probably depend on several generalizations:

I. *Gardnerella vaginalis* (formerly *Corynebacterium vaginale, Hemophilus vaginalis*) is probably responsible for most cases of nonspecific vaginitis.

   While this remains somewhat controversial,[39, 82–87] it has been shown that this gram-negative rod is cultured in most women with nonspecific vaginitis,[39, 81, 87] that the symptoms and physical findings may be transmitted to normal women inoculated with a pure culture of this organism,[88] and that clinical resolution of symptoms and signs after (metronidazole) antibiotic therapy correlates closely with microbiologic eradication of *Gardnerella vaginalis.*[39] Some investigators suggest that the story may be more complicated: that various anaerobic organisms that produce characteristic organic acids may also play a (perhaps synergistic) role.[87] From a practical viewpoint, however, anaerobic cultures and other methods to identify these other organisms are not usually recommended, since metronidazole therapy (which is even more effective in vitro against anaerobes than against *Gardnerella*) is so successful. It is hoped that future research will clarify the theoretic uncertainties here, but practical conclusions include:

   A. There is much evidence that *Gardnerella vaginalis* is sexually transmitted.[39, 81, 89] The (usually asymptomatic) male partners of women with nonspecific or *Gardnerella* vaginitis are very commonly infected. Treatment is thus generally recommended for the patient and her partner, but, as yet, there is no study that demonstrates that this will improve treatment results or lessen the incidence of recurrent reinfection.

   B. The most impressive treatment results follow use of metronidazole 500 mg bid for 7 days, but it may be that other schedules of metronidazole are also effective (see page 324 for the treatment of *Trichomonas* infection, for example).

      Metronidazole appears to be clearly superior to sulfa drugs, ampicillin, or tetracycline.

   C. Ampicillin should be used in the pregnant woman with *Gardnerella vaginalis* vaginitis,[90] since metronidazole definitely should be avoided during pregnancy.

      Some of the newer cephalosporins may also be effective (see Table 7–4)—this requires further study.

D. The *Gardnerella* organism will be missed on many routine cultures, since an environment high in carbon dioxide content is most propitious for growth.

Some authorities suggest that differential hemolysis of human blood agar (90 per cent of *Gardnerella* strains hemolyze this medium) versus sheep blood agar (most strains do not hemolyze this medium) may be a reasonable screening procedure, with subsequent subcultures to chocolate agar.[6, 38] Others suggest that thioglycolate, Casman broth, or chocolate agar medium at 37° in a candle jar will give best results.

E. The question of when to culture for *Gardnerella vaginalis* is more complicated.

In the woman strongly suspected of having infectious vaginitis who has a homogeneous malodorous vaginal discharge, a negative KOH preparation for fungi, a negative wet mount for trichomonads (and especially if the wet mount shows clue cells and KOH liberates a fishy amine odor), it can be argued that *Gardnerella vaginalis* is so likely that metronidazole should be prescribed and that culture results are superfluous (see page 323).[86] On the other hand, such a woman who is pregnant or suffers from refractory/recurrent vaginitis of uncertain etiology should certainly be cultured.

II. Anaerobic vaginitis may well be a significant entity,[87] and further research is needed.

Practically, however, our approach would not change from that discussed above unless inexpensive diagnostic methods become available and drug therapy with medications other than metronidazole are found to be superior.

III. Other bacterial infections have been anecdotally assumed to cause vaginitis,[7] but this is nearly impossible to prove.

Streptococci, staphylococci, *Escherichia coli,* and other organisms are commonly grown on vaginal cultures—whether they are ever pathogenic (except in puerperal infections) is unclear.

IV. Whether mycoplasmas or chlamydiae are responsible for infectious vaginitis remains unresolved.

Pending further studies, it sometimes makes sense to prescribe tetracycline or erythromycin for the woman with unexplained vaginitis whose symptoms do not resolve with the treatments described in Table 7–4. This is unusual.

REFERENCES

1. Komaroff, AL, et al.: Management strategies for urinary and vaginal infections. Arch Intern Med 138:1069–1073, 1978.
2. Conte, JE, Jr: Urinary tract infection/vaginitis protocol. Use in a walk-in clinic. West J Med 129:181–187, 1978.
3. Josey, WE: Vaginitis. Reducing the number of refractory cases. Postgrad Med 62:171–174, 1977.
4. Rogers, RE: Vaginal discharge. Guide to diagnosis and management. Hosp Med 11:68–79, 1977.
5. Palmer, A: Vaginitis. Practitioner 214:666–672, 1975.
6. Hurd, JK, Jr: Vaginitis. Med Clin North Am 63:423–432, 1979.
7. Gardner, HL, Kaufman, RH: Benign Diseases of the Vulva and Vagina. St. Louis: C. V. Mosby, 1969, pp. 1–23.
8. Ridley, CM: The Vulva. Philadelphia, W. B. Saunders, 1975, pp. 246–249.
9. Gardner, HL, Kaufman, RH: Benign Diseases of the Vulva and Vagina. St. Louis: C. V. Mosby, 1969, pp. 107–110.
10. Eschenbach, DA, Holmes, KK: Acute pelvic inflammatory disease: Current concepts of pathogenesis, etiology and management. Clin Obstet Gynecol 18:35–56, 1975.
11. Chow, AW, et al.: The bacteriology of acute pelvic inflammatory disease. Am J Obstet Gynecol 122:876–879, 1975.
12. Eschenbach, DA, et al.: Polymicrobial etiology of acute pelvic inflammatory disease. N Engl J Med 293:166–171, 1975.
13. Jacobson, L. Westron, L: Objective diagnosis of acute pelvic inflammatory disease. Diagnostic and prognostic value of routine laparoscopy. Am J Obstet Gynecol 105:1088–1098, 1969.
14. Cunningham, FG, et al.: Evaluation of tetracycline or penicillin and ampicillin for treatment of acute pelvic inflammatory disease. N Engl J Med 296:1380–1383, 1977.
15. Fisher, CJ, Jr, et al.: The clinical spectrum of toxic shock syndrome. West J Med 135:175–182, 1981.
16. Goodpasture, HC, Voth, DW: Toxic shock syndrome—additional perspectives. JAMA 247:1464, 1982.
17. Bennett, JV: Toxins and toxic shock syndrome. J Infect Dis 143:631–632, 1981.
18. Rein, MF, Chaple, TA: Trichomoniasis, candidiasis, and the minor venereal diseases. Clin Obstet Gynecol 18:73–88, 1975.
19. McCormack, WM, et al.: Clinical spectrum of gonococcal infection in women. Lancet 1:1182–1185, 1977.
20. Handsfield, HH, et al.: Asymptomatic gonorrhea in men. Diagnosis, natural cause, prevalence and significance. N Engl J Med 290:117–123, 1974.
21. Holmes, KK: Screening and the detection of gonorrhea. West J Med 123:367–371, 1975.
22. Ridley, CM: The Vulva. Philadelphia: W. B. Saunders, 1975, pp. 39–53.
23. Brown, ZA, et al.: Clinical and virologic course of herpes simplex genitalis. West J Med 130:414–421, 1979.
24. Corey L, et al.: Genital herpes simplex virus infections: Clinical manifestations, course and complications. Ann Intern Med 98:958–972, 1983.
25. Corey L, Holmes KK: Genital herpes simplex infection: Current concepts in diagnosis, therapy and prevention. Ann Intern Med 98:973–983, 1983.
26. Symposium on Acyclovir. Am J Med July 20, 1982.
27. Ridley CM: The Vulva. Philadelphia: W. B. Saunders, 1975, pp. 77–78.
28. Josey, WE, et al.: Corynebacterium vaginale (Hemophilus vaginalis) in women with leukorrhea. Am J Obstet Gynecol 126:574–578, 1976.
29. Wentworth BB, et al.: Isolation of viruses, bacteria, and other organisms from venereal disease clinic patients: Methodology and problems associated with multiple isolations. Health Laboratory Science 10:75–81, 1973.
30. McLennan, MT, et al.: Diagnosis of vaginal mycosis and trichomoniasis. Reliability of cytologic smear, wet smear and culture. Obstet Gynecol 40:231–234, 1972.
31. Holmes, KK, Stamm WE: Chlamydial genital disease: A growing problem. Hosp Pract 105–117 (Oct.), 1979.
32. Oriel, JD, et al.: Infection of the uterine cervix with Chlamydia trachomatis. J Infect Dis 137:443–451, 1978.
33. McCormack, WM, et al.: Fifteen months follow-up study of women infected with Chlamydia trachomatis. N Engl J Med 300:123–125, 1979.
34. Schachter, JL: Chlamydial infection. N Engl J Med, 298:428, 490, 540, 1978.
35. Riccardi, NB, Felmen, YM: Laboratory diagnosis in the problem of suspected gonococcal infection. JAMA 242:2703–2705, 1979.
36. Klaus, BD, et al.: Gonorrhea detection in posthysterectomy patients. JAMA 240:1360–1361, 1978.
37. Grys, E: Topografin Rzesistkowicaez Wharzndzie rodnym Kobiety. Wiad Parazytol 10:122, 1964.
38. Greenwood, JR, Pickett, MJ: Salient features of hemophilus vaginalis. J Clin Microbiol 9:200–204, 1979.
39. Pheiffer, TA, et al.: Nonspecific vaginitis. Role of hemophilus vaginalis and treatment with metronidazole. N Engl J Med 298:1429–1434; 1978.
40. Edelin K et al.: What's causing the patient's vaginitis? Patient Care, 15–52, (Apr.), 1982.
41. Keighley, EE: Trichomoniasis in a closed community: Efficacy of metronidazole. Br Med J 1:207–209, 1971.
42. Catterall, RD, Nicol CS: Is trichomonal infection a venereal disease? Br Med J 1:1177, 1960.
43. Lal, S: Metronidazole in the treatment of alcoholism. Q J Study Alcohol 30:140, 1969.
44. Cibley, LJ, Kasdon, SC: A New Look at Vulvovaginitis. Chicago: G. D. Searle, 1971.
45. Hager, WD, et al.: Metronidazole for vaginal trichomoniasis. Seven day vs. single day regimen. JAMA 244:1219–1220, 1980.
46. Underhill, RA, Peck, JE: Causes of therapeutic failure after treatment of trichomonal vaginitis with

metronidazole: Comparison of single dose treatment with a standard regimen. Br J Clin Pract 28:134–136, 1974.

47. Rustia, M, Shubik, P: Induction of lung tumors and malignant lymphoma in mice by metronidazole. J Natl Cancer Inst 48:721–726, 1972.

48. Voogd, CE, et al.: The mutagenic action of nitroimidazoles. I. Metronidazole nimorazole, dimetridazole, and ronidazole. Mutat Res 26:483–490, 1974.

49. Is Flagyl dangerous? Med Lett Drugs Ther 17:53–56, 1975.

50. Beard, CM, et al.: Lack of evidence for cancer due to use of metronidazole. N Engl J Med 301 519–522, 1979.

51. Jirovec, O, Petic, M: Trichomonas vaginalis and trichomoniasis. Adv Parasitol 6:117, 1968.

52. Vorherr, H, et al.: Vaginal absorption of povidone-iodine. JAMA 244:2628–2629, 1980.

53. Robertson, WH: A concentrated therapeutic regimen for vulvovaginal candidiasis. JAMA 244:2549–2550, 1980.

54. Robertson, WH: Vulvovaginal candidiasis treated with clotrimazole cream in seven days compared with fourteen day treatment with miconazole cream. Am J Obstet Gynecol 132:321, 1978.

55. Pace, HR, Schantz, SI: Nystatin (mycostatin) in the treatment of monilial and nonmonilial vaginitis. JAMA 162:268–271, 1956.

56. Van Slyke, KK, et al.: Treatment of vulvovaginal candidiasis with boric acid powder. Am J Obstet Gynecol 141:145–148, 1981.

57. Gilpin, CA: Resistant monilial vaginitis: The male aspect. J Fla Med Assoc 54:337–338, 1967.

58. Davis, BA: Vaginal moniliasis in private practice. Obstet Gynecol 34:40–45, 1969.

59. Drake, TE, Maibach, HI: Candida and candidiasis. Postgrad Med 53:83, 120, 1973.

60. Rohatiner, JJ: Relationship of Candida albicans in the genital and anorectal tracts. Br J Vener Dis 42:197, 1966.

61. Miles, MR, et al.: Recurrent vaginal candidiasis. Importance of an intestinal reservoir. JAMA 238:1836–1837, 1977.

62. Gardner, HL, Kaufman, RH: Benign Diseases of the Vulva and Vagina. St. Louis: C. V. Mosby, 1969, pp. 216–229.

63. Rigg, LA, et al.: Absorption of estrogens from vaginal creams. N Engl J Med 298:195–197, 1978.

64. Gardner, HL, Kaufman, RH: Benign Diseases of the Vulva and Vagina. St. Louis: C. V. Mosoy, 1969, pp. 208–215.

65. Rigg, LA, et al.: Absorption of estrogens from vaginal creams. N Engl J Med 298:195–197, 1978.

66. Friedrich, EG, Jr: Vulvar pruritus—A symptom, not a disease. Postgrad Med 61:164–171, 1977.

67. Gardner, HL, Kaufman, RH: Benign Diseases of the Vulva and Vagina. St. Louis: C. V. Mosby, 1969, pp. 149–208.

68. Ridley, CM: The Vulva. Philadelphia: W. B. Saunders, 1975, pp. 242–292.

69. Janovski, NA, Douglas, CP: Diseases of the Vulva. Hagerstown: Harper & Row, 1972, pp. 39–49.

70. Green, TH, Jr: Gynecology: Essentials of Clinical Practice, 3rd ed. Boston: Little, Brown, 1977, pp. 238–245.

71. Orkin, M, et al.: Treatment of today's scabies and pediculosis. JAMA 236:1136–1139, 1976.

72. Green TH, Jr: Gynecology: Essentials of Clinical Practice, 3rd ed. Boston: Little, Brown, 1977, pp. 224.

73. Friedrick, EG: Lichen sclerosis. J Reprod Med 17:147–154, 1976.

74. Janovski, NA, Douglas, CP: Diseases of the Vulva. Hagerstown: Harper & Row, 1972, pp. 57–62.

75. Gardner, HL, Kaufman, RH: Benign Diseases of the Vulva and Vagina. St. Louis, C. V. Mosby, 1969, pp. 121–138.

76. Green, TH, Jr: Gynecology: Essentials of Clinical Practice, 3rd ed. Boston. Little, Brown, 1977, pp. 514–516.

77. Kaufman, RH: Hyperplastic dystrophy. J Reprod Med 17:137–145, 1976.

78. Woodniff, JF, et al.: The contemporary challenge of carcinoma in situ of the vulva. Am J Obstet Gynecol 115:677–686, 1973.

79. Ridley, CM: The Vulva. Philadelphia: W. B. Saunders, 1975, pp. 152, 204.

80. Tumulty, PA: The Effective Clinician. Philadelphia: W.B. Saunders, 1973, pp. 125–136.

81. Amsel, R, et al.: Nonspecific vaginitis: Diagnostic criteria and microbial and epidemiologic associations. Am J Med 74:14–22, 1983.

82. Gardner, HL, Dukes, CD: Hemophilus vaginalis vaginitis—A newly defined specific infection previously classified "nonspecific vaginitis." Am J Obstet Gynecol 69:962, 1955.

83. McCormack, WM, et al.: Vaginal colonization with Corynebacterium vaginale (Hemophilus vaginalis) J Infect Dis 136:740–745, 1977.

84. Heltai, A, Talegany, P: Nonspecific vaginal infections. A critical evaluation of Hemophilus vaginalis. Am J Obstet Gynecol 77:144, 1959.

85. Delabra, EC, et al.: Incidence and significance of Hemophilus vaginalis in nonspecific vaginitis. Am J Obstet Gynecol 89:996, 1964.

86. Kaufman, RH: The origin and diagnosis of nonspecific vaginitis. N Engl J Med 303:637–638, 1980.

87. Spiege, CA, et al.: Anaerobic bacteria in nonspecific vaginitis. N Engl J Med 303:601–607, 1980.

88. Criswell, BS, et al.: Hemophilus vaginalis: Vaginitis by inoculation from culture. Obstet Gynecol 33:195–199, 1969.

89. Gardner, HL, Dukes, CD: Hemophilus vaginalis vaginitis. Ann NY Acad Sci 83:280–289, 1959.

90. Lee, LL, Schmale, JD: Ampicillin therapy for Corynebacterium vaginale (Hemophilus vaginalis) vaginitis. Am J Obstet Gynecol 115:786–788, 1973.

8

MALE GENITO-URINARY INFECTIONS

SYMPTOMS AND SIGNS........................... 342

URETHRITIS...................................... 349

   Gonococcal versus Nongonococcal
     Urethritis 350
   Treatment of Gonococcal Urethritis........... 353
   Treatment of Nongonococcal Urethritis....... 357
   Recurrent Nongonococcal Urethritis 360

BACTERIAL URINARY INFECTIONS 363

RECURRENT URINARY INFECTIONS 365

   Prostatitis................................... 366
   Localization Studies.......................... 367
   Summary 374

APPENDIX   I: URINARY SYMPTOMS AND
               FEVER 375

          II: SYPHILIS: TESTS AND
               TREATMENT 378

        III: "PERSONAL" DISEASES ARE
               PUBLIC PROBLEMS 382

REFERENCES...................................... 384

Don D., a 24-year-old truck driver, enters the clinic with the complaint "I guess I have the clap." Always in good health previously, Don has never suffered from any venereal infections or other genitourinary problems. One week before, he noted a "burning" discomfort during urination, which has persisted. For the past 4 days, he has found "mucus on the penis and my underwear."

There is no history of fever, joint pains, skin rash, eye symptoms, genital sores, or swollen groin nodes.

Examination reveals a healthy, afebrile young male. Inspection and palpation of the groin, scrotum, rectum, and prostate are entirely normal. There are no penile lesions, but a moderate amount of spontaneous mucopurulent discharge is evident at the urethral meatus and staining the underwear.

Dysuria in the adult male is most often caused by an infection localized in one (or more) of several anatomic sites in the genitourinary tract. Differential diagnosis may, at times, be complicated because similar clinical syndromes may result from infection of the kidneys, bladder, prostate, urethra, epididymis, or external genitalia by many different types of agents. Specific treatment may be elusive because it is not always possible to precisely localize the site of infection or to identify the offending microorganism and because sometimes noninfectious disorders will mimic these various infections.

Most often, however, a careful history and physical examination will help localize the site of infection. Serious acute diseases can usually be differentiated easily from less threatening problems, and further steps can then be taken to distinguish among those common and uncommon disorders that affect the anatomic site involved.

SYMPTOMS AND SIGNS

CONSIDER

1. The patient is afebrile. Fever in the adult male with dysuria is always worrisome. Of greatest concern are acute prostatitis, acute pyelonephritis, disseminated gonococcal infection, syphilis, postobstructive urinary infection, and localized genitourinary abscesses. These are discussed briefly in Appendix I.

2. There is no other evidence of systemic illness. Characteristic skin rashes may be seen with Reiter's syndrome, gonococcemia, or secondary syphilis. Joint pains—arthralgias, tenosynovitis, or arthritis—may also occur with disseminated gonococcal infection, Reiter's syndrome, or secondary syphilis. Concurrent conjunctivitis suggests Reiter's syndrome.

3. There are no visible or palpable abnormalities of the penis, groin, scrotum, or prostate. Many venereal diseases will present with characteristic

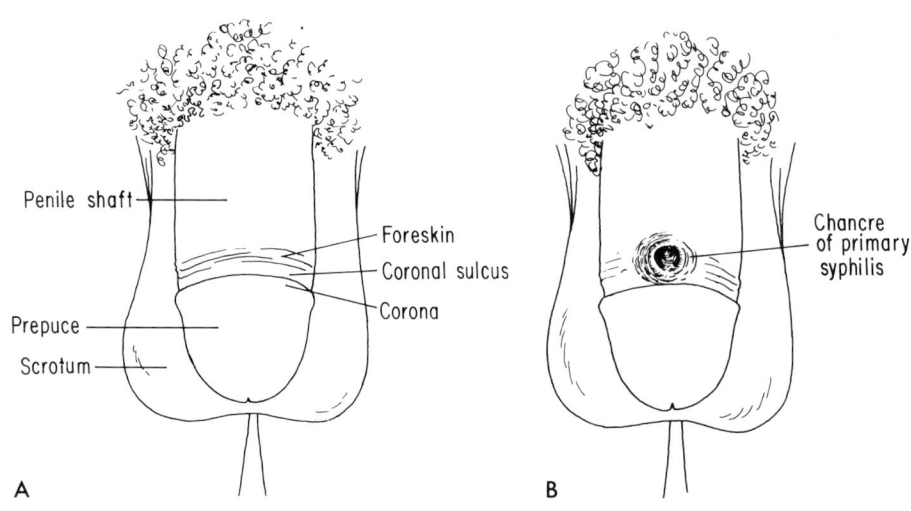

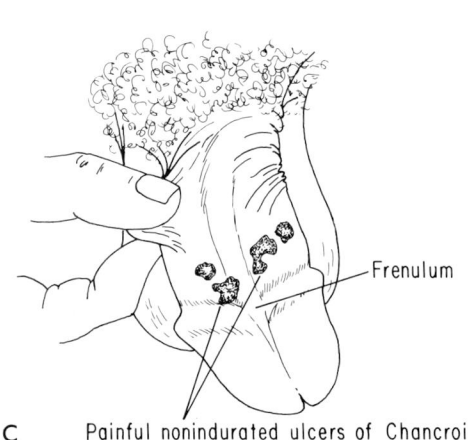

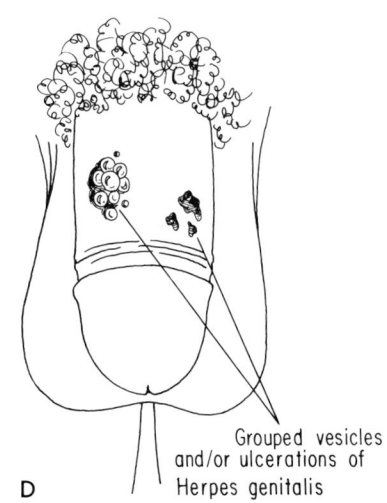

FIGURE 8–1. Normal anatomy (A) and genital ulcerations. B, Chancre of primary syphilis. C, Chancroid. D, Herpes genitalis.

visible or palpable abnormalities of the external genitalia. Thus, familiarity with normal genital anatomy is crucial when approaching such problems.

Figure 8–1 illustrates the normal surface anatomy of the penis, as well as common locations for the characteristic lesions of three venereal infections—primary syphilis, chancroid, and herpes genitalis—all of which usually present as penile ulcerations (Table 8–1). Figure 8–2 illustrates common "genital bumps" whose diagnosis is usually based on gross appearance alone (Table 8–2).

Figure 8–3 illustrates common groin rashes—gross appearance is helpful here as well, but definitive diagnosis depends on KOH preparation of the scrapings from the rash to diagnose tinea or candidiasis, Wood's light (black light) examination for the fluorescence of erythrasma, and examination of the entire patient for evidence of nongenital dermatitis (Table 8–3). Occasionally, rash or swelling involves only the penis (Table 8–3); various venereal diseases may cause balanitis (swelling of the glans penis), balanoposthitis (swelling of the foreskin and glans), or penile edema, but careful examination and follow-up must exclude early neoplastic lesions as well.

Genital infestations (Fig. 8–4, Table 8–4) usually present with intense penile or pubic pruritus. Pubic lice may occasionally be seen crawling among the pubic hairs; more often, only the nits (eggs) will be visible, clinging to the

TABLE 8–1. GENITAL ULCERATIONS[1, 2]

DISEASE	GROSS APPEARANCE	PRESUMPTIVE DIAGNOSIS	DEFINITIVE DIAGNOSIS	TREATMENT
Herpes genitalis[3, 4] (herpes simplex)	Multiple, grouped painful vesicles and/ or superficial ulcerations (Incubation: average 6 days, range 1–45 days)[3]	Gross appearance	Tzanck test of vesicle fluid: multinucleated giant cells; viral cultures[4]	First attack: Acyclovir 5% ointment in polyethylene glycol 4–6 times a day × 7–14 days. Recurrent attacks: expectant therapy
Primary syphilis (*Treponema pallidum*)	Painless, indurated, usually single ulceration with heaped-up border; adenopathy common (incubation: 10–90 days)	Gross appearance; darkfield microscopy: motile spirochetes	Darkfield microscopy and serology test for syphilis (Appendix II)	Benzathine penicillin 2.4 million U IM; ? repeat dose in 1 week; penicillin allergic: tetracycline 500 mg qid × 12–15 days
Chancroid[5, 113] (*Hemophilus ducreyi*)	Painful, often multiple and nonindurated genital ulcerations with purulent exudate (incubation: 10 days)	Gross appearance and Gram's stain of exudate from genital lesions: *Hemophilus*	Culture: *Hemophilus ducreyi*	Tetracycline 500 mg qid × 3 weeks or sulfa 1 gm qid × 2–3 weeks or trimethoprim-sulfamethoxazole 160 mg/800 mg bid × 2–3 weeks* or streptomycin 1 gm IM × 6 days
Lymphogranuloma venereum (*Chlamydia trachomatis*)[6]	Painless, single, transient ulcer (often not seen)	Inguinal and/or sinus tract lymphadenitis (nonspecific)	Chlamydial cultures of swollen lymph node; complement fixation test	Similar to chancroid

Occasionally: herpes zoster, Behçet's disease, bullous diseases, bites, trauma, carcinoma, erythema multiforme, contact dermatitis

*Short courses of therapy for chancroid—either single dose (640 mg/3200 mg) or five day (160 mg/800 mg bid ×5 days) regimens—have been found effective when using trimethoprim-*sulfametrole*.[113]

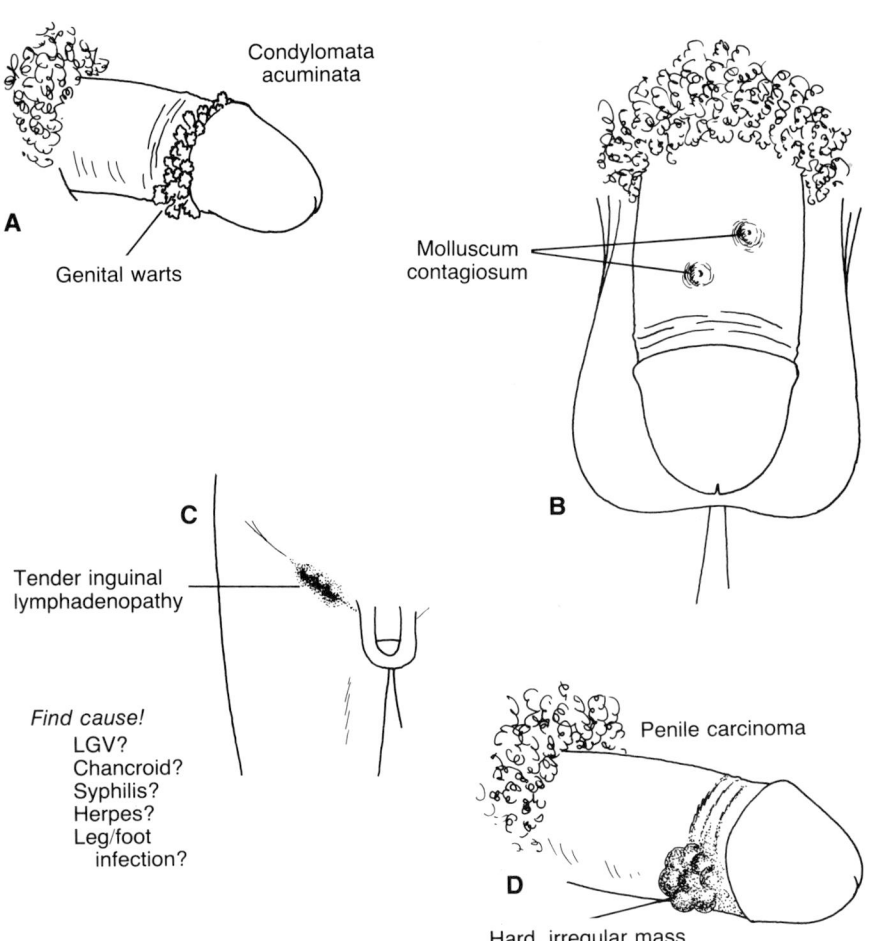

FIGURE 8–2. Genital "bumps." *A*, Genital warts. *B*, Molluscum contagiosum. *C*, Inguinal lymphadenopathy. *D*, Penile carcinoma.

TABLE 8–2. GENITAL "BUMPS"[7]

Disease	Gross Appearance	Presumptive Diagnosis	Definitive Diagnosis	Treatment
Condyloma acuminata (Genital warts)	Pink, frond-like excrescence, often multiple	Gross appearance	Biopsy (rarely necessary)	Topical podophyllin in benzoin or liquid nitrogen or topical trichloroacetic acid
Molluscum contagiosum	Multiple, smooth round papules, 3–10 mm diameter with central dimpling (umbilication)	Gross appearance	Biopsy (rarely necessary); Lipschütz cells in expressed discharge of lesions	Expectant or topical 0.7% cantharidin or topical trichloroacetic acid
Lichen planus	Pruritic violaceous papules; may coalesce into annular, silver-lace lesions	Gross appearance Often, nongenital lesions coexist (hands, extremities, buccal mucosa)	Biopsy (rarely necessary)	Topical steroids
Penile carcinoma	Irregular, firm growth, may ulcerate	Gross appearance	Biopsy	Surgery (usually)
Inguinal adenopathy	Firm and/or tender swellings of groin	Remember: herpes, syphilis, chancroid, LGV, leg/foot infection	Biopsy?	First find cause!

Tinea

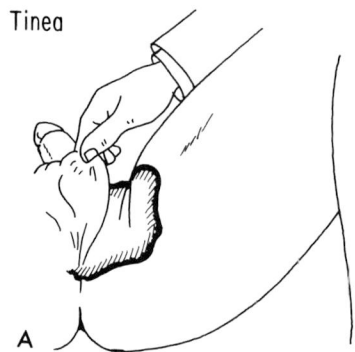

Erythrasma

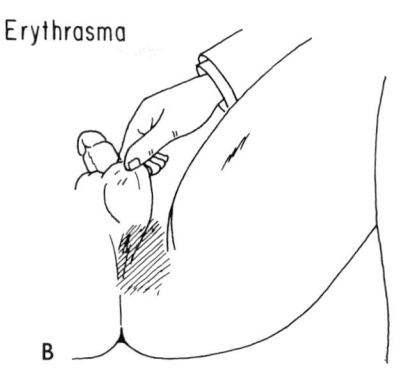

Candidiasis

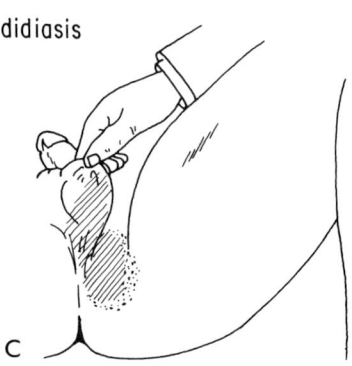

FIGURE 8–3. Genital rashes. A, Tinea. B, Erythrasma. C, Candidiasis (see Table 8–3).

TABLE 8–3. GENITAL RASHES

DISEASE	GROSS APPEARANCE	PRESUMPTIVE DIAGNOSIS	DEFINITIVE DIAGNOSIS	TREATMENT
Groin Rash[8]				
Tinea cruris	Pale, pink, slightly scaly rash of inner thigh(s), often sparing scrotum; central clearing	Gross appearance KOH "prep": fungi	Fungal culture (rarely necessary)	Topical clotrimazole or haloprogin or miconazole nitrate bid × 3 weeks
Candidiasis	Scaly, fiery-red erythema of thigh and scrotum; peripheral "satellite lesions"	Gross appearance KOH prep: budding yeast and hyphae	Fungal culture (rarely necessary)	Nystatin, clotrimazole, haloprogin, or miconazole nitrate bid × 2–3 weeks
Erythrasma	Erythematous plaque-like thigh, scrotal rash	Gross appearance KOH prep; Wood's light: coral red fluorescence	Culture: *Corynebacterium minutissimum* (rarely necessary)	Oral erythromycin 250 mg qid × 2 weeks

Remember: allergic dermatitis, contact dermatitis, psoriasis, intertrigo, seborrhea, drug eruptions

		Penile Rash		
Balanitis[10]	Inflammation, swelling of glans penis (balanoposthitis: foreskin, too)	Consider: retained smegma, contact irritants, candidiasis, Reiter's syndrome, diabetes mellitus	Exclude: syphilis, gonorrhea, herpes, chancroid	Penile soaks in glass of warm saline and/or potassium permanganate solution tid; ?topical nystatin; ?topical steroids
Penile venereal edema[11]	Painless, subcutaneous boggy edema of prepuce and distal shaft of penis	Exclude: gonorrhea (40%), NGU (20%), herpes (12%), scabies (12%)		Treat balanitis (above) and treat associated venereal disease (if any)
Neoplastic, preneoplastic lesions[9]:	Bowen's disease, erythroplasia of Queyrat, balanitis obliterans, epidermoid carcinoma, basal cell carcinoma, Kaposi's sarcoma			

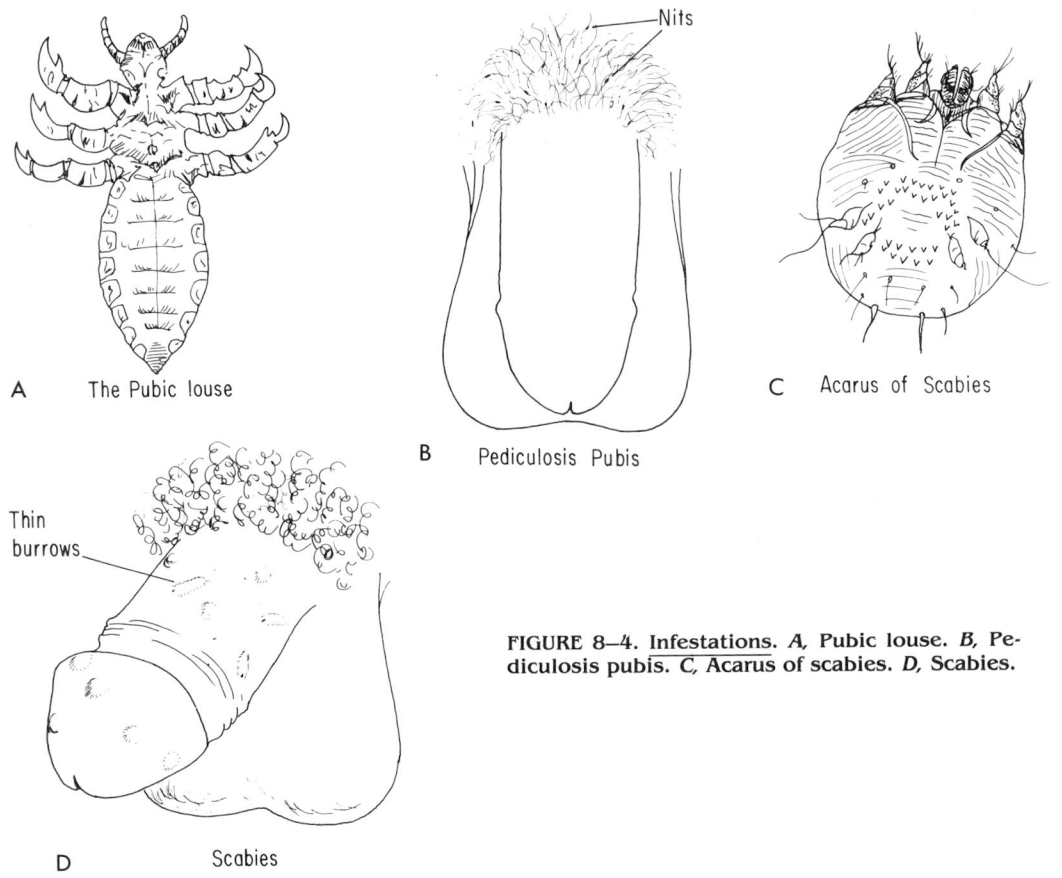

FIGURE 8–4. Infestations. *A*, Pubic louse. *B*, Pediculosis pubis. *C*, Acarus of scabies. *D*, Scabies.

TABLE 8–4. GENITAL INFESTATIONS[12]

DISEASE	GROSS APPEARANCE	PRESUMPTIVE DIAGNOSIS	DEFINITIVE DIAGNOSIS	TREATMENT
Pediculosis pubis (crabs)	Tiny, squat, crab-shaped creature, clinging to skin at base of pubic hair (or nits on hair)	Gross appearance	Examine hair shaft under microscope for nit or mature crab	Gamma benzene hexachloride (Kwell) 1% lotion applied to all hair areas—rinse after 24 hours and repeat; launder bedclothes
Scabies	1–10 mm, needle-thin burrows in genital, pubic skin; interdigital burrows too?	Gross appearance	Examine scraping of unroofed burrow under microscope for mite or its eggs. (Use mineral oil.)	Kwell (as above) or crotamiton topically

hair shaft. Scabies infestation causes severe itching and a variety of visible clues—papules, burrows, and excoriated areas of pseudofolliculitis may be seen. The mature organism (the acarus) is only occasionally found; the diagnosis is thus often presumptive.

Figure 8–5 illustrates the palpable anatomy of normal scrotal contents. All males with genitourinary symptoms (dysuria, urinary hesitancy, penile discharge, genital or groin pain) should undergo careful manual examination of the groin, scrotum, and prostate. Epididymitis (Figs. 8–6 and 8–7) is a common cause of scrotal pain and dysuria; orchitis and testicular torsion (Fig. 8–8) are rare, but very serious, causes of scrotal pain. A variety of other scrotal swellings are benign (hydrocele, varicocele, spermatocele—Fig. 8–9), but swelling of (or a mass within) the testis itself is a urologic emergency—testicular cancer must be excluded. Routine examination of

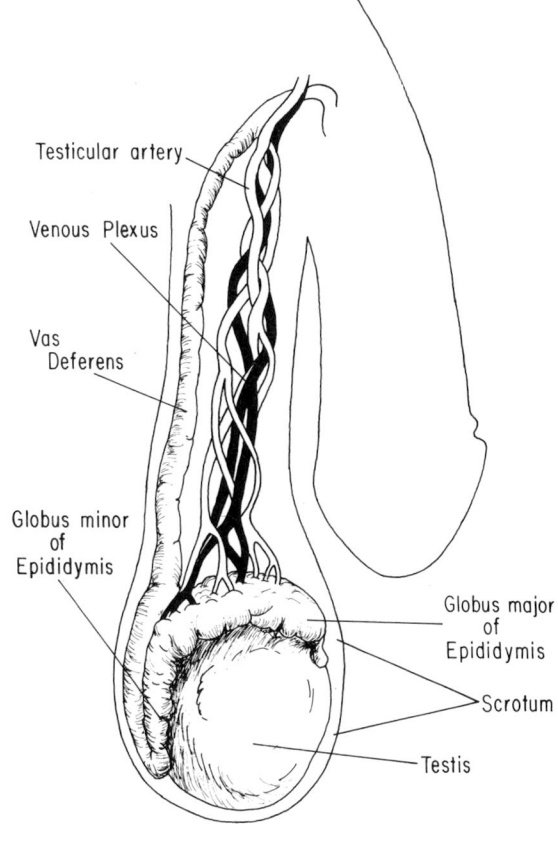

FIGURE 8–5. Normal scrotal contents.

The scrotum is a pendulous sac that normally contains four paired structures: testis, epididymis, vas deferens, and the vasculature of the spermatic cord.

The testis hangs vertically in the scrotum; its longitudinal axis is 4 to 5 cm long, and its width and anteroposterior diameter are about 3 cm each.

The epididymis is a tubular structure that hugs the superior and posterior testis—the globus major (the head of the epididymis) lies atop the testis, and the globus minor (the tail) enlarges at the lower pole of the testis.

The vas deferens is a duct that emerges from the tail of the epididymis and runs cephalad, together with the arterial and venous supply of the testis and epididymis within the spermatic cord. These structures run the length of the scrotum, from the lower testis into the inguinal canal.

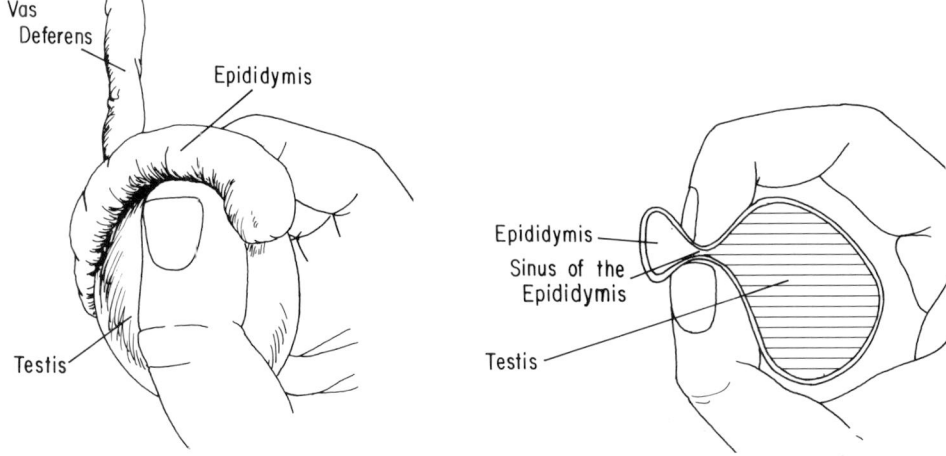

FIGURE 8–6. Palpation of testis and epididymis. The examining finger separates the firm, anterior, oval testis from the soft, tubular posterior epididymis by gently pinching the sinus of the epididymis.

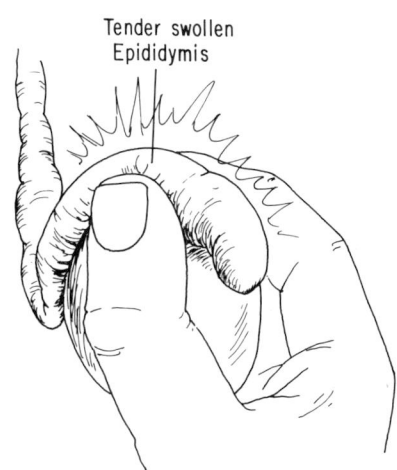

FIGURE 8–7. Epididymitis refers to swelling and inflammation of the epididymis due to bacterial (or other) infection, trauma, or other poorly understood factors (reflux of urine through ejaculatory ducts, for example). The epididymis itself is usually thickened and tender in the presence of infection (while visible erythema or swelling of the entire scrotum, or both, are occasionally seen with severe infection). In young males, chlamydial infection is a common cause;[14] in men older than 35, gram-negative bacilli are probably more common. (Gonorrhea is a much less common cause of epididymitis today than previously—but urethral cultures for gonorrhea should be obtained.) Treatment usually involves broad-spectrum antibiotics (tetracycline when chlamydial disease is suspected; cephalexin [Keflex] or ampicillin when gram-negative infection is more likely); bedrest with scrotal elevation, and analgesics.

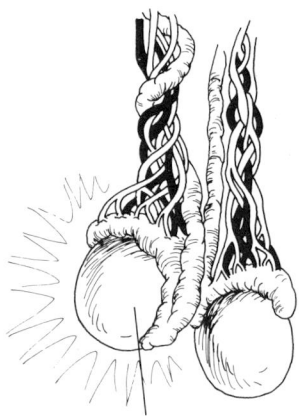

Tender swollen testicle

FIGURE 8–8. Testicular torsion usually occurs in men under the age of 30, but any (usually sudden) onset of scrotal pain, associated with extreme testicular tenderness, must initiate concern about a twisting of the spermatic cord (and blood supply)—torsion—with impending testicular infarction. When in doubt, a urologist must be consulted immediately, since surgery must be performed within several hours if infarction is to be avoided. Careful palpation is crucial. With torsion, it is the testis that is tender (not just the epididymis). Sometimes the involved testicle will sit higher in the scrotum owing to foreshortening of the twisted spermatic cord (see figure). Sometimes the epididymis may be situated anteriorly (instead of its usual posterior location), also suggesting the diagnosis. Tenderness is often so extreme that palpation is difficult—testicular ultrasound will help here, as may nuclear scans or Doppler studies.[114]

Orchitis, acute infection of the testis, is sufficiently rare today to warrant great caution in making this diagnosis. Epididymitis will sometimes also involve the testis (epididymo-orchitis); in this case, the epididymis is abnormal to palpation, too. Acute pyogenic orchitis is very rare, but high fever with an extremely tender, swollen (sometimes fluctuant) testicle, with or without visible scrotal erythema and edema, should always raise this suspicion. Recent epididymitis, urinary tract infection, urinary catheterization, or other instrumentation is sometimes the underlying cause. Trauma, mumps infection, and a variety of other infections may occasionally produce a similar picture. When in doubt, the urologist should be consulted immediately, primarily because testicular torsion should never be missed.

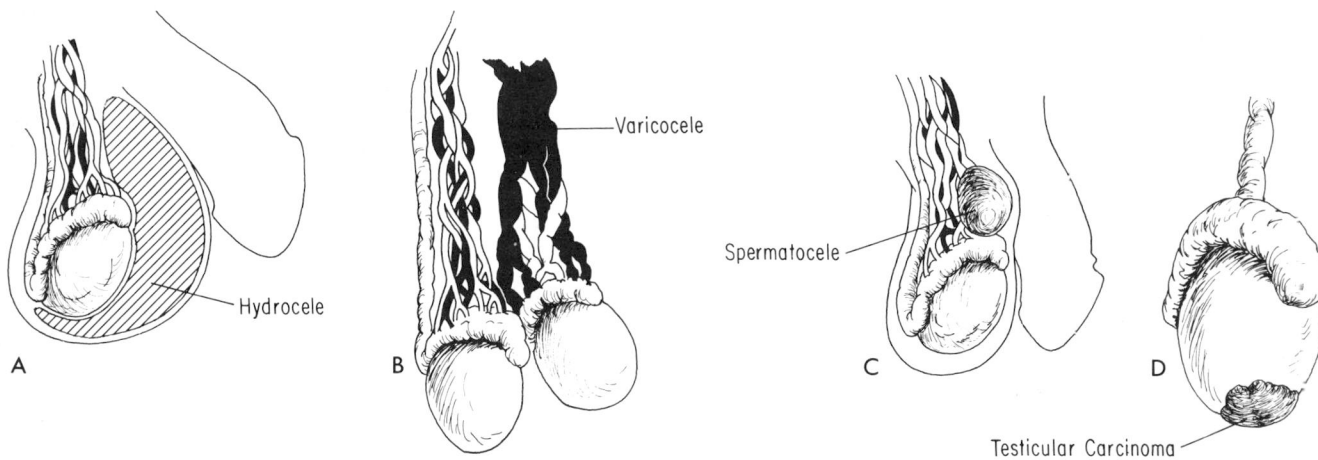

FIGURE 8–9. A, A hydrocele is a cystic accumulation of clear fluid within (usually) the tunica vaginalis—a remnant of peritoneal "tongue" that migrates into the testis during embryological descent of the testis and that covers the testis, separating it from the epididymis. Hydroceles present as painless swellings of the scrotum. The amount of fluid present determines whether the swelling is tense or soft and whether the testis is palpable through the hydrocele. Transillumination always reveals the cystic nature of the mass. Aspiration of the cystic contents is almost never advisable (fluid will reaccumulate), except in the very rare instance of acute pyogenic orchitis that ruptures into the tunica vaginalis, producing pyocele.

Hydrocelectomy is necessary only if the swelling is large and uncomfortable, if it is associated with an inguinal hernia that also requires repair, or if it is cosmetically disturbing.

B, A varicocele is a dilated plexus of scrotal veins, situated above the testis, resembling a "bag of worms" on palpation. These dilated vessels are usually nontender and asymptomatic. They tend to be most prominent when the patient is standing and least prominent when the patient is supine. Varicoceles usually deserve no further attention unless male infertility is an associated problem, or, very rarely, if the varicocele arises acutely in an older male on the right side and will not deflate in the supine position. In the former situation, varicocelectomy may improve fertility (for obscure reasons). In the latter situation, a renal neoplasm with involvement of the inferior vena cava must be excluded (but this is very rare).

C, A spermatocele is a cyst containing sperm that usually feels like a small, nontender ball lying above the testis and that does transilluminate. Spermatoceles are usually asymptomatic, but careful palpation must document that the mass is separate from the testis, to distinguish it from a testicular neoplasm. Treatment is usually unnecessary.

D, Testicular tumors are usually malignant neoplasms that arise in young men. They are usually painless, hard swellings of all or part of the testis itself. They do not transilluminate.

Any localized or diffuse swelling of the testis itself must be assumed to be a malignant tumor, especially in a young man. Testicular ultrasound will often be helpful when palpation cannot clearly distinguish a testicular mass from swellings of the epididymis or other contiguous structures.

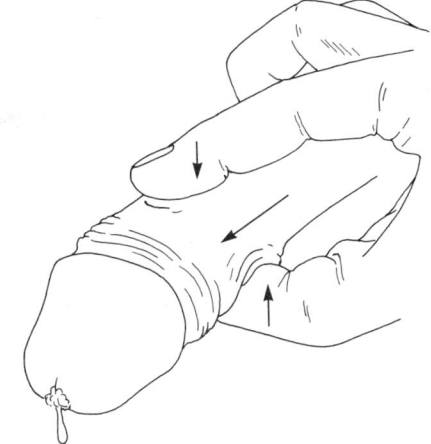

FIGURE 8–10. Urethral stripping.

male genitalia will so familiarize the clinician with normal variants that these different disorders are usually easy to recognize.

4. There is no prior history of genitourinary problems. It is always helpful to inquire about similar episodes in the past. Whatever the site or etiology of the present problem, chronic or recurrent symptoms or a known history of prior genitourinary disease (especially renal failure, nephrolithiasis, prostate disease, or recent urethritis) will raise specific questions more immediately (see below).

5. In Don's case, urethral discharge is present. This is the most helpful clue to the cause of this patient's problem. While dysuria and discharge may occur with prostatitis or epididymitis, for example, the majority of men with both dysuria and urethral discharge suffer from one of the different types of urethritis. In the absence of palpable abnormalities of the prostate or epididymis, and with the lack of other prostatitis symptoms (back pain, testicle pain, urinary frequency—see page 366), urethritis is the diagnosis until proven otherwise.

The diagnostic importance of this finding necessitates that the examiner look very carefully to determine the presence or absence of urethral discharge. When the male patient complaining of dysuria does not describe (or demonstrate) spontaneous discharge, the examiner should "strip" the urethra for expressible secretions. Urethral stripping involves squeezing the urethra (on the underside of the penis) sequentially from the proximal to the distal penile shaft, trying to "milk" secretions from the urethral orifice (Fig. 8–10). Discharges are often thereby quantititated (primarily for purposes of clinical investigation):[15, 16] spontaneous urethral discharge $(3+)$; no spontaneous discharge but moderate discharge following penile stripping $(2+)$; slight discharge after stripping $(1+)$; no discharge (0) even after stripping. Quantitation is not diagnostically useful.

Dysuria in the absence of any expressible discharge may still be caused by urethritis (see page 360), but most male urethritis is accompanied by some discharge,[13, 14] and its absence should then raise other questions (see below).

URETHRITIS

Urethritis may be due to gonorrhea or a variety of other infectious nongonococcal causes. Probably at least one half of cases of nongonococcal urethritis (NGU) are due to chlamydial infection,[17-20] while other rarer or undiscovered agents are responsible for the remainder (see below). NGU is now probably more common than gonococcal urethritis.[21–23]

Gonococcal versus Nongonococcal Urethritis

A simple stepwise approach to the patient with suspected urethritis will usually distinguish gonococcal from nongonococcal urethritis (see also Fig. 8–13). While the clinical history and examination may be suggestive of one or the other, specific diagnostic separation depends on the urethral Gram's stain or urethral culture or both.

CONSIDER

I. Clinical findings.

Gonococcal urethritis typically presents after a brief episode (lasting a week or less) of dysuria, accompanied by spontaneous purulent urethral discharge. The incubation period from the time of venereal exposure to the onset of symptoms usually ranges from 2 to 14 days.

Nongonococcal urethritis (NGU) often presents with more indolent and prolonged symptoms (more than 1 week). Discharge is less often spontaneous (but about 80 per cent will have some discharge after stripping). The discharge of NGU is more often mucoid or watery in appearance. Occasionally patients with NGU will demonstrate discharge only when the bladder is full (upon arising in the morning).

These clinical distinctions are nonspecific, however. There is clearly some overlap between the clinical presentations of NGU and gonococcal urethritis. Some patients with gonorrhea will present with discharge that is more prolonged in duration or that is mucoid in appearance. (Only a few will have no discharge at all.) On the other hand, NGU may present with acute purulent discharge. Clinical distinctions are even less clear when gonorrhea and NGU coexist. Both gonococci and chlamydiae are occasionally isolated from the same patient.[16, 24]

Therefore,

II. The urethral Gram's stain is essential.

Spontaneous or "stripped" urethral discharge can be smeared directly on a microscopic slide. When discharge is absent or is difficult to

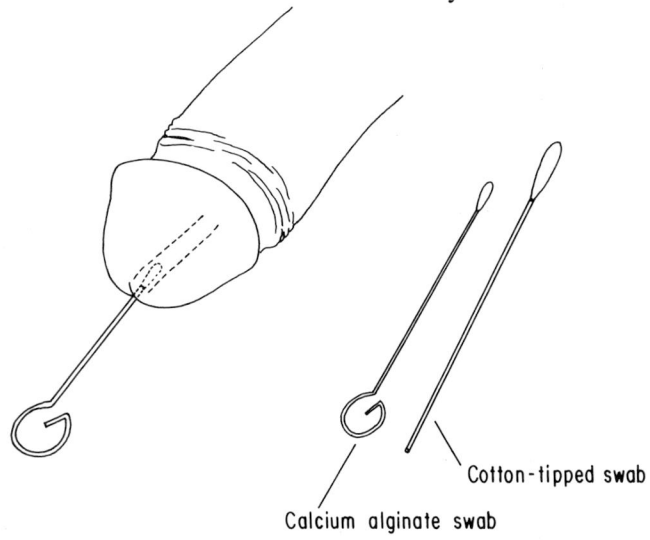

Calcium alginate swab

Cotton-tipped swab

FIGURE 8–11. Urethral swabs. The calcium alginate swab is smaller and more flexible than the usual cotton-tipped swab. The former is always preferable in obtaining urethral specimens.

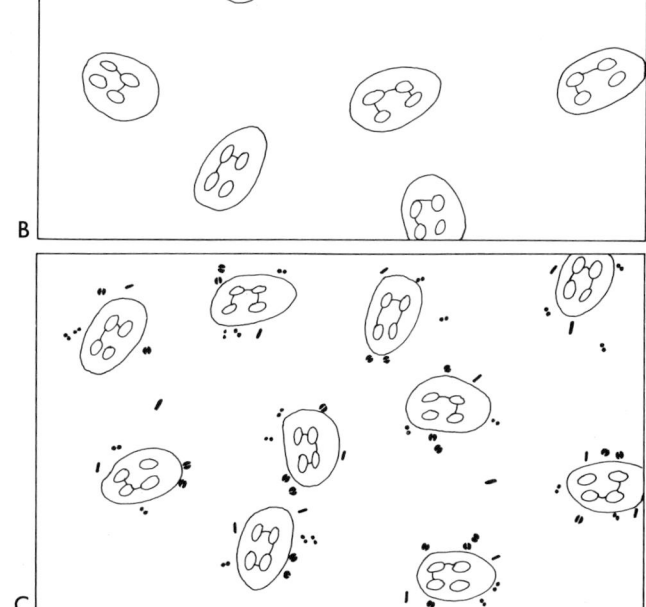

FIGURE 8–12. The urethral Gram's stain. *A*, Typical intracellular gram-negative kidney bean–shaped diplococci are depicted. This is a "positive" gonococcal (GC) smear. *B*, Inflammatory cells without microorganisms are demonstrated. This is a GC-negative smear—typical of nongonococcal urethritis. *C*, Inflammatory cells and a variety of microorganisms are see here, none of which are intracellular gram-negative diplococci but some of which are extracellular gram-negative diplococci. This is a "borderline" GC smear.

express, a urethral swab is inserted 2 cm into the anterior urethra and then "rolled" over a slide (Fig. 8–11). Gram's stains of these specimens will be helpful only if the stain is well prepared and the examiner knows what to look for.[15, 25] The results of urethral Gram's stains can be divided into three categories (Fig. 8–12):

A. GC (gonococcus) positive.

    Gram-negative diplococci that are typical in appearance (rounded external contours with flattened, apposing internal contours—likened to kidney beans) are found within polymorphonuclear leukocytes.

B. GC negative.

    No typical gram-negative diplococci are found.

C. Borderline.

    Gram-negative diplococci are found, but all are either extracellular or atypical in appearance.

GC-positive smears correlate highly (90 to 95 per cent) with subsequent positive cultures for gonorrhea, while GC-negative smears have been highly predictive of negative cultures (assuming prior antibiotic therapy has not interfered). However, these diagnostic Gram's stain findings are found in only about 85 per cent of all patients: about 15 per cent of patients will show borderline Gram's stains. Most patients with borderline smears are culture negative for gonorrhea,[25] but in some (about 10 per cent) gonococci will grow on subsequent cultures.

The value and shortcomings of the urethral Gram's stain are depicted schematically in Table 8–5. Given 100 hypothetical males with urethritis (of whom 40 are subsequently proven to have gonorrhea and the remaining 60 to have NGU), perhaps 40 will have positive GC smears, but in a few of these gonococci will not be subsequently grown on culture. Such culture-negative, smear-positive cases may represent observer error (false positive Gram's stains in patients with NGU); failure to grow gonococci because of inadequate specimen procurement, plating techniques, or laboratory errors; or even, rarely, *Neisseria meningitidis* urethritis.[26, 27] As Table 8–5 illustrates, however, a positive GC smear is an excellent test in the presumptive diagnosis of gonococcal urethritis.

Among our 60 hypothetical patients with either borderline or negative GC smears, an occasional patient will be found in whom subsequent culture grows *Neisseria gonorrhoeae*. The frequency of such cases will vary with the examiner's skill in procuring and interpreting Gram's stains as well as with the incidence of borderline smears in a given patient population.

Therefore the urethral Gram's stain is usually an excellent guide to presumptive diagnosis, and initial therapy is usually based on the results of this test. Since misdiagnoses do occasionally occur, gonococcal cultures should be obtained regardless of Gram's stain results.*

III. Urethral cultures.

Cultures of spontaneous discharge or urethral swabs should be plated immediately on warm (room temperature) Thayer-Martin culture medium. Culturettes (transport media) may also be used if they are sent to the laboratory for plating within an hour or two, but maximal yield will be guaranteed by immediate plating after specimens are obtained.

---

*Some would argue that cultures are unnecessary if the Gram's stain is unequivocally positive since treatment is then not affected.

TABLE 8–5. GRAM'S STAIN AND GONOCOCCAL CULTURE IN 100 HYPOTHETICAL MALES WITH URETHRITIS

URETHRAL GRAM'S STAIN		GONOCOCCAL CULTURE	
		Positive	*Negative*
Positive (typical intracellular gram-negative diplococci)	40	37	3
Borderline or indeterminate (atypical or extracellular gram-negative diplococci)	15	2	13
Negative (no gram-negative diplococci)	45	1	44
Total	100	40	60

When urethral swabs cannot be used (for whatever reason),* sterilely collected fresh urine specimens can be cultured—good yields for *N. gonorrhoeae* have been reported.[28, 29]

In the male homosexual, cultures should also be obtained from the pharynx (swab the posterior pharynx) and anorectal area (insert the swab a few centimeters into the anal canal without contaminating the swab with feces). Even when the homosexual male has symptoms only of urethritis, concomitant asymptomatic pharyngeal or rectal gonorrhea is not rare,[30-32] and the site(s) of infection may have therapeutic implications (see Table 8–6).

Cultures for chlamydiae, ureaplasmas, and other organisms are not readily available in most practice settings and only rarely need be obtained in the male with urethritis.

Don's clinical symptoms are believed to be suggestive of gonorrhea. A Gram's stain of urethral discharge reveals many polymorphonuclear leukocytes with both intracellular and extracellular gram-negative diplococci that are typical morphologically of *Neisseria* organisms. The discharge is cultured immediately on Thayer-Martin medium.

Don admits sexual intercourse with three different women in the past 2 weeks, none of whom had any known genitourinary symptoms. He denies any homosexual activity but admits to cunnilingus with two of his three "contacts." There has been no history of any penile sores, and Don has never had a serologic test for syphilis. There is no history of penicillin allergy.

What does this mean?

1. Don must be assumed to have gonorrhea and should be treated accordingly. As noted above, false positive gonococcal Gram's stains may occur, but it is always difficult to prove whether the Gram's stain is falsely positive or the subsequent culture falsely negative. Positive Gram's stains mandate treatment for gonorrhea.

2. It may be worthwhile to culture the pharynx, but the relation of cunnilingus to oropharyngeal gonorrhea is unclear.[30]

3. Any or all of Don's three sexual consorts could have gonorrhea, whether symptomatic or not, and thus all should be traced, examined, and treated for presumed gonorrhea. (Often, it makes sense to await absolute proof—positive cultures—before initiating contact tracing and treatment. Had Don needed to inform an unsuspecting and asymptomatic wife about his problem, for example, he might understandably demand such proof.)

Male homosexual contacts must be traced as diligently as female contacts. Asymptomatic male gonorrhea is not rare.[33, 34]

4. A serologic test for syphilis should be obtained. The results of this test and the antibiotic regimen prescribed for gonorrhea will determine the need for subsequent surveillance for coexistent, incubating syphilis (see below and Appendix II).

Treatment of Gonococcal Urethritis

Many different antibiotic regimens will cure gonococcal urethritis.[35] In many settings, penicillin remains the drug of choice, but a specific antibiotic

---

*An occasional patient will refuse or simply be unable to cooperate.

TABLE 8–6. TREATMENT OF GONORRHEA

	PENICILLIN, (IM) PROCAINE	AMPICILLIN (ORAL)	AMOXICILLIN (ORAL)	TETRACYCLINE (ORAL)
Dose	4.8 million U plus 1.0 gm oral probenecid	3.5 gm plus 1.0 gm oral probenecid	3.0 gm plus 1.0 gm oral probenecid	500 mg qid × 5 days (10 gm total)
Cost	$2 (plus $2)*	$3 (plus $2)	$3 (plus $2)	$4
Duration	Single dose	Single dose	Single dose	5 days
Efficacy (good†; poor‡)				
Genital	Good	Good	Good	Good
Pharyngeal	Good	Poor	Poor	Good
Anorectal, female	Good	Good	Good	Good
Anorectal, male	Good	Good	Good	Poor
Cure of incubating syphilis	Yes	Probable	Probable	Yes
Effect on NGU/PGU	Poor	Poor	Poor	Good
Safety in pregnancy[36]	Yes	Yes	Yes	No
Drug of choice?	Often	Often	Often	Often
Disadvantages	Penicillin allergy	Suspected pharyngeal infection?	Suspected pharyngeal infection?	Noncompliance?
	Painful injection			Male homosexual?
	Postgonococcal urethritis	Postgonococcal urethritis	Postgonococcal urethritis	

regimen should be chosen only after considering different host factors, site(s) of infection (urethra, rectum, pharynx), patient compliance, drug costs, and side effects. The effect of a specific treatment regimen on possible coexistent incubating syphilis or on subsequent development of postgonococcal urethritis should also be considered. Table 8–6 outlines some of the advantages and disadvantages of different antibiotic regimens.

Penicillins. In general, the three penicillin regimens (intramuscular procaine penicillin, oral ampicillin, oral amoxicillin) are recommended for urethritis, because they are well tolerated, are highly (and equally) effective, and the penicillin can be given as a single dose. Because ampicillin and amoxicillin are not as effective for pharyngeal gonorrhea[37–39] and have not been as clearly proven to reliably cure incubating syphillis and anorectal gonorrhea,[39] parenteral procaine penicillin is often favored,* especially in the male homosexual. All treatment regimens include 1 gm of oral probenecid, which delays renal excretion of penicillins.

Postgonococcal urethritis (see below) is more commonly encountered after successful penicillin treatment than after some other treatment regimens (especially tetracycline).[40]

It is probably safe to resume sexual activity within 3 to 4 days after penicillin therapy.

The only definite contraindications to these penicillin regimens is an unequivocal history of penicillin allergy.

Tetracycline. Tetracycline is desirable for many reasons. It is highly effective[41, 42] (except in male anorectal infection, in which failure rates approximate 15 per cent[43, 44]), well tolerated, effective against incubating syphilis, and the most successful drug in preventing postgonococcal urethritis. The only major disadvantage is potential patient noncompliance since the drug must be taken qid for 5 consecutive days. (A loading dose is unnecessary.)

Tetracycline is certainly the drug of choice when clinical findings are equivocal (i.e., borderline urethral Gram's stain) and treatment is initiated before culture results are available, or when the patient is penicillin allergic.

Other Drugs. Trimethoprim-sulfamethoxazole has been evaluated less thoroughly but appears to be highly effective in gonococcal urethritis.[45] It is

*The physician favors penicillin injections much more than the patient does—procaine penicillin injected intramuscularly hurts!

TABLE 8–6. TREATMENT OF GONORRHEA (Continued)

	SPECTINOMYCIN (IM)	TRIMETHOPRIM-SULFAMETHOXAZOLE (ORAL)	CEFOXITIN (IM)	ERYTHROMYCIN (ORAL)
Dose	2.0 gm	80 mg/400 mg, 4 tablets bid × 2 days	2.0 gm (reconstituted w/ 4 ml 0.5% lidocaine) plus 1.0 gm probenecid	10 gm total (500 mg qid × 5 days)
Cost	$12	$5	$18	$5
Duration	Single dose	2 days	Single dose	5 days
Efficacy (good†; poor‡)				
Genital	Good	Good	Good	Poor
Pharyngeal	Poor	Good	Uncertain	Poor
Anorectal, female	Good	Uncertain	Uncertain	Poor
Anorectal, male	Good	Uncertain	Uncertain	Poor
Cure of incubating syphilis	Uncertain	Uncertain	Uncertain	Uncertain
Effect on NGU/PGU?	Poor	Uncertain	Uncertain	Good
Safety in pregnancy[36]	Probably	Uncertain	Probably	Yes
Drug of choice?	Uncommon§ (PPNG)	Rarely§	Rarely§	Almost never§
Disadvantages	Syphilis? Pharyngeal infection? Postgonococcal urethritis	Incompletely studied	Cost Painful Incompletely studied	Lower efficacy Noncompliance?

*If prepackaged (e.g., Wycillin) in syringes, cost is much higher ($12.00).
†Good implies greater than 90% cure rate.
‡Poor implies less than 90% cure rate.
§See text.

attractive because it can be administered orally for only 2 days, and thus compliance may be enhanced. Its effects on pharyngeal and anorectal infection, incubating syphilis, and subsequent postgonococcal urethritis are incompletely studied, however.

Erythromycin[46] is almost never the drug of choice in urethritis, although it may occasionally have a role in treatment of disseminated gonococcal infection[47] (or in nongonococcal urethritis[48]—see page 357).

Spectinomycin and cefoxitin[49] are usually reserved for the (currently) rare instances of urethritis caused by penicillinase-producing *N. gonorrhoeae* (PPNG) or when infection is recurrent or apparently refractory to other drugs. PPNG should be especially suspected when infection is acquired in areas of the world where PPNG now flourishes—the Far East primarily, but PPNG is expected to become an increasing problem in the United States as well. Spectinomycin is not highly effective against pharyngeal gonorrhea[40] or incubating syphilis.[50] Cefoxitin injections are painful, and the drug has not been as well studied as spectinomycin.

> Don is treated with 1 gm oral probenecid and 4.8 million units procaine penicillin G—2.4 million units intramuscularly in each buttock. Blood is drawn for a serologic test for syphilis (VDRL). Don is told he should refrain from sex for the next few days, preferably until he returns to the clinic in 1 week for repeat cultures. He is told that his female sex partners should be notified and that they need to be examined and treated, even if they are asymptomatic.
>
> Don is not pleased. He is a long-distance trucker and explains that two of his three recent sex partners are "far away and I'll probably never see them again" and complains that it will be inconvenient for him to return for follow-up examination.

NOTE

1. Whenever possible, follow-up gonococcal cultures should be obtained (3 to 7 days following completion of therapy) from all sites that were

originally culture positive. This may seem overly compulsive when one considers that antibiotic-resistant gonococci are (currently) rare in the United States and that cure rates with most drug regimens exceed 90 per cent. It is true that positive post-treatment cultures usually imply venereal reinfection rather than antibiotic failure, but no drug regimen is 100 per cent effective, and penicillinase-producing (or other resistant) gonococci will likely become a more common problem in the future (see Appendix III).

2. Contact tracing (initiated by the patient) is often difficult, embarrassing, and inconvenient. For these reasons, state departments of public health often play an active role here, but, allowing the patient the opportunity to "break the news" is often more humane. The frequency of asymptomatic gonorrhea must be emphasized (to the patient), as must the potential serious consequences (especially to women) of untreated gonorrhea: disseminated gonococcemia,[51] salpingitis, endocarditis,[52] and subsequent female sterility are among the many possible consequences. Most male patients will respond to such "scare tactics" and aid in contact tracing of their sexual consorts.

3. Penicillin reactions are rare[53] but must be remembered. Any patient given a parenteral dose of penicillin should be observed for a half-hour or hour thereafter, so that rare but potentially lethal anaphylactic reactions can be treated immediately.

> One week later, Don returns for his follow-up appointment. Urethral cultures were positive for penicillin-sensitive *N. gonorrhoeae*. VDRL was nonreactive. (Don says he is "fine," and notes no symptoms or discharge.) Examination is normal, but "stripping" the urethra reveals a few drops of clear to mucoid discharge that is cultured again on Thayer-Martin medium. Don is told that, if the culture is now negative and he continues to be asymptomatic, no further treatment or surveillance is necessary.
>
> Don's local girlfriend, Connie, accompanies him. She is asymptomatic, has a normal pelvic, pharyngeal, and rectal examination, and cultures for *N. gonorrhoeae* are taken from all three sites. Probenecid and procaine penicillin are administered to Connie, and a VDRL test is obtained. Don says that he has notified his other two female partners and that treatment will be administered in their local areas.
>
> Subsequently, all cultures from Don and Connie are reported negative. Connie's VDRL is also nonreactive. Connie is told that repeat cultures are unnecessary and that she was "never infected." She is greatly relieved.

NOTE

1. While Don is asymptomatic after treatment, he continues to show evidence of urethritis (discharge). This is not at all uncommon following successful eradication of gonorrhea[54]—such persistent discharge may represent postgonococcal urethritis,[54] concomitant NGU,[24] or simply delayed clinical resolution of adequately treated gonococcal urethritis.

2. Negative VDRL serologic tests imply that no further surveillance for syphilis is necessary in either Don or Connie. If, however, different antibiotic regimens had been used initially (see Table 8–6), a repeat VDRL test in the next 1 to 3 months would be worthwhile, since incubating syphilis will sometimes not provoke seropositivity for up to 3 months after exposure (and the symptomatic stage of primary syphilis can be inapparent).

If the VDRL were positive here, it should be confirmed with an FTA-ABS test, and syphilis chemotherapy should be given in addition to gonorrhea therapy (see Appendix II).

3. Connie is treated for gonorrhea before culture results are available

(and in spite of the fact that they are subsequently negative). False negative gonorrhea cultures do occur (see above); all sexual contacts of a patient with proven gonorrhea should be treated. Why then bother to obtain cultures in these patients? Cultures are obtained here to document infection and thus to advise post-treatment cultures should initial cultures return positive. Such matters should be explained to the patient.

> Two weeks later, Don returns to the clinic saying, "I guess I've got it again." For the past 4 days, Don has noted dysuria and discharge, both less prominent than previously, but otherwise "just like before." Don admits to sexual activity with Connie and another woman in a remote town, both in the past 2 weeks. Neither woman is symptomatic, to his knowledge.

> Examination is normal except for a mucopurulent urethral discharge apparent only after urethral stripping. Gram's stain reveals 10 polymorphonuclear leukocytes per high-power field, but no microorganisms are seen. A specimen is sent for gonococcal cultures.

Treatment of Nongonococcal Urethritis

Nongonococcal urethritis is now probably more common than gonorrhea, but its specific causes are incompletely understood.[21-23] The etiology of one half or more of cases of NGU is unknown. Genital mycoplasmas have been implicated by some investigators,[19, 55, 56] and evidence is mounting to support their etiologic role in some cases of NGU.[57] The role of other infectious agents (for example, *Corynebacterium genitalium* type I), is undecided.[58] There is substantial evidence that *Chlamydia trachomatis*—an intracellular bacterium, which in some ways resembles a virus—causes up to one half of the cases of NGU.[17-20] The frequent incidence of chlamydial infection in clinical studies of NGU and the response of chlamydial infection to antibiotic therapy form the basis for the therapeutic approach to NGU.

Most cases of NGU (whatever the specific microbial cause) are responsive at least initially to tetracycline therapy,[59] but recurrence of NGU after tetracycline therapy is quite common. This recurrence after treatment is least common in (proven) chlamydial urethritis, more common in (proven) mycoplasma urethritis, and most common in NGU in which neither chlamydiae nor mycoplasmas are isolated.[59]

Unfortunately, culture techniques to isolate chlamydiae and mycoplasmas are available only in large centers or reference laboratories and are not currently practical in most settings.* Thus our ability to predict response to therapy, or to prove the cause of therapeutic failure, is often limited.

Given these uncertainties, what should be done with our patient?

1. Because isolation techniques for chlamydiae and mycoplasmas are not practical in our setting, the most specific diagnosis we can make is nongonococcal urethritis (NGU). (Whether postgonococcal urethritis (PGU) is different from NGU is unknown. Many patients who develop NGU following gonococcal urethritis—previously termed PGU—are shown to have had simultaneous initial infection with both gonococci and chlamydiae, the latter infection persisting and becoming symptomatic after penicillin therapy.)

2. Tetracycline is the drug of choice in NGU,[60] but the precise dose, preparation, and duration of therapy are debatable. At least 7 days' therapy is advised, and almost all patients will improve within 7 to 10 days of initiating

---

*Immunofluorescent antibody staining for diagnosis of chlamydial urethritis may provide more rapid and inexpensive identification. These techniques had not received FDA approval at the time of this writing.

TABLE 8–7. ANTIMICROBIAL SPECTRUM OF TREATMENTS FOR
NONGONOCOCCAL URETHRITIS*

	N. Gonorrhoeae/Chlamydiae/Ureaplasmas		
Tetracycline[60] 500 qid × 7–21 days	+	+	±
Minocycline[59] 100 mg qid × 7–21 days	±	+	±
Erythromycin[48] 500 mg qid × 7–21 days	±	+	±
Sulfisoxazole[56] 500 mg qid × 7–21 days	−	+	−
Spectinomycin[56] 2 gm IM, 1 or 2 doses	+	−	+
Rifampin[62](?)	±	+	−

*Clinical studies do not allow more precise quantitative estimates of efficacy than usually (+), unpredictably (±), not usually (−).

treatment. Recurrence of symptoms and signs of urethritis is common (about 30 per cent) in the subsequent 4 to 8 weeks, and, while prolonged initial treatment with tetracycline (21 days) delays recurrent urethritis, 3 weeks of initial tetracycline treatment are probably no more successful than 1 week of treatment in achieving permanent "cure."[59]

Tetracycline hydrochloride 500 mg qid for 7 days is thus recommended in NGU.[60] (This regimen is also curative for urethral gonorrhea.) Doxycycline may be less effective than tetracycline,[61] while minocycline is as effective but is more expensive and more likely to cause side effects.[59]

Erythromycin is the alternative drug of choice in patients who cannot use tetracycline, but sulfonamides or rifampin may occasionally be effective too. In almost all patients with NGU, however, either tetracycline or erythromycin is the drug of choice. Table 8–7 lists drugs that have been evaluated in the treatment of either NGU or other infections with chlamydiae or mycoplasmas.

3. The need for treatment of the sexual partners of men with NGU is uncertain. Recurrent NGU probably is often due to reinfection by an asymptomatic sexual partner, but current data do not permit recommendations for routine antibiotic therapy of all sex partners of all men with their first bout of NGU. There is certainly sufficient theoretic reason to believe that female partners of men with culture-proven *Chlamydia* urethritis should be treated[22, 23, 59] (but, again, we usually do not have definitive microbiologic proof in most clinical practices).

Treatment of sexual partners is recommended here.

4. There are other causes of urethritis in males (*Trichomonas*, herpes, *Candida*), but these are unusual. When a female sex partner is known to have vaginitis or genital lesions, these entities should be searched for routinely in the male with NGU. Otherwise, such searches will rarely be fruitful, although in recurrent or refractory NGU, they must be remembered (see page 360).

Don is told that his recurrent symptoms are probably not due to gonorrhea again, but a result of "the other kind of infectious urethritis," which can feel just the same. It is explained that cultures will be sent to test for gonorrhea to make absolutely sure, but the new treatment will cover gonorrhea anyway.

Tetracycline, 500 mg qid for 7 days followed by 250 mg qid for 7 days, is prescribed. Don is told that similar treatment for Connie may help prevent this from recurring. Don says that he would rather not involve Connie unless it is absolutely necessary. We suggest but cannot insist. Don refuses.

Subsequent gonococcal cultures are negative.

NOTE

1. There is no "scientific" rationale for 14 days' tetracycline therapy. It is chosen here as a compromise between 7-day and 21-day therapy in the (unfounded) hope that it will prevent (or at least delay) recurrent NGU.

2. As noted above, gonorrhea cultures should be obtained even when the clinical diagnosis is NGU and even when adequate therapy for gonorrhea is prescribed. Figure 8–13 illustrates the general approach to the patient with suspected urethritis.

> Eight weeks pass before Don returns to the clinic saying, "Can't we get rid of this damned thing once and for all?"
>
> Dysuria and discharge had resolved before he completed the 2 weeks' tetracycline therapy, and Don remained asymptomatic for the next 5 weeks. For the past week, however, Don has again noted dysuria but has not seen any discharge. Don has been sexually active only with Connie for the past 2 months. Connie is apparently asymptomatic.
>
> Examination is normal. No discharge can be stripped from the urethra, but a swab of the anterior urethra reveals numerous polymorphonuclear leukocytes per high-power field, without microorganisms. Gonococcal cultures are obtained, and additional urethral swabs are also examined by adding a few drops of saline to one swab (wet mount) and a drop of KOH to another (KOH "prep") and examining these slides for trichomonads and candidae respectively (see Chapter 7, "Vulvovaginal Disorders"). No such organisms are observed. Subsequent gonococcal cultures are negative again.

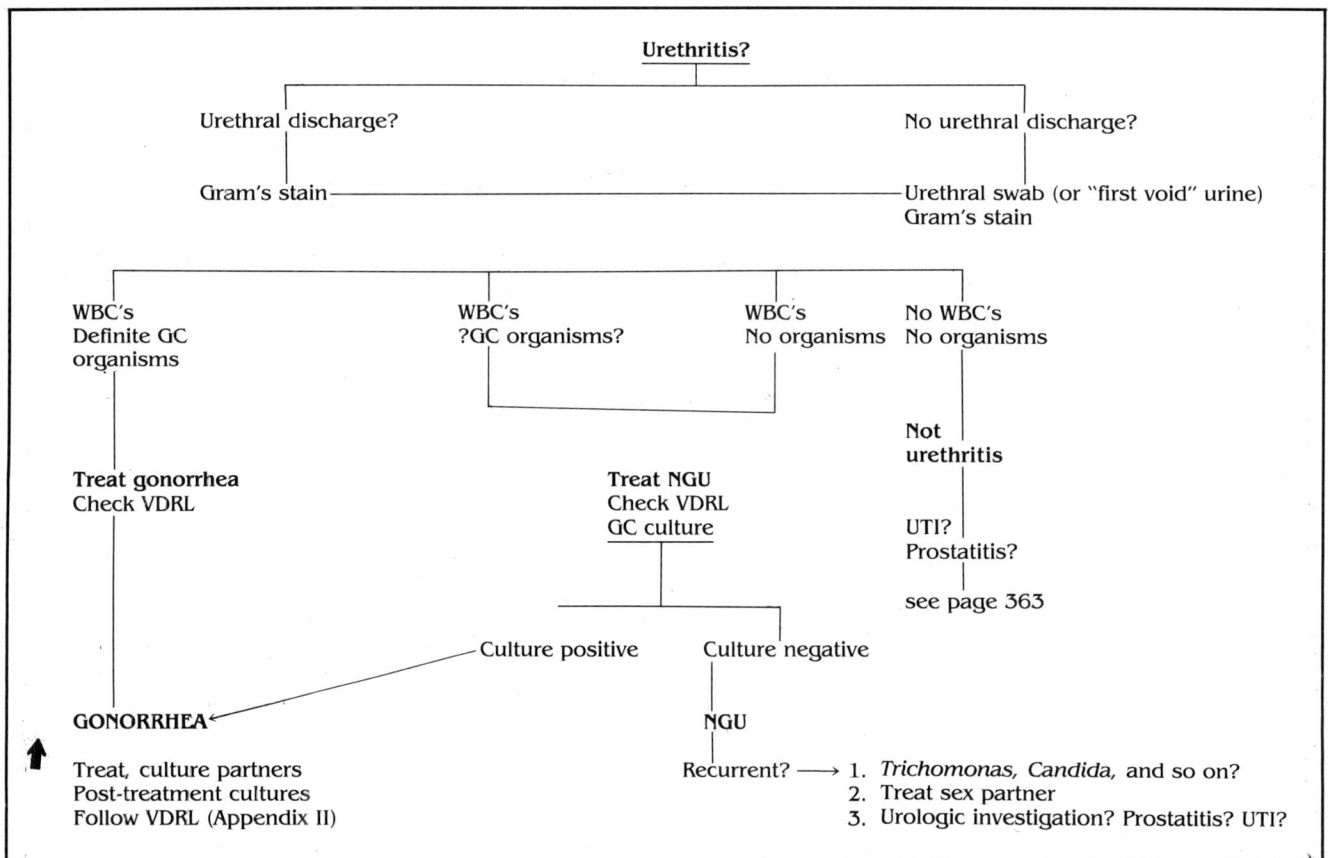

FIGURE 8–13. The approach to suspected urethritis.

Recurrent Nongonococcal Urethritis

As noted above, recurrent nongonococcal urethritis is not rare. This is probably most often the result of venereal reinfection, rather than relapse of the original infection.

In Don's case,

NOTE

1. While there is no urethral discharge, urethritis is likely, given the presence of symptoms and inflammatory cells noted on urethral swab examination. (Various criteria have been advocated to define urethritis even in the absence of symptoms—for example, quantitative pyuria[59]: greater than 4 white blood cells per high-power field on urethral Gram's stain.[16]) When urethral polymorphonuclear leukocytes are not found, other causes of urinary symptoms must be sought—urinary tract infection or prostatitis (see Figures 8–13 and 8–14). Urine cultures will be helpful here (see page 363).

2. Recurrent urethritis is one situation in which trichomonads or candidae should be sought. *Candida* infection in the male is usually accompanied by balanoposthitis (Table 8–3) and is more common in the uncircumcised male. Often there is visible erythema and inflammation of the penile head—a KOH preparation performed on a scraping will reveal fungal hyphae, and brief treatment with topical antifungal agents (Table 8–3) will be curative.

Trichomonas urethritis is uncommon, but it may be present even though examination of the external genitalia is normal. Metronidazole is the treatment of choice for *Trichomonas* infection (see Chapter 7, "Vulvovaginal Disorders").

(If candidiasis or *Trichomonas* had been found, Connie would, of course, have to be examined and treated as well.)

3. While it is difficult to prove, Connie should be suspected as the source of Don's recurrent urethritis. Don and Connie should both be treated with tetracycline, perhaps for 3 weeks. (Again, optimal duration of therapy is unknown and has not been studied in recurrent urethritis.) Cultures for chlamydiae should be considered when symptoms persist in spite of treatment.

4. When recurrent urethritis persists in spite of repeated therapy, a few other possibilities should be remembered. Traumatic urethritis may occur in patients who repeatedly milk the urethra (especially when overly concerned about recurrence of prior urethritis, to "see if it's cured"), those who engage in unusual sexual practices (flagellation, use of foreign bodies, for example), or who have recently undergone urethral instrumentation.

A urethral diverticulum is an outpouching of the anterior or posterior urethra that may cause a variety of syndromes—urinary infection, prostatitis, incontinence, dribbling, obstruction—and is usually diagnosed by simple palpation. Compression of the bulging mass along the course of the urethra usually expels urine retained in the diverticulum. Most diverticula need not be repaired, but urologic consultation is indicated in the setting of recurrent urethritis.

Periurethral abscess is a rare condition, usually following acute gonococcal urethritis, in which a painful, fluctuant swelling along the course of the urethra may be palpated.

Urethral strictures are not uncommon but usually do not produce any palpable abnormality. These are usually discovered when a catheter cannot be passed into the bladder or when obstructive symptoms develop. Causes include trauma (stricture developing in months), infection (stricture following gonorrhea only after many years, if at all), and various congenital types.

Reiter's syndrome should be remembered when recurrent urethritis is puzzling, especially when other systemic symptoms coexist (rash, arthritis, fever).

It is always important to remember that either prostatitis (page 366) or epididymitis (Fig. 8–7) may be the underlying cause of recurrent urethritis.

> Don is given two prescriptions, one for himself and one for Connie, each for tetracycline 500 mg qid for 21 days. Don is told that Connie should not take this if there is any chance of pregnancy. Don is told that, as long as both he and Connie are treated simultaneously, there need be no avoidance of sexual intercourse, but that he should abstain from sex with other women, at least until completely treated.

Proscription of sexual intercourse is probably unnecessary when both partners are treated; at least a condom is advisable when treatment is not simultaneous.

> Don is not heard from again until 6 months later. He enters the clinic and explains "I need more of that tetracycline—I've got it again." Don says he had done well following his last treatment, noting only occasional mild dysuria from time to time, but had been asymptomatic until 3 days ago when he noted the onset of urinary urgency, dysuria, vague suprapubic discomfort, and urinary frequency. He has noted no discharge, fever, or back pain. He has been sexually active with several different women, none of whom he suspects of venereal disease or infection, but "who knows?"
>
> Examination is entirely normal. Don is afebrile. There is no flank, prostate, or scrotal tenderness, and no discharge can be stripped from the urethra. A swab of the urethra reveals no cells or microorganisms on Gram's stain.
>
> Urinalysis reveals more than 50 white blood cells per high-power field and many visible bacilli.
>
> Don denies any urethral instrumentation. He repeats that he has never had bladder or kidney infections, even in childhood.

Several facts deserve emphasis here:

1. Don's symptoms now are not so suggestive of urethritis. Urinary symptoms in the male may be highly nonspecific. Dysuria, for example, may be the initial symptom in infections of the urethra, bladder, prostate, kidney, or epididymis. Nevertheless, most men with uncomplicated urethritis (with or without discharge) do not complain of urinary frequency, urgency, or suprapubic discomfort—these symptoms are much more common in bladder, kidney, and prostate infections.

2. Despite the prior history of urethritis, there is no evidence of urethritis now. The absence of both urethral discharge and urethral inflammation (on Gram's stain) is a compelling reason to investigate other possibilities. (Urethral cultures for gonorrhea might be obtained anyway, given the not-so-rare incidence of asymptomatic gonorrhea in the promiscuous male.)

3. There is no fever, evidence of systemic illness, or visible/palpable genitourinary abnormality.

4. A bacterial urinary infection is likely. The symptoms and urinalysis strongly support this hypothesis.

Figure 8–14 summarizes the general approach to urinary symptoms in the male.

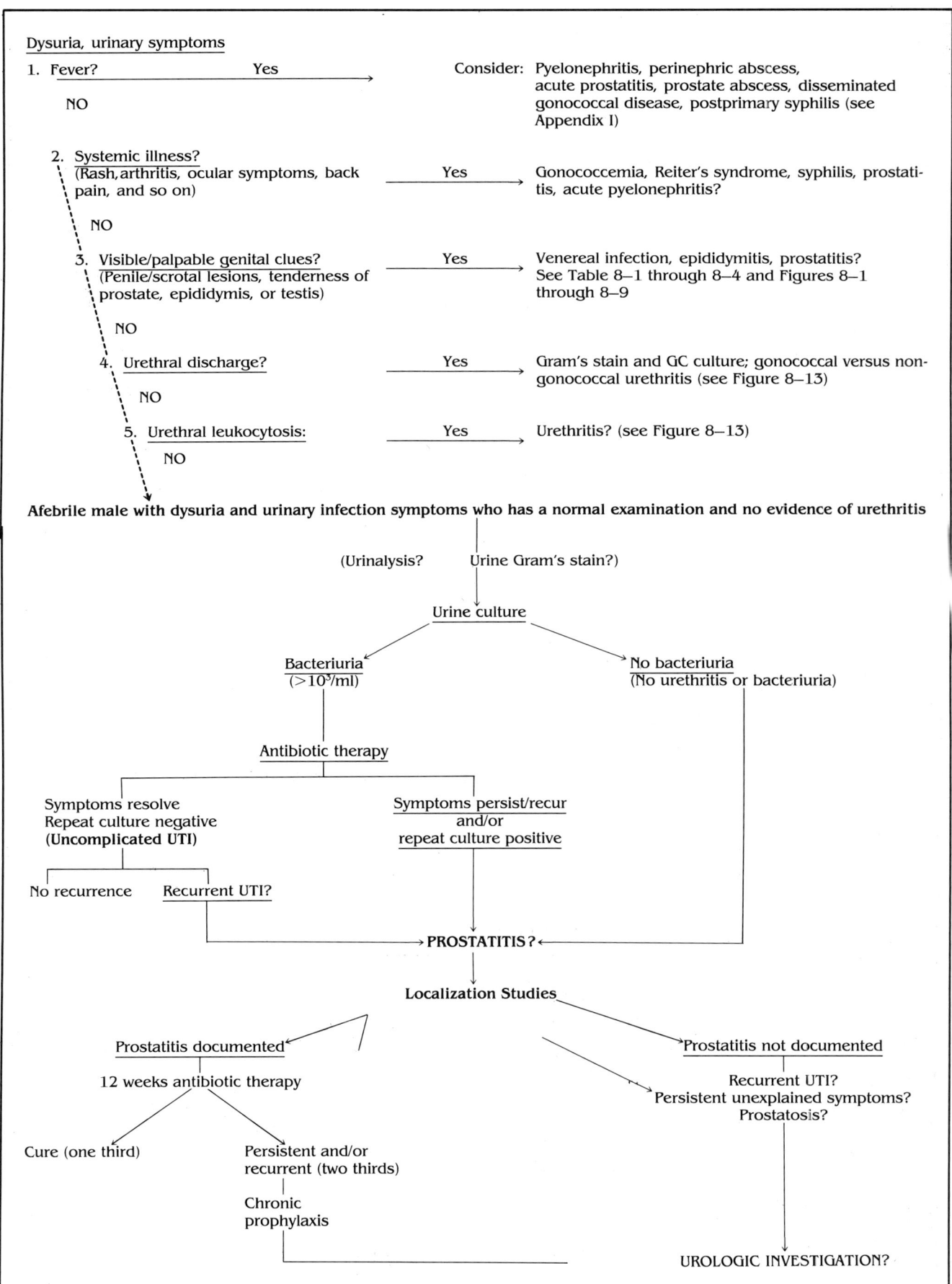

Dysuria, urinary symptoms

1. Fever?   Yes   →   Consider: Pyelonephritis, perinephric abscess, acute prostatitis, prostate abscess, disseminated gonococcal disease, postprimary syphilis (see Appendix I)

NO

2. Systemic illness?
(Rash, arthritis, ocular symptoms, back pain, and so on)   Yes   →   Gonococcemia, Reiter's syndrome, syphilis, prostatitis, acute pyelonephritis?

NO

3. Visible/palpable genital clues?
(Penile/scrotal lesions, tenderness of prostate, epididymis, or testis)   Yes   →   Venereal infection, epididymitis, prostatitis? See Table 8–1 through 8–4 and Figures 8–1 through 8–9

NO

4. Urethral discharge?   Yes   →   Gram's stain and GC culture; gonococcal versus nongonococcal urethritis (see Figure 8–13)

NO

5. Urethral leukocytosis: Yes   →   Urethritis? (see Figure 8–13)

NO

Afebrile male with dysuria and urinary infection symptoms who has a normal examination and no evidence of urethritis

(Urinalysis?   Urine Gram's stain?)

Urine culture

Bacteriuria ($>10^5$/ml)   No bacteriuria (No urethritis or bacteriuria)

Antibiotic therapy

Symptoms resolve
Repeat culture negative
(Uncomplicated UTI)

Symptoms persist/recur
and/or
repeat culture positive

No recurrence   Recurrent UTI?

→ **PROSTATITIS?** ←

Localization Studies

Prostatitis documented   Prostatitis not documented

12 weeks antibiotic therapy   Recurrent UTI?
Persistent unexplained symptoms?
Prostatosis?

Cure (one third)   Persistent and/or recurrent (two thirds)

Chronic prophylaxis

UROLOGIC INVESTIGATION?

FIGURE 8–14. Male urinary tract infections.

BACTERIAL URINARY INFECTIONS

It is widely believed that bacterial infection of the bladder or kidney is uncommon in the adult male, and, when documented, is sufficient reason to initiate urologic investigations to identify (and, it is hoped, reverse) the underlying cause of infection. While this is certainly true of infants, adolescent boys, and adult men with documented recurrent urinary infections, we know surprisingly little about single episodes of acute urinary infection in the healthy adult male. Most studies of male urinary infection deal with middle-aged or older men who experience recurrent or refractory infection and have a high incidence of underlying structural and functional genitourinary disease.[63-65] Whether these studies apply to all men with single episodes of urinary infection is unknown.

Most urologists, however, do advocate the notion that urinary tract infection in the male is abnormal and should suggest "complicated" infection: prostatitis most often, but bacteriuria superimposed on underlying urorenal disease as well. Urinary infection in the male often thus leads to various urologic investigations: in most cases, cystoscopy and intravenous pyelography.

Many men who consult urologists about urinary infection, however, comprise a selected population: usually, those who have recurrent infections or who do not improve with initial antibiotic therapy (see page 365). Should all men with a documented urinary infection consult a urologist? Probably not. Several facts are pertinent here:

1. Certainly not all men with urinary tract infections have structural or functional urorenal disease. The yield of routine urologic investigation of all males after one urinary tract infection is unknown. Even in studies of older men with recurrent infection, however, a substantial minority have a normal urologic work-up.[63-65]

2. Some men with urinary tract infection treated with a short course of appropriate antibiotics will be cured,[63-65] i.e., symptoms resolve and long-term follow-up demonstrates no recurrence of bacteriuria (symptomatic or not). (This outcome is especially common after treatment of infections that result from urinary instrumentation. Cystoscopy or bladder catheterization, performed for other reasons, is probably the single most common cause of male UTI.)

Spontaneous urinary infection in a male with recent symptoms, no prior history of urinary infections, and normal renal function (serum creatinine and normal IVP) often is cured with a brief course of antibiotics, when infection is due to *Escherichia coli* (the most common organism).[63]

3. Many urologists believe that urinary infection in the male is commonly associated with (sometimes "silent") prostatitis. This is clearly the case in men with recurrent urinary infections and is usually the explanation for recurrent UTI when extensive urologic investigation is otherwise unrevealing. However, the prevalence of prostatitis among males with a single episode of urinary infection is unknown. Thus, the treatment of an isolated urinary infection in the male need not necessarily be identical to treatment of prostatitis (see below), but the possibility of prostatitis should always be remembered in this setting.

What, then, should be done now?

A clean-catch urine specimen is obtained for culture (and a urethral swab is cultured for gonococci). Don is begun on a course of ampicillin 250 mg qid for 7 days.

Two days later Don is asymptomatic. Urine culture grows 10,000 *E. coli* sensitive to ampicillin, while the gonococcal culture is negative. Serum creatinine is normal, as is the IVP (there is no postvoiding residual urine or radiographic evidence of prostate abnormality).

Don is told to complete his course of ampicillin and to return 3 to 4 days after antibiotic therapy is finished to provide a urine specimen for follow-up cultures.

NOTE

1. Don has a bacterial UTI, but the site of infection (bladder, kidney, or prostate) is undetermined. A "positive" urine culture in the male is not defined by the traditional criterion of growth of greater than or equal to 10^5 bacteria per ml (nor is it so in the female—see Chapter 6, "Female Urinary Tract Infections"). A carefully obtained clean-catch urine specimen that grows greater than or equal to 10^3 bacteria per ml should be considered documentation of infection (especially if confirmed with a repeat culture, whenever this is practical).

Localizing the site of infection is sometimes of therapeutic importance, but such localization studies are not reliable when the routine urine culture is positive (see page 367).

2. It makes sense here to treat the urinary infection with a brief course of antibiotics and then to reassess the situation. Even if prostatitis or some underlying urologic disorder is responsible for the current infection, antibiotics will be needed. Unless "serious UTI" is suspected clinically (see Appendix I), initial antibiotic choices may be somewhat arbitrary (see Table 6–6) since most (isolated, nonrecurrent) urinary infections in males are due to *E. coli* (occasionally *Enterococcus, Staphylococcus saprophyticus*, and various gram-negative bacteria). Such infections usually respond symptomatically and bacteriologically to broad-spectrum antibiotics, at least temporarily.

Since at least some male urinary infections reflect prostatic infection, the ability of certain antibiotics to penetrate the prostate should be noted when initially treating male urinary infections. Trimethoprim, trimethoprim-sulfamethoxazole, and tetracycline are often the initial antibiotics of choice for male urinary infections, since these drugs are favored in the treatment of documented bacterial prostatitis (see page 371).

Failure to improve symptomatically, persistence of infection bacteriologically, and recurrence of symptomatic infection are the hallmarks of "complicated" infection (Fig. 8–15), and thus initial antibiotic therapy is as much a diagnostic test as it is therapeutic intervention. When complicated infection is thus suspected, further investigation is always needed.

3. Intravenous pyelography and serum creatinine determination are helpful studies in males with urinary infections because the absence of renal failure or obvious obstructive disease (hydronephrosis, calculi, postvoiding bladder residual, or prostatic obstruction) is reassuring about the importance of bacteriuria per se. As in the female (see Chapter 6, "Female Urinary Tract Infections"), bacteriuria per se is a significant health hazard primarily when underlying (especially obstructive) urorenal disease is present (or, of course, if the patient is very ill with serious UTI—see Appendix I). In other words, "it is far better to have a well-drained tract in the presence of infection

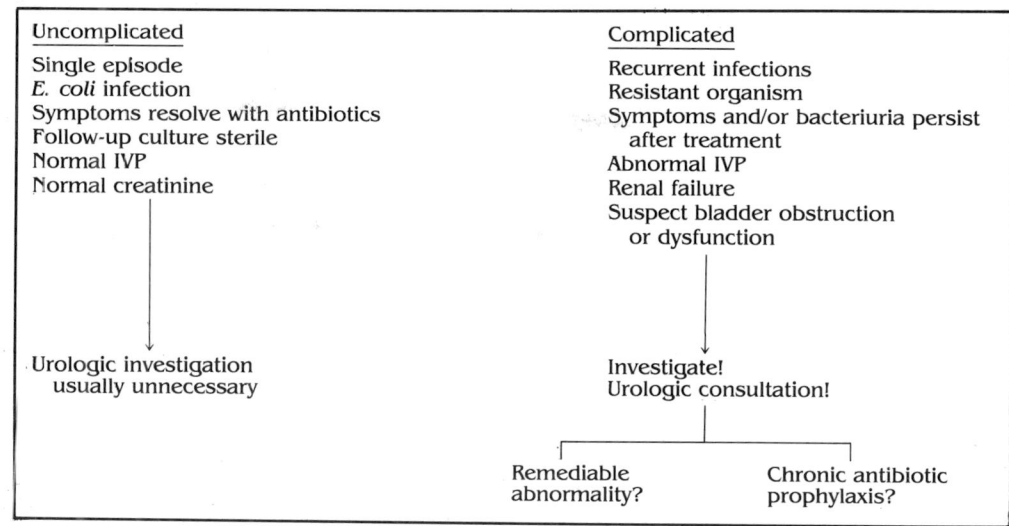

FIGURE 8–15. Male UTI: Complicated or uncomplicated?

than an obstructed system with sterile urine."[66] (Whether an intravenous pyelogram (IVP) and serum creatinine determination are necessary in all males with their first urinary infection is unknown. A cost-benefit clinical study addressing this issue should be performed.)

The urologist certainly should be consulted when infection persists or is refractory to therapy (see below), when bladder dysfunction (e.g., neurogenic bladder) or obstruction (e.g., prostatic hypertrophy) is suspected, and when the IVP reveals abnormalities that either themselves require treatment (hydronephrosis, for example) or that may predispose to refractory infection (e.g., calculi, diverticula)—see also Table 8–10.

4. Follow-up urine cultures should be obtained in all men treated for urinary infection. Failure to achieve bacteriologic cure is a helpful diagnostic marker for complicated infection. We do not know how often recurrent (symptomatic or asymptomatic) bacteriuria in men represents repeated reinfection (as in most women) versus relapse of a refractory (temporarily suppressible) focus of infection. Nevertheless, the latter is probably much more common in males than in females—prostatitis is the usual culprit—and this has diagnostic and therapeutic implications (see below).

Don does not return for post-treatment urine cultures.

Six weeks later, Don calls to say that his symptoms have returned. He had remained completely asymptomatic after treatment until 1 week ago, when he again noted mild dysuria and urinary frequency, which have persisted. He denies fever, back, flank, or perineal pain, and there is no urethral discharge.

Examination at this time is normal, except for equivocal tenderness of the prostate, which is otherwise normal in contour and consistency.

Urinalysis reveals more than 20 white blood cells per high-power field with visible bacilli. Subsequent urine culture grows greater than 10^5 E. coli with similar antibiotic sensitivities as previously.

RECURRENT URINARY INFECTIONS

Virtually all cases of recurrent urinary infection in males will fall into one or more of four categories:

I. Iatrogenic infections occur after repeated urologic instrumentation—periodic cystoscopy for bladder tumor checks, for example—or when an indwelling catheter is present.

In the former situation, prophylactic antibiotics immediately following instrumentation will usually prevent symptomatic infection, while in the latter situation, bacteriuria is usually impossible to prevent or eradicate as long as the catheter remains. (Removal of the catheter is always desirable but is not always possible. Treatment of the patient undergoing long-term catheterization is usually reserved for symptomatic infection with fever and toxicity.)

II. Urologic dysfunction.

As noted above, a normal IVP does not exclude all urologic dysfunctions that may result in recurrent or refractory urinary tract infection. Cystoscopy, voiding cystourethrography, and urodynamic testing (for example, cystometrography) are important when underlying bladder/urethral dysfunction is suspected. Obstructive symptoms—urinary hesitancy, dribbling, incontinence, frequent nocturia, or urinary retention—usually suggest the need for such studies.

III. Upper tract bacteriuria.

As in some women, urinary infections in men may be localized to the upper urinary system (ureter, kidney) in the absence of known anatomic or functional upper tract urorenal abnormality (stones or hydronephrosis, for example). Such upper tract bacteriuria—this entity has not been as carefully studied in men as in women—is very different from acute pyelonephritis (see Appendix I and Chapter 6, "Female Urinary Tract Infections"), but symptoms, when present at all, are not distinctive: dysuria, urinary urgency, and frequency without fever are typical and are often indistinguishable from symptoms of bladder or prostate infection. Like prostate infection (see below) upper tract bacteriuria is often refractory to short courses (10 days) of antibiotic therapy.[64] Prolonged antibiotic therapy (12 weeks) is often necessary when upper tract infection is present. Unfortunately the test that often distinguishes upper tract from lower tract infection in women (the antibody-coated bacteria [ACB] test) does not distinguish upper tract bacteriuria from prostatitis in men (it is positive in both). From a practical viewpoint, this is not a great problem since the patient with (proven or suspected) chronic prostatitis should also be treated with prolonged antibiotic regimens (see page 371). Thus, a positive ACB test in the male with recurrent UTI usually implies the need for prolonged initial therapy.

Prostatitis*

In the male without demonstrable urologic dysfunction whose UTI is not related to urologic instrumentation, upper tract bacteriuria is probably much less common than:

IV. Chronic prostatitis.

Chronic prostatitis may present in one of three ways:

A. When asymptomatic bacteriuria is detected, for whatever reason.
B. When recurrent symptomatic urinary infections occur.

Symptoms are nonspecific—urinary frequency, hesitancy, and

*Acute prostatitis is briefly discussed in Appendix I.

dysuria are common, but "terminal dysuria" (discomfort only at the end of urination) is sometimes a clue.

C. Even in the absence of clear-cut urinary tract infection (by urine culture criteria), when (often vague) genitourinary symptoms occur/recur: intermittent dysuria; perineal, back, or suprapubic pain; testicular pain; urinary frequency.[67]

Chronic bacterial prostatitis is usually an indolent infectious process, often localized in the "peripheral zone" of the prostate tissue,[68] and most frequently caused by gram-negative aerobic bacilli (usually *E. coli*) or enterococci.[69, 70] Mixed infections are not rare, but the role of other (especially gram-positive) bacteria[71] (*Staphylococcus aureus, Staph. epidermidis,* streptococci, diphtheroids) is controversial.[72]

Unfortunately, chronic bacterial prostatitis is difficult to diagnose and even more difficult to treat (see page 371). In fact, chronic bacterial prostatitis has even been difficult to define because the history, physical examination, microscopic analysis of prostate secretions, cystoscopy, and even biopsy and culture of prostate tissue itself may not clearly separate chronic bacterial prostatitis from nonbacterial prostatitis, sometimes called prostatosis.[69] Since prostatosis is probably as common a problem as chronic bacterial prostatitis but does not respond to antibiotic therapy (see below), the diagnostic dilemma is a real one. Microbial localization studies[69] will often help.

Localization Studies. (Fig. 8–16)

Bacterial localization studies, originally described by Meares and Stamey,[70] involve sterile procurement for culture of samples of urethral urine, bladder urine, prostate secretions, and residual ("prostate") urine with subsequent comparison of quantitative culture results from each site (urethra, bladder, and prostate). The study involves several steps:

1. After carefully cleansing the glans penis and retracting the foreskin, the patient voids and collects the first 10 to 15 ml of urine in a sterile container—this is labeled VB_1 (urethral urine).

2. After the patient has voided another (perhaps) 150 cc of urine into

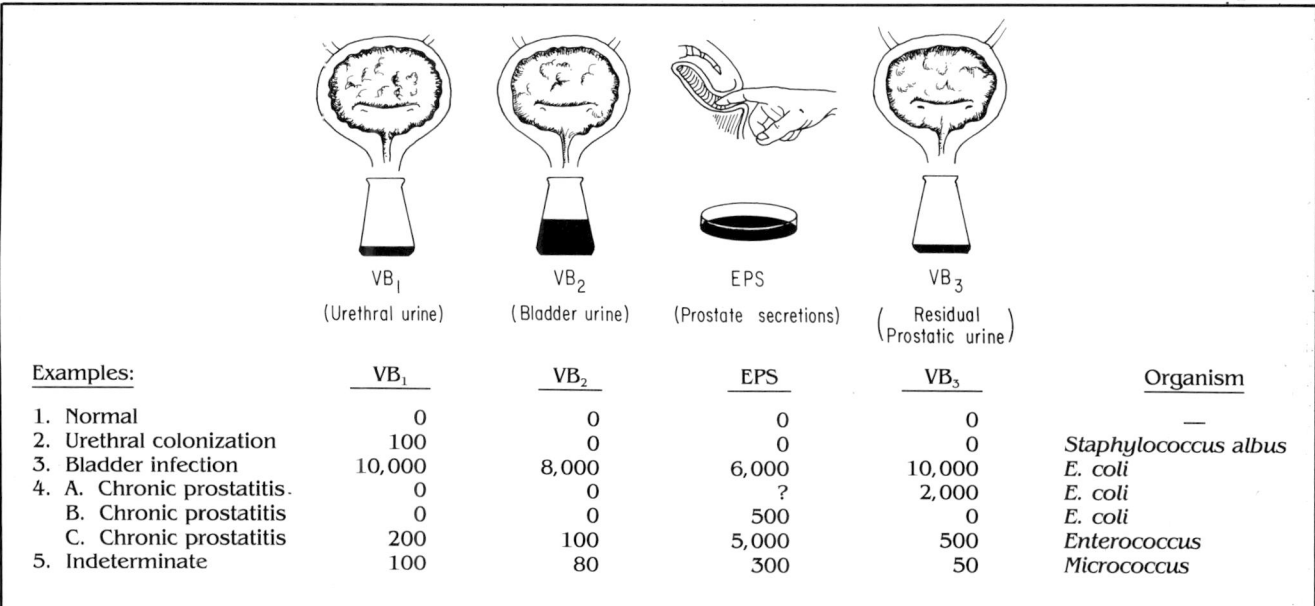

Examples:	VB_1	VB_2	EPS	VB_3	Organism
1. Normal	0	0	0	0	—
2. Urethral colonization	100	0	0	0	*Staphylococcus albus*
3. Bladder infection	10,000	8,000	6,000	10,000	*E. coli*
4. A. Chronic prostatitis.	0	0	?	2,000	*E. coli*
B. Chronic prostatitis	0	0	500	0	*E. coli*
C. Chronic prostatitis	200	100	5,000	500	*Enterococcus*
5. Indeterminate	100	80	300	50	*Micrococcus*

FIGURE 8–16. Localization studies: examples.

the toilet, collect another 10 to 15 cc of midstream urine in a sterile container labeled $\underline{VB_2}$ (bladder urine). Then instruct the patient to stop urinating when the bladder feels empty but not to void the last few drops.

3. The patient then bends forward, holding the penis in one hand and a sterile container in the other, directly beneath the urethral meatus. The physician then massages the prostate gland—side to side and then rostrocaudally. The few drops of prostate secretions that emit from the urethra are then collected and labeled $\underline{EPS}$ (expressed prostatic secretions).

4. The patient then voids again (any residual urine) into a sterile container labeled $\underline{VB_3}$ (prostatic urine).

These four specimens (there may be only three if EPS cannot be obtained) are inoculated immediately onto culture media.

Figure 8–16 shows a few typical examples of the results of such studies. Several points deserve emphasis here:

1. A normal study consists of all specimens being sterile (example 1) or small quantities of (probably) nonpathogenic organisms colonizing the urethra alone (example 2). Example 2 emphasizes the need for strict aseptic technique in collection of specimens to avoid urethral urine contamination.

2. Localization tests are invalid if bladder urine is infected (example 3). Bladder infection may be but is not always the result of prostatitis, and no conclusions can be drawn about localization of infection unless bladder urine (VB_2) is sterile or nearly so (Example 4C).

3. Prostatic infection is suggested when VB_1 and VB_2 are sterile but EPS or VB_3 is infected with organisms known to produce prostatitis (examples 4A and 4B). Sometimes, more than 10^3 organisms will be grown, but even a few hundred colonies in EPS may be significant if other specimens are sterile. As such, the microbiology laboratory must be alerted that precise quantitation is desired, since such low colony counts are often disregarded by the laboratory in routine urine cultures.

4. The EPS specimen is very important, since the number of bacteria within the prostatic secretions may be very small (example 4B) or their collection only in the residual urine specimen (VB_3) may dilute the bacterial count so greatly that significant infection may be disregarded (or the study may appear "indeterminate"). Note example 4C in which the EPS specimen is very helpful.

5. Sometimes the study will be nondiagnostic (example 5), either because the different specimens are not quantitatively distinguishable or because the cultured organism is of uncertain significance. (Most studies suggest that gram-negative bacilli or enterococci are almost exclusively the pathogens in prostatitis, but the etiologic role of "nonpathogenic" gram-positive organisms has been tellingly argued as well.[71])

The value of taking the trouble to specifically diagnose or exclude chronic bacterial prostatitis thus derives from several considerations:

1. When bacterial prostatitis is documented, this is itself a sufficient explanation for recurrent symptomatic urinary infection, and often sophisticated urologic testing can at least be postponed while antibiotic therapy is attempted. When bacterial prostatitis cannot be documented, full urologic investigation is necessary in the male with recurrent urinary infection.

2. When bacterial prostatitis is known to be the problem, antibiotics may be curative in a substantial minority (about one third).[72] Other specific therapies may be helpful when standard antibiotic therapy fails[74-77] (see page 371).

3. Chronic bacterial prostatitis is still a consideration in the male with urinary symptoms who does not have a documented urinary infection on routine urine culture. Familiarity with the diagnostic techniques (localization studies), then, is important when vague urinary symptoms (but negative urine cultures) suggest occult prostatitis or prostatosis.

4. Prostatosis[69, 73] is important because it is so common and because treatment is quite different from that of prostatitis (Table 8-8). Practicing urologists who take the trouble to carefully distinguish prostatitis from prostatosis by means of localization studies note that the two entities are equally common. Patients with prostatosis usually complain of vague back and perineal discomfort, perhaps mild dysuria, urgency, or urinary frequency, but definite bacteriologic evidence of infection (past or present) is always lacking. Rectal examination may reveal a mildly tender prostate gland, but the prostate is usually normal to palpation (as it is in many cases of chronic infectious prostatitis). Expressed prostatic secretions may indicate inflammation (greater than 10 white blood cells per high-power field), but cultures for bacteria, mycoplasmas, viruses, and gonorrhea are negative (by definition).

Urologic investigation of such patients is always indicated, since the symptoms are so nonspecific and other urologic problems may present similarly.

The treatment of prostatosis is even more difficult than treatment of prostatitis (see page 371). Occasional patients may respond to several weeks of tetracycline therapy (is chlamydial prostatitis a subset of prostatosis?),* but antibiotics usually do not help at all.

Periodic prostatic massage may result in symptomatic improvement of prostatosis, suggesting that prostatic congestion is somehow a factor in pathogenesis; regular sexual activity may achieve the same benefit as massage, but this recommendation has an obvious placebo effect (often occasioning the smirking rejoinder: "Can I have a prescription for that, Doc?"). Other treatment suggestions include anticholinergic drugs, elimination of caffeine and alcohol, avoidance of prostatic trauma (horseback riding, bicycles), and frequent voiding.

Nevertheless, many of these regimens often are ineffective, and some

---

Ureaplasma prostatitis, responsive to tetracycline treatment, has also been described.[115]

TABLE 8–8. PROSTATOSIS

SYMPTOMS	DIAGNOSIS	TREATMENT
Vague, recurrent urinary problems Perineal discomfort Dysuria	Palpation: prostate usually normal or mildly tender Cultures: urine, semen, urethra normal Prostatic secretions: >10 WBC/high-power field (inflammation) or normal Urologic investigation normal	Tetracycline (chlamydial infection?)* Anticholinergic drugs Elimination of caffeine, alcohol Avoidance of prostatic trauma Prostatic massage

Ureaplasma prostatitis, responsive to tetracycline treatment, has also been described.[115]

patients with prostatosis become baleful "doctor-shoppers," looking for cure, finding only frustation (and sometimes psychiatric consultation). Transurethral resection of the prostate is occasionally reported to be helpful in prostatosis, but surgery should be considered only as a last resort.

<u>What then should be done for Don?</u> There are three options:

1. <u>Defer further diagnostic study and begin empiric therapy with antibiotics known to be effective against both prostatic and nonprostatic urinary infection.</u> When there is no other reason to suspect underlying urologic disease that would require urologic consultation, this is often a reasonable initial approach. Many antibiotics have been found effective (to greater and lesser degrees) in both prostatitis and urinary infection. For various reasons, trimethoprim-sulfamethaxozole (160 mg/800 mg bid) is the initial drug of choice (see below). While prolonged treatment (12 weeks) is most successful, one or two shorter (2 to 6 weeks) courses may be attempted first. <u>If this approach is chosen, follow-up bacteriologic studies are essential.</u>

2. <u>Refer Don to a urologist.</u> This is a common and reasonable decision, especially when the generalist physician is not comfortable with this type of problem. Actually, many urologists are not expert in (or advocates of) the bacterial localization studies that attempt to establish a specific diagnosis. Very often the urologist in this situation will perform cystoscopy, intravenous pyelography, and perhaps urodynamic studies—in all of which the results are frequently normal—and will then prescribe antibiotics anyway.

<u>This option is clearly preferred when other indications for urologic investigation are present:</u> prostate enlargement in the elderly male; obstructive symptoms (such as hesitancy, dribbling, overflow incontinence); or other medical problems that are associated with neurogenic bladder dysfunction (diabetes, neurologic disease, after perineal or spinal surgery, for example).

3. <u>Perform bacterial localization studies to document or exclude chronic bacterial prostatitis.</u> If chronic bacterial prostatitis is documented, specific antibiotic treatment can then be initiated (see below). If this diagnosis cannot be made in the patient with recurrent urinary infections, urologic investigation is warranted to rule out other structural causes of recurrent urinary infection.

> Don is given a 4-day prescription for ampicillin 250 mg qid. On the fourth day of treatment, he is brought back for bacterial localization studies, and further antibiotics are withheld, pending culture results, since Don is now asymptomatic.
>
> Forty-eight hours later, specimens VB_1 and VB_2 are sterile, while VB_3 grows 1000 *E. coli* sensitive to many different antibiotics. An EPS specimen result is not available since it could not be obtained during prostate massage.
>
> Don is told that his infection is in his prostate gland and that prolonged treatment is needed. Trimethoprim-sulfamethoxazole bid is prescribed for the next 12 weeks.
>
> A urine culture is sterile 10 days after the beginning of treatment with trimethoprim-sulfamethoxazole, and Don is asymptomatic. He agrees to continue antibiotics for 3 months.

NOTE

1. <u>Bladder urine must be sterilized before localization studies are attempted.</u> A few days' treatment with an antibiotic that is effective against

the etiologic organism, but that does not penetrate the prostate gland (see below), will usually render bladder urine temporarily sterile even when the prostate remains infected. Localization studies can then be performed.

2. Prostatitis is documented.* Heavy *E. coli* growth in specimen VB_3 with sterile VB_1 and VB_2 specimens is diagnostic, even when an EPS specimen cannot be obtained.

Semen cultures[78] (with simultaneous cultures of clean-catch urine) may also be useful in the diagnosis of prostatitis.

3. Urologic consultation can be deferred, since chronic bacterial prostatitis is well documented and since there are no other reasons to suspect complicating urologic conditions.

Treatment of Chronic Bacterial Prostatitis. Antibiotic therapy is the mainstay of treatment for chronic bacterial prostatitis. It is possible to eradicate the prostatic focus of infection permanently in only a minority of patients, but it is usually possible to sterilize the urine and thereby at least to suppress symptoms. The reasons for this paradox include:

1. The relation between asymptomatic chronic bacterial prostatitis and the development of urinary symptoms is poorly understood. The usual scenario probably involves acquisition of initially asymptomatic prostatic infection (by unknown means—it may be related to sexual activity in some), with subsequent development of dysuria and other urinary symptoms when infection "spreads" to the bladder or urethral urine. Symptomatic improvement after antibiotic sterilization of the urine is then common, but recurrent symptomatic episodes then follow because a persistent infection within the prostate gland itself has not been eradicated.

2. The ideal antibiotic for prostatic infection has not yet been found.[79, 80] Trimethoprim-sulfamethoxazole is theoretically the most desirable available drug, but even prolonged courses (12 weeks or more) of treatment result in bacteriologic cure of prostatitis in at most one third of patients.[81, 82] Occasionally other antibiotics may succeed[74, 83–85] (see Table 8–9—the tetracyclines are probably the best alternative drug).

3. The desirability of permanently eradicating the prostate infection can be argued from many different angles. The risk of recurrent symptomatic cystitis, acute pyelonephritis, epididymitis, acute prostatitis, prostatic abscess, or even bacteremia and osteomyelitis[86] in patients with intractable prostatitis is small but real.

While the theoretic importance of eradicating asymptomatic bacterial prostatitis cannot be disputed, the fact is that, practically, this is often impossible.

---

*Remember that acute prostatitis—see Appendix I—is usually obvious on physical examination; localization studies are useful primarily in the patient with subacute or chronic prostatitis.

TABLE 8–9. ANTIBIOTIC REGIMENS FOR CHRONIC PROSTATITIS

Trimethoprim-sulfamethoxazole[64, 81–83]: 80 mg/400 mg, 2 tablets bid × 4–12 weeks
Tetracycline hydrochloride: 500 mg qid × 2–6 weeks(?)
Minocycline[83, 84]: 100 mg bid (50 mg qid) × 2–6 weeks(?)
Doxycycline[84]: 100 mg bid × 2–6 weeks(?)
Erythromycin[85]: 500 mg qid × 2 weeks plus sodium bicarbonate 650 mg qid
Aminoglycoside[74]: Parenteral (IM) gentamicin daily for 1 week

The need for prolonged or repetitive courses of antibiotic therapy for chronic bacterial prostatitis underlines the importance of establishing a correct diagnosis. Most studies of prostatitis do not clearly distinguish among acute prostatitis (see Appendix I), chronic bacterial prostatitis, prostatosis (or nonbacterial prostatitis), and "prostatodynia."[73] The few studies that have employed rigorous diagnostic standards have shown that documented chronic bacterial prostatitis can sometimes be cured and almost always controlled (symptomatically) with antibiotic therapy.[81, 82]

> Don remains well for the 3 months of trimethoprim-sulfamethoxazole therapy. A routine urine culture at the conclusion of therapy is sterile.
>
> Four weeks later, urinary urgency, dysuria, and frequency recur, and urine culture reveals 100,000 *E. coli* sensitive to most antibiotics.
>
> Don begins taking ampicillin for 7 days, and a urologic consultation is arranged for 1 week hence.

NOTE

I. Recurrence is the rule, not the exception, in antibiotic-treated chronic bacterial prostatitis.

Often the goal of therapy is simply the prevention of symptoms and of bladder bacteriuria—this usually can be accomplished with long-term daily prophylaxis with low-dose antibiotics (for example, trimethoprim-sulfamethoxazole 40/200 mg qd).[81, 82] Recurrence rates remain high after discontinuance of (even) many months of daily suppressive therapy.

II. A urologist's opinion should be obtained now.

In general (even when prostatitis is well documented), recurrent infection in the male deserves urologic consultation for two reasons (see also Table 8–10):

A. To exclude any other urologic abnormality that might predispose to recurrent infection.

Urethral strictures, diverticula, phimosis, and bladder calculi should be excluded—cystoscopy is helpful here. Careful urodynamic studies—cystometrography, voiding cystourethrography—may be helpful even when intravenous pyelography and cystoscopy are normal, since specific pharmacologic therapy is available for some disorders of bladder control (for example, neurogenic bladder).[87, 88]

B. Sometimes recurrent prostatitis requires surgical intervention.

When the prostate is significantly enlarged or there is evidence of bladder outlet obstruction, prostatectomy may be indicated.[77] Occasionally prostatic calculi may be responsible for recurrent infection, and these must be removed to effect cure (Fig. 8–17).[75, 76]

Generally prostatectomy is reserved for those patients with chronic prostatitis who have evidence of obstructive upper tract

TABLE 8–10. REASONS FOR UROLOGIC CONSULTATION IN MALE GENITOURINARY INFECTIONS

Recurrent unexplained UTI
Suspected bladder dysfunction or obstruction
Documented upper tract abnormalities on IVP—such as calculi, hydronephrosis
To differentiate prostatitis from prostatosis
Suspected perinephric abscess, acute prostatitis, prostatic abscess? (see Appendix I)
Possibility of testicular tumor, torsion, or infection

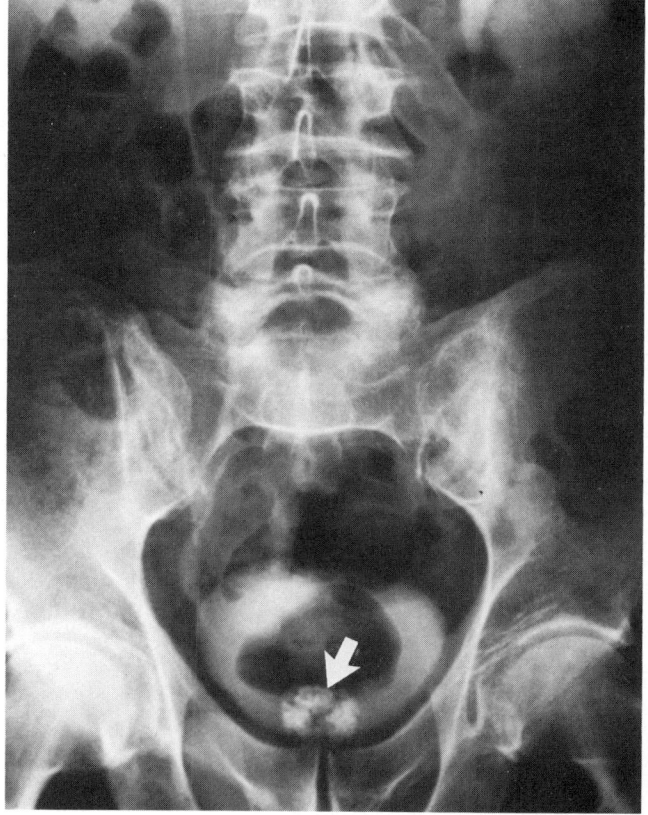

FIGURE 8–17. This 62-year-old man developed recurrent urinary infections, localized to the prostate by microbiologic methods, which failed to respond to multiple courses of antibiotic therapy and chronic prophylaxis. The x-ray demonstrates an extraordinary number of prostatic calculi. Prostatectomy resulted in cure of recurrent infection.

dysfunction (hydronephrosis), disabling lower obstructive symptoms (hesitancy, bladder distention, dribbling, frequent nocturia), or those whose recurrent urinary infections are truly intractable or dangerous (the patient with a prosthetic heart valve who develops bacteremia, for example).

Otherwise, prostatectomy for chronic bacterial prostatitis is a procedure of last resort and is not usually effective anyway.

On examination of the prostate the urologist finds it to be "slightly boggy." Repeat localization studies at this time reveal 1000 *E. coli* in the EPS specimen and VB$_3$ specimen, with sterile cultures of specimens VB$_1$ and VB$_2$.

IVP, cystometrogram, cystoscopy, and voiding cystourethrogram are all normal.

Trimethoprim-sulfamethoxazole 40 mg/200 mg qd is begun and continued for 6 months. Don does well during this time. Recurrent symptoms (and bacteriuria) develop 2 months after discontinuation of antibiotics, and daily trimethoprim-sulfamethoxazole is prescribed indefinitely thereafter.

NOTE

1. Recurrent chronic bacterial prostatitis has been well documented.

2. Urologic evaluation is normal. This is the rule, not the exception, in patients with chronic prostatitis.

3. Long-term prophylaxis is indicated but should be interrupted after varying intervals to assess the need for continued therapy. Permanent resolution after months or years of therapy does sometimes occur. (Recent

reports describing the emergence of antibiotic-resistant enterobacteria in patients treated with long-term trimethoprim-sulfamethoxazole therapy also bear notice.[89])

4. Other antibiotic regimens may occasionally be worth a try when oral regimens are unsuccessful. (Anecdotal reports of occasional success with daily parenteral gentamicin for 7 to 10 days are of interest here.)

Summary

The treatment of recurrent urinary infections in males may be frustrating, whether prostatitis is the culprit or not. Important generalizations include:

1. If possible, localize the infection. Sometimes prostatitis requires a different approach from other UTIs.

2. Search for and, when possible, correct any urologic dysfunction that may predispose the patient to recurrent urinary infections or render urinary infections more dangerous or refractory in that patient.

3. Whatever the site of infection, chronic suppressive antibiotic therapy will limit symptomatic episodes of urinary infection, but recurrence rates are high when antibiotics are stopped. Such suppression is important when (especially irreversible) urologic disease complicates the situation (since chronic infection may contribute to renal failure in this setting).

Some patients will not benefit from long-term antibiotic therapy (especially those with indwelling catheters.).

Inoperable calculous disease of the upper tract, renal failure, longstanding infection, and mixed infections are often associated with a poor response to antibiotic therapy[63] (but often treatment is still worth a try).

4. Most patients can be helped. Therapeutic approaches must be individualized. While the initial goal of therapy is always cure, symptomatic control and prevention of life-threatening infection are often more pragmatic "end points."

Urinary Symptoms and Fever

Fever is always an important finding in the male with symptoms of urinary infection (Figs. 8–14 and 8–18). While low-grade fever may occur (rarely) with uncomplicated cystitis or urethritis, temperature elevation should always suggest the following:

1. Acute pyelonephritis.

Most men with acute pyelonephritis will be obviously sick—febrile with chills, nausea, anorexia, and back or flank pain. Such findings in a male with dysuria or urinary frequency but a normal prostate examination should always suggest acute pyelonephritis.

Documentation of bacteriuria and pyuria on urinalysis will be helpful initially, but urine culture, blood cultures, and radiographic examination of the urinary tract are mandatory. Unlike women (see Chapter 6, "Female Urinary Tract Infections"), the majority of men who develop acute pyelonephritis will have some underlying structural (stones, hydronephrosis) or functional (neurogenic bladder, for example) urinary disorder, and all should be investigated fully. Urinary tract obstruction should be ruled out immediately—intravenous pyelography is usually safe, but ultrasound examination is often adequate to rule out hydronephrosis and is the procedure of choice in patients who are diabetic, dehydrated, or have some other contraindication to the dye used in intravenous pyelography[90] (multiple myeloma, iodine

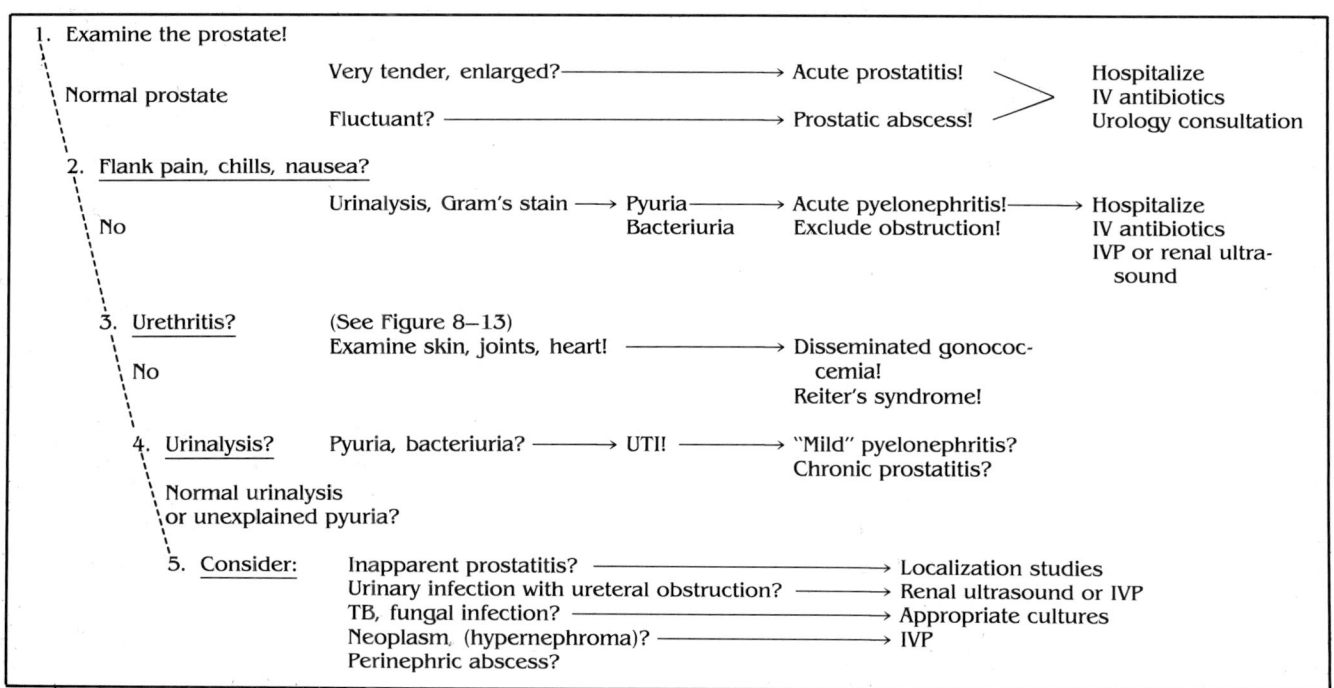

FIGURE 8–18. The male with urinary symptoms and fever.

sensitivity, for example). Obstructive infection will not improve until the obstruction is relieved. In the absence of obstruction, parenteral antibiotics will produce clinical improvement within 48 to 72 hours, and oral antibiotics are usually continued for 2 to 3 weeks thereafter (see also Chapter 6, "Female Urinary Tract Infection").

Perinephric abscess[91] may present with a similar clinical picture, but the diagnosis often requires more sophisticated diagnostic techniques—gallium scanning, CT, or angiography. In the patient with clinical acute pyelonephritis (especially if a diabetic) who does not improve within a few days of appropriate parenteral antibiotic therapy, this entity must be seriously considered.

2. Acute prostatitis.[92, 93] Gentle digital examination of the prostate is crucial in all men with urinary symptoms and fever. Unlike chronic prostatitis, the diagnosis of acute prostatitis is usually obvious. Patients present with fever, chills, dysuria, urinary frequency or hesitancy, usually with severe back or perineal pain, and "jump off the table" when the "boggy and edematous" prostate is palpated. While vigorous and repeated palpation of the prostate is contraindicated—it may precipitate bacteremia—rectal examination usually makes the diagnosis and excludes the (rarer) possibility of a prostatic abscess (see below). Hospitalization is usually necessary.

Fortunately antibiotic therapy is usually highly successful in acute prostatitis, perhaps because the prostate's "epithelial barrier" is rendered more permeable to antibiotics by the extensive inflammation; antibiotics do, therefore, achieve adequate concentrations within the gland (unlike the usual case of chronic prostatitis). Initial antibiotic therapy is usually based on the Gram's stain of urine or prostate secretions. Gram-negative bacilli are most common—aminoglycosides with or without ampicillin are the usual drugs of choice, at least until microbial sensitivities are determined. Gram-positive cocci on Gram's stain should prompt treatment for both enterococci and staphylococci—cephalosporins, vancomycin, or various antibiotic combinations (nafcillin plus ampicillin, for example) will be helpful until culture results are available. Subsequent culture results then allow specific therapy.

Urinary retention is occasionally so severe in the patient with acute prostatitis that (sometimes suprapubic) catheter drainage of the bladder may be necessary during the acute stage. Treatment is usually continued for several weeks with oral antibiotics after defervescence occurs with parenteral administration of antibiotics. Chronic prostatitis, epididymitis, recurrent urinary tract infections, or frank prostatic abscess may ensue, even if treatment is optimal.

3. Prostatic abscess.[94–96]

Prostatic abscess is not always obvious at the initial presentation, but localized swelling and fluctuance of the prostate should always raise this question. The patient with acute prostatitis who responds slowly to antibiotic therapy should undergo daily, gentle prostate palpation if early detection of the "occult" abscess is to be accomplished. Ultrasound examination (or even CT scan) may sometimes point to this diagnosis. Parenteral antibiotic therapy is necessary, but, while spontaneous abscess rupture occasionally occurs, surgical drainage is usually indicated. The urologist should be consulted whenever prostatic abscess is suspected, since these patients are often very sick and require surgical drainage.

4. Disseminated gonococcemia.[51, 97]

This disease is more common in women than in men, but it should always be carefully sought when symptoms and signs of urethritis are associated with fever. There are probably two stages of disseminated gonococcemia: the first, when fever coexists with polyarthralgias, polyarthritis, tenosynovitis, and characteristic skin lesions (usually of the distal upper extremities); the second, when monoarticular arthritis supervenes. The first phase may be immune complex–mediated, but gonococci can occasionally be demonstrated in the vesiculopustular skin lesions or in the blood cultures. In the second phase, gonococci localize to one joint and cause frank septic arthritis. Endocarditis[52] may rarely ensue.

The documentation of fever is often the crucial diagnostic step, since the manifestations of disseminated gonococcemia may be surprisingly subtle. Fever is often low grade and unaccompanied by other septic symptoms—chills, nausea, toxicity, for example. Skin lesions may be few and may be easily overlooked unless carefully searched for. The rheumatic complaints are often nonspecific, especially in the first stage (see above), and may not even be brought to the physician's attention when the patient assumes some traumatic cause for his tenosynovitis and fails to make any connection between a wrist or ankle "sprain" and burning on urination.

Careful examination, then, is a must. The diagnosis of gonococcemia is clinical. At times, no organism is recovered, in spite of obtaining appropriate cultures from urethra, pharynx, rectum, blood, skin lesions, and joint fluid, but the clinical syndrome is distinctive,[51, 97] and antibiotics should be begun immediately. Several days of intravenous administration of high-dose penicillin is usually recommended, but this may be no more efficacious than oral treatment at home.[47] Hospitalization may or may not be necessary, depending upon the certainty of diagnosis and the degree of the patient's disability. Frank gonococcal arthritis (a purulent joint effusion) should always be treated in the hospital.

5. Others.

Fever may be a manifestation of secondary or tertiary syphilis. The VDRL test is always positive in the former and usually positive in the latter (see Appendix II).

Whenever fever (usually with chills and flushing) follows the penicillin treatment of urethritis, the Jarisch-Herxheimer reaction[98] should be remembered, and results of syphilis serologic tests analyzed.

Reiter's syndrome may be associated with fever, but usually only when other systemic manifestations (arthritis, skin lesions) are present to suggest the diagnosis.

Localized venereal infection with prominent inguinal lymphadenopathy will sometimes induce low-grade fever—for example, herpes simplex and lymphogranuloma venereum may cause fever.

Finally, unusual infections—tuberculosis, fungal infections—should be remembered when fever and urinary symptoms occur and other diagnoses have been excluded. Rarely, upper tract infection proximal to ureteral obstruction (by stone, stricture, or neoplasm) will cause fever and nonspecific urinary symptoms, and perinephric abscess or xanthogranulomatous pyelonephritis (see Chapter 6, Appendix I) may be associated with a normal urinalysis and nonspecific symptoms. Renal cell carcinoma may also cause fever.

Syphilis: Tests and Treatment[99-101]

Syphilis is today an uncommon disease and is usually diagnosed in its early stages—primary syphilis when a genital (or other) chancre appears, secondary syphilis when a characteristic rash and lymphadenopathy arise. Sometimes syphilis is diagnosed purely on the basis of serologic tests—this is termed early latent syphilis when negative serologic tests have only recently (within 1 year) converted to positive, or late latent syphilis when the interval between documented seronegativity and subsequent seropositivity exceeds 1 year. Symptomatic forms of late syphilis—called tertiary syphilis, which may involve virtually any part of the body—are rare today. Neurosyphilis may cause a variety of clinical syndromes; asymptomatic neurosyphilis usually refers to positive serologic tests of the CSF, while active neurosyphilis is associated with clinical symptoms, positive CSF serologic findings, as well as (usually) pleocytosis and increased protein in the CSF.

Figure 8–19 summarizes the clinical classifications of syphilis as well as the expected serologic results and treatment recommendations for each. Serologic tests for syphilis include nontreponemal tests and treponemal tests. The nontreponemal tests include VDRL (Venereal Disease Research Laboratory), ART (automated reagent test), and RPR (rapid plasma reagin)—these tests measure patients' serum reaginic antibody to a prepared cardiolipin-lecithin antigen. The nontreponemal tests are highly sensitive (and are

	Early syphilis			Late syphilis
	Primary	Secondary	Early latent	Late latent tertiary neurosyphilis
RPR				
Reactivity (at the time of diagnosis)	70 per cent	99 per cent	75 per cent	80 per cent
Serologic response to therapy	Greater than 95 per cent revert to negative in 12 months	Greater than 95 per cent revert to negative in 24 months	Often remains positive	Often remains positive
FTA-ABS				
Reactivity	85 per cent	99 per cent	95 per cent	95 per cent
Serologic response to therapy	—— OFTEN REMAINS POSITIVE INDEFINITELY ——			
TREATMENT				
Preferred	Benzathine penicillin, 2.4 million units IM, single dose (Some authorities repeat dose 1 week later.)			Benzathine penicillin, 2.4 million units IM weekly × 3 consecutive weeks (7.2 million units total)
				Active neurosyphilis? (high-dose IV penicillin)
Penicillin allergy?	Tetracycline[102] (or erythromycin) 500 mg qid × 12 to 14 days			Tetracycline or erythromycin, 500 mg qid × 30 days

FIGURE 8–19. Syphilis: tests and treatment.

thus used as screening tests), but they are sometimes falsely positive and thus require confirmation with the more laborious and expensive treponemal tests—the FTA-ABS (fluorescent treponemal antibody absorption) test is most widely used—that measure antibody to the treponeme itself.

Both nontreponemal and treponemal tests are reported quantitatively. (We will use the RPR and FTA-ABS tests in this discussion.) The RPR is reported in titers (1:4, 1:32, for example). Rising titers over time are best indicators of recent infection. False positive tests are usually (but not always) positive in low titers (1:8 or less). Significant positive titers are usually greater than 1:8. In primary and secondary syphilis the RPR rises and falls with infection and treatment—the RPR is thus used to follow the results of treatment (and it usually eventually reverts to normal after treatment).

The FTA-ABS test is reported as nonreactive, borderline, and variously positive (1+ through 4+). Borderline or weakly reactive tests (1+, 2+) are equivocal. Strongly reactive (3+, 4+) tests are rarely falsely positive. (In the discussion below a positive FTA-ABS test refers to a strongly reactive result.) Since the FTA-ABS test often remains positive indefinitely despite treatment, this test cannot be used to follow the patient.

Despite its decreasing incidence, syphilis is indeed the great masquerader. Syphilology cannot be given its due in this brief discussion. Nevertheless, in the diagnosis and treatment of syphilis, three clinical situations constitute the majority of diagnostic and therapeutic problems:

I. When the patient demonstrates a genital lesion suggestive of primary syphilis.

    A. Figure 8–1 illustrates a typical syphilitic chancre.

        When such a lesion is present, darkfield microscopy of exudate scraped from the base of the chancre will usually confirm the diagnosis of syphilis—visualization of the motile, corkscrewing treponeme is diagnostic. In this setting, serologic tests are also performed, initially to confirm the diagnosis and subsequently to document return to seronegativity after treatment. Both the treponemal and nontreponemal tests will turn positive within 1 month after appearance of the chancre (in most cases); within the first week or two, however, these tests will sometimes be negative. Thus, if the initial serologic test is negative, the RPR and FTA-ABS tests should be repeated 1 month later; 6 to 12 months thereafter, follow-up RPR is obtained to document return to seronegativity. At least 95 per cent of patients adequately treated for primary syphilis will have a negative RPR test after 12 months elapse.[103] (Remember: The nontreponemal tests are used for follow-up, since the treponemal tests often remain positive indefinitely.)

    B. Darkfield microscopy is not always available, or the clinician may be inexperienced in its performance and interpretation.

        When this is the case, the diagnosis of primary syphilis depends on the gross appearance of the chancre and the results of serologic tests for syphilis. In the patient with a suspicious lesion whose RPR and FTA tests are both positive, primary syphilis should be assumed and treatment given. When only one of the tests is positive, treatment should be given, but serologic tests repeated after 1 month. When both serologic tests are initially negative, immediate treatment is determined by how suspicious the lesion is—certainly, if repeat serologic tests are positive 1 month later, treatment is indicated at that time.

Follow-up serologic tests are useful in several ways. Repeatedly negative tests usually exclude early syphilis. Persistently positive tests may simply reflect persistent seropositivity or indicate chronic false positive reactions when the RPR test is positive but the FTA-ABS test is negative. A continued false positive RPR test is seen among drug addicts, the elderly, and patients with autoimmune or immunologic disorders. A brief false positive RPR test result occurs after vaccination or other acute infections (mononucleosis, hepatitis, for example) but reverts to normal within 6 months.

Figure 8–20 illustrates the sequence of diagnostic testing and interpretation of various results in the patient with suspected primary syphilis.

II. When secondary syphilis is suspected.

Six weeks or more after the initial venereal contact, secondary syphilis may occur (and often without a history of a primary syphilitic lesion). A diffuse maculopapular rash involving palms and soles (with or without fever, lymphadenopathy, and arthralgias) is the usual clue. The RPR (or other nontreponemal) test is "always" positive in this situation, and the diagnosis is thus achieved. Almost all patients with secondary syphilis will become (RPR) seronegative after treatment, but some not before 24 months have elapsed.

III. When serologic tests for syphilis are done as screening tests.

Serologic tests for syphilis are often obtained routinely in patients admitted to the hospital, when there is a recent or remote history of

	Day 1	Day 2	1 Month Later	6 to 12 Months Later	Interpretation
			RPR ⊖ FTA ⊖		False ⊕ dark field exam but adequately treated anyway, or, false-negative serology with primary syphilis
	(A) Dark field ⊕ (Treatment now)	RPR ⊖	RPR ⊕ FTA ⊕		
		RPR ⊕	(No test)	RPR ⊖	Primary syphilis treated (>95 per cent)
Chancre?				Repeat RPR	
		RPR ⊕ (Treatment now) FTA ⊕	(No test)	RPR ⊕	Primary syphilis, treated, persistently seropositive (<5 per cent)
			RPR ⊕ (Treatment now) FTA ⊕		
	(B) Dark field ⊖ or dark field exam not done	RPR ⊖ FTA ⊖			
			RPR ⊖ FTA ⊖		No syphilis (not treated)
		RPR ⊕ FTA ⊖ (Treatment now)	RPR ⊖ FTA ⊖		False ⊕ RPR, acute, OR primary syphilis (treated)
				RPR ⊖	
			RPR ⊕ FTA ⊖	Repeat RPR RPR ⊕ FTA ⊖	Chronic false ⊕ RPR OR primary syphilis (treated), persistently seropositive
				RPR ⊕ FTA ⊕	Early syphilis (treated)
	Day 1	Day 2	1 Month Later	6 to 12 Months Later	

FIGURE 8–20. Serologies and chancres.

380

(+) RPR

(A) — (+) FTA
- A1 — History chronic sero-positivity — Treat only if titer is rising
- A2 — No recent "contact" or prior serology — Tertiary syphilis? / Latent syphilis? / Neurosyphilis? → Lumbar puncture → Active neurosyphilis? / Normal spinal fluid—treat for late latent syphilis
- A3 — Recent "contact" — Lumbar puncture? — Treat primary syphilis, follow

(B) — (−) FTA
- B1 — Recent "contact" — Repeat tests 1 month —
  - (+) RPR, (+) FTA — Treat primary syphilis, follow
  - (+) RPR, (−) FTA — ? False (+) RPR—follow Treat anyway!
  - (−) RPR, (−) FTA — False (+) RPR, acute No treatment indicated
- B2 — No recent "contact" — Repeat tests 6 to 12 months —
  - (−) RPR, (−) FTA — False (+) RPR, acute
  - (+) RPR, (+) FTA — Treat early syphilis
  - (+) RPR, (−) FTA — False (+) RPR, chronic Treat anyway?

FIGURE 8–21. When the "screening test" is positive.

exposure to syphilis, when a patient's sexual lifestyle imposes risk of asymptomatic syphilis (male homosexuals are commonly afflicted), or when other venereal infections are diagnosed and treated (since syphilis may coexist with other venereal infections).

Figure 8–21 illustrates that the approach to the patient with a positive screening RPR test depends on the simultaneous results of the FTA-ABS test, any history of a recent (possible) exposure to syphilis (contact), and the past history of positive serologic tests for syphilis.

The patient who has had a recent contact and whose tests (RPR) are seropositive (Fig. 8–21 A3 or B1) should be treated for primary syphilis, especially when the FTA-ABS test is positive (initially or within 1 to 2 months thereafter).

The patient with no known exposure to syphilis in whom both RPR and FTA-ABS tests are seropositive (Fig. 8–21 A2) may have either early (primary, secondary, or early latent) or late (late latent, tertiary, or neurosyphilis) syphilis.* Since the treatment of early syphilis is different from that of late syphilis (Fig. 8–19), the prior history and results of a careful examination for evidence of tertiary syphilis (dementia, aortitis, spinal myelitis, visible gummas) or neurosyphilis (cerebrospinal fluid should be examined) must be reviewed. When it is not possible to distinguish early from late syphilis, treat for the latter.

When neurosyphilis is "active" (symptomatic and/or associated with inflammatory cerebrospinal fluid), high dose intravenous penicillin should be given in hospital.[104, 105] This is now recommended by most authorities, especially since benzathine penicillin may not produce sufficient treponemicidal activity in the central nervous system.[106, 107]

Conversely, the patient with a positive RPR but negative FTA-ABS test usually has a false-positive RPR (Figure 8–21, B2). Rarely, the FTA-ABS will convert to positive several months later, and such patients should then be treated for early syphilis.

---

*An exception is the patient with known chronic seropositivity (Fig. 8–21 A1). Treatment should be initiated here only if titers are rising or the patient has been exposed to (possible) syphilis again.

APPENDIX III

"Personal" Diseases Are
Public Problems

In 1943 gonorrhea was regularly cured with a single dose of 160,000 units of penicillin.[108] The following three decades saw the gradual emergence of different chromosomal mutations that imparted increasing antibiotic resistance to the modern gonococcus, such that a 30-fold higher dose of penicillin is now recommended for uncomplicated gonorrhea. The past decade has witnessed a new mechanism of antibiotic resistance—plasmid-mediated penicillinase production—that threatens to render penicillin treatment of gonorrhea a mere historical footnote. The specter of potentially untreatable gonorrhea has quickened the pulse of more than a few public health officials recently.

During this same time, new venereal diseases (or, more likely, old diseases with new names) have surfaced. Chlamydial infection, for example, is now known to cause many cases of nongonococcal urethritis and probably a variety of other communicable diseases as well.[22, 23] As with gonorrhea, treatment of documented chlamydial infection is usually successful at the present time. Because diagnostic facilities for such documentation are not widely available, treatment for presumed chlamydial infection is usually presumptive—broad-spectrum antibiotics that cover several diagnostic possibilities, chlamydiae included. Will chlamydial and other communicable pathogens develop antibiotic resistance precisely <u>because</u> of the frequency and ease with which we now cure them with broad-spectrum antibiotics?

The potential nightmare of rampant antibiotic-resistant gonococcal or chlamydial disease fortunately remains in the province of science fiction, and it is hoped will remain so. The pharmaceutical industry has proven itself very resourceful in keeping a few steps ahead of most modern infectious diseases. (The modern history of the gonococcus has also resulted in crisis intervention research whose elucidation of host defense mechanisms[109, 110] and microbial virulence factors[111, 112] may one day help produce the ultimate weapon—the gonococcal vaccine.) Nevertheless, there is good reason for at least mild paranoia about the (relatively) benign venereal diseases. The current epidemic of genital herpes is a case in point—the medical and sociocultural implications of untreatable venereal disease deserve notice. If potentially invasive pathogens—like the gonococcus—become untreatable, the "herpes generation" will be considered fortunate by comparison.

For the individual health practitioner, such fears may be difficult to put into perspective. When one considers the excellent cure rates for gonococcal and nongonococcal urethritis with any of several different antibiotic regimens, it often seems somewhat academic to compulsively distinguish gonorrhea from NGU, to pursue contact tracing, to monitor for antibiotic resistance with cultures and sensitivity testing, or to prove cure with follow-up cultures. In the midst of growing public pressure for cost-conscious medical care (and next door to a busy waiting room), the practicing physician is often tempted to treat the male patient with dysuria with broad-spectrum antibiotics without bothering to establish specific diagnoses or causes. The purist will argue that this is sloppy medicine, but in fact there is much to recommend such an approach, at least from the individual patient's point of view (he usually gets better).

The fact is that these "academic compulsions" are much more important to the public health than to the outcome of most individual patient encounters. The purist's objection to empiric diagnosis and treatment of common disorders is more telling when the practitioner recalls the duty to be public defender as well as personal healer. Until preventive therapy of venereal disease becomes a reality, easily treatable venereal diseases deserve more haunting reputations despite (perhaps even because of) the very ease with which we cure them. Only by remaining academic and compulsive in these areas will the individual practitioner fully do his part in controlling communicable disease. Hence:

1. Careful documentation, reporting, and surveillance for communicable diseases must achieve a high priority for the individual practicing physician.

2. To accomplish this, reliable and accessible aids must be made available to practitioners. While most state health departments will provide gonorrhea culture services free of charge, many physicians do not use them. Such services are sometimes slow, inefficient, and poorly publicized. More rapid transportation of specimens and reporting of results as well as clear identification of official responsibility for contact tracing are crucial to improving the utility of these services for the practitioner. Waiting a week for gonorrhea culture results frustrates clinician and patient alike and surely contributes to negligence and the use of more convenient (and more costly) proprietary laboratories.

3. The Centers for Disease Control* until recently provided free of charge its weekly "Morbidity and Mortality Weekly Report" to interested physicians. This excellent publication, at the very least, heightens our awareness and keeps us up to date on recent trends in communicable health problems. Inflation notwithstanding, this publication should be subsidized again and made available to us all.

4. Practicing clinicians must make known their needs to the research community. Too many widely quoted clinical studies involve selected patient populations catered to by research facilities. Practical mundane issues must be addressed with the same intensity as are the quests for revolutionary biologic breakthroughs. Diagnostic and therapeutic strategies that are easily available to all practicing physicians should be studied and refined. For example, studies that recommend urethral cultures for chlamydiae or ureaplasmas or other fastidious organisms are not currently very helpful for most practicing physicians. (When such cultures do become routinely available, their cost effectiveness and utility in clinical practice should be scrutinized carefully. It may well be that a simple urethral Gram's stain is in fact the best diagnostic test!)

---

*United States Department of Health, Education and Welfare; Public Health Service; Centers for Disease Control; Atlanta, Georgia 30333.

REFERENCES

1. Nickel, WR, Plumb, RT: Other infections and inflammations of the external genitalia. *In* Harrison, J. H., et al. (eds.): Campbell's Urology, 4th ed. Philadelphia: W. B. Saunders, 1978, pp. 640–692.
2. McCormack, WM: Sexually transmissible diseases. Postgrad Med 58:179–186, 1975.
3. Corey, L, et al.: Genital herpes simplex virus infections: Clinical manifestations, course and complications. Ann Intern Med 98:958–972, 1983.
4. Corey, L, Holmes, KK: Genital herpes simplex infection: Current concepts in diagnosis, therapy and prevention. Ann Intern Med 98:973–983, 1983.
5. Fitzpatrick, JE, et al.: Treatment of chancroid. Comparison of trimethoprim-sulfamethoxazole with recommended therapies. JAMA 246:1804–1805, 1981.
6. Schachter, J, Dawson, CR: Lymphogranuloma venereum. JAMA 236:915–916, 1976.
7. Burns, E, Thompson, I: Infections and inflammation of the male genital tract: Penis and urethra. *In* Harrison, J, et al. (eds): Campbell's Urology, 3rd ed. Philadelphia: W. B. Saunders, 1970, pp. 513–553.
8. Millikan, LE: Superficial and cutaneous fungal infections. Diagnosis and treatment. Postgrad Med 60:52–58, 1976.
9. Consultant pp 221–225 (Oct), 1980 (photographs).
10. Persky, L: Balanoposthitis. Medical Aspects of Human Sexuality. pp 105–106 (Jan) 1980.
11. Wright, RA, Judson, FN: Penile venereal edema. JAMA 241:157–158, 1979.
12. Orkin, M, et al.: Treatment of today's scabies and pediculosis. JAMA 236:1136–1139, 1976.
13. Gott, LJ: Common scrotal pathology. Am Fam Physician 15:165–173 (May) 1977.
14. Berger, RE, et al.: Chlamydia trachomatis as a cause of idiopathic epididymitis. N Engl J Med. 298:301–304, 1978.
15. Jacobs, NF, Kraus, SJ: Gonococcal and nongonococcal urethritis in men. Clinical and laboratory differentiation. Ann Intern Med 82:7–12, 1975.
16. Swartz, SL, et al.: Diagnosis and etiology of nongonococcal urethritis. J Infect Dis 138:445–454, 1978.
17. Dunlop, E, et al.: Chlamydial infection: Incidence in "nonspecific" urethritis. Br J Vener Dis 48:425–428, 1972.
18. Richmond, SJ, et al.: Chlamydial infection: Role of Chlamydia subgroup A in nongonococcal and post-gonococcal urethritis. Br J Vener Dis 48:437–444, 1972.
19. Holmes, KK, et al.: Etiology of nongonococcal urethritis. N Engl J Med 292:1199–1205, 1975.
20. Bowie, WR: Etiology and treatment of nongonococcal urethritis. Sex Transm Dis 5:27–33, 1978.
21. Schachter, J, et al.: Are chlamydial infections the most prevalent venereal disease? JAMA 231:1252–1255, 1975.
22. Guze, PA, et al.: Spectrum of human chlamydial infections. West J Med 135:208–225, 1981.
23. Schachter, J: Chlamydial infections. N Engl JMed 298:427–434, 1978.
24. Oriel, JD, et al.: The lack of effect of ampicillin plus probenecid given for genital infections with Neisseria gonorrhoeae on associated infections with Chlamydia trachomatis. J Infect Dis. 133:568–570, 1976.
25. Arnold, AJ, Kleris, GS: The "borderline" smear in men with urethritis. JAMA 244:157–159, 1980.
26. Williams, DC, et al.: Neisseria meningitidis urethritis: Probable pathogen in two related cases of urethritis, epididymitis, and acute pelvic inflammatory disease. JAMA 242:1653–1654, 1979.
27. Miller, MA, et al.: Neisseria meningitidis urethritis: A case report. JAMA 242:1656–1657, 1979.
28. LaBreque, DR: Diagnosis of gonorrhea (Letters). JAMA 244:238, 1980.
29. Luciano, AA, Grubin, L: Gonorrhea screening. Comparison of three techniques. JAMA 243:680–681, 1980.
30. Wiesner, PJ, et al.: Clinical spectrum of pharyngeal gonococcal infection. N Engl J Med. 288:181–185, 1973.
31. Klain, E, et al.: Anorectal gonococcal infection. Ann Intern Med 86:340–346, 1977.
32. Janda, WM, et al.: Prevalence and site-pathogen studies of Neisseria meningitidis and Neisseria gonorrhoeae in homosexual men. JAMA 244:2060–2064, 1980.
33. Merino, HI, Richards, JB: An innovative program of venereal disease case finding, treatment, and education for a population of gay men. Sex Transm Dis 4:50–52, 1977.
34. Roberts, RB (ed.): The Gonococcus. New York: John Wiley and Son, 1977.
35. Goodhart, GL: Treatment of uncomplicated genital gonorrhea. Sex Transm Dis 6 (Suppl.):126–142 (April–June), 1979.
36. Goodrich, JT: Treatment of gonorrhea in pregnancy. Sex Transm Dis 6 (Suppl):168–173 (April–June), 1979.
37. Kraus, SJ: Incidence and therapy of gonococcal pharyngitis. Sex Transm Dis 6 (Suppl.):143–148 (April–June), 1979.
38. U. S. Department of HEW: Gonorrhea. CDC recommended treatment schedule, 1979. Ann Intern Med 90:809–811, 1979.
39. McCormack, WM: Treatment of gonorrhea (editorial). Ann Intern Med 90:845–846, 1979.
40. Karney, WW, et al.: Spectinomycin versus tetracycline for the treatment of gonorrhea. N Engl J Med 296:889–894, 1977.
41. Kaufman, RE, et al.: National gonorrhea therapy monitoring survey. Treatment results. N Engl J Med. 294:1–4, 1976.
42. Jaffe, HW, et al.: National gonorrhea therapy monitoring study. In vitro antibiotic susceptibility and its correlation with treatment results. N Engl J Med 294:5–9, 1976.
43. Sands, M: Treatment of anorectal gonorrhea infection in men. JAMA 243:1143–1144, 1980.
44. Lebedeff, DA, Hochman, EB: Rectal gonorrhea in men: Diagnosis and treatment. Ann Intern Med 92:463–466, 1980.

45. Sattler, FR, Ruskin, J: Therapy of gonorrhea. Comparison of trimethoprim-sulfamethoxazole and ampicillin. JAMA 240:2267–2270, 1978.
46. Brown, ST, et al.: Comparison of erythromycin base and estolate in gonococcal urethritis. JAMA 238:1371–1373, 1977.
47. Thompson, SE, et al.: Gonococcal tenosynovitis-dermatitis and septic arthritis. Intravenous penicillin versus oral erythromycin. JAMA 244:1101–1102, 1980.
48. Felman, YM, Nikitas, JA: Nongonococcal urethritis. A clinical review. JAMA 245:381–386, 1981.
49. Berg, SW, et al.: Cefoxitin as a single-dose treatment for urethritis caused by penicillinase-producing Neisseria gonorrhoeae. N Engl J Med 301:509–511, 1979.
50. McCormack, WM, Finland, M: Spectinomycin. Ann Intern Med 84:712–716, 1976.
51. Holmes, KK, et al.: Disseminated gonococcal infection. Ann Intern Med 75:979–993, 1971.
52. Cooke, DB, et al.: Gonococcal endocarditis in the antibiotic era. Arch Int Med. 139:1247–1250, 1979.
53. Rudolph, AH, Price, EV: Penicillin reactions among patients in venereal disease clinics. A national survey. JAMA 223:499–501, 1973.
54. Holmes, KK, et al.: Studies of venereal disease. II. Observations on the incidence, etiology, and treatment of the postgonococcal urethritis syndrome. JAMA 202:131–137, 1967.
55. Bowie, WR, et al.: Etiology of nongonococcal urethritis. Evidence for Chlamydia trachomatis and Ureaplasma urealyticum. J Clin Invest 59:735–742, 1977.
56. Bowie, WR, et al.: Differential response of chlamydial and ureaplasma-associated urethritis to sulphafurazole (sulfisoxazole) and aminocyclitols. Lancet 2:1276–1278, 1976.
57. Taylor-Robinson, D, McCormack, WM: The genital mycoplasmas. N Engl J Med 302:1003–1010, 1980.
58. Furness, G, et al.: Corynebacterium genitalium (nonspecific urethritis corynebacterium): Biologic reactions differentiating commensals of the urogenital tract from the pathogens responsible for urethritis. Invest Urol 15:23–27, 1977.
59. Bowie, WR, et al: Therapy for nongonococcal urethritis. Double-blind randomized comparison of two doses and two durations of minocycline. Ann Intern Med 95:306–311, 1981.
60. Holmes, KK, et al.: Studies of venereal disease. III. Double-blind comparison of tetracycline hydrochloride and placebo in treatment of nongonococcal urethritis. JAMA 202:138–140, 1967.
61. Arya, OP, et al.: Management of nonspecific urethritis in men. Evaluation of six treatment regimens and effect of other factors including alcohol and sexual intercourse. Br J Ven Dis 54:414–421, 1978.
62. Confalik, ED, et al.: Treatment of nongonococcal urethritis with rifampicin as a means of defining the role of ureaplasma urealyticum. Br J Vener Dis 55:36–43, 1979.
63. Freeman, RB, et al.: Long-term therapy for chronic bacteriuria in men. U.S. Public Health Service cooperative study. Ann Intern Med 83:133–147, 1975.
64. Smith, JW, et al.: Recurrent urinary tract infections in men: Characteristics and response to therapy. Ann Intern Med 91:544–548, 1979.
65. Gleckman, R, et al.: Therapy of recurrent invasive urinary tract infections in men. N Engl J Med 301:878–880, 1979.
66. Kunin, CM: Long-term therapy of urinary tract infections. Ann Intern Med 83:273–274, 1975.
67. Drach, GW: Prostatitis: Man's hidden infection. Urol Clin North Am 2:499–520, 1975.
68. Blacklock, NJ: Anatomical factors in prostatitis. Br J Urol 46:47–54, 1974.
69. Meares, EM: Bacterial prostatitis versus "prostatosis." A clinical and bacteriological study. JAMA 224:1372–1375, 1973.
70. Meares, EM, Stamey, TA: Bacteriologic localization patterns in bacterial prostatitis and urethritis. Invest Urol 5:492–518, 1968.
71. Drach, GW: Problems in diagnosis of bacterial prostatitis: Gram-negative, gram-positive, and mixed infections. J Urol 111:630–636, 1974.
72. Zinner, NR: The perplexing problem of prostatitis. Postgrad Med 58:96–104, 1975.
73. Drach, GW, et al.: Classification of benign diseases associated with prostatic pain: Prostatitis or prostatodynia? (Letters). J Urol 120:266, 1978.
74. Pfau, A, Sachs, T: Chronic bacterial prostatitis: New therapeutic aspects. Br J Urol 48:245–253, 1976.
75. Meares, EM: Infection stones of prostate gland. Laboratory diagnosis and clinical management. Urology 4:560–566, 1974.
76. Eykyn, S, et al.: Prostatic calculi as a source of recurrent bacteriuria in the male. Br J Urol 46:527–532, 1974.
77. Smart, CJ, Jenkins, JD: The role of transurethral prostatectomy in chronic prostatitis. Br J Urol 45:654–662, 1973.
78. Mobley, DF: Semen cultures in the diagnosis of bacterial prostatitis. J Urol 114:83–85, 1975.
79. Stamey, TA, et al.: Chronic bacterial prostatitis and the effusion of drugs into prostatic fluid. J Urol 103:187–194, 1970.
80. Fair, WR, et al.: A reappraisal of treatment in chronic bacterial prostatitis. J Urol 121:437–441, 1979.
81. Drach, GW: Trimethoprim-sulfamethoxazole therapy of chronic bacterial prostatitis. Br J Urol 111:637–639, 1974.
82. Meares, EM: Long-term therapy of chronic bacterial prostatitis with trimethoprim-sulfamethoxazole. Can Med Assoc J 112:225–255, 1975.
83. Paulson, DF, White, RD: Trimethoprim-sulfamethoxazole and minocycline hydrochloride in the treatment of culture-proved bacterial prostatitis. J Urol 120:184–185, 1978.
84. Brannan, W: Treatment of chronic prostatitis. Comparison of minocycline and doxycycline. Urology 5:626–631, 1975.
85. Mobley, DF: Erythromycin plus sodium bicarbonate in chronic bacterial prostatitis. Urology 3:60–62, 1974.

86. Genster, HG, Andersen, M: Spinal osteomyelitis complicating urinary tract infections. J Urol 107:109, 1972.
87. Khanna, OP: Disorders of micturition. Neuropharmacologic basis and results of therapy. Urology 8:316–328, 1976.
88. Wein, AJ, et al.: Management of neurogenic bladder dysfunction in the adult. Urology 8:432–443, 1976.
89. Murray, BE, et al.: Emergence of high level trimethoprim resistance in fecal Escherichia coli during oral administration of trimethoprim or trimethoprim-sulfamethoxazole. N Engl J Med 306:130–135, 1982.
90. Byrd, L, et al.: Radiocontrast-induced acute renal failure. Medicine 58:270–279, 1979.
91. Thorley, JD, et al.: Perinephric abscess. Medicine 53:441, 1974.
92. Meares, EM: Prostatitis: A review. Urol Clin North Am 2:3, 1975.
93. Meares, EM, Stamey, TA: The diagnosis and management of bacterial prostatitis. Br J Urol 44:175, 1972.
94. Trapnell, J, Roberts, M: Prostatic abscess. Br J Surg 57:565–569, 1970.
95. Pai, MG, Bhat, HS: Prostatic abscess. J Urol 108:599–600, 1972.
96. Bartlett, JG, et al.: Prostatic abscess as involving anaerobic bacteria. Arch Int Med 138:1369–1371, 1978.
97. Handsfield, HH, et al.: Treatment of gonococcal arthritis dermatitis syndrome. Ann Intern Med 84:661–667, 1976.
98. Editorial: The Jarisch-Herxheimer reaction. Lancet 1:340–341, 1977.
99. Sparling, PF: Diagnosis and treatment of syphilis. N Eng J Med 284:642–653, 1971.
100. Jaffe, HW: The laboratory diagnosis of syphilis. Ann Int Med 83:846, 1975.
101. Lee, TJ, Sparling, PF: Syphilis. An algorithm. JAMA 242:1187–1189, 1979.
102. Fiumara, NJ: Treating syphilis with tetracycline. Am Fam Physician July 1982:131–133.
103. Fiumara, NJ: Treatment of primary and secondary syphilis. Serologic response. JAMA 243:2500–2502, 1980.
104. Simon, RP: Neurosyphilis: An update. West J Med 134:87–91, 1981.
105. Hotson, JR: Modern neurosyphilis: A partially treated chronic meningitis. West J Med 135:191–200, 1981.
106. Rothenberg, R: Treatment of neurosyphilis. J Am Ven Dis Assoc 3:153–158, 1976.
107. Ducas, J, Robson, HG: Cerebrospinal fluid penicillin levels during treatment for latent syphilis. JAMA 246:2583–2584, 1981.
108. Mahoney, JF, et al.: The use of penicillin sodium in the treatment of sulfonamide-resistant gonorrhea in men: A preliminary report. Am J Syph Gonorrhea Ven Dis 27:525–528, 1943.
109. Ofek, I, et al.: Resistance of Neisseria gonorrhoeae to phagocytosis: Relationship to colonial morphology and surface pili. J Inf Dis 129:310–316, 1974.
110. Rice, PA, et al.: Natural serum bactericidal activity against Neisseria gonorrhoeae isolates from disseminated, locally invasive, and uncomplicated disease. J Immunology 124:2105–2109, 1980 (May).
111. Sparling, PF: Antibody-cleaving Neisseria. N Eng J Med 290:1011–1012, 1978.
112. Mulks, MH, Plaut, AG: IgA protease production as a characteristic distinguishing pathogenic from harmless Neisseriaceae. N Eng J Med 299:973–976, 1978.
113. Plummer, FA, et al.: Single dose therapy of chancroid with trimethoprim-sulfametrole. N Eng J Med 309:67–71, 1983.
114. Haynes, BE, et al.: The diagnosis of testicular torsion. JAMA 249:2522–2527, 1983.
115. Branner, H, et al.: Studies on the role of Ureaplasma urealyticum and Mycoplasma hominis in prostatitis. J Infect Dis 147:807–813, 1983.

9

SHOULDER PAIN

INITIAL APPROACH............................... 387

SYMPTOMS AND SIGNS 388

    Examination of the Shoulder................... 393

PERIARTICULAR SHOULDER DISORDERS.......... 407

    Diagnosis..................................... 410
    Treatment 416
        Pain Relief................................. 416
        Anti-inflammatory Measures............... 417
        Injections 418
        Exercise Therapy.......................... 418
        When the Patient Does Not Improve 423

THE SHOULDER AND THE HAND.................. 426

PRACTICAL NEUROLOGY OF THE UPPER
EXTREMITY.. 431

APPENDIX   I: SHOULDER BIOMECHANICS AND
                 ANATOMY....................... 441

           II: TRAUMATIC SHOULDER PAIN...... 447

          III: THORACIC OUTLET SYNDROMES.. 451

REFERENCES...................................... 454

Sheldon Shoulder, a 47-year-old accountant, enters the clinic complaining of shoulder pain. Sheldon was awakened this morning with moderately severe aching pain in the anterolateral aspect of the left shoulder, which has worsened over the ensuing several hours. He needed assistance to dress and bathe this morning and now has difficulty using the shoulder at all.

Sheldon says he has been healthy all his life and has no prior history of shoulder problems, "except the usual aches and pains." He denies any recent injury, fever, neck pain, or neurologic symptoms or any cardiopulmonary or systemic complaints. Sheldon, who is left-handed, admits that he is usually quite sedentary, but last week spent 3 days painting the ceilings and walls of his living and dining rooms, with much unaccustomed shoulder and arm activity.

When asked to locate the pain, he points to the anterolateral deltoid area; he denies radiation into the neck or hand but says that the pain sometimes hurts halfway down the arm, above the elbow.

INITIAL APPROACH

Acute shoulder pain is usually the result of one of several mechanical shoulder disorders. The history, examination, and subsequent clinical course in such patients usually allow accurate diagnosis and successful therapy, as

TABLE 9–1. CAUSES OF REFERRED SHOULDER PAIN

Most common cause	Uncommon causes
Cervical spine disease	Vascular claudication
	Aneurysm
Most serious causes	Vasculitis
Myocardial infarction	Thrombophlebitis
Aortic dissection	Mediastinal neoplasm
Pulmonary embolism	Esophagitis and/or esophageal spasm
Ruptured abdominal viscus (duodenal	Subphrenic abscess
ulcer, colonic diverticulum)	Hepatic hematoma or abscess
Splenic rupture	Splenic infarction
Ectopic pregnancy	Peptic ulcer
	Pancreatitis
Other common causes	Splenic flexure syndrome
Angina pectoris	Hepatic flexure syndrome
Pneumothorax	Pancoast tumor
Pericarditis	Mesothelioma
Pneumonia	Spinal cord lesions
Pleuritis	Brachial plexus disease
Cholecystitis	Entrapment neuropathy

discussed on pages 404 to 426. These mechanical disorders (see below) are so common, in fact, that the clinician must beware of developing the "telescopic vision" that will miss less common but more serious disorders. This can be avoided if the clinician, even before examining the patient, remembers a few simple concepts (see also Fig. 9–6).

SYMPTOMS AND SIGNS

I. The great majority of shoulder pains are due to periarticular and articular disorders, but the shoulder is a common location for referred pain.

Because the shoulder and arm are innervated by neural segments (C4-T2) that also innervate structures in the neck, great vessels, heart, lungs, mediastinum, diaphragm, and upper abdomen, pain from many of these areas may be referred to the shoulder/arm area. Some of the common and uncommon diseases that may present with acute pain referred to the shoulder are noted in Table 9–1.

Most of these disorders produce symptoms and signs that clearly distinguish them from local musculoskeletal shoulder disorders. However, always allow the patient to describe in his or her own words the location and radiation of pain and any associated symptoms (cough, fever, paresthesias, dyspnea). Remember:

A. Disorders of the neck are the most common cause of referred shoulder pain.

Even when radicular symptoms are absent and the neurologic examination is completely normal (see page 431), pain in the deltoid muscle, trapezius muscle, and scapular or interscapular area is very often referred from the cervical spine (Fig. 9–1). For this reason, examination of neck range of motion—flexion, extension, rotation, and lateral flexion—should be performed in all patients with shoulder pain (Fig. 9–2).

B. Very abrupt onset of shoulder pain in the absence of trauma or strain should suggest one of the serious disorders listed in Table 9–1.

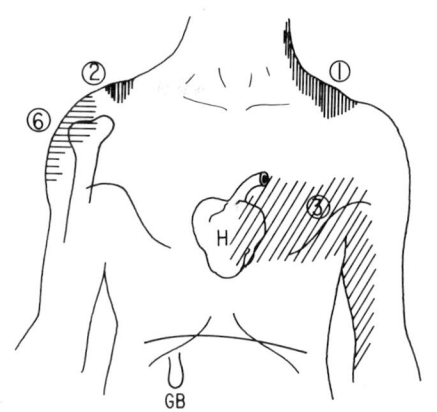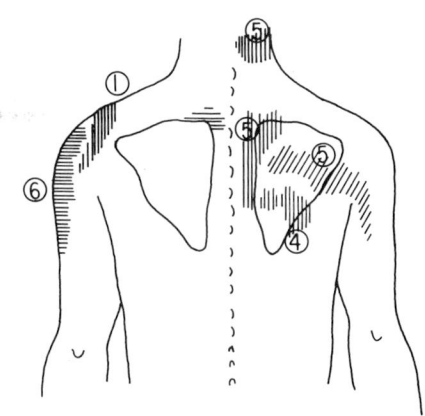

FIGURE 9–1. Referred shoulder pain.

1. Trapezius ridge—a common site of pain referred from the diaphragm. The pain of pleuritis, pericarditis and subdiaphragmatic diseases may be felt here.

2. The acromioclavicular area—sometimes diaphragmatic or subdiaphragmatic diseases will refer pain to this area. Acute cholecystitis is one example.

3. Cardiac pain usually involves the left chest and inner arm (but may be highly variable in location—see Chapter 13).

4. Gallbladder disease commonly refers pain to the lower scapula.

5. Cervical spine disease often causes pain in the back of the neck, interscapular areas, and posterior shoulder.

6. Most articular and periarticular disorders of the shoulder cause pain over the deltoid area.

A few patients with a ruptured abdominal viscus (perforated ulcer [Fig. 9–3] or colonic diverticulum), ectopic pregnancy, or cardiac emergency will so present.

C. Location of pain sometimes suggests a specific visceral disease.

Diaphragmatic irritation often causes pain in the trapezius ridge. Pleuritis, pericarditis, subphrenic abscess, splenic infarction, and other diaphragmatic problems may be announced by pain in the trapezius area. Pain just in the acromioclavicular area is sometimes caused by subdiaphragmatic disease (cholecystitis, hepatic abscess, splenic rupture). Gallbladder disease commonly causes pain in the scapula. Cardiac pain, when it involves the shoulder, is usually referred to the pectoral and inner arm area.

D. Listen carefully to the patient.

Apparently unrelated symptoms may be important. The classic example is that of the splenic flexure syndrome,[1] in which left shoulder pain is due to distention of the splenic colon, and the patient (or physician) ignores the fact that constipation, flatulence, or mild left abdominal discomfort is associated with the shoulder pain.

Similarly, not all pain that occurs "when I use my arm" is mechanical shoulder pain. A more precise history may reveal that physical exercise without specific exercise of the shoulder itself precipitates the shoulder pain: suspect coronary insufficiency. Shoulder exercise that tires the arm or causes discomfort during repetitive shoulder exercises (for example, cleaning upper windows) should prompt careful examination for vascular claudication (Fig. 9–4). (Ask the patient to lift a light weight overhead repetitively for several minutes with the symptomatic arm. Then inquire about symptoms,

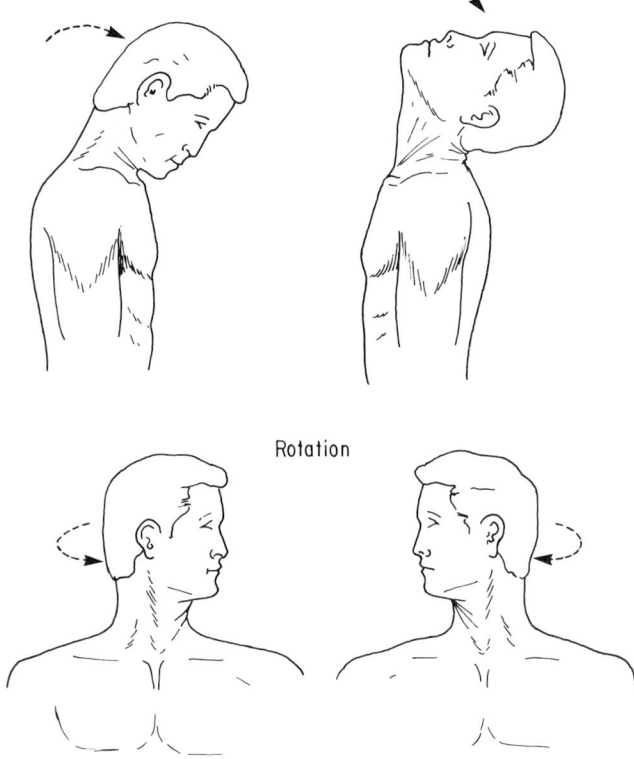

Flexion

Extension

Rotation

Lateral Flexion

FIGURE 9–2. Range of motion of the cervical spine.

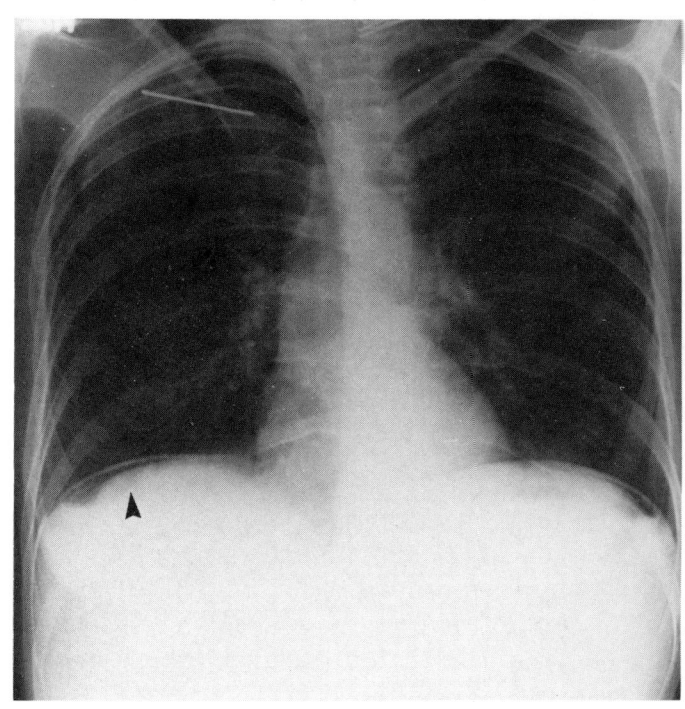

FIGURE 9–3. This 40-year-old woman complained of abrupt onset of very severe right shoulder pain. Examination of the shoulder was entirely normal. X-ray demonstrates free air under the diaphragm, due to perforation of a duodenal ulcer.

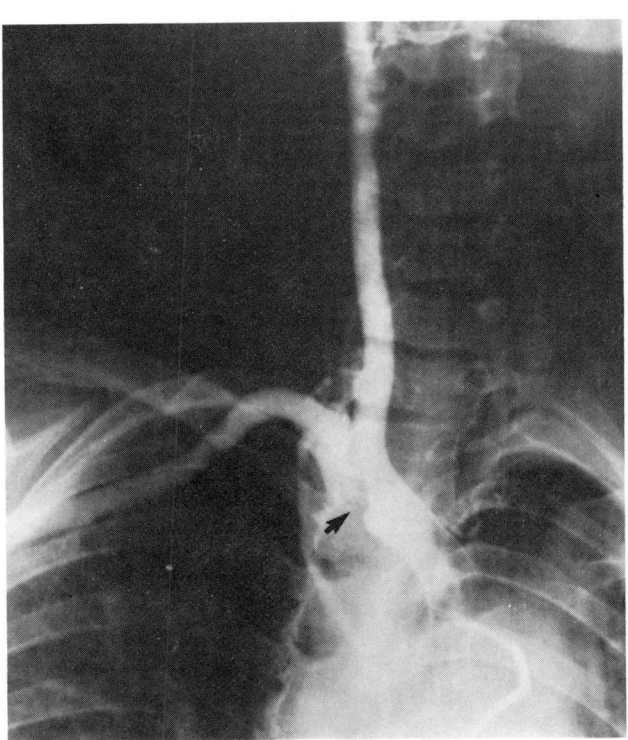

FIGURE 9-4. This 55-year-old man complained of shoulder pain, most prominent during repetitive abduction exercise of the right shoulder. Examination of the shoulder was completely normal except for a slightly diminished right radial pulse. Repetitive exercise of the shoulder demonstrated fatigue of the shoulder and arm muscles and reproduced the patient's pain. This arteriogram demonstrates stenosis of the right subclavian artery (arrow). Vascular reconstruction ameliorated the patient's symptoms.

examine the brachial and radial pulses, and listen for supraclavicular or axillary bruits.)

Especially when careful local examination of the shoulder is normal (see below), these referred disorders must be suspected.

II. Fever is rare in the patient with shoulder pain, but always record the patient's temperature!

Septic shoulder arthritis is rare but is an emergency. The patient with sepsis of the shoulder (glenohumeral) joint will invariably demonstrate extreme limitation of any shoulder motion (see below), but the patient who is elderly or immunosuppressed may have only low-grade fever and mild pain. Any patient with fever and extreme acute limitation of shoulder motion will require diagnostic arthrocentesis[2] to exclude sepsis. (Occasionally gout, pseudogout, or rheumatoid arthritis will so present.) Glenohumeral arthrocentesis can be performed via the anterior or posterior approach (Fig. 9–5). Strict aseptic technique is essential.

Joint fluid should be cultured immediately on appropriate culture media and should be analyzed at least for differential cell counts and crystals; Gram's stain should be done.

(Aspiration of acromioclavicular and sternoclavicular joints is much less commonly necessary, but these articulations are quite superficial, and arthrocentesis is generally quite simple—see also page 398.)

III. Chronic or recurrent shoulder pain often results from the same "degenerative" mechanical events that underlie various acute mechanical shoulder problems (see page 408).

Nevertheless, chronic shoulder pain and disability usually imply a distinctive differential diagnosis. Degenerative arthritis is usually apparent on examination and x-ray (see Fig. 9–16). Adhesive capsulitis, chronic rotator cuff tears, and impingement syndromes are equally common, often overlap clinically, and may be associated with normal x-rays (see page 423).

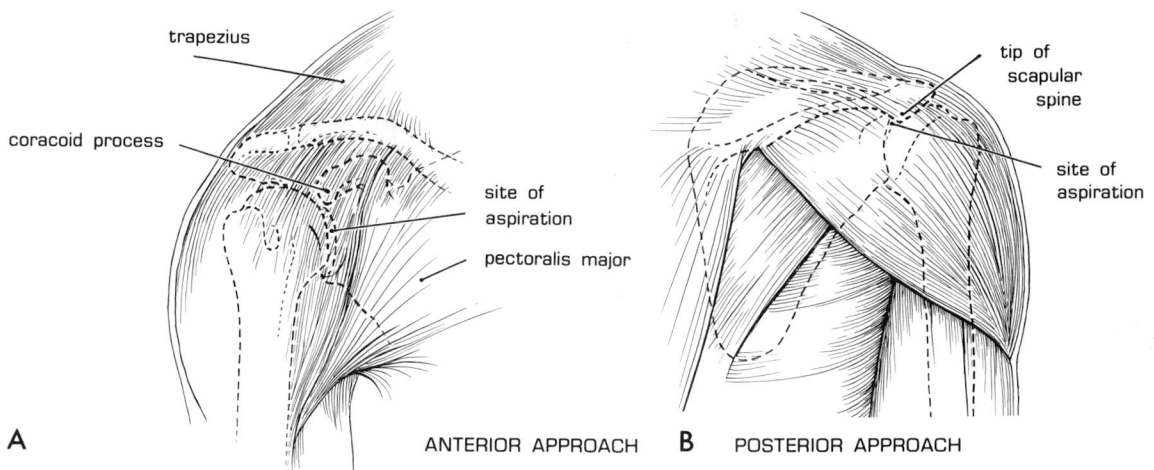

FIGURE 9–5. Shoulder arthrocentesis.

A, The anterior approach to shoulder injection and aspiration. A point is located just inferior and lateral to the coracoid process (and just medial to the head of the humerus). The needle (at least 1½ inches long) is directed posteriorly and slightly superolaterally. Usually a slight "give" is appreciated when the joint space is entered. Normally, no fluid will be aspirated unless blood (traumatic hemarthrosis), pus, or inflammatory synovial fluid is present.

B, The posterior approach involves standing behind the patient, palpating the tip of the scapular spine, and directing a needle 1 to 2 cm inferior to the scapular tip anteriorly toward the coracoid process (which should be simultaneously palpated with the opposite hand). (Reproduced with permission from Weiss, J: The painful shoulder. In Kelley, WN, Harris, ED, Jr, Ruddy, S, and Sledge, CB: Textbook of Rheumatology. Philadelphia: WB Saunders Co., 1981, pp. 439, 440.)

IV. Any history of trauma to the shoulder, whether direct or indirect, should be noted.

Fractures, dislocations, and subluxations usually follow obvious shoulder injuries. Most, but not all, of these require immediate orthopedic attention (see Appendix II).

Otherwise, mild mechanical trauma—falls on an outstretched arm, forceful distraction of the shoulder, lifting heavy objects overhead, or simple overuse of the shoulder—may contribute to various other acute mechanical shoulder disorders. Always inquire about such a history in the patient with acute shoulder pain.

V. Systemic, neurologic, and neoplastic diseases only rarely begin with shoulder pain, but the history will usually suggest these problems.

Relentless, progressively worsening shoulder pain for weeks or months must be carefully investigated. Primary or metastatic neoplasms of bone (for example, multiple myeloma or metastases from breast, lung, thyroid, kidney, or prostate carcinoma) or local infiltrative neoplasms (for example, Pancoast tumor of the lung—see page 405)—must be suspected.

Cervical root syndromes are common causes of radicular arm and shoulder pain, but the distribution of pain and the physical examination are usually diagnostic (see page 427). Rarely, disorders of the spinal cord—myelitis, syringomyelia, primary spinal neoplasms, arachnoiditis—will cause relentless, puzzling, atypical shoulder pain. Hence the importance of the neurologic examination in some patients with shoulder pain (see pages 423 and 431).

A few systemic disorders will cause prominent shoulder pain as part of a more generalized illness. Thyroid disease,[3] diabetes mellitus,[4] amyloidosis,[5] muscular dystrophies, inflammatory myopathies, connective tissue diseases, and even drug reactions (isoniazid[6]) may be responsible for unexplained shoulder pain.

Polymyalgia rheumatica (with or without associated temporal arteritis) is especially important to remember in the elderly patient. Discomfort is usually bilateral, stiffness is often more prominent than pain (and is notoriously worse in the morning), and the proximal areas of the legs and lower back are often involved as well as the neck and shoulders.

Figure 9–6 outlines some of the important historical features that help distinguish the very common acute mechanical shoulder syndromes from the less common referred, serious, neurologic, or systemic disorders. Thereafter, an informed physical examination will facilitate further differential diagnosis of acute mechanical shoulder pain.

Sheldon denies any history suggestive of cardiac, pulmonary or intra-abdominal disorders, and there are no associated systemic or neurologic symptoms. Prior "aches and pains" have occurred, usually in the left shoulder the day after unaccustomed exercise (throwing, lifting, for example), but have always been transient and mild. There is no history of direct or indirect shoulder trauma other than the recent painting spree.

Temperature and other vital signs are normal. Brief examination of the neck, heart, lungs, and abdomen is normal. Attention is turned to examination of the shoulder.

Examination of the Shoulder[7–11]

Physical examination of the patient with shoulder pain should always attempt to answer these basic questions (Fig. 9–6):

1. Is range of motion of the shoulder normal (full and painless) or abnormal (restricted or painful)? Most mechanical disorders cause impaired shoulder mobility.

2. Are any palpable structures tender (or abnormal visually), and does palpation reproduce the patient's pain? Many mechanical disorders cause localized tenderness.

3. Is the neurologic examination of the upper extremity normal? Mechanical shoulder disorders do not cause neurologic compromise.

I. Shoulder range of motion.

Full and painless range of motion of the shoulder depends upon coordinated interaction among several shoulder joints and their various periarticular structures, powering muscle groups, and interposed soft tissues. Those readers unfamiliar with the mechanics of shoulder motion should review Appendix I in which pertinent anatomic biomechanics of the shoulder are discussed.

The shoulder moves in seven different directions (and their various combinations)—flexion, extension, abduction, adduction, internal rotation, external rotation, and elevation (Fig. 9–7). These movements can be quickly assessed by asking the patient to raise both arms directly overhead, palms touching (elevation with flexion and abduction); then, to touch both hands to the opposite shoulder blades behind and below the neck (abduction and external rotation); finally, to lower the hands to the sides (adduction) and reach behind the back to touch the opposite shoulder blades from below, as high up as possible (adduction, extension, and internal rotation). The painful shoulder should be compared with the normal shoulder.

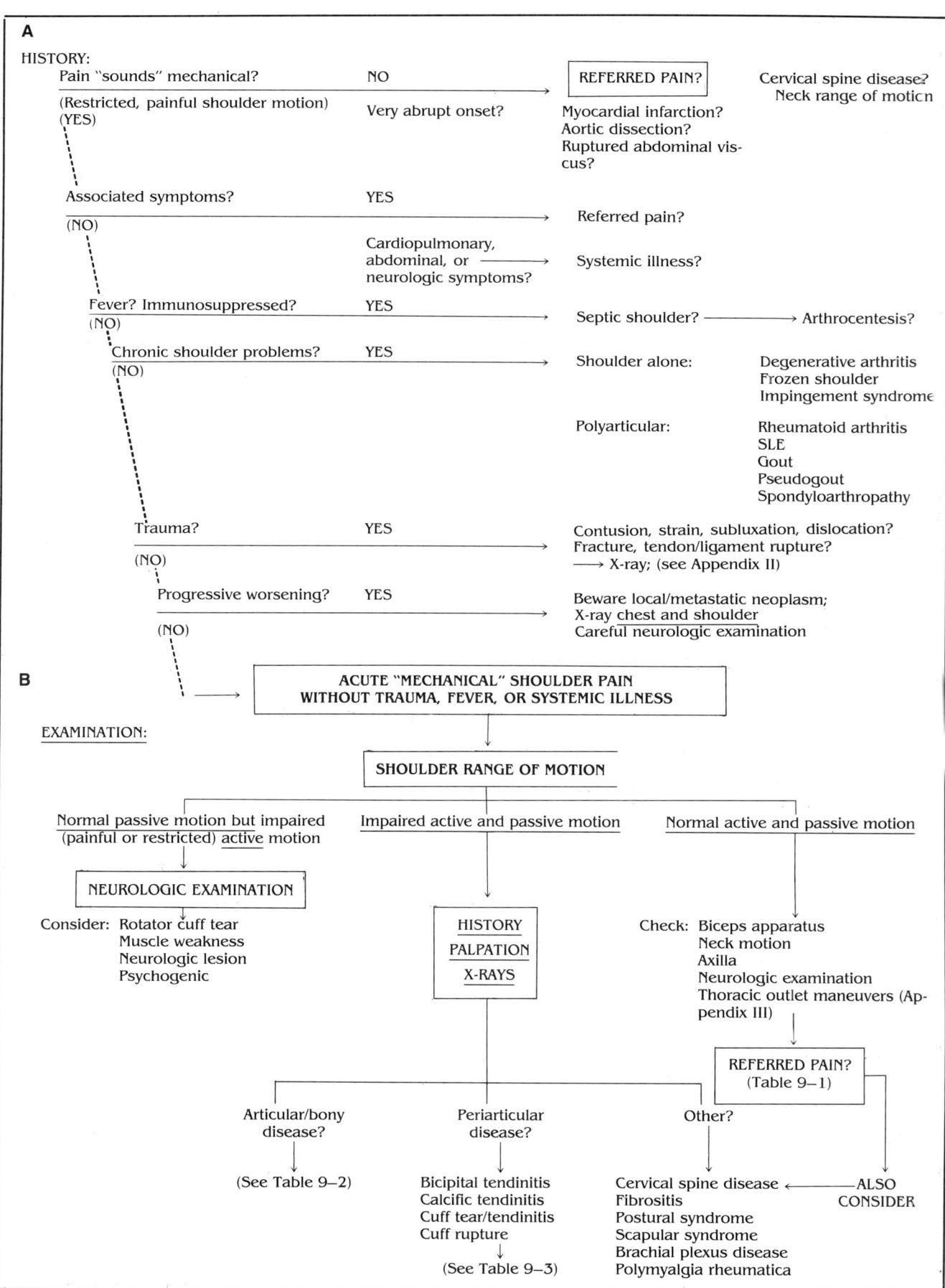

FIGURE 9–6. Diagnosis of acute shoulder pain.

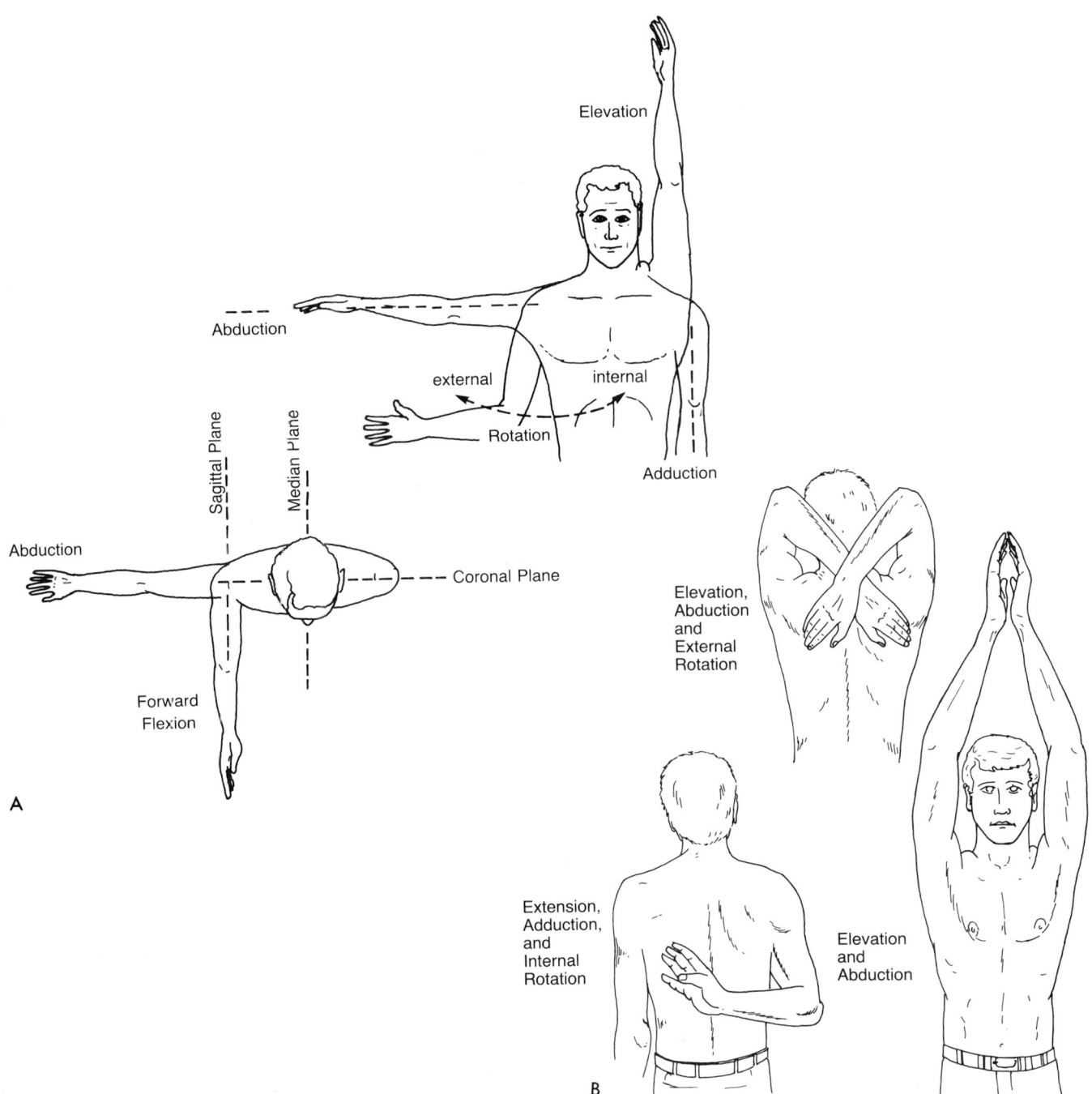

FIGURE 9–7. Shoulder range of motion. *A,* The planes of shoulder movement. *B,* Quick assessment of shoulder range of motion.

Such range-of-motion testing will reveal one of three results (Figure 9–6):

A. When active range of motion is full, symmetric, and painless, a primary mechanical shoulder disorder is less likely to be the source of pain, and a careful search for referred pain will be important.

   Especially important here are examination of the neck, axilla, thoracic outlet, and the neurologic findings (see below).

   Problems with the biceps apparatus may not impair the range of movement depicted in Figure 9–7, but further testing will be helpful here (see page 411).

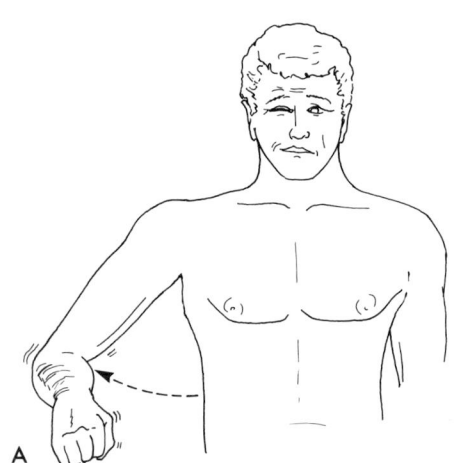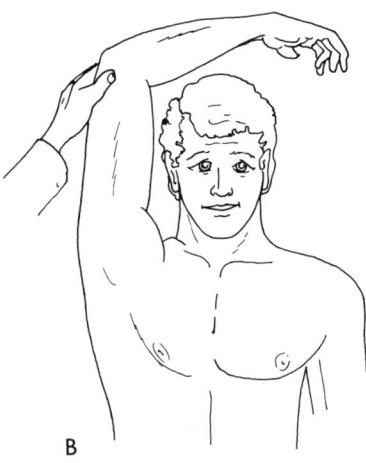

FIGURE 9–8. Active and passive range of motion. *A,* Impaired active range of motion. *B,* Normal passive range of motion (the examiner moves the shoulder).

B. When active range of motion is impaired or painful, passive range of motion should then be tested (Fig. 9–8).

The patient attempts to relax shoulder and arm muscles to allow the examiner to passively move the shoulder through the same arcs of motion, especially those noted to be impaired on active motion testing. Passive testing allows the examiner to ignore variations in the patient's own muscle power and, it is hoped, to detect whether impaired movement results from weakness rather than some mechanical restrictive pathologic condition (joint or bone disease or periarticular disorder—see page 404).

When passive range of motion is normal while active testing is abnormal (Fig. 9–6), a muscular disorder is most likely—this may represent primary musculotendinous weakness (tendon rupture, myopathy) or neurogenic weakness (see page 425).

C. When limitation of motion is demonstrated on both active and passive testing, attempts should be made to better localize the restrictive process.

First, decide whether the glenohumeral joint is the site of restriction by manually immobilizing the scapula while (actively or passively) abducting the shoulder (Fig. 9–9A). Since scapulothoracic motion (see Appendix I) alone can achieve almost 90 degrees of

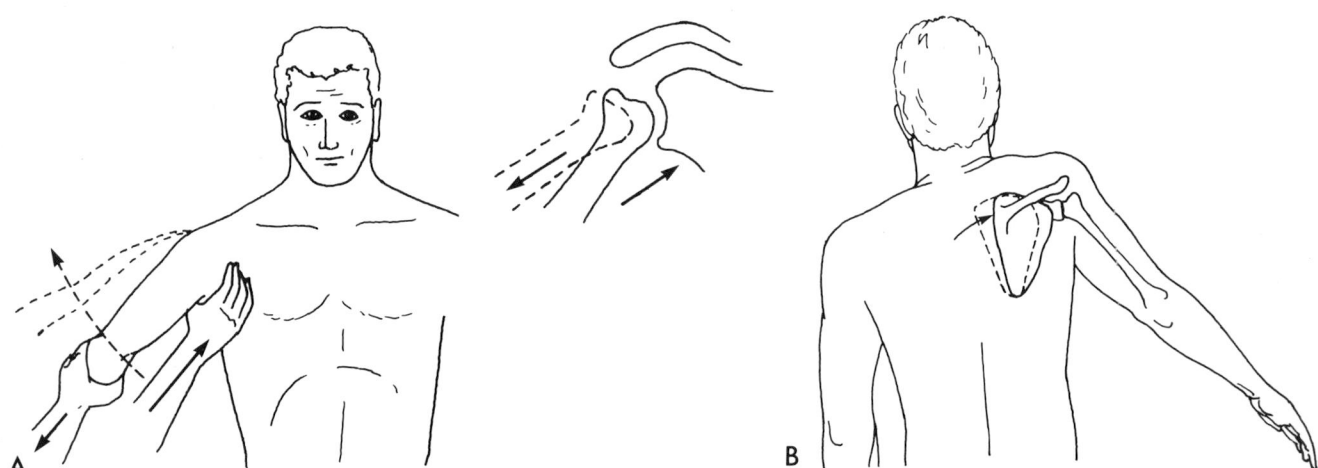

FIGURE 9–9. Assessment of shoulder motion. *A,* Immobilization of the scapula to assess glenohumeral motion. The scapula is stabilized so that glenohumeral movement alone can be examined. *B,* The "shoulder shrug," wherein the shoulder moves owing to scapular motion, not glenohumeral motion (see also Appendix I).

shoulder abduction even when the glenohumeral joint is frozen (the shoulder "shrugs" upward without glenohumeral motion—Figure 9–9B), immobilizing the scapula will help determine whether the glenohumeral joint is the site of restricted motion. When this maneuver suggests that the glenohumeral apparatus is restricted (the most common situation), then feel the structure of the shoulder as movement is undertaken. Bony or intra-articular restriction (due to degenerative arthritis,[12] most often) seems inflexible, and motion ends abruptly—"the bones block each other"; much more commonly, extra-articular restriction (due to periarticular disorders of tendons, bursae, and muscles—page 407) "gives" slightly with pressure and is restricted by pain and muscle spasm rather than palpable blockage. Simultaneous palpation for crepitus, local tenderness, and swelling will also be helpful (see below).

Thus, simple range-of-motion testing usually allows the examiner to distinguish mechanical from nonmechanical (referred) shoulder pain; often to differentiate musculotendinous (or neurogenic) weakness from structural restrictive disorders (see page 404); and sometimes to localize the site of this restriction to the glenohumeral joint itself or to the periarticular structures (see page 407). These diagnostic features are summarized in Figure 9–6.

Once range-of-motion testing has initially suggested one of these different possibilities, palpation of different shoulder structures can then provide further information.

> Sheldon sits on the examining table, arm at his side, elbow flexed, hand in lap. There is no obvious bony asymmetry of the shoulder or neck, and posture is otherwise normal. Attempted active range of motion of the shoulder elicits pain in the deltoid area at 60 degrees of abduction, 90 degrees of flexion, 60 degrees of extension, and 30 degrees of external or internal rotation. Passive range-of-motion testing elicits pain at similar positions, but there is no palpable blockage of motion, and the impression is that further motion is possible, but that pain is the limiting factor. Scapular immobilization suggests that glenohumeral movement is painfully limited, and much of Sheldon's shoulder motion involves scapular shrugging.

Thus active and passive range-of-motion testing here suggests a painful restrictive process involving the glenohumeral joint or periarticular structures.

II. Palpation of the shoulder: bones and muscles.[7]

Many important shoulder structures are not discretely palpable—the glenohumeral joint space and capsule, the rotator cuff muscles and tendons, the ligaments of the glenohumeral-coracoid apparatus. Nevertheless, some understanding of shoulder mechanics (see Appendix I) and familiarity with other palpable landmarks often permit indirect examination of even these impalpable structures. Moreover, many shoulder problems can be diagnosed by simple palpation and manipulation of superficial, palpable structures.

Brief visual inspection of the shoulder, neck, and arm should begin the examination. Careful inspection may detect localized muscle atrophy, structural asymmetry, abnormal posture, and localized swelling or deformity.

The lateral tip of the acromion is a helpful initial orientation point

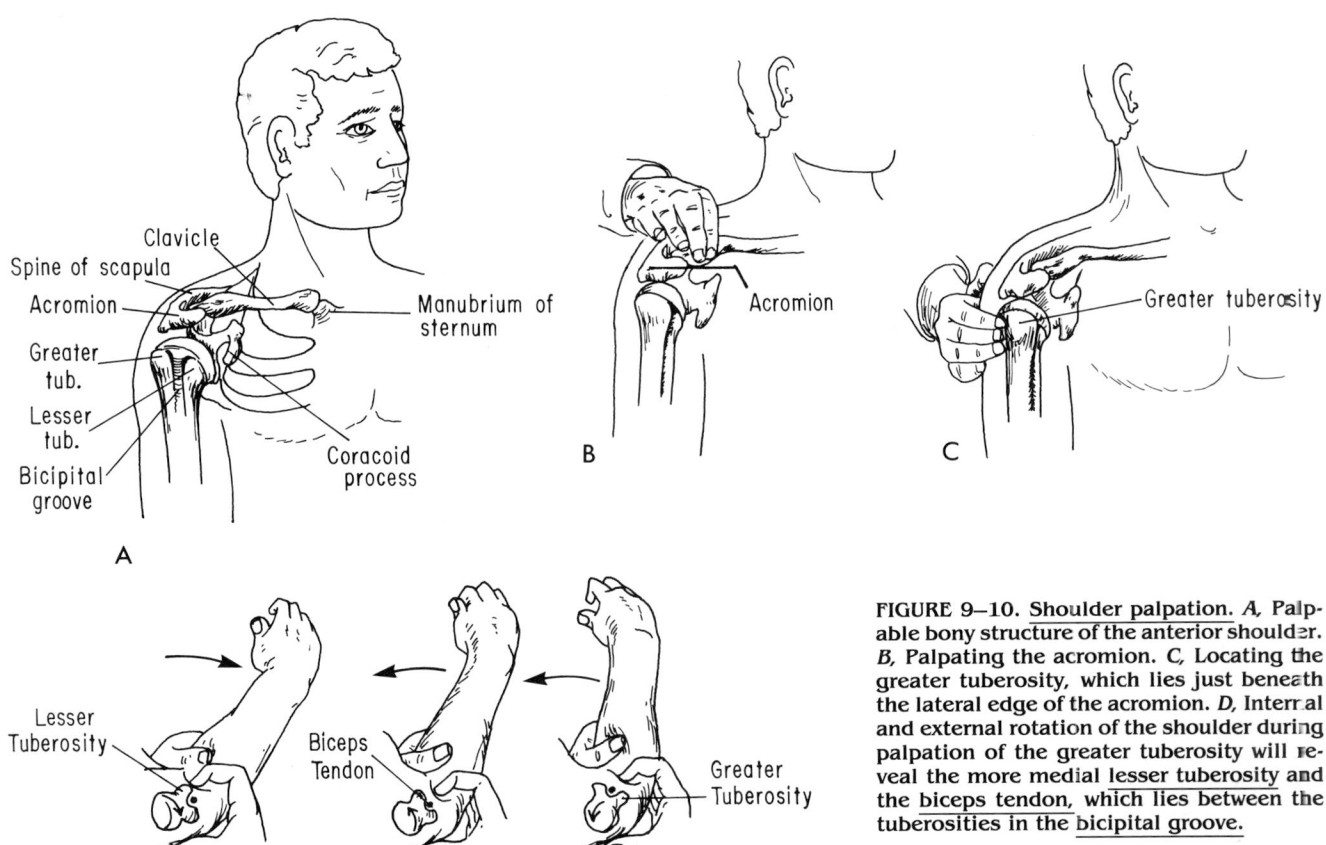

FIGURE 9–10. Shoulder palpation. *A*, Palpable bony structure of the anterior shoulder. *B*, Palpating the acromion. *C*, Locating the greater tuberosity, which lies just beneath the lateral edge of the acromion. *D*, Internal and external rotation of the shoulder during palpation of the greater tuberosity will reveal the more medial lesser tuberosity and the biceps tendon, which lies between the tuberosities in the bicipital groove.

for shoulder palpation (Fig. 9–10). The acromion is the triangular-shaped extension of the scapula that forms the bony hood of the glenohumeral shoulder joint. Immediately below the lateral acromion is the humerus, whose greater tuberosity lies about an inch below the acromial tip and which can be felt to rotate medially and laterally as the humerus itself is internally and externally rotated respectively. The lesser tuberosity lies an inch medial to the greater tuberosity, while the long head of the biceps tendon runs through the bicipital groove (the "valley") between these tuberosities. Since the rotator cuff muscles insert their tendons on these tuberosities (the supraspinatus, infraspinatus, and teres minor on the greater tuberosity; the subscapularis on the lesser tuberosity), palpation of this subacromial area allows direct or indirect examination of the key structures of the "suprahumeral joint" that are so commonly the cause of periarticular shoulder disorders (see page 407). One inch medial to the lesser tuberosity is the coracoid process of the scapula (where the short head of the biceps tendon and the pectoralis minor muscle insert).

Returning to our orientation point (the acromial tip), we can easily delineate other palpable structures: 1 inch medial to the acromial tip and 1 inch superior to the coracoid process is the acromioclavicular joint (where a slight depression can be felt and joint movement appreciated as the shoulder is abducted). Because of its superficial location, disorders of the acromioclavicular joint are usually easy to diagnose. Point tenderness over the joint (see Fig. 9–24) and palpable crepitus on movement of the joint will usually be apparent when acromioclavicular separation (see page 447) or acromioclavicular degenerative arthritis is the cause of shoulder pain. Often acromioclavicular pain is more prominent when the shoulder is abducted beyond 90 degrees (while most periarticular shoulder disorders cause pain at lesser degrees of abduction). Figure 9–11 illustrates one method of localizing pain and tenderness to the acromioclavicular joint.

The clavicle then runs medially from the acromioclavicular joint to the sternoclavicular joint, where the articulation of the medial clavicle and sternal manubrium can also be palpated during shoulder movement. The clavicle itself bows posteriorly (concave) at its lateral one third, while its medial two thirds are directed anteriorly (convex) before articulating with the sternum.

The scapula (Fig. 9–12) is best appreciated in all its peculiar shape and protuberances by returning again to the acromial tip. "Finger-follow" the acromial tip posteriorly and then medially as it becomes the scapular spine, a horizontal bony ridge that gradually fades beneath overlying musculature as it is followed medially toward the thoracic vertebrae. The scapular spine separates the upper scapula (where the supraspinatus muscle originates) from the lower scapula or shoulder blade (from which the infraspinatus and teres minor muscles originate).

These bony landmarks are partially obscured by overlying musculature, but even the heavily muscled shoulder usually allows accurate bony palpation. Palpation of the scapula and overlying muscles (see below) is especially important when shoulder pain is posterior.

Scapular syndromes are common but often go unrecognized (Fig. 9–12).

Figure 9–13 illustrates Cailliet's depiction of the origin and insertion of shoulder muscles. Only a few of these muscles are directly palpable (Figs. 9–12 and 9–14).

The deltoid muscle is the large, muscular hood of the shoulder that originates from the anterior, lateral, and posterior acromion (and the clavicle) and inserts into the upper one third of the humerus in its anterior, lateral, and posterior components. Shoulder flexion, abduction, and extension respectively allow palpation of these three components of the deltoid muscle.

As one moves medially from the acromion along the clavicle, the two heads of the sternocleidomastoid muscle are palpable at the sternoclavicular area—this muscle originates above from the styloid process behind the ear. The supraclavicular fossa—the location of important neurovascular structures (as well as the apex of the lung)—is thus bounded medially by the sternocleidomastoids, anteriorly by the clavicle, and laterally by the acromion. The posterior border of the supraclavicular space is formed by the large trapezius muscle, which blends with the deltoid anterolaterally along the clavicle and acromion, but is much more prominent itself along its posterior attachment to the spine of the scapula and its medial attachments to the cervicothoracic vertebral spine (Figs. 9–12 and 9–14*B*). The trapezius thus covers much of the posterior shoulder area. Rhomboid muscles can be palpated by having the patient adduct and internally rotate the shoulder (Fig. 9–7) while placing the hand behind the back (as if to fasten a bra). The patient then offers posteriorly directed resistance with this hand against the examiner's hand. The rhomboids will contract along the vertebal border of the scapula. Other palpable muscles form the borders of the axilla—ante-

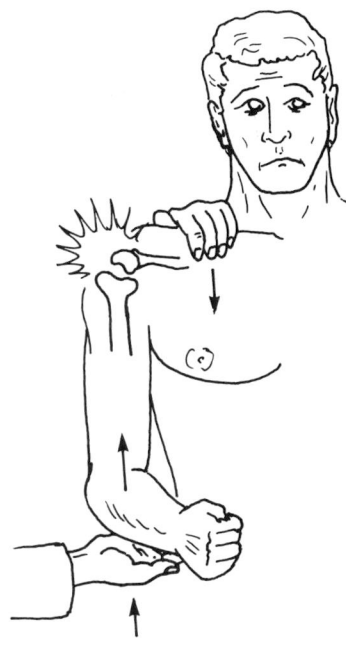

FIGURE 9–11. Elicitation of pain due to acromioclavicular disease. The clavicle is pushed down while the acromion is pushed up without moving the glenohumeral joint at all. The humerus is pushed vertically upward, along its longitudinal axis.

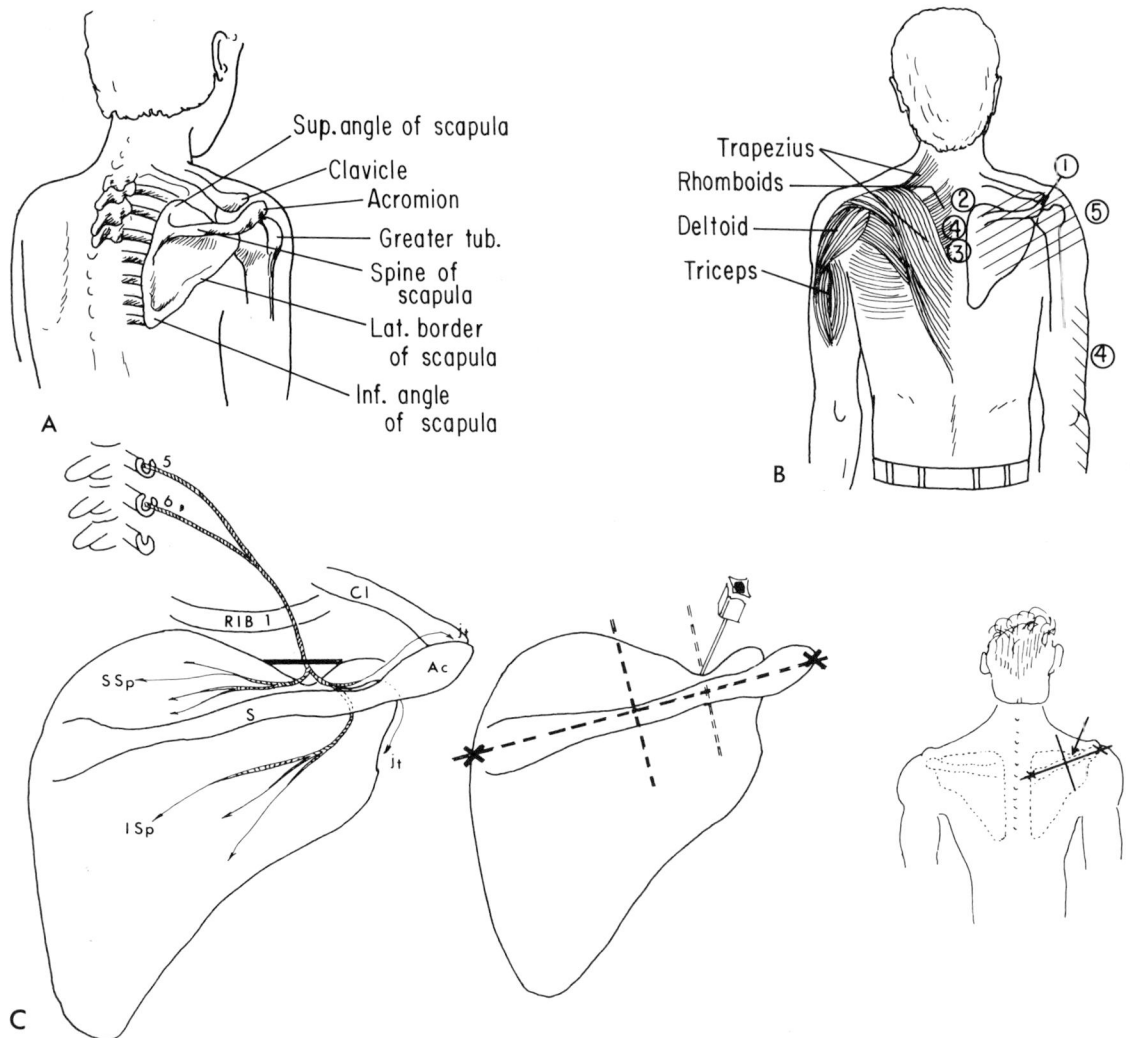

FIGURE 9–12. The scapula and "scapular syndromes."

A, The posterior aspect of the shoulder bone structure.

B, The posterior shoulder muscles (*left*) and the location of tenderness or pain in various scapular syndromes (*right*):

1. Disorders of the acromioclavicular joint may refer pain to the posterior shoulder.

2. Scapular spurs may develop at the superior scapular angle, resulting in a painful snapping as the scapula moves across the posterior chest wall during shoulder motion. Radiographic views of the scapula (including profile views) may reveal the bony spur at the superomedial scapular border. Resection of the spur will relieve the pain. Scapulocostal syndrome[13] is similar to the scapular spur syndrome, but a spur cannot be located. Here there is pain and tenderness at the superomedial scapular border, where the impalpable levator scapulae muscles insert (see Fig. 9–13). Local anesthetic infiltration, anti-inflammatory drugs, and occasionally a brief period of figure-of-8 shoulder harness (see Appendix II) will help in this case.

3. Scapulocostal tendinitis refers to (alleged) inflammation along the inner border of the medial scapula where the ribs abut the anterior scapula. Anesthetic injection of local points of tenderness will often relieve the pain that tends to occur with scapular motion. There is often tenderness along the medial scapular border. Local heat and exercise are also helpful.

4. Dorsal scapular nerve entrapment[14] may also cause pain along the medial scapula and lateral arm and forearm. Pressure over the anterior scalene muscle (in the supraclavicular fossa just lateral to the sternocleidomastoid muscle) will be tender and cause radiation of pain in a similar distribution.

5. Suprascapular nerve entrapment[15] may cause vague, diffuse pain over the posterolateral shoulder that tends to worsen when the affected arm is adducted across the anterior chest (to touch the opposite shoulder).[16] The suprascapular nerve innervates both the acromioclavicular and the glenohumeral joints, and thus temporary amelioration of shoulder pain by local anesthetic infiltration of this nerve is nonspecific.

C, Suprascapular nerve block. *Left*, The anatomy and course of the suprascapular nerve, originating from C5–6. The motor nerve to the supraspinatus, SS_p, and infraspinatus, IS_p, and the sensory branches to the acromioclavicular joint and the shoulder joint, jt, are shown. *Right*, Bisection of a line drawn along the scapular spine with the site of the groove and of needle insertion. (*C* reproduced with permission from Cailliet, R: Shoulder Pain. Philadelphia: F.A. Davis Co., 1966, p. 49.)

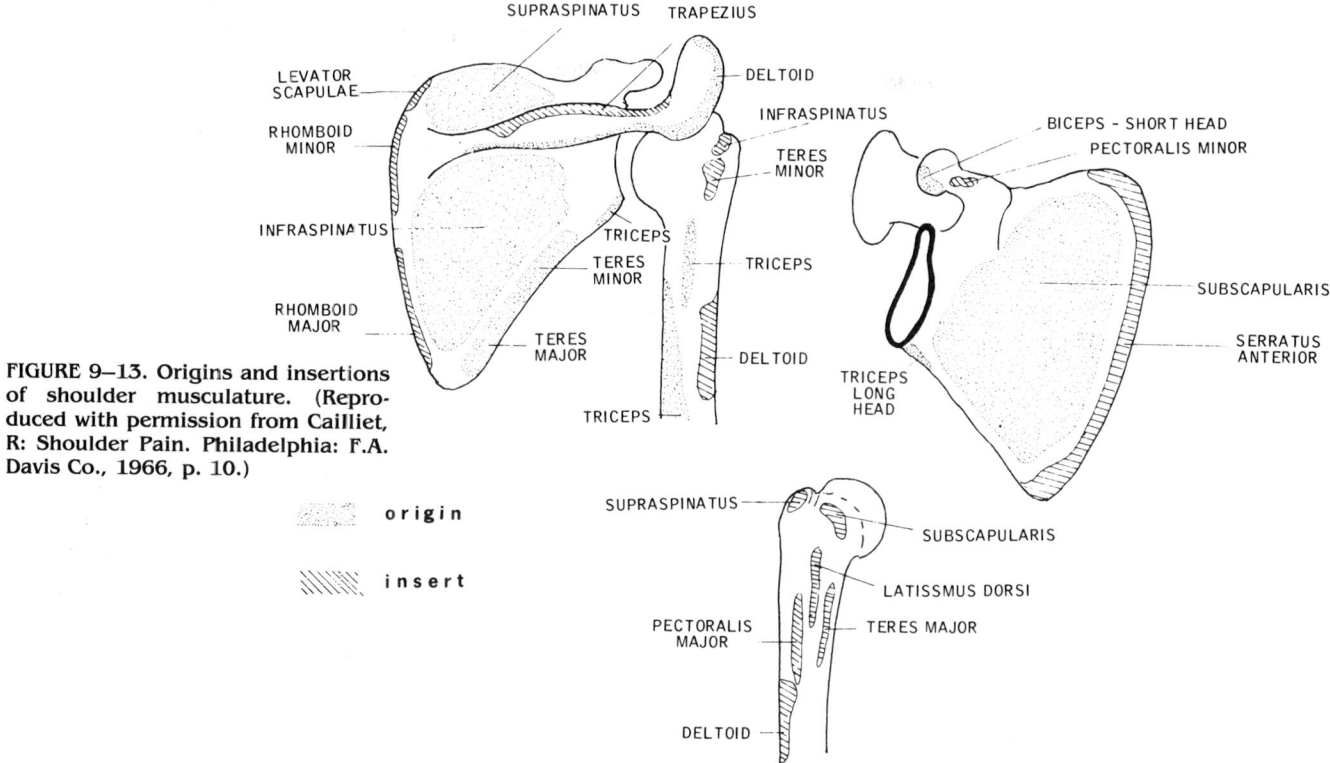

FIGURE 9–13. Origins and insertions of shoulder musculature. (Reproduced with permission from Cailliet, R: Shoulder Pain. Philadelphia: F.A. Davis Co., 1966, p. 10.)

origin

insert

riorly the pectoralis major; posteriorly the latissimus dorsi; and medially the serratus anterior, which overlies the rib cage (Fig. 9–14).

Familiarity with shoulder musculature is important for several reasons.

A. Fibrositis[17–20] is a poorly understood phenomenon.

Patients complain of shoulder pain and stiffness that are poorly

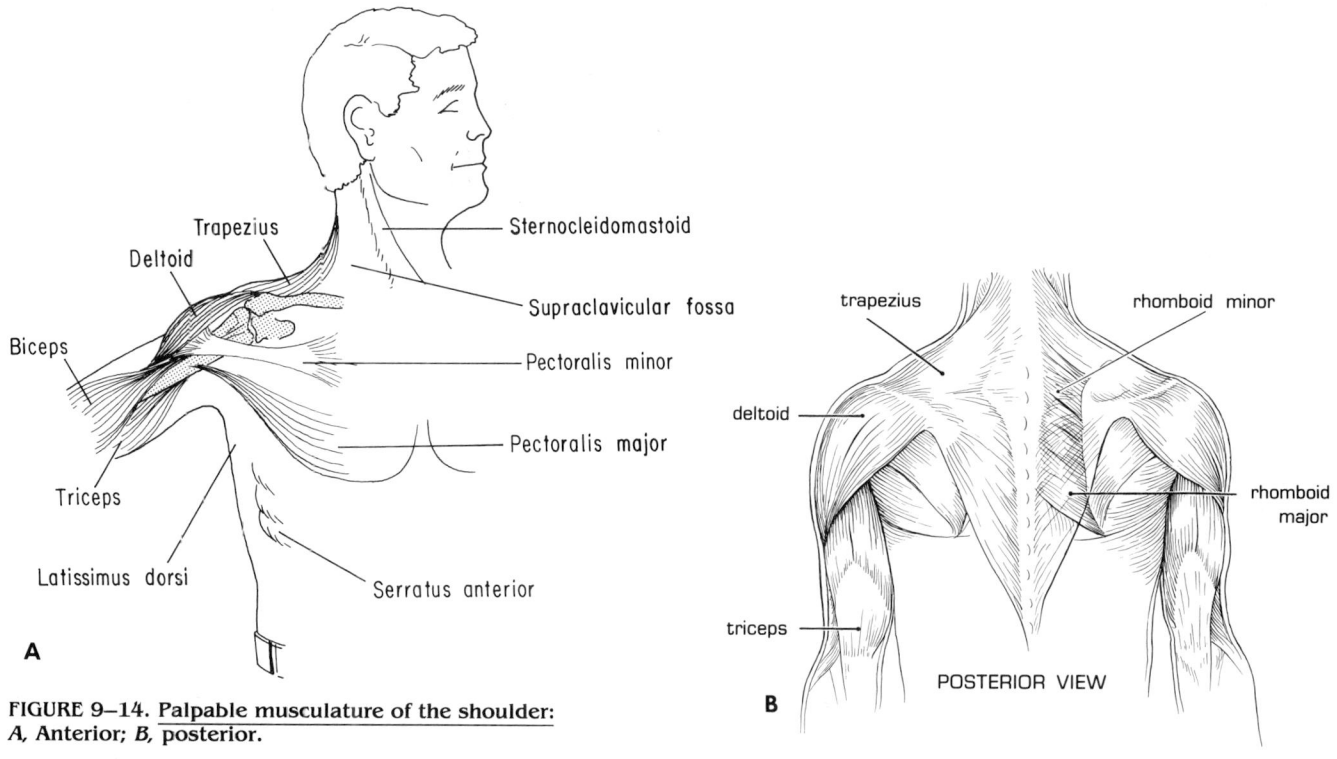

FIGURE 9–14. Palpable musculature of the shoulder: A, Anterior; B, posterior.

localized by history but that commonly involve the upper trapezius, medial scapular, and interscapular areas. A trigger point—an area of point tenderness (and sometimes induration or nodularity) whose palpation reproduces the pain—will be found in one or more of these areas. Direct instillation of a local anesthetic into the tender fibrositic nodule will often relieve the pain permanently.

Psychophysiologic complexities (and sleep disorders)[18] are common here, and a careful approach is important both to establish a correct diagnosis and to help the patient. Cervical spine disease very commonly accompanies fibrositis in these areas. Bennett's[18] approach to fibrositis is both comprehensive and balanced. Sometimes, tricyclic antidepressants are needed.[18]

B. Postural disorders are often responsible for vague neck, shoulder, and scapular discomfort or pain.

Examination is usually unremarkable, but local muscle tenderness may be noted (especially in the trapezius area). The slumped shoulder posture is a common denominator in the young and middle-aged (sometimes associated with poor general physical conditioning or depression) while degenerative kyphoscoliosis may cause similar problems in the elderly. Shoulder exercises (see page 420 and Appendix III), proper postural corrections (advising the secretary who sits hunched over the typewriter), and physiotherapy usually help.

C. Muscle weakness or paralysis, especially of the trapezius or serratus anterior muscle, may cause persistent shoulder discomfort because of the abnormal shoulder contours and mechanics that result.

Familiarity with motor examination of these specific muscle groups (Fig. 9–15) will allow quick assessment in recognizing scapular tilting (trapezius muscle weakness) or scapular winging (serratus muscle weakness). Lesions of the long thoracic nerve (C5-7) are not rare and will cause serratus anterior weakness.

In Sheldon's case:

Palpation of the shoulder reveals normal bony landmarks without localized tenderness of acromioclavicular or sternoclavicular joints or of the scapula, acromion, or humeral tuberosities. There is vague, poorly localized tenderness of the entire subacromial area anteriorly and laterally down to the midhumerus, but pointed palpation of the subacromial bursa, coracoid process, tuberosities, and biceps tendon does not indicate discrete tenderness. There is mild generalized tenderness of the deltoid and the trapezius muscles.

Thus palpation is not very helpful in Sheldon's case.

III. Neurologic examination.

Since disorders of cervical nerve roots, brachial plexus, and peripheral nerves may be the primary causes of shoulder pain (see page 431) since these structures can themselves be damaged secondarily by mechanical shoulder disorders—especially fractures and dislocations—(and since, as noted above, muscular weakness or imbalance may be the *cause* of disordered shoulder mobility), at least a brief screening neurologic examination of the upper extremities should be recorded in all patients with shoulder pain. Primarily because of the complexity of the brachial plexus, neurologic examination of the upper extremity can be confusing, even to the experienced neurologist. This examination is discussed in

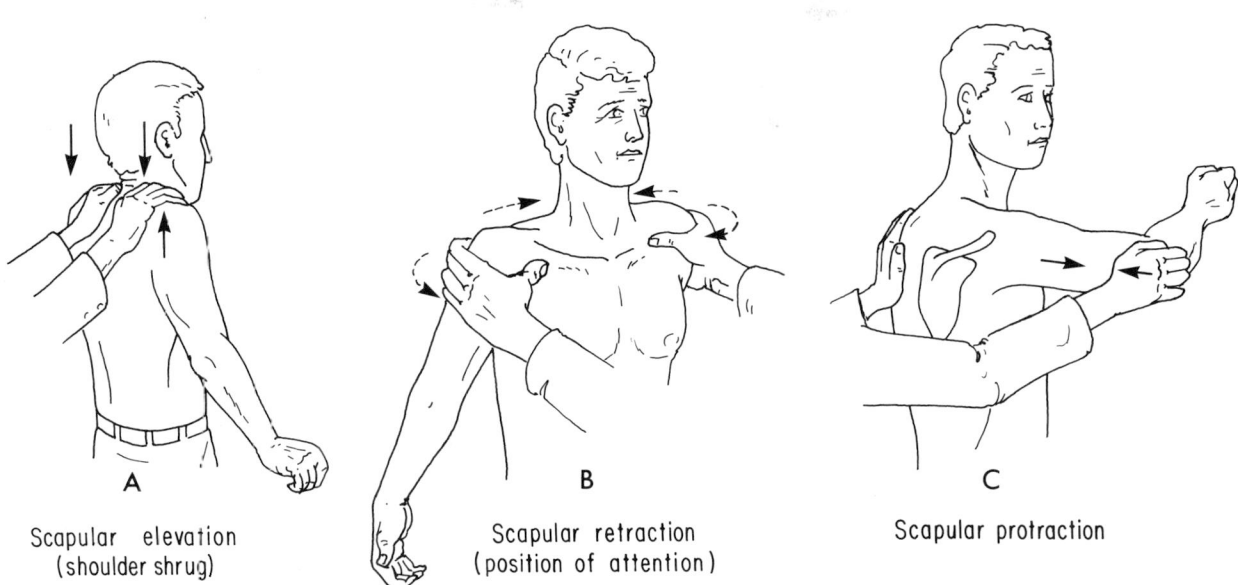

A
Scapular elevation
(shoulder shrug)

B
Scapular retraction
(position of attention)

C
Scapular protraction

FIGURE 9–15. Scapular muscle testing. *A,* Scapular elevation (shoulder shrug) requires movement of the trapezius (cranial nerve XI) and levator scapulae muscles (dorsal scapular nerve, C3–5). Unilateral weakness will cause scapular "tilting"—an "asymmetric shrug." *B,* Scapular retraction (position of attention) involves movement of the rhomboids (dorsal scapular nerve, C5); the examiner attempts to "break" the position of attention. *C,* Scapular protraction (reaching) involves movement of the serratus anterior muscle (long thoracic nerve, C5–7). Weakness causes the scapula to "wing"—a hollow appears along its vertebral border (where the examiner's hand rests in the figure).

greater detail beginning on page 431, but a screening neurologic examination should always include:

A. Range of motion of the neck (Fig. 9–2)—to detect cervical spine disorders, which are the usual cause of neurologic problems in the shoulder (see also page 427).

B. Muscle testing of the trapezius and serratus anterior (Fig. 9–15) as well as brief examination of motor strength of the deltoid, biceps, triceps, wrist extensors and flexors, and digits (see also page 435).

When mechanical shoulder disorders are painful, muscle testing of the upper arm—especially around the deltoid, trapezius and biceps—may be impossible, i.e., limited by pain. Since weakness of muscle groups distant from the shoulder (for example, triceps or wrist) should not occur with uncomplicated mechanical shoulder disorders, a brief examination of these muscle groups is always important.

C. Deep tendon reflexes—the biceps (C5), brachioradialis (C6), and triceps (C7).

D. Sensory examination should be informed by anatomic knowledge of both spinal dermatomes and peripheral nerves (see page 434).

Comparison of light touch on selected areas of each arm and hand is sufficient.

In most patients, this screening examination—muscle testing against resistance, reflexes, and brief sensory (touch) analysis—can be performed in just 2 minutes. While muscle weakness or limitation does not always imply a primary neurologic disorder, abnormal reflexes or sensation should not occur with uncomplicated mechanical shoulder disorders—hence, reflex or sensory abnormalities (or weakness distant from the painful shoulder, as above) raise important diagnostic questions (see p. 426).

CONSIDER

> Neck range of motion is normal. Palpation of the supraclavicular space and axilla are normal. Shoulder shrug (trapezius muscle) and deltoid muscle testing are difficult because of Sheldon's pain, but motor testing, reflexes, and touch sensory examination of the upper extremity are otherwise normal.

What does this mean?

1. Acute mechanical shoulder pain is apparently the problem. Pain that is clearly related to shoulder motion and associated with restricted movement usually excludes referred pain as a consideration. (An exception is when spasm of the shoulder musculature occurs in response to some local nonmechanical disorder—for example, a primary neurologic event or a local mass. There is, however, no evidence of such a disorder here.)

2. The mechanical disorder appears to involve the glenohumeral apparatus and could be either articular or periarticular. Since passive range of motion is as consistently painful and limited as active range of motion, muscle weakness alone is not the problem. The glenohumeral apparatus has been implicated by immobilizing the scapula during the examination and demonstrating that pain and restriction do apparently involve the glenohumeral apparatus.

3. There is no compelling reason to consider a primary articular (or bony) disorder here. Glenohumeral arthritis[12] or bone disease would be unusual in a healthy, middle-aged patient with no history of trauma, fever, chronic shoulder disability, or polyarthritis and when there is no insidiously progressive history suggestive of neoplastic disease (Fig. 9–6). Some of the common articular and bony disorders of the shoulder are enumerated in Table 9–2 and Figures 9–16 through 9–21. (Detailed discussion is beyond the scope of this text.) It can be seen that the clinical history and examination, together with shoulder x-rays, will usually exclude (or implicate) such disorders. When infection or neoplasm is clinically suspected, but the x-ray is nondiagnostic, a bone scan will usually help.

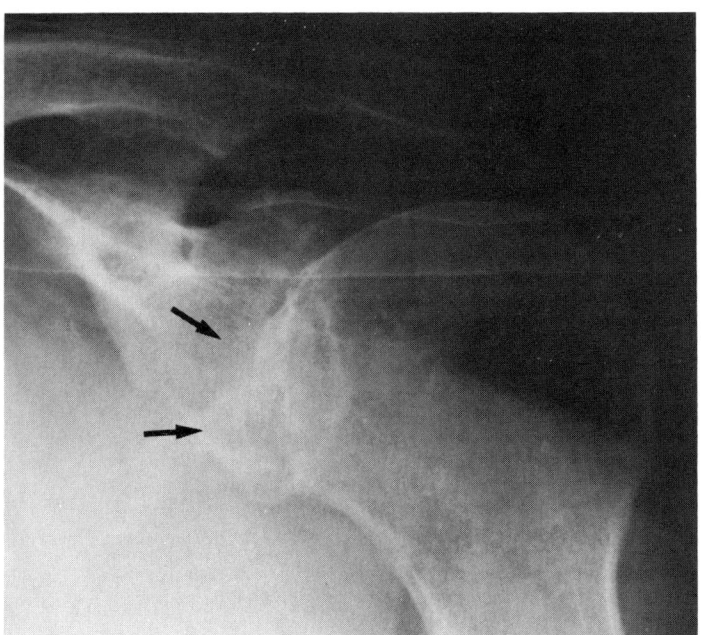

FIGURE 9–16. Degenerative arthritis of the glenohumeral joint. Note that the joint space is obliterated by proliferative sclerotic bone bridging the glenohumeral joint (arrows). This 60-year-old man described progressively worsening limitation of left shoulder mobility over several years. There was a prior history of recurrent shoulder dislocations.

TABLE 9–2. SOME ARTICULAR AND BONY DISORDERS OF THE SHOULDER

DIAGNOSIS	CLINICAL CLUES	CONFIRMATION
Degenerative arthritis		
Glenohumeral	Older patient;* history of trauma; bony restriction on examination	X-ray (Fig. 9–16)
Acromioclavicular	Palpable crepitus and point tenderness of acromioclavicular joint (Fig. 9–24); chronic history; prior dislocation?	Examination; x-ray may or may not help.
Sternoclavicular	Palpable crepitus and point tenderness of sternoclavicular joint; history of trauma; chronic symptoms	Examination; x-ray often not helpful.
Aseptic necrosis of humeral head	Underlying disease: Steroid therapy; diabetes; systemic lupus; sickle cell disease; renal transplant; alcoholism	X-ray (Fig. 9–17)
Trauma		
Fracture	History	Examination; x-ray
Dislocation	History	Examination; x-ray
Subluxation	History	Examination; x-ray
Bacterial arthritis	Fever; extreme tenderness; extremely limited motion	Joint aspiration (Fig. 9–5)
Inflammatory arthritis		
Gout	Male, usually; history of podagra and/or polyarthritis; diuretic therapy?	Clinical setting; arthrocentesis: uric acid crystals
Pseudogout	Elderly patient; X-ray: chondrocalcinosis	Clinical setting; arthrocentesis: calcium pyrophosphate crystals
Rheumatoid arthritis	Longstanding polyarticular involvement	Clinical setting; serologic tests; arthrocentesis; x-ray changes (Fig. 9–18)
Other connective tissue disease (e.g., SLE)	Clinical symptom complex	Clinical setting; serologic tests; arthrocentesis; x-ray changes
Paget's disease		X-ray (Fig. 9–19)
Neoplasms[35]		
Primary, benign Chondroblastoma Giant cell tumor Aneurysmal bone cysts Others	Insidious history; constant, progressively worsening pain	X-ray changes; exploration for tissue diagnosis
Primary, malignant Osteogenic sarcoma Ewing's sarcoma Others	Insidious history; constant, progressively worsening pain	X-ray changes (Fig. 9–20); exploration for tissue diagnosis
Malignant, systemic Lymphoma Metastatic neoplasm	Insidious history; constant, progressively worsening pain; history of malignant disease	X-ray changes (Fig. 9–20); clinical setting; bone scan
Multiple myeloma	Insidious history; ESR; anemia	Bone marrow study; serum and protein electrophoresis; x-ray (Fig. 9–21)

*Degenerative arthritis in the younger patient is almost always post-traumatic, but it should also (rarely) suggest a neuropathic joint, ochronosis, sickle-cell disease, Gaucher's disease, or hemophilia.

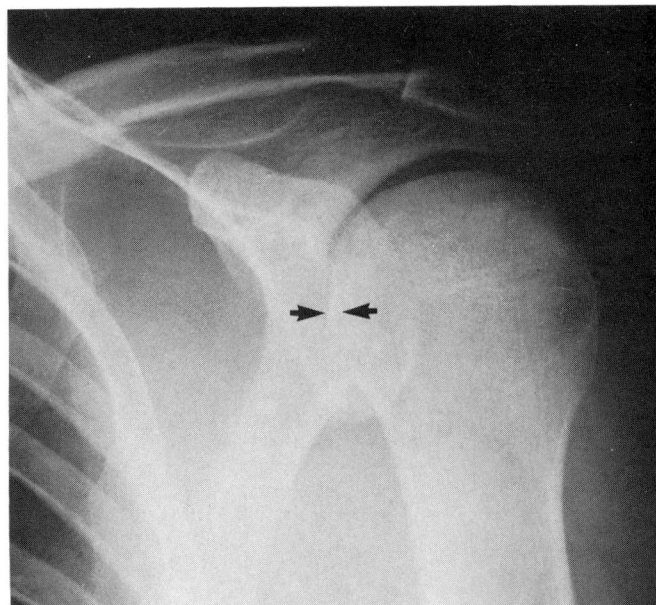

FIGURE 9–17. Aseptic necrosis of the humerus. This 39-year-old woman, on high-dose corticosteroids for systemic lupus erythematosus, developed subacute severe left shoulder pain. The x-ray demonstrates flattening of the humeral head on its medial side, parallel to the long axis of the humerus (arrows).

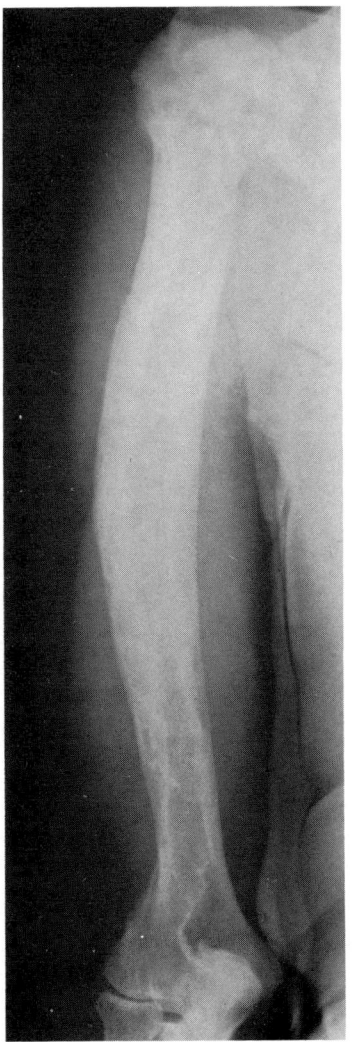

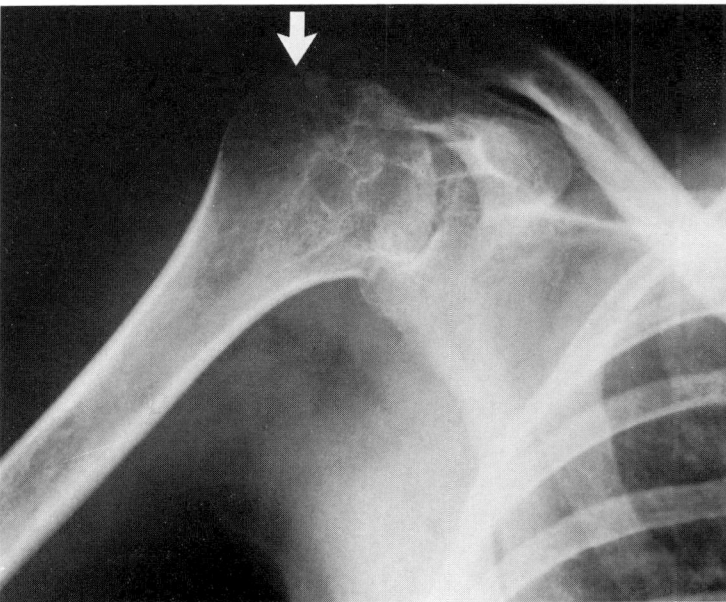

FIGURE 9–18. Rheumatoid arthritis of the shoulder. X-ray demonstrates marked joint space narrowing, cystic destruction of the humeral head (arrow) and marked periarticular osteopenia. This joint was one of many involved in this patient with severe polyarticular rheumatoid arthritis.

FIGURE 9–19. This 72-year-old man described progressive pain in the right shoulder and along the entire course of the upper arm. X-ray demonstrates extensive osteoblastic changes characteristic of Paget's disease.

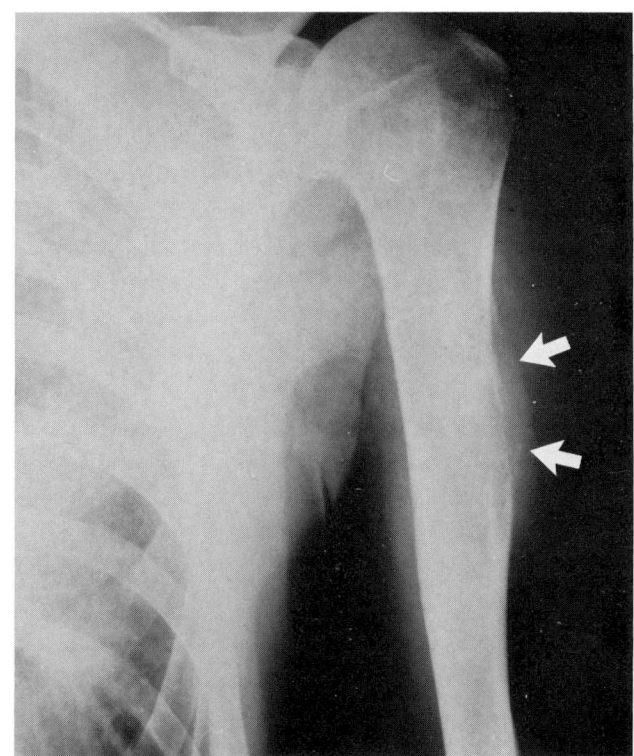

FIGURE 9–20. Malignant neoplasm of the humerus. This 64-year-old man with worsening left shoulder pain was originally thought to have a primary neoplasm of the shaft of the humerus. Subsequent evaluation demonstrated that this was, in fact, a metastatic lesion (*arrows*) from a primary carcinoma in the lung.

4. Thus, in Sheldon's case, an acute periarticular disorder is most likely. Acute periarticular disease probably accounts for 90 per cent of acute nontraumatic shoulder pain.

PERIARTICULAR SHOULDER DISORDERS

The musculotendinous and other soft-tissue structures that surround the glenohumeral joint comprise a complex, interdependent group of mechanisms that are tightly packed into one small area that has been (mis)named the suprahumeral "joint." In fact not a joint at all, this space (Fig. 9–22) is bounded by the glenoid fossa medially, the humeral head inferiorly, and the

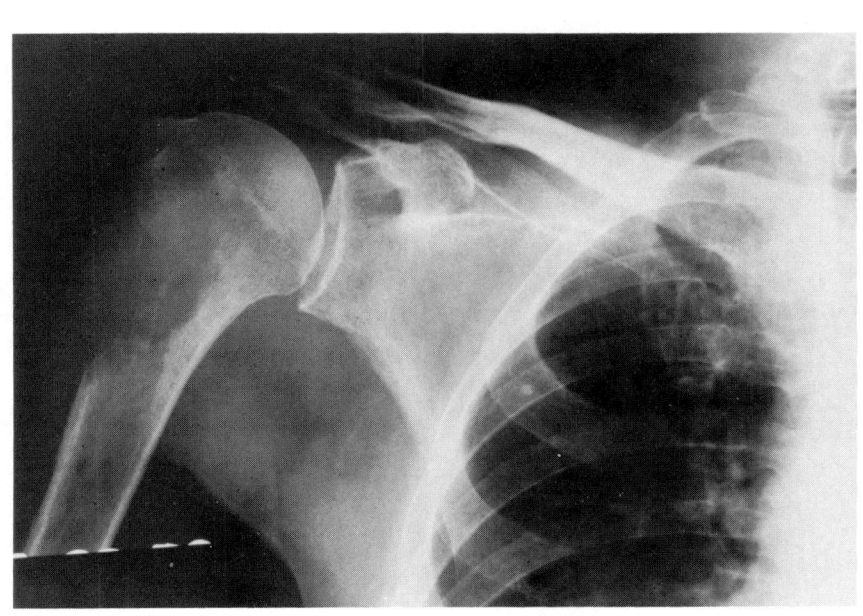

FIGURE 9–21. This 72-year-old woman complained of insidious, progressively worsening right shoulder pain. X-ray demonstrates extensive bony destruction of the proximal humerus. Multiple myeloma was diagnosed and treated.

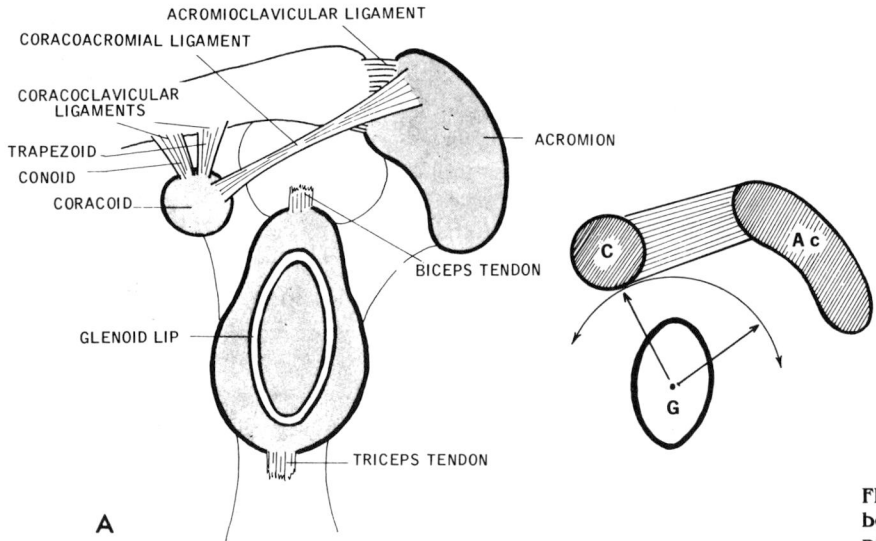

ACROMIOCLAVICULAR LIGAMENT
CORACOACROMIAL LIGAMENT
CORACOCLAVICULAR LIGAMENTS
TRAPEZOID
CONOID
CORACOID
GLENOID LIP
ACROMION
BICEPS TENDON
TRICEPS TENDON

A

C   Ac

G

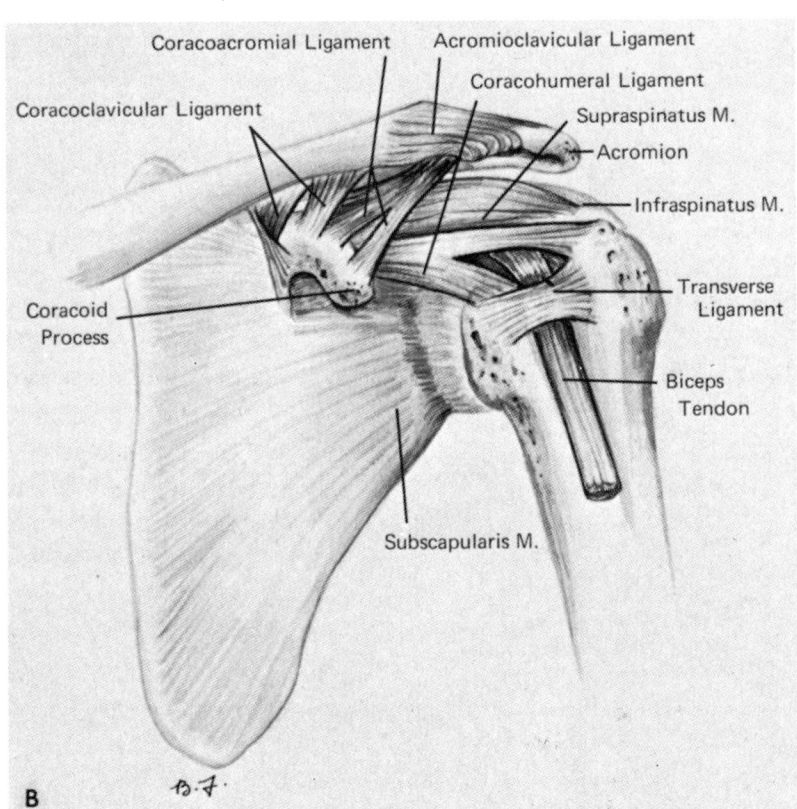

Coracoacromial Ligament
Coracoclavicular Ligament
Coracoid Process
Acromioclavicular Ligament
Coracohumeral Ligament
Supraspinatus M.
Acromion
Infraspinatus M.
Transverse Ligament
Biceps Tendon
Subscapularis M.

B

FIGURE 9–22. The suprahumeral joint. A, The bony acromiocoracoid arch. The diagram depicts the shape of the glenoid fossa and its relationship to the acromial process, the coracoid process, and the coracoacromial ligament. In essence, this diagram shows the socket of the glenohumeral joint and portrays the relationship of the suprahumeral "joint."

B, The ligamentous and muscular structures of the suprahumeral "joint." (*A,* reproduced with permission from Cailliet, R: Shoulder Pain. Philadelphia: F.A. Davis Co., 1966, p. 3; *B* reproduced with permission from DePalma, AT: Surgery of the Shoulder, 2nd ed. Philadelphia, J.B. Lippincott Co., 1973, p. 59.)

acromion, coracoacromial ligament, and coracoid process superiorly, while the deltoid muscle occupies its lateral aspect. This suprahumeral space includes several important structures:

1. The superior aspect of the glenohumeral joint capsule and its associated glenohumeral ligaments (not depicted in Fig. 9–22).

2. The long head of the biceps tendon, which traverses the groove between the tuberosities, invaginates the synovial capsule (but remains extra-articular) and inserts into the superior glenoid fossa.

3. The tendinous insertion of the rotator cuff muscles (see also Fig. 9–13).

4. The subacromial bursa, which interposes itself between the underlying

supraspinatus muscle and the overlying coracoacromial ligament, acromion, and deltoid (Fig. 9–23). The subcoracoid bursa is probably not a separate structure from the subacromial bursa—both are said to comprise the subdeltoid bursa—but the subcoracoid aspect of this bursa separates the deep subscapularis muscle from the overlying coracoid process and coracoacromial ligament.

5. Interposed fatty and connective tissue.

Relationships among these structures are schematically outlined in Figures 9–22 and 9–23.

With the exception of acute shoulder injuries that may directly or in-

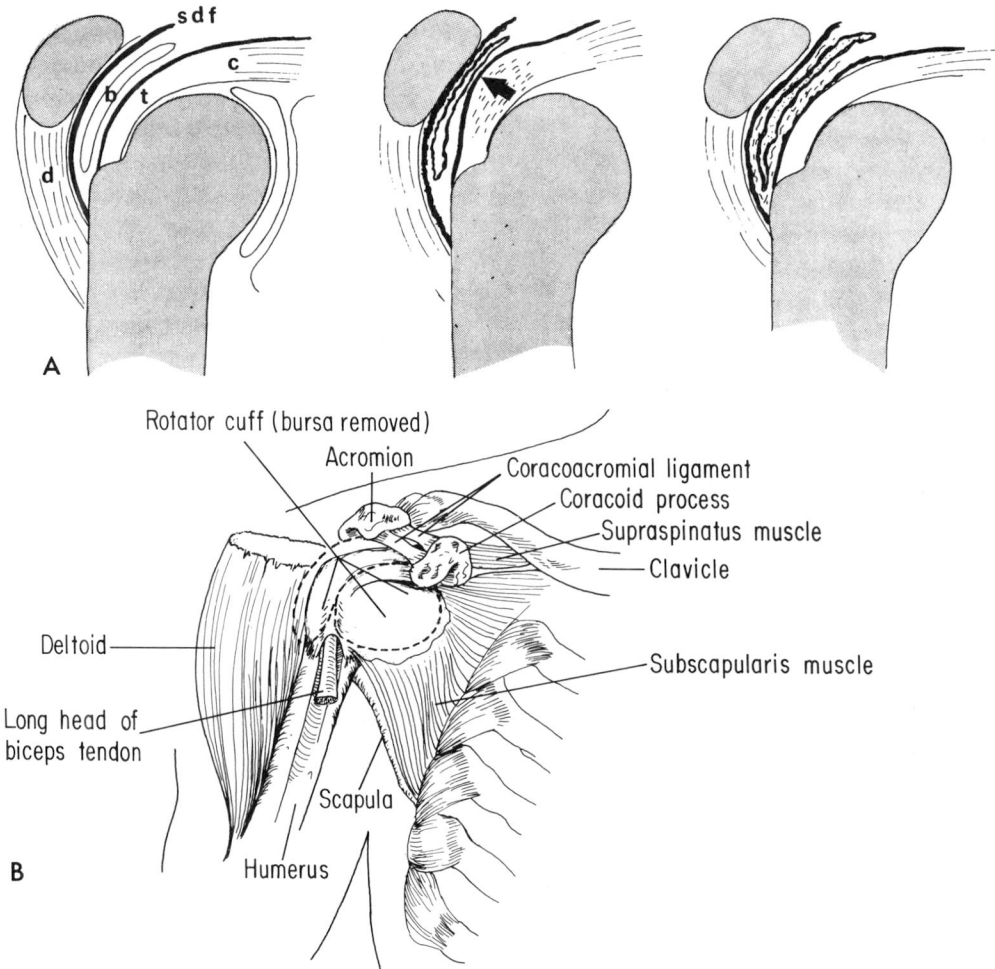

FIGURE 9–23. Acute tendinitis and inflammation of contiguous structures. *A,* Cailliet's depiction of suprahumeral inflammatory conditions, originating in the rotator cuff tendons and "spreading" to involve the subdeltoid bursa and fascia. (A), The tissues contained between the rotator cuff, **c,** and its tendons, **t,** and the subdeltoid fascia, **sdf,** lining the undersurface of the deltoid muscle, **d.** The subdeltoid fascia is rich in blood vessels and sympathetic nerves that originate in the stellate ganglia. Between the subdeltoid fascia and the fascia covering the cuff is loose connective tissue within which is located the subdeltoid bursa, **b.** (B) Acute bulging of the tendon compresses and causes inflammation and swelling of the fascial tissues and the bursa. This is the acute mechanical phase, during which there is severe pain and mechanical limitation of motion. (C) The bulging of the tendon has subsided, but the resultant fascia and bursal inflammation persists, causing stiffness of the shoulder. (A) can go to (B) and then to (C) and reverse through the entire phase back to (A). The tendon remains frayed, and degenerative changes remain.

B, The rotator cuff. The subdeltoid bursa (dotted lines) has been "removed," the deltoid muscle has been retracted posteriorly, and the pectoral muscles have been eliminated. The economy of space in the suprahumeral area is obvious here—difficulty in precise anatomic localization of inflammation (*A*) and tenderness (Fig. 9–24) is understandable. (*A* reproduced with permission from Cailliet, R: Shoulder Pain. Philadelphia: F.A. Davis Co., 1966, p. 39.)

directly damage these structures, most periarticular disorders arise when overuse or misuse of the shoulder is superimposed on an ongoing degenerative process within the rotator cuff, biceps apparatus, or both. These degenerative changes are probably universal and occur as a natural aging phenomenon,[21] (analogous to the wear and tear degenerative arthritis of the hip and knee) and probably underlie most clinical cases of calcific tendinitis, subacromial bursitis, and rotator cuff tendinitis, tears, and ruptures (see below).[22] Aging (as well as minor repetitive traumatic events over the years) results in a loss of strength and elasticity of the cuff tendons—often in a "critical zone" where local ischemia may contribute—with resulting attrition, susceptibility to tears, and often calcific scarring. Superimposed stretching or unaccustomed overuse of these structures may then result in tearing (or complete ruptures) or inflammation of these tendons, the overlying subacromial bursa, and, sometimes, the contiguous biceps tendon as well. Precise pathogenesis of these different events remains controversial,[23] but these facts, as well as the extreme economy of space within the suprahumeral joint, emphasize several important facts.

Diagnosis

1. Most of these problems occur in the middle-aged. Young patients with periarticular shoulder disorders usually have a clear history of recent trauma or indirect injury.

2. Figure 9–23 demonstrates that, while each structure in the suprahumeral area may be damaged or inflamed individually, often several structures are involved simultaneously. Subacromial bursitis, for example, is only rarely a primary phenomenon (as in gout, tuberculosis, sepsis, rheumatoid arthritis) and usually results from primary inflammatory changes in the rotator cuff or biceps tendons.

3. It is sometimes difficult to precisely distinguish one syndrome from another (see Table 9–3), since there is so much structural overlap and contiguous inflammation. Figure 9–24 illustrates the close relationship of various periarticular structures that may be tender on examination.

4. Nevertheless, physical examination following a careful history, and sometimes with the use of x-rays, will often allow the examiner to make a specific anatomic diagnosis.

The most common syndromes include the following (see Table 9–3):

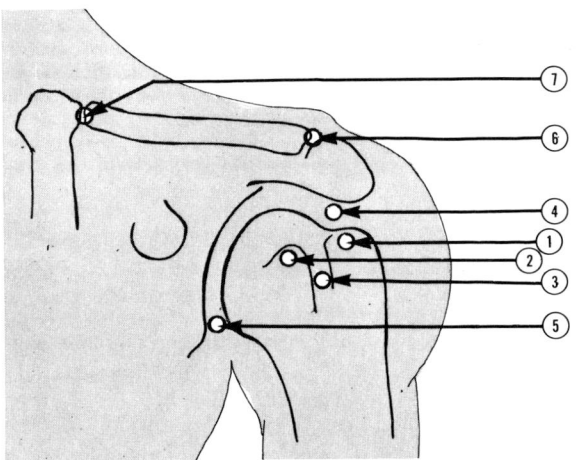

FIGURE 9–24. Palpable areas of tenderness of the shoulder. 1, The greater tuberosity and the site of supraspinatus tendon insertion. 2, Lesser tuberosity, site of subscapularis muscle insertion. 3, Bicipital groove in which glides the bicipital tendon. 4, Site of the subdeltoid bursa. 5, Glenohumeral joint space. 6, Acromioclavicular joint. 7, Sternoclavicular joint. (Reproduced with permission from Cailliet, R: Shoulder Pain. Philadelphia: F. A. Davis Co., 1966, p. 41).

I. Bicipital tendinitis[24, 25] refers to inflammation of the long head of the biceps tendon.

The acute disorder usually follows some form of minor trauma—strenuous or prolonged biceps exercise (shoveling, for example) or a fall on the elbow—but the patient may be unaware of any such event. Pain is usually localized to the anterior and inner aspect of the shoulder but may radiate to the biceps, forearm, or even the neck or scapula. Sleeping on the shoulder is often painful. Diagnosis depends on physical findings, which usually include:

A. Tenderness on palpation of the bicipital groove (Figs. 9–10, 9–24, and 9–25A).

B. Pain during maneuvers that specifically stress the long head of the biceps tendon. Yergason's test (Fig. 9–25A) is most helpful here.

The patient's arm relaxes at the side with the elbow flexed to 90 degrees. The patient is asked to forcefully supinate the forearm against the examiner's active resistance. Precipitation of (usually

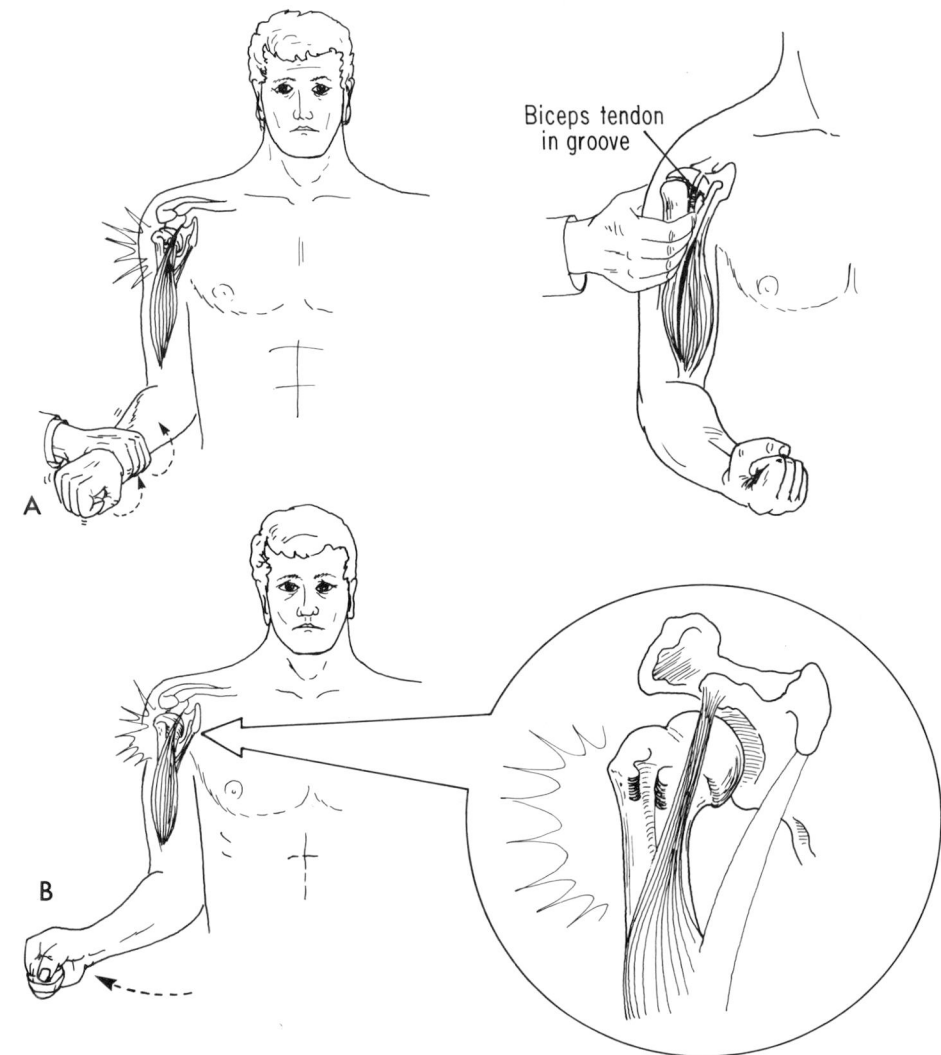

FIGURE 9–25. *A*, Bicipital tendinitis. Pain along the anterior shoulder will be precipitated by palpation of the biceps tendon within the bicipital groove and/or by the Yergason test—the patient attempts to supinate the forearm against resistance (the shoulder is not moved at all during this maneuver).

B, Bicipital subluxation. External rotation of the shoulder, against resistance, will precipitate subluxation of the biceps tendon (medially) out of the bicipital groove (inset) in susceptible patients.

anterior) shoulder pain suggests inflammation of the biceps tendon. (Note that this maneuver does not require any true shoulder motion).

Yergason's test also refers to a maneuver that will diagnose recurrent biceps tendon subluxation (Fig. 9–25B), which is occasionally the cause of tendinitis. The examiner palpates the bicipital groove as the patient forcefully externally rotates the shoulder against resistance with the elbow flexed and the arm at the side. Recurrent subluxation (the tendon slips out of the bicipital groove) will be palpable as the biceps tendon moves (painfully and) medially during this maneuver. (Note that this maneuver does move the shoulder and may cause pain when other periarticular disorders are the problem. See below.)

C. Relatively painless and full shoulder range of motion.

If there is isolated inflammation of the biceps tendon, shoulder range of motion (Fig. 9–7) may be normal. Contiguous inflammation of the subdeltoid bursa or other suprahumeral structures is common, however, and range of motion is often impaired.

Treatment of bicipital tendinitis includes brief rest (a few days in a sling), anti-inflammatory drugs, and early mobilization with exercise therapy (see below). Corticosteroid injections (20 to 40 mg prednisone equivalents) directly into the tendon sheath are sometimes necessary (see Fig. 9–28). Conservative therapy is usually quite effective (see page 416), and surgery is rarely necessary unless bicipital subluxation is the primary problem.

Another bicipital disorder that may cause acute shoulder pain is acute rupture of the biceps tendon. In young patients this is unusual unless there is very forceful injury. In the older patient, rupture may occur spontaneously or during mild biceps exercise (lifting, for example). A sudden snapping pain down the upper arm with visible/palpable distal bulging of the ruptured muscle mass above the antecubital fossa constitutes the typical clinical picture.

Surgery is usually not undertaken in the elderly patient unless severe pain and dysfunction persist (this is unusual). In the young athlete, surgical repair is indicated, usually as soon as possible.

II. Calcific tendinitis/"bursitis."[23, 26, 27]

This entity is often incorrectly called subacromial or subdeltoid bursitis. In fact, as we have seen, degenerative and inflammatory processes in the rotator cuff are probably the primary problem, with the overlying bursa involved only secondarily (Fig. 9–23). This entity usually afflicts patients between the ages of 30 and 50 years when calcific deposits form at sites of prior inflammation or degeneration in the rotator cuff (the supraspinatus tendon most often). These deposits are often asymptomatic when small and not impinging upon the overlying tendon fibers or bursae (Fig. 9–23). (Asymptomatic calcifications noted radiographically are common at this stage.) Gradual growth of the calcific deposits, frictional trauma against the overlying acromion during arm motion, or sudden strain may then induce further acute or subacute inflammatory reactions that cause pain and dysmobility. There are two distinct syndromes:

A. The subacute syndrome is most common.

Pain is initially felt intermittently during sudden movements of the shoulder, especially abduction and rotation, but then gradually increases in severity (over several days to weeks) until muscle spasm results in more severe and painfully limited motion. These episodes will resolve spontaneously, only to recur again and again.

B. The acute syndrome (Fig. 9–26) begins quite abruptly, sometimes in the middle of the night, and severe, painful limitation of motion is obvious from the start.

There is usually exquisite point tenderness (Fig. 9–10 and 9–24) over the subacromial bursa (which is tensely draped over the inflamed calcific deposit—Figure 9–23) or over the greater tuberosity (where the most commonly involved tendon—the supraspinatus—inserts). Abduction and rotation are most seriously impaired, but all shoulder motions may be restricted and painful. Spontaneous resolution will usually occur after 1 to 2 weeks, but therapy is almost always necessary since the pain and limitation are so severe.

Treatment of calcific tendinitis involves the usual conservative measures (see page 416).

Local injection therapy is probably more effective here than in all of the other periarticular disorders. Needle aspiration of the swollen subdeltoid bursa is worth a try, since occasionally calcific debris can be aspirated, but more often the needle simply decompresses the tensely swollen bursa. Especially when there is highly localized and very painful point tenderness, local injection of 20 to 40 mg corticosteroid can be attempted (see Fig. 9–28).

Surgical therapy is rarely necessary.

III. Rotator cuff tendinitis/tear.[28]

The distinction between calcific tendinitis/bursitis and this entity is partly semantic. In each, the suprahumeral space is inflamed, and rotator cuff tendons are involved. Previous (symptomatic or asymptomatic) attritional degeneration of the cuff tendons may be the antecedent

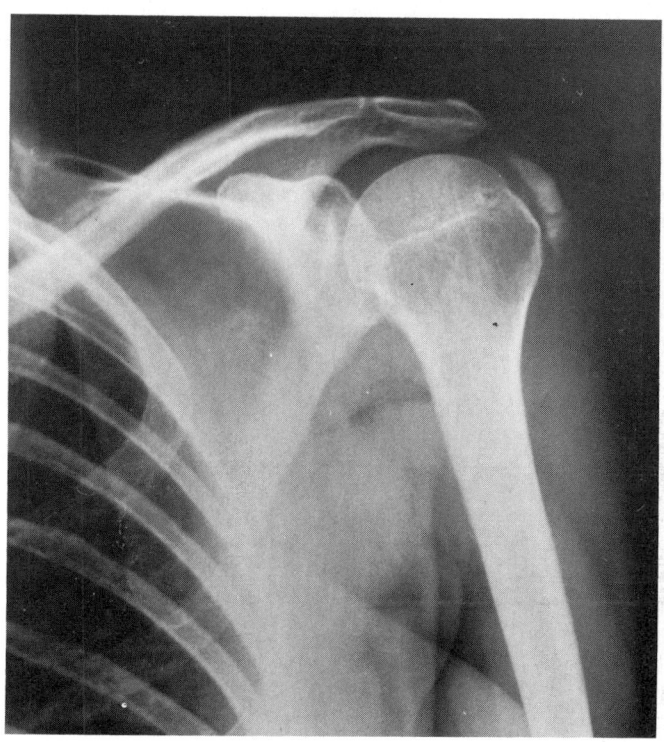

FIGURE 9–26. Calcific tendinitis. This 42-year-old man complained of acute onset of extremely severe shoulder pain, associated with marked tenderness of the subacromial area and extremely painful limited range of motion. The x-ray reveals extensive calcification of the suprahumeral space.

pathologic event in each, while overuse or unaccustomed shoulder exercise in the middle-aged patient is a common precipitant of the acute process.

Rotator cuff tendinitis here refers to one of two syndromes. The first is a clinical syndrome identical to calcific tendinitis, but without visible calcification on x-ray. (In other words, the absence of x-ray calcification by no means excludes tendinitis/bursitis.) The second syndrome is an incomplete traumatic tear of the rotator cuff tendon(s)—a fall on the outstretched arm or a forceful abduction/external rotation injury to the shoulder is a common mechanism of such injury. In each syndrome there is limitation of shoulder motion (especially abduction and external rotation) as well as tenderness of the subacromial area, sometimes precisely localized over the specific tendon insertion (the greater or lesser tuberosity).

Tendinitis or incomplete rotator cuff tear usually heals uneventfully with simple conservative therapy (page 416). Frank rupture of the rotator cuff often requires surgery, however. The key diagnostic feature that distinguishes full cuff rupture from a partial tear is the degree of shoulder weakness demonstrated on neurologic examination (see below). Very often, pain and muscle spasm around the shoulder will inhibit shoulder motion to such an extent that it is not possible to accurately assess motor strength of the shoulder girdle in these situations. Infiltration of a local anesthetic directly into the painful area will temporarily eliminate local pain and muscle spasm so that motor function can be more precisely assessed.

Often, careful examination a few days after the initial encounter allows more precise diagnosis, when conservative therapy has reduced swelling, local tenderness, and muscle spasm. When there is any question about the distinction between tendinitis and more severe rotator cuff injury, the patient must be examined again a few days later.

IV. Rotator cuff rupture.[29–32]

Rotator cuff rupture refers to a full-thickness tear of the musculotendinous apparatus, sometimes involving all cuff muscles, more often involving just the supraspinatus or subscapularis. Such massive cuff ruptures are somewhat uncommon but usually present with a very typical history: A fall on the outstretched arm or sudden weighted hyperabduction injury results in immediate "tearing" pain in the shoulder that may lessen over the next few hours (perhaps because of capsular hemorrhage), only to recur with a vengeance 6 to 12 hours later, with associated marked loss of shoulder power. Examination usually reveals severe pain and tenderness of the cuff tendon insertions, marked weakness of shoulder abduction, and (sometimes) a cracking/popping sensation on palpation of the moving shoulder joint. Experienced examiners are sometimes able to actually palpate the cuff tear.

Lesser tears of the cuff may also produce marked disability, however, and some authorities believe that the site and extent of tear are not so important as is the mechanical relationship of the cuff muscles with the deltoid (see also Appendix I). Manual laborers or athletes with powerful deltoid action may be disabled by small cuff tears; the sedentary adult with less developed shoulder musculature may tolerate a larger cuff tear with less apparent disability; and vice versa. The point is that, while it may be difficult to distinguish clinically different degrees of cuff injuries, Moseley's warning pertains:

Any patient, especially 50 years of age or older, who has a forceable strain or fall injuring the shoulder, and who suffers pain with inability to abduct the arm and whose x-ray is negative for fracture, dislocation, or calcium deposits has almost certainly a rupture of the rotator cuff.[33]

It must be remembered that the strain may be quite minor, especially in the elderly, and the brief fall or momentarily painful heavy lifting may not even be recalled by the patient. Major trauma need not occur to raise suspicion of a serious cuff tear in the elderly, but such a trauma history is usually present in the young.

Arthrography is necessary to diagnose tears and ruptures of the rotator cuff. Demonstration of extravasation of contrast material from the glenohumeral joint into the subdeltoid bursa is diagnostic of rotator cuff tear (Fig. 9–27, A through D). An orthopedist should be consulted when cuff rupture is suspected.

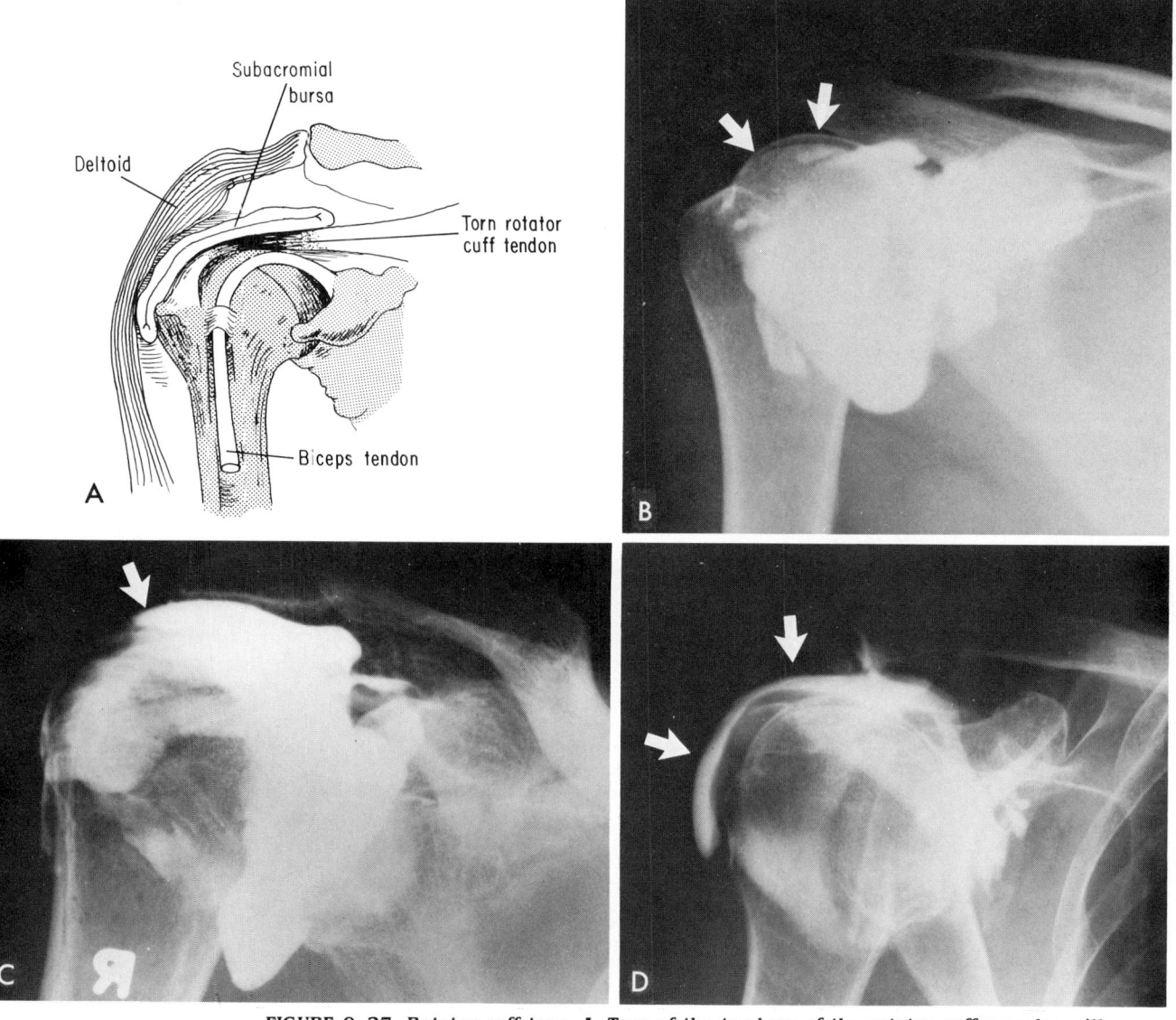

FIGURE 9–27. Rotator cuff tear. A, Tear of the tendons of the rotator cuff muscles will cause inflammation of the overlying subacromial (subdeltoid) bursa or communication of the glenohumeral joint space with the bursa or both. B, The normal arthrogram demonstrates dye filling the glenohumeral joint (where the dye is injected) but not communicating into the subdeltoid bursa (arrows). C, D, This patient sustained a fall on his outstretched arm and complained of inability to use his shoulder. Examination revealed normal passive range of motion but markedly impaired active abduction. The arthrogram reveals extravasation of dye into the suprahumeral space (arrow) and dye outlining the entire subdeltoid bursa (arrows). Surgical repair was successful.

The young patient with an obvious complete rupture of the rotator cuff confirmed by arthrography will often undergo surgery immediately, especially if complete use of that shoulder is crucial to the patient's occupation. Results of surgical therapy are, in general, good, but an experienced orthopedist is always conservative about the indications for operative repair.[34] The elderly patient, even with a severe rotator cuff tear, may be managed conservatively unless ongoing painful disability persists. In general, conservative therapy of even complete ruptures of the rotator cuff probably does not prevent a good surgical result (i.e., successful operation may be undertaken months after the injury).

Table 9–3 enumerates some of the differential diagnostic points in evaluating acute periarticular shoulder disorders.

Further examination of Sheldon's shoulder reveals no abnormality of the biceps apparatus, and Yergason's test is negative. The acromioclavicular joint appears normal. Sheldon is able to hold his shoulder at 60 degrees of abduction, but only with extreme pain. Anteroposterior, lateral, and axillary x-ray views of the shoulder are normal.

NOTE

The clinical picture here does not precisely conform with any of the specific syndromes—either periarticular or articular—discussed above. This is not uncommon, since there is a broad spectrum of severity of each of these lesions, and clinical overlap among them is frequent.

While the patient will be treated for a presumed periarticular inflammatory process, it should be remembered that a precise diagnosis has not been documented (yet).

Treatment

Pain Relief. Analgesics are usually necessary, especially during the first few days of acute calcific tendinitis or bicipital tendinitis. In such instances,

TABLE 9–3. MUSCULOTENDINOUS (PERIARTICULAR) DISORDERS OF THE SHOULDER

	HISTORY	EXAMINATION	X-RAYS	POSSIBLE SEQUELAE
Bicipital tendinitis	Anterior shoulder pain; biceps stretch, exercise, or overuse	Tender bicipital groove; Yergason's test*; shoulder range of motion may be normal	Normal	Subacute/chronic tendinitis; tendon rupture; frozen shoulder
Calcific tendinitis	Recurrent (subacute) episodes and/or sudden, acute syndrome of pain and tenderness in subacromial area	Extremely painful point tenderness (Fig. 9–24); limited abduction/ rotation; shoulder power normal (but pain renders testing difficult)	Calcific deposit	Impingement syndrome; ruptured rotator cuff; frozen shoulder; chronic tendinitis (see p. 423)
Rotator cuff tendinitis/tear	History of overuse, fall, or shoulder distraction	Limitation of motion; tenderness over tendon insertion; shoulder power normal (can maintain abduction)	Normal	Impingement syndrome; ruptured rotator cuff; frozen shoulder; chronic tendinitis (see p. 423)
Massive cuff rupture	Fall; sudden abduction trauma; severe pain— temporarily better, then worse	Severe pain and limitation of motion; cannot maintain abduction even when pain-free (prominent shoulder weakness)	Normal (but arthrography is diagnostic)	Marked disability if not repaired

*Exclude recurrent biceps subluxation (Fig. 9–25B).

narcotics are not infrequently required, but, after the first several days, potent analgesics are rarely necessary and should be avoided.

Local anesthesia, via needle infiltration of periarticular structures with topical anesthetics, is often helpful but may also be abused. Local injections are most helpful when acute calcific tendinitis is associated with severe, reproducible point tenderness. (As discussed above, occasionally local anesthetic infiltration is a helpful diagnostic maneuver when pain and muscle spasm so limit shoulder mobility that range-of-motion testing will not allow adequate examination of the rotator cuff.)

When topical anesthetic agents or corticosteroids are injected into periarticular structures (Fig. 9–28)—a common practice in the treatment of calcific tendinitis, fibrositis, scapular syndromes, and acromioclavicular joint disease—the patient must be warned that the immediate pain relief derives from the local anesthetic, but that pain may recur within just a few hours after injection. The corticosteroid is usually the main therapeutic ingredient (and often requires 24 to 48 hours to take effect). An exception is the patient with fibrositis—the local anesthetic alone will often be therapeutic.

Anti-inflammatory Measures. In the first 24 to 48 hours, ice packs are probably as effective as any drug. Early application of local heat may stimulate vasodilatation and actually increase local swelling and pain. After the first 2 to 3 days, local heat is often soothing and may have mild therapeutic benefit.

Since the natural history of most of these entities is that of slow but spontaneous resolution, the argument is often advanced that anti-inflammatory drugs are superfluous. However, anecdotal experience suggests that anti-inflammatory drugs are useful as analgesics (alone or in combination with primary analgesics) and allow more comfortable exercise therapy, presumably by reducing local edema and inflammation. There is no controlled scientific

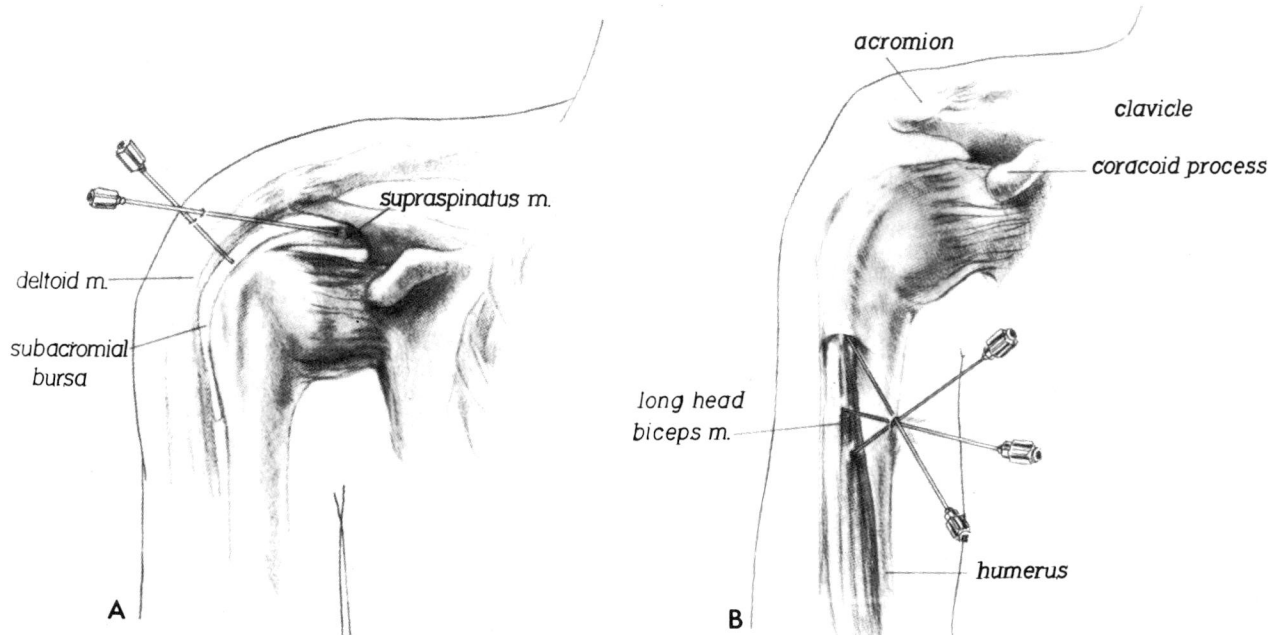

FIGURE 9–28. Injection therapy. A, Diagram of subacromial bursa and supraspinatus tendon injection. The precise area of point tenderness (Fig. 9–24) is usually injected first, followed by injection of the anatomic site of the bursa and/or the anatomic course of the involved rotator cuff tendon. B, Diagram of bicipital tendon sheath injection. The long head of the biceps tendon is carefully palpated, and injection into the (superficial) sheath of the tendon is then performed. (Reproduced with permission from Owen, DS: Aspiration and injection of joints and soft tissues. In Kelley, WN, Harris, ED, Jr, Ruddy, S, and Sledge, CG: Textbook of Rheumatology. Philadelphia: W. B. Saunders Co., 1981, p. 565.)

documentation of this or of the value of locally injected corticosteroids as primary anti-inflammatory therapy.[36] Aspirin is the least expensive oral drug (see Table 1–4) and is usually as effective as most of the other nonsteroidal anti-inflammatory drugs.[37] Short courses of oral corticosteroids (6-day Medrol Dosepak) are more often dramatically effective and are favored here when acute periarticular disease is the diagnosis (and when there are no contraindications to oral steroids).

Injections. As noted above, injection of corticosteroids locally is occasionally helpful. Strict aseptic technique is essential. Repeated tendon injections should be avoided, since tendon rupture may result.

(Intra-articular injection into the glenohumeral joint (Fig. 9–5) is never necessary in the treatment of these extra-articular disorders, yet such practices are not uncommon,[38] and may be associated with serious complications.[39, 40] Occasionally the patient with rheumatoid arthritis will benefit from intra-articular injection when shoulder involvement is the limiting problem, despite systemic anti-inflammatory therapy [this is rare]. Similarly the patient with intractable degenerative arthritis of the glenohumeral or acromioclavicular joints may occasionally benefit from intra-articular steroid therapy. In general, familiarity with needling the glenohumeral joint is important only when septic arthritis must be excluded by arthrocentesis or when arthrography is performed.)

Exercise Therapy.[8, 22] When to rest the painful shoulder and when to exercise it are a common source of confusion (and error). In general, mobilization of the shoulder should be begun as early as possible in acute, nontraumatic periarticular disorders. (Traumatic injuries usually require different and specific durations of immobilization as primary therapy—see Appendix II.) A compromise must be struck: Further damage to inflamed/torn tissues by "too early" active exercise therapy must be avoided, but restitution of full shoulder use as soon as possible is a high priority. Thus the difference between (and timing of) passive exercise therapy and active exercise therapy must be clearly understood by physician and patient.

Passive shoulder exercises (Fig. 9–29) involve moving the glenohumeral joint through its full range of motion without active contraction of any of the musculotendinous structures of the shoulder girdle (some of which are inflamed, torn, or in spasm as a result of the primary process). If properly performed, these passive exercises should not instigate further damage or inflammation and, thus, can be initiated very early (within the first 48 hours). In the patient with a severely painful shoulder (usually acute calcific tendinitis) an arm sling may be helpful during the first few days, but daily passive exercises should be encouraged, nevertheless. As illustrated in Figure 9–29, Codman's pendulum exercises allow multidirectional movement at the glenohumeral joint without active use of the shoulder girdle itself. Precise directions here, preferably with a demonstration, are crucial. A posture must be assumed that allows the arm and hand to dangle freely, perhaps with the hand holding a light weight, such that the arm may move side to side, forward and back, and then circularly, simply by the action of the patient's trunk and legs (and without the use of the shoulder itself). True passive movement must be emphasized here, since improper performance of these exercises will hurt the tender, swollen periarticular structures.

(When pendulum exercises cannot be performed — by the very elderly patient in a wheelchair, for example—a wall-climbing exercise may be done passively, but, again, careful instructions are crucial. The patient faces the wall and, using only the muscles of the hand and forearm, "climbs the wall"

FIGURE 9–29. Passive glenohumeral exercises. Pendular glenohumeral exercise (so-called Codman exercises). 1, the posture to be assumed to permit the arm to "dangle" freely, with or without a weight. 2, The arm moves in forward-and-back sagittal plane, in forward and backward flexion. Circular motion in the clockwise and counterclockwise directions is also done in ever-increasing large circles. 3, The front view of the exercise showing lateral pendular movement actually in the coronal plane. The lower right diagram shows the effect of gravity, G, upon the glenohumeral joint, ghj, with an immobile scapula, s. The p-to-p arc is the pendular movement. (Reproduced with permission from Cailliet, R: Shoulder Pain. Philadelphia: F. A. Davis Co., 1966, p. 45.)

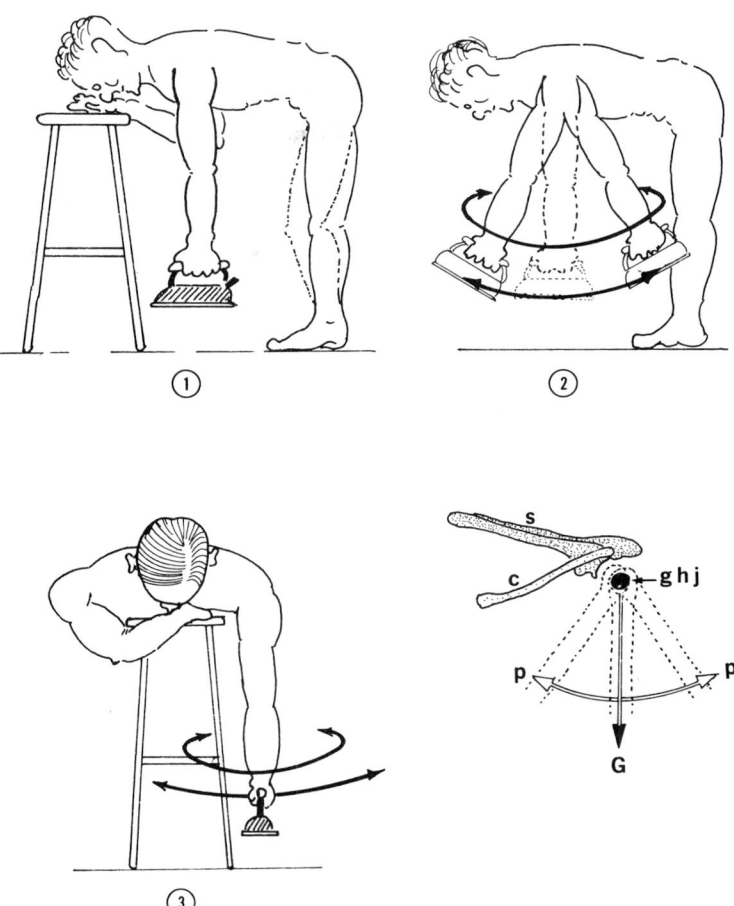

with the hand "pulling" the arm gradually up the wall [Fig. 9–30]. The exercise is begun facing the wall, since shoulder flexion alone is usually less painful than abduction, but gradual turning away from the wall as the hand climbs allows passive abduction as well. This is not an exercise that is easy to master as a passive maneuver [try it], but most can master it if properly instructed.)

Passive exercises, passively performed, prevent the vicious cycle of painful movement → progressive muscle spasm → persistent immobility → soft-tissue contracture → frozen shoulder (see below).

Active range-of-motion exercise (Fig. 9–30) is begun when severe pain has resolved and pendulum exercises can be performed without difficulty; in general, the earlier the better. Many exercises are helpful, but the most valuable are those that achieve full range of motion in all planes but that especially emphasize abduction and external rotation. Figure 9–30 illustrates some of these exercises.

Broomstick maneuvers are the simplest to communicate (Fig. 9–30*F* and *G*). A broomstick (baseball bat, yardstick, or the like) is held in both hands at the level of the knees. With the elbows straight, the stick is elevated directly overhead (full flexion/elevation). The elbows are then bent, and the broomstick is placed behind the neck (abduction and external rotation) and then returned to the overhead position. While it is overhead, the stick is then moved laterally from one side to the other (adduction and abduction). One hand then releases the stick; that hand is placed behind the back to grab the stick from below (this shoulder is now extended and internally rotated). The stick is then alternately pulled from above and below to exercise the upper arm and the lower arm simultaneously.

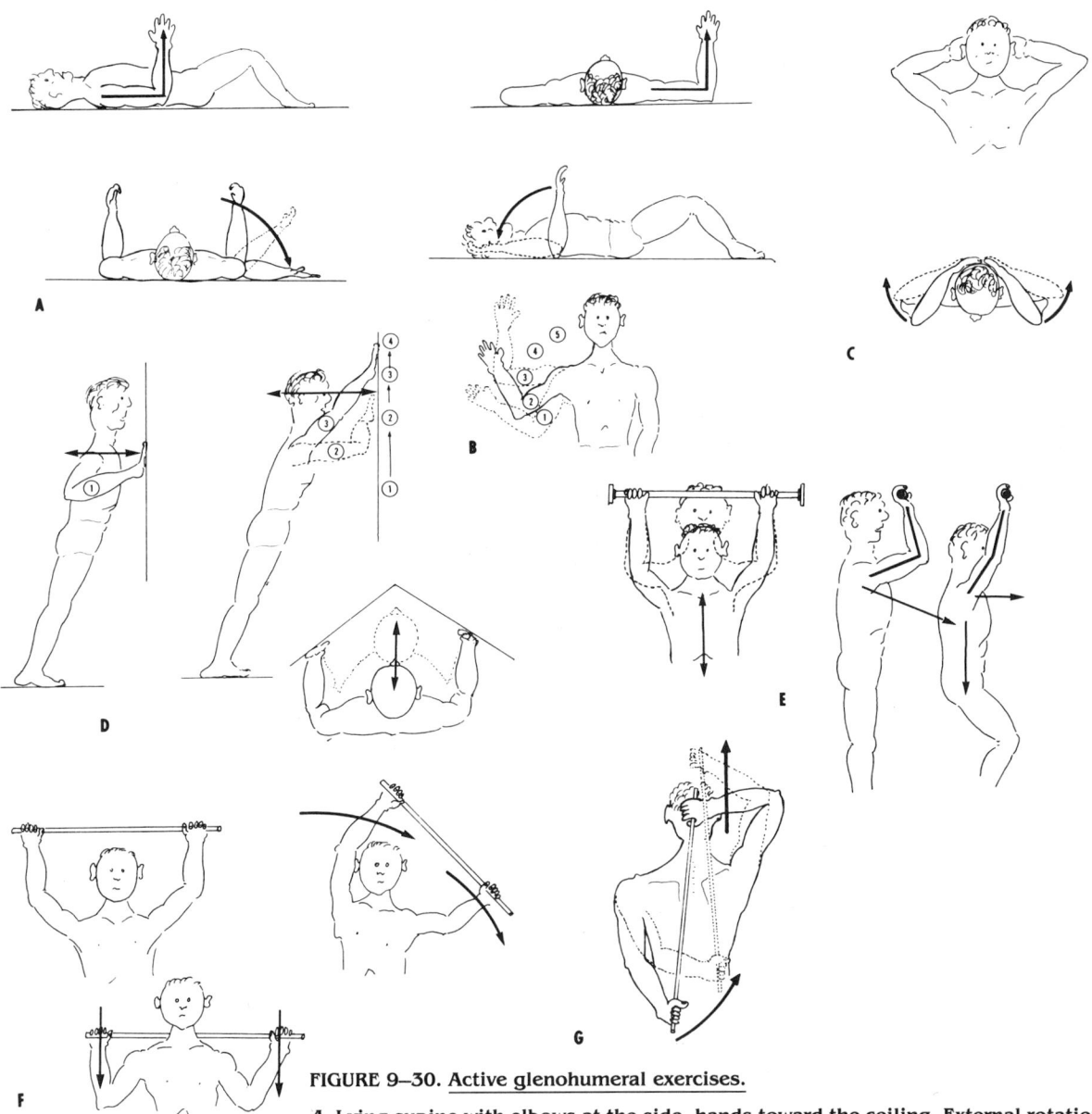

FIGURE 9–30. Active glenohumeral exercises.

A, Lying supine with elbows at the side, hands toward the ceiling. External rotation is attempted actively by the patient and passively by the therapist. Resistance may be applied when range permits. This exercise can be performed in the upright position against the wall.

B, Similar exercise to *A,* but with increasing abduction of the arm through positions 1 to 5.

C, Hands behind head, the movement is backward motion of the elbows, to the floor when supine and to the wall when erect. This motion may be assisted by a therapist and may be resisted.

D, "Push-ups" from the wall performed in a corner. The exercise starts with hands at waist level; then the hands "climb" until they are fully extended overhead, still apart. The anterior capsule is stretched, as are the pectorals. Rhythm is necessary. Avoid arching the back and the neck.

E, with a "chinning bar" (between the door frames) that is adjustable, begin with the bar at face level and gradually elevate the bar, either by changing the position in the door frame or by doing a deep knee bend. Ultimately the bar should be above and behind the head.

F, Similar to *E,* except that a "wand" or wooden dowel is held by both hands. This exercise is more active than in *E,* the ultimate object being to place the wand behind the head from a fully extended overhead position. Lateral motion with arms overhead should attempt movement of arms behind the head.

G, Wand behind the back. In the illustration the wand is elevated by the right hand to bring the left (involved) arm up behind the back, which stretches the anterior capsule and the external rotators.

H, Placing hands behind the back upon a table, parallel bars, or sink and doing deep knee bends. (From Cailliet, R: Shoulder Pain. Philadelphia: F. A. Davis Co., 1966, pp. 50–51).

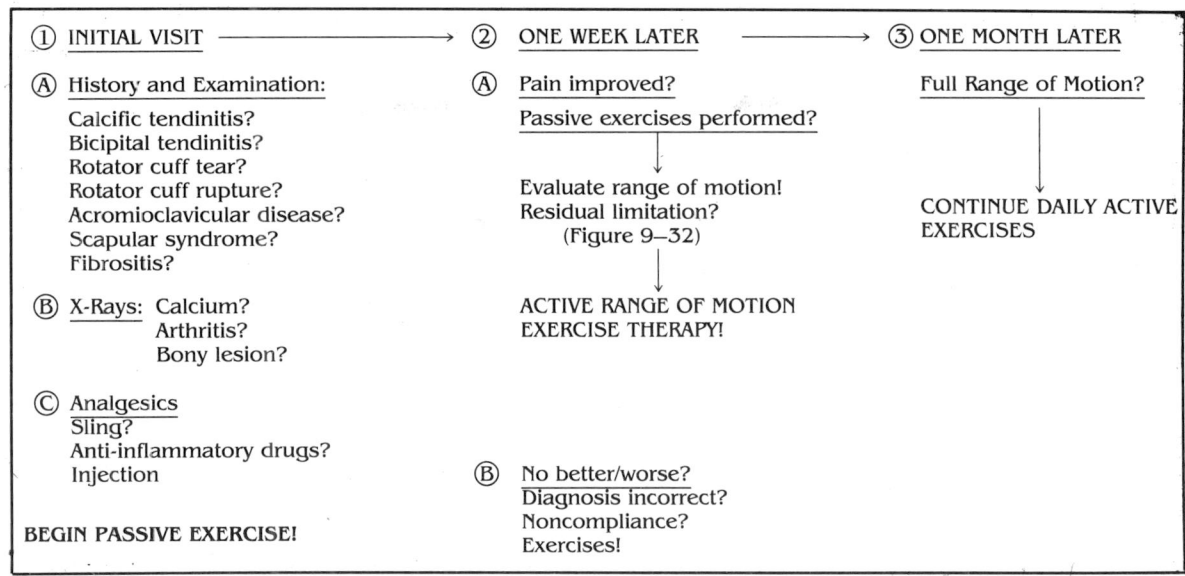

FIGURE 9–31. Acute periarticular shoulder pain.

Very frequently, active exercise will be uncomfortable or restricted. It must be emphasized that all ranges of motion must be returned to normal if an optimal result is to be achieved. At times, specific ranges of motion should be stressed. External rotation alone, for example, can be performed with the elbows at the sides, by gradually rotating the forearm outwardly to touch the floor, bed, or wall behind (Fig. 9–30A).

Repeat examination of shoulder range of motion should be analyzed by the physician after 1 week and, finally, 1 month later (Figs. 9–31 and 9–32).

> Sheldon is told that his problem is most likely tendinitis of the shoulder cuff muscles, perhaps precipitated by his recent physical overuse. He is told that rest and anti-inflammatory measures will reduce the swelling for the first few days, but that exercises must be begun early to insure that scar tissue does not form and that the shoulder returns to normal function as soon as possible. Local ice application for the first 48 hours, before and after frequent daily pendulum exercises, should be begun, and prescriptions are given for prednisone (40 mg qd for 2 days, 30 mg qd for 2 days, 20 mg qd for 2 days, 10 mg qd for 2 days) and codeine. Sheldon is instructed that pendulum exercises should be painless within the first 4 to 5 days, and that sequential active exercises (Fig. 9–30) should then be begun.
>
> A return appointment is scheduled for 7 days hence (Fig. 9–31).

NOTE

I. When periarticular disorders are the problem, specific instructions are crucial, and the rationale for treatment should be explained.

The sequence of therapeutic measures must be clearly understood by the patient, and the need for early exercise therapy must be emphasized. While the precise scientific rationale for different treatments is unclear, the concept of inflammation with possible subsequent formation of scar tissue is a helpful one for the patient.

II. Return appointments and follow-up examinations are always worthwhile.

Most cases of acute periarticular disease will improve over 1 to 2 weeks, with or without treatment. Failure to improve completely, however, has two important implications:

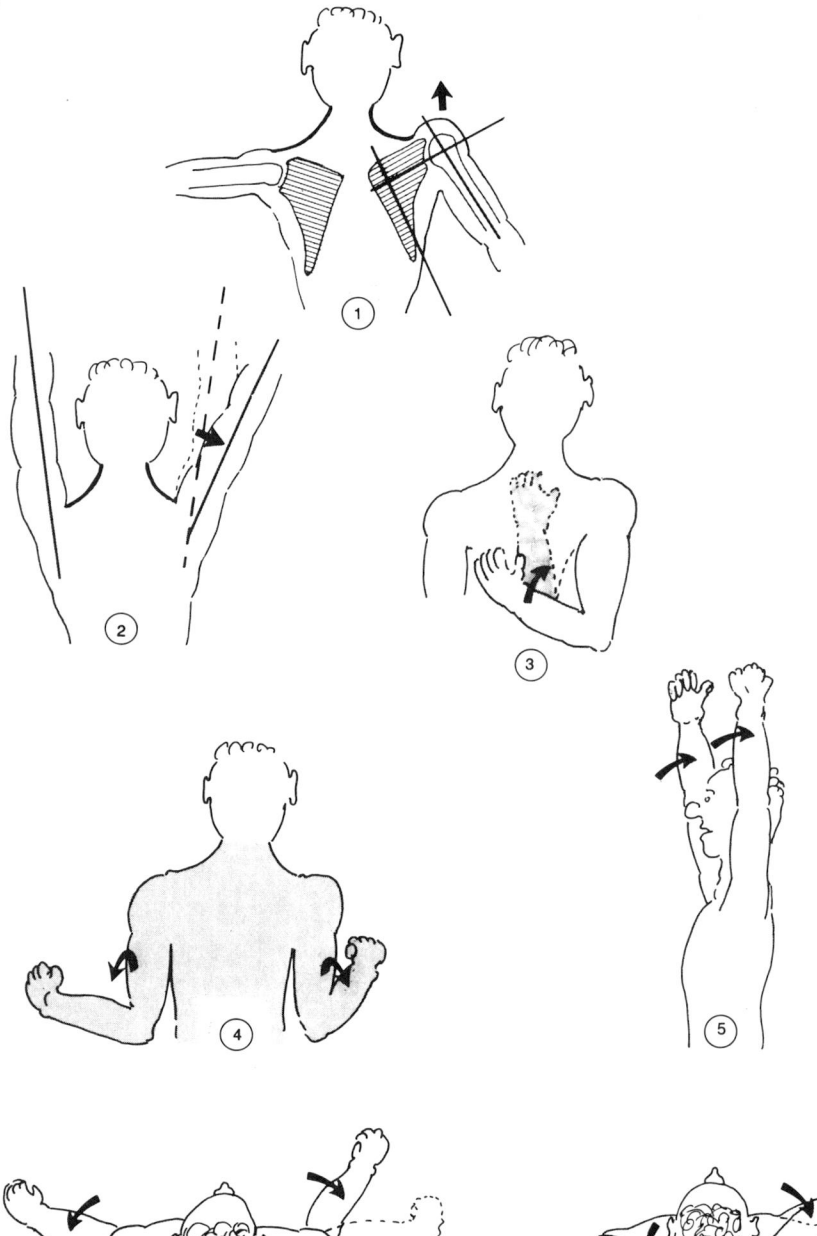

FIGURE 9–32. Subtle signs of shoulder limitation. 1, Shrugging with excessive scapular rotation and limited glenohumeral abduction. 2, Limited right arm overhead elevation. Arm "away" from head and ear. 3, Limited posterior flexion and internal rotation. Hand fails to reach normal interscapular distance of reach. 4, Limited external rotation of right arm, done with flexed elbow. 5, Overhead elevation of right arm limited in posterior direction compared with normal, viewed from side. 6, External rotation as viewed from above. 7, With hands behind head, right arm fails to fully extend posteriorly. (Reproduced with permission from Cailliet, R: Soft Tissue Pain and Disability. Philadelphia: F. A. Davis Co., 1977, pp. 164–165.)

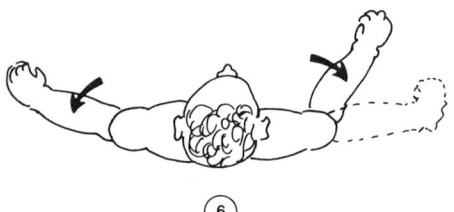

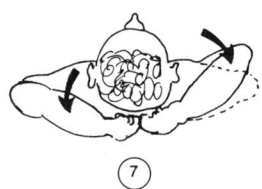

A. Another diagnosis or complication of the initial process must then be considered (see below).
B. Most of the time the initial diagnosis will be correct, but signs of residual periarticular disability may be fairly subtle and are often ignored by the patient (Fig. 9–32).

    Chronic recurrent periarticular disorders are very common—at least some of these result from incompletely healed acute processes that do not receive optimal treatment and reconditioning. Relief of pain and return of the involved shoulder to full symmetric elevation, rotation, and abduction are the ultimate goals of therapy—less than this implies residual disability and the need for further exercise therapy. After 1 to 2 weeks then, even if the patient feels fine, the shoulder should be reexamined, compared with its opposite, and its range of motion tested (Fig. 9–32).

When the Patient Does Not Improve

It is hoped that prevention of prolonged immobilization, documented restoration of normal shoulder motion, and ongoing exercise therapy will prevent some cases of subsequent chronic periarticular shoulder disability. The most common of these include:

1. Impingement syndrome refers to "catching" of the suprahumeral structures beneath the coracoacromial arch during attempted elevation/abduction of the shoulder beyond 60 to 90 degrees. This is usually the result of chronic cuff tendinitis or bursitis, and prolonged conservative therapy (exercises) is usually the treatment of choice, but resection of the acromion or coracoacromial ligament or both is sometimes necessary. Associated degenerative arthritis of the acromioclavicular joint is not rare, and rotator cuff tears may also coexist.[41]

2. As noted above, rotator cuff tears may be missed in the acute stage or not be associated with any obvious traumatic precipitating event. The (usually middle-aged or elderly) patient who complains of a chronically stiff and painful shoulder may have a significant rotator cuff tear without the classic findings of cuff rupture (see above). Tears of the anterior glenohumeral capsule[42] may cause similar nonspecific symptoms and yet worsen insidiously.

3. Sometimes termed adhesive capsulitis,[43] "frozen shoulder" refers to a poorly understood but specific clinical entity, usually afflicting patients in middle age, wherein progressive (and usually, but not always, painful) immobilization of the shoulder develops over the course of weeks to months.

The initial pathogenetic events underlying adhesive capsulitis[44] are debatable. Dense pericapsular adhesions are found surgically in some patients[40] but not in others;[45] local autonomically mediated ischemia[46] may play a critical role in the final common pathway, which results in a shrunken, contracted joint capsule that limits shoulder mobility. These events may be the end result of an acute periarticular disorder (especially calcific or bicipital tendinitis) but may also follow myocardial infarction, cerebrovascular accident, or prolonged shoulder immobilization due to any cause.

Examination usually reveals extreme passive and active limitation of motion, especially of abduction and rotation, without much localized tenderness. Routine shoulder x-rays are usually normal (except perhaps for "disuse osteoporosis"). Specific diagnosis may require arthrography,[47] which delineates the contracted capsular configuration and helps exclude other diagnoses (e.g., rotator cuff tears).[48] (Arthrography is sometimes *therapeutic* for adhesive capsulitis since it distends the joint space.) The subacute or chronic clinical course, normal x-rays, and severe limitation of motion on active and passive testing usually confirm this diagnosis on purely clinical grounds without the need for arthrography.

Treatment of true frozen shoulder is controversial, and, while controlled studies are scant, some authorities suggest that the natural history is one of slow but spontaneous recovery.[49] This fact underlies the importance of aggressive but conservative therapy: Some combination or sequence of exercise therapy, corticosteroid injections and manipulations[45, 50, 51] will usually be successful, and open surgical therapy is only rarely indicated.

These chronic shoulder disorders may be difficult to distinguish one from another and, in fact, commonly coexist. Impingement syndromes may result from rotator cuff tears. Rotator cuff tears may initiate the frozen shoulder. Adhesive capsulitis may cause a dramatic impingement syndrome. An orthopedist should always be consulted when acute periarticular disorders do not resolve completely, when any form of chronic disability persists, or when suspected rotator cuff tear causes ongoing difficulty for the patient. Decisions about the need for arthrography, arthroscopy, manipulation, or surgical exploration under anesthesia are the orthopedist's province.

(Many causes of chronic shoulder pain are not periarticular but are due to disease of the bones or joints. These have been briefly outlined in Table 9–2.)

Shoulder disorders that cause recurrent, but not chronic, ongoing disability may also require the orthopedist, but several are easily suspected by the nonorthopedist.

Recurrent bicipital tendon subluxation is discussed above—Yergason's test will help here.

Recurrent glenohumeral subluxation/dislocations (see Appendix II) usually are anterior humeral displacements that occur when the shoulder is abducted and externally rotated (the usual patient thus learns to avoid such movement). The "apprehension test" involves positioning the patient's arm in that abducted/externally rotated posture—the patient with recurrent dislocations will not allow this (Fig. 9–33).

Degenerative arthritis of the acromioclavicular or sternoclavicular joint may cause palpable/audible crepitus on shoulder movement, and such patients may complain of intermittent "locking" or "catching" in certain positions.

> Sheldon returns 10 days later. His pain persists but is "definitely better." Pendulum exercises have been performed without difficulty for several days, but active exercise is more troublesome. Sheldon says that the shoulder "feels weak," and he finds that "my arm and back have to do the work of my shoulder."
>
> Physical examination reveals several changes. Palpation is unremarkable, except for mild diffuse tenderness of the subacromial area, and the lateral deltoid area "feels funny." There is marked impairment of shoulder abduction, and there appears to be more scapular than glenohumeral movement when abduction is attempted (the shoulder shrugs). These movements are not impaired because of pain but feel genuinely "weak." Passive range of motion is normal, except for very mild discomfort after full passive abduction and elevation. Sheldon is unable to hold the arm at 90 degrees of abduction against even mild resistance once it is passively elevated to that position.
>
> Repeat neurologic examination is otherwise normal, except for a questionably diminished triceps and brachioradialis reflex.

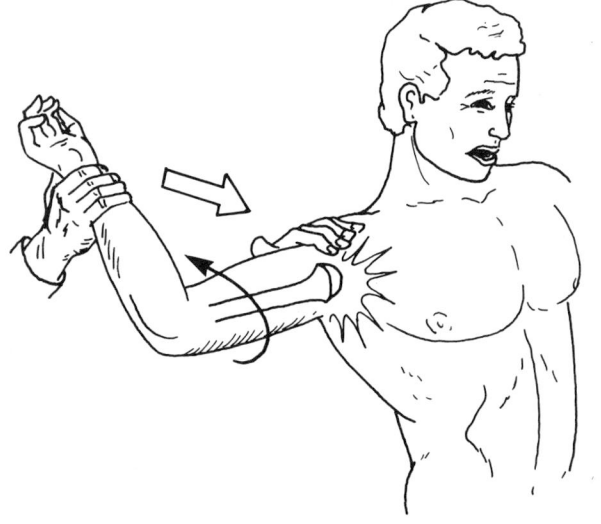

FIGURE 9–33. The apprehension test for recurrent glenohumeral subluxation.

What does this mean?

I. The critical findings are that passive range of motion is normal, while active range of motion is significantly impaired, and pain does not appear to be the limiting factor.

These facts imply that inflammation, swelling, or muscle spasm of the articular or periarticular structures cannot be the only problem here, since restriction of motion by articular or periarticular disorders should be apparent on both passive and active testing (or be limited by pain and spasm).

II. Therefore, muscular weakness of some kind is a likely explanation for the current shoulder problem.

This may be the result of one of two basic processes:

A. Rupture of the rotator cuff.

The absence of specific trauma in a relatively young patient argues strongly against this diagnosis, but, again, in any patient with a painful shoulder who is (or becomes) unable to maintain abduction of the shoulder, rotator cuff rupture must be suspected. Therefore, an arthrogram may be indicated.

B. A primary neuromuscular disorder must be considered.[52–55]

Various neurologic or primary myopathic disorders may begin with shoulder pain. Direct contusions of the deltoid muscle or axillary nerve, cervical radiculopathies, brachial plexus lesions, and systemic muscle disease (muscular dystrophy, inflammatory myositis) may all result in both shoulder pain and weakness. Careful observation and palpation of the shoulder during attempted abduction may be helpful in distinguishing rotator cuff rupture from primary muscle weakness: Impaired abduction despite apparently forceful and palpable deltoid contraction suggests an articular or periarticular disorder (e.g., rotator cuff injury), while visible/palpable lack of deltoid contraction implicates a deficiency of the deltoid muscle itself (or its innervation).

In practice, clear differentiation between these two entities may not be so easy, since the deltoid is a large muscle and visible/palpable muscle contractions often coexist with frank muscular weakness. Usually the setting in which the problem occurs is most helpful. Primary neuropathic or myopathic shoulder disorders are usually subacute or chronic or are associated with other evidence of neuromuscular disease (see page 431). The rotator cuff rupture is usually traumatic.

Arrangements for an orthopedic consultation and arthrography are made for 1 week hence. Sheldon is encouraged to continue at least passive exercises until that time.

NOTE

1. An arthrogram[56] (Fig. 9–27, *B* through *D*) may be diagnostically useful in a variety of situations. The diagnosis of rotator cuff tear, synovial capsule tear, and frozen shoulder (adhesive capsulitis) may depend on it, while lesions of the bicipital apparatus and other suprahumeral structures may often be recognizable as well. Arthroscopy is now preferred by some orthopedists in certain circumstances.[57]

2. The timing of orthopedic consultation and arthrography depends on the clinical situation. As noted previously, conservative therapy (for a few weeks) of even a (suspected) large rotator cuff may be the best course in the elderly patient. In the young, healthy patient with an obvious traumatic rotator cuff injury, there is no point in delaying consultation since the orthopedic surgeon is the ultimate arbiter in choosing when and if to operate.

3. In Sheldon's case, consultation and arthrography are indicated for both diagnostic and therapeutic purposes. The diagnosis is in doubt. Documentation of rotator cuff tear will allow more effective treatment planning.

> The next day Sheldon calls to say that his shoulder is "about the same, but my wrist and hand feel funny." Since his orthopedic appointment is still a week away, "Can I do anything to help it in the meantime?" Sheldon is told to return to the clinic where repeat examination reveals new changes.
>
> At this time, passive shoulder motion remains full and painless, while active abduction is very weak, and passive abduction cannot be maintained with even great effort. In addition, there is now demonstrable weakness of the triceps muscle and extensors of the wrist and fingers, as well as impaired touch sensation over the lateral deltoid area. The brachioradialis reflex is absent; the triceps reflex is diminished.

What does this mean?

There are now unequivocal neurologic abnormalities affecting structures distant from the shoulder. More precise testing is indicated (see below), but our original diagnosis must now be discarded since acute periarticular disorders alone cannot cause such findings. Many diverse pathologic entities can produce pain, disability, or neurologic symptoms in the shoulder and hand simultaneously. Certain problems should be considered before one reviews the neurologic examination in greater detail (page 431).

THE SHOULDER AND THE HAND

When the shoulder and the hand are impaired simultaneously (or sequentially) in the patient who presents with shoulder pain, several entities should be considered. Careful physical examination and selected x-rays will usually allow an early correct diagnosis (Table 9–4).

Mechanical shoulder disorders can affect the hand and forearm in several ways. Periarticular or articular disease of the shoulder may produce pain that is felt down the arm, sometimes even into the hand. In such instances the pain usually is best localized to the shoulder, and hand/forearm pain is clearly related to shoulder motion. Neurologic examination of the hand and forearm should be normal. (An association has been noted between periarticular shoulder disorders and median nerve entrapment— carpal tunnel syndrome.[58] How these disorders are pathogenetically related, if at all, is unclear— perhaps two common disorders serendipitously coexist in some patients—but treatment must be directed to each separate problem.)*

Trauma to the shoulder[59] may damage neurovascular structures in proximity to the shoulder, resulting in mechanical shoulder problems associated with neurologic impairment of the arm and hand. Glenohumeral dislocation may compress structures in the brachial plexus (especially the posterior or medial cords) or peripheral nerves (especially the axillary nerve or the radial nerve—see Figure 9–35). Proximal fractures of the humerus less commonly produce this same picture. Direct trauma to the clavicle or

---

*Occasionally, shoulder pain may be the primary complaint in the patient with carpal tunnel syndrome.

TABLE 9–4. DIAGNOSIS OF SHOULDER/HAND SYNDROMES

SHOULDER DISORDER	HAND INVOLVEMENT	DIAGNOSIS
Acute Mechanical Shoulder Disorders		
Nontraumatic		
Acute periarticular disorders	Referred pain; ? associated carpal tunnel; ? associated cubital tunnel (Table 9–7)	Clinical examination; carpal and cubital tunnel signs; neurological examination normal unless associated entrapment neuropathy
Traumatic		
Glenohumeral subluxation, dislocation, fracture	Neurovascular compression in axilla	Clinical examination; x-rays of shoulder
Neck injury	Cervical root disorder (Table 9–6)	Clinical examination; x-rays of cervical spine
Traction injury	Brachial plexus traction (Table 9–5)	Clinical examination; electrical studies
Reflex sympathetic dystrophy		
Frozen shoulder	Swelling, periarticular pain, and vasomotor instability of hand	Clinical findings; response to steroids and/or sympathectomy
Shoulder immobilization		
Cervical spine disease		
Cervical spondylosis	Root syndromes (Table 9–6)	Clinical examination; x-rays (Fig. 9–34)
Disc disease	Usually C5-6, C6-7	Myelogram; CT scan
Neoplasms; syrinx		CT scan; myelogram
Thoracic outlet syndrome (Appendix III)		
Scalenus anticus syndrome		
Costoclavicular syndrome	Dysesthesias, usually C8-T1; rarely, vascular compromise	History; Adson test; hyperabduction test; military test
Hyperabduction syndrome		
Nontraumatic brachial plexus disease		
Pancoast tumor		Chest x-ray (Fig. 9–36)
Subclavian aneurysm	Neurologic changes depend on site of lesion	Clinical examination; ? arteriography
Brachial neuritis		Neurodiagnostic studies

supraclavicular space may damage both shoulder mechanics and the brachial plexus, while traction injuries (due to falls or positioning under general anesthesia) may simultaneously damage the shoulder (dislocations, rotator cuff tears), and the brachial plexus.

The shoulder/hand syndrome[60, 61] is a poorly understood condition in which impaired shoulder mobility is associated with pain, swelling, and vasomotor instability of the ipsilateral hand. Although the syndrome is sometimes seen following myocardial infarction, cerebrovascular accidents, or prolonged bedrest/immobilization, many cases are "idiopathic." Overactivity of the sympathetic nervous system (hence the term reflex sympathetic dystrophy syndrome —RSDS) is probably partly responsible for the characteristic swelling of the hand and the autonomic disturbance of the hand seen in this syndrome. Fluctuations in ambient temperature (while the patient is taking a bath, for example) will cause extreme erythema of the hand, alternating with intermittent pallor, associated with disturbances of sweating and often severe periarticular pain and tenderness of the hand and fingers. (The neurologic examination is usually normal, but muscle testing may be difficult in the full-blown syndrome).

Sometimes RSDS is relieved with surgical sympathetic blockade, but local heat, physical therapy, and oral corticosteroids often help. Chronic disability, refractory to all therapeutic methods, does occur in a few patients.

Cervical spine disease is a very common cause of pain in the shoulder. This pain may be primarily referred muscular pain (Fig. 9–1) or frank radicular pain with dermatomal sensory symptoms (paresthesias) and neurologic impairment of the spinal root involved (see Fig. 9–37 and Table 9–6).

Cervical spondylosis or acute disc disease is the most common cause of cervical radiculopathy. Neck pain is often associated, and when radicular syndromes are present, neck flexion, extension, and lateral rotation (Fig. 9–2) will usually exacerbate symptoms (and traction may relieve them). When cervical spine diseases cause involvement of the forearm or hand, the clinical syndrome is characteristic, and one can usually localize the problem to one specific cervical root.[62] Nerve roots most commonly involved are C6 (neural compression at C5–6) and C7 (neural compression at C6–7). C6 root compression causes pain and stiffness in the neck and shoulder with dysesthesias along the radial arm and forearm and into the thumb and first finger. Note that this may superficially resemble the carpal tunnel syndrome, but in C6 nerve root disease the Tinel/Phalen signs at the wrist are negative (see page 433), the biceps muscle may be weak, and the brachioradialis reflex may be depressed. C7 root compression causes neck and shoulder pain with dysesthesias of the posterior arm and forearm into the middle finger with weakness of the triceps muscle and a depressed triceps reflex (see Table 9–6).

Cervical spine films usually reveal degenerative changes (Fig. 9–34) or narrowing of the intervertebral foramina on oblique views when cervical spondylosis is the problem. Acute cervical disc herniation is often associated with normal x-rays–CT or myelography is necessary here.

Disorders of the brachial plexus (Fig. 9–35) may result from various traumatic events, as noted above. Nontraumatic brachial plexus disorders that may cause shoulder and hand problems include:

1. Thoracic outlet syndromes. Shoulder and hand discomfort in association with dysesthesias of the forearm and hand, as well as symptoms of vascular compromise (Raynaud's phenomenon, arm claudication, or edema),

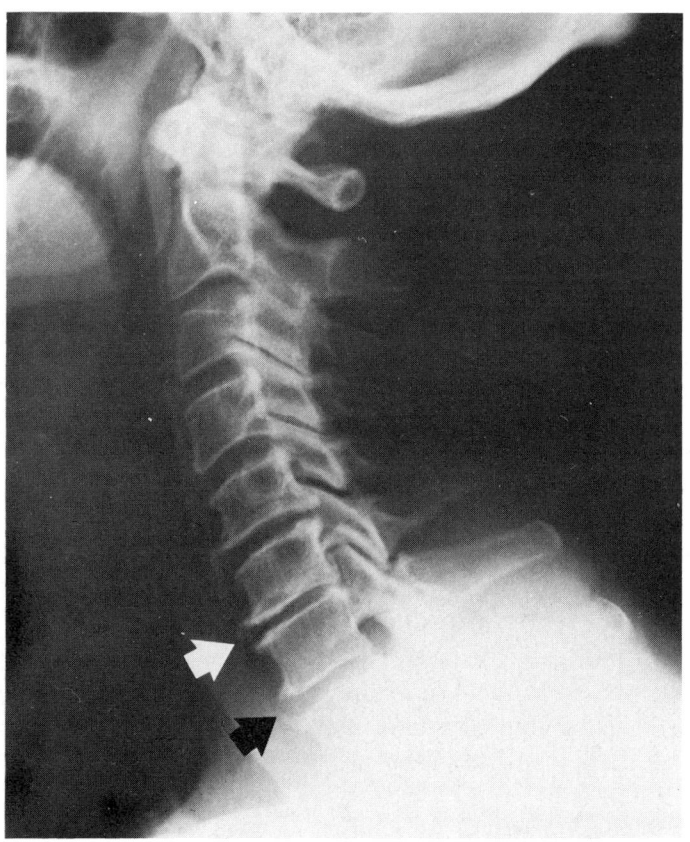

FIGURE 9–34. This 68-year-old man described the subacute onset of pain in the left shoulder and arm with occasional dysesthesias of the hand (principally the thumb and radial forearm). Examination revealed limitation of motion of the neck, slight weakness of the biceps and brachioradialis muscles, and a diminished brachioradialis reflex. The diagnosis of C6 radiculopathy was made, and these x-rays demonstrate cervical spondylosis with narrowing of the disc space, especially at C6–7 and C7–T1 (arrows). Heat, traction, and physical therapy relieved the patient's symptoms. A myelogram was thus not performed.

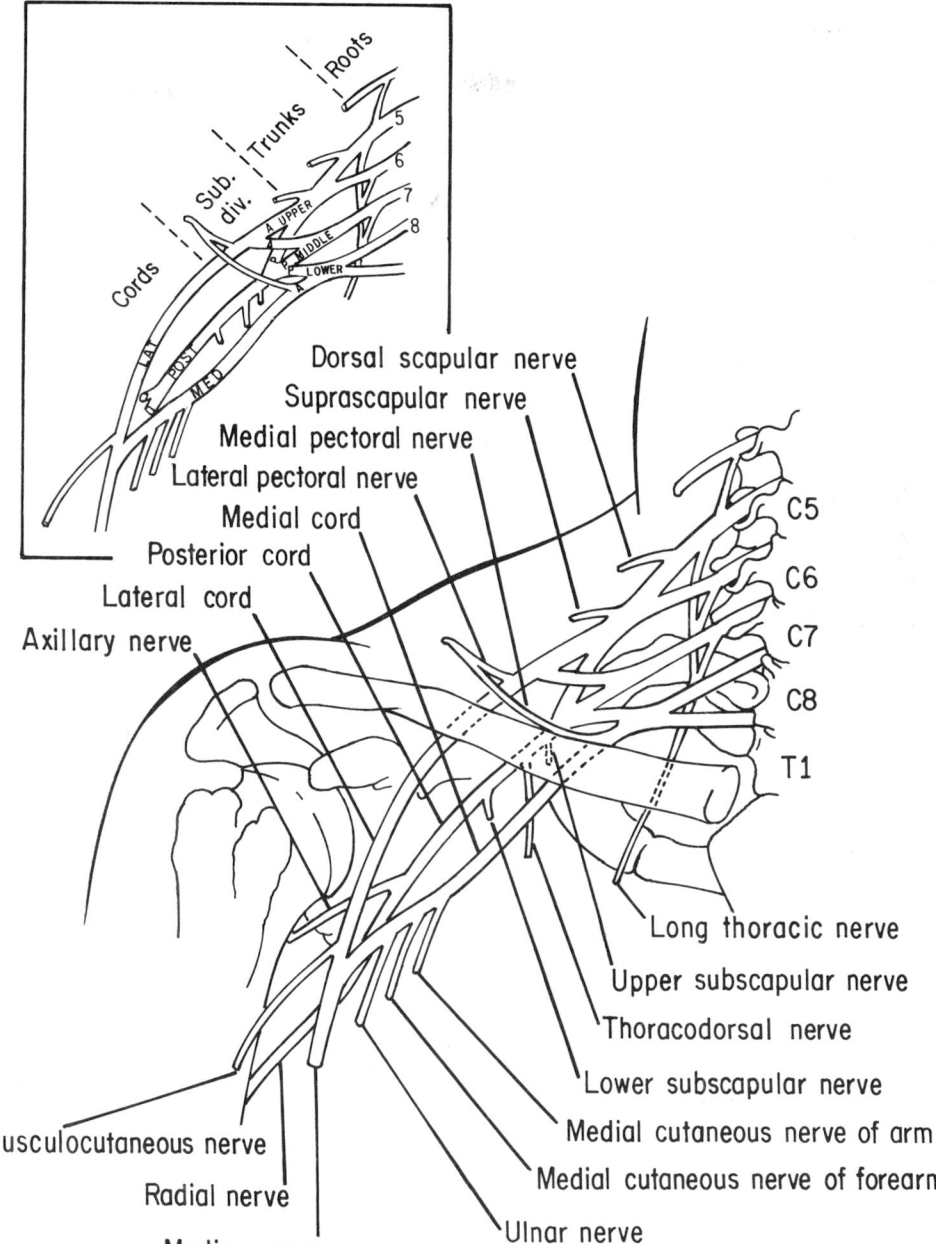

FIGURE 9–35. The brachial plexus. (Adapted with permission from DeJong, RN: The Neurologic Examination, 4th ed. New York, Harper and Row, 1979, p. 570.)

may result from compression of the neurovascular bundle in the supraclavicular or axillary space. Symptoms are often intermittent and postural, frank motor weakness is rare, and the lower brachial plexus (C8-T1) is most often involved, with dysesthesias primarily in the ulnar forearm and the fourth and fifth digits. The history and various diagnostic maneuvers will usually help localize the problem quite precisely. Treatment is usually conservative. These various disorders are discussed in more detail in Appendix III.

2. Neoplasms may infiltrate the brachial plexus (Fig. 9–36). Most common is the Pancoast tumor,[63, 64] a malignant neoplasm (usually squamous cell) of the apex of the lung that involves the upper chest wall as well as (usually) the lower brachial plexus (C8–T1). Pain is usually in the chest wall, and shoulder pain is most often localized to the axilla, "inside" the arm, and down into the fourth and fifth fingers. The diagnosis is made by chest x-ray; apical lordotic views are occasionally necessary. Confusing or atypical shoulder and arm pain requires a chest x-ray, especially in the smoker.

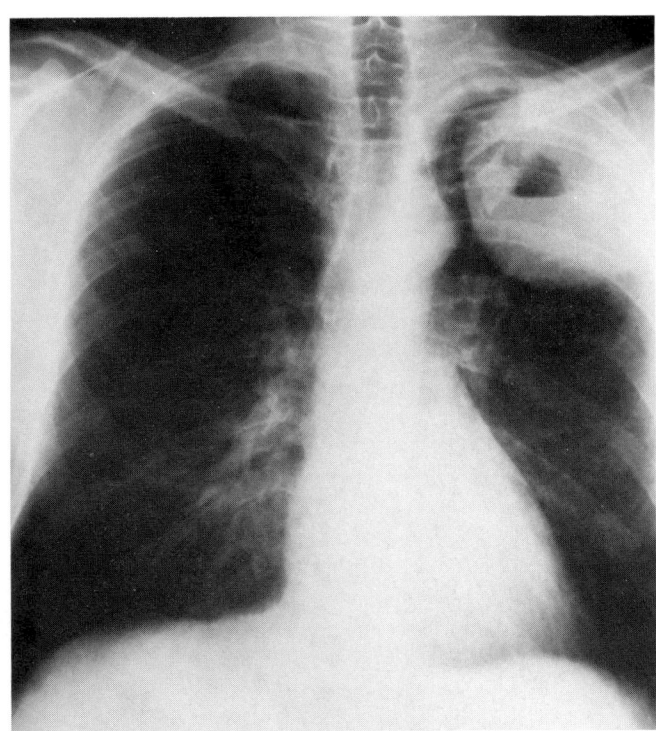

FIGURE 9–36. This unfortunate 52-year-old man complained of vague but progressively worsening left shoulder pain for 6 months before the correct diagnosis was made. Multiple x-rays of the shoulder and neck were obtained before this chest x-ray demonstrated a cavitating Pancoast tumor of the left lung. He died 8 months later.

3. Brachial neuritis[65-67] is a peculiar disorder with a well-described clinical picture. Middle-aged males are most commonly afflicted by severe (often acute) pain in the shoulder or neck or both, often worsened by movements of the shoulder and neck, but initially without evidence of neurologic compromise. Hence, initially the disorder is often mistaken for a mechanical shoulder or neck problem. Days to weeks thereafter, however, dysesthesias and motor weakness appear, the specific sensorimotor deficits varying with the segments of the brachial plexus or peripheral nerves involved. Most commonly involved are axillary, suprascapular, and radial nerves. Spontaneous resolution is the rule but may be delayed for months (or, rarely, years). The cause in most cases is unknown (except when the disorder is clearly due to radiation therapy or herpes zoster or is a rare heredofamilial variety), but cases following immunization, systemic infectious illness, and serum sickness have been described.

> Sheldon again denies any traumatic event, neck pain, hand swelling, or vasomotor symptoms.
>
> Range of motion of the neck is normal, except for mild discomfort in the shoulder during lateral neck rotation. The supraclavicular fossa, axilla, and chest are normal to palpation and auscultation. All pulses are normal, and the Adson, hyperabduction, and costoclavicular maneuvers are unremarkable (see Appendix III). Examination of the hand and forearm reveals no swelling, local tenderness or vasomotor changes; there is no evidence of carpal tunnel disease.
>
> Detailed neurologic examination reveals marked weakness of shoulder abduction, flexion, and extension, and active deltoid contraction is visibly weak during testing. There is also definite but milder weakness of elbow, wrist, and proximal finger extension. The grip is subjectively weaker on the left, but elbow, wrist, and finger flexion are normal. Reflexes are normal, except for absence of the brachioradialis response and diminished triceps jerk. Sensory examination reveals an area of impaired touch sensation over the upper outer deltoid and perhaps subjective sensory loss over the lower radial forearm.
>
> The right arm and both legs are normal. There are no long tract signs.

Problems of this kind will require the assistance of an experienced neurologist or neurosurgeon. However, the generalist physician can usually arrive at a likely diagnosis by gaining familiarity with the following.

PRACTICAL NEUROLOGY OF THE UPPER EXTREMITY

Usually, neurologic complaints associated with shoulder problems will be due to one of the shoulder/hand disorders discussed above and in Table 9–4. Cervical spine disease is by far the most common: cervical spondylosis in the middle-aged and elderly patient and acute disc herniation in the younger patient population. The initial diagnostic approach is centered around one crucial consideration: Do the clinical history and neurologic examination suggest a disorder of the spinal cord, nerve root(s), brachial plexus, or peripheral nerves?

One look at the complexity of the brachial plexus (Fig. 9–35) may prompt the non-neurologist to call for help immediately. In fact, systematic analysis of the area of pain or sensory disturbance, the integrity of deep tendon reflexes, and the location of motor weakness will usually answer the question and prompt a reasonable differential diagnosis. The pathologic lesion responsible for various root, nerve, and plexus syndromes will be suggested by the specific neurologic abnormality (Tables 9–5 through 9–7)— and, of course, the clinical setting.

CONSIDER

I. Pain or sensory symptoms.

When cervical nerve roots are responsible for pain in the shoulder and arm, there are usually symptoms other than pain. Careful questioning often reveals that pain refers to prickling, lancinating, or electric discomfort, frequently associated with pins and needles sensations in a similar distribution. Nevertheless, pain may be the predominant symptom, and,

TABLE 9–5. BRACHIAL PLEXUS LESIONS

LOCATION	AREA OF PAIN	SENSORY LOSS	MOTOR LOSS	REFLEX CHANGES	COMMON CAUSATIVE LESIONS
Total plexus	Often none	Entire upper extremity	Complete paralysis of arm and hand	All absent	Vehicular trauma
Upper trunk	Supraclavicular; shoulder area	Very variable	Deltoid; rotator cuff; biceps	Diminished biceps	Fall; traction; stab wound; anesthesia pressure palsy
Lower trunk	Axilla; inner arm	Ulnar hand, forearm	Small muscles of hand	—	Shoulder fracture/ dislocation; thoracic outlet syndrome; Pancoast tumor
Lateral cord	Lateral forearm and hand (thumb)	Over area of pain	Biceps; forearm pronation	—	Shoulder fracture/ dislocation; clavicle injury; brachial neuritis; retro- clavicular or axillary mass (adenopathy, Pancoast tumor)
Medial cord	Combined ulnar and median nerve (Table 9–7)			—	
Posterior cord	Combined axillary and radial nerve (Table 9–7)			Decreased triceps and brachioradialis	

TABLE 9–6. NERVE ROOT LESIONS

Root	Area of Pain	Sensory Loss	Motor Loss	Reflex Changes	Common Causative Lesions
C5	Upper anterior arm, forearm pain and/or dysesthesias	Often none	Deltoid; rotator cuff; rhomboids; ± biceps	Diminished biceps	Cervical spondylosis
C6	Radial arm, forearm, thumb pain and/or dysesthesias	Often none	Biceps; brachioradialis; wrist extensors; ± deltoid	Diminished brachioradialis	Cervical spondylosis; acute cervical disc herniation (C6-7)
C7	Posterior arm, forearm, middle finger pain and/or dysesthesias	Often none	Triceps; wrist flexors; finger extensors	Diminished triceps	Cervical spondylosis; acute cervical disc herniation (C7-8)
C8	Ulnar arm, forearm, little finger pain and/or dysesthesias	Often none	Wrist, finger flexors; finger extensors		Cervical rib; thoracic outlet syndromes; Pancoast tumor; deep cervical mass (lymphadenopathy)
T1	Axilla, inner arm, forearm pain and/or dysesthesias	Often none	Small hand muscles		

TABLE 9–7. PERIPHERAL NERVE LESIONS

Root	Area of Pain	Sensory Loss	Motor Loss	Reflex Changes	Common Causative Lesions
Axillary	Lateral acromion, upper deltoid dysesthesias	Small area, lateral deltoid	Deltoid	—	Fractured/dislocated humerus; IM injections
Radial	Dorsal forearm and dorsal radial hand (backs of thumb and index fingers) dysesthesias	Often none	Triceps; wrist, finger extensors; brachioradialis	Diminished triceps, brachioradialis	Crutch palsy; hyperabduction (Saturday night) palsy
Median	Palmar thumb, index, middle finger dysesthesias	Over area of pain	Finger flexors (except small finger); thumb abduction, palmar; thumb opposition; wrist flexors (if nerve is affected above the wrist—rare)	—	Carpal tunnel syndrome
Ulnar	Ulnar hand, little finger, ulnar half of ring finger—palmar and dorsal aspect	Over area of pain	Wrist, little finger flexors; thumb adductors; little finger opposition, abductors	—	Cubital tunnel syndrome at elbow (due to trauma); occasionally local damage at ulnar wrist

when this is the case, the location and distribution of pain, as well as the relation of pain to neck motion, will often suggest the diagnosis. In root disorders, sensory symptoms are usually obviously dermatomal, and neck range of motion and Valsalva maneuvers (which increase intraspinal pressure and irritate nerve roots) will exacerbate the symptoms. The precise location of pain and dysesthesias will vary with the specific nerve root involved (Table 9–6).

When only one root is involved (a common situation in cervical spine disease), pain and sensory symptoms are much more prominent than objective sensory loss or motor weakness, since there is dermatomal overlap in skin innervation (not illustrated in Figure 9–37) and since virtually all muscle groups are innervated by several different nerve roots simultaneously (Table 9–8). Analysis of reflexes will be very helpful, however, since diminution of the biceps, brachioradialis, and triceps reflex is common in lesions of C5, C6, and C7 respectively.

When pains (or, more often, sensory dysesthesias) do not conform to dermatomal patterns, the peripheral cutaneous sensory system must be considered (Fig. 9–37), especially when other clinical findings do not suggest spinal or nerve root disease. As Table 9–7 indicates, differential diagnosis of these peripheral nerve disorders is very different from that of cervical root disorders. Unlike the root disorders, sensory peripheral nerve disorders usually produce dysesthesias rather than pain. Disorders of the median and ulnar nerves are probably the most common causes of sensory disturbances in the upper extremity.

The median nerve is usually entrapped in the carpal tunnel of the wrist (Fig. 9–38). Dysesthesias and pain involve the palmar aspect of the hand and the first three fingers. Tapping the carpal tunnel often elicits the patient's symptoms (a positive Tinel's sign), while forced wrist flexion sustained for 30 to 60 seconds by the patient often does the same (positive Phalen's sign). Motor weakness (Table 9–7) is a late finding—therapy attempts to prevent motor loss. Wrist splints and anti-inflammatory drugs are helpful temporarily—in a minority of cases, surgical decompression of the carpal tunnel is required. Electrical studies should be performed

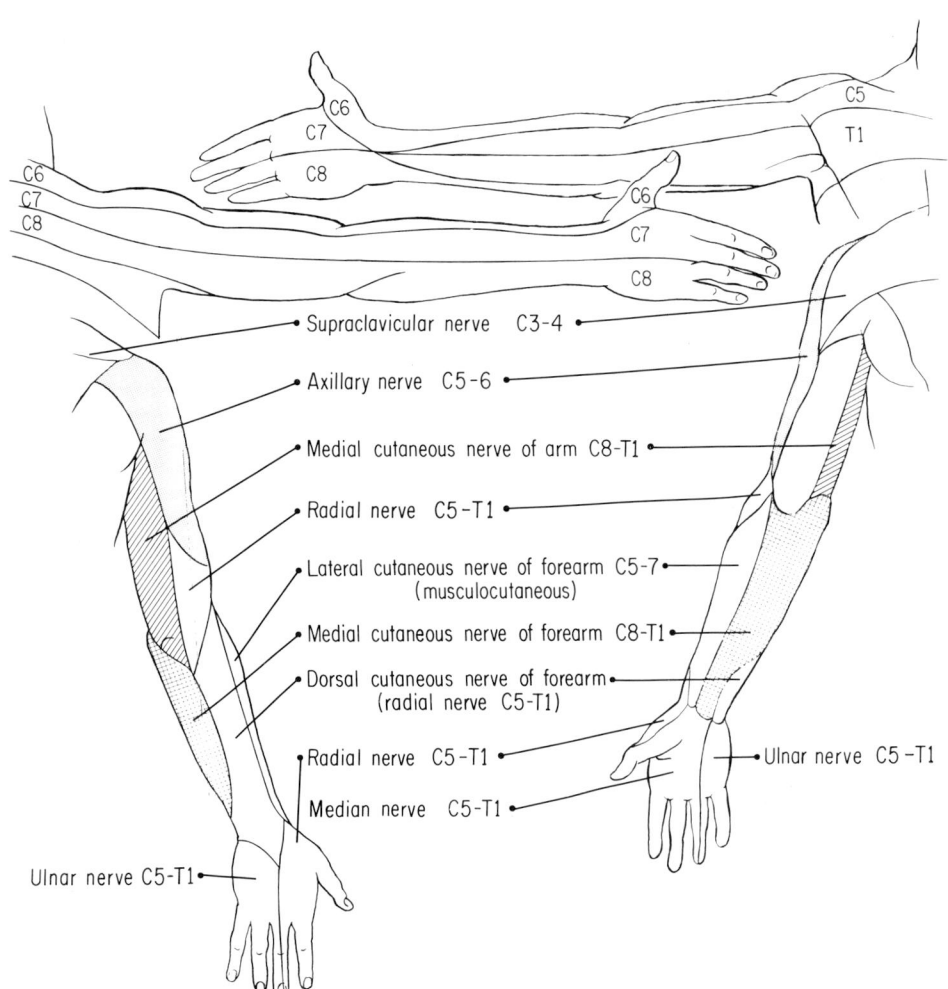

FIGURE 9–37. Dermatomes of the upper extremity and the cutaneous innervation of the arm by the peripheral sensory nerves (see also Fig. 9–35).

Supraclavicular nerve C3-4

Axillary nerve C5-6

Medial cutaneous nerve of arm C8-T1

Radial nerve C5-T1

Lateral cutaneous nerve of forearm C5-7 (musculocutaneous)

Medial cutaneous nerve of forearm C8-T1

Dorsal cutaneous nerve of forearm (radial nerve C5-T1)

Radial nerve C5-T1

Median nerve C5-T1

Ulnar nerve C5-T1

Ulnar nerve C5-T1

before surgery is recommended—root syndromes (especially C6) may mimic carpal tunnel syndrome, and, rarely, the median nerve may be entrapped at the forearm, not the wrist. Not uncommonly there are predisposing causes: (occupational) trauma, hypothyroidism, acromegaly, rheumatoid arthritis, amyloidosis, and many others. Many cases of carpal tunnel syndrome, however, are idiopathic.

The <u>ulnar nerve</u> may also be compressed at the wrist (Fig. 9–38)—the

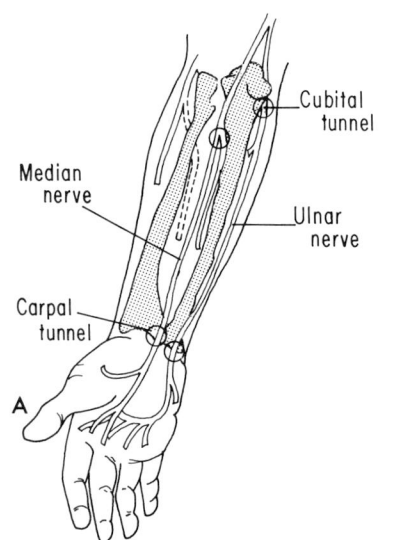

Cubital tunnel

Median nerve

Ulnar nerve

Carpal tunnel

A

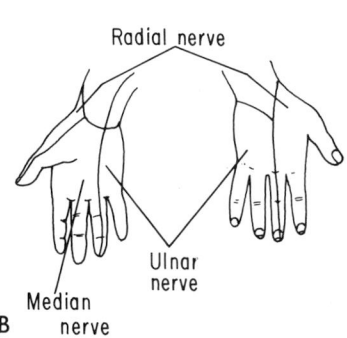

Radial nerve

Ulnar nerve

Median nerve

B

FIGURE 9–38. *A,* Peripheral entrapment of the median nerve (usually at the wrist, rarely in the forearm—see circles) or ulnar nerve (usually at the elbow, occasionally at the wrist) is the most common cause of sensory disturbances (paresthesias, tingling) in the hand. *B,* Sensory innervation of the hand—note that the median nerve supplies primarily the <u>palmar</u> surface of the hand.

patient with rheumatoid arthritis is a common victim—but much more often the site of entrapment is the medial epicondyle of the elbow (the funny bone), where manipulation of the palpable ulnar nerve as it encircles the epicondyle will elict the patient's symptoms (positive Tinel's sign at the elbow). Electrical studies should be performed before any attempted surgical decompression (root disorders—especially C8-T1— may be mistaken for ulnar nerve disease).

Radial nerve disorders cause significant motor weakness (see below) but minimal sensory changes.

Local trauma to the shoulder/deltoid area will sometimes cause local axillary nerve damage, resulting in a small dysesthetic area over the deltoid.

II. Weakness.

When shoulder/arm weakness is the presenting problem, analysis of any associated sensory symptoms will help suggest the level and site of the responsible lesion, but specific motor testing is most useful. Extreme focal motor weakness is more often the result of plexus (Table 9–5) or peripheral nerve (Table 9–7) involvement than of single root disease. When motor weakness is prominent, clinical analysis must decide:

A. Which shoulder, arm, or hand movements are weak (for example, shoulder abduction, elbow flexion, wrist extension)?
B. Which specific muscles participate in the weakened motor function?
C. What is the innervation—via brachial plexus, nerve roots, and peripheral nerves—of those specific muscles?
D. Do other clinical findings—the clinical setting and history, sensory symptoms or loss, reflex changes, and pertinent local physical examination (of the neck, axilla, chest)—point to nerve root, brachial plexus, or peripheral nerve disorders?

If weakness alone is the problem, could a primary myopathy or a local musculotendinous lesion be responsible, rather than a primary neurologic event?

Analysis of motor weakness of the shoulder, arm, and hand is briefly outlined in Table 9–8. These tables are not complete, and full discussion of upper extremity innervation is far beyond the scope of this text.[68] Nevertheless, this brief tabular outline will allow testing of specific muscle groups and identification of those that appear weak. This will often permit a tentative (differential) diagnosis based on the cervical nerve root(s), brachial plexus locale(s), or peripheral nerves(s) that could be responsible for such weakness. In general, a single unifying localization that can explain all (motor, sensory, and reflex) findings is most reliable (see below). Once this clinical localization of the lesion is at least tentatively decided, the common causes of such lesions can be suggested by a review of Tables 9–5, 9–6, and 9–7.[69-71]

While more sophisticated testing by a neurologist may then be necessary (electromyography, nerve conduction studies, for example[72]), the generalist physician can often make an educated guess whether root, plexus, or nerve is involved and thence undertake the indicated preliminary diagnostic studies (chest x-ray, cervical spine x-rays) that will help substantiate the correct diagnosis.

TABLE 9–8. ANALYSIS OF MOTOR WEAKNESS OF SHOULDER, ARM, AND HAND

MOVEMENT	TEST	PRIMARY MOVERS	NERVE	PLEXUS	ROOT
Shoulder abduction	Abduct arm 90 degrees	Deltoid Supraspinatus Other abductors: trapezius, rhomboids, serratus anterior, subscapularis, infraspinatus	Axillary Suprascapular	Posterior cord Upper trunk	C5-6 C4-6
Shoulder adduction	Adduct horizontally, vertically	Latissimus dorsi Pectoralis major Other adductors: biceps, triceps, coracobrachialis, deltoid, rotator cuff	Thoracodorsal Anterior thoracic	Posterior cord Upper and lower subdivisions	C6-8 C5-T1
Shoulder external rotation	Elbow at side, rotate forearm externally (Fig. 9–7)	Infraspinatus Teres minor	Suprascapular Axillary	Upper trunk Posterior cord	C4-6 C5-6
Shoulder internal rotation	Elbow at side, rotate forearm internally (Fig. 9–7)	Subscapularis Teres major Other rotators: deltoid, latissimus dorsi, pectoralis major. biceps	Subscapular Lower subscapular	Posterior cord Posterior cord	C5-7 C5-7
Shoulder flexion	Forward elevation (Fig. 9–7)	Deltoid Pectoralis major Coracobrachialis Other flexors: biceps, subscapularis	Axillary Medial and lateral pectoral nerve Musculocutaneous	Posterior cord Upper and lower subdivisions Lower lateral cord	C5-6 C5-T1 C6-7
Shoulder extension	Backward elevation (Fig. 9–7)	Deltoid Latissimus dorsi Other extensors: triceps, teres major	Axillary Thoracodorsal	Posterior cord Posterior cord	C5-6 C6-8
Elbow flexion	Flex arm at elbow	Biceps Brachialis Brachioradialis Other flexors: pronator teres, flexor carpi radialis, palmaris longus	Musculocutaneous Musculocutaneous Radial	Lower lateral cord Lower lateral cord Posterior cord	C5-6 C5-6 C5-6
Elbow extension	Extend arm at elbow	Triceps	Radial	Posterior cord	C6-8
Elbow supination	Turn forearm palm up	Biceps Brachioradialis Supinator brevis	Musculocutaneous Radial Radial	Low/lateral cord Posterior cord Posterior cord	C5-6 C5-6 C5-7
Elbow pronation	Turn forearm to palm-down position	Pronator teres Pronator quadratus	Median Median	Lower cord Lower cord	C6-7 C7-T1

Abduction / Adduction

Movement	Action	Muscle	Nerve	Cord	Roots
Wrist flexion	Flex wrist, palm up	Flexor carpi radialis	Median	Lower cord	C6-8
		Flexor carpi ulnaris	Ulnar	Lower cord	C7-T1
		Other flexors: palmaris longus, flexor digitorum, flexor pollicis			
Wrist extension	Extend wrist, palm down	Extensor carpi radialis	Radial	Posterior cord	C6-8
		Extensor carpi ulnaris	Radial	Posterior cord	C6-8
		Other extensors: extensor digitorum communis			
Thumb abduction Radial	Abduct thumb in palmar plane	Abductor pollicis longus	Radial	Posterior cord	C6-8
		Extensor pollicis brevis	Radial	Posterior cord	C6-8
Palmar	Abduct thumb at right angles from palm	Abductor pollicis brevis	Median	Lower cord	C8-T1
Thumb adduction Ulnar	Adduct thumb in palmar plane	Adductor pollicis	Ulnar	Lower cord	C8-T1
Palmar	Adduct thumb at right angles to palm				
Thumb opposition	Cross thumb over palm to touch little finger	Opponens pollicis	Median	Lower cord	C8-T1
Little finger opposition	Cross little finger over palm toward thumb	Opponens digiti minimi	Ulnar	Lower cord	C8-T1

Table continues on following page

TABLE 9–8. ANALYSIS OF MOTOR WEAKNESS OF SHOULDER, ARM, AND HAND (Continued)

Movement	Test	Primary Movers	Nerve	Plexus	Root
Little finger abduction	Abduct little finger from 4th finger in plane of palm	Abductor digiti minimi	Ulnar	Lower cord	C8-T1
Finger flexion Index, middle	Flex distal	Flexor digitorum profundus	Median	Lower cord	C7-T1
	Flex proximal	Flexor digitorum superficialis	Median	Lower cord	C7-T1
		Interossei	Ulnar	Lower cord	C8-T1
		Lumbricales (1, 2)	Median	Lower cord	C7-T1
Ring, little	Flex distal	Flexor digitorum profundus	Ulnar	Lower cord	C7-T1
	Flex proximal	Flexor digitorum superficialis	Median	Lower cord	C7-T1
		Interossei	Ulnar	Lower cord	C8-T1
		Lumbricales (3, 4)	Ulnar	Lower cord	C8-T1
Finger extension	Extend distal	Lumbricales (1, 2)	Median	Lower cord	C7-T1
		Lumbricales (3, 4)	Ulnar	Lower cord	C8-T1
		Interossei	Ulnar	Lower cord	C8-T1
	Extend proximal	Extensor digitorum communis	Radial	Posterior cord	C6-8

CONSIDER

1. Sheldon's pain is not radicular, the neck is clinically normal, and there is prominent motor weakness. All these facts argue against (isolated) nerve root disease.

Sheldon's sensory loss is suggestive of a possible C6 root distribution, but a look at the cutaneous distribution of peripheral nerves (Fig. 9–37) indicates that similar dysesthesias may occur with involvement of the axillary nerve or the dorsal forearm branch of the radial nerve. Thus the subjective sensory symptoms alone cannot localize the lesion. Symptomatic cervical spine disease seems unlikely: Thus, one should remember the peripheral nerves and the brachial plexus.

2. Sheldon's motor weakness involves abduction, flexion, and extension of the shoulder as well as weakness of the extensors of the elbow, wrist, and fingers. Perusal of Table 9–8 would then suggest involvement of the deltoid, triceps, and extensor carpi muscles, as well as the extensor digitorum muscles. The nerve root innervation of these different muscle groups involves C5 through C8 inclusive. Peripheral nerves that innervate these muscles include (primarily) the axillary and radial nerves. As noted above, disorders of these peripheral nerves could also produce Sheldon's sensory symptoms. Finally, the posterior cord of the brachial plexus is the one single location that could account for all these neurologic findings.

3. As such, our attention should be directed to the posterior brachial plexus. A lesion here would explain all of Sheldon's motor, sensory, and reflex changes.

In the absence of a history of trauma, we must be concerned about mass lesions in the axillary and retroclavicular areas as well as idiopathic brachial neuritis (see above and Table 9–5).

4. Careful physical examination of the neck, axilla, and clavicular areas is thus indicated, as are radiographic examinations of these areas (cervical spine, apical lordotic x-ray).

> Careful palpation of the axilla and clavicular and neck areas reveals no abnormalities.
>
> X-rays of the cervical spine (posteroanterior, lateral, and oblique) and of the chest (with lordotic view) are completely normal.

5. Neurologic consultation should be obtained. This is certainly not necessary in many situations in which there is a peripheral neurologic disorder of the upper extremity.

Symptomatic cervical spine disease (disc herniation in the young and middle-aged; spondylosis in the older patient) is usually treated conservatively with physical therapy (temporary collars, massage, heat, and neck traction), anti-inflammatory drugs, and neck exercises. The neurologist or neurosurgeon is usually needed only when conservative therapy fails, when motor weakness is prominent, and/or when a disease other than cervical spondylosis or disc herniation is suspected (for example, spinal cord tumor).

Thoracic outlet syndromes are usually remarkably improved after 6 to 8 weeks of exercise therapy (see Appendix III). An occasional patient may require resection of local impinging structures (cervical rib, scalenus anticus muscle, for example).

Peripheral entrapment neuropathies (of the median nerve at the wrist, of the ulnar nerve at the elbow) occasionally require surgery to release the entrapped nerve, but more often prevention of repetitive pressure at the elbow (leaning on the medial epicondyle often compresses the ulnar nerve), a temporary wrist splint, or a change in occupation/avocation (the carpal tunnel syndrome is frequently temporary and remediable) will often work wonders.

Here, however, motor weakness is pronounced, symptoms are worsening, and the diagnosis is far from obvious.

> The neurologic consultant finds clinical and electrodiagnostic evidence for a combined radial and axillary nerve disorder and suggests that brachial neuritis is the most likely diagnosis.
>
> Physical therapy and the passage of time (4 months) result in complete recovery without subsequent disability or recurrence.

Not all patients with brachial neuritis recover uneventfully, just as some patients with cervical spondylopathy, entrapment neuropathy, or a thoracic outlet syndrome will require specific surgical therapy. The point is simply that careful examination will often suggest a specific diagnosis, even in a complicated clinical presentation, and thus will allow the generalist physician to begin appropriate evaluations and institute indicated consultations.

Shoulder Biomechanics and Anatomy[8, 73]

The shoulder joint is in fact many joints. Full painless range of motion of the shoulder depends upon a coordinated interaction of seven "joints" (Fig. 9–39) as well as the multiple muscle groups, ligaments, and soft-tissue structures that subserve these joints. Two of these "joints"—the suprahumeral and the scapulocostal—are not joints at all but are pseudoarticulations that also must be well understood if the mechanics of the true "joints"—the glenohumeral, acromioclavicular, and sternoclavicular—are to be appreciated. (The costosternal and costovertebral joints are noted here for the sake of completeness, but the other five joints will be emphasized more.)

While the shoulder moves in seven different directions (Fig. 9–7), detailed analysis of shoulder abduction illustrates important mechanical concepts. The normal shoulder abducts to 180 degrees (directly overhead). This movement is accomplished by the simultaneous action of two component mechanisms: the glenohumeral mechanism and the scapulothoracic mechanism. The former refers to the arc of motion between the humerus and the glenoid fossa—this glenohumeral joint allows about 120 degrees of abduction. The remaining 60 degrees of shoulder abduction result from the scapulothoracic mechanism—movement of the glenoid fossa itself as the scapula (of which the glenoid fossa is a part) rotates on the thoracic wall to achieve full (180 degrees) shoulder abduction.

Before the glenohumeral and scapulothoracic mechanisms are analyzed in more detail, it must be emphasized that each mechanism shares in all degrees of shoulder motion, i.e., the initial 120 degrees is not accomplished solely by glenohumeral motion any more than the latter 60 degrees is entirely scapulothoracic. As noted in Cailliet's geometric representation (Fig. 9–40),

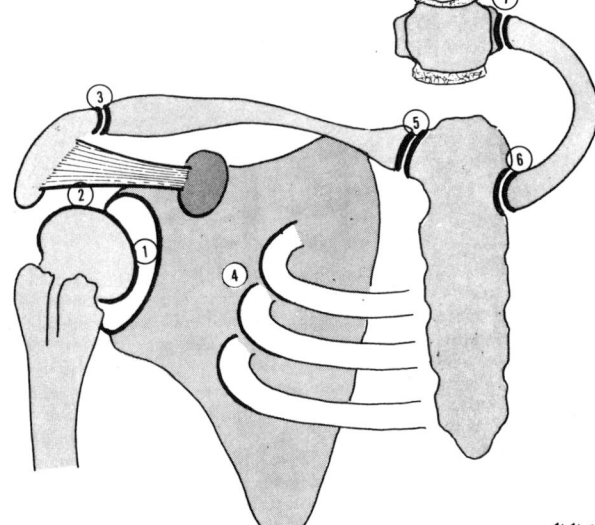

FIGURE 9–39. Composite drawing of the shoulder girdle and its seven "joints." (Reproduced with permission from Cailliet, R: Shoulder Pain. Philadelphia: F. A. Davis Co., 1966, p. 2.)

Key:
1 = Glenohumeral
2 = Suprahumeral
3 = Acromioclavicular
4 = Scapulocostal
5 = Sternoclavicular
6 = Costosternal
7 = Costovertebral

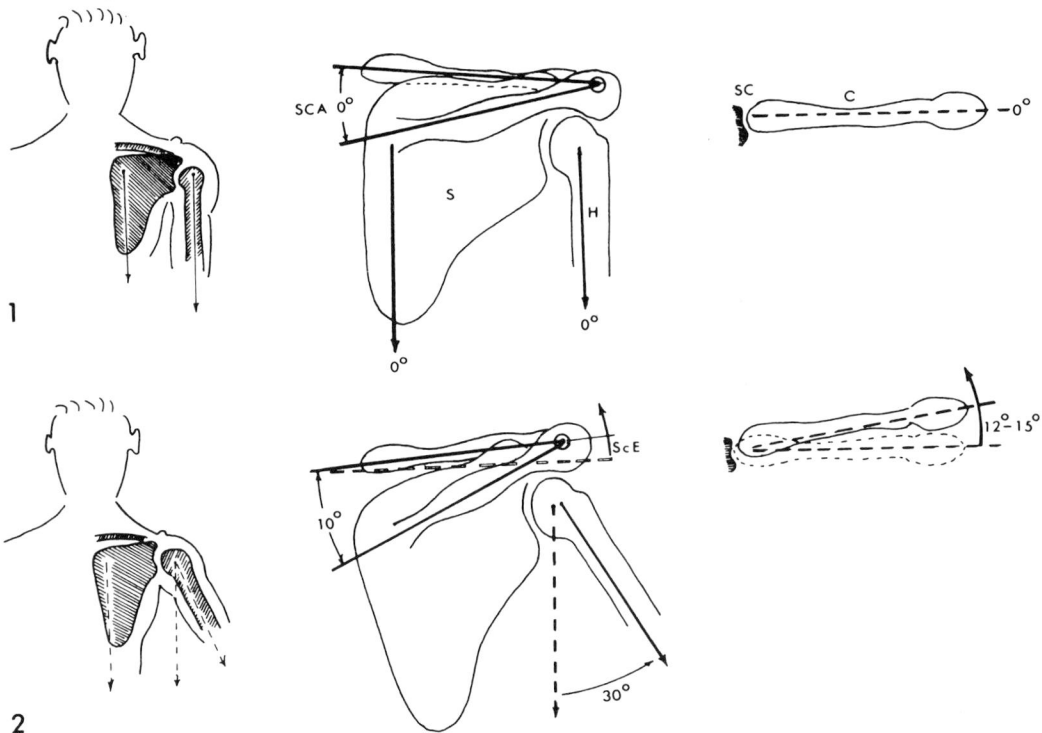

FIGURE 9—40. The composite movements of the glenohumeral and scapulothoracic mechanisms during shoulder abduction. Movement of the arm through all phases of abduction involves all joints of the shoulder girdle in a synchronous manner.

Phase 1: The resting arm: 0 degrees scapular rotation, S; 0 degrees spinoclavicular angle, SCA; 0 degrees movement at the sternoclavicular joint, SC; no elevation of the outer end of the clavicle, C; no abduction of the humerus, H.

Phase 2: Humerus abducted 30 degrees: outer end of clavicle elevated 12 to 15 degrees with no rotation of the clavicle; elevation occurs at the sternoclavicular joint; some movement occurs at the acromioclavicular joint, as seen by increase of 10 degrees of the spinoclavicular angle (angle formed by the clavicle and the scapular spine).

Illustration continues on opposite page.

all phases of motion involve synchronous movement of both component mechanisms. For each 30 degrees of shoulder abduction, an arc of approximately 20 degrees is achieved by glenohumeral motion and an arc of approximately 10 degrees by scapulothoracic motion throughout the entire 180 degrees of abduction (a 2:1 ratio throughout).

The glenohumeral mechanism involves the glenohumeral articulation and the suprahumeral joint. The glenohumeral joint is peculiar because the surface area of the glenoid fossa (the "female aspect" of the joint) is very small when compared with the surface area of the humeral head (the "male aspect"). Unlike other large joints, only a small part of the humerus articulates with the glenoid fossa at any one time. This allows greater range of motion (for example, compared with the "ball and socket" hip arrangement) but also demands extensive muscular and ligamentous support to maintain stability and prevent dislocation. This support is provided by three "layers" of structures: the glenohumeral capsule and ligaments, the suprahumeral structures or "joint", and the overlying sling of shoulder girdle musculature.

The perimeter of the glenoid fossa is encircled by a fibrous fold—the

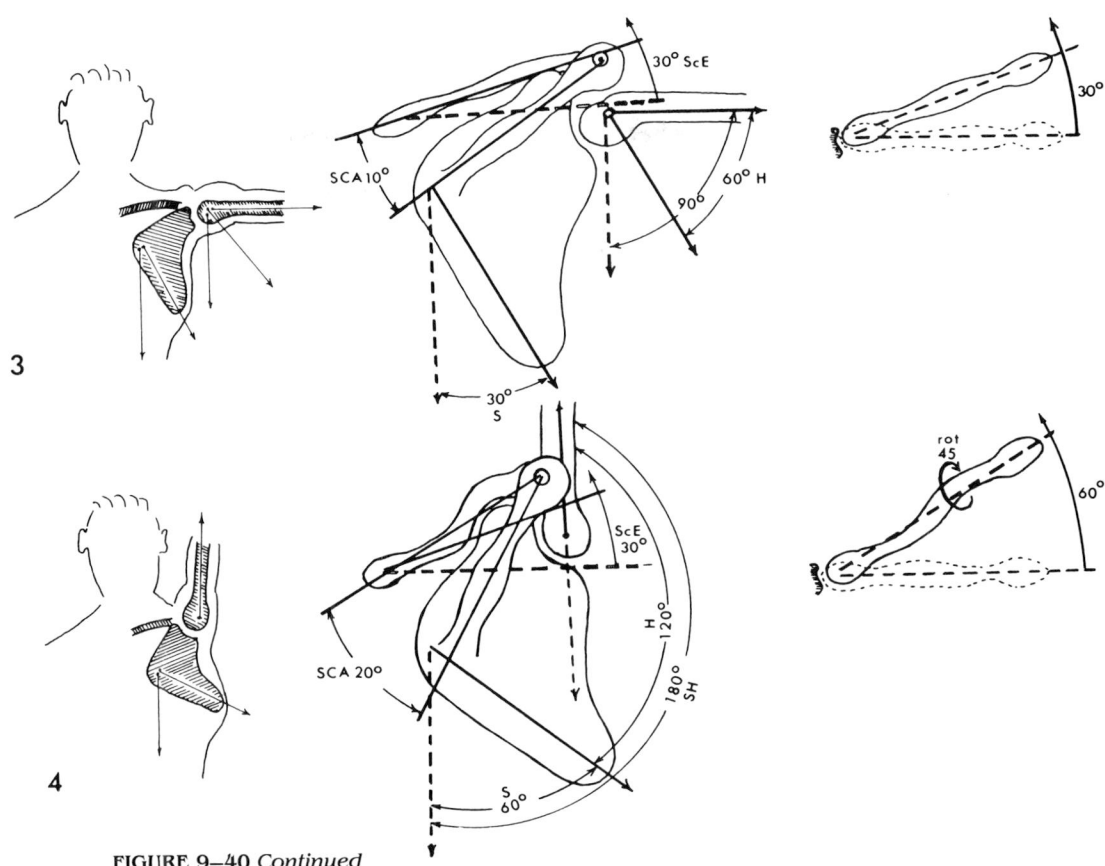

FIGURE 9–40 *Continued*

Phase 3: Humerus, H, abducted to 90 degrees (60 degrees glenohumeral, 30 degrees scapular): clavicle elevated to its final position, 30 degrees; no rotation of clavicle as yet—all movement at the sternoclavicular joint; no change in the SCA.

Phase 4: Full overhead elevation (SH 180 degrees, H 120 degrees, S 60 degrees): outer end of clavicle has not elevated further (at the sternoclavicular joint), but the SCA has increased (to 20 degrees). Because of the clavicle's rotation and its "cranklike" form, the clavicle elevates additional 30 degrees. The humerus through this phase has rotated, but this has not influenced the degrees of movement. (Reproduced with permission from Cailliet, R: Shoulder Pain. Philadelphia: F. A. Davis Co., 1966, pp. 30–31.)

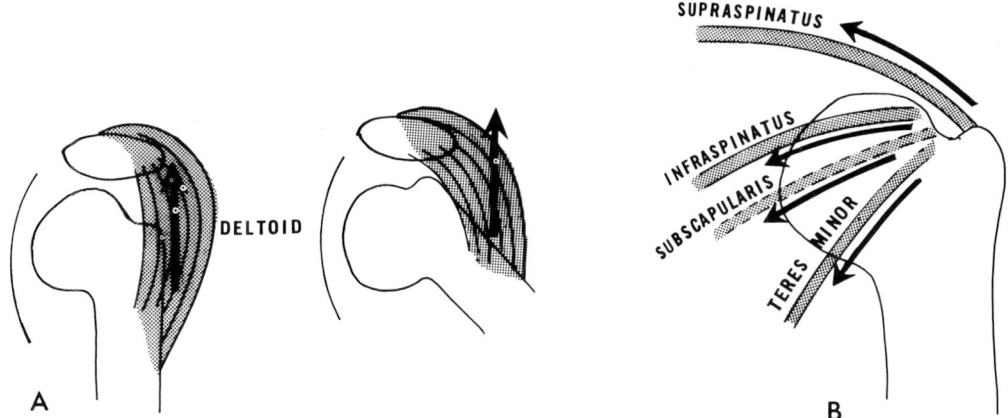

FIGURE 9–41. Deltoid function and rotator cuff function. *A,* Deltoid function. *Left,* With the arm dependent, the deltoid acts along the longitudinal axis of the humerus during elevation of the arm. *Right,* With some abduction initiated by the cuff, the deltoid pulls at an angle to the humerus, becoming the prime mover of abduction. *B,* Rotator cuff mechanism. The supraspinous (supraspinatus) muscle pulls the head of the humerus into the glenoid and slightly rotates the humerus into abduction. The infraspinous (infraspinatus) muscle also rotates the head and slightly pulls it down. The teres minor muscle pulls in a more downward direction. The subscapular (subscapularis) muscle pulls the head into the glenoid, but its main rotatory action is to rotate internally the humerus about its longitudinal axis. (Reproduced with permission from Cailliet, R: Soft Tissue Pain and Disability. Philadelphia: F. A. Davis Co., 1977, p. 151).

glenoid labrum (Fig. 9–22)—that deepens the "cup" of the shallow glenoid fossa itself. The synovial capsule of the joint attaches to the perimeter of the glenoid and also inserts around the neck of the humerus. The joint capsule is thin walled but is reinforced anteriorly by three glenohumeral ligaments that are actually folds of the capsule itself.

The suprahumeral structures (Figs. 9–22 and 9–23) overlie the glenohumeral capsule and ligaments. The coracohumeral ligament arises from the base of the coracoid process and inserts into the greater and lesser tuberosities of the humerus. The musculotendinous rotator cuff structures—the supraspinatus, infraspinatus, teres minor, and subscapularis (or SITS) muscles—originate from different parts of the scapula and cover the humeral head before inserting into the humeral tuberosities. The bony acromion and coracoid process and the interposed coracoacromial ligament form a hood over the humeral head, while subacromial and subcoracoid bursae are interposed between the deeper cuff structures and the more superficial coracoacromial hood structures.

Finally, the deltoid muscle forms the overlying shoulder girdle muscle sling that is the primary mover of the glenohumeral mechanism. Originating from the anterior, lateral, and posterior aspects of the scapular acromion and the clavicle, and inserting into the upper one third of the humerus in anterior, lateral, and posterior components (Figs. 9–13 and 9–14), the deltoid elevates the humerus parallel to its long axis, such that its isolated action would impinge the humeral head up into the suprahumeral ligamentous hood (Fig. 9–41). Only when deltoid action is coordinated with rotator cuff muscle action can true abduction be achieved at the glenohumeral joint. The SITS muscles rotate, depress, and adduct the humeral head into the glenoid fossa, thereby changing the muscular torque of the deltoid, such that it becomes the abductor force for the glenohumeral mechanism.

Glenohumeral abduction, then, requires the coordinated action of the deltoid and rotator cuff muscles, the unhindered movement of the glenohumeral articulation, as well as the integrity of the suprahumeral structures. Thus abduction may be impaired by neurogenic muscular dysfunction, isolated deltoid weakness, rotator cuff tears, restricted articular motion, periarticular swelling or impingement, or instability of the supporting structures. Differentation among these various disorders is outlined in the text proper.

The scapulothoracic mechanism is also somewhat complicated but can best be understood by considering the anatomy of the scapula and its prime muscular movers. The scapula is a broad blade of bone that has at its superolateral aspect two bony projections (the acromion and coracoid) and the concavity of the glenoid fossa—these three structures form the apices of a rough triangle (Fig. 9–22). The fixed relationship among these structures illustrates that for the glenoid fossa to move upward (to help achieve shoulder abduction), so must the acromion, coracoid, and entire scapular blade move upward—or more precisely, rotate in the coronal plane.

Scapular rotation (and thus glenoid elevation) occurs via two coordinated mechanisms. First, the trapezius and serratus anterior muscles rotate the blade of the scapula such that the medial border is depressed, the lateral border is elevated, and the acromion, coracoid, and glenoid fossa rotate upward and medially (Fig. 9–42A). Simultaneously the clavicle—which forms the only bony articulation with the scapula (at the acromioclavicular joint)—is elevated at the sternoclavicular joint by the sternocleidomastoid and trapezius muscles (Fig. 9–42B). The coracoclavicular ligaments (Fig. 9–22)

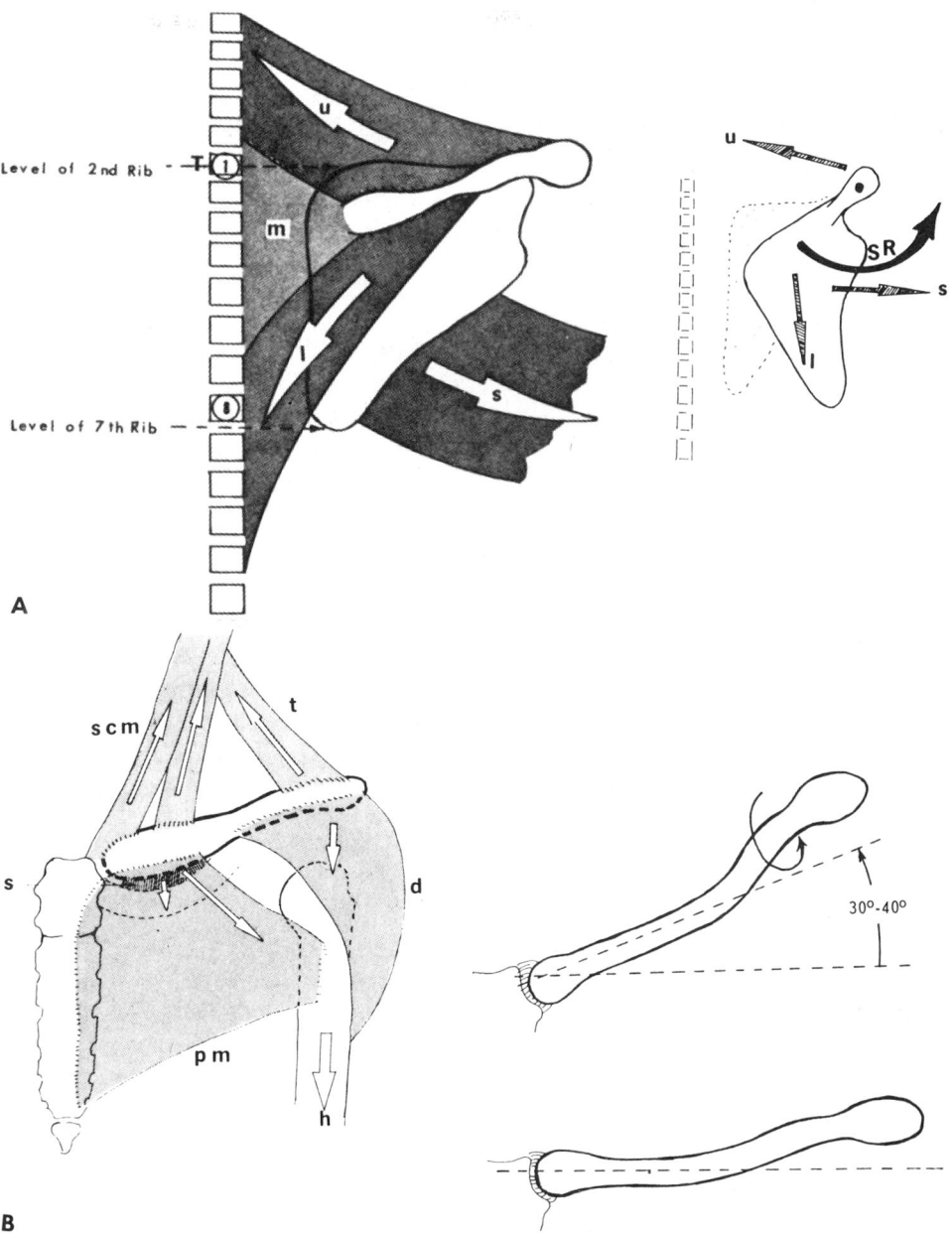

FIGURE 9–42. The scapulothoracic mechanism. *A,* Scapular musculature: rotators. The scapular muscles forming the rotator phase of the scapulohumeral rhythm are shown with the upper trapezius fibers elevating the outer border of the spine, the lower fibers of the trapezius depressing the medial border of the spine, and the serratus pulling the lower portion of the scapula forward from its position under the blade. The combined action moves the scapula in orbit around the acromioclavicular center of rotation.

u = upper ⎫	s = serratus anterior
m = middle ⎬ trapezius	SR = scapular rotation
l = lower ⎭	

B, Muscles acting upon the clavicle. The major muscles acting upon the clavicle are shown, their direction of pull indicated by arrows: scm, sternocleidomastoid; t, trapezius; d, deltoid; s, subscapularis; and pm, pectoralis major. The gravity pull of the arm itself is represented by h. The muscles that act indirectly upon the clavicle are not shown. (Reproduced with permission from Cailliet, R: Shoulder Pain. Philadelphia: F. A. Davis Co., 1966, pp. 19, 28.)

maintain a fixed relationship between clavicle and scapula throughout the arc of scapular motion (i.e., there is no rotation of the scapula on the clavicle). Thus, the scapula pivots about the acromioclavicular joint as the clavicle is elevated at the sternoclavicular joint. In addition, the shape of the clavicle and the integrity of the coracoclavicular ligaments allows further scapular rotation as the crank-shaped clavicle rotates during abduction, elevating the scapula even further without additional sternoclavicular movement (Fig. 9–42B).

The reverse action (downward scapular rotation with adduction of the shoulder) involves downward scapular rotator muscles—the rhomboids, levator scapulae, pectoralis major, and latissimus dorsi (Fig. 9–14)—and reversal of clavicular elevation and rotation at the sternoclavicular joint.

The integration of the glenohumeral and scapulothoracic mechanisms, then, depends upon the coordinated function of many different structures. Impaired shoulder movement must be analyzed from the perspective of these biomechanical features. Impaired shoulder mobility may result from disorders of the clavicle, scapula, glenohumeral joint, acromioclavicular joint, sternoclavicular joint, the various ligaments and muscles (and tendons) surrounding these bones and joints, the nerves that innervate those muscles or disorders of other soft-tissue structures (bursae, for example) that impede the action of these structures. The examination of the shoulder, then, depends on analyzing which mechanisms are impaired; where; and why.

Traumatic Shoulder Pain[74]

Even a superficial discussion of traumatic shoulder injuries is far beyond the scope of this book. Nevertheless, while many shoulder injuries require orthopedic consultation, some do not, and a brief overview of various traumatic disorders may allow a more efficient and rational use of orthopedic consultants.

Whether the traumatic incident is direct (fall, forceful traction, direct blow) or indirect (for example, a throwing injury), shoulder x-rays should always be obtained. These should always include (at least) anteroposterior, lateral, and axillary views and sometimes tangential or rotatory views. (Axillary x-rays are important to exclude a posterior dislocation that might otherwise be missed on routine films.)

An orthopedist should be consulted immediately when:

1. X-rays reveal fracture(s). While some clavicular and scapular fractures may be treated conservatively (for example, splinted and immobilized), this general rule holds.

2. X-rays reveal dislocation(s). In general, all patients with acute or recurrent glenohumeral dislocations[75, 76] require orthopedic attention.

Acute glenohumeral dislocations are usually of the anterior variety (Fig. 9-43B and C), and prompt reduction is most important. Many methods are used by different orthopedists, but the Stimson maneuver is often successful and is easy for the nonorthopedist to implement. Figure 9-43 demonstrates the patient with an anterior dislocation lying prone or on the side (usually under mild sedation) with the arm dangling toward the floor (perhaps with a light weight attached to the wrist). Maintenance of this position for 10 to 15 minutes will often reduce the dislocation as muscle spasm relaxes and the humerus falls back into place. If relocation is successful, immobilization of the shoulder in a splint for a few weeks is usually indicated, but an orthopedist should be consulted in any event.

Acromioclavicular dislocations are common (usually following a fall on the tip of the shoulder). Frank dislocation refers to an obvious visible upriding of the distal clavicle, clearly apparent on both examination and x-rays (Fig. 9-44C and D). This usually implies rupture of both the acromioclavicular and coracoclavicular ligaments and often requires operative repair (grade III). Lesser degrees of acromioclavicular separation are usually treated conservatively. A grade I sprain is associated with normal x-rays but tenderness over the acromioclavicular joint. Grade II sprain refers to a slight upriding of the distal clavicle but without complete separation at the acromioclavicular joint on x-ray. These injuries can be managed conservatively by simple reduction of the joint and application of a sling that maintains the appropriate position (usually for 3 or 4 weeks) (Fig. 9-44).

Sternoclavicular dislocations are much less common but are also sometimes more difficult to diagnose. X-rays may not be very helpful, and, in general, any traumatic injury that results in significant pain and tenderness

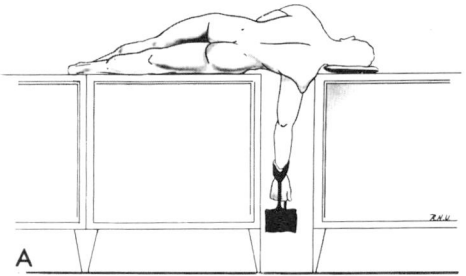

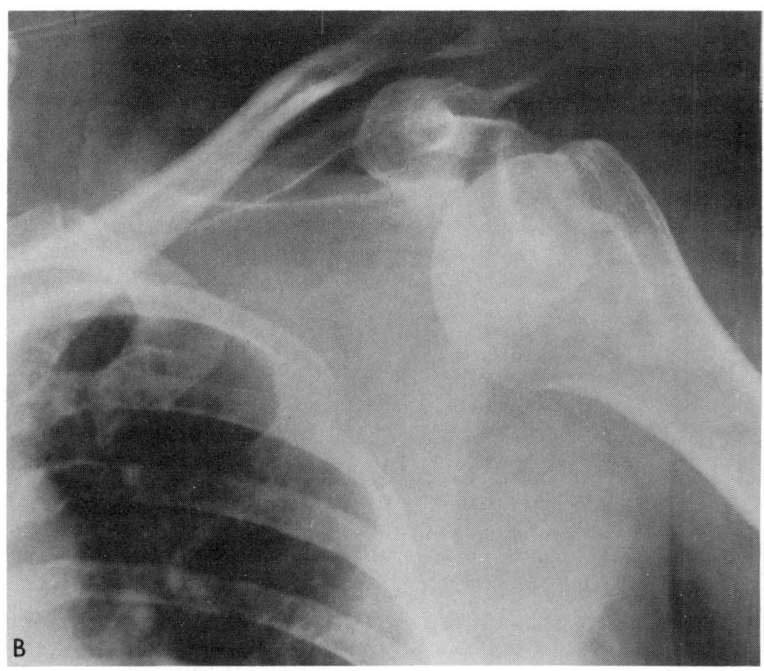

FIGURE 9–43. A, The traction method (Stimson) of reduction of the dislocated shoulder. B, C, Anterior dislocation of the humerus. This patient suffered from recurrent dislocation. X-rays demonstrate humeral position before (B) and after reduction (C) of the dislocation. (A reproduced with permission from Rowe, CR: Acute and recurrent anterior dislocation of the shoulder. Orthop Clin North Am 11:257, 1980.)

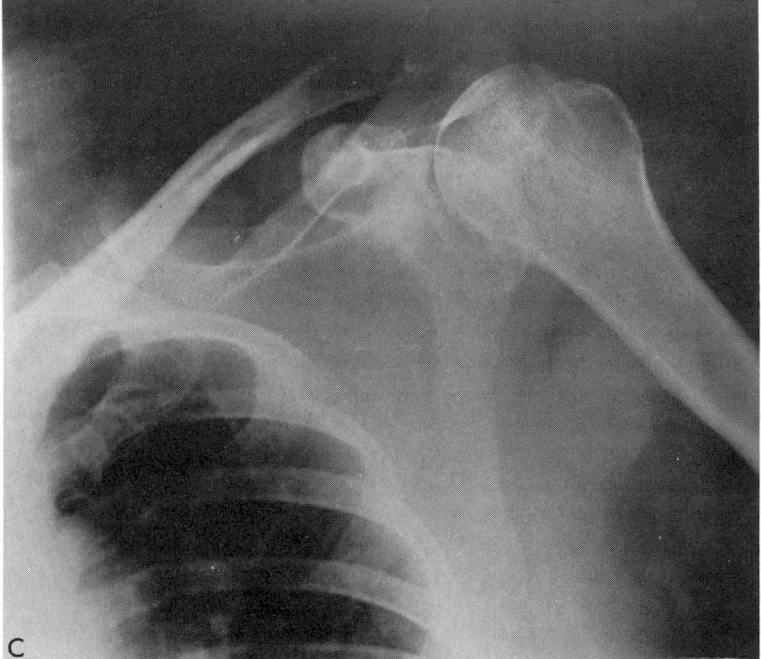

about the sternoclavicular joint (even with normal x-rays) merits at least a conversation with an orthopedist.

3. Even when x-rays are normal, the patient who is unable to move the shoulder following shoulder trauma deserves orthopedic attention. Especially if relief of local pain (with local anesthetics or systemic analgesics) does not allow resumption of shoulder mobility, several disorders must be considered, and a more experienced examiner should be consulted: These disorders include ruptures of the rotator cuff, unsuspected (especially posterior) glenohumeral dislocations, inapparent scapular fractures, synovial capsular tears, and intra-articular hemarthrosis.

Otherwise, for shoulder injuries in which x-rays are normal and shoulder mobility is largely preserved (even if painful), a few points deserve emphasis:

1. The mechanism of trauma and a precise history will help diagnose the problem. Falls on the tip of the shoulder often injure the acromioclavi-

cular or sternoclavicular joint or both. Falls on the outstretched hand are more likely to injure the rotator cuff or the biceps tendon but may also produce glenohumeral subluxation/dislocation. Direct trauma to isolated structures may cause muscle or nerve injury: Deltoid or trapezius contusions are common, as are injuries to the musculocutaneous nerve and axillary nerve.

2. Not all rotator cuff tears are associated with obviously impaired shoulder mobility. As noted in the text proper, any patient who develops weakness of the shoulder following trauma and whose x-rays are unremarkable must be suspected of rotator cuff injury. Immediate orthopedic consultation is certainly not required for all suspected rotator cuff injuries, but the patient must be followed carefully to document restitution of full shoulder mobility and strength.

3. Throwing injuries are common causes of traumatic shoulder pain. While they are most common in baseball players, they may occur in many different sports and activities. Most such injuries involve strains of the musculotendinous structures of the shoulder girdle, and a knowledge of individual muscle origins and insertions (Fig. 9–13) will be very helpful here.

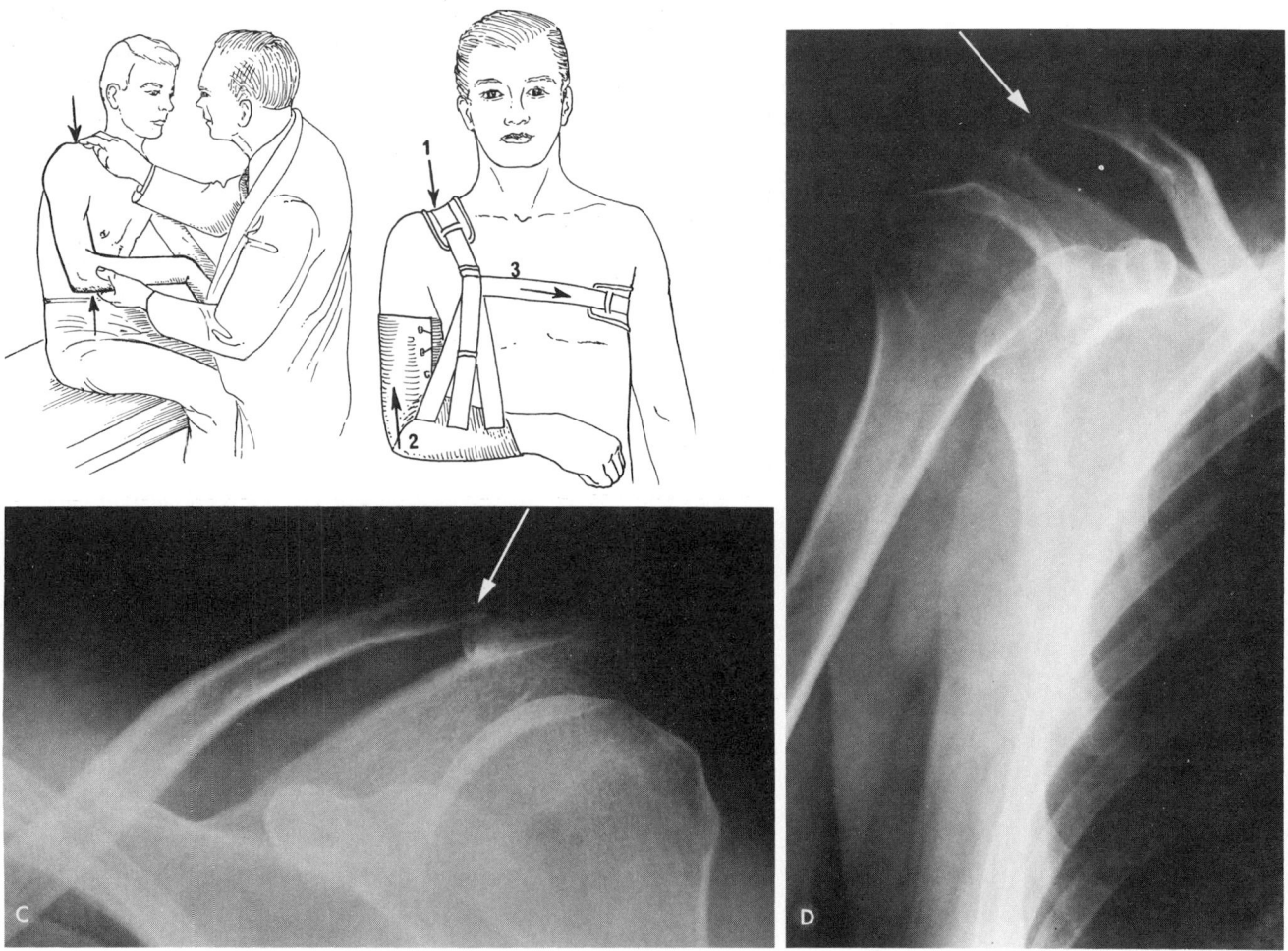

FIGURE 9–44. Reduction of sprain of the acromioclavicular joint. This is advisable with grades I and II dislocations. A, Reduction of grade II sprain of the acromioclavicular joint. Downward pressure on the clavicle and upward pressure on the forearm readily corrects the displacement. B, Kenny-Howard sling. The shoulder strap is applied over a piece of felt; it holds the clavicle down (1). The sling supports the forearm and keeps the acromion in an elevated position (2). The halter pulls both the shoulder strap and the sling inward (3). C, D, Acromioclavicular separation (grade III). These injuries require orthopedic attention. (A and B reproduced with permission from DePalma, AF: Surgery of the Shoulder, 2nd ed. Philadelphia: J. B. Lippincott Co., 1973, p. 318.)

In general, knowledge of the point in the throwing motion when pain began, as well as careful examination for localized tenderness and swelling of musculotendinous structures, will usually reveal the diagnosis. As noted by DePalma:

> Pain on the anterior aspect of the shoulder during the entire stage of forward movement of the body indicates either a tearing of the fibers of insertion of the anterior deltoid or the pectoralis major or both, or an injury to the biceps tendon . . . On the other hand, pain in the posterior aspect of the shoulder during the follow-through phase of throwing implicates the insertion of the posterior deltoid into the spine of the scapula or the tendon of insertion of the long head of the triceps into the scapula just beneath the glenohumeral joint or the insertion of the rhomboid major into the vertebral border of the scapula.[77]

Figure 9–45 demonstrates common areas of tenderness following such throwing injuries. It must be remembered that glenohumeral subluxation/dislocation, rotator cuff injuries, and injuries to the biceps apparatus may also occur following throwing injuries.

When x-rays are normal, when the neurovascular status is intact, and when either traumatic musculotendinous strain or joint sprain (without subluxation/dislocation) is most likely, conservative treatment can usually be initiated without orthopedic consultation.

Conservative treatment involves application of ice to the injured area for the first 24 to 48 hours and sling support of the arm, followed by heat and active shoulder motion after a variable period. In simple musculotendinous injuries, recovery is commonly rapid, and active shoulder motion often may be begun after just 3 to 4 days. (Throwing, however, must be discontinued until all pain, tenderness, and swelling disappear and until active range of motion is completely normal.) On the other hand, acromioclavicular or sternoclavicular sprains usually require more prolonged immobilization in specific types of slings (Fig. 9–44), but ongoing exercise of the hand and forearm during this interval (ranging from 3 to 6 weeks) is most important. Physical therapy following the period of immobilization must be stressed.

In all instances of traumatic shoulder pain, the mechanism of injury will enlighten our approach to the patient. Simultaneous injuries to the hand, wrist, elbow, neck, and other areas may be overshadowed by more prominent shoulder pain. Careful attention to the entire examination is crucial.

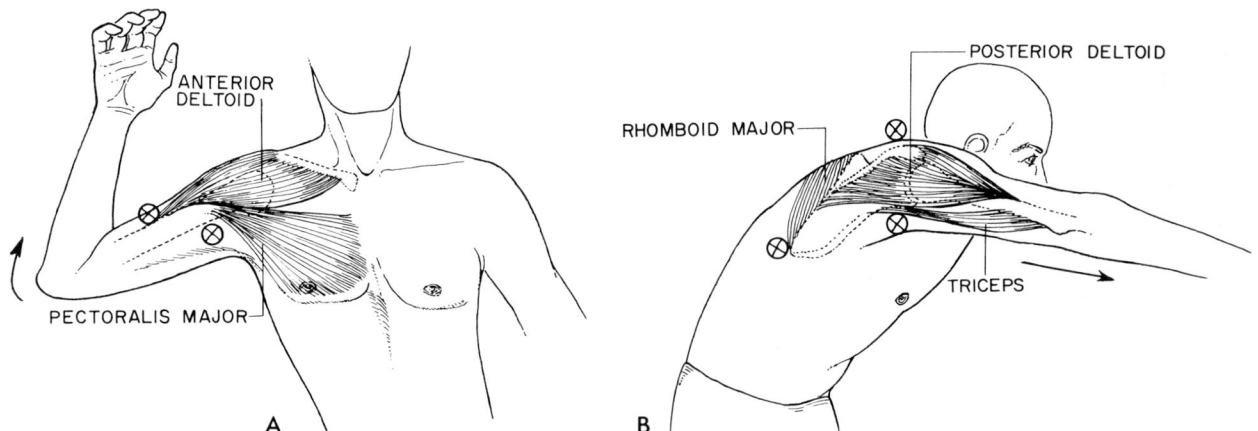

FIGURE 9–45. Throwing injuries. *A,* During the preparatory phase of the throwing act when the arm has reached the extremes of abduction, extension and external rotation, the anterior deltoid and the pectoralis major are at their maximal length. With forward movement of the body, more tension is applied to the muscle-tendon units, and injury may result at their insertions. *B,* During the follow-through phase, the posterior muscle-tendon units reach their maximum tension and elongation; these are the posterior deltoid, the triceps, and the rhomboid major. A powerful pitch may overpower the muscle units, causing an injury to their insertions. (Reproduced with permission from DePalma, A. F.: Surgery of the Shoulder, 2nd ed. Philadelphia: J. B. Lippincott Co., 1973, pp. 271, 273.)

Thoracic Outlet Syndromes[78-80]

The thoracic outlet refers to the area traversed by the brachial plexus, subclavian artery, and subclavian vein in their passage from the neck to the upper extremity. The artery and nerve plexus travel together, passing through three areas of potential entrapment: (1) through the scalene triangle (formed by the scalenus anticus muscle anteriorly, scalenus medius muscle posteriorly, and the first rib inferiorly); (2) arching over the first rib (and behind the clavicle); and (3) into the axilla behind the insertion of the pectoralis minor tendon on the coracoid process. The subclavian vein traverses the same path, but usually begins its course superficial to the scalene triangle (and thus lies anterior to the scalenus anticus muscle).

Compression of the nerve plexus or great vessels may occur at any of these three locations. Specific signs and symptoms vary with the site of compression as well as the cause.

Most patients with thoracic outlet syndrome do not complain primarily of shoulder pain. Most describe pain or dysesthesias of the hand and forearm as the initial complaint, and almost all admit to neurologic (paresthesias, lancinating pains) or vascular symptoms (pallor, cyanosis, edema) at sites distant from the shoulder even when shoulder pain is part of the presenting complaint. Diagnosis depends on recognizing the characteristic symptom complex (usually dysesthesias in the C8-T1 dermatomes), which is usually episodic and which can be reproduced by maneuvers on physical examination that further exaggerate the neurovascular compression. There are three common syndromes:

1. Scalenus anticus syndrome. Here the subclavian artery and neural plexus are compressed within the scalene triangle (the vein is less often involved because it does not usually traverse this triangle). Compression is most often the result of anomalous cervical ribs or anatomic variations in the scalene muscles themselves (thickened ligamentous insertions, bifid muscle bellies, an accessory scalenus minimus muscle, for example). Maneuvers that further restrict the area of the scalene triangle—by elevating the first rib and tensing the scalenus anticus muscle—will then reproduce symptoms.

The Adson maneuver (Fig. 9–46A) is performed with the patient sitting, both arms at sides, the examiner palpating the radial pulse and prepared to auscultate for vascular bruits in the ipsilateral supraclavicular area. The patient is instructed to take and hold a deep breath, simultaneously hyperextend the neck, and turn the chin toward the involved arm (sometimes abduction of the ipsilateral arm is performed as well). A positive (abnormal) test includes reproduction of the patient's symptoms together with diminution (or loss) of the palpated radial pulse (sometimes associated with development of a transient supraclavicular bruit and thrill).

2. The costoclavicular syndrome. Here, the neurovascular bundle is compressed between the first rib posteriorly and the clavicle anteriorly. Abnormalities of rib or clavicle (old fractures with callus formation, exos-

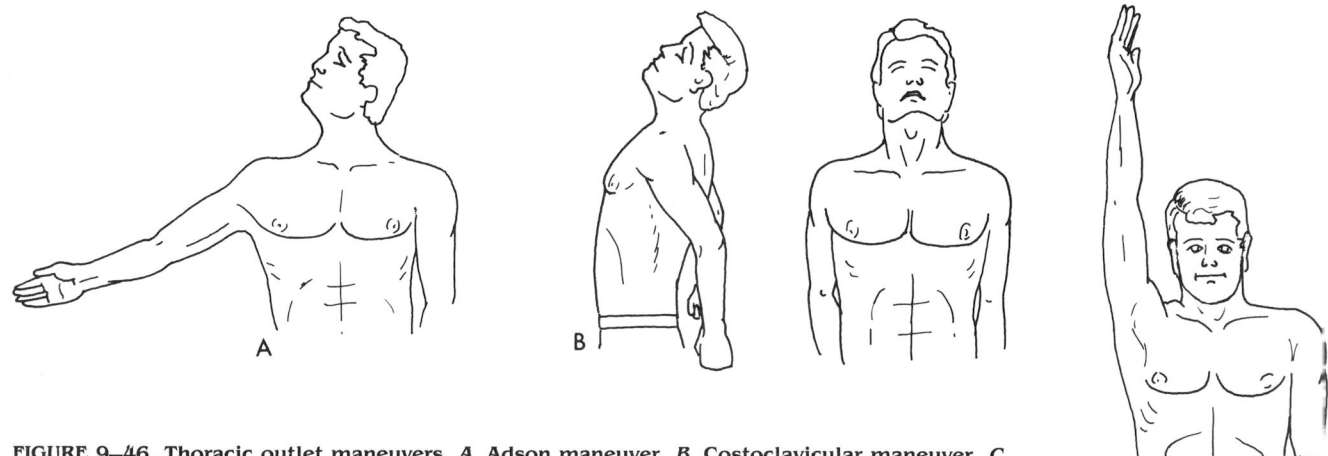

FIGURE 9–46. Thoracic outlet maneuvers. *A*, Adson maneuver. *B*, Costoclavicular maneuver. *C*, Hyperabduction maneuver.

toses, masses) that further narrow the costoclavicular space will induce symptoms that are often postural and intermittent (carrying heavy objects with arms at sides, sleeping with arms overhead, carrying a back pack).

The costoclavicular maneuver (Fig. 9–46B) is performed with the patient sitting, hands in lap, examiner poised to palpate the radial pulse and auscultate above. The patient then is instructed to throw the shoulders back and down—exaggerated military position. Reproduction of symptoms and obliteration of the radial pulse (with or without a bruit) is a positive (abnormal) test.

3. Hyperabduction syndrome. Here, the neurovascular bundle is compressed before it enters the axilla, usually where the tendon of the pectoralis minor muscle inserts onto the coracoid process. Most patients experience symptoms during sleep (the patient is often unaware that he or she sleeps with arms overhead and hyperabducted), but persons whose occupation or avocation requires frequent assumption of this position may also be afflicted during the day—painters, mechanics, gymnasts, for example.

The hyperabduction maneuver (Fig. 9–46C) is performed with the patient sitting, arms at sides. The arm is then elevated directly overhead (in full shoulder flexion) and backward while the examiner palpates the pulse and auscultates for axillary or infraclavicular bruits. A positive test involves diminished pulsation and reproduction of symptoms.

These maneuvers are easy to perform and always worth the effort when vague, intermittent shoulder/arm symptoms are associated with neurovascular symptoms in the arm and hand. A few words of caution:

1. In many asymptomatic people the radial pulse will be obliterated or diminished with any or all of these maneuvers. The symptom complex must be reproduced or exacerbated by the maneuvers if pulse changes are to be considered of diagnostic importance.

2. These syndromes are often distressing, but almost never threatening. Serious complications—acute arterial or venous thrombosis, subclavian aneurysm, distal gangrene (ischemic or embolic), chronic venous insufficiency—do occur, but these are very rare. Most often, simple conservative therapy suffices (Table 9–9), and surgery is only uncommonly necessary.

3. It is just as easy to overdiagnose these syndromes as to miss them.

TABLE 9–9. SHOULDER GIRDLE EXERCISES FOR THORACIC OUTLET SYNDROME

At the beginning, each exercise is done 10 times in succession twice a day. As the shoulders and neck gain strength, the number of times each exercise is done consecutively can be increased. The six exercises follow:

1. Stand erect with the arms at the sides, holding in each hand a 2-pound weight (sandbags, or bottles, jars, or sacks filled with sand). (a) Shrug the shoulders forward and upward. (b) Relax. (c) Shrug the shoulders backward and upward. (d) Relax. (e) Shrug the shoulders upward. (f) Relax and repeat.

2. Stand erect with the arms out straight from the sides at shoulder level; hold a 2-pound weight in each hand (palms should be down). (a) Raise the arms sideward and up until the back of the hands meet above the head (keep elbows straight). (b) Relax and repeat. **Note:** As strength improves.and exercises 1 and 2 become easier, weights should be made heavier; increase to 5 and later to 10 pounds.

3. Stand facing a corner of the room with one hand on each wall, arms at shoulder level, palms forward, elbows bent and abdominal muscles contracted. (a) Slowly let the upper part of the trunk lean forward and press the chest into the corner. Inhale as the body leans forward. (b) Return to the original position by pushing out with the hands. Exhale with this movement.

4. Stand erect with the arms at the sides. (a) Bending the neck to the left, attempt to touch the left ear to the left shoulder without shrugging the shoulder. (b) Bending the neck to the right, attempt to touch the right ear to the right shoulder without shrugging the shoulder. (c) Relax and repeat.

5. Lie face down with the hands clasped behind the back. (a) Raise the head and chest from the floor as high as possible while pulling the shoulders backward and the chin in. Hold this position for a count of three. Inhale as the chest is raised. (b) Exhale and return to the original position. (c) Repeat.

6. Lie down on the back with arms at the sides, with a rolled towel or small pillow under the head. (a) Inhale slowly and raise the arms upward and backward overhead. (b) Exhale and lower the arms to the sides. (c) Repeat 5 to 20 times.

(Reproduced with permission from Allen, EV, Barker, NW, and Hines, EA: Neuromuscular compression syndromes of the thoracic outlet and shoulder girdle. *In* Peripheral Vascular Diseases, 3rd ed. Philadelphia: W. B. Saunders Co., 1966.)

Great care should be taken initially to exclude other conditions that may mimic thoracic outlet syndromes (and that as a group are much more common). These include carpal tunnel syndromes, Raynaud's phenomenon, ulnar entrapment neuropathy (usually at the elbow), cervical spondylosis, spinal cord lesions, Pancoast tumors (or other axillary/supraclavicular tumor masses), and atherosclerotic or vasculitic arterial disease (Fig. 9–4).

4. Conservative therapy depends on identifying the clinical site of compression, addressing postural/occupational stresses that worsen compression, and initiating shoulder girdle exercises. Symptoms predominantly during sleep may require loose binding of the wrists to the waist or legs to prevent full hyperabduction during sleep.

The exercises described in Table 9–9 should be performed ten times each at least twice a day; benefits should not be expected for at least several weeks (and sometimes several months). The great majority of patients with thoracic outlet syndromes will improve symptomatically simply by following these exercise programs and by redressing any postural or occupational contributing factors. Failure to improve usually suggests that the diagnosis is in error, but more sophisticated testing (arteriography, nerve conduction studies) may be needed.

REFERENCES

1. Dworkin, H, et al.: Supradiaphragmatic reference of pain from the colon. Gastroenterology 22:272, 1952.
2. Owen, DS: Aspiration and injection of joints and soft tissues. In Kelley, WN, et al. (eds.): Textbook of Rheumatology. Philadelphia: W. B. Saunders, 1981, Chap. 37.
3. Golding, DN: Hypothyroidism presenting with musculoskeletal symptoms. Ann Rheum Dis 29:10–14, 1970.
4. Bridgeman, JF: Periarthritis of the shoulder and diabetes mellitus. Ann Rheum Dis 31:69–71, 1972.
5. Katz, JA, et al.: The shoulder pad signs—a diagnostic feature of amyloid arthropathy. New Engl J Med 288:354–355, 1973.
6. Good, AE, et al.: Rheumatic symptoms during tuberculosis therapy—a manifestation of isoniazid toxicity? Ann Intern Med 63:800–807, 1965.
7. Hoppenfeld, S.: Physical Examination of the Spine and Extremities. New York: Appleton-Century-Crofts, 1976, pp 1–34.
8. Cailliet, R.: Shoulder Pain. Philadelphia: F.A. Davis, 1966, pp 1–32.
9. Davies, GJ, et al.: Functional examination of the shoulder girdle. Physician Sports Med 9:82–104 (June), 1981.
10. DePalma, AF: Surgery of the Shoulder. Philadelphia: J.B. Lippincott, 1973, pp 42–79.
11. Moseley, HF: Shoulder Lesions. Edinburgh: E & S Livingstone, 1969, pp 22–30.
12. Master, R, et al.: Arthritis of the glenohumeral joint. Unique clinical and radiographic features and a favorable outcome. Arthritis Rheum 20:1500–1506, 1977.
13. Michele, AA, et al.: Scapulocostal syndrome (fatigue—postural paradox). NY J Med 50:1353–1356, 1950.
14. Kopell, PH, Thompson, WAL: Peripheral Entrapment Neuropathies. Baltimore: Williams and Wilkins, 1963, pp 144–154.
15. Kopell, PH, Thompson, WAL: Peripheral Entrapment Neuropathies. Baltimore: Williams and Wilkins, 1963, pp 130–142.
16. Clein, LJ: Suprascapular entrapment neuropathy. J Nuerosurg 44:337–340, 1975.
17. Smythe, HA: Fibrositis and other diffuse musculoskeletal syndromes. In Kelley, WN, et al. (eds.): Textbook of Rheumatology. Philadelphia: W.B. Saunders, 1981, pp 485–493.
18. Bennett, RM: Fibrositis: Misnomer for a common rheumatic disorder. West J Med 134:405–413, 1981.
19. Brown, BB Jr: Diagnosis and therapy of common myofascial syndromes. JAMA 239:646, 1978.
20. Simons, DG: Muscle pain syndromes. Am J Phys Med 54:289; 55:15, 1976.
21. DePalma, AF: Surgery of the Shoulder. Philadelphia: J.B. Lippincott, 1973, pp 100–137.
22. Cailliet, R: Soft Tissue Pain and Disability. Philadelphia: F.A. Davis, 1977, pp 149–153.
23. Uhthoff, HK, et al.: Calcifying tendinitis. A new concept in its pathogenesis. Clin Orthop 118:164–168, 1976.
24. Moseley, HF: Shoulder Lesions. Edinburgh: E & S Livingstone, 1969, pp 88–98.
25. Cailliet, R.: Shoulder Pain. Philadelphia: F.A. Davis, 1966, pp 71–73.
26. Moseley, HF: The natural history and clinical syndrome produced by calcified deposits in the rotator cuff. Surg Clin North Am 43:1489–1494, 1963.
27. Moseley, HF: Shoulder Lesions. Edinburgh: E & S Livingstone, 1969, pp 99–118.
28. DePalma, AF: Surgery of the Shoulder. Philadelphia: J.B. Lippincott, 1973, pp 433–440.
29. Nixon, JE, DeStefano, V: Rupture of the rotator cuff. Orthop Clin North Am 6:423–448, 1975.
30. Samilson, R, Binder, WF: Symptomatic full thickness tears of the rotator cuff: An analysis of 292 shoulders in 276 patients. Orthop Clin North Am 6:449–466, 1975.
31. DePalma, AF: Surgery of the Shoulder. Philadelphia: J.B. Lippincott, 1977, pp 440–450.
32. Moseley, HF: Shoulder Lesions. Edinburgh: E & S Livingstone, 1969, pp 60–87.
33. Moseley, HF: Shoulder Lesions. Edinburgh: E & S Livingstone, 1969, p 76.
34. Rowe, CR: Rupture of the rotator cuff: Selection of cases for conservative treatment. Surg Clin North Am 43:1531–1534, 1963.
35. Marcove, RC: Neoplasms of the shoulder girdle. Orthop Clin North Am 6:541–552, 1975.
36. Richardson, AT: The painful shoulder. Proc R Soc Med 68:731–736, 1975.
37. Simon, LS, Mills, JA: Nonsteroidal anti-inflammatory drugs. N Engl J Med 302:1179–1185, 1237–1243, 1980.
38. Fitzgerald, RJ, Jr.: Intrasynovial injection of steroids. Uses and abuses. Mayo Clin Proc 51:655, 1976.
39. Chandler, GN, Wright, V: Deleterious effect of intra-articular hydrocortisone. Lancet 1:661, 1958.
40. Sweenam, R: Corticosteroid arthropathy and tendon rupture (Editorial). J. Bone Joint Surg 51B:33–97, 1969.
41. Kessel, L, Watson, M: The painful arc syndrome. Clinical classification as a guide to management. J Bone Joint Surg 59B:166–172, 1977.
42. Kummel, BM: The syndrome of anterior capsular derangement of the shoulder. Orthop Rev 1:7, 1972.
43. Neviaser, JS: Adhesive capsulitis and the stiff and painful shoulder. Orthop Clin North Am 11:327–331, 1980.
44. Neviaser, JS: Adhesive capsulitis of the shoulder. Med Times 90:783, 1962.
45. Lundberg, BJ: The frozen shoulder. Acta Orthop Scand (Suppl) 119:1–59, 1969.
46. Bland, JH, et al.: The painful shoulder. Semin. Arthritis Rheum 7:21, 1977.
47. Weiss, JJ, et al.: Arthrography and the diagnosis of shoulder pain and immobility. Arch Phys Med Rehabil 55:205–209, 1974.
48. Neviaser, JS: Arthrography of the shoulder joint—a study of the findings in adhesive capsulitis of the shoulder. J Bone Joint Surg 44A:321, 1962.
49. Reeves, B.: The natural history of the frozen shoulder syndrome. Scand J Rheumatol 4:193, 1975.

50. Steinbrocker, O, Argyros, T: The frozen shoulder: Treatment by local injection of depot corticosteroids. Arch Phys Med Rehabil 55:209–213, 1974.
51. Weiser, HI: Painful primary frozen shoulder mobilization under local anesthesia. Arch Phys Med Rehabil 58:406–408, 1977.
52. Bateman, JE: Neurological causes of cervicobrachial pain. Surg Clin North Am 43:1679–1684, 1963.
53. Bateman, JE: Nerve lesions about the shoulder. Orthop Clin North Am 11:307–326, 1980.
54. Moseley, HF: Shoulder Lesions. Edinburgh: E & S Livingstone, 1969, pp 260–281.
55. Coventry, MB: Problem of the painful shoulder. JAMA 151:177–185, 1953.
56. Neviaser, JS: Arthrography of the shoulder. Orthop Clin North Am 11:205–218, 1980.
57. Johnson, LL: Arthroscopy of the shoulder. Orthop Clin North Am 11:197–204, 1980.
58. Phalen, GS: The carpal tunnel syndrome. Seventeen years' experience in diagnosis and treatment of 654 hands. J Bone Joint Surg 48A:211–228, 1966.
59. D'Aubigne, RM: Nerve injuries in fractures and dislocations of the shoulder. Surg Clin North Am 43:1685–1689, 1963.
60. Steinbrocker, O: The shoulder-hand syndrome. Associated painful homolateral disability of the shoulder and hand with swelling and atrophy of the hand. Am J Med 3:402–407, 1947.
61. Kozin, F, et al.: The reflex sympathetic dystrophy syndrome. I & II. Am J Med 60:321–331, 332–338, 1976.
62. Yoss, RE, et al.: Significance of symptoms and signs in localization of involved roots in cervical disc protrusions. Neurology 7:673–683, 1957.
63. Paulson, DL: Carcinoma of the superior pulmonary sulcus. J Thorac Cardiovasc Surg 70:1095–1104, 1975.
64. Miller, JI, et al.: Carcinoma of the superior pulmonary sulcus. Ann Thorac Surg 28:44–47, 1979.
65. Tsairis, P, et al.: Natural history of brachial plexus neuropathy. Report on 99 patients. Arch Neurol 27:109–117, 1972.
66. Bacevich, BB: Paralytic brachial neuritis. J Bone Joint Surg 58A:262–263, 1976.
67. Flagman, PD, Kelly, JJ: Brachial plexus neuropathy. An electrophysiologic evaluation. Arch Neurol 37:160–164, 1980.
68. De Jong, RN: The Neurologic Examination. Hagerstown, Md: Harper & Row, 1979, pp 334–374; 569–573.
69. Adams, RD, Victor, M: Principles of Neurology. New York: McGraw-Hill, 1981, pp 917–922.
70. De Jong, RN: The Neurologic Examination. Hagerstown, Md: Harper & Row, 1979, p 547.
71. Omer, GE: Physical diagnosis of peripheral nerve injuries. Orthop Clin North Am 12:207–228, 1981.
72. Bralliar, F: Electromyography: Its use and misuse in peripheral nerve injuries. Orthop Clin North Am 12:229–238, 1981.
73. DePalma, AF: Surgery of the Shoulder. Philadelphia: J.B. Lippincott, 1973, pp 80–99.
74. DePalma, AF: Surgery of the Shoulder. Philadelphia: J.B. Lippincott, 1973, Chap 9.
75. Rowe, CR: Acute and recurrent anterior dislocations of the shoulder. Orthop Clin North Am 11:253–270, 1980.
76. May, VR: Posterior dislocation of the shoulder: Habitual, traumatic and obstetrical. Orthop Clin North Am 11:271–286, 1980.
77. DePalma, AF: Surgery of the Shoulder. Philadelphia: J.B. Lippincott, 1973, Chap. 8.
78. Allin, EV, Barker, NW, Hines, EA: Neurovascular compression syndromes of the thoracic outlet and shoulder girdle. In Peripheral Vascular Diseases, 3rd ed. Philadelphia: W.B. Saunders, 1966, Chap. 9.
79. Lord, JW, Rosati, LM: Thoracic outlet syndromes. Ciba Clin Symp 23:3–32, 1971.
80. Urschel, HC Jr., Razzuk, MA: Management of thoracic outlet syndrome. N Engl J Med 286:1140–1143, 1972.

CLASSIFYING DIZZINESS	456
DIZZINESS SIMULATION TESTS	461
DISEQUILIBRIUM	463
(PRE)SYNCOPE	471
Common Causes	471
General Approach	473
Orthostatic Hypotension	478
Diagnostic Categories of Syncope	480
Neurologic Causes	481
Cardiac Causes	483
VERTIGO	486
Peripheral Versus Central Vertigo	486
Peripheral Vestibular Disease	493
LIGHT-HEADEDNESS	502
APPENDIX I: SYNCOPE: IS THE CAUSE A CARDIAC ARRHYTHMIA?	509
APPENDIX II: EVALUATION OF VESTIBULAR FUNCTION	512
Nystagmus	512
Nylen-Bárány Test	515
Caloric Testing	516
APPENDIX III: AUDITORY TESTING	519
Bedside Hearing Tests	519
Technologic Testing	522
APPENDIX IV: COSTS OF TESTS THAT MAY BE USEFUL IN EVALUATING DIZZINESS	524
REFERENCES	525

10

DIZZINESS

Derwood, a 72-year-old man, enters the clinic complaining, "I'm dizzy all the time." Derwood says that "for quite some time now I've been dizzy and it seems to be getting worse. I can't get around as well as I used to because I get so dizzy. I know I am getting old, but do I have to be like this?"

Derwood's daughter, who accompanies him and appears distraught, interjects that her father has always been a healthy, vigorous man who has never had any medical problems and that "this dizziness has been getting much worse, and I do not trust him to be alone anymore."

CLASSIFYING DIZZINESS

Dizziness is a word used by different people to describe many different phenomena. Dizziness may refer to weakness, light-headedness, fainting, vertigo, difficulty in walking, seeing, or hearing, and various combinations thereof. It is not surprising then that the differential diagnosis of dizziness is, in fact, a series of differential diagnoses, depending upon the precise meaning of dizziness in each individual case. Before we proceed any further, every attempt must be made to define the patient's symptoms more precisely.

Ask the patient to describe the symptoms without using the word "dizziness." Do not initially provide hints or ask for a choice among other synonymous terms—faintness or light-headedness, for example—simply ask the patient to describe what he or she feels, in his or her own words.

> Derwood is told that dizziness means different things to different people. When asked to describe what he feels, he says, "I just get dizzy, that's all." Derwood is alert, but his responses seem slow and he seems to concentrate hard to answer each question:
>
> "Can you describe what you mean with words other than 'dizzy'?"
>
> "Well, I feel out of balance. I feel like I might even fall down. I haven't yet, but I get awful woozy when I walk."
>
> "Do you have this feeling right now?"
>
> "No, I feel all right now, but, just a minute ago when I came in here, I was pretty dizzy."
>
> "Is it mainly when you walk, then, that you have trouble or do you get this feeling sometimes when you are sitting or resting, too?"
>
> "I guess it is mainly when I am up and around."
>
> "Can you tell me, then, how you feel bad when you walk? Try not to say 'dizzy.'"
>
> "Well, I feel unsure of myself. I can't trust my walking."
>
> "Do the room or your surroundings spin or move, or do you feel spinning inside your head?"
>
> "No, not exactly."
>
> "Do you feel like you are going to faint?"
>
> "I feel like I will fall, not faint. I do feel a little light-headed."
>
> "Do you think the problem is in your head or in your legs?"
>
> "Well, both I guess. I just can't trust myself."

NOTE

I. The patient's own description of the symptoms provides the most important clinical information when one is analyzing complaints of dizziness.

   A detailed, painstaking history will make the diagnosis in the majority of cases.

II. The most common specific symptoms that are vaguely labeled "dizziness" include the following:

   A. Vertigo—a definite rotational sensation or a sense of environmental motion.

      Either the patient's environment seems to spin (or sway, oscillate, tip or move), or the patient senses movement or rotation within his or her head. The sensation that follows rapid pirouettes or getting off a merry-go-round or a rotating chair are examples to which most people can relate.

   B. (Pre)syncope—actual loss of consciousness (syncope) or the sensation that loss of consciousness is about to happen (presyncope).

      The common momentary presyncopal sensation that follows

rising to the standing position after a prolonged squat is an example of presyncope that many patients have experienced. Some patients will remember fainting in the past, and that experience can then serve as a reference point.

C. Disequilibrium—the sensation that balance (especially during ambulation) is impaired, but usually without the sensation of vertigo or near fainting.

D. Light-headedness—this word may be as vague a term as dizziness itself, but it refers here to a head sensation that is nonvertiginous and nonsyncopal.

   Such patients note "fuzziness," an imprecise feeling of being "not right in the head" or "feeling like my head is not attached to the rest of me."

E. Other symptoms—especially weakness, fatigue or anxiety—may initially be described as dizziness, but closer questioning will usually distinguish these from vertigo, syncope and disequilibrium, if not always from light-headedness.

   These different types of dizziness will be discussed in detail in the remainder of the chapter. While the initial approach to the dizzy patient must involve an attempt to distinguish among these various types of dizziness, remember:

III. It is not always possible to classify the patient's symptoms into only one category.

   There is some overlapping among these different subjective perceptions, and even the observant, articulate patient will not always be able to distinguish clearly among them. The sensations of vertigo and disequilibrium are commonly confused (or coexist), while the experience of presyncope may be difficult to distinguish from nonspecific light-headedness. The patient who communicates poorly or who is not a reliable observer is even less likely to be precise in his or her description.

   Nevertheless, it is usually possible to narrow the field during the history—subsequent physical examination and dizziness simulation tests (see below) will then permit greater precision, leading to a specific diagnosis, or at least a more specific differential diagnosis in most cases. It is crucial to emphasize that the initial classification of the patient's symptoms based on the history must be treated as a hypothesis—each hypothesis must be tested.

IV. Derwood appears to be describing primarily disequilibrium, with some element of nonspecific light-headedness.

Let us test the hypothesis.

Further history reveals that the problem has been present for 6 to 10 months and is worsening. The symptoms are fairly predictable in that walking and, especially, turning seem to cause most of the problems. Derwood cannot remember the symptoms occurring when he is supine or sitting, and there are no associated symptoms of nausea or vomiting, hearing problems or tinnitus, diplopia, speech difficulties, or dysesthesias. Derwood admits that "my eyes are failing a little."

Prior medical history is completely unremarkable. Derwood is a nonsmoker, does not drink alcohol, uses no drugs or medicines, and has never been hospitalized.

Physical examination reveals an impassive, elderly man who moves and talks slowly. Vital signs are normal, as is his general physical examination,

except for wax in both ears, early cataracts bilaterally, and a faint right carotid bruit. Neurologic examination reveals normal but slow mental status responses, intact cranial nerves without nystagmus (vision is 20/40 bilaterally, there are early cataracts), full symmetric muscle strength, normal reflexes and sensation (without regressive reflexes), and slow but accurate coordination of hands and feet. There is a slight resting tremor of the left hand (which improves with use) and a suggestion of increased muscle tone of both arms. Romberg testing is normal, but Derwood complains of dizziness when asked to walk down the corridor and especially when turning back to retrace his steps. His gait is short-stepped and shuffling, arms motionless at his sides, and his trunk bent over; the turn is negotiated very slowly with short, hesitant steps, and Derwood says, "There it is; I am dizzy now." At this time, blood pressure and pulse are normal, and there is no nystagmus.

What does this mean?

1. Dizziness in this case does appear to be of the disequilibrium variety, and it can be reproduced by simple ambulation and turning. The differential diagnosis is thus narrowed considerably (see Fig. 10–1).

2. The extent and focus of the physical examination of the dizzy patient are determined by the subjective type of dizziness. Otologic and neurologic testing are most important in the patient with vertigo (page 486). Hemodynamic (blood pressure, pulse, orthostatic changes) and cardiac examination must be emphasized in the patient with a history of impending or actual loss of consciousness (presyncope or syncope—page 471). Patients complaining of disequilibrium or light-headedness require very thorough general and neurologic examinations since these complaints are often multifactorial in etiology or psychosomatic.

Especially when dizziness remains vague and a specific type cannot be easily assigned, complete examination combined with dizziness simulation tests (see below) is essential.

Here, physical findings suggest parkinsonism. This is one of many neurologic disorders that may induce the sensation of disequilibrium (see below and Table 10–2, page 468).

3. Simulating or recreating the patient's symptoms is crucial. Usually this requires performance of a simple battery of dizziness simulation tests during physical examination. These tests should be performed even when one type of dizziness (or a specific disease) is identified beforehand, since other types of dizziness may coexist.

Figure 10–1 illustrates the highly successful approach to the dizzy patient developed by Drachman and Hart over a decade ago.[1] In this study, patients complaining of dizziness were referred to a university hospital "dizziness clinic," where a probing history was elicited and a thorough general and neurologic examination performed. Thereafter, a battery of dizziness simulation tests (Table 10–1) was performed in an attempt to recreate the patient's symptoms, thereby more precisely identifying the general type of dizziness and (sometimes) demonstrating physical findings characteristic of specific disease entities. This landmark study today remains the basis for the generalist physician's clinical approach to the dizzy patient. This study illustrates several pertinent facts:

1. The majority of dizzy patients suffer from one of a very few common disorders: labyrinthine (or peripheral vestibular) dysfunction (25 per cent), hyperventilation (23 per cent), and various gait/equilibrium disorders (19 per

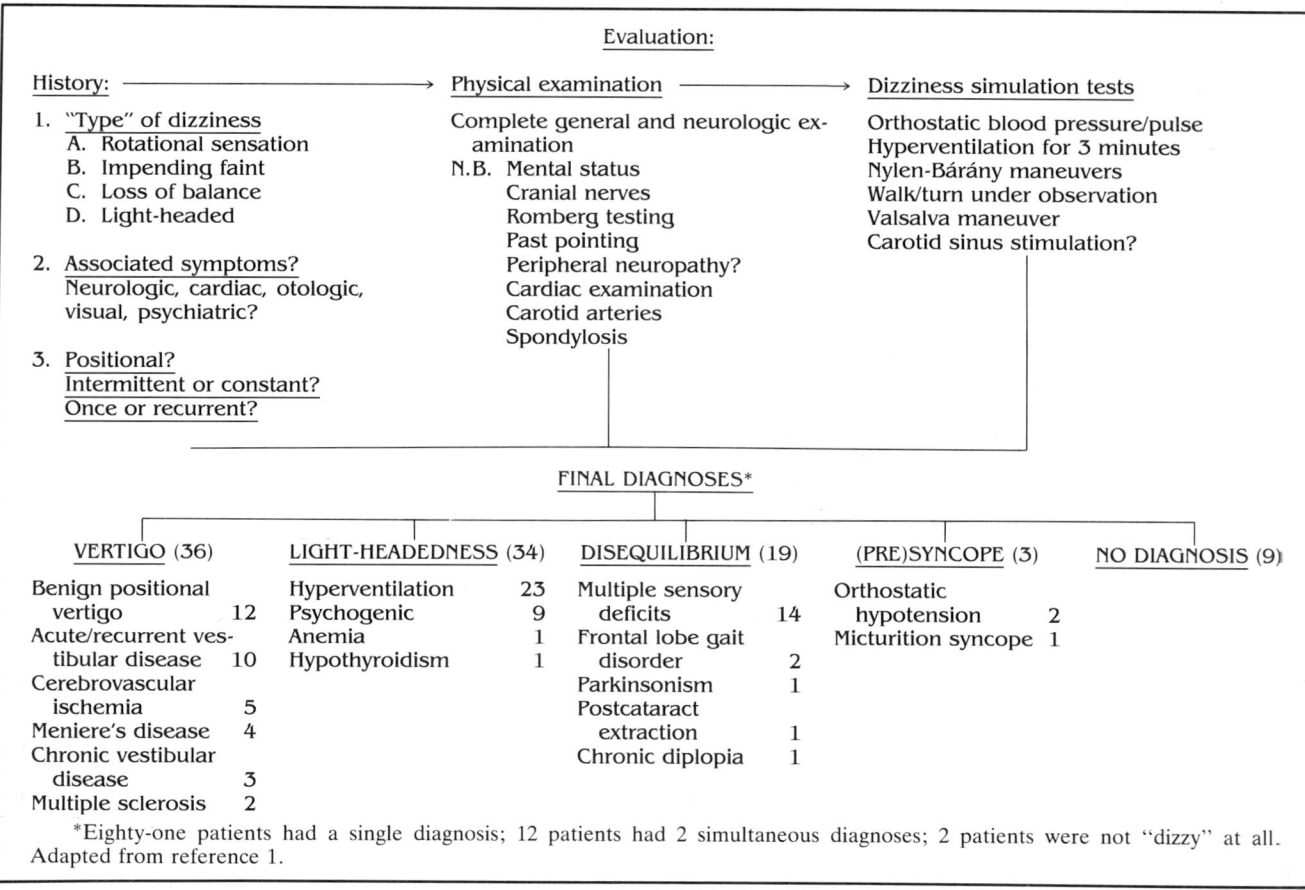

Evaluation:

History: ————————→ Physical examination ————————→ Dizziness simulation tests

1. "Type" of dizziness
   A. Rotational sensation
   B. Impending faint
   C. Loss of balance
   D. Light-headed

2. Associated symptoms?
   Neurologic, cardiac, otologic,
   visual, psychiatric?

3. Positional?
   Intermittent or constant?
   Once or recurrent?

Complete general and neurologic examination
N.B. Mental status
     Cranial nerves
     Romberg testing
     Past pointing
     Peripheral neuropathy?
     Cardiac examination
     Carotid arteries
     Spondylosis

Orthostatic blood pressure/pulse
Hyperventilation for 3 minutes
Nylen-Bárány maneuvers
Walk/turn under observation
Valsalva maneuver
Carotid sinus stimulation?

FINAL DIAGNOSES*

VERTIGO (36)		LIGHT-HEADEDNESS (34)		DISEQUILIBRIUM (19)		(PRE)SYNCOPE (3)		NO DIAGNOSIS (9)
Benign positional vertigo	12	Hyperventilation	23	Multiple sensory deficits	14	Orthostatic hypotension	2	
Acute/recurrent vestibular disease	10	Psychogenic	9	Frontal lobe gait disorder	2	Micturition syncope	1	
Cerebrovascular ischemia	5	Anemia	1	Parkinsonism	1			
Meniere's disease	4	Hypothyroidism	1	Postcataract extraction	1			
Chronic vestibular disease	3			Chronic diplopia	1			
Multiple sclerosis	2							

*Eighty-one patients had a single diagnosis; 12 patients had 2 simultaneous diagnoses; 2 patients were not "dizzy" at all. Adapted from reference 1.

FIGURE 10–1. One hundred and four "dizzy" patients.

cent). Nevertheless, the differential diagnosis of each type of dizziness is often very extensive, and there are many other disorders that may cause vertigo, light-headedness, disequilibrium, or presyncope that were not identified in Drachman and Hart's patient population. (In addition, syncope and presyncope are not uncommon problems—they are under-represented in this study.) Subsequent sections of this chapter discuss further the differential diagnosis of each type of dizziness. Familiarity with the diagnosis of the most common disorders will allow more ready recognition of the unusual case.

2. Some patients are dizzy for more than one isolated reason. Twelve of the 104 patients studied (Fig. 10–1) suffered from a combination of two coexisting types of dizziness. In addition, some of the specific types of dizziness often have multifactorial causes. This is especially the case in

TABLE 10–1. DIZZINESS SIMULATION TESTS

Always
   Observe gait, ambulation, turning
   Measure blood pressure and pulse with patient supine, sitting, and standing
   Observe patient during 3 minutes of voluntary hyperventilation
   Perform Nylen-Bárány maneuvers
   Romberg testing (eyes open and closed)

Occasionally helpful
   Valsalva maneuver
   Carotid sinus massage
   Past pointing
   Fistula test
   Caloric testing (see Appendix II)

patients with disequilibrium and light-headedness. This emphasizes the necessity of thorough examination of all dizzy patients, since one immediately apparent diagnosis may not be the "whole story," and successful therapy always depends on precise diagnosis.

3. In some patients, no diagnosis can be reached. In 9 per cent of Drachman and Hart's series, no diagnosis was established. Any practicing clinician will admire this low "failure rate," since dizziness is often a confusing clinical complaint.

A variety of laboratory tests may be helpful in the dizzy patient, but specific tests are chosen for specific purposes. There is no routine laboratory assessment. The extent of laboratory testing is always determined by purely clinical findings—the history, clinical setting, and physical examination. The cost of various diagnostic tests that may be needed in the evaluation of the dizzy patient is given in Appendix IV. No patient needs all these tests. Many patients require no laboratory tests at all, but all patients require dizziness simulation tests.

DIZZINESS SIMULATION TESTS

Dizziness simulation tests (Table 10–1) are an essential component of the clinical evaluation of all dizzy patients. These tests are helpful in three general ways:

I. The most common causes of dizziness (Fig. 10–1) can be quickly diagnosed by reproducing the patient's symptoms with one or more of these tests.

Hence the following are important: observation of gait, ambulation, and turning (page 463); orthostatic blood pressure and pulse recordings (page 478); Nylen-Bárány positional testing for vertigo (page 515); and voluntary hyperventilation (page 505).

Each of these standard tests should be performed in every dizzy patient. Each must be performed and interpreted according to very specific guidelines that are outlined in subsequent sections of this chapter. All of these tests can be performed in less than 10 minutes (total).

II. Some tests provide experiential examples of the different types of dizziness.

When the patient is unable to more precisely define the symptoms, the type of dizziness can sometimes be better categorized after dizziness simulation testing. For example:

A. Voluntary hyperventilation will simulate light-headedness (see page 505).

B. Voluntary Valsalva maneuvers can simulate (pre)syncope.

The Valsalva maneuver requires that the patient expire forcefully into a sphygmomanometer tube until a pressure of 40 to 50 mm of mercury is achieved; the patient is then asked to hold that pressure for 10 to 15 seconds. (This maneuver can be potentiated—the potentiated Valsalva maneuver—by having the patient squat for 30 seconds before performing the Valsalva maneuver.) This maneuver reduces venous return to the heart (see page 472) and transiently impairs cardiac output, thus simulating impaired cerebral perfusion (and presyncope). Such maneuvers should be performed cautiously

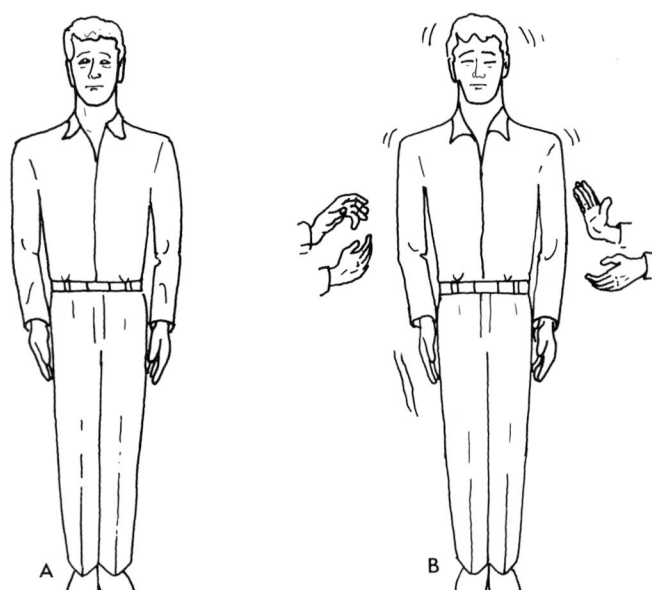

FIGURE 10–2. The Romberg test. The patient stands upright, feet together, arms at sides. The examiner should stand next to the patient. *A*, With his eyes open, the patient is able to stand unsupported without difficulty. *B*, With his eyes closed, the patient loses his balance. This test result suggests peripheral neuropathy or vestibular dysfunction or both. Cerebellar disease more often results in inability to maintain this posture with the eyes either open or closed.

(if at all) in any patient with suspected cardiopulmonary or cerebrovascular disease.

C. Caloric testing of the ears will cause vertigo (see Appendix II).

D. Romberg testing, walking and turning with eyes closed, can sometimes simulate disequilibrium.

Figure 10–2 illustrates the Romberg test. This is most helpful in the patient with suspected disequilibrium. The test is performed in two steps: with the patient's eyes open and with eyes closed. (Even the normal patient may experience subjective disequilibrium and waver with the eyes closed during the Romberg test, and thus the Romberg test may simulate disequilibrium in some normal patients.) Cerebellar disease will cause an abnormal Romberg test with eyes open or closed. In general, disorders that cause proprioceptive sensory loss (for example, peripheral neuropathy, subacute combined degeneration due to vitamin B_{12} deficiency) or vestibular imbalance allow the patient to perform the Romberg test normally when the eyes are open, but the test is abnormal when such patients' eyes are closed.

III. A few tests may confirm a suspected diagnosis but are useful only uncommonly.

Carotid sinus massage should be attempted only under controlled circumstances, often in hospital. (Carotid sinus syncope is an unusual cause of episodic or impending loss of consciousness—see Fig. 10–5.) The elderly patient should be tested with extreme caution: Always palpate and auscultate both carotid arteries before testing—massage of one carotid when the contralateral carotid is occluded or severely diseased may cause cerebrovascular ischemia. Vigorous massage can even cause cerebral embolization from the carotid artery. Continuous ECG recording during massage is necessary to adequately document events.

The fistula test involves introducing air under pressure into the patient's ear (with a pneumatic otoscope) when a cholesteatoma or other cause of perilymph fistula is suspected as the cause of vertigo (Table 10–8). This test will precipitate acute vertigo under these circumstances.

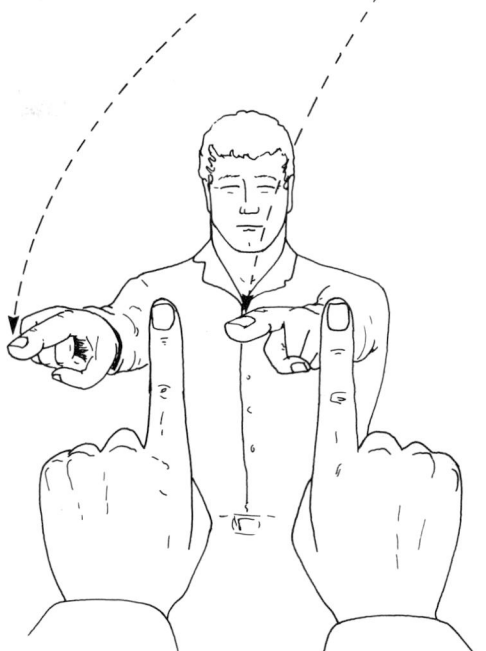

FIGURE 10–3. Past pointing. The patient is asked to raise his hands over his head and then, with his eyes closed, touch the examiner's fingers before him. This figure illustrates abnormal past pointing to the right— past pointing often points toward the side of the vestibular lesion (see Table 10–7).

Past pointing—Figure 10–3—sometimes helps in the diagnosis of vestibular and proprioceptive dysfunction. The normal patient can perform this test without difficulty, sometimes after a few practice attempts. Especially the patient with vestibular disease will have difficulty with past pointing (Table 10–7).

Derwood's blood pressure is 140/80 when he is supine and 145/75 when he is standing. The supine pulse is 80 and does not change upon standing. Nylen-Bárány maneuvers do not elicit dizziness or nystagmus. Hyperventilation induces a dry mouth, numbness in the fingers and toes, and a feeling of floating dizziness that is different from Derwood's own symptoms.

Romberg testing is unremarkable, but ambulation clearly reproduces Derwood's symptoms. He says, "There it is, I am dizzy, I'm not sure of myself," especially when walking and turning.

DISEQUILIBRIUM

Some patients complain of dizziness that, when more precisely defined, in fact represents a disturbance in balance, coordination, or equilibrium such that confident ambulation is impaired. Symptomatically, some such patients readily admit that "the problem is in my legs," but many others feel "dizzy in the head, too" or cannot decide whether the problem is "in the legs or in the head." Common to all, however, is the perception that ambulation either causes the problem or clearly makes matters worse.

Human locomotion requires the constant input of visual, vestibular, and proprioceptive information (the afferent arc); the processing of this constantly changing spatial orientation data at all levels of the nervous system—the cerebral cortex, the cerebellum, the brain stem, the spinal cord, and peripheral neuromuscular system (the integrative mechanism); and the voluntary and involuntary motor responses and adaptations to such data (the efferent arc). Disturbances of locomotion then may result from one or more dysfunctions at one or more levels of this entire complicated system (Fig. 10–4). Thus, disequilibrium may result from perceptual distortions of spatial orientation—most commonly visual impairment, cochleovestibular imbalance, or

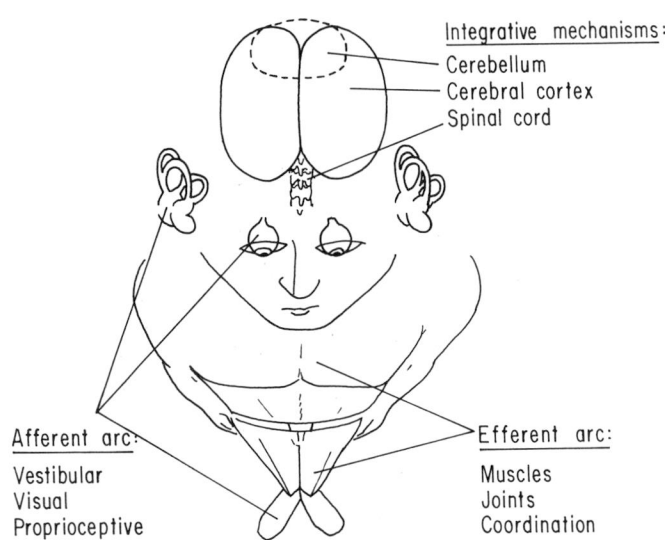

Integrative mechanisms:
— Cerebellum
— Cerebral cortex
— Spinal cord

Afferent arc:
Vestibular
Visual
Proprioceptive

Efferent arc:
Muscles
Joints
Coordination

FIGURE 10–4. The afferent, integrative and efferent components of the equilibrium system.

peripheral (proprioceptive) neuropathy; from disintegration of the integrative mechanisms—most commonly diffuse cortical or cerebellar disease; or, from efferent motor disability—usually muscle weakness, joint disease, or impaired motor control (extrapyramidal diseases, cortical apraxias).

The complexity of these locomotor systems emphasizes the importance of a thorough general and neurologic examination for all dizzy patients, but especially those with disequilibrium. While severe isolated defects may sometimes cause greatly disabled equilibrium and ambulation—severe peripheral neuropathy, blindness, advanced cerebellar ataxia, for example—these are uncommon and are usually obvious when present. Much more often the disability of the patient with disequilibrium relates directly to the number of different sensory, integrative, and locomotor deficits that afflict the patient simultaneously.

It should not be surprising, then, that the most common cause of disequilibrium is the syndrome of multiple sensory deficits. Various combinations of visual impairment (for example, cataracts), cochleovestibular dysfunction (for example, deafness or labyrinthine disease), peripheral neuropathy (the elderly diabetic or alcoholic is a common victim), muscle weakness, or orthopedic disorders (most often spinal and extremity degenerative arthritis) summate to cause disability in walking, turning, and maintaining balance.

Unless the peripheral neuropathy component is extremely severe, such patients usually do not seem frankly ataxic. Instead, their gait appears hesitant or apprehensive—they are unsteady on their feet. Turning is difficult—it is slow, short stepped, and wavering. Often the patient's distress is partly relieved by supplying additional "sensory information"—a cane or a companion's arm may be dramatically helpful. Such patients may then seek medical help "because I can't get around on my own anymore."

The key to successful treatment of multiple sensory deficit disequilibrium is the identification of all of the multiple components that together result in disability. When all contributing factors are identified, treatment of predominant or reversible disorders often will tip the balance toward more confident walking. A few problems can be cured (for example, visual correction). More often, each problem can be rendered less of a handicap by a combination of supportive devices (hearing aids, eyeglasses, walkers), physical therapy, pharmacologic therapy of underlying medical conditions (diabetes, arthritis), and patient education about what can and cannot be corrected. A common example involves the elderly diabetic afflicted with peripheral neuropathy, degenerative spinal and hip arthritis, and cataracts. Diabetic control, treatment of arthritis, and use of a cane or walker will help, but cataract surgery may be the key to success. (Temporary worsening of disequilibrium immediately after cataract surgery is yet another example of the influence of altered sensory input on equilibrium—gradual adjustment to aphakia results in gradual improvement of equilibrium.)

Consultation with various specialists then will often be necessary, depending upon the specific deficit.

Most patients with multiple sensory deficits are elderly. The elderly patient complaining of disequilibrium should never be dismissed with the hasty conclusion: "It's your age, you'll just have to live with it."[5]

Other common causes of disequilibrium include (see Table 10–2, page 468):

1. Atypical presentations of vestibular disorders. Vestibular disease does not always cause frank vertigo—poor balance or coordination may be a more prominent subjective description of vestibular symptoms, especially among the elderly. Vestibular disorders, however, usually cause symptoms when the patient changes head and neck positions—this may occur during walking and turning but will also be noted when the patient turns over in bed or looks over his or her shoulder. A careful history for such clues will usually distinguish vestibular disease from other types of disequilibrium. Moreover, "central vestibular" disorders (page 489)—especially multiple sclerosis, acoustic nerve tumors, and cerebrovascular disease—commonly produce vague symptoms that do resemble disequilibrium more than vertigo.

Thus, testing vestibular function is always important in the dizzy patient—to exclude vestibular disorders that present atypically as the solitary cause of dizziness and to assess the contribution of vestibular dysfunction to the sum of other sensory deficits.

2. Metabolic disturbances may cause disequilibrium. The most common metabolic cause, by far, is drug side effects or intoxication. Alcohol, barbiturates, other sedatives, and tranquilizers are the common culprits, but any drug used by the patient should be suspected. Hypothyroidism[6] may cause different types of dizziness, but vague disequilibrium is probably most common. Hypoglycemia may produce similar symptoms but usually impairs mental functioning more than equilibrium alone and is (except rarely) very episodic.

3. Frontal lobe apraxia.[7,8] These patients walk slowly with short, hesitant steps, often stopping and appearing unable to start again (as if stuck to the floor). Turning is difficult and is sometimes accomplished by pivoting around one stationary foot, the opposite foot slowly encircling its fellow. (Some have likened this gait to walking on ice.) The initiation of walking is especially difficult—these patients may be deceptively well when accompanied by a companion who "gets them going" with a gentle nudge at the elbow.

While this apraxia occasionally antedates other objective evidence of frontal lobe disease (dementia, placidity, regressive reflexes, mental slowing, inattention, mood lability, pseudobulbar palsy[7]), careful neurologic examination usually supports the diagnosis of diffuse cortical dysfunction even when sensory, motor, and cerebellar testing is normal. Diffuse cortical atrophy is the common cause. CT scanning is often indicated, especially when frontal lobe signs are predominant or of recent onset, since cerebral neoplasms, subdural hematomas, normal pressure hydrocephalus, and multiple infarct states can also be responsible for a similar clinical picture.

4. Senile gait. This is an unpleasant term for a gait disturbance commonly described in the elderly.[9] The patient walks slowly when unsupported, often bent forward, and may have difficulty initiating the first step. Turning is precarious, and fear of falling always adds to the elderly patient's disequilibrium. Minimal support usually permits confident, apparently fluid, ambulation. The togetherness of the elderly couple who always walk arm in arm is a "touching" example.

This gait disorder may be an early manifestation of frontal lobe apraxia, since other evidence of diffuse cortical dysfunction may be apparent after careful neurologic examination. However, the precise etiology in some elderly patients is unclear. This gait disturbance is *not* necessarily a precursor of dementia.

Many elderly people do not have gait disturbance,[5] and, as noted above, disequilibrium in the elderly should not be carelessly dismissed as an old age phenomenon. Careful general and neurologic examination are crucial in the elderly patient complaining of disequilibrium, since senile gait alone is never severely disabling (but may be one of the components adding up to cause disability—see above).

5. Parkinson's disease.[10] This disorder (and other less common extrapyramidal disorders) not infrequently presents with a vague sensation of disordered equilibrium and ambulation, and such complaints may occasionally precede by many months other neurologic findings (e.g., tremor and cogwheel rigidity) that are typical of this disorder. Even at such an early stage, however, there are often other subtle clues: impassive (masked) facies, muscle "tightness," deterioration of handwriting, and infrequent blinking. It is this more subtle early presentation of parkinsonism that is easy to miss, but pharmacologic therapy may be especially helpful at this early stage.

In its advanced form the parkinsonian gait is festinating: The steps are short and rigid, the feet shuffle along, the trunk is bent forward, and the arms hang motionless at the sides—the appearance is that of the lower body shuffling frantically forward to catch up with the upper body. At this stage the diagnosis is usually obvious. Different neurologic variants of parkinsonism (progressive supranuclear palsy,[11] for example) should be remembered, as should the fact that various drugs (especially phenothiazines, reserpine, and antidepressants) may induce a similar picture.

6. Cerebellar disease. Gait disorders due to cerebellar disease are usually gross, not subtle. The patient reels unsteadily in short, irregular steps with a wide-based gait, often lurching from side to side or falling, especially when attempting to stop, sit, or turn around.

In adults, cerebellar ataxias can usually be conceptually divided among acute, subacute, and chronic varieties.[12]

Acute cerebellar ataxia may be the result of intoxication (alcohol, barbiturates, anticonvulsants, heavy metals), primary or metastatic tumors, infection, demyelinating disease, or vascular accidents (infarct or hemorrhage). Usually other cerebellar signs are obvious on physical examination—dysmetria, dysdiadochokinesia, hypotonia—and such findings may often be predominantly unilateral.

Subacute cerebellar disease may be caused by slow-growing tumors (primary gliomas, cerebellopontine angle tumors) but is more often due to alcoholic cerebellar degeneration. In the latter disorder, the legs are always more involved than the arms, and this may occasionally cause confusion—the gait is disproportionately impaired in relation to other tests of coordination: malingering is even sometimes suspected. Rarely, subacute cerebellar degeneration announces an otherwise inapparent distant cancer: Here the arms are more disabled than the legs, and both nystagmus and dysarthria are more common than in the alcoholic variety.

Chronic cerebellar disease is usually heredofamilial[12] or alcoholic in origin.

Disequilibrium due entirely to cerebellar disease of the acute, subacute, or chronic form is usually obvious on physical examination, and subsequent efforts are directed toward establishing the cause.

7. Sensory ataxia. While peripheral neuropathy is a frequent component of the multiple sensory deficit syndrome, an isolated peripheral neuropathy is only uncommonly the sole cause of disequilibrium. Such patients literally must see to walk. The usual gait is characteristic: The legs are held apart, each foot is flung out and forward, often higher than necessary, and stomped to the ground (this gait has been likened to that of a circus clown walking in oversized shoes), all as the patient bends forward to carefully watch the feet interact with the ground. The gait disturbance is hence much worse in the dark or with the eyes closed—the basis for the Romberg test. Sensory ataxia is always associated with severe impairment of foot/toe proprioceptive testing.

8. Psychogenic* disequilibrium. Patients who are ataxic when walking or standing and yet have otherwise normal neurologic examinations, including full control and coordination of the legs in the sitting and supine positions, should be suspected of psychogenic gait disorders, but the examiner must be very careful here. Several of the disorders noted above may produce disequilibrium and impaired ambulation in spite of what otherwise appears to be a relatively normal neurologic examination: apraxia, early Parkinson's disease, and midline cerebellar disease (alcoholic or carcinomatous) must be remembered.

Usually the psychogenic gait disturbance is bizarre, intermittent, or inconsistent (for example, the patient has no difficulty indoors but is unable to walk outdoors). Interviewing family members or other observers is often useful when this problem is suspected.

Table 10–2 enumerates some of the common and uncommon causes of disequilibrium. Obviously, different patient populations will include different proportions of these disorders. Disequilibrium in young, otherwise healthy adults is most often drug induced, due to vestibular disease, the result of anxiety or hyperventilation (see page 503), or hysterical. Multiple sensory deficits are much more common in the elderly, sometimes in combination with senile gait, cortical apraxias, or mild extrapyramidal disease. The alcoholic population is more likely to suffer from cerebellar degeneration or severe peripheral neuropathy.

Note in Table 10–2 that disequilibrium may be caused by disorders that are usually grouped among the differential diagnoses of other types of dizziness (Fig. 10–1). Vestibular disease and hyperventilation, for example, are common causes of disequilibrium even though these disorders are more commonly encountered in patients complaining of vertigo and light-headedness, respectively. This must be a recurrent theme throughout any discussion of dizziness in general: There is frequently symptomatic overlap among the different types of dizziness, and one specific disease may cause different

---

*"Psychogenic" is a nonspecific item. Anxiety and depression are the common underlying disorders (see also page 506).

TABLE 10–2. CAUSES OF DISEQUILIBRIUM

CAUSE	GAIT	NOTE
Multiple sensory deficits	Hesitant, apprehensive; often remarkably better with sensory assist (cane, companion)	Peripheral neuropathy? cervical spondylosis? vestibular dysfunction? poor vision? deafness? weakness? orthopedic problems?
Hyperventilation (see p. 503)	Intermittent, vague "loss of control"	Reproduce with voluntary hyperventilation.
Vestibular disease (see p. 486)	Often veers to one side repeatedly; symptoms when head or body turns, i.e., not just gait related.	Nystagmus? neurologic abnormality? Nylen-Bárány maneuvers?
Senile gait	Unassisted: slow, "scared" Assisted: fluid, easy ambulation	Exclude other contributing factors
Remember metabolic disorders: drugs, hypothyroidism, hypoglycemia		
Parkinsonism	Early: slow, diminished arm swing, difficulty turning Later: "festinating"	Early: impassive facies, poor handwriting, muscle tightness, slow Later: tremor, cogwheeling, drooling Remember drug-induced parkinsonism: phenothiazines, reserpine, antidepressants
Frontal lobe apraxia	Not ataxic but apraxic; "walking on ice"; difficulty initiating walking and turning ("stuck to the floor")	Dementia? regressive reflexes? mood lability? (Evaluate! CT scan!)
Cerebellar ataxia	Lurching, reeling, wide-based gait— sudden, irregular gross loss of motor control, especially when attempting to sit, turn, or stop; Romberg abnormal with eyes open and closed	Other unilateral cerebellar findings— dysmetria, disdiadochokinesia: vascular? mass lesion? Midline?: alcoholic? neoplastic? Heredofamilial?
Peripheral neuropathy (sensory ataxia)	"Circus clown" walk; must see to walk; Romberg abnormal with eyes closed	Proprioceptive loss in feet/legs; look for other sensory deficits; rarely the only cause
Hysterical/psychogenic	Unpredictable, intermittent, or bizarre	Normal examination; interview family, other observers

types of dizziness in different patients. Uncommon presentations of common disorders (Fig. 10–1) will be seen more often than will uncommon or rare disorders. For example, atypical symptoms of vestibular disease are more common than is dizziness due to severe cerebellar disease. Table 10–2 lists causes of disequilibrium in approximate order of frequency (in my experience).

Treatment of disequilibrium, then, obviously depends on the nature of the etiologic process. Sensory-assist devices (canes, walkers, eyeglasses, for example), treatment of remediable sensory deficits (vestibular, orthopedic, neuropathic, or ocular), antiparkinsonian drug therapy, reversal of metabolic disorders (hypothyroidism, drug reactions, alcoholism), attention to treatable cortical disease (normal pressure hydrocephalus, subdural hematomas, for example), and psychiatric consultation are among the many possible approaches.

> Derwood is told that he has most likely developed Parkinson's disease and that "the stiffness in your muscles causes the problem in walking that makes you feel dizzy." Parkinsonism is explained in some detail to Derwood and his daughter, and L-Dopa, 500 mg qd, increasing by 500 mg per week, is begun. Derwood is told that a cane might be useful until the medicine improves his condition. Daily low-dose aspirin is suggested because of the asymptomatic carotid bruit, and a consultation is arranged with an ophthal-

mologist to evaluate the early cataracts. Wax is removed from both ears, and Derwood's hearing thereafter appears normal.

A return appointment is scheduled in 3 weeks.

NOTE

Even when a specific cause of dizziness is identified and treated, other potentially contributory factors should be addressed, especially in the elderly who are most susceptible to the multiple sensory deficit syndromes. For example, mild parkinsonism may be much less problematic when vision, hearing, and other senses are intact.

Two weeks later, Derwood's daughter calls to say that her father has "passed out" twice and is "much worse."

Derwood is brought into the clinic in a wheelchair. He is alert and looks well. He says he feels "fine now, but the last few days I have been a lot dizzier than before I saw you." Derwood says that he feels well, "except when I walk—then I get real dizzy, more than before, and I guess I have fainted a couple of times." Derwood's daughter confirms this and says that her father has passed out at least twice and has bruises on his elbow and forehead to prove it. Derwood is currently taking L-dopa, 500 mg tid.

"Sylvia, can you describe what you saw when Derwood passed out?"

"The first time, he woke me up in the middle of the night—he was moaning on the floor of the bathroom and had hit his elbow against the bathtub. I guess he got up in the night to urinate and passed out. He looked pale and sweaty when I got there, and he was very dizzy when I tried to get him back to bed—he almost passed out again—but he seemed okay after I put him back to bed."

"Did you take his pulse at the time?"

"No, I didn't."

"Derwood, do you remember fainting?"

"No, I guess I just passed out. I can't remember that one. The next time, though, I was just walking into my bedroom after the late movie on TV, and all of a sudden—boom!—I just went down and out. I woke up on the floor, and Sylvia got me into bed."

"Had you just gotten up when you fainted?"

"Yes."

"Did you feel any warning that you would pass out before you went down?"

"No, I just blacked out, that's all."

"How long were you out?"

"Just a few seconds, I think." (Sylvia confirms this.)

"How did you feel when you woke up?"

"Still dizzy walking, but otherwise okay."

"How do you feel in between these spells?"

"Like I might pass out again. I am dizzy when I walk or stand up."

"Have you felt short of breath, had pains in the chest, palpitations or any fainting spells in between these two spells?"

"I just feel faint and dizzy—more than before."

NOTE

After careful questioning it seems clear that this is a different kind of dizziness. The patient describes the sensation of impending loss of conscious-

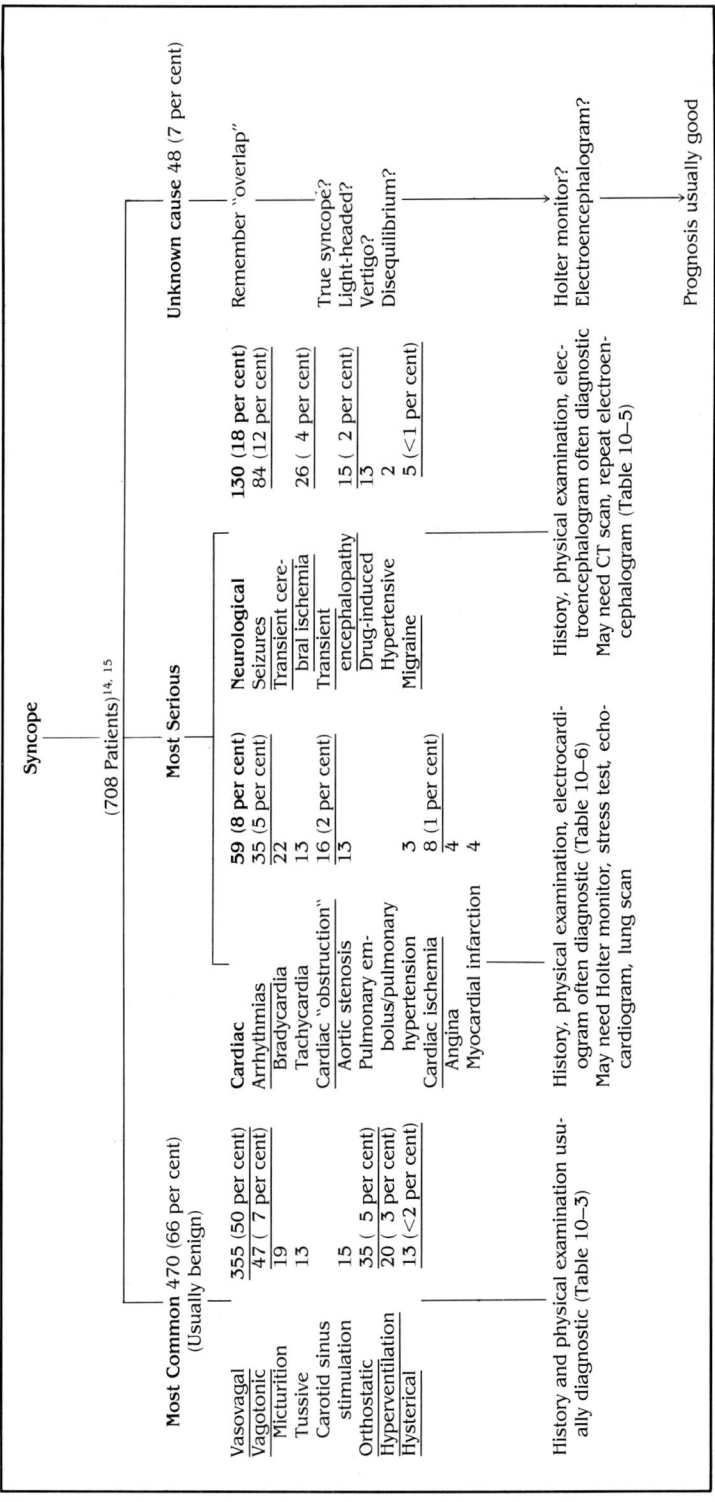

FIGURE 10–5. Combined results of two studies of the etiology of syncope among 708 patients.[14]

ness—"beginning to pass out"—and, in fact, he has actually lost consciousness twice.

When true syncope (actual loss of consciousness)* occurs, a specific, but lengthy, differential diagnosis applies[13] (Fig. 10–5). In such circumstances, the patient usually complains of fainting or blacking out rather than dizziness.

However, dizziness often is used to describe the sensation of presyncope—feelings of light-headedness, weakness, visual blurring ("graying out"), and apprehension—that may precede actual syncope or resolve without occurrence of syncope. The nonspecificity of these presyncopal symptoms emphasize that it is often difficult to distinguish presyncope from other types of dizziness. Light-headedness (page 502), for example, is commonly confused with presyncope. Thus, dizziness that "feels like I am going to pass out," but is never associated with actual loss of consciousness, is a nonspecific symptom. In such cases, various causes of actual syncope (Fig. 10–5) may still be the problem, but further history and dizziness simulation tests must attempt to exclude the other (more common) causes of dizziness.†

(PRE)SYNCOPE

Figure 10–5 illustrates the combined results of two studies of the etiology of syncope in large numbers of patients studied two decades apart (Wayne in 1961[14] and Day et al. in 1982[15]). With few exceptions, there is remarkable similarity between these two studies in the incidence of various etiologic diagnoses. Figure 10–5 illustrates three important facts about the diagnostic approach to syncope:

Common Causes

1. Most syncopal episodes are not due to any serious disease.[16, 17] Transient impairment of venous return to the heart is responsible for most episodes of (pre)syncope. There are many possible causes (Table 10–3).

Vasovagal syncope (the common faint) is by far the most common cause. Engel[18] has suggested that this form of syncope results from some primordial physiologic response to fear or injury ("flight or fight").‡ Precipitating factors often include emotional stress, fear, apprehension, or pain from some real or threatened trauma. Vasovagal syncope is thus not an uncommon event in a dentist's office or a phlebotomy laboratory.

Symptoms almost invariably occur with the patient in the upright position (usually standing), and there are frequently (but not always) exogenous vasodilatory influences: a hot or close environment, fever, excessive alcohol intake, vasodilator drug ingestion, prolonged motionless standing without exercise (for example, the soldier at attention). Some patients are well known

---

*By definition, syncope refers to transient loss of consciousness with loss of motor control.

†Unfortunately, no simulation test reliably mimics presyncope and distinguishes it from other types of dizziness. The potentiated Valsalva maneuver sometimes will do so (see page 461) but not usually.

‡Sudden peripheral arterial vasodilatation (Engel's preparation for flight) accompanies the "fright," but venous return is impaired ("flight" does not occur—muscle exercise thus does not accelerate venous return) or cardiac output does not increase to compensate for vasodilatation. Paradoxical bradycardia may be seen in the cardioinhibitory variety; hypotension without bradycardia is often called the vasodepressor variety. Loss of consciousness, then, usually results from transiently impaired cerebral perfusion.

TABLE 10–3. COMMON (USUALLY BENIGN) SYNCOPE/PRESYNCOPE RESULTING FROM IMPAIRED VENOUS RETURN TO THE HEART

CAUSE*	SETTING	PRODROME	OBSERVATION	DIAGNOSIS
Vasovagal (common faint; vasodepressor syncope)[19]	Emotional stress; warm, crowded room; pain or injury; almost always begins with patient in upright position	Usually pallor; nausea; sweating; epigastric distress; weakness	Pallor; sweating; resolves quickly when patient supine; brief duration; bradycardia?	Clinical setting and history usually diagnostic; examination normal
Postural hypotension (see Table 10–4)	Immediately or soon after standing; may occur during prolonged motionless standing	Usually similar to vasovagal symptoms; sometimes abrupt, without warning	Always positional; relief (or prevention) by lying down	Orthostatic blood pressure recordings; many possible causes
Hyperventilation	See p. 503	Paresthesias; sighing respirations; light-headedness; dry mouth; palpitations	Actual loss of consciousness unusual; eyewitness account always helps; if syncope occurs, usually very brief	History; reproduced with voluntary hyperventilation
Vagotonia/Valsalva Mechanisms				
Voluntary Valsalva[20]	Straining; weight lifting[20]			
Cough syncope[21]	COPD†/severe coughing			
Micturition syncope[22]	During (often nocturnal) urination			
Glossopharyngeal neuralgia[23]	Episodic, severe pain in throat, ears, neck			
Swallowing, diving, stretching			Brief duration; onset usually when upright; clinical setting characteristic; transient bradycardia common	
Painful visceral disease	Esophageal disease; mediastinal disease; pleuropulmonary disease; gallbladder disease; acute glaucoma			
Iatrogenic	Prostate or pelvic examination; thoracentesis; venipuncture; bronchoscopy; esophagoscopy			
Carotid sinus syncope[2–4]	Tight collar; head turn; neck pressure; usually upright	May be sudden	Three types: bradycardiac; hypotensive; cerebral	Reproduce with carotid sinus stimulation and ECG monitor (beware carotid occlusion)

*The first three disorders are the most common.
†Chronic obstructive pulmonary disease.

"easy fainters." (As Table 10–3 suggests, certain specific precipitants may also cause excessive vagotonia with identical clinical results—cough syncope and micturition syncope are the most common of these.)

The common faint is usually announced by warning symptoms (prodrome) before actual loss of consciousness occurs. Seconds (or a few minutes) of vague nausea, epigastric queasiness, sweating, clamminess, light-headedness, generalized warmth, blurred vision, and pallor (if observed) precede the common faint. During the period of unconsciousness—which is usually very brief (seconds to a few minutes) once the patient reaches the supine position*—the patient may be observed to be pale and diaphoretic with a slow or even unobtainable pulse. Immediately following the resumption of consciousness, the patient is often nervous, weak, nauseated or dizzy, but residual symptoms beyond 30 minutes after such a faint are usually due to anxiety rather than any persistent physiologic dysfunction.

*Fainting in a phone booth may, theoretically, be fatal.

Syncope is always frightening. Bodily injury may result, the severity of which depends on the setting in which loss of consciousness occurs. Such bodily injury (a bruise on the head or worse) often indirectly indicates that true loss of consciousness has in fact occurred. Nevertheless, the cause of syncope is most often benign.

2. It is not rare for the cause of an isolated episode of syncope to remain undiscovered. In one study, in which syncope was sufficiently worrisome to warrant hospitalization in an intensive care unit, almost one half of the patients studied left the hospital without a specific diagnosis.[24] The prognosis in such undiagnosed cases is usually good.

There are no routine laboratory tests for all patients who experience one isolated syncopal episode. In general, the ECG is probably worthwhile, but in young, healthy patients with classic vasovagal syncope and a normal physical examination, the ECG will almost always be normal. Serum electrolytes, urea nitrogen, glucose, calcium, and arterial blood gas values are useful when the patient has had a suspected or definite seizure or when there is a history of diabetes or some underlying problem (uremia, parathyroidectomy, diuretic therapy, severe lung disease, for example). X-rays rarely help (but skull x-rays are often performed when head trauma results from syncope). Lumbar puncture is almost never necessary (but will exclude the very rare case of transient syncope due to subarachnoid hemorrhage). CT scan in the absence of focal neurologic findings is rarely helpful. The EEG may be helpful, but usually only when a seizure disorder is suspected from the history (see Table 10–5).

Recurrent syncope is another matter. When carefully evaluated, most patients with a documented history of repeated episodes of syncope will have a demonstrable cause. As Figure 10–6 and Table 10–3 suggest, however, it is often the history—not laboratory tests—that make the diagnosis.

3. A careful history and physical examination will usually suggest the correct diagnosis. The patient's description of warning (presyncopal) symptoms and postsyncopal symptoms, to which the physician must pay painstaking attention; any observer's description of the patient during and after loss of consciousness; and a thorough physical examination (almost always performed after the event has resolved—the clinician only rarely is on hand during the syncopal event) are the most valuable pieces of diagnostic information.

Detailed reconstruction of the setting in which syncope occurred is always helpful. Physical examination must include dizziness simulation tests (especially orthostatic blood pressure recordings and voluntary hyperventilation), as well as a careful cardiopulmonary and neurologic examination.

General Approach

How, then, do we decide whether a syncopal episode is serious or benign? Which questions in the clinical history are most helpful? What observations are most important in the examination of the patient during and after a syncopal episode?

Figure 10–6 outlines a general approach to the clinical analysis of syncope. Consider Derwood's problem (page 469) in the light of this outline:

1. Loss of consciousness definitely occurred. When an eyewitness is not available, the patient must be questioned very carefully about actual loss of

1. DID LOSS OF CONSCIOUSNESS ACTUALLY OCCUR?　　　　　NO　————————→　Consider other types of dizziness
　　Dizziness simulation tests!

YES

2. CONSIDER THE CLINICAL SETTING!　　　　　　　Clues:

A. Patient profile:	B. Medications?	C. Precipitating event:	
Known seizure disorder?	Iatrogenic:	Cough syncope?	
Known cardiac disease?	Orthostatic hypotension?	Micturition	
Diabetic?	Cardiac arrhythmias?	syncope?	
Psychotic?	Seizures?	Arising to stand:	orthostatic?
Hyperventilator?	Hypoglycemia?		
"Easy fainter"?		Turning head:	vestibular disease?
			carotid sinus disease?
			vertebrobasilar TIA?
		Arm exercise:	subclavian steal syndrome?
		Physical exertion:	cardiac arrhythmia?
			cardiac ischemia?
			aortic stenosis?
		Positional but	atrial myxoma?
		unpredictable:	hydrocephalus?
			vestibular?

　　N.B. WORRY WHEN SYNCOPE OCCURS WITH PATIENT SUPINE!!
　　　　　　　Often:　　　　seizure, arrhythmia!
　　　　　　　Sometimes:　　hyperventilation, hysteria?
　　　　　　　Rarely:　　　　vasovagal

3. ANALYZE PRODROME (WARNING SYMPTOMS)!

　　N.B. SUDDEN SYNCOPE (NO WARNING AT ALL)　————————→　WORRY!
　　　　　　　　　　　　　　　　　　　　　　　　　　　　　　　　Often:　　　　seizure, arrhythmia!
　　　　　　　　　　　　　　　　　　　　　　　　　　　　　　　　Sometimes:　orthostatic hypotension, carotid sinus
　　　　　　　　　　　　　　　　　　　　　　　　　　　　　　　　　　　　　　syncope, hysteria?

Palpitations?　————————→　Arrhythmia? Also: hypoglycemia, hyperventilation?
Chest pain?　————————→　Angina? Myocardial infarction? Pulmonary embolus? Arrhythmia? Aortic dissection?
Dyspnea?　————————→　Myocardial infarction? Pulmonary embolus? Hyperventilation? Pneumothorax?
Neurologic symptoms?　————————→　Diplopia, dysarthria, dysphagia, dysesthesia, dizziness: vertebrobasilar ischemia? (5Ds)
Automatisms: temporal lobe epilepsy?
Focal seizures: central nervous system mass lesion, intracerebral catastrophe, hyperglycemia?
Headache: Subarachnoid hemorrhage?

Vague, prolonged presyncope/altered
　mental status　————————→　Hypoxemia, hypoglycemia, hypothyroidism, hypotension?
Hysteria? Hyperventilation? (6 Hs)

4. SYNCOPAL EVENT OBSERVED?　————————→　True loss of consciousness?　　　　Hysterical (p. 476)?
Grand mal seizure (versus nonspecific brief clonic movements)?
N.B. Pallor, clamminess, and　　　　Pulse during event: extreme tachycardia: (heart rate >160 beats/min)—primary arrhythmia
　　　brief clonic "jerking,"　　　　　　extreme bradycardia? (heart rate <40 beats/min)—primary arrhythmia
　　　are nonspecific　　　　　　　　　　versus vasovagal?
Witnessed in medical setting? Electrocardiogram, blood gases, glucose! Careful examination!

WORRY!　Cyanotic, respiratory distress?
　　　　　Definite focal or grand mal seizure?
　　　　　No heartbeat (apical or carotid) or extreme tachycardia (heart rate >160 beats/min) documented?

FIGURE 10–6. Clinical analysis of syncope.　　　　　　　　　　　　*Illustration continued on opposite page*

consciousness. Often the patient will describe vague, distant awareness of the environment throughout the "syncopal" event. This is not true syncope. The patient who "thinks" he or she "was out for 1 to 2 seconds" probably was not.

Here we have a reliable eyewitness who documents true syncope. Moreover, the patient has ongoing symptoms that seem to point to impending recurrence of syncope.

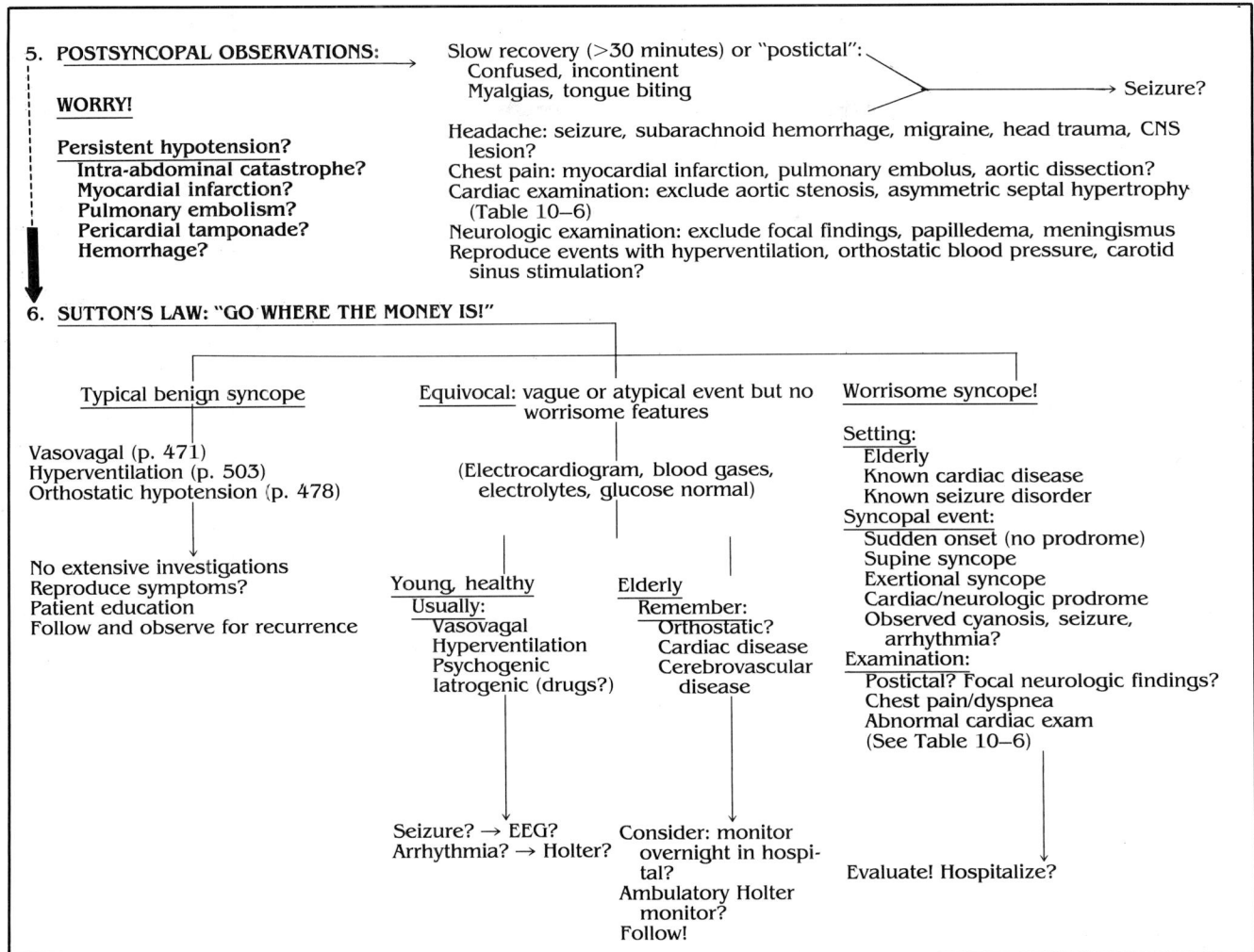

Figure 10–6. *Continued*

2. The clinical setting suggests the possibility of micturition syncope (the first episode) or orthostatic hypotension (both syncopal events have occurred in the upright position; Derwood is dizzy when up but well when supine; and both parkinsonism and L-dopa therapy may cause orthostatic hypotension—see Table 10–4, pages 482, 484, and 485).

Derwood's age and known vascular disease (i.e., carotid bruit) should also suggest the possibility of a cardiac or cerebrovascular cause (Tables 10–5 and 10–6, pages 482, 484, and 485).

The second syncopal event occurred while he was walking. This should at least suggest exertional (usually cardiac) syncope, but orthostatic hypotension may also cause such an event when symptoms occur soon after arising.

Supine syncope (which did not occur here) is always worrisome, since vasovagal and orthostatic syncope almost always occur with the patient in an upright position. Syncope during exertion is always worrisome.

3. Syncope appears to have occurred suddenly, without any warning symptoms (or prodrome). Most benign syncope is heralded by typical prodromal symptoms that are characteristic of vasovagal (page 471) or, less commonly, hysterical or hyperventilation syncope (page 476). When syncope occurs without any warning at all, cardiac arrhythmias and seizure disorders

should be given special consideration. Orthostatic hypotension, carotid sinus syncope,[21-23] and hysteria may also cause such events.

Most cardiac causes of syncope do present with prodromal symptoms: palpitations in the patient with tachyarrhythmias, chest pain or dyspnea in the patient with myocardial infarction or pulmonary embolism, or syncope that is clearly exertional when due to cardiac outflow obstruction (Table 10–6).

Seizure disorders typically cause sudden syncope, but usually other clues will suggest the possibility of seizures (see page 481 and Table 10–5).

Vertebrobasilar ischemia (or, rarely, other cerebrovascular events) may cause syncope, but this is uncommon and is usually associated with typical neurologic prodromes (the five Ds of vertebrobasilar ischemia: diplopia, dysarthria, dysphagia, dysesthesias, dizziness).

Prodromal symptoms that are very vague, prolonged (hours), or associated with symptomatic mental status impairment (confusion, drowsiness, hallucinations) are usually indicators of metabolic or psychosomatic disorders (the 6-Hs—Figure 10–6, 3: hypoxemia, hypoglycemia, hypothyroidism, hypotension, hysteria, hyperventilation).

4. We have an eyewitness account of the syncopal event(s). Observers should always be asked about the patient's color, pulse, respirations, and (any) seizure activity.

Cyanosis and respiratory distress should suggest a primary cardiopulmonary event. Remember pallor and clamminess will occur with any type of syncope.

Repetitive tonic-clonic seizure activity (page 481) usually implies a true seizure—this may be a primary event (idiopathic epilepsy), secondary to a neurologic lesion, or due to prolonged hypoxia, hypotension, or other metabolic insults. Pseudoseizures—brief, clonic jerking movements—are utterly nonspecific and are common when syncope of any kind lasts for 15 seconds or more. (In such circumstances, however, incontinence, tongue biting, and postictal confusion—commonly seen with true seizures—are unusual.)

Extreme bradycardia (or even pulselessness) may be due to a primary cardiac arrhythmia or simply a severe vasovagal event. Absence of a carotid or apical pulse recorded by an experienced observer (a nurse, for example) is always worrisome, but many cases of transient "cardiac arrest" are in fact vasovagal.

When the syncopal event is witnessed by medical personnel, an ECG and blood glucose and blood gas values may be very helpful, since cardiac arrhythmias, hypoglycemia, and severe hypoxemia require immediate therapy.

Even an experienced medical observer may be fooled by the hysterical patient with "seizures" or syncope—very careful observation during the event is often diagnostic, as Adams and Victor describe:

> The lack of aura, initiating cry, hurtful fall and incontinence; the presence of peculiar movements such as grimacing, squirming, biting, striking at or resisting those who offer assistance; the retention of consciousness during a motor seizure which involves both sides of the body; the long duration of the seizure and the abrupt termination by strong sensory stimulation are all typical of the hysterical attack.[25]

In Derwood's case, our history can only document that syncope did in fact occur, that it was of brief duration, and that neither cyanosis nor seizure activity occurred. In addition,

5. Observation of the patient immediately after the syncopal event did not suggest a postical state or a primary neurologic disorder. The syncopal episodes were brief, Derwood was not confused or complaining of neurologic or cardiopulmonary symptoms after the event, and he was well after returning to bed.

In addition, careful neurologic and cardiac examinations do not suggest structural neurologic or cardiac disease as the cause.

6. Orthostatic hypotension is the most likely diagnosis. All symptomatic events can be explained on this basis.

If Derwood's physical examination fails to reveal orthostatic hypotension, cardiac arrhythmias should also be considered because of his age, his known vascular disease, the absence of any prodromal symptoms during the event about which we have the most information (the second) and the possibility of exertional provocation of syncope in that instance.

> Derwood's blood pressure is 140/80 when he is supine, 115/75 when he is sitting, and 85/60 when he is standing. The pulse increases from 80 to 110 from the supine to standing position. Ten seconds after standing, Derwood says, "There it is, I am dizzy now, I have to lie down." Resumption of the supine position relieves the dizziness within 30 seconds, although Derwood looks a little pale and sweaty. His blood pressure returns to 140/80 within 1 minute. The remainder of the physical examination is unchanged. The ECG is normal.

> Derwood is questioned further about any possible excessive fluid or blood losses (diarrhea, melena, polyuria), which he denies. Stool is heme negative and abdominal examination is benign. Hemoglobin, urea nitrogen, and electrolytes are normal.

NOTE

The presence of postural hypotension is verified. Exact reproduction of the patient's symptoms at the time of demonstrated postural hypotension documents that this is the current problem.

Only if postural blood pressure is recorded carefully will this common problem not be missed. Normally, rising from the supine to standing position will slightly elevate the blood pressure or not change it, and the pulse will increase no more than 10 beats per minute. Postural hypotension is usually most apparent within 30 seconds after assumption of the standing position (when severe, it may be obvious in the sitting position as well). However, brachial blood pressure should be recorded sequentially in the supine, sitting, and standing position and checked again after 1 to 3 minutes with the patient still standing, if symptoms do not occur sooner and the blood pressure does not drop more quickly. Occasionally, onset of orthostatic hypotension will be delayed for 2 to 5 minutes. Pulse rates should be recorded in each position.

Orthostatic Hypotension

The patient with orthostatic hypotension, upon assuming the upright position, usually feels weak, light-headed and mildly nauseated—syncope may be averted by lying down, but the patient then often sweats and looks pale. The pulse usually increases at the time of hypotension (as a compensatory hemodynamic mechanism), and the patient may thus also note palpitations.

Orthostatic hypotension is usually due to one of several common, easily identified problems (Table 10–4). Drug side effects, various causes of

TABLE 10–4. ORTHOSTATIC HYPOTENSION

CAUSE	EXAMPLES	FINDINGS	TREATMENT
Drugs			
Diuretics	Thiazides, furosemide	Orthostatic tachycardia	
Vasodilators	Nitrates, hydralazine, prazosin, minoxidil	Orthostatic tachycardia	
Antidepressants	Tricyclics, MAO inhibitors	Orthostatic tachycardia	
Antihypertensives	Methyldopa, reserpine, guanethidine	± Pulse rise*	Withdraw drug or reduce dose
Antipsychotics	Chlorpromazine HCl, thioridazine HCl	Orthostatic tachycardia	
L-DOPA		± Pulse rise*	
Sedative/hypnotics	Barbiturates	Orthostatic tachycardia	
Intravascular volume depletion	Blood loss, fluid loss (diarrhea, sweat, polyuria), decreased colloid (hypoalbuminemia), adrenal insufficiency	Orthostatic tachycardia	Volume replacement; treat specific disease entity
Neurologic disease[26]			
Diffuse neuropathy	Diabetes, alcohol, amyloid, porphyria, Guillain-Barré syndrome, beriberi, tabes, syringomyelia, familial dysautonomia	No orthostatic tachycardia; sensorimotor neuropathy plus impotence, anhidrosis, pupillary change, sphincter disturbance/incontinence	Treat underlying condition; stockings/sodium/fludrocortisone acetate
Primary dysautonomia Acute/subacute[27]	Guillain-Barré–like illness with only autonomic neuropathy		Resolves spontaneously; steroid therapy?
Postganglionic[28]	Middle-aged/elderly patient with gradual onset of autonomic neuropathy	Impotence, anhidrosis	Stockings/sodium/fludrocortisone acetate
Chronic preganglionic[29, 30]	Associated CNS disease: parkinsonism, Wernicke's disease, multiple infarct state	Autonomic disease plus other CNS signs	Tyramine?[31] MAO inhibitors?[30] Propranolol? Indomethacin[32]
Miscellaneous			
Pregnancy	Third trimester		Parturition
Varicose veins	Only in severe cases		Stockings/surgery
Prolonged recumbency	Hospitalization		Conditioning
Sympathectomy (surgical)			Stockings/sodium/fludrocortisone acetate
Severe anemia			Blood
Pheochromocytoma[33]		Labile or fixed hypertension	Surgery/drugs
Mitral valve prolapse[34]		Cardiac click—murmur	Propranolol?
Hypoaldosteronism[35]		Usually diabetic with renal failure; hyperkalemia	Fludrocortisone acetate[36]
Idiopathic		More common in elderly patients with cerebrovascular disease	Stockings, salt tablets, fludrocortisone acetate; avoid prolonged bedrest, dehydration/diminished salt intake, drugs, alcohol; elevate head of bed Indomethacin? Dihydroergotamine? Midodrine? Clonidine?

*The failure of the pulse to accelerate often indicates autonomic dysfunction as the cause of orthostatic hypotension — sometimes, this is drug-induced.

intravascular volume depletion, and a few miscellaneous disorders (pregnancy, prolonged recumbency) comprise the great majority. Patients who are febrile, mildly dehydrated, anemic, or otherwise systemically ill are probably more susceptible to these common insults.

Less commonly, diseases of the autonomic nervous system are responsible. Dysautonomia may occur as an isolated phenomenon or in association with various peripheral neuropathies or diffuse cortical or extrapyramidal diseases (Table 10–4). Because the autonomic system is broadly impaired in these circumstances there are usually other clues: coexisting impotence, sweating disorders, pupillary changes, sphincter disturbances with urinary/fecal incontinence or retention, and the absence of compensatory tachycardia when hypotension is induced by standing (or sitting). This phenomenon—failure of cardioacceleration—is diagnostically useful (it suggests autonomic dysfunction) and may also explain why many patients with autonomic failure faint without any prodromal symptoms (unlike patients with the more common causes of postural hypotension—Table 10–4).

Treatment of orthostatic hypotension, then, depends on:

1. Establishing the etiologic mechanism: As can be seen in Table 10–4, many different disorders may cause (or contribute to) orthostatic hypotension, and sometimes several causes can be identified in the same patient. Consider, for example, the diabetic hypertensive patient with Parkinson's disease: The primary disease (parkinsonism, diabetic neuropathy), treatment thereof (diuretics, antihypertensive drugs, L-dopa), or other unrelated events (diarrhea, fever, prolonged bedrest) may induce orthostatic hypotension.

2. Whenever possible, therapy should be specific. Specific therapy may be as straightforward as discontinuing certain medications, completing a pregnancy, or treating diarrhea, but it may also involve specific pharmacologic replacement (cortisol, aldosterone, blood), drug therapy of specific disorders (for example, propranolol in mitral valve prolapse or corticosteroids in acute pandysautonomia), or even surgery (for example, in pheochromocytoma or very severe varicose veins). Common sense and understanding of basic pathophysiology are essential. For example, a low-salt diet in the patient with chronic renal failure and "obligate" daily urinary sodium wasting may induce persistent, puzzling, but easily treatable orthostasis due to volume depletion (thus, liberalize the excessive salt restriction).

3. Often, however, therapy must be nonspecific. This is especially true when the underlying condition is irreversible (for example, diabetes), untreatable (for example, postsympathectomy), or of unknown cause (various primary dysautonomias and idiopathic postural hypotension).

In general, the most helpful nonspecific therapy includes prescription elastic stockings (which are expensive—they must be individually fitted), salt supplements (over-the-counter salt tablets are quite inexpensive), and fludrocortisone acetate[36] (Florinef), a mineralocorticoid preparation. This drug is usually effective at a dose of 0.5 to 2 mg qd or bid (maximum 6 to 10 mg a day), but its expansion of extracellular fluid volume may precipitate edema, congestive heart failure, or supine hypertension, especially in the elderly. (Concomitant treatment with beta blockade drugs—see Chapter 13, "Chest Pain"—often dampens supine hypertension while Florinef relieves orthostatic hypotension.*) As such, body weight and supine blood pressure should be monitored after initiation of therapy.

---

*This is controversial. Some authorities report that beta blockers can raise blood pressure in these patients.

Equally important are general physical conditioning (especially in the patient whose orthostatic hypotension results from prolonged recumbency/hospitalization/deconditioning) and patient education. The need to avoid dehydration, nonessential drugs, and rapid positional changes must be emphasized. Alcohol (a vasodilator) and, when possible, extremes of environmental heat should be avoided. Raising the head of the bed on 6-inch blocks may be distressing at first (and thus requires gradual elevation over time), but this often allows safer conditions for arising in the morning or during the night, and may also prevent recumbency diuresis,[109] which may play a role in the pathogenesis of idiopathic postural hypotension.

4. When a treatable cause cannot be identified and when these nonspecific measures fail, several vasoactive drugs may be tried. Many such agents have been advocated—none is uniformly effective. Ephedrine and methylphenidate hydrochloride (Ritalin) occasionally help, but their side effects (palpitations, insomnia, urinary retention) often limit their usefulness. Tranylcypromine,[37] indomethacin[32] and dihydroergotamine[38] have been touted by some investigators. Midodrine[39] and clonidine[40] appear promising but require further investigation.

> Derwood's L-dopa is discontinued, and Derwood's daughter, Sylvia, is warned that Derwood will be dizzy upon arising for another few days, but that this is a benign side effect of the medication. Sylvia is skeptical and wants Derwood hospitalized. Derwood refuses.
>
> Three days later, Derwood is able to rise and walk without dizziness, but "my balance isn't very good." Carbidopa/levodopa (Sinemet) 10/100 mg in gradually increasing doses is tolerated well without orthostatic hypotension. Monthly return visits demonstrate improvement in bradykinesia and tremor, but Derwood's daughter calls frequently with many questions and worries. Neurologic consultation is arranged. The diagnosis of parkinsonism is confirmed, and therapy is continued. Derwood's daughter is only somewhat relieved.

Diagnostic Categories of Syncope

Because syncope is by definition a transient phenomenon, establishing a cause is not always so easy as in this case. This is particularly true when only one syncopal event occurs or when recurrent syncope is very infrequent, when the patient is a poor historian, when there are no eyewitnesses, and when the patient's physical examination is normal between (or after) the event(s). Such situations are, in fact, quite common.

As Figure 10–6 suggests, at the conclusion of a careful history, physical examination (and perhaps simple laboratory tests—an ECG for example), all cases of syncope should be placed in one of three diagnostic categories:

1. Most patients will have had typical benign syncope, as suggested by the findings in Table 10–3. These patients often require no further evaluation.

2. A minority (about 25 per cent in one study[24]) will have worrisome syncope in which various historical or physical findings suggest a serious (usually cardiac or neurologic) diagnosis. Under most circumstances these patients are admitted to hospital and monitored—either electrocardiographically or with a variety of tests that aim to diagnose or exclude arrhythmias, cardiac disease, or neurologic disorders.

3. Finally, some will constitute a group with clinically equivocal syncope: Either the history is vague or nonspecific or the physical examination (or

ECG) discloses findings that might cause syncope but that are otherwise nonspecific (for example, a heart murmur, extrasystoles on the ECG, an undocumented history of seizures). Among this group, the young, healthy patient will usually not require hospitalization, but ambulatory electrocardiography or echocardiography or electroencephalography may be needed, depending upon the particular circumstances (see Table 10–5 and 10–6). The elderly patient with unexplained (but not specifically worrisome) syncope will often best be served by brief hospitalization, 24-hour electrocardiographic monitoring, and observation. In general, diagnostic testing is more likely to be helpful in the elderly than in the young, but each clinical situation requires an individualized approach.

As noted previously, sometimes a specific diagnosis cannot be made. In general, however, the clinician at least attempts to exclude serious syncope. A few generalizations may be helpful here:

1. Syncope that occurs very frequently is usually the easiest to diagnose. Syncopal episodes that occur daily or several times per week and that are of recent onset (weeks) are usually caused by cardiac arrhythmias, seizures, postural hypotension, hyperventilation, or hysteria. In such patients, then, dizziness simulation tests, ECG monitoring, or electroencephalography after a careful history and physical examination will often make the diagnosis. Hospitalization is often worthwhile, since observing and examining the patient during a syncopal event is always helpful (Fig. 10–6).

Frequent syncopal episodes that abate during hospitalization, that occur only when the patient is alone, or that elude diagnosis for many years are often psychogenic.

Conversely, hysterical syncope or hysterical seizures often occur only when the patient is "on stage"—careful questioning of observers is always helpful here (see page 476).

Neurologic Causes

2. Neurologic causes of syncope can almost always be excluded (or suggested) by a careful history. The most common neurologic causes of serious syncope are epilepsy and cerebrovascular disease.

Epilepsy[41, 42] can be subdivided into many different classifications, but for our present purposes the distinctions in Table 10–5 are most helpful. Partial seizures may result in loss of consciousness if the focal seizure or psychomotor seizure progresses to a generalized seizure, but the premonitory symptoms (i.e., the partial seizure) before loss of consciousness will usually suggest these diagnoses. Psychomotor seizures may mimic many other conditions (and may be very difficult to diagnose), but at least it is usually easy to distinguish these from simple syncope or other types of dizziness. Note also that petit mal epilepsy is a disease of childhood. Many adults are diagnosed as suffering from petit mal epilepsy when recurrent syncopal events elude better definition: This diagnosis is almost always in error.

Most seizures, then, that cause actual loss of consciousness are generalized seizures. Typical grand mal seizures cause a typical sequence of events— since the seizure is rarely observed by the clinician, familiarity with the typical events allows more fruitful questioning of observers who have witnessed the event. Sometimes preceded by a vague aura of "not feeling well," loss of consciousness occurs abruptly, and the patient slumps to the ground. In 5 to 15 seconds, the tonic phase induces stiffening of all muscles (and

TABLE 10–5. NEUROLOGIC CAUSES OF SYNCOPE

TYPE	CHARACTERISTICS	REMEMBER
Epilepsy[41, 42] Generalized Grand mal	Abrupt loss of consciousness; tonic phase 5–15 sec; clonic phase 1–2 min; gradual awakening in 5–10 min; postictal headache, myalgias, confusion	Duration several minutes EEG may be normal between seizures Usually idiopathic May be caused by drug withdrawal, uremia, CNS infection, hypoxic or metabolic encephalopathy, especially in patients over age 50
Akinetic	Abrupt loss of consciousness; minimal motor activity; unconscious for several minutes; postictal symptoms	Abrupt onset and postictal state—different from other causes of syncope EEG may be normal between seizures
Petit mal	Brief episodes (30 sec) of staring or "absence" and automatisms (e.g., lip smacking, clucking)	Onset "always" before puberty
Partial (may progress into generalized seizures or terminate spontaneously) Focal	Focal neurologic symptoms without initial loss of consciousness; unilateral motor activity, paresthesias, vertigo, visual patterns, aphasia, smell/taste—all suggest specific cerebral focus	Partial focal or psychomotor phenomena usually distinguish these seizures from other kinds of syncope Often structural neurologic disease is cause
Psychomotor (rare)	Bizarre behavior, hallucinations, illusions, automatisms	
Cerebrovascular Disease[6, 43, 44] Vertebrobasilar transient ischemia	Syncope almost always preceded by symptoms of brain stem ischemia—diplopia, dysarthria, dysphagia, dysesthesias, dizziness; must distinguish syncope from "drop attacks" or transient global amnesia	Beware treatable precipitants: Low cardiac output Hyperviscosity Vasculitis Anemia Polycythemia Hypoglycemia Hypoxemia Migraine[45] Subclavian steal[46]
Carotid ischemia	Does not cause syncope unless bilateral carotid stenosis or carotids supply vertebrobasilar system as collaterals	
Vascular spasm (rare)	Underlying cause—subarachnoid hemorrhage, migraine, hypertensive encephalopathy, severe hypocapnia—usually obvious	
Hypoglycemia		

often tongue biting)—the legs are usually fully extended, the arms in varying positions. The tonic phase then elides into the clonic phase, during which mild trembling is followed by rhythmic but often violent jerking of the entire body (and apnea), which gradually subsides over the next 1 to 2 minutes. Finally, all movement gradually ceases, and over the following 5 to 10 minutes, the patient groggily emerges from deep coma, usually confused, often incontinent of urine, and frequently complaining of headache, myalgias, or the traumatic effects of the fall.

Careful descriptions of generalized seizures are not often confused with other types of dizziness or syncope. (Akinetic seizures are atypical grand mal seizures in that the characteristic sequence of major motor activity is inapparent: Only minimal twitching may occur, but the abrupt loss of consciousness and postictal state should suggest the diagnosis.)

Of great importance is the fact that the EEG may be normal between seizures. A normal EEG does not exclude epilepsy—unless it is obtained during the event—any more than an abnormal EEG confirms epilepsy. (Many nonepileptic patients will have nonspecific EEG abnormalities of no consequence.) When the EEG is obtained while the patient is asymptomatic, findings that *might* explain episodic loss of consciousness are spike and wave activity, focal sharp waves, or focal slowing. A neurologist should be consulted in these circumstances.

In young patients, epilepsy is usually idiopathic. In the patient whose seizures begin after the age of 50 years, a primary neurologic cause—vascular disease, neoplasms, metabolic disturbances—is much more frequent.

While cerebrovascular disease is epidemic in prevalence, syncope is not a common symptom of transient cerebral ischemia. When vascular syncope does occur, it is usually due to vertebrobasilar ischemia[43] and is almost always preceded by more specific neurologic symptoms of brain stem ischemia—the "five Ds" mentioned earlier. Transient vertebrobasilar ischemia must be distinguished from drop attacks in which consciousness is preserved ("the legs give way"), from transient global amnesia (in which amnesia for minutes to hours is not associated with any loss of consciousness), and from other types of dizziness that may mimic "brain stem symptoms" (especially hyperventilation and vertigo—see below).

As a rule, unilateral carotid disease does not produce syncope. Rarely, transient loss of consciousness may result from bilateral carotid stenosis, aortic arch disease, or diffuse cerebrovascular spasm (due to migraine, subarachnoid hemorrhage, hypertensive encephalopathy, for example).

Other disorders of the central nervous system (intermittent hydrocephalus with tumors of the third or fourth ventricle, for example) are very rare causes of recurrent syncope.

Recurrent hypoglycemia usually causes impaired mentation or dizziness rather than syncope, but this problem is so treatable that it must always be remembered.

Cardiac Causes

3. Some cardiac arrhythmias are difficult to document, but most cardiac syncope will be apparent (or strongly suspected) on the basis of the history and physical examination. Cardiac syncope occurs when cardiac output is sufficiently reduced to impair cerebral perfusion.

Engel[16] has shown that complete asystole (absence of cardiac output) results in loss of consciousness within 12 to 15 seconds when the patient is supine but within 5 to 6 seconds when the patient is upright. (This may explain lack of warning symptoms in some upright patients who develop transient loss of cardiac output.) Transient asystole or severe bradycardia usually implies sinoatrial arrest (due to sick sinus syndrome or bradycardia-tachycardia syndrome), ventricular fibrillation, or advanced atrioventricular block (the classic Stokes-Adams attack). Thus, asystole or sudden severe bradycardia may result in abrupt sudden syncope.

Most tachyarrhythmias will cause prodromal palpitations, "skipping," and gradual "gray-out" of vision before loss of consciousness occurs. The duration of these warning symptoms will depend on the rate of the tachycardia

TABLE 10–6A. MOST COMMON CARDIAC CAUSES OF SYNCOPE

TYPE	CHARACTERISTICS	TREATMENT
Cardiac Arrhythmias[47]*		
Bradycardia		
Advanced (second degree, third degree) AV heart block (Stokes-Adams attacks)	Usually elderly	Withdraw offending drugs? (digitalis, beta blockers, verapamil); pacemaker usually
Sick sinus syndrome	Sinus arrest Slow, fixed junctional rhythm Often exertional syncope	Anticholinergic drugs?; pacemaker usually
<u>Reflex</u> asystole or severe bradycardia	Excessive vagotonia Usually brief Setting obvious (see Table 10–3)	Anticholinergic drugs?; pacemaker rarely
Tachycardias		
Ventricular tachycardia	Palpitations, gray-out	Antiarrhythmic drugs; pacemaker rarely
Supraventricular tachycardia	Palpitations, gray-out	Antiarrhythmic drugs; pacemaker rarely
Ventricular fibrillation	Palpitations, gray-out	Antiarrhythmic drugs; resuscitation
Bradycardia/tachycardia	Rapid SV tachycardia, followed by asystole with loss of consciousness, followed by arousal in sinus rhythm	Antiarrhythmic drugs plus pacemaker

*Remember intermittent arrhythmias may be difficult to document—repeated monitoring, and/or electrophysiologic studies may be needed (see Appendix I).

(greater than 160 beats per minute is usually symptomatic) as well as the degree of underlying cardiac disease (i.e., how well is cardiac output maintained despite tachycardia)?

These different arrhythmias are certainly the most common cause of cardiac syncope. As Table 10–6 indicates, the therapeutic approach to such patients obviously will depend on the type of arrhythmia responsible for an individual patient's symptoms. ECG documentation of the arrhythmia is thus crucial. Very often the initial ECG or a brief period of ECG monitoring (often in hospital[24]) will detect the arrhythmia. Less often, but not at all uncommonly, continuous ECG monitoring will not detect transient but potentially life-threatening arrhythmias. This problem is briefly discussed in Appendix I.

Structural cardiac disorders that transiently impair cardiac output may also cause syncope. Valvular aortic stenosis is the most common of these, but Table 10–6 emphasizes that a careful history, cardiopulmonary examination, and noninvasive testing (ECG or echocardiogram or both) will usually suggest these different disorders.

Cardiac ischemic events may cause syncope. Syncope during myocardial infarction is usually caused by arrhythmias or pump failure with hypotension. Classic angina pectoris or coronary artery spasm may also be associated with transient arrhythmias or hypotension (especially when left main disease or three-vessel disease jeopardizes extensive areas of myocardium during the ischemic event). Rarely, spasm of the coronary arteries supplying the atrioventricular node may cause transient extreme bradycardia with syncope. Almost always, however, the history (and, if possible, the ECG during the event) will suggest these diagnoses.

Four months later, Derwood's daughter calls about her father. She is frantically upset and says that Derwood is "worse than ever. He's so dizzy he can't stand up."

Derwood arrives, looking pale and diaphoretic, holding his head in both hands. He is very unsteady on his feet and begins to fall when attempting

TABLE 10–6B. LESS COMMON CARDIAC CAUSES OF SYNCOPE

TYPE	HISTORY	EXAMINATION/ECG*	CONFIRM DIAGNOSIS
Cardiac Outflow Obstruction			
Valvular aortic stenosis	Usually exertional	Aortic systolic murmur with basal thrill; delayed carotid upstroke (pulsus parvus et tardus); ECG: LVH	Echocardiography and/or angiography
Asymmetric septal hypertrophy	Usually exertional	Apical systolic murmur, increased with Valsalva maneuver; double peak carotid upstroke (pulsus bisferiens); ECG: high voltage, deep Q waves, LVH	Echocardiography and/or angiography
Severe pulmonary hypertension: primary (rare) or due to pulmonary disease, atrial septal defect, mitral stenosis	Usually exertional	Right ventricular heave, increased S_2P; ECG: RVH	Echocardiography and/or angiography
Valvular pulmonic stenosis	Usually exertional	Pulmonic systolic murmur with thrill; pulmonic ejection click; right ventricular heave; wide S_2 split or soft S_2P; ECG: RVH	Echocardiography and/or angiography
Tetralogy of Fallot	Usually exertional	Onset usually in infancy; often cyanotic	Echocardiography and/or angiography
Pericardial tamponade	Usually exertional	Pulsus paradoxicus; faint heart sounds; pericardial rub?; ECG: low voltage	Echocardiography
Atrial myxoma	Positional and/or exertional syncope	Normal examination or "tumor plop" sound; ECG: usually normal	Echocardiography and/or angiography
Pulmonary embolism (massive or submassive)	Predisposing factors (see Chap. 13)	Normal examination, or increased S_2P, elevated JVP; ECG: normal, or acute RAD	Lung scans and/or angiography
Remember also: aortic dissection, tension pneumothorax, prosthetic valve dysfunction			
Cardiac Ischemia			
Myocardial infarction	Usually some antecedent or postsyncopal cardiopulmonary symptoms: e.g., chest pain, dyspnea, palpitations, nausea, diaphoresis	ECG: usually (but not always) ischemic (see Chap. 13)	Hospitalization; cardiac enzymes determination
Angina pectoris	Only rarely is syncope only symptom (angina equivalent); occasionally angina induces cardiac arrhythmia, causing syncope; very rarely Prinzmetal's angina causes syncope	ECG: usually ischemic (see Chap. 13)	Document event with electrocardiography during symptoms; Holter monitor?; hospitalization?

*LVH, left ventricular hypertrophy; RVH, right ventricular hypertrophy; JVP, jugular venous pressure; RAD, right axis deviation.

to stand or walk. He says, "Everything is spinning around and I can't stop it."

Derwood says he had been doing well until this morning "when the dizziness started in as soon as I woke up." He admits vomiting twice today, but denies difficulty with his speech, swallowing, strength, or sight except that "I feel wobbly when I walk and my eyes keep spinning." He denies headache, trauma, falling, fever, hearing loss, and the use of any drugs other than Sinemet. He denies use of alcohol, tobacco, or caffeine.

Vital signs and general examination are normal. Brief neurologic examination reveals normal mental status and sensorimotor status. There is jerky nystagmus of both eyes; attempts to stand up result in near falls, usually to the right. Coordination of the hands and legs appears normal.

VERTIGO

In this instance, Derwood's dizziness is, in fact, vertigo—the illusion of environmental motion, usually described as spinning or whirling. Vertigo may be perceived as internal—"I, or my head, or my eyes are moving"—or, more commonly, as external—"the world or the room or the ground is moving." Disorientation in space and some sense of illusory motion are the common denominators here. The sense of motion is usually rotatory—"like getting off a merry-go-round"—but may be linear—"the ground tilts up and down, like being on a boat at sea." Similarly the spatial disorientation may be obviously vertiginous—"everything is turning"—or more vague—"my balance is off." The patient's description, then, may be so idiosyncratic or imprecise as to be misleading, but a careful history will usually allow at least a tentative diagnosis of vertigo. This is crucial, since there are so many other types of dizziness and because the differential diagnosis of vertigo is so discrete (see below).

All vertigo reflects dysfunction at some level of the vestibular system. The vestibular system, however, is extremely complex (Fig. 10–7). The ear, the vestibular and cochlear divisions of the acoustic (eighth cranial) nerve, the vestibular and cochlear nuclei in the medulla of the brain stem, and their connections with the temporal lobe of the cerebral cortex are only the rudiments of the system: Afferent and efferent connections with cerebellum, brain stem, oculomotor and visual apparatus, and spinal cord are also critical components. The assessment of vertigo, then, can be humbling even for the otoneurologist with his proliferating technologic capabilities (see Appendices II and III). Nevertheless, the cause of vertigo can usually be diagnosed by following several simple guidelines.[48-52]

Peripheral versus Central Vertigo

In general, vertigo is classified as peripheral or central. Peripheral vertigo is much more common than central vertigo. Distinguishing peripheral vertigo from central vertigo is of great clinical importance since most peripheral disorders can be treated by the nonspecialist without difficulty, while central vertigo often implies serious neurologic disease. The clinical distinction between the two usually depends simply on the clinical history and the physical examination (especially the neurologic findings and the evaluation of associated nystagmus).*

---

*Those not familiar with descriptions, pathophysiology, and clinical interpretation of the various types of nystagmus should read Appendix II as a supplement to the following discussion.

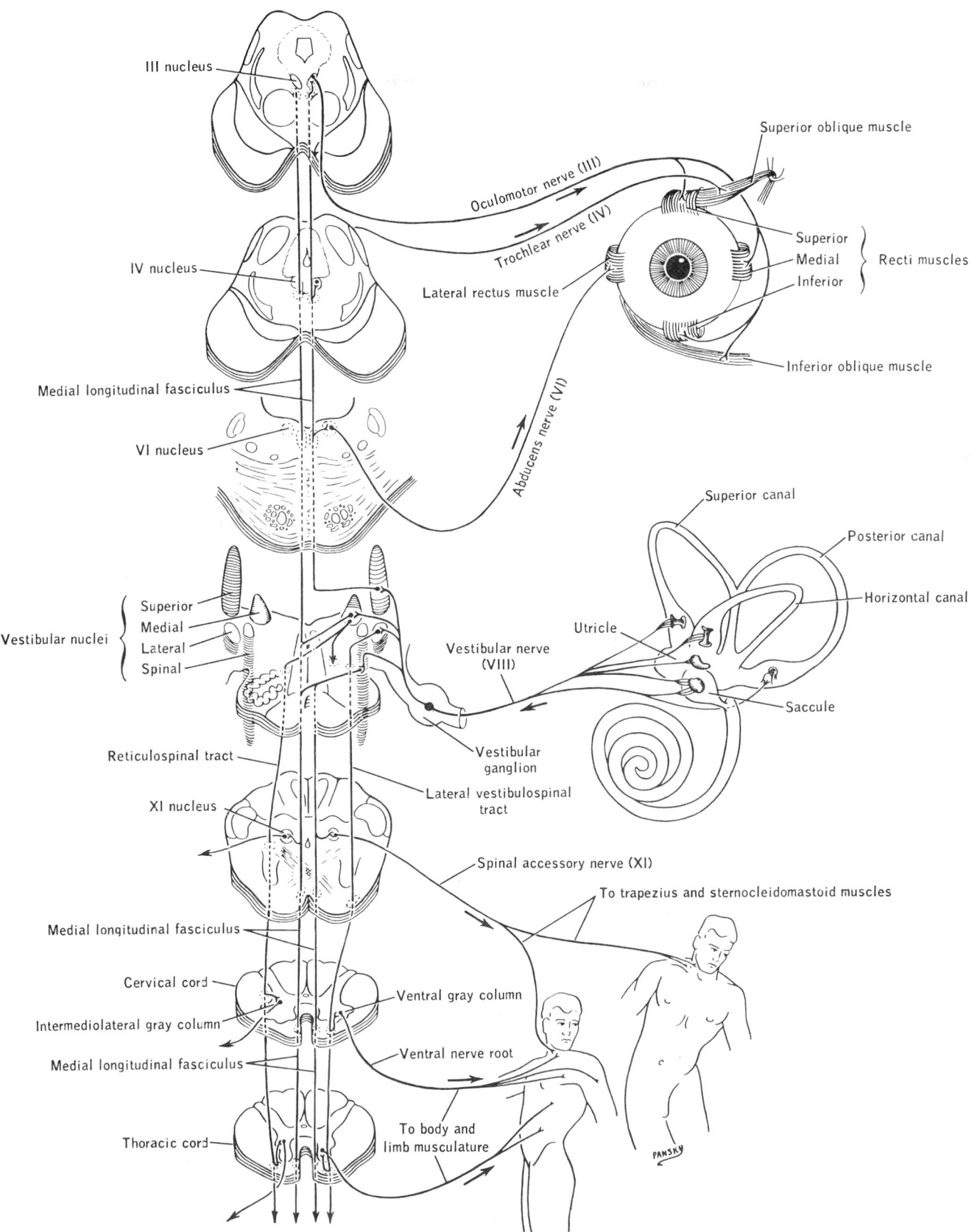

Simple vestibular reflex pathways.

FIGURE 10–7. The vestibular reflex pathways. (Reproduced with permission from House, E. L., et al.: A Systematic Approach to Neuroscience. New York: McGraw-Hill, 1979, p. 240.)

TABLE 10–7. DIFFERENCES BETWEEN PERIPHERAL AND CENTRAL VESTIBULAR DYSFUNCTION*

SYMPTOM/SIGN	PERIPHERAL	CENTRAL
Severity of vertigo	Marked	Mild
Nystagmus	Bilateral Unidirectional Rotatory/horizontal Never vertical Fast-phase usually opposite to side of lesion	Bilateral or unilateral Bidirectional or unidirectional May be vertical
Direction of environmental spin	Toward fast phase of nystagmus	Variable
Direction of past pointing; direction of Romberg fall	Toward slow phase of nystagmus	Variable
Tinnitus/deafness	Often present	Usually absent
Common causes	Positional vertigo Labyrinthitis Meniere's disease (See Table 10–8)	Multiple sclerosis Vertebrobasilar ischemia Drug-induced (See Fig. 10–11)

*Adapted from reference 50.

Table 10–7 indicates some of the differences between peripheral and central vestibular disorders that can be recognized with a careful history and physical examination.

Peripheral vestibular disease refers to dysfunction of the (external, middle or inner) ear or vestibular end-organ (semicircular canals, utricle, saccule) with or without involvement of the contiguous auditory end-organ, the cochlea. These peripheral diseases usually cause prominent vertigo, which is usually unmistakable and which may be quite severe—nausea, vomiting, and marked disequilibrium are often associated with the vertigo. The nystagmus that accompanies peripheral disorders may be either spontaneous (apparent with simple observation of eye movements) or positional (apparent or heightened after precipitation of nystagmus by assuming particular head/body positions).

When nystagmus is spontaneous, those characteristics illustrated in Table 10–7 usually denote peripheral nystagmus—and thus peripheral disease. Peripheral nystagmus affects both eyes equally (bilateral), is unidirectional (the direction of fast and slow components of nystagmus remains fixed, regardless of gaze direction), and is horizontal or rotatory (clockwise or counterclockwise). Figure 10–8 illustrates basic nomenclature used in describing nystagmus in this text; Figure 10–9 illustrates examples of peripheral nystagmus.

When nystagmus is positional only, i.e., is demonstrable only during the Nylen-Bárány maneuver (see Appendix II), different criteria help distinguish peripheral from central nystagmus. Other clinical findings associated with peripheral vertigo—the direction of past pointing, environmental movement

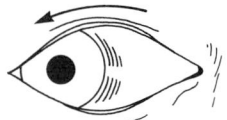 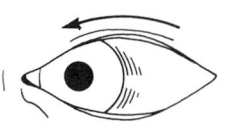

The fast component of nystagmus is depicted by the solid arrow.

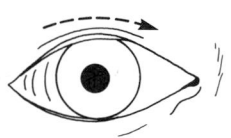 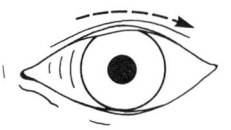

The slow component of nystagmus is depicted by the broken arrow

FIGURE 10–8. (Fast) nystagmus to the right. The appearance of the eyes is that of "frantic," jerky eye movements to the right—the direction of the fast component. In Figures 10–9 and 10–10, the nomenclature depicted here will be used.

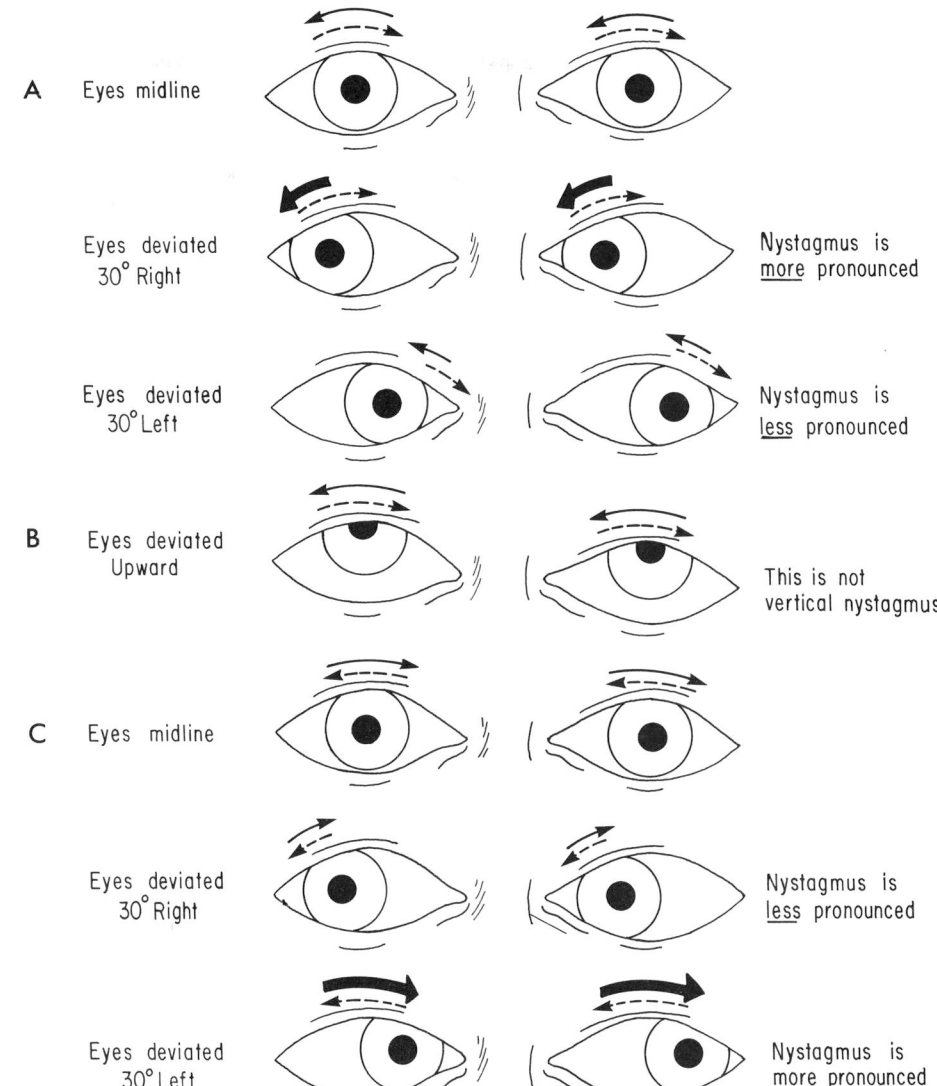

A   Eyes midline

Eyes deviated
30° Right

Nystagmus is
more pronounced

Eyes deviated
30° Left

Nystagmus is
less pronounced

B   Eyes deviated
Upward

This is not
vertical nystagmus

C   Eyes midline

Eyes deviated
30° Right

Nystagmus is
less pronounced

Eyes deviated
30° Left

Nystagmus is
more pronounced

FIGURE 10–9. Peripheral nystagmus. A, In this case, nystagmus (fast right) affects each eye equally (bilateral), is unidirectional (the direction of fast and slow components stays the same in all gaze directions), and is horizontal and rotatory (i.e., the eyes move in the horizontal plane and in a counterclockwise direction during nystagmus). B, Remember that horizontal/rotatory nystagmus, which occurs on vertical gaze, is not vertical nystagmus. C, In this instance, nystagmus (fast left) is horizontal/rotatory, unidirectional (fast component is always to the left), and bilateral.

in relation to nystagmus directions (Table 10–7)—are also briefly discussed in Appendix II.

The most common causes of peripheral vertigo are benign positional vertigo, "vestibular neuronitis," and various forms of labyrinthitis (page 497). Benign positional vertigo causes intermittent, brief episodes of vertigo always (and only) related to sudden changes in head and body position. Vestibular neuronitis or labyrinthitis usually causes a circumscribed period of persistent vertigo (usually lasting a few days) that then resolves. Very often the distinction between benign positional vertigo and vestibular neuronitis/labyrinthitis is made simply on the basis of this difference in the course and timing of symptoms.

Other specific causes of peripheral vertigo (Table 10–8, page 494) will usually be suspected after careful examination of the ear itself or specific audiologic testing (see Appendix II), since associated cochlear symptoms—hearing loss and tinnitus—are expected in some diseases of the vestibular apparatus. Table 10–8 summarizes some of these differential points (page 494).

Central vestibular dysfunction[53] refers to disorders of the central nervous system (usually the brain stem). Figure 10–11 (page 492) illustrates the most common pathologic conditions that affect vestibular nuclei in the brain stem or their various central connections with the visual, oculomotor, cortical,

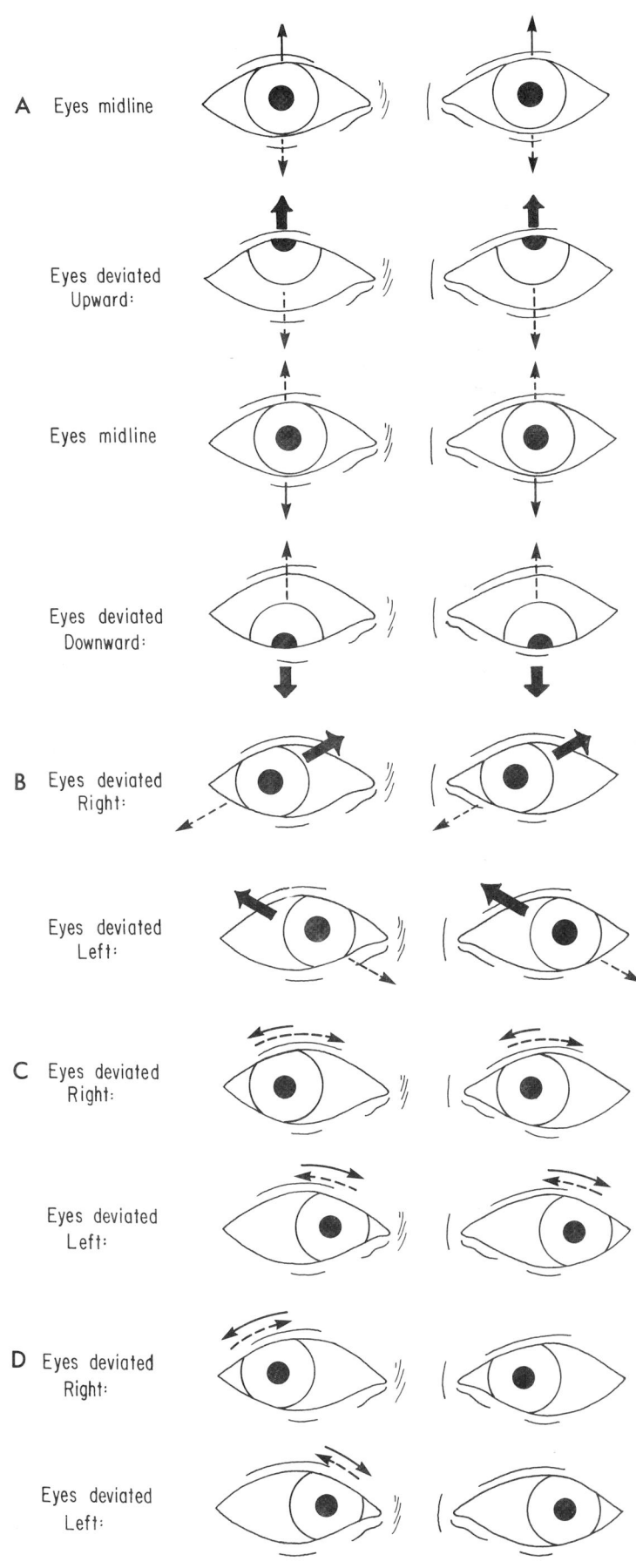

A Eyes midline

Eyes deviated
Upward:

Eyes midline

Eyes deviated
Downward:

B Eyes deviated
Right:

Eyes deviated
Left:

C Eyes deviated
Right:

Eyes deviated
Left:

D Eyes deviated
Right:

Eyes deviated
Left:

FIGURE 10–10. Central nystagmus. *A,* Vertical nystagmus. In the upper panel, the fast (upward) component of vertical nystagmus is more prominent on upward gaze. In the lower panel, the fast component of vertical nystagmus is "downbeating" and is even more prominent on downward gaze. *B,* Vertical nystagmus may persist on horizontal eye movements as well—this is still vertical nystagmus. *C,* Bidirectional nystagmus. The fast and slow components in this case change direction in different gaze directions *D,* Unilateral nystagmus. Nystagmus in this instance affects only the right eye (and also changes direction—it is bidirectional as well).

cerebellar, and spinal systems that integrate and interpret vestibular information. Drug-induced vertigo (and nystagmus) is certainly the most common cause of central vertigo, but concern about vertebrobasilar vascular insufficiency, demyelinating diseases, and various tumors more often results in medical consultation. All of these central disorders are decidedly rare when compared with the peripheral vestibular disorders.

As Table 10–7 suggests, central vertigo is usually subjectively milder and less disabling than peripheral vertigo, and nonspecific dizziness or disequilibrium, rather than frank vertigo, may be a more prominent subjective complaint among such patients. The diagnosis is usually suspected on the basis of the clinical history and a thorough neurologic examination: Evaluation of the type of nystagmus that accompanies the complaints of vertigo is crucial. Spontaneous nystagmus that is vertical, bidirectional (the direction of slow and fast components varies in different gaze positions), or unilateral (nystagmus of one eye only or where conjugate gaze is dissociated in some way) is usually central in origin. Figure 10–10 shows examples of vertical, bidirectional, and unilateral nystagmus.

As in peripheral vestibular disease, central vertigo will sometimes be entirely positional, i.e., there is no spontaneous nystagmus. Analysis of nystagmus during positional testing (see Appendix II) will then be most helpful.

How then should we approach the patient with vertigo?[54] Figure 10–11 outlines one general approach. This approach particularly emphasizes the importance of evaluating nystagmus, but it must be emphasized that the clinical history and other elements of the physical/neurologic examination are equally essential components of the evaluation. Since peripheral vertigo is much more common than central vertigo, very often the presenting symptoms alone will suggest a specific diagnosis (Table 10–8). The scheme illustrated in Figure 10–11 emphasizes that most patients complaining of vertigo will fall into one of several subsets:

1. The patient who is experiencing ongoing vertigo and demonstrates spontaneous nystagmus on examination.

2. The patient with ongoing or intermittent vertigo who does not demonstrate spontaneous nystagmus but in whom positional nystagmus can be elicited by Nylen-Bárány maneuvers (see Appendix II).

In these two common situations, a systematic diagnostic approach based on the history and physical findings (and especially, evaluation of nystagmus) will at least allow differentiation between peripheral and central vertigo. A more specific diagnosis can then usually be achieved by considering the differential diagnosis of each type of vertigo—outlined in Figure 10–11 and Table 10–8.

3. The patient with ongoing or intermittent vertigo in whom neither spontaneous nor positional nystagmus can be demonstrated. There are several factors that may explain the absence of demonstrable nystagmus in the patient complaining of vertigo.

First, as noted in Appendix II, spontaneous but mild nystagmus may be missed by the observer's naked eye. Visual aids are helpful here. Also, the test for positional nystagmus (Nylen-Bárány maneuvers) may be improperly performed (page 515).

Second, the patient's so-called vertigo may in fact be a different type of dizziness entirely—the history must always be carefully reviewed in the patient complaining of vertigo in whom nystagmus cannot be demonstrated.

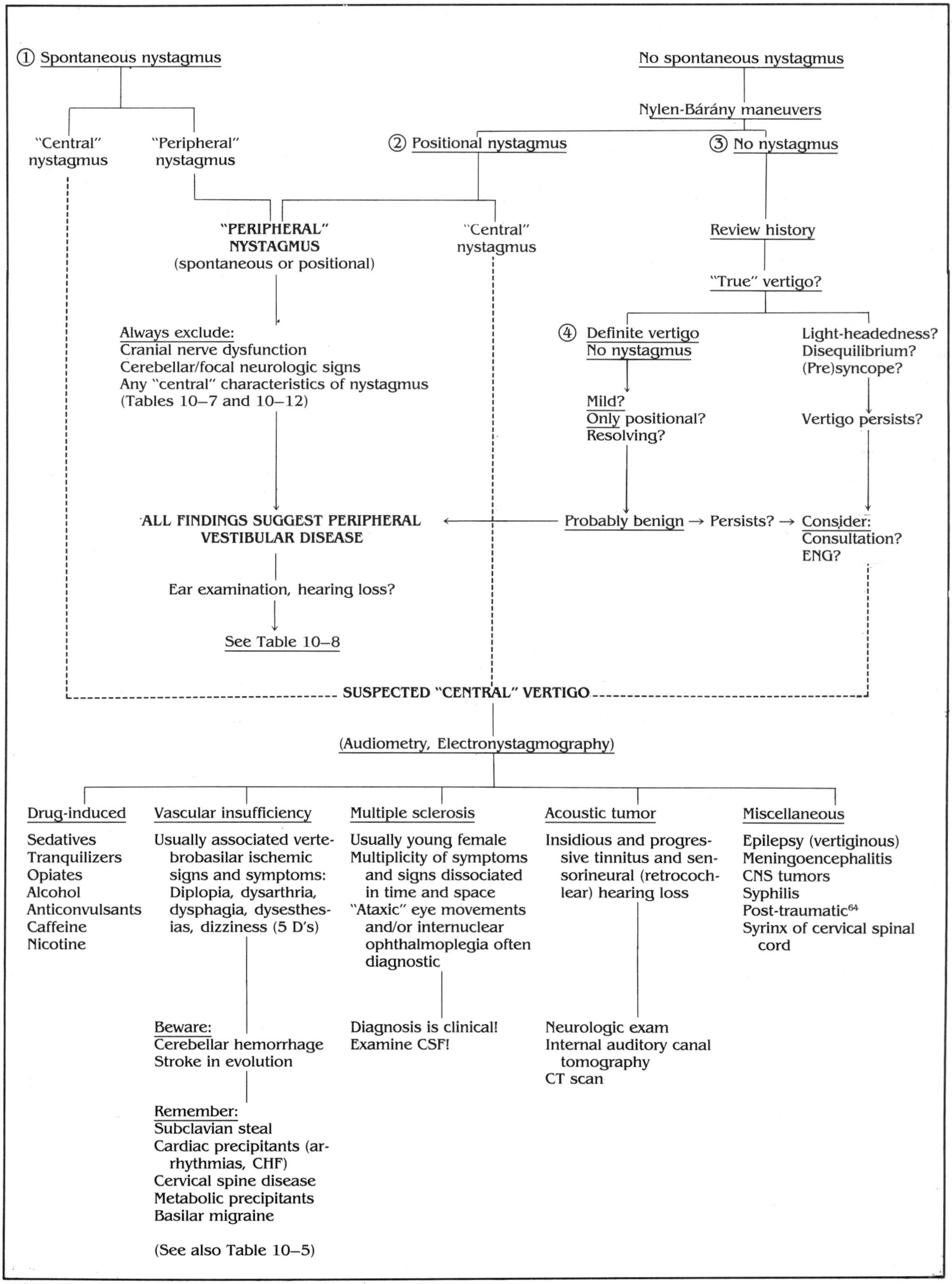

① Spontaneous nystagmus

No spontaneous nystagmus

Nylen-Bárány maneuvers

"Central" nystagmus "Peripheral" nystagmus ② Positional nystagmus ③ No nystagmus

"PERIPHERAL" NYSTAGMUS (spontaneous or positional)

"Central" nystagmus

Review history

"True" vertigo?

④ Definite vertigo No nystagmus

Light-headedness? Disequilibrium? (Pre)syncope?

Always exclude:
Cranial nerve dysfunction
Cerebellar/focal neurologic signs
Any "central" characteristics of nystagmus
(Tables 10–7 and 10–12)

Mild?
Only positional?
Resolving?

Vertigo persists?

ALL FINDINGS SUGGEST PERIPHERAL VESTIBULAR DISEASE ← Probably benign → Persists? → Consider: Consultation? ENG?

Ear examination, hearing loss?

See Table 10–8

SUSPECTED "CENTRAL" VERTIGO

(Audiometry, Electronystagmography)

Drug-induced	Vascular insufficiency	Multiple sclerosis	Acoustic tumor	Miscellaneous
Sedatives Tranquilizers Opiates Alcohol Anticonvulsants Caffeine Nicotine	Usually associated verte-brobasilar ischemic signs and symptoms: Diplopia, dysarthria, dysphagia, dysesthes-ias, dizziness (5 D's)	Usually young female Multiplicity of symptoms and signs dissociated in time and space "Ataxic" eye movements and/or internuclear ophthalmoplegia often diagnostic	Insidious and progres-sive tinnitus and sen-sorineural (retrococh-lear) hearing loss	Epilepsy (vertiginous) Meningoencephalitis CNS tumors Syphilis Post-traumatic[64] Syrinx of cervical spinal cord
	Beware: Cerebellar hemorrhage Stroke in evolution	Diagnosis is clinical! Examine CSF!	Neurologic exam Internal auditory canal tomography CT scan	
	Remember: Subclavian steal Cardiac precipitants (ar-rhythmias, CHF) Cervical spine disease Metabolic precipitants Basilar migraine (See also Table 10–5)			

FIGURE 10–11. The clinical analysis of vertigo.

Third, psychogenic vertigo is not rare and should at least be considered when complaints of vertigo are not attended by demonstrable nystagmus. Psychogenic vertigo is usually accompanied by other clues[55-57] (peculiar somatic complaints accompanied by entirely subjective, i.e., "internal" vertigo*) but sophisticated technologic testing (electronystagmography [ENG],[58] auditory brain stem responses,[59]—see Appendix II) are now available to help distinguish psychogenic from "organic" vertigo.

4. The patient whose vertigo has subsided, in whom neither nystagmus nor vertigo can be elicited on examination. Here, differential diagnosis is largely based on the clinical history. Such patients will be served best by the clinician with a clear understanding of the natural history and clinical course of the common causes of intermittent vertigo (see Figure 10–11 and Table 10–8).

Let's look at Derwood more closely:

> When Derwood is in the sitting position and with his eyes looking straight ahead, spontaneous nystagmus is obvious. (Derwood's nystagmus is similar to that depicted in Figure 10–9C.) Viewing through an ophthalmoscope, it can be appreciated that both eyes rotate together, the fast component clockwise (to the patient's left), the slow component counterclockwise (to the patient's right). Derwood is asked to move both eyes a little to his right (no more than 30 degrees): In this position the nystagmus is less intense, but the fast and slow components move in the same directions as previously. Voluntary deviation of both eyes 30 degrees to the left intensifies the nystagmus, greatly worsens the vertigo (Derwood retches), but there is no directional change in the components of nystagmus. There is no vertical nystagmus. Derwood says the room is spinning to his left.

> The remainder of the neurologic examination is unchanged from previously, except that there is past pointing to the right and a tendency to fall to the right on Romberg testing. Examination of the ears is normal. Hearing appears normal bilaterally (to watch tick).

What does all this mean?

1. Acute vertigo is associated with spontaneous nystagmus that has all the characteristics of a peripheral disorder (Table 10–7): The nystagmus is bilateral, rotatory, and unidirectional; the vertigo is intense, is associated with nausea and vomiting, and is clearly worsened by head and eye position.

2. The only neurologic abnormalities are completely consistent with a peripheral vestibular disorder—past pointing and an abnormal Romberg test (Figs. 10–2 and 10–3) are common among patients with peripheral vestibular disease. Considering Table 10–7 and Figure 10–11, there is no reason to suspect a central lesion, except perhaps for the patient's age and the realization that underlying cerebrovascular disease is common in this age group (and Derwood has a carotid bruit). It must be remembered that when any component of the evaluation is inconsistent with a peripheral disorder, further consideration of (more serious) central vertigo is in order.

Peripheral Vestibular Disease

Table 10–8 enumerates the most common peripheral vestibular disorders that cause vertigo and/or dizziness. Acoustic nerve tumors and highly localized vascular events involving the internal auditory artery and the brain stem

---

*As noted above, internal vertigo refers to illusory movement or rotation "in my head," not in the environment. Internal vertigo is not synonymous with psychogenic vertigo, but psychogenic vertigo is more often internal than external.

TABLE 10–8. PERIPHERAL VESTIBULAR DISORDERS CAUSING VERTIGO AND DIZZINESS

CAUSE	PRESENTING SYMPTOMS	HEARING LOSS	USUAL COURSE	DIAGNOSIS	TREATMENT
Sinusitis	Sinus congestion, mild vertigo	Conductive (if any)	Resolution with specific treatment	**ENT examination**	Antibiotics and/or decongestants
Otitis					
Otitis media	Earache				Antibiotics
Serous otitis	Earache, "pop," fullness	Conductive (if any)	Resolution with specific treatment	**Ear examination**	Decongestants
Wax	Fullness, decreased hearing				Wax removed
External otitis	Itch, pain, swelling				Local drops (polymyxin B-neomycin-hydrocortisone) cortisporin otic solution
Cholesteatoma	Vertigo, tinnitus usually following persistent chronic otitis or tympanic membrane perforation	Conductive	Slow progression; labyrinthine invasion; worsening symptoms	**Ear examination; fistula test,** x-rays (mastoid and auditory canal)	Surgery
Meniere's disease[60]	Episodic (duration: hours); severe vertigo, tinnitus, ear pressure, and hearing loss	Always during attack; sensorineural: low tones early	Episodic recurrence; well between attacks; progressive hearing loss; ± constant tinnitus	**Clinical story; audiometry;** rule out treatable causes	Treat allergy, syphilis, endocrine disease?[61]; medical and/or surgical therapy
Acoustic neuroma*	Persistent unilateral tinnitus; insidious unilateral hearing loss; vertigo often absent or mild	Progressive sensorineural	Progression to disequilibrium, facial hemiparaesthesias, facial weakness, other cranial nerve involvement	**Clinical story; audiometry;** tomography, CT scan of auditory canal	Surgery
Internal auditory artery infarction*	Sudden deafness, tinnitus, vertigo	Sensorineural	Permanent hearing loss; resolution of vertigo in several days	**Clinical story; audiometry**	Watch for other ischemic symptoms; aspirin
Cogan's syndrome (very rare)[62, 63]	Ocular keratitis; tinnitus deafness	Sensorineural	Deafness persists; multisystem disease	**Clinical picture;** vasculitis common	Steroids?
Vestibular neuronitis	Acute onset vertigo; tinnitus ±; preceding URI ±; continuous vertigo, may be positional but is not only positional	No	Monophasic illness: acute vertigo resolves in few days; positional vertigo for weeks (months); thereafter eventual full recovery	**Clinical story; normal hearing**	Rest; antiemetics; motion drugs (see Table 10–9); adaptation (see Table 10–10)
Labyrinthitis	Similar to vestibular neuronitis	No	Depends on cause—trauma: cervical whiplash, labyrinthine trauma, hemorrhage; toxic: alcohol, quinidine, salicylates, loop diuretics, aminoglycosides; infection: viral; severe otitis media	**Clinical story; normal hearing**	Eliminate cause, if any (e.g., allergy, drug); antiemetics; motion drugs; adaptation
Benign positional vertigo	Vertigo entirely positional ("When I turn over in bed")	No	Polyphasic illness: intermittent symptoms for days to weeks, slow regression, may recur intermittently	**Clinical story; Nylen-Bárány maneuvers**	Motion drugs; adaptation; antiemetics
Labyrinthine apoplexy* (infarction? of labyrinthine branch of internal auditory artery)	Sudden tinnitus, vertigo	No	Permanent labyrinthine destruction, but vertigo subsides	**Clinical story**	? (syndrome not pathologically documented)
Head trauma[64]	Vertigo following trauma; blood/spinal fluid in ear?; positive fistula test?	Often (may be conductive or sensorineural)	Symptoms often persist	**Clinical and x-ray findings** (exclude fracture of temporal bones)	Refer to otologist

*Acoustic neuroma, internal auditory infarction, and labyrinthine apoplexy may be considered either peripheral or central.

are included here, because these may be considered either central or peripheral, depending on the specific clinical circumstances. For example, a small acoustic neuroma will not cause any neurologic impairment and will affect only the peripheral VIII cranial nerve. Similarly, infarction or transient ischemia of a small area of the lateral medulla of the brain stem usually causes the lateral medullary syndrome, accompanied by prominent brain stem neurologic symptoms, but may also occasionally cause only sudden deafness and vertigo.

NOTE

I. Occasionally, peripheral causes of vertigo will be apparent on routine examination of the ear. For example, in various forms of infectious or inflammatory otitis, the diagnosis is easy. A cholesteatoma is usually visible with the otoscope. The patient with acute or recurrent sinusitis often experiences disequilibrium and vertigo; serous otitis frequently coexists.

II. Documentation of any associated hearing loss and assessment of the type of hearing loss (conductive or sensorineural) are always important.
As can be seen in Table 10–8, Meniere's disease and acoustic neuromas are virtually always associated with (sensorineural) hearing loss. Diseases of the external and middle ear are associated with hearing loss that is conductive. The most common causes of peripheral vertigo— benign positional vertigo, vestibular neuronitis/labyrinthitis (see page 497)—are not associated with any hearing loss at all. The evaluation of hearing is briefly discussed in Appendix III.

III. An understanding of the typical clinical history of serious causes of peripheral vertigo (and their expected associated physical findings) usually will allow a presumptive diagnosis and guide further testing (if any).

CONSIDER

A. Meniere's disease[60, 61, 65] (endolymphatic hydrops) is probably over-diagnosed.
In part, this is because its clinical manifestations may be highly variable (especially early in its course), but more so because there is no specific confirmatory diagnostic test or procedure (short of attempts at curative surgery). Most patients, however, describe a characteristic symptom complex: episodic attacks lasting usually 1 to 3 hours (rarely, for a day or more), during which the patient notes fullness or pressure in the ear as well as unilateral tinnitus, diminished hearing, and severe (often violent) vertigo. During an attack, spontaneous peripheral nystagmus is usually obvious. Between attacks, most patients are well and dread the next recurrence.
Ninety per cent of Meniere's disease is unilateral. Audiometry usually reveals sensorineural hearing loss (often low tones early in the course of the disease)[65] of the cochlear variety (see Appendix III). Pulec has suggested that a substantial minority (36 per cent) of patients will have remediable underlying causes[61] (allergies, syphilis, hypothyroidism). Otherwise, treatment of this condition is extremely variable and controversial: Vitamins, diet, diuretics, antihistamines,

vasodilators, and neuroleptics have all been ascribed varying successes, but the frequency of spontaneous remissions in this disorder makes all drug evaluations difficult.

Several types of surgical therapy have been advocated.[52] These should be reserved for patients in whom medical therapy fails and who are seriously incapacitated. Because the therapeutic implications of the diagnosis of Meniere's disease may be extreme (i.e., medical therapy is frustrating and surgical therapy is controversial), evaluation by specialists experienced in the technologic diagnosis (see Appendices II and III) and treatment of these patients is always worthwhile.

B. Acoustic neuromas[66–69] only uncommonly (10 to 20 per cent) present with vertigo.

Much more often, slowly progressive and unremitting unilateral tinnitus and sensorineural hearing loss are the dominant symptoms. Initially, when the tumor (most often, a schwannoma; rarely, a neurofibroma) is small the neurologic examination is normal, (there may be either peripheral or central nystagmus or there may be no nystagmus), but the tumor slowly destroys the eighth nerve and ultimately compresses adjacent neural structures as it enlarges. Thus, auditory symptoms and signs predominate early, but a diminished unilateral corneal reflex, (central) nystagmus, facial dysesthesias, or facial weakness may be the earliest hint of brain stem compression by an enlarging tumor mass. (Cranial nerves VII and V are usually first affected by mass extension.[70, 71]) The earlier the diagnosis, the better the prognosis. Hence, vague dizziness or vertigo associated with hearing loss must always be thoroughly investigated: Audiometry that reveals sensorineural loss of the retrocochlear variety (see Appendix III) always necessitates tomography of the internal auditory canal or a CT scan.

C. Infarction involving the internal auditory artery in the brain stem is not, in fact, a peripheral disorder but is commonly confused with the entities described above.

This represents vertebrobasilar ischemic disease,[42, 72] but only the small branch to the vestibular/cochlear nuclei and nerves is involved. The middle-aged and elderly are most often affected. There is usually sudden onset of (usually permanent) sensorineural deafness, together with vertigo (and central nystagmus), which itself gradually resolves over several days. The diagnosis is difficult to prove initially, and it may be confused with a first bout of Meniere's disease. This event may be a warning of more extensive vertebrobasilar infarction to come, but such is not the usual course. The persistence of unilateral (retrocochlear) sensorineural deafness with gradually resolving vertigo in the absence of any other neurologic findings (and without recurrent episodes suggestive of Meniere's disease) usually will make the diagnosis.

Consultation with an otologist, audiologist, neurologist, or neurosurgeon is always indicated for patients suspected of cholesteatoma, acoustic neuroma, or Meniere's disease. The patient with persistent post-traumatic vertigo or hearing loss should also consult a specialist.[64] Otherwise, most disease entities that cause peripheral vertigo do not require specialist consultation. These comprise the great majority of patients with vertigo. For example:

D. Vestibular neuronitis[73] is a poorly understood condition.

Investigations[74] suggest that it may be a form of cranial polyneuritis, but associated neurologic findings have not been widely reported (perhaps because they are so subtle and transient[73]). This disorder may follow an upper respiratory or herpes infection, but the etiology in many cases is unclear.

Vestibular neuronitis is usually a monophasic illness. Vertigo usually begins suddenly (or the patient awakens with vertigo), and symptoms are constant or occur very frequently through the day. (The vertigo is not *just* positional—as in benign positional vertigo—but positional changes do frequently *exacerbate* it). Spontaneous peripheral nystagmus is usually obvious. The constant severe vertigo usually resolves within a few days, but mild entirely positional vertigo may then supervene, slowly resolving over days to weeks (see page 499). Hearing is normal, but caloric testing (if performed) may reveal a hypoactive labyrinth (see Appendix II).

E. Labyrinthitis[52] is often considered synonymous with vestibular neuronitis, but some make the distinction that both audiometry and caloric testing are normal in labyrinthitis.

This distinction is usually not clinically important, except that labyrinthitis, which is usually idiopathic, is sometimes induced by drugs (e.g., aminoglycosides, loop diuretics, salicylates), trauma, shellfish allergies, or tobacco, and thus the etiology may have a bearing on treatment and the subsequent clinical course (e.g., unrecognized drug toxicity may cause permanent damage). As noted in Table 10–8, labyrinthitis and neuronitis are usually self-limited, and most often only symptomatic therapy is needed (see Tables 10–9 and 10–10, pages 499 and 500).

F. Benign (paroxysmal) positional vertigo[75–77] (BPV) causes brief episodes of vertigo (30 seconds) that are only and always positional, i.e., symptoms occur intermittently in response to sudden changes in head and body position, but the patient usually can find a position in which symptoms do not occur.

Turning over in bed, looking up or down, arising from a chair, looking over a shoulder, negotiating a corner or curve are among the many maneuvers that will precipitate symptoms. Positional vertigo* can persist for a few months, during which time symptoms may wax and wane, and occasionally the illness will recur several months later—the illness may be polyphasic. BPV is thought often to be due to cupulolithiasis, in which inorganic deposits accumulate in the cupula of the semicircular canal, rendering it more sensitive to gravitational and directional stimuli.[77] Occasionally, local ear disease, head trauma, or cervical spine disease[78] will cause similar symptoms. As noted above, vestibular neuronitis and labyrinthitis may also cause positional vertigo after the acute stage has resolved (see below).

CONSIDER Table 10–8:

1. As noted above, a normal ear examination usually rules out local infectious, inflammatory, or obstructive ear disorders (otitis, wax, for exam-

---

*Positional vertigo (and nystagmus) is present only when certain positions are assumed. Positioning vertigo (and nystagmus) means that changes in position augment nystagmus and vertigo already present at rest.

ple). Rarely a cholesteatoma may not be apparent on simple ear inspection. A fistula test with a pneumatic otoscope will help (see page 462).

2. The absence of hearing loss and tinnitus usually excludes a tumor of the cerebellopontine angle (acoustic neuroma, most often), Meniere's disease, and localized vascular infarction of the internal auditory artery.

3. Considering Derwood's clinical findings, then (page 493), the most likely diagnosis is some form of labyrinthitis or vestibular neuronitis (see below).

> Derwood denies any other drug use, known food allergies, recent falls or trauma, or any upper respiratory infection.
>
> Derwood is told that a virus infection of the inner ear is causing his troubles and that medicine can relieve his symptoms, but the virus will have "to run its own course." Derwood and his daughter are told that the worst symptoms usually last only a few days, and that brief hospitalization might help since Derwood is so incapacited by his symptoms. Derwood refuses hospitalization. His daughter is very angry. Derwood asks for "medicine to get me through the worst part."
>
> Derwood is told to rest and is given prescriptions for meclizine 25 mg bid and trimethobenzamide hydrochloride (Tigan) antiemetic suppositories (Table 10–9). He is told to return in 4 or 5 days, but to call if any visual symptoms, speech/swallowing problems, or sensorimotor symptoms develop beforehand.

NOTE

I. In Derwood's case, hospitalization makes sense for two reasons:

A. Derwood is vomiting, is unable to walk, and his daughter appears less than enthusiastic about caring for him at home.

Even when the cause of vertigo is benign, symptoms may be incapacitating enough to require hospitalization.

B. Especially in the elderly, one must always be concerned about atypical presentations of (especially vascular) neurologic catastrophe.

Vertigo alone may be the initial manifestation of vertebrobasilar ischemia[72] (uncommonly)—when this is so, other manifestations of brain stem dysfunction usually ensue within the next few weeks. The consistently peripheral nature of Derwood's vertigo and nystagmus makes this very unlikely, but the associated symptoms of past pointing and Romberg falling sometimes can be confused with the neurologic signs of brain stem or cerebellar disease. The experienced examiner can usually differentiate peripheral from central disorders, but in the patient who is ill, elderly, or atypical, caution is always prudent.

II. Drug therapy of peripheral vestibular disease is only sometimes helpful.

Table 10–9 lists commonly useful drugs. Meclizine and cyclizine produce less sedation than the antihistamines and are, therefore, more often useful in ambulatory patients. Transdermal scopolamine is very helpful for motion sickness and may become the drug of choice in benign positional vertigo and labyrinthitis. When parenteral drug administration is desirable (for example, in the vomiting or hospitalized patient), other drugs may be more useful (Table 10–9).

Helpful adjunctive measures include minor tranquilizers and antiemetics (the latter are especially needed when the vertigo is severe).

TABLE 10–9. DRUGS USED TO TREAT VERTIGO[79-81]

	TRADE NAME	DOSE	SIDE EFFECTS	ROUTE	COST*/ AMOUNT
Specific Therapy					
Meclizine	Antivert; Bonine	25–50 mg bid	Few	Oral	$4/30
Cyclizine	Marezine	50 mg qid	Few	Oral, rectal, IM	$4/40
Promethazine	Phenergan	25 mg qid	Sedation	Oral, rectal, IM, IV	$9/40 pills
Dimenhydrinate	Dramamine	50 mg qid	Sedation	Oral, rectal, IM, IV	$4/40
Diphenhydramine	Benadryl	50 mg qid	Sedation	Oral, IM, IV	$4/40
Scopolamine (transdermal)	Transderm-V	One adhesive patch every 2–3 days	Few	Dermal patch	$13/5 patches
Adjunctive Therapy					
Tranquilizers					
Diazepam	Valium	2–10 mg qid	Sedation	Oral, IM, IV	$9/30 (5 mg)
Antiemetics					
Prochlorperazine	Compazine	5–15 mg qid	Dystonia	Oral	$6/30 (10 mg)
		25 mg q6h		Rectal	
		10–25 mg q6h		Parenteral	
Trimethobenzamide	Tigan	250 mg qid		Oral	$8/30 (250 mg)
		100–200 mg qid		Rectal	
Perphenazine	Trilafon	2–4 mg q4–6h		IM, oral	$8/30 (2 mg)

*Costs are those of the generic preparations, which are less expensive.

In addition, since peripheral vertigo tends to improve with ocular fixation (while central vertigo worsens), instructing the patient to avoid the natural inclination to close the eyes is worthwhile. Since peripheral disorders also tend to fatigue (see Appendix II), intermittent voluntary induction of vertigo (by sudden head turning, for example) may thereafter relieve vertigo (temporarily). These instructions are termed adaptation maneuvers (Table 10–10); they are most useful for the patient with persistent (chronic) vestibular disorders.

III. Careful follow-up is indicated.

A presumptive diagnosis is often confirmed or refuted by the subsequent clinical events.

Derwood's daughter calls each of the next 3 days to complain that her father is not better. There are no new symptoms, and the medication controls his vomiting so that he is able to eat. Derwood is content to "wait it out."

Five days later, Derwood walks into clinic "feeling a lot better." The vertigo has subsided "most of the time, but I still get it when I turn over in bed or look the wrong way."

There is now no spontaneous nystagmus, past pointing, or unstable Romberg testing. Hearing is normal. Cranial nerves are normal.

Nylen-Bárány maneuvers (see Appendix II) elicit nystagmus with the left ear downward: The nystagmus is rotatory, fast-phased to the left, begins 5 seconds after assuming the head-down position, produces moderately intense vertigo, lasts 15 seconds, and cannot be reproduced when the maneuver is attempted again.

What does this mean?

1. Derwood now has positional vertigo and nystagmus that are clearly peripheral in origin—the Nylen-Bárány maneuver here reveals nystagmus that demonstrates latency, fatigue, and habituation (see Appendix II). Positional nystagmus[82] (and vertigo) is usually due to a peripheral vestibular disorder, but central lesions may also produce positional vertigo: Careful

TABLE 10–10. VESTIBULAR ADAPTATION EXERCISES

AIMS OF EXERCISE

1. To loosen the muscles of the neck and shoulders; to overcome the protective muscular spasm and tendency to move "in one piece."
2. To train movement of the eyes, independent of the head.
3. To practice balancing in everyday situations with special attention to developing the use of the eyes and muscle senses.
4. To practice head movements that cause dizziness and thus gradually overcome the disability.
5. To become accustomed to moving about naturally in daylight and in the dark.
6. To encourage restoration of self-confidence and easy spontaneous movement.

All exercises are started in exaggerated slow time and gradually progress to more rapid time. The rate of progression from the sitting exercises to standing exercises depends upon the dizziness in each individual case.

SITTING EXERCISES—WITHOUT ARM RESTS

1. Eye exercises—at first slowly then quickly.
   a. Up and down.
   b. Side to side.
   c. Repeat a and b, focusing on finger at arm's length.
2. Shrug shoulders and rotate 20 times.
3. Bend forward and pick up objects from the ground, 20 times.
4. Rotate head, shoulders, and trunk with eyes open, then closed, 20 times.
5. Rotate head and shoulders slowly, then fast, 20 times.

STANDING EXERCISES

1. Repeat 1.
2. Repeat 5.
3. Change from a sitting to standing position with eyes open, then closed.
4. Throw a ball from hand to hand above eye level.
5. Throw a ball from hand to hand under knees.
6. Change from sitting to standing and turn around in between.
7. Repeat 4.

WALKING

1. Walk across the room with eyes open, then closed, 10 times.
2. Walk up and down a slope with eyes open, then closed, 10 times.
3. Play any games involving stooping or stretching and aiming, such as bowling, shuffleboard.
4. Stand on one foot with eyes open, then closed.
5. Walk with one foot in front of the other with eyes open, then closed.

Courtesy of Glenn Johnson, M.D., Hitchcock Clinic, Hanover, N.H.

evaluation of the Nylen-Bárány maneuvers allows these distinctions. Any central characteristics of positional nystagmus (see Appendix II) warrant further investigation for neurologic lesions.

2. Treatment is similar to that described above, but drugs are less often needed here; reassurance and adaptation maneuvers often suffice.

Derwood is told to continue taking meclizine if he finds it helpful and is warned about the relation of rapid head movements to symptoms. Adaptation and ocular fixation are explained briefly again. He is told that he may have symptoms for weeks or a few months, but that he will gradually improve over time. Derwood seems relieved and reassured.

Sylvia, Derwood's daughter, is uncharacteristically silent until they prepare to depart when she asks, "Is this contagious?" She is told that it is probably not, but, when asked the purpose of her question, she says, "Well, I've been awful dizzy myself lately, and I wonder if I caught it." Sylvia is asked to return later that day to be examined more fully.

Sylvia is a 32-year-old single woman who works as a secretary and is finishing college at night. She lives alone with Derwood, who is a widower—she is his only child.

Sylvia says that, for the past few weeks, she has experienced increasingly frequent "dizzy spells."

"At first, they happened only once in a while, but now I feel a little dizzy all the time, and then it scares me when I get a real bad spell on top of it."

Sylvia is asked to describe exactly what she feels, without saying "dizzy."

"I'm spaced out, sort of light-headed, like I'm there, but I'm not all there. I'm sort of outside my own body. It's like what happens if I take Valium— I get a floating feeling, like I'm weightless or something. I get real weak and tired, and when a bad dizzy spell comes, I feel weird all over."

"When did you last feel this way?"

"Well, I feel it a little bit now, all the time. My last bad spell was last night. It woke me up."

"Describe exactly what you felt last night."

"I woke up scared. I was sweating, and my mouth was dry, and I felt terrible. I was very dizzy—I mean light-headed. It lasted about an hour—I got back to sleep by watching a late movie on TV."

"Is that a typical spell?"

"Yes, they're all more or less the same, but they're getting worse. They happen all the time now."

"Does anything else happen during a spell?"

"I don't think so. That's about it."

"How do you feel now?"

Sylvia sighs, deeply. "Tired. Dizzy. Am I going to have Parkinson's disease, too?"

NOTE

1. Again, the value of asking the patient to describe the symptoms without using the word "dizziness" cannot be overemphasized. Initially the patient should be given no clues at all—ask what happens, when it happens, what it "feels like." If symptoms are intermittent, ask the patient to describe the last spell in as much detail as possible. The patient's own, untutored description is by far the most important piece of clinical information.

2. While the precise diagnosis will require further history and examination, Sylvia's initial description identifies the symptom as light-headedness. Since all forms of dizziness may overlap in symptomatology and description, this initial impression should be confirmed. We must be certain that disequilibrium, syncope or presyncope, vertigo, or other symptoms are not being imprecisely described as light-headedness. This should be attempted only after the patient speaks freely.

"Sylvia, when you feel dizzy, do you feel like you're going to pass out?"

"Sort of, but not exactly. Maybe when it starts, but then it goes on and on, and I never faint."

"Does the room spin around or move?"

"No, not really. I spin a little, maybe."

"Do you have trouble with your walking or balance?"

"Well, I feel a little off when I walk when I'm dizzy. It feels more like maybe my legs are moving on their own, and I'm up there just watching them."

"You say this is similar to the feeling Valium gives you? Do you take Valium now?"

"No, I took it after my mother died, but it made me a little like this, so I stopped. I don't take any medicine or drugs."

"This light-headed feeling—do you relate it to anything? Can you guess when it will happen to you?"

"No, it happens any time. Day or night. Sometimes at work, sometimes at home. I can't figure it out."

Sylvia denies any significant past medical problems. Her dizziness is unrelated to physical exertion, the time of day, or meals. It can happen lying down as well as sitting or standing. There is no history of hearing loss, tinnitus, or cardiopulmonary symptoms, except that "my heart races and I feel a little breathless sometimes when I'm dizzy. I feel that way now, too."

Sylvia sighs again, deeply.

LIGHT-HEADEDNESS

Light-headedness is difficult to define in "nondizzy" terms. It usually refers to a dizzy sensation "in the head" that is not vertiginous, presyncopal, or due to disequilibrium. This vague "negative definition" emphasizes two paradoxical diagnostic points. On the one hand, the light-headed patient's description is usually imprecise, and even articulate patients are frustrated by the clinician's request to describe the problem without saying "dizzy." "Floating," "giddiness," "dreaming," or "unreality"—"flying," "stoned," "spaced-out," or "high" in more recent vernacular—are examples of such descriptions. In some patients then, very vague descriptions may actually be a helpful clue to the diagnosis. On the other hand, the differential diagnosis of light-headedness is rather brief (hyperventilation, with or without associated psychiatric disorders, is usually the cause—see below). For this reason alone, dizziness simulation testing should always be performed to exclude the possibility that the patient's symptoms are actually atypical descriptions of vertigo, presyncope, or disequilibrium, since, as we have seen, these types of dizziness require a very different approach.

Most difficult to distinguish from nonspecific light-headedness is presyncope. Symptoms are superficially similar, and dizziness simulation testing may not clearly distinguish one from another: Some patients cannot appreciate a difference between symptoms evoked by hyperventilation (see below) and those provoked by the potentiated Valsalva maneuver (page 461). Since the elderly are most subject to the serious cardiac and neurologic causes of presyncope (but are certainly not immune to anxiety, depression, and hyperventilation), it is often necessary to exclude serious disease (arrhythmias, transient ischemic attacks) in the elderly patient with episodic (presyncopal?) light-headedness. Similarly, certain vestibular symptoms, especially in the elderly, are not always obviously vertiginous; however, the history, combined with a careful neurologic examination and Nylen-Bárány maneuvers (see Appendix II), usually will distinguish vague vestibular symptoms from light-headedness. (Acoustic neuromas and cerebrovascular ischemic events are the most important vestibular causes of nonspecific light-headedness, but there are almost always other clues to these problems: deafness, tinnitus, brain stem symptoms, for example—see above.)

Usually, however, the symptom of light-headedness can be differentiated from other types of dizziness by simply listening to the patient and performing a careful examination.

Sylvia's general physical and neurologic examinations are normal. Dizziness simulation testing reveals:

Blood pressure is 110/70, supine and standing.

Gait, coordination, and ambulation appear normal.

Nylen-Bárány maneuvers elicit no symptoms or nystagmus.

Potentiated Valsalva maneuver causes light-headedness, but, "No, that's not the same."

Hyperventilation for 3 minutes is attempted: Within 30 seconds, Sylvia is flushed, eyes fluttering, chest heaving, and she says, "Oh, I'm so dizzy, I can't go on. That's it."

Hyperventilation is stopped. Sylvia is asked to describe exactly what she feels.

"It's what I get. I am real dizzy, and my mouth is dry, and I'm weak all over."

"Is that all?"

"My chest feels tight, and I have prickly feelings around my lips and in my left hand, too."

"Is that a familiar feeling, too?"

Sylvia begins to cry. "Yes, I forgot, that happens too. What's the matter with me? Am I crazy?"

Hyperventilation[83-85] is probably the single most common cause of dizziness in the general population (Fig. 10–1). Most physicians are well acquainted with acute hyperventilation, since it is usually dramatic and obvious: Hyperpnea, tachycardia, obvious anxiety and tremulousness, peripheral and circumoral paresthesias, sometimes progressing to frank tetany with carpopedal spasm are the hallmarks familiar to most clinicians. In such circumstances the only diagnostic uncertainty involves excluding uncommon but serious organic precipitants of acute hyperventilation (which are usually apparent): Sepsis, metabolic acidosis, hepatic encephalopathy, salicylate intoxication, and primary neurologic or cardiopulmonary events all may present initially as tachypnea with respiratory alkalosis and apparent anxiety. Other physical illnesses that cause pain, distress, or anxiety may also result in secondary hyperventilation, while various underlying metabolic disturbances (especially, hypokalemia and hypocalcemia) often potentiate the symptoms of hyperventilation.

This acute hyperventilation syndrome is just the "tip of the iceberg,"[84] however. Even more common is chronic hyperventilation,[85] whose clinical manifestations can be amazingly protean. Table 10–11 lists just some of the panoply of symptoms that may be caused by hyperventilation. Familiarity with such symptoms is important because dizziness due to chronic hyperven-

TABLE 10–11. SYMPTOMS OF HYPERVENTILATION

Cardiovascular: Palpitations, tachycardia, precordial pain, Raynaud's phenomenon	*Respiratory:* Shortness of breath, chest pain, sighing respirations, yawning	*Musculoskeletal:* Muscle spasms, tremors, twitching, tetany
Neurologic: Dizziness, paresthesias, unsteadiness, impaired memory and/or concentration, slurred speech	*Gastrointestinal:* Globus hystericus, dryness of mouth, dysphagia, bloating, belching/flatulence, abdominal pain	*Psychic:* Tension, anxiety, depression, apprehension
General: Fatigue, diffuse weakness, insomnia, nightmares		

tilation is usually accompanied by one or more of these symptoms—a valuable clue to the diagnosis of hyperventilation is the simultaneous occurrence of puzzling combinations of diverse symptoms in association with dizziness. The dizzy patient who describes associated dry mouth, tremors, a "lump in my throat," and bilateral foot paresthesias is a typical example.

Most nonspecific light-headedness is due to chronic hyperventilation and is psychogenic in origin—usually associated with anxiety (especially in the young) or depression (especially in the elderly). Light-headedness that is constant, "always there," or, conversely, "comes and goes in a split second" is almost always psychogenic, especially when physical examination is normal. Episodic light-headedness that is totally unpredictable and yet distinguishable from other types of dizziness will usually be reproduced by hyperventilation or be associated with other evidence of psychologic distress or frank psychiatric illness.

On the other hand, episodic light-headedness that is at all predictable must alert the clinician to other possibilities. Postural light-headedness is usually orthostatic (page 478) but may be vestibular or rarely vascular (carotid sinus syncope). Exertional light-headedness may be due to anemia, cardiac disease, or cerebrovascular ischemia. Symptoms that reliably occur at certain times of the day or night may suggest various types of hypoglycemia; this disorder, however, is overdiagnosed in "epidemic" proportions.[86]

Thus, failure to listen carefully to the patient causes most diagnostic errors, but the diagnosis of hyperventilation may be a problem for several other reasons:

1. As can be seen from Table 10–11, hyperventilation may mimic many organic diseases. Usually the concurrence of symptoms in various organ systems, the paucity of physical findings, and the reproduction of complaints by voluntary hyperventilation make the diagnosis. Two more difficult situations are common: the patient who presents with only cardiopulmonary symptoms, and the patient who presents with only neurologic symptoms. Usually, careful questioning, examination, and voluntary hyperventilation will be diagnostic here as well, but because hyperventilation may also cause objective disturbances in arterial blood gases (hypocapnia but never hypoxemia), the ECG (usually nonspecific ST-T wave changes), or the EEG (nonspecific slowing), the situation can become confusing.

Thus, prudence is always more important than making an immediately correct diagnosis: The patient with chest pain, tachycardia, shortness of breath, and an abnormal ECG usually requires observation, often in the hospital (to exclude myocardial infarction, for example), even when hyperventilation alone is the likely diagnosis. Similarly the patient with obvious hyperventilation who describes actual loss of consciousness, seizures, or unilateral neurologic symptoms deserves very careful attention. Actual syncope is unusual in hyperventilation (but it does occur—Figure 10–5): Other diagnoses must be considered. So-called seizures in hyperventilation are usually simple tremulousness, muscle spasms, or actual tetany (without loss of consciousness): When definite syncope with seizures occurs, one must remember that hyperventilation and seizure disorders may coexist, and in fact, hyperventilation may trigger otherwise latent seizure foci. Finally, it is not rare for hyperventilation to induce apparently focal neurologic symptoms (*unilateral* paresthesias are common),[87] but such symptoms must always suggest more serious diagnoses as well.

2. Hasty overdiagnosis is too common. Most normal people will develop

light-headedness or other physical symptoms (Table 10–11) when they voluntarily hyperventilate for 3 minutes. This is one reason hyperventilation is an important part of dizziness simulation testing: It mimics light-headedness and, it is hoped, aids in the differentiation of various types of dizziness. For this very reason, however, attributing a patient's symptoms to hyperventilation simply because voluntary hyperventilation causes light-headedness in that patient is dangerously simplistic. When hyperventilation does not clearly reproduce all of the patient's symptoms, the diagnosis is in doubt. For these reasons it is essential that:

3. The voluntary hyperventilation maneuver must be performed and interpreted according to very specific guidelines. The patient should be supine and comfortable. Without any explanatory cues or expressed expectations, the patient is instructed to breathe deeply and rapidly through the mouth for 3 minutes. It is often necessary to demonstrate the desired depth and rate of hyperventilation (full deep breaths, approximately 30 per minute). During the maneuver, it is sometimes helpful to feign examination of specific bodily areas—lungs, heart, pulses—to distract the patient from our true purpose: to observe the pattern and coordination of thoracic excursions, and to be alert for signs of psychic or physical distress. Most patients with chronic hyperventilation develop symptoms and distress rapidly (within 1 minute) and appear to breathe abnormally—such panicky, awkward intercostal breathing is easily distinguished from normal smooth, diaphragmatic breathing.

Following hyperventilation, the patient should simply be asked what he or she felt. No suggestions should be offered. When the patient volunteers that all the symptoms have been exactly reproduced by voluntary hyperventilation, the diagnosis is usually confirmed. Very often the symptomatic patient will hesitate or answer slowly—the fact that the examiner has reproduced the spells is very confusing or embarrassing to some patients. Allow the patient the time to describe all the symptoms. Finally, the reluctant patient should be asked, "Do these feelings remind you of what happens to you when you are dizzy?"

The emphasis in the evaluation of voluntary hyperventilation must be on allowing the patient to make the connection between spontaneous symptoms and induced symptoms, without prompting or cues from the examiner.

4. Hyperventilation is only rarely a diagnosis unto itself. While organic physical illness may present as hyperventilation (see above), the underlying problem is almost always anxiety or depression. Occasionally a patient will appear to have primary hyperventilation in which recurrent or chronic hyperventilation is alleviated simply by breathing training (see below). This is rare, however, and too often patients are done a disservice by the physician who says "It's all nerves," or "It's all in your head," and, therefore, "Go home, don't worry about it." This is often as good as not making the diagnosis at all. The underlying problem must be uncovered.

In Sylvia's case, the diagnosis of hyperventilation syndrome is clear.

Sylvia is told that her dizziness and other symptoms are caused by hyperventilation. She is told that hyperventilation is a very common problem among healthy people and that she herself is generally healthy. It is explained that hyperventilation lowers the carbon dioxide level in the blood because the lungs "breathe it all out during the heavy breathing," and this chemical change affects the brain and the nerves and the heart in such a way that various symptoms result. Sylvia is told that many people won't believe this because they are often not aware that they are overbreathing when their symptoms occur (and that sometimes it's hard to tell even

if someone else were to watch them). Sylvia is told that her sighing is a sign of this, and she admits that she often has the feeling that she "can't get a good breath, and I need to take one good deep one to satisfy myself." This, she is told, is a manifestation of chronic hyperventilation.

Sylvia is told that a few blood tests are in order, but that these will probably be normal because the cause of hyperventilation is usually some type of emotional stress. Sylvia says that this is impossible because her symptoms do not occur when she is worried or upset about anything, and "it even happened in the middle of the night." It is explained that this is usually the case: Hyperventilation symptoms often occur at unpredictable times, but almost always there is some ongoing worry, pressure, or ambivalence at the root of the problem, and unless that is recognized, she will not get better. Sylvia is impressed by the reproduction of her symptoms with hyperventilation, but appears genuinely reluctant to accept this explanation.

NOTE

The successful treatment of hyperventilation depends on three general principles:

1. The patient must be convinced of the diagnosis. This often takes time and may not be accomplished in a single visit. That hyperventilation is the cause of symptoms is usually "brought home" to the patient by reproduction of symptoms during voluntary hyperventilation and by demonstrating that the patient can control or abort symptoms by interrupting the pathophysiologic mechanism. Rebreathing into a paper bag to prevent hypocapnia is a common approach here, but this device is not acceptable to many patients: It is inconvenient, looks and feels "silly," and allows the patient to think that the problem cannot be controlled "naturally." More satisfying to many is instruction about how to breathe in such a way that they can control their own problem without external devices.

The patient is instructed to practice (twice a day for 2 weeks), 5 minutes of voluntary, controlled slow, regular breathing. Sitting quietly before a clock with a second hand, the patient is told to breathe no more than five times every 60 seconds for 5 consecutive minutes, slowly in and slowly out, without holding the breath or breathing too deeply. The patient is told that this is not easy and takes practice, but that in 2 weeks most people master it without difficulty. Thereafter, whenever hyperventilation symptoms begin, the patient is told to sit down and begin the slow, regular breathing that he or she has practiced—the symptoms will subside.

Many patients do not bother to follow through with this exercise since simple explanation and reassurance are treatment enough for many. Those who do practice breathing exercises, though, often achieve two goals: (1) the hyperventilation symptoms are voluntarily controlled when they occur; and (2) such slow, regular breathing is a relaxing maneuver in itself.[88] (Sometimes, formal behavioral modification therapy or biofeedback training may be helpful as well.)

Such exercises control the symptoms of hyperventilation, not the cause. Thus:

2. Serious underlying psychiatric disorders must be recognized. Anxiety neuroses of various types requiring various treatments are the underlying problem in many (especially young, healthy) patients.[89] A review of the monograph by Wheeler et al. on neurocirculatory asthenia[90]—one end of the anxiety/chronic hyperventilation spectrum—is instructive and emphasizes the

chronic, frustrating, but physically benign course of such patients over time. Rosenbaum's review of the drug treatment of anxiety is also helpful.[91]

Depression should be especially considered when hyperventilation symptoms develop for the first time in the middle-aged or elderly. Weight loss, anorexia, insomnia, loss of libido, and constipation are among the biologic signs of depression that may intermingle with those of hyperventilation. Suicidal ideation or intent must always be questioned. Pharmacologic therapy or psychiatric evaluation is indicated here.

Hypochondriasis is not an uncommon associate of hyperventilation, and Adler describes well the underpinnings of the very difficult patient/physician therapeutic interaction needed here.[92]

Hysteria and malingering are sometimes difficult to differentiate from each other, but such patients usually do not complain of dizziness alone. They more often manifest dramatic, visible, or objective signs (hysterical paralysis, for example) or present with intractable pain problems. Hysterical syncope or feigned seizures can usually be recognized easily if witnessed (see page 476).

Psychosis may result in dizziness of all types—disequilibrium, vertigo, syncope, light-headedness. Schizophrenia usually begins in the young; light-headedness here is often characterized by bizarre symptom complexes suggesting depersonalization or delusions ("I'm dizzy because my father is controlling my mind, and so I can't control my legs!").

Many patients with chronic hyperventilation, however, have no definable psychiatric disorder. In such cases,

3. Underlying emotional issues must be exposed, if they cannot always be resolved. Many patients develop the symptoms of hyperventilation in response to life stresses that are unavoidable and unalterable. Commiseration, encouragement, and an open door for return visits help most.

Many patients, however, are unaware of the very real impact of covert stress or are simply in need of common-sense advice about how better to cope with obvious personal dilemmas (see also Chapter 4, Headache).

All patients with chronic hyperventilation should be told that symptoms often do not correlate temporally with some obvious stress or anxiety-producing confrontation. The critical importance of subliminal stress—which the patient often has accepted as an unavoidable fact of life—must be emphasized to these patients. Interpersonal or marital conflicts, ambivalence about career or sexuality, and other ongoing psychodynamic issues that are deeply important but seemingly insoluble to the patient are the common denominators here. These areas must be probed. Unless this is done, patients' skepticism about the diagnosis will be the rule, not the exception.

> **Sylvia admits that she is worried about her father, especially since he has been ill and "I am all he has to lean on." She denies any biologic symptoms of depression, suicidal intent, hallucinations, or evidence of psychotic illness. She agrees that her working, going to school, and caring for her father is a "full-time deal" but says she has been doing this for years and is not sure why this would cause problems now. It is emphasized again that hyperventilation usually happens when a person is forced to deal with a situation that is stressful but unavoidable: a job one hates, a lover who is not free, a burdensome family obligation. Sylvia is asked to think about these things and to practice controlled slow breathing.**

> **Blood count and chemistry are determined and are normal. Sylvia is reassured that her father's parkinsonism will probably not progress very rapidly or affect her and that otherwise his (and her) general health is good.**

> **Sylvia and Derwood are both asked to return in 2 weeks.**

REMEMBER

1. <u>Reasonable goals must be established.</u> Patients who hyperventilate because of emotional conflicts that are likely to persist must be told that the symptoms probably will happen again. Often, recognition of the basic problem and symptomatic control are most important. Permanent cure is rare: Insight and coping mechanisms are the goal in most cases.

2. <u>Ongoing care and follow-up are essential.</u> The chronic hyperventilator is only sometimes reassured and permanently helped by a brief explanation and reassurance. More often, the underlying anxiety neurosis persists or emotional stress reaccumulates. Occasionally a previously inapparent depression (or, rarely, psychosis) becomes more obvious over time.

Continuing care by one physician is crucial for such patients: Hyperventilation symptoms so often mimic organic symptoms (Table 10–11) that repeated hospitalizations to rule out serious illnesses are common among these patients whose physicians do not understand them. When consultations are requested (usually by the patient) for second opinions, the primary physician should document for the consultant the objective evidence for hyperventilation. If this is not done, consultants will often initiate extensive investigations that can fuel the patient's anxiety and subvert the primary physician's therapeutic approach (which most often will be behavioral and nontechnologic). Not a few consultants will miss the diagnosis of hyperventilation, and the patient who is provided with conflicting diagnoses is much more difficult to manage.

> **Sylvia returns 2 weeks later, feeling well but "a little ashamed of myself." Symptoms have recurred several times, but Sylvia has been able to control them easily with her breathing exercises. Sylvia is much relieved that Derwood is now doing so well, and he is now independent again and less in need of her constant attention. Sylvia has decided to postpone school for one semester "to get my head together."**

Syncope: Is the Cause a Cardiac Arrhythmia?

In general, intermittent cardiac arrhythmias should be suspected as possible causes of syncope in several settings:

I. When the patient is elderly or has known cardiac disease or a history of prior arrhythmias or uses cardioactive drugs.

II. When syncope is worrisome (Fig. 10–6)—i.e., it occurs abruptly (without any warning at all), during or immediately after physical exertion, or in the supine position, or, if cyanosis or definite arrhythmias are documented by observers during the syncopal event.

III. When palpitations, "skipped beats," or other cardiac symptoms immediately precede loss of consciousness.

IV. When the resting ECG does not document an arrythmia but does suggest a predisposition to arrhythmias.

Documentation of preexcitation syndromes (short P-R interval, Wolff-Parkinson-White syndrome), frequent extrasystoles, or advanced conduction system disease is valuable information. The last deserves elaboration. Bifascicular conduction disease—either left bundle branch block (LBBB), right bundle branch block (RBBB) with left anterior hemiblock (LAH), or RBBB with left posterior hemiblock (LPH)—and trifascicular conduction disease (alternating LBBB/RBBB, or RBBB with alternating LAH/LPH) in and of themselves are not an indication for any specific therapy or intervention.[93–96] Syncope in such patients may be of many different types,[97] and most of these disorders are not treatable with cardiac pacemakers. However, syncope in such patients certainly warrants careful study and may require invasive electrophysiologic procedures to document whether pacemaker therapy or antiarrhythmic drugs are indicated (see below).

When a cardiac arrhythmia is suspected, the first diagnostic step after the history, physical examination, and resting ECG should be continuous ECG monitoring.[98–100] Continuous 24-hour (or longer) monitoring will then result in one of several outcomes (Figs. 10–12 and 10–13):

A. As Figure 10–12 demonstrates, when typical symptoms occur during the period of ECG monitoring, the monitor may reveal either a normal or an abnormal rhythm. In the former situation it can usually be assumed that symptoms are not the result of cardiac arrhythmias (A3, Fig. 10–12). In the latter situation (A1, Fig. 10–12), the type of arrhythmia will dictate specific therapy.

Occasionally, ischemic changes may be documented at the time of typical symptoms (A2, Fig. 10–12)—classic angina or coronary artery spasm may thus be suggested.

B. Conversely, as Figure 10–13 illustrates, typical symptoms often do not occur during ECG monitoring.

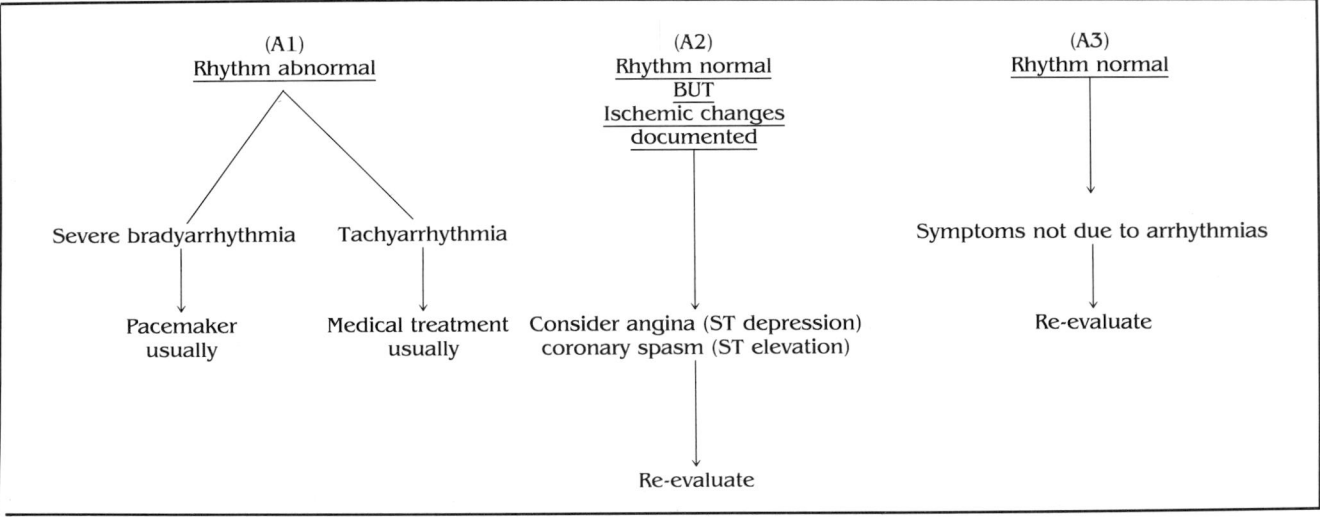

FIGURE 10–12. When "typical" syncope or dizziness occurs during ECG monitoring.

When this is the case, arrhythmias are usually not documented (B1, Fig. 10–13), and subsequent investigation must then be individualized.

Occasionally a serious arrhythmia will be documented even in the absence of typical symptoms (B2, Fig. 10–13)—the relationship of these arrhythmias to the patient's symptoms must then be in doubt, even when specific antiarrhythmic therapy is necessary (because of the seriousness of the arrhythmia). In these patients the response to antiarrhythmic therapy then determines whether syncopal symptoms are related or not.

When ECG monitoring does not reveal a specific cause of suspected cardiac arrhythmias, more sophisticated (and invasive electrophysiologic) studies may occasionally be very helpful.[101] Studies[94, 102, 103] document the value of such procedures, but only when patients are very carefully selected:

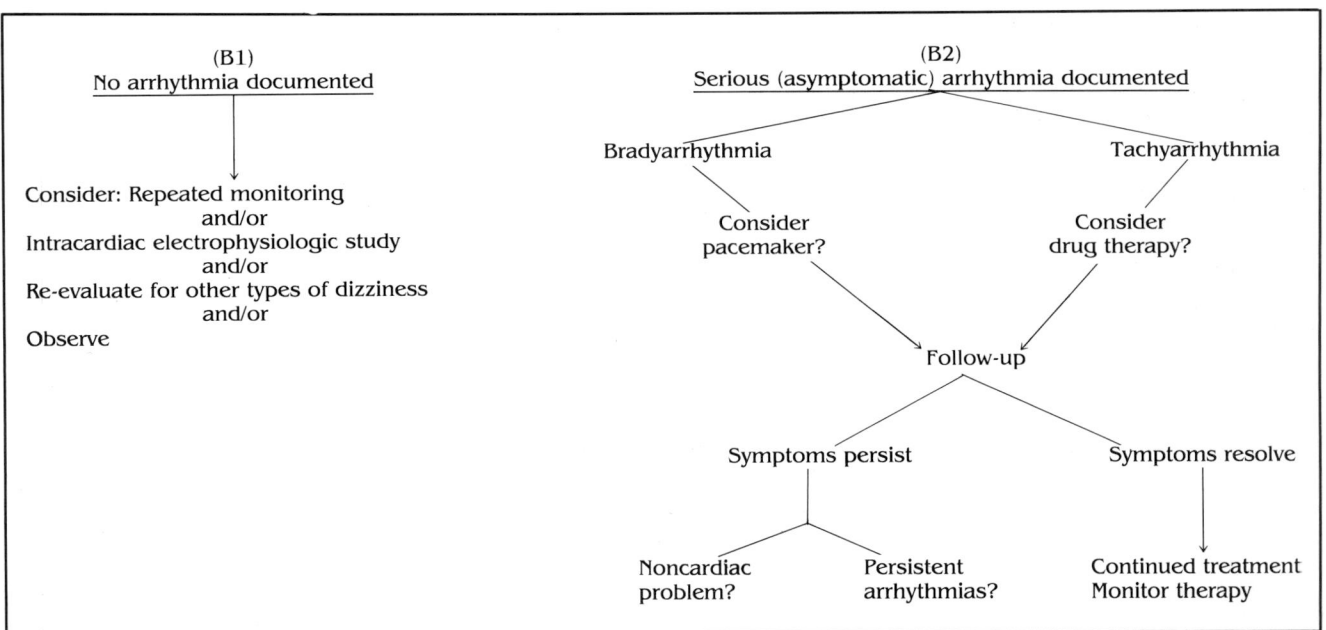

FIGURE 10–13. When "typical" syncope and dizziness do not occur during ECG monitoring.

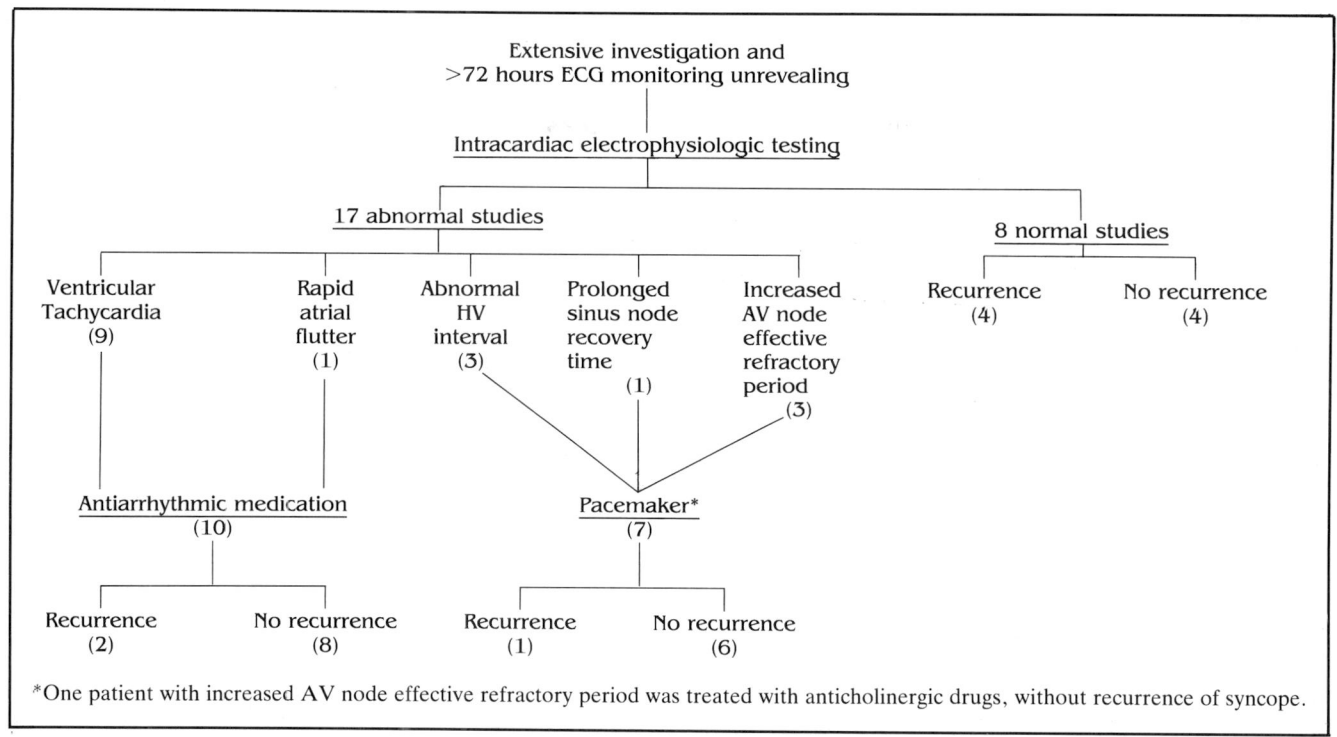

FIGURE 10–14. Twenty-five patients, recurrent syncope.[103]

1. Patients with recurrent worrisome syncope (Fig. 10–6) that remains unexplained despite extensive medical, neurologic, and noninvasive cardiac investigation.

2. Patients with severe structural cardiac disease (for example, cardiomyopathy, severe valvular disease, ventricular aneurysms) or known conduction system disease (for example, bifascicular disease or preexcitation syndromes on the resting ECG).

Such electrophysiologic studies usually include cardiac catheterization and intracardiac ECG monitoring with measurement of sinus node recovery time, atrioventricular node effective refractory period, atrio–His bundle–ventricular intervals, atrial and ventricular pacing, premature atrial and ventricular stimulation, and evaluation of various pharmacologic/pacemaker interventions for documented abnormalities. Obviously only cardiac specialists experienced in such studies should be consulted. These studies are quite safe under those circumstances.[104]

Very few patients with syncope need undergo such studies. In carefully selected high-risk patients, however, these studies can certainly be valuable. Figure 10–14 illustrates diagnoses in 25 such carefully selected patients in whom recurrent unexplained syncope was thus evaluated.[103] Abnormal studies were documented in 17 of 25 (68 per cent). Of these 17 patients, 14 suffered no further recurrence after initiation of appropriate antiarrhythmic or pacemaker treatment. Among the 8 patients with normal electrophysiologic studies, syncope recurred in half.

APPENDIX II

Evaluation of Vestibular Function

Nystagmus

Since nystagmus is such an important sign in the dizzy patient, some basic understanding of its pathophysiology is essential.

First, nystagmus that is visible to the naked eye* is abnormal, but only if extraocular motion is properly tested (Fig. 10–15). "Normal nystagmus" may be noted when the eyes are moved into extreme horizontal deviation (end-point nystagmus), or when the examiner's finger is moved too quickly or jerkily in directing the patient's gaze (a few nystagmoid beats will be seen); or when the examiner's finger is held too close to the patient (here, ocular conversion causes brief nystagmus). Proper testing for nystagmus requires that the examiner's fingers be held at least 12 inches from the patient and moved slowly and steadily through a 60-degree arc—30 degrees to one side and 30 degrees to the other—spontaneous pathologic nystagmus will usually be apparent on such testing.

Second, it must be remembered that nystagmus is not always due to (peripheral or central) vestibular dysfunction. Pendular nystagmus, for example, refers to a constant oscillation or wobbling of the eyes that is usually equal in amplitude and speed (no fast and slow phases) in both horizontal directions and that is asymptomatic—vertigo does not occur. This is most often congenital or related to a severe visual deficit. Extraocular muscle weakness (due to neuromuscular diseases) or cerebellar disorders will often

---

*More sophisticated testing such as electronystagmography may demonstrate nystagmus in normal subjects.

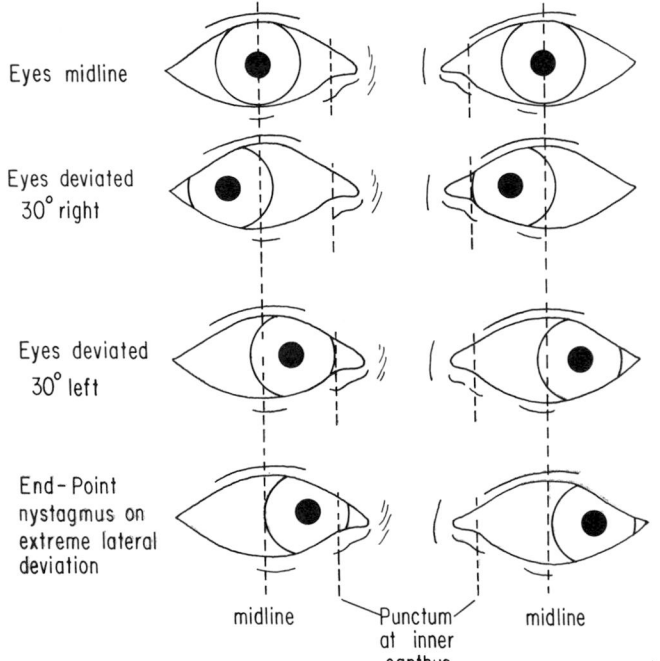

Eyes midline

Eyes deviated 30° right

Eyes deviated 30° left

End-Point nystagmus on extreme lateral deviation

midline   Punctum at inner canthus   midline

FIGURE 10–15. Testing for spontaneous nystagmus. The eyes are first examined in the midline. The eyes are then deviated 30 degrees to either side. The eyes should not deviate beyond the punctum of the inner canthus—beyond this point, spontaneous (normal) end-point nystagmus is commonly seen and may have no significance.

cause nystagmus too. Hence the importance of careful examination of cranial nerves and cerebellar function in the patient with nystagmus.

Third, sometimes nystagmus is expected. Sedatives, alcohol, and anticonvulsants often cause bilateral (and sometimes even vertical) nystagmus—most of these circumstances, however, are obvious and do not present diagnostic problems. Head injuries with concussion often cause transient nystagmus during recovery. Fracture of the petrous bone (with or without hemorrhage into the labyrinth) may cause persistent nystagmus as well as vertigo and hearing loss. (A specialist should be consulted whenever trauma affects the auditory/vestibular system.[64])

To understand better the testing of vestibular function, consider the normal function of the vestibular-ocular interaction:

Figure 10–16 simplistically illustrates the relationship of the vestibular system and the neurologic mechanisms for conjugate lateral gaze. Pathologic nystagmus results from weakness or imbalance somewhere within this system.

In general, when the eyes fixate on an object, they try to maintain this fixation despite disruptive input from the vestibular system. For example, when the head is turned to the left, the eyes tend to look right to maintain their prior fixation. How does this happen? When the head is turned to the left, the left labyrinth is stimulated and the right labyrinth is relatively suppressed (by rotational flow of endolymph in the semicircular canals). Stimulation of the hair cells in the ampulla excites the vestibular division of the (left) eighth cranial nerve, which then stimulates the ipsilateral vestibular nuclei in the medulla. The contralateral (right) sixth nerve nucleus is then activated (thus moving the right eye laterally—abducting it to the right) while simultaneously the ipsilateral (left) third nerve nucleus is stimulated via the medial longitudinal fasciculus (thus moving the left eye medially—adducting

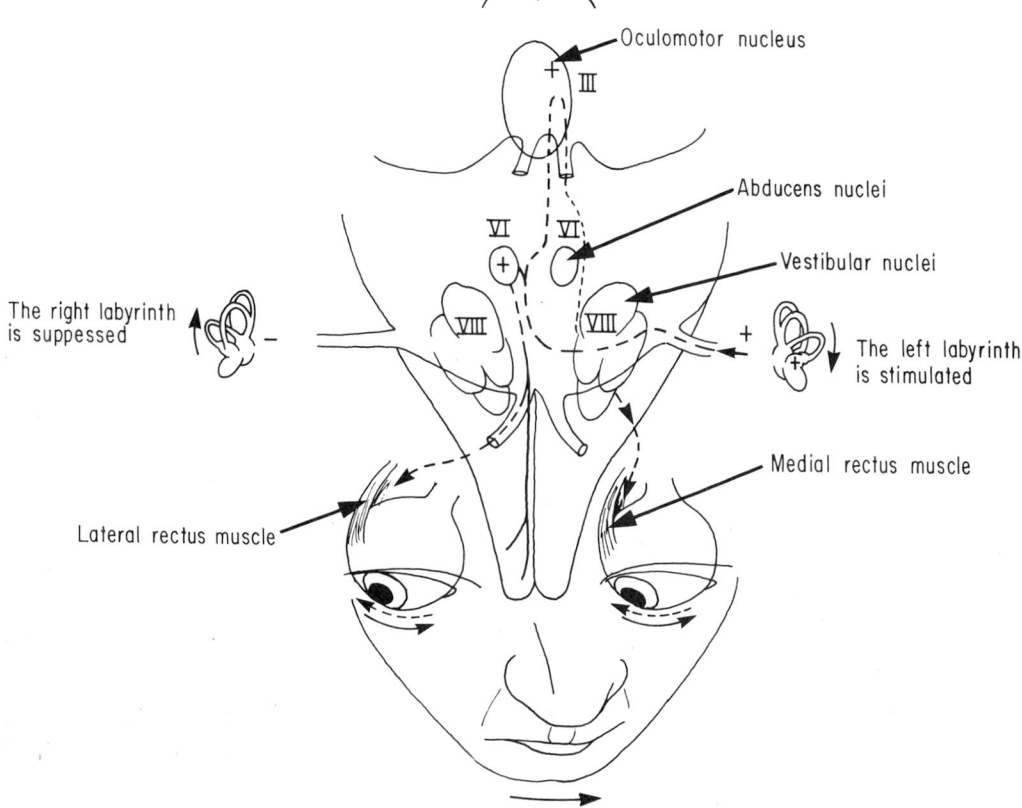

FIGURE 10–16. A simplistic diagram of the vestibular-oculomotor interaction. In this case, the patient turns his head to the left and attempts to maintain visual fixation on an object before him. Such a patient would demonstrate nystagmus—the fast component to the left, the slow component to the right—as the left labyrinth is stimulated and the right labyrinth is suppressed.

The right labyrinth is suppessed

The left labyrinth is stimulated

Oculomotor nucleus

Abducens nuclei

Vestibular nuclei

Medial rectus muscle

Lateral rectus muscle

The head turns left

it to the right). Under normal circumstances, then, turning the head left moves both eyes conjugately to the right to fixate gaze. If the head continues to rotate to the left (in a revolving chair, for example), inhibitory influences (from the cerebral cortex and the brain stem) then reverse the process, stimulating the left sixth nerve and right third nerve to move the eyes back to the left (simplistically, to "see where we're going"). The initial eye movement (toward the right in this case) is usually slow, while the return movement (to the left) is fast. This is an example of normal nystagmus during "eye pursuit," with its fast and slow components. Note that the fast component of nystagmus is directed toward the overactive left labyrinth, the slow component toward the (relatively) underactive right labyrinth.

Vestibular disorders usually render the diseased labyrinth hypoactive. In acute labyrinthitis (see page 497), then, the diseased side discharges subnormally, and thus the unaffected labyrinth appears overactive; the normal synchrony and balance of the labyrinths are upset. When, for example, the right labyrinth is diseased and hypoactive, the situation described above will occur spontaneously. The normal (but now overactive) left labyrinth will stimulate slow rightward deviation of both eyes (the slow component toward the diseased side), followed by a quick return to the left (the fast component away from the diseased side). Horizontal or rotatory nystagmus results: slow right, fast left.

Consider what the patient experiences in these circumstances: The eyes move right initially in response to illusory environmental movement to the left (because the left labyrinth is relatively hyperactive and senses—or actually creates—the perception of environmental movement to the left). This illusion of leftward environmental motion results in past pointing to the right and a tendency to fall to the right on Romberg testing (Table 10–7). (This may seem paradoxical, but try it. Sit on a revolving chair and spin rightward—clockwise—until vertigo occurs. Then look straight ahead at an object before you, close your eyes, and try to point your finger at that object. The object seems to move to the left, and your finger misses the object, off to the right. If you spin long enough, you will fall—to the right.)

These relationships apply only to peripheral vestibular diseases, and there are two important clinical exceptions:

1. When a labyrinth has been completely destroyed, nystagmus may not occur at all, since the absence of any input from that side often results in central compensatory mechanisms. This may occur in end-stage Meniere's disease, vascular infarction of the labyrinth, or severe drug toxicity, for example.

2. Benign positional vertigo, a very common entity (see page 497), is an exception in that the diseased labyrinth may be hyperactive. Phenomena just opposite to those described above may then be seen in such patients.

Conversely, central (usually brain stem) disease induces changes that are, in varied ways, inconsistent with the events expected in peripheral vestibular disease. For example, environmental spin may be directed toward the slow phase of nystagmus; past pointing or falling may veer toward the fast phase of nystagmus.

When nystagmus is spontaneous, the relationships and distinctions between central and peripheral nystagmus noted in Table 10–7 will be helpful. When spontaneous nystagmus is not present, the Nylen-Bárány maneuvers (see below) attempt to induce positional nystagmus—other clinical criteria then distinguish central positional nystagmus from peripheral positional nystagmus (Table 10–12). <u>Any characteristics of spontaneous or positional nystagmus that appear central must be noted: When any feature is not consistent with peripheral disease, central disease should be excluded with further testing.</u>

NYLEN-BÁRÁNY TEST[1] (Table 10–12)

The patient is first observed, seated, with the eyes straight ahead. Any spontaneous nystagmus at rest, on horizontal gaze (no more than 30 degrees from the midline), or on vertical gaze is noted and analyzed. Extraocular movements are tested.

The patient turns the head 30 to 45 degrees to one side and is then lowered backward to the supine position, such that the head is extended down over the end of the examining table to about a 30-degree subhorizontal angle (figure in Table 10–12).[53] The patient is now lying down, head turned to one side and inclined backward, one ear toward the floor, with the examiner supporting the patient's head and neck. This position is maintained for 30 seconds. The patient's eyes are observed while in the midline and while looking down toward the floor. Induction of nystagmus is often accompanied by the onset of vertigo and a frantic urge to get up (especially when peripheral vestibular disease is the problem). The patient is then brought back to the upright position, the eyes are observed for 30 to 60 seconds (nystagmus may then occur again), and the maneuver is repeated, turning the head now down to the opposite side.

TABLE 10–12. CHARACTERISTICS AND CAUSES OF POSITIONAL NYSTAGMUS

	PERIPHERAL	CENTRAL
Intensity of vertigo	Severe	Mild or absent
Latency of onset	Yes; but nystagmus usually begins within 2–10 sec	None; nystagmus begins immediately
Fatigue of nystagmus	Yes; nystagmus gradually abates	No; nystagmus persists
Habituation	Yes; cannot elicit nystagmus (or nystagmus lessens) after one or more maneuvers	No; nystagmus reproducible repetitively
Common causes	Labyrinthitis; otitis; benign positional vertigo (Table 10–8)	Multiple sclerosis; brain stem tumor; brain stem ischemia (Fig. 10–11)

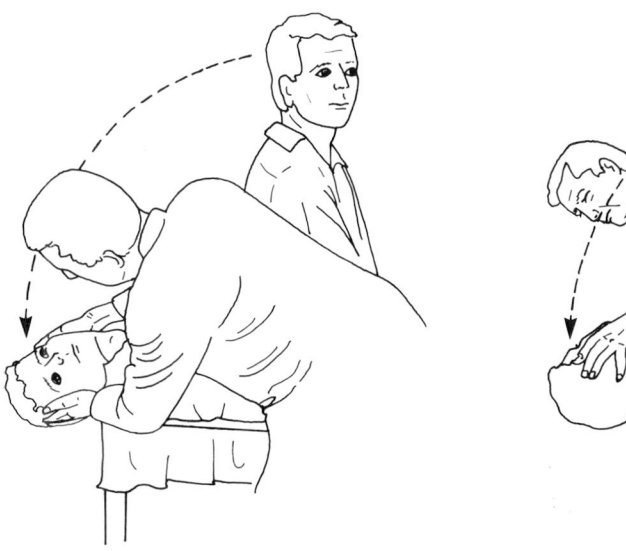

During the Nylen-Bárány maneuver, remember:

I. Positional nystagmus should be observed for:
A. Direction of slow/fast components.
B. The head position that elicits nystagmus.
C. The latency of onset of nystagmus (the time between assumption of the head position and the onset of nystagmus).
D. The persistence or fatigue of nystagmus.
Does nystagmus wane as the head position is maintained, or does it continue unabated?
E. The intensity of vertigo induced.
F. The presence or absence of habituation.
Does repeating the test in the vulnerable position cause a lesser or absent nystagmus response—habituation—or does nystagmus develop with equal intensity and duration on repetitive testing—absence of habituation?

As noted in Table 10–12, peripheral nystagmus is usually accompanied by severe vertigo, begins a few to several seconds after assumption of the head-down position (latency), gradually fatigues (lasts several to 20 seconds, and then resolves), and demonstrates habituation on repeated testing. Any central characteristics (Table 10–12) merit further consideration of CNS disorders (Fig. 10–11).

II. Nystagmus is not always easy to detect with the naked eye.
This is one reason electronystagmography has been a major advance (see below). Otherwise, during testing, observation of the optic disc with an ophthalmoscope is often helpful, especially when subtle rotatory nystagmus is present; or Frenzl's glasses can be used—these contain 20-diopter lenses with internal illumination that allow better visualization by the examiner and inhibit ocular fixation by the patient since he or she cannot focus through the lenses (ocular fixation will suppress peripheral vestibular nystagmus).

CALORIC TESTING

Caloric stimulation involves irrigating the tympanic membrane with cool or warm water to assess the vestibular/oculomotor response to such stimulation. This is a time-honored diagnostic technique that may be helpful in expert, experienced hands but that has many practical limitations. It requires a lot of time (up to an hour), may be uncomfortable for the patient, and is often difficult to interpret.

For the nonspecialist, caloric testing is rarely worthwhile, but it may be helpful in two ways:

1. When the patient's dizziness sounds vertiginous, but we cannot be sure (and positional testing is normal), caloric stimulation will induce nystagmus and vertigo in most normal patients. The patient can then compare this induced vertiginous sensation with his or her own symptoms. This is rarely necessary.

2. When labyrinthine dysfunction is suspected and confirmation is desired. (In many referral centers, electronystagmography has replaced this technique, but electronystagmography is not universally available.) The results of caloric testing must always be interpreted in light of other clinical information, since the diagnostic sensitivity and specificity of caloric testing vary with each specific disease entity. For example, caloric testing is almost always abnormal in cases of acoustic tumors but is often normal in labyrinthitis and in a few cases of Meniere's disease.

Proper caloric testing[105] (Fig. 10–17) requires that the patient lie supine, head elevated 30 degrees above the horizontal, and that the ears be examined otoscopically so that any debris (wax) can be removed, and to assure the integrity of the tympanic membranes. Ideally, the patient should wear Frenzl's glasses. A 20-cc syringe is filled with cool water (30°C) that is slowly (1 cc per second) instilled into the external canal toward the tympanic membrane. The expected response is movement of both eyes toward the cold water, followed by rapid phase nystagmus away from the irrigated ear. (Cold water renders the labyrinth hypoactive—as noted above, the slow phase of nystagmus moves toward the lesion or hypoactive side.) The direction and duration of nystagmus are recorded—usually nystagmus lasts from 30 seconds to 2 minutes. After a wait of 5 to 10 minutes, the opposite ear is irrigated with water of 30°C and similar observations are recorded.

Warm water (44 to 48°C) may then be used to test each ear sequentially (5 to 10 minutes apart)—some say a wait of 30 minutes is wise before switching temperatures. Since warm water renders the normal labyrinth hyperactive (and the nonirrigated ear relatively hypoactive), the slow nystagmus phase moves toward the opposite ear, and the fast phase moves back toward the warmly irrigated ear. The mnemonic COWS is used to indicate the direction of fast-phase nystagmus in a normal ear after Cold irrigation (fast-phase Opposite) or Warm irrigation (fast-phase to Same side).

The importance of testing with both cold and warm water is apparent when one considers the interpretation of caloric testing (Fig. 10–18). If only cold water is used and irrigation of the right ear, for example, elicits more

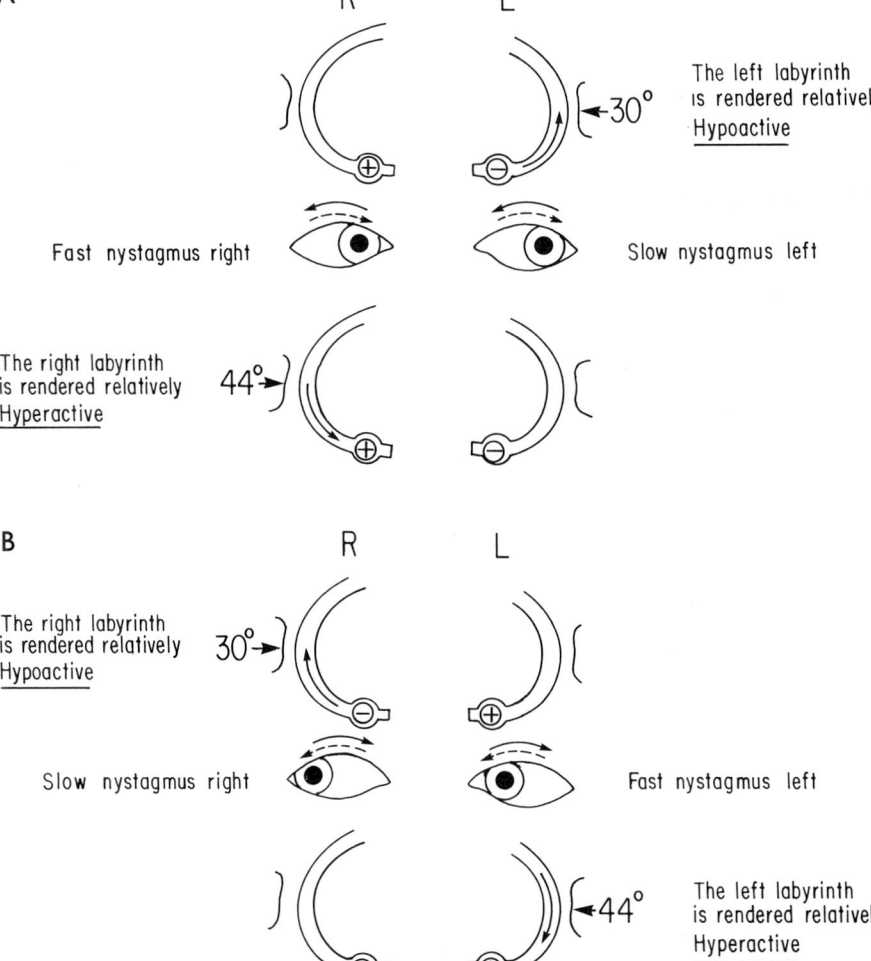

FIGURE 10–17. Normal caloric testing. A, Either of two caloric stimuli will normally induce fast nystagmus to the right and slow nystagmus to the left: when the left ear is irrigated with cold water or when the right ear is irrigated with warm water. B, Fast nystagmus to the left and slow nystagmus to the right normally will be induced by either of two stimuli: cold water irrigation of the right ear or warm water irrigation of the left ear.

prolonged nystagmus than irrigation of the left ear, one might suppose that the left labyrinth is defective. If, however, we then elicit more prolonged nystagmus after irrigating the left ear with warm water than after irrigating the right ear with warm water, our conclusions might be reversed. Such a response, called left directional preponderance (both stimuli that induce fast nystagmus to the left are predominant), implies that the peripheral vestibular apparatus and nerve endings are normal bilaterally, but that the brain stem gaze direction mechanisms are somehow unequal, one side predominating. This result may be seen in various disease entities, but normal persons may also show some degree of directional preponderance, too, and thus this is nonspecific. Figure 10–18C illustrates left directional preponderance.

On the other hand, if both cold and warm irrigation of the right ear elicit more prolonged nystagmus than both cold and warm irrigation of the left ear, defective left vestibular apparatus is implied. Such a result, called left canal paresis (Fig. 10–18B) (or right canal dominance) implies disease somewhere in the left peripheral vestibular apparatus. (Unilateral canal paresis does not precisely localize the lesion. Any disorder of the peripheral vestibular system—including the eighth nerve—may cause such a finding.)

Figures 10–17 and 10–18A illustrate the typical responses to cold and warm irrigation of each ear. The normal caloric response (Fig. 10–18A) is equal nystagmus to all four stimuli, lasting approximately 2 minutes. Graphic examples of left canal paresis and left directional preponderance are illustrated in the Figures 10–18B and 10–18C.

The difficulty of accurately performing and interpreting these tests makes caloric testing very impractical for the generalist physician, especially since other clinical information (see text proper) will usually provide the crucial clues to diagnosing peripheral or central vestibular disease. When in doubt:

Electronystagmography[58, 106] quantitates much more objectively the vestibular testing that is so subject to misinterpretation during simple caloric testing. During electronystagmography, eye movements are recorded graphically from electrodes placed around both eyes, as different maneuvers (caloric stimulation, visual tracking, positional testing, opticokinetic testing) attempt to stimulate the vestibular system. This technique requires sophisticated (and expensive) equipment but has proven very useful in documenting and localizing vestibular dysfunction. Central causes of vertigo/nystagmus are more easily diagnosed with this method. Psychogenic vertigo is more easily distinguished from elusive organic disorders (multiple sclerosis, for example) that may present as atypical vertigo: Complaints of vertigo during normal electronystagmography testing help document hysterical or psychogenic vertigo.

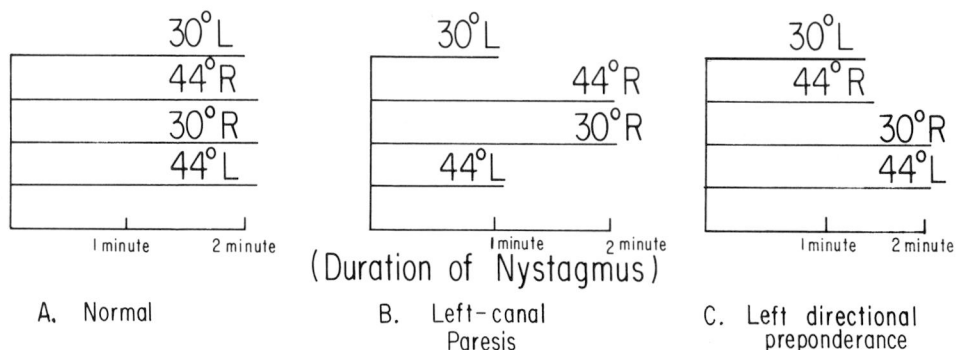

FIGURE 10–18. Results of caloric testing. A, Normally, both ears respond equally to warm and cold irrigation. B, Left canal paresis. This implies disease somewhere in the left peripheral vestibular apparatus. C, Left directional preponderance. This is a nonspecific finding.

Auditory Testing[107, 108]

Dizzy patients, especially those with vertigo, often require hearing tests. There are two basic reasons for this:

1. The simple presence or absence of hearing loss is often of initial diagnostic importance. For example, the patient whose dizziness appears to be primarily a disequilibrium problem but who also has unilateral hearing loss will require testing to exclude an acoustic neuroma. Similarly, vertigo associated with hearing loss suggests different diagnoses from vertigo with normal hearing (Table 10–8).

It is, then, important to be able to easily and confidently exclude hearing loss among dizzy patients. Simple bedside hearing tests usually suffice here (see below).

2. Once hearing loss is suspected or documented, the type of hearing loss (conductive versus sensorineural) and the anatomic site of impairment (middle ear, cochlea, retrocochlear organs) must be established. While the type of hearing loss (conductive versus sensorineural) can often be decided at the bedside, technologic testing is required to document the type and site of disease.

Conductive hearing loss points to disorders peripheral to the cochlea (i.e., in the external or middle ear)—for example, canal obstruction with wax, otitis media, or otosclerosis. Conversely, the patient with sensorineural hearing loss must have disease of either cochlea or structures central to the cochlea (eighth cranial nerve, brain stem)—the latter disorders are termed retrocochlear. Thus, while the vertiginous patient with cochlear hearing loss will often have Meniere's disease, the diagnosis of retrocochlear hearing loss must raise other (primarily neurologic) questions.

The general approach to the question of hearing loss as it relates to the patient with vertigo is described in Figures 10–19 and 10–20.

BEDSIDE HEARING TESTS (Figs. 10–19 and 10–20)

The watch tick test is very simple: A simple wristwatch is held near the patient's ear (the opposite ear covered by the patient's hand). The distance (in inches away from the ear) at which the patient can hear the sound of the watch is recorded and then compared with similar testing of the opposite ear. When the examiner has used the same watch with many patients and tested himself or herself, the normal watch tick distances will be established (for that watch). Unilateral hearing loss is easiest to detect; for example, the right ear hears the watch at 12 inches, the left at only 5 inches—further bedside tests will then help decide what is wrong with the left ear. Bedside audiometry (with a small portable console and headphone) is more sensitive than the watch tick test but is not always available and takes more time.

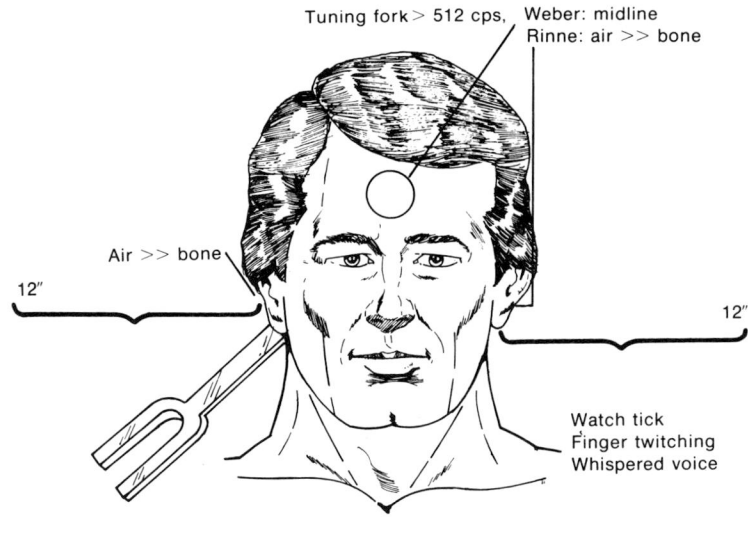

NORMAL

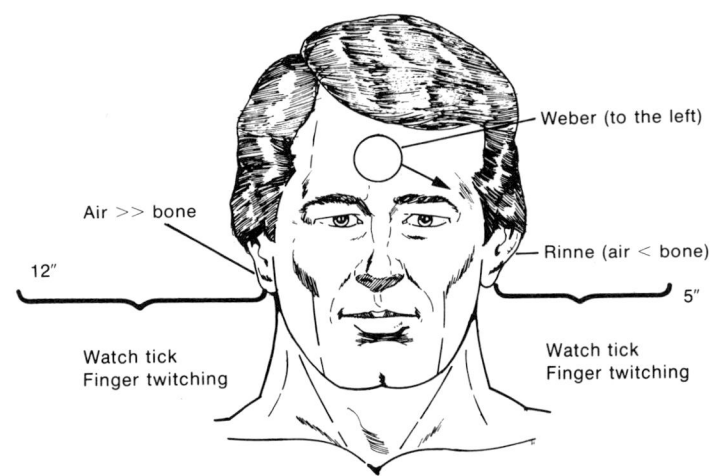

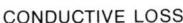

CONDUCTIVE LOSS

FIGURE 10–19. Bedside hearing tests. (Reproduced with permission from Branch, W. T., and Funkenstein, H. H.: Vertigo. *In* Branch, W. T. (ed.): Office Practice of Medicine. Philadelphia: W. B. Saunders Co., 1982, p. 341.)

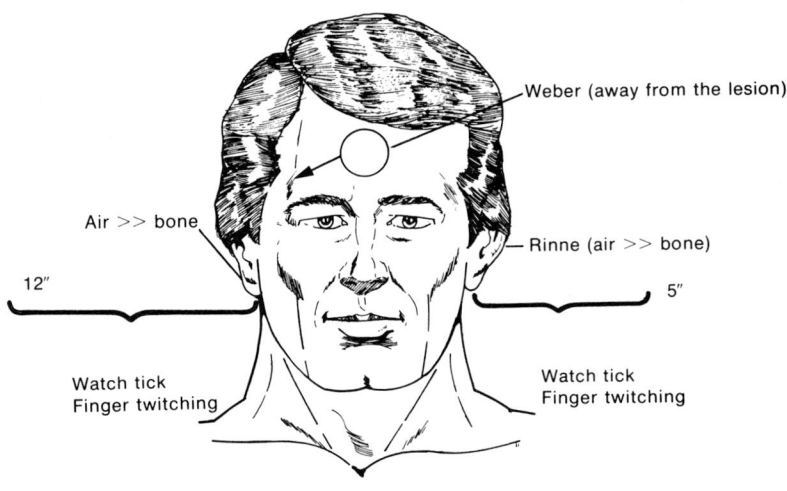

SENSORINEURAL LOSS

The Rinné test and Weber test are then used together to decide which type of hearing loss is the problem. The Rinné test distinguishes conductive from sensorineural hearing loss for each ear; the Weber test compares each ear to the other ear. Thus the two tests are used in tandem.

The Rinné test involves lightly striking a tuning fork of 256 or 512 Hz and placing its handle against the patient's mastoid process behind the ear (this tests bone conduction). When the sound becomes inaudible to the patient, the tuning fork is moved off the mastoid bone, and its prongs are held at the external ear (this tests air conduction). A normal ear will hear sound via air conduction louder and longer than via bone conduction (Fig. 10–19A). Since sensorineural hearing loss affects the end-organ (cochlea or retrocochlear structures), both air conduction and bone conduction will be impaired by sensorineural hearing loss, but sound via air conduction will remain louder and longer than that via bone conduction (in both ears). Thus the patient with unilateral sensorineural hearing loss will have a normal Rinné test, even in the impaired ear (Fig. 10–19C). In conductive (or non-neural) deafness, the reverse is true: sound heard by air conduction is not louder and longer than that by bone conduction, because external or middle ear disease primarily interferes with air conduction. The patient with conductive hearing loss will have an abnormal Rinné test: the tuning fork will be heard better (louder, longer) over the mastoid than next to the ear (Fig. 10–19B).

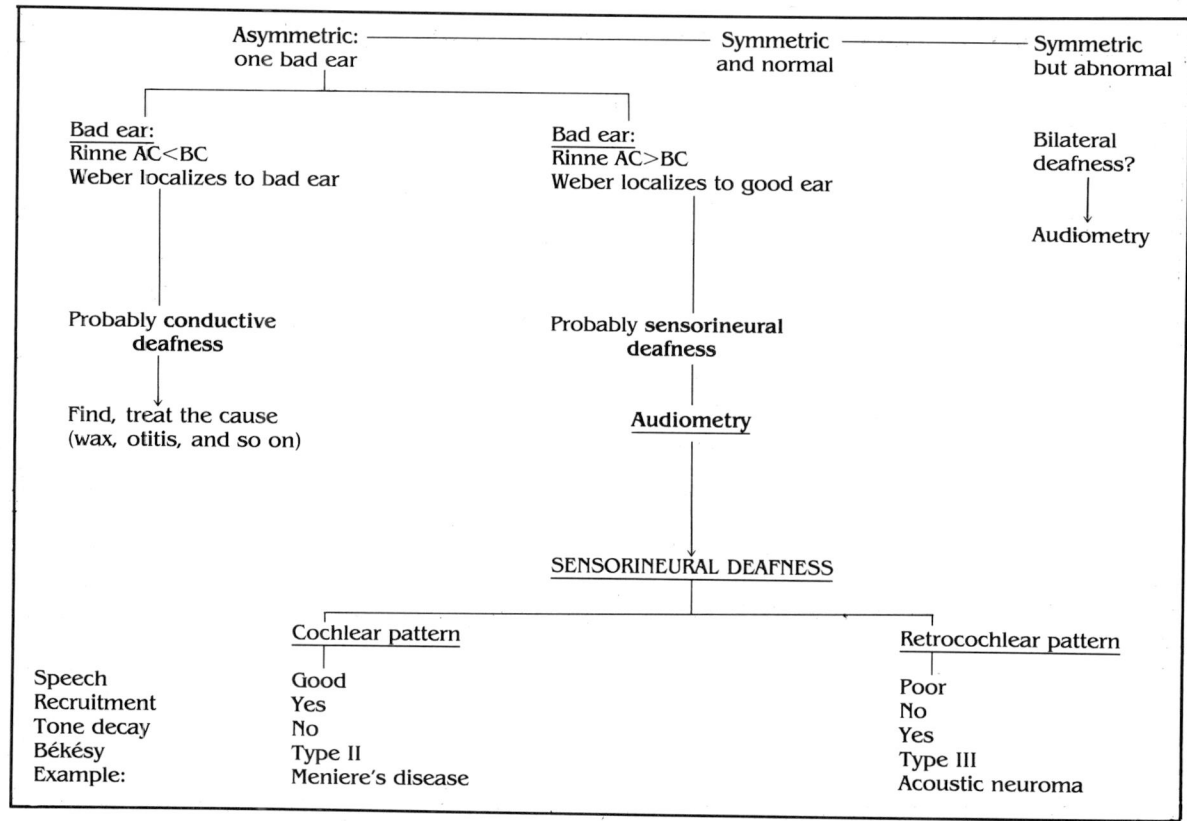

FIGURE 10–20. Watch tick test for hearing loss.

The Weber test compares ears. The tuning fork is struck and placed on the vertex of the skull or elsewhere in the midline: the forehead, the bridge of the nose, or the point of the chin. When hearing is equal on both sides (i.e., both are normal) the midline tuning fork sound is heard by the patient in the midline (Fig. 10–19A). When hearing is unequal, the sound lateralizes to one side. Since conductive deafness "improves" bone conduction (in relation to air conduction), the Weber test sound will lateralize to the deaf ear if conductive loss is the problem (Fig. 10–19B). The Weber test sound will lateralize to the normal ear if sensorineural loss is the problem (Fig. 10–19C), since in this case (both) bone (and air) conduction are diminished in the deaf ear.

Consider the patient whose watch tick test suggests impaired hearing on the left (5 inches/12 inches left, 12 inches/12 inches right). If Rinné testing of the good right ear reveals air conduction greater than bone conduction, but Rinné testing of the bad left ear reveals air conduction less than bone conduction, this implies conductive hearing loss on the left, and the Weber test should lateralize to the bad left ear (Fig. 10–19B). In such a situation, the external ear and tympanic membranes should be carefully examined, and causes of conductive hearing loss (otitis, otosclerosis, for example) evaluated.

When the Rinné and Weber tests suggest sensorineural loss (i.e., air conduction greater than bone conduction in both ears, sound in the Weber test lateralizing to the good right ear—Figure 10–19C), further testing would be needed to establish whether cochlear or retrocochlear disease is the problem in the left ear.

A word of caution: Sensorineural deafness in one ear may occasionally result in a Rinné test result that suggests conductive deafness, when the opposite (good) ear actually hears the tuning fork over the contralateral mastoid process. In this situation, the Rinné test would falsely suggest conductive loss (in the bad ear), but sound in the Weber test would lateralize to the good ear. Such results would be inconsistent and impossible to interpret. "This false impression of a conductive deafness can be avoided by asking in which ear the sound was heard and by applying a masking noise to the opposite ear."[52]

TECHNOLOGIC TESTING

Pure tone audiometry quantitates the patient's hearing threshold for tones at different frequencies and compares these results with normal standards. Because sensorineural deafness impairs bone conduction and air conduction, audiometry will reveal equal depression of bone conduction and air conduction in the deaf ear. Since conductive deafness impairs air conduction (through the external and middle ear) but does not affect the end-organ or central connections, air conduction will be abnormal and bone conduction normal: There will be an "air-bone gap" on audiometry.

There are many possible audiometry results: Bilateral loss, mixed conductive and sensorineural loss, unilateral conductive and contralateral sensorineural loss are all possible. Pure tone audiometry is needed to document the type and degree of hearing loss.

While certain disease entities may produce typical audiometry profiles (for example, low-frequency sensorineural loss is common in Meniere's disease), audiometry alone cannot make a specific diagnosis.

To differentiate cochlear from retrocochlear hearing loss (when audiometry documents sensorineural deafness), a battery of audiologic tests is often helpful. These tests include:

1. Speech discrimination. Various methods are standardized to assess the patient's ability to recognize spoken words. When speech recognition is markedly impaired (out of proportion to hearing loss), retrocochlear disease is usually the cause. Cochlear disease will impair speech discrimination much less (while conductive deafness will not affect it at all).

2. Recruitment. In cochlear disease, the deaf ear will be abnormally sensitive to small increments in the loudness of sounds above its perception threshold (recruitment). This is not the case with retrocochlear problems, in general. Recruitment can be measured with the short increment sensitivity index or the alternate binaural loudness balance test. A known sound increment on the good side is compared with the increase in loudness required by the patient to subjectively equal this loudness in the bad ear, i.e., the patient adjusts the loudness on the bad side until the sound on each side is perceived as equally augmented. When small increments in the bad ear are perceived as equal to larger increments on the good side, recruitment is present, and cochlear disease is more likely.

3. Tone decay. In a simplistic sense, tone decay is the opposite of recruitment. A continuous tone just above hearing threshold is offered to each ear. In retrocochlear disease the tone will decay into inaudibility over 5 to 10 seconds; in general, cochlear lesions do not cause decay, and the tone continues to be (barely) audible.

4. Von Békésy tests measure the patient's comparative ability to perceive continuous versus intermittent tones of varying loudness and frequency. A special continuous frequency audiometer records hearing thresholds for interrupted tones of fixed or varying frequencies and for uninterrupted tones of fixed or varying frequencies. There are four general types of von Békésy results. In general, patients with retrocochlear disorders have more difficulty with uninterrupted tones (similar to tone decay)—usually a so-called Type III pattern.

All of these specialized tests are both insensitive and nonspecific. There is so much overlap between responses to the various tests in cochlear and retrocochlear diseases that one must always interpret the results with extreme conservatism and in view of the other clinical findings. Typical cochlear and retrocochlear patterns on these various tests can be misleading. As with nystagmus (see text proper), any atypical findings must be investigated. The patient with unilateral sensorineural deafness who shows *any* retrocochlear responses must be further investigated (for example, CT scan for acoustic neuroma), depending on the clinical situation. In the patient with a classic history of Meniere's disease whose testing is consistently cochlear there is less of a diagnostic problem.

Auditory brain stem evoked response[59] is currently the most sophisticated auditory localization test. Recording electrodes are placed on the forehead and ears, and auditory stimuli are then presented to each ear. The evoked neural responses from the cochlea through the auditory nerve and thence up the brain stem are then recorded as a series of wave forms, each wave form originating at a different level of the central auditory connections. Analysis of these wave forms can then localize the site (but not the cause) of hearing impairment. This is especially helpful in infants and children, but uncooperative adults or suspected malingerers/hysterics may also be good candidates.

APPENDIX IV

Costs of Tests That May Be Useful in Evaluating Dizziness

TEST	TYPE OF DIZZINESS*	COST
Hemoglobin	D, S, L	$ 4
VDRL	D, V	$ 6
B$_{12}$ level	D	$ 21
T$_4$ and T$_3$ resin uptake	D, L, V	$ 33
BUN	D, L	$ 4
Electrolytes	D, L, S	$ 20
Cortisol	L, S	$ 36
Alcohol level	D, L, S, V	$ 30
Toxicology screen	D, L, S, V	Variable
5-hour Glucose tolerance test	D, L, S	$ 42
Arterial Po$_2$	D, S	$ 17
Electrocardiography	D, S, L	$ 45
Electroencephalography	S, V	$100
Cervical spine x-rays	D, V	$ 75
Tomography of internal auditory canal	D, V	$ 90
24-hour Holter ECG monitor	D, S, L	$130
Lung scan (ventilation/perfusion)	S	$300 ($180/120)
Echocardiography (2D and M-mode)	D, S, L	$230 ($170 + 60)
Carotid battery	D, S, L	$210
Exercise test, ECG	S	$175
Exercise test, thallium	S	$300
Audiometry, basic (screening)	D, V	$ 25
Audiometry, complete	D, V	$ 50
Electronystagmography	V	$120
Auditory brain stem responses	V	$200
Intracardiac electrophysiology	S	$700
Psychometric testing (Halstead-Reitan battery)	D, S, L, V	$240
CT scan of brain	D, V	$400
Hospital bed/ECG monitoring	D, S, L	$300 (per day)
ICU bed/ECG monitoring	D, S, L	$600 (per day)

*D, disequilibrium; S, syncope (presyncope); V, vertigo; L, light-headedness.

REFERENCES

1. Drachman, DA, Hart, CW: An approach to the dizzy patient. Neurology 22:323–334, 1972.
2. Weiss, S, Baker, JP: The carotid sinus reflex in health and disease: Its role in the causation of fainting and convulsions. Medicine 12:297, 1933.
3. Engel, GL: Fainting, 2nd ed. Springfield, Ill.: Charles C Thomas, 1962, pp 130–138.
4. Bahl, OP, et al.: Treatment of carotid syncope with demand pacemaker. Chest 59:262–265, 1971.
5. Kokman, E, et al.: Neurological manifestations of aging. J Gerontol 32:411–419, 1977.
6. Swanson, JW, et al.: Neurologic aspects of thyroid dysfunction. Mayo Clin Proc 56:504–512, 1981.
7. Adams, RD, Victor, M: Principles of Neurology, 2nd ed. New York: McGraw-Hill, 1981, pp 85, 302.
8. Adams, RD, Victor, M: Principles of Neurology, 2nd ed. New York: McGraw-Hill, 1981, pp 298–304.
9. Critchley, M: Neurologic changes in the aged. J Chronic Dis 3:459–477, 1956.
10. Adams, RD, Victor M: Principles of Neurology, 2nd ed. New York: McGraw-Hill, 1981, pp 807–812.
11. Richardson, JC, et al.: Supranuclear ophthalmoplegia, pseudobulbar palsy, nuchal dystonia and dementia. Trans Am Neurol Assoc 88:25, 1963.
12. Dreyfus, PM, et al.: Cerebellar ataxia: Anatomical, physiological and clinical implications. West J Med 128:499–511, 1978.
13. Lee, JE, et al.: Episodic unconsciousness. *In* Barondess, JA (ed.): Diagnostic Approaches to Presenting Syndromes. Baltimore: Williams and Wilkins, 1971, pp 133–166.
14. Wayne, HH: Syncope. Physiological considerations and an analysis of the clinical characteristics in 510 patients. Am J Med 30:418–438, 1961.
15. Day, SC, et al.: Evaluation and outcome of emergency room patients with transient loss of consciousness. Am J Med 73:1524, 1982.
16. Murdoch, BD: Loss of consciousness in healthy South African men. Incidence, causes and relationship to EEG abnormality. S Afr Med J 57:771–774, 1980.
17. Dermskian, G, Lamb, LE: Syncope in a population of healthy young adults. Incidence, mechanism and significance. JAMA 168:1200–1207, 1958.
18. Engel, GL: Fainting, 2nd ed. Springfield, Ill.: Charles C Thomas, 1962.
19. Engel, GL: Fainting, 2nd ed. Springfield, Ill.: Charles C Thomas, 1962, pp 7–27.
20. Compton, D, et al.: Weightlifter's blackout. Lancet 2:1234–1237, 1973.
21. Skolnick, JL, Dines, DE: Tussive syncope. Minn Med 2:1609–1613, 1969.
22. Haldane, JH: Micturition syncope: Two case reports and a review of the literature. Can Med Assoc J 101:712–713, 1969.
23. Kong Y, et al.: Glossopharyngeal neuralgia associated with bradycardia, syncope and seizures. Circulation 30:109–113, 1964.
24. Silverstein, MD, et al.: Patients with syncope admitted to medical intensive care units. JAMA 248:1185–1189, 1982.
25. Adams, RD, Victor, M: Principles of Neurology, 2nd ed. New York: McGraw-Hill, 1981, p 1022.
26. Wichser, J, et al.: Dysautonomia—its significance in neurologic disease. Calif Med 117:28–37 (Oct), 1972.
27. Young, RR, et al.: Pure pan-dysautonomia with recovery. Description and discussion of diagnostic criteria. Brain 98:613–636, 1975.
28. Ziegler, MG, et al.: The sympathetic nervous system defect in primary orthostatic hypotension. N Engl J Med 296:293–297, 1977.
29. Shy, GM, Drager, GA: A neurological syndrome associated with orthostatic hypotension. Arch Neurol 2:511–527, 1960.
30. Meyer, JS, et al.: Cerebral dysautoregulation in central neurogenic orthostatic hypotension (Shy-Drager syndrome). Neurology 23:262–273, 1973.
31. Diamond, MA, et al.: Idiopathic postural hypotension: Physiologic observations and report of a new mode of therapy. J Clin Invest 49:1341–1348, 1970.
32. Kochar, MS, Istskovitz, HD: Treatment of idiopathic orthostatic hypotension (Shy-Drager syndrome) with indomethacin. Lancet 1:1011–1014, 1978.
33. Manger, WM, Gifford, RW: Current concepts of pheochromocytoma. J. Cardiovasc Med, 3:289, 1978.
34. Santos, AD, et al.: Orthostatic hypotension: A commonly unrecognized cause of symptoms in mitral valve prolapse. Am J Med 71:746–750, 1981.
35. Schambelan, M, et al.: Isolated hypoaldosteronism in adults. A renin-deficiency syndrome. N Engl J Med 287:573–578, 1972.
36. Hickler, RB, et al.: Successful treatment of orthostatic hypotension with 9α-fluorohydrocortisone. N Engl J Med 261:788–791, 1959.
37. Seller RH: Idiopathic orthostatic hypotension: Report of successful treatment with a new form of therapy. Am J Cardiol 23:838–844, 1969.
38. Jennings, G, et al.: Treatment of orthostatic hypotension with dihydroergotamine. Br Med J 2:307, 1979.
39. Schirger, A, et al.: Midodrine. A new agent in the management of idiopathic orthostatic hypotension and Shy-Drager syndrome. Mayo Clin Proc 56:429–433, 1981.
40. Robertson, D, et al.: Clonidine raises blood pressure in severe idiopathic orthostatic hypotension. Am J Med 74:193–200, 1983.
41. Treiman, DM, Delgado-Escueta, AV: How to evaluate and treat episodic loss of consciousness. Drug Ther 5:112, 1980.
42. Adams, RD, Victor M: Principles of Neurology, 2nd ed. New York: McGraw-Hill, 1981, pp 211–230.

43. Burns, RA: Basilar-vertebral artery insufficiency as a cause of vertigo. Otolaryngol Clin North Am 6:287–300, 1973.
44. Adams, RD, Victor, M: Principles of Neurology, 2nd ed. New York: McGraw-Hill, 1981, pp 529–592.
45. Bickerstaff, ER: Impairment of consciousness in migraine. Lancet 2:1057–1059, 1961.
46. Patel A, Toole JF: Subclavian steal syndrome—reversal of cephalic blood flow. Medicine 44:289–303, 1965.
47. D'Amato, AN: Cardiac arrhythmia. *In* Cecil's Textbook of Medicine, 15th ed. Philadelphia: W.B. Saunders, pp 1238–1268.
48. Busis, SN: Diagnostic evaluation of the patient presenting with vertigo. Otolaryngol Clin North Am 6:3–23, 1978.
49. Holt, GR, Thomas, JR: Vertigo. Am Fam Physician 14:84–92, 1976.
50. Daroff, RB: Vertigo. Am Fam Physician 16:143–150, 1977.
51. Barber, HO: Current ideas on vestibular diagnosis. Otolaryngol Clin North Am 11:283–300, 1978.
52. Wolfson, RJ, et al.: Vertigo. CIBA Clin Symp 33(6):1–32, 1981.
53. Frederick, MW: Central vertigo. Otolaryngol Clin North Am 6:267–285, 1973.
54. Smith JD: Vertigo: Key to correct diagnosis. Consultant 141–147 (Oct), 1980.
55. Cappon, D: Psychiatric problems: Dizziness. Postgrad Med 48:317, 1970.
56. Tiwari, S, Bakris, GL: Psychogenic vertigo: A review. Postgrad Med 70:69–77, 1981.
57. Afzelius, LE, et al.: Vertigo and dizziness of functional origin. Laryngoscope 90:649–656, 1980.
58. Barber, HO, Stockwell, CW: Manual of Electronystagmography. St. Louis: CV Mosby, 1976.
59. Musiek, F, Porcelli, AV: Using new auditory/visual tests. Patient Care 69–77 (Jan 15), 1981.
60. Wolfson, RJ, Dave, V: Meniere's disease. *In* English, G (ed.): Otolaryngology. New York: Harper & Row, 1979, Chap 29, pp 1–31.
61. Pulec, JL: Meniere's disease: Etiology, natural history and results of treatment. Otolaryngol Clin North Am 6:189–228, 1973.
62. Cheson, BD, et al.: Cogan's syndrome: A systemic vasculitis. Am J Med 60:549–555, 1976.
63. Cogan, DG: Syndrome of nonsyphilitic interstitial keratitis and vestibuloauditory symptoms. Arch Ophthalmol 33:144, 1945.
64. Healy, GB: Hearing loss and vertigo secondary to head injury. N Engl J Med 306:1029–1031, 1982.
65. Eliachar, I, et al.: Basic audiometric findings in Meniere's disease. Otolaryngol Clin North Am 6:41–52, 1973.
66. Hitselberger, WE: Tumors of the cerebellopontine angle in relation to vertigo. Arch Otolaryngol 85:95, 1967.
67. Shiffman, F, et al.: The diagnosis and evaluation of acoustic neuromas. Otolaryngol Clin North Am 6:25–40, 1973.
68. Pulec, JL, et al.: A system of management of acoustic neuroma based on 364 cases. Trans Am Acad Ophthalmol Otolaryngol 75:48–55, 1971.
69. Wortzman, G, et al.: The role of CT scanning in the diagnosis of acoustic neuroma. J Otolaryngol (Suppl) 3:63–72, 1977.
70. Ojemann RG: Acoustic neuroma. *In* Contemporary Neurosurgery, lesson 20. Baltimore: Williams and Wilkins, 1979.
71. Ojemann, RG, et al.: Evaluation and surgical treatment of acoustic neuroma. N Engl J Med 287:895, 1972.
72. Fisher, CM: Vertigo in cerebrovascular disease. Arch Otolaryngol 85:529–534, 1967.
73. Clemis, JD, Becker, GW: Vestibular neuronitis. Otolaryngol Clin North Am 6:139–155, 1973.
74. Adour, KK, et al.: Vestibular vertigo. A form of polyneuritis? JAMA 246:1564–1567, 1981.
75. Aschan, G: The pathogenesis of positional nystagmus. Arch Otolaryngol 159(suppl):90, 1961.
76. Dix, MR, Hallpike, CS: The pathology, symptomatology and diagnosis of certain common disorders of the vestibular system. Proc R Soc Med 45:341–354, 1942.
77. Baloh, RW: Benign paroxysmal positional vertigo. West J Med 137:311–312, 1982.
78. Jongkees, LBW: Cervical vertigo. Laryngoscope 79:1473–1484, 1969.
79. Cone, AM: Evaluation and management of the dizzy patient. South Med J 68:584–590, 1975.
80. Wood, CD, Graybiel, A: The antimotion sickness drugs. Otolaryngol Clin North Am 6:301–313, 1973.
81. DiGregorio, GJ, Fruncillo, RJ: Antiemetics. Am Fam Physician 26:200–202, 1982.
82. Barber, HO: Positional vertigo and nystagmus. Otolaryngol Clin North Am 6:169–187, 1973.
83. Lewis, BI: Hyperventilation syndrome. Ann Intern Med 38:918–927, 1953.
84. Lum, LC: Hyperventilation: The tip and the iceberg. J Psychosom Res 19:375–383, 1975.
85. Waites, TF: Hyperventilation—chronic and acute. Arch Intern Med 138:1700–1701, 1978.
86. Yager, J, Young, RT: Non-hypoglycemia is an epidemic condition. N Engl J Med 291:907–908, 1974.
87. Tavel, ME: Hyperventilation syndrome with unilateral somatic symptoms. JAMA 187:301–303, 1964.
88. Benson, H: The Relaxation Response. New York: William Morrison, 1975.
89. Pincus, GH, Tucker, GJ: Behavioral Neurology, 2nd ed. New York: Oxford University Press, 1978, Chap 6.
90. Wheeler, EO, et al.: Neurocirculatory asthenia (anxiety neurosis, effort syndrome, neurasthenia). JAMA 142:878–889, 1950.
91. Rosenbaum, JF: The drug treatment of anxiety. N Engl J Med 306:401–404, 1982.
92. Adler, G: The physician and the hypochondriacal patient. N Engl J Med 304:1394–1396, 1981.
93. McAnulty, JH, et al.: A prospective study of sudden death in "high risk" bundle branch block. N Engl J Med 299:209–215, 1978.
94. Castor, JA: Cardiac electrophysiology: Hemiblocks and stopped hearts. N Engl J Med 299:249–250, 1978.

95. Dhingra, RC, et al.: Prospective observations in patients with chronic bundle branch block and marked H-V prolongation. Circulation 53:600–604, 1976.
96. McAnulty JH, et al.: Natural history of "high risk" bundle branch block. Final report of a prospective study. N Engl J Med 307:137–143, 1982.
97. Dhingra, RC, et al.: Syncope in patients with chronic bifascicular block. Significance, causative mechanisms and clinical implications. Ann Intern Med 81:302–306, 1974.
98. Lipski, J, et al.: Value of Holter monitoring in assessing cardiac arrhythmias in symptomatic patients. Am J Cardiol 37:102–107, 1976.
99. Samet, P, et al.: Syncope of circulatory origin: Clinical evaluation and therapeutic approach. Primary Cardiol 4:114, 1978.
100. Castle, L: Primary work-up of patients with suspected cardiac syncope. Mod Med 24–40 (Mar), 1980.
101. DiMarco, JP, Ruskin, JN: Recurrent unexplained syncope: Use of intracardiac electrophysiology. Primary Cardiol 8:21–32, 1982.
102. Greene, HL: Clinical applications of His bundle electrocardiography. JAMA 240:258–260, 1978.
103. DiMarco, JP, et al.: Intracardiac electrophysiologic techniques in recurrent syncope of unknown cause. Ann Intern Med 95:542–548, 1981.
104. DiMarco, JP, et al.: Complications in patients undergoing cardiac electrophysiologic procedures. Ann Intern Med 97:490–493, 1982.
105. Branch, WT, Funkenstein, H: Clinical evaluation of vertigo. Primary Care 4:267–282 (June), 1977.
106. Ruben, W: Electronystagmography and its value in the diagnosis of vertigo. Otolaryngol Clin North Am 6:95–117, 1973.
107. Page, JM: Audiologic tests in the differential diagnosis of vertigo. Otolaryngol Clin North Am 6:53–71, 1973.
108. Martin, FN: Introduction to Audiology. Englewood Cliffs, NJ: Prentice-Hall, 1975.
109. Wilcox, C.S.: Current therapy for orthostatic hypotension. J Cardiovasc Med 8:292, 1983.

11
ABDOMINAL PAIN

ACUTE ABDOMINAL PAIN 530
    History.. 530
    Physical Examination.......................... 539
    Tests.. 549
    Acute Right Lower Quadrant Pain 560
    Acute Right Upper Quadrant Pain 568

CHRONIC/RECURRENT ABDOMINAL PAIN......... 575
    Chronic/Recurrent Lower Abdominal Pain...... 577
      Presumptive Diagnosis and Treatment of
        Chronic Lower Abdominal Pain 583
    Chronic/Recurrent Upper Abdominal Pain...... 594

SEVERE CENTRAL ABDOMINAL PAIN 608
APPENDIX: AMBULATORY TREATMENT OF
    PEPTIC ULCER DISEASE 619
    REFERENCES....................................... 624

Abdominal pain is often considered the province of the general surgeon, and for good reason. The exploratory laparotomy always will remain the most instructive clinicopathologic exercise of all, and only the surgeon has this regular opportunity to sharpen his or her clinical skills by comparing preoperative diagnoses with palpable disease on the operating table. Similarly, it is always the surgeon who is the ultimate arbiter in differentiating surgical from nonsurgical abdominal pain: The experienced surgeon knows best when to wait, when to worry, and when to cut.

Nevertheless, it is often the nonsurgeon who first examines the patient complaining of abdominal pain, and in fact, most such patients do not require the operative skills of a surgeon. Figure 11–1 illustrates the final diagnoses among 1000 consecutive patients evaluated in an emergency room for abdominal pain.[1] Only about one fourth (274) of these patients required hospitalization—little more than half of whom (150) underwent laparotomy. The great majority of patients (726) could be treated or followed as outpatients—many of these had abdominal pain that remained unexplained (413) but was self-limited (and presumably benign); one third of the nonsurgical group (242) had pelvic or urinary disorders; the remainder had an assortment of medical gastrointestinal disorders.

Hence, the diagnostic approach to the patient with abdominal pain requires a broad clinical perspective. Disease in the thorax, pelvis, genitourinary organs, skeletal and neuromuscular systems may cause abdominal pain. The abdominal surgeon's expertise is needed less often in such circumstances.* Nevertheless, clinical questions confronting the nonsurgeon always include: Is this a "surgical abdomen"? Should the surgeon be consulted? In

---

*We will not consider the patient with traumatic abdominal pain. The approach of Botsford and Wilson[2] to such patients is an excellent introduction to that subject.

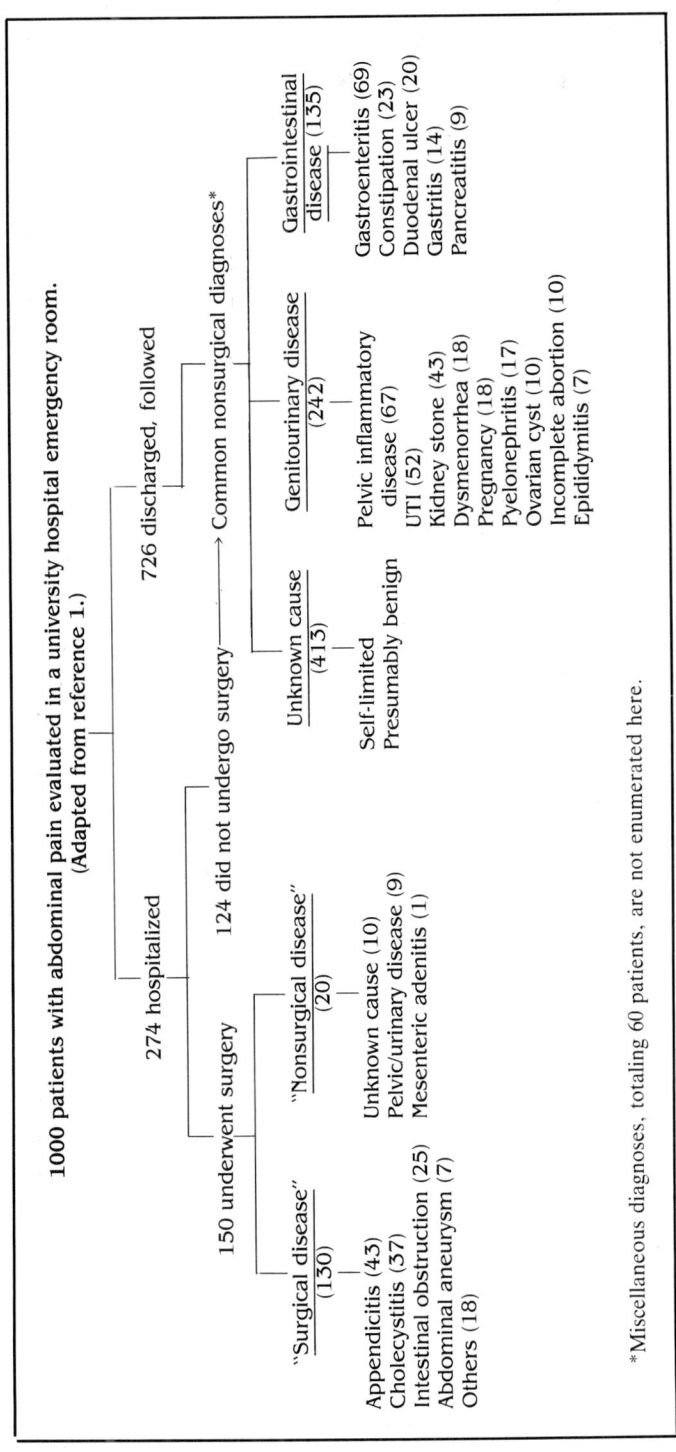

1000 patients with abdominal pain evaluated in a university hospital emergency room. (Adapted from reference 1.)

274 hospitalized

726 discharged, followed

150 underwent surgery

124 did not undergo surgery → Common nonsurgical diagnoses*

"Surgical disease" (130)
Appendicitis (43)
Cholecystitis (37)
Intestinal obstruction (25)
Abdominal aneurysm (7)
Others (18)

"Nonsurgical disease" (20)
Unknown cause (10)
Pelvic/urinary disease (9)
Mesenteric adenitis (1)

Unknown cause (413)
Self-limited
Presumably benign

Genitourinary disease (242)
Pelvic inflammatory disease (67)
UTI (52)
Kidney stone (43)
Dysmenorrhea (18)
Pregnancy (18)
Pyelonephritis (17)
Ovarian cyst (10)
Incomplete abortion (10)
Epididymitis (7)

Gastrointestinal disease (135)
Gastroenteritis (69)
Constipation (23)
Duodenal ulcer (20)
Gastritis (14)
Pancreatitis (9)

*Miscellaneous diagnoses, totaling 60 patients, are not enumerated here.

FIGURE 11-1.

fact, the generalist physician can often diagnose, treat, or confidently observe the patient with abdominal pain.

CONSIDER

> Sally S., a 25-year-old waitress, enters the clinic complaining of 24 hours' abdominal pain. The day before, Sally noted the onset of mild "middle" abdominal pain (she places her hand over the umbilicus) that has progressively worsened since then. She slept fitfully during the night because of the pain. Sally is slightly nauseated and anorectic today, but there has been no vomiting, diarrhea, constipation, or fever. Sally denies any urinary or vaginal symptoms and has just completed a normal menstrual period. There is no history of prior abdominal surgery or other significant medical illnesses.
>
> Sally does have a history of dysmenorrhea, "but that always starts before my period; this is different."

ACUTE ABDOMINAL PAIN

History

In general, the helpful historical clues in the initial approach to the patient with acute abdominal pain are the location of pain, the severity of pain, and the timing of pain. Associated symptoms, prior medical history, and the specific clinical setting are always important as well, but the location, severity, and timing are the keys to correct diagnosis. (Clinical features that alleviate or exacerbate symptoms are also important, of course, but more so in the patient with chronic/recurrent pain than in the patient with acute abdominal pain.)

I. Where is the pain?

The clinicopathologic importance of the location of abdominal pain is best understood by considering that the innervation of most intra-abdominal viscera is bilateral. Pain arising in abdominal viscera is transmitted to the spinal cord and brain via bilateral autonomic sensory nerves. Such pain is thus usually perceived in the midline.[3]

There are three general zones of midline abdominal pain: epigastric, periumbilical, and hypogastric.[4] Epigastric pain is mediated by the celiac sympathetic plexus and some parasympathetic fibers that also innervate the thoracic structures. Midline epigastric pain should thus suggest disorders of the thorax (heart, lungs, esophagus, and mediastinum), stomach, duodenum, pancreas, liver, and biliary system. Periumbilical pain, mediated by celiac and superior mesenteric ganglia, usually implies disease of the small intestine or the cecum (and appendix). Hypogastric pain, mediated by the inferior mesenteric ganglia and pelvic parasympathetic fibers, usually implicates the colon, rectum, or pelvis. Figure 11–2 illustrates these clinical correlations. Such midline abdominal pain, mediated by the autonomic nervous system, is visceral in quality, i.e., deep, dull, diffuse (within a zone) and not precisely localized (with one finger, for example) by the patient or by the examiner (see below).

When disease of intra-abdominal viscera causes irritation of contiguous parietal peritoneum, the resulting pain is not visceral, but parietal (or somatic or peritoneal). Such parietal pain is usually sharp and much more precisely localized, often directly over the anatomic location of the

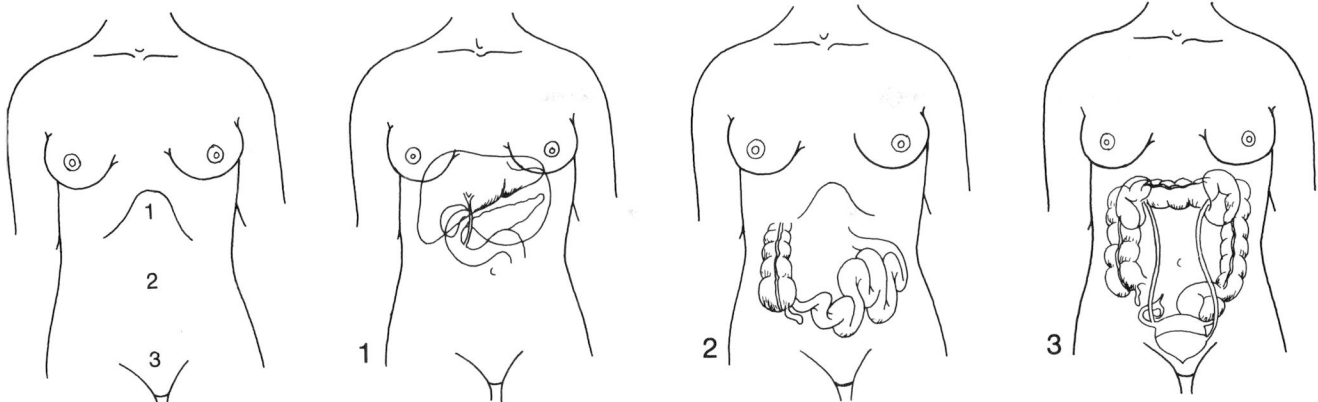

FIGURE 11–2. "Visceral" abdominal pain: deep, dull, diffuse. The three general localizations of midline "visceral" abdominal pain: epigastric, periumbilical, hypogastric. 1. Epigastric pain usually suggests disease of the thorax, stomach, duodenum, pancreas, liver, or gallbladder. 2. Periumbilical pain usually implies disease of the small intestine or cecum or both. 3. Hypogastric pain usually implicates the large intestine, pelvic organs, or urinary system.

(usually inflamed or perforated) viscus. Pain often worsens with movement and cough and is accompanied by localized tenderness on examination directly over the site of pain (see below). Such pain occurs because, unlike the viscera themselves, the parietal peritoneum is innervated *unilaterally* by peripheral (nonautonomic) nerves that travel to the spinal cord at segmental (dermatomal) levels T6 through L1.[3]

While the location of parietal pain may be epigastric, periumbilical, or hypogastric (when, for example, parietal peritoneum is irritated by an epigastric gallbladder, a periumbilical strangulated hernia, or a hypogastric pelvic abscess, respectively), most parietal pain lateralizes to one of four quadrants: right upper quadrant, left upper quadrant, right lower quadrant, or left lower quadrant. Thus, when parietal pain appears to be the problem, knowledge of anatomic location of intra-abdominal organs subjacent to the involved quadrant of peritoneum is crucial to diagnosis, as is appreciation of the typical "path of perforation" when an intra-abdominal viscus ruptures and causes localized peritonitis (see below). Figure 11–3 illustrates differential diagnoses of localized peritonitis.

These two types of abdominal pain emphasize a few generalizations about the location of pain:

A. When parietal pain (with peritoneal signs—see page 539) appears to be the problem, a disease process involving an intra-abdominal, intraperitoneal organ is usually responsible.

Conversely, visceral abdominal pain may be due to disease of intra-abdominal intraperitoneal organs in which the peritoneum is not involved; disease of intra-abdominal extraperitoneal organs—pancreas, kidneys, ureters, great vessels, and pelvic organs; or disease of extra-abdominal organs (thorax, spine, hips, for example) in which pain is referred to the abdomen. Thus, visceral pain in the *upper* abdomen may be referred from the thorax or spine, may reflect disease of epigastric organs (Fig. 11–2), or may imply disease of more "occult" intra-abdominal organs—especially the retroperitoneal (or, rarely, pelvic) structures. Similarly, visceral pain in the *lower* abdomen may be referred from the spine, hips, or pelvic bones, may reflect disease of the colon or rectum (Fig. 11–2) or may indicate disease in the pelvis, urinary organs, or retroperitoneum. (Only

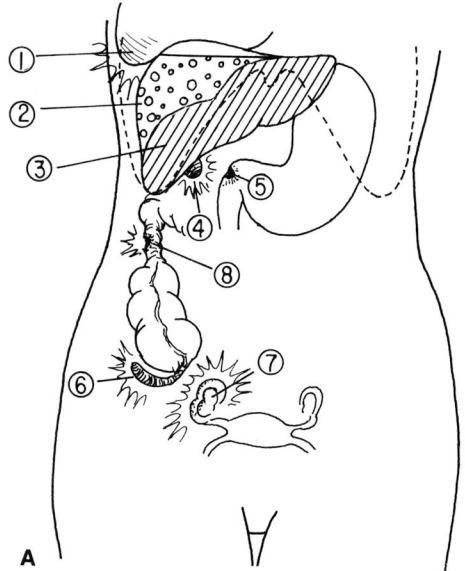

A

1. Pleurisy
2. Subdiaphragmatic abscess
3. (Peri) hepatitis
4. Cholecystitis
5. Perforated duodenal ulcer
6. Appendicitis
7. Ectopic pregnancy, tuboovarian hemorrhage, abscess, or rupture
8. Perforated colon (cancer or diverticulum)

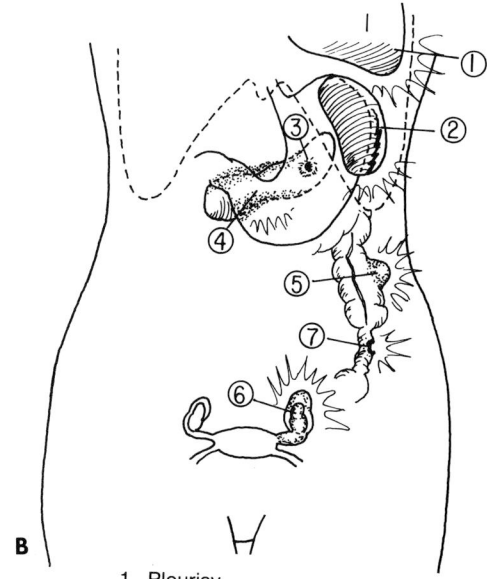

B

1. Pleurisy
2. Splenic rupture
3. Perforated gastric ulcer
4. Pancreatitis
5. Diverticulitis (splenic flexure)
6. Ectopic pregnancy, tuboovarian hemorrhage, abscess, or rupture
7. Perforated colon Carcinoma

FIGURE 11–3. Common and uncommon conditions that may cause "parietal" pain and localized peritonitis in the various quadrants of the abdomen: *A,* Right upper quadrant. *B,* Left upper quadrant. *C,* Right lower quadrant. *D,* Left lower quadrant.

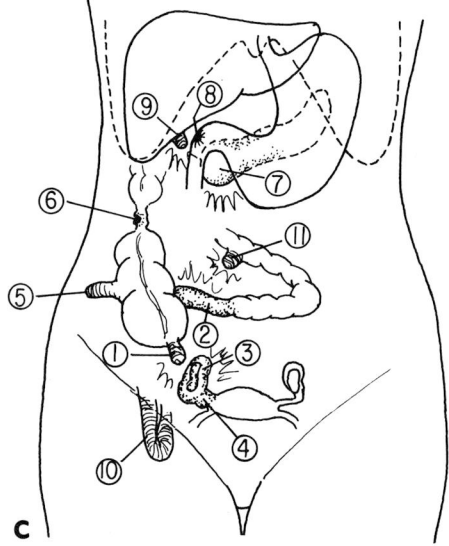

C

1. Appendicitis
2. Acute Crohn's disease
3. Ectopic pregnancy, tuboovarian abscess, or ovarian torsion/hemorrhage
4. Pelvic inflammatory disease
5. Cecal diverticulitis
6. Colon cancer (perforation)
7. Acute pancreatitis and/or pseudocyst
8. Perforated duodenal ulcer
9. Acute cholecystitis
10. Incarcerated inguinal hernia
11. Meckel's diverticulitis

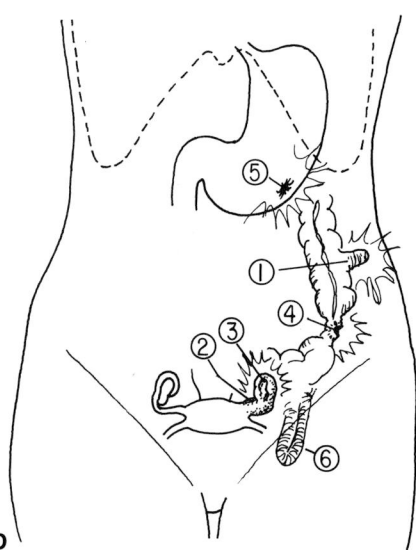

D

1. Sigmoid diverticulitis
2. Pelvic inflammatory disease
3. Ectopic pregnancy, tuboovarian abscess, or ovarian torsion / hemorrhage
4. Perforated sigmoid carcinoma
5. Perforated gastric ulcer
6. Incarcerated inguinal hernia

rarely is lower abdominal pain due to disease in the thorax or upper abdominal organs.) Finally, visceral pain in the *central* abdomen may be referred from the spine, thorax, or pelvis; reflect disease of periumbilical organs (early appendicitis, for example); or suggest disease of the pancreas or mesenteric vasculature.

B. <u>Visceral pain may become parietal pain.</u>

In fact, progression from deep, dull, midline visceral pain to sharp, severe, highly localized parietal pain is characteristic of several common (and serious) intra-abdominal diseases.

The pain of acute appendicitis often begins as visceral pain in the periumbilical area (or may be generalized), when inflammation involves only the appendix and not (yet) the overlying parietal peritoneum.[5] Progression of the inflammatory process to involve the peritoneum produces localized peritonitis (see page 539) with parietal pain and tenderness precisely localized over the anatomic location of the appendix.

The pain of acute cholecystitis often begins in the epigastrium. This visceral pain may terminate spontaneously—called an attack of biliary colic[6, 7]—but may also progress to parietal pain and localized peritonitis in the right upper quadrant directly over the inflamed gallbladder, beneath the irritated parietal peritoneum.

The pain of acute diverticulitis may begin as diffuse visceral hypogastric pain but then moves (usually) to the left lower quadrant when a pericolonic abscess, the result of diverticular inflammation and perforation, irritates the overlying peritoneum.[8]

Thus, <u>the march of visceral pain in one location to parietal pain in another is often highly suggestive of one specific disease.</u> Certainly such a sequence narrows the differential diagnosis.

C. <u>Visceral, parietal, or referred pain may radiate.</u>

Radiation of pain is not synonymous with temporal progression of pain from one site to another. Rather, when pain is perceived to be located primarily in one site but to simultaneously involve a secondary site, the pain is said to radiate from the first site to the second. Occasionally the precise path of such radiation is diagnostically helpful.

Pain due to <u>intra-abdominal disease may radiate extra-abdominally.</u> The pain of acute cholecystitis sometimes radiates to the subscapular area, since the gallbladder is innervated by spinal segments T6 through T9. The pain of ureteral colic may radiate into the testicle or upper leg, along a T12–L2 distribution. The pain of acute pancreatitis often radiates directly through the midabdomen into the back.

Pain due to <u>extra-abdominal disease may radiate into the abdomen.</u> Spinal nerve root irritation (due to degenerative arthritis, compression fractures, diabetes, or rare thoracic spinal discs or neoplasms) may radiate around the abdomen in a dermatomal distribution. Hip disease may cause lower abdominal pain, as may epididymitis, prostatitis, or iliofemoral thrombophlebitis. Diseases of the chest (especially pneumonia, pleuritis, pericarditis, and myocardial infarction) may radiate into the abdomen.

Pain due to <u>intra-abdominal disease may radiate to different parts of the abdomen.</u> The pain of dissecting aortic aneurysm typically "rips" or "tears" from the chest (or epigastrium) down the back or into the lower abdomen. The pain of gastroenteritis typically migrates from one part of the abdomen to another, sometimes in concert with peristalsis.

Thus, the question, "Where is the pain?" is really three different questions: "Where was the pain initially?" "Where is the pain now?" "Does the pain spread or radiate to other sites?" The answers to these questions are of great importance in diagnosis. Usually the quality of pain—visceral or parietal—becomes apparent during assessment of its location.

Sally says that the pain began the day before in the area of the umbilicus, or just below it. Today the pain seems more prominent in the right lower quadrant and suprapubic area. The pain remains dull, deep, and aching, and Sally cannot localize it with just one finger, but places both hands over the (hypogastric) area of the discomfort. The pain does not radiate.

Coughing and moving about do not seem to greatly worsen Sally's pain.

What does this mean?
1. The pain sounds visceral, but only careful abdominal examination (see below) will exclude parietal pain (with so-called peritoneal signs).

    In the absence of such localizing findings, it will also be important to exclude extra-abdominal (referred) pain—examination of the back, hips, pelvis, groin, and other structures will especially help, since the pain is in the lower abdomen (see page 560).
2. The initial (periumbilical) location of the pain suggests disease of the small intestine (or cecum), but the current location in the hypogastric area is more suggestive of disease of the colon, rectum, or pelvis (Fig. 11–2).
3. The location of pain allows a more directed review of systems.

    Special attention here must be paid to any associated bowel, urinary, menstrual, or gynecologic symptoms, since pain appears to be visceral and hypogastric (Fig. 11–2).

II. The timing of abdominal pain is often helpful.

The most important factors to consider are the manner of onset of pain, the course of pain since its inception, and the total duration of pain at the time of clinical presentation.

When the onset of pain is very abrupt, the patient can often recall exactly what he or she was doing at the moment pain began. ("I was fine one minute, and then bam! There it was!") In general, very abrupt onset of pain should suggest perforation of an abdominal viscus (most commonly, a duodenal/gastric ulcer or a colonic diverticulum) or a pelvic organ (ruptured ectopic pregnancy, perforated uterus); obstruction of a nonintestinal viscus (for example, a bile duct or ureter); or an acute vascular event (infarction of bowel, kidney, heart, lung, or spleen; leaking aortic aneurysm; dissecting aortic aneurysm).* Usually such pain is very severe. Because the physical examination may be relatively unimpressive in a few such patients (and laboratory tests and x-rays may be nondiagnostic), this history alone is of great importance—pain of abrupt onset and great severity is always serious (see page 608), whatever the physical examination reveals.

---

*Occasionally, acute pancreatitis will begin with sudden abruptness.

Gradual onset of pain usually suggests an inflammatory process (appendicitis, diverticulitis, gastroenteritis, salpingitis, pneumonia, pyelonephritis) or intestinal obstruction. It is important to remember that when an inflammatory process follows visceral obstruction (for example, appendicitis with a fecalith, pyelonephritis "behind" a ureteral stone, cholangitis with a common duct biliary stone), onset of pain may be more abrupt. Similarly, pain of gradual onset due to an inflammatory process will become abruptly much more severe if perforation follows inflammation—sudden worsening of pain will announce perforation of the appendix, gallbladder, or colon following gradual onset of appendicitis, cholecystitis, or diverticulitis, for example.

The pain of intestinal obstruction varies with the site and mechanism of obstruction (see Table 11–5, page 543). In general, the more distal the site of obstruction, the more slowly pain begins and progresses. Thus, colonic obstruction may cause very little pain until late in its course; acute gastric volvulus will cause abrupt, severe pain. Similarly, obstructive processes that quickly threaten infarction or perforation will cause more rapid progression of pain—closed-loop obstruction due to volvulus and an incarcerated hernia are typical examples.

Acute abdominal pain whose onset awakens the patient from sleep usually proves to be a significant problem.

Knowledge of the course and duration of pain since its inception is also helpful. Steady, severe, progressively worsening pain is always worrisome. Pain that comes and goes, i.e., the patient is pain free between salvos of abdominal pain, is usually due to intestinal peristalsis with partial bowel obstruction or simple gastroenteritis. Occasionally the pain of biliary or ureteral obstruction will also be colicky,[6] but this is unusual: The pain of biliary or ureteral "colic" is, in fact, usually steady and persistent.

Most causes of abdominal pain that prove to require surgery will be apparent on physical examination (see below) within 24 to 48 hours of the onset of pain. When pain has already been present for 2 to 3 days, but physical examination does not reveal evidence of localized peritonitis, palpable masses, or abdominal distention (see page 543), a "surgical abdomen" is much less likely. Common disorders like appendicitis, cholecystitis, bowel obstruction, diverticulitis, and acute vascular events are only rarely more indolent in onset and progression. Occasionally, large-bowel obstruction, serious pelvic disease, and subacute mesenteric ischemia may be more insidious in onset (several days) or associated with relatively benign examinations.

Conversely, when ongoing pain has been present for less than 24 hours, many surgical problems may be "brewing" despite the absence of dramatic physical findings. The pain of appendicitis is a typical example in which, for the first 12 hours (or occasionally longer), pain may be centrally located and entirely nonspecific. Acute onset of abdominal pain within the previous 12 to 24 hours always requires continuing observation (see page 557) whatever the results of the physical examination. How the patient is observed usually depends on:

III. The severity of pain.

As noted above, when pain is abrupt in onset and very severe or when pain is more gradual in onset but suddenly or progressively becomes very severe, serious disease is likely.

On the other hand, the subjective severity of pain is remarkably variable among individuals. Denial of severe pain by the patient whose pain began very abruptly or whose examination suggests a surgical abdomen (see page 568) is not reassuring; a totally normal examination in the patient complaining of terrible pain usually is reassuring (usually, but not always—see page 608). The latter patient still deserves careful observation (see page 613), but objective findings on physical examination are usually more reliable predictors than just the subjective severity of pain.

Sally says that her pain did not begin abruptly, but came on gradually over the course of several hours the day before. She had been completely well 2 days ago.

Sally's pain has worsened during the past 12 hours. The pain is constant and has now been present for a total of 24 hours. Sally describes her pain as "very uncomfortable but not unbearable."

What does this mean?
A. The gradual onset of pain suggests an inflammatory process, while early intestinal obstruction is also possible.
B. The constancy of pain and its increasing severity must inspire caution, however mild the pain may be subjectively.

Many of the common benign causes of abdominal pain—acute gastroenteritis, constipation, dysmenorrhea, urinary infection—cause pain that is inconstant, crampy, waxing and waning. Unrelenting pain that worsens always deserves careful attention.

Thus, in Sally's case the location, timing, and severity of pain suggest an inflammatory process in the small or (more likely) large intestine or pelvis, while early intestinal obstruction is also possible.

Brief consideration of any associated symptoms and the overall clinical setting then often help to further narrow the differential diagnosis. (None of these historical findings can be interpreted until the history is correlated with the results of the physical examination—see page 539. Careful analysis of the history alone, however, should always precede physical examination.)

Sally had a normal bowel movement 8 hours ago. She denies any recent diarrhea or constipation. She has just completed (4 days ago) a menstrual period, which was normal in duration and quality and which was preceded by another normal period her usual 28 days before. Sally denies any vaginal discharge or itching, dysuria or urinary complaints, fever or chills. Sally last had sexual intercourse about 10 days ago—she denies any dyspareunia. Her pain appears unrelated to defecation, urination, or skeletal movement.

Sally is vaguely queasy and perhaps mildly anorectic, but there has been no vomiting.

NOTE

1. Diarrhea in association with acute abdominal pain is most often due to infectious gastroenteritis, but acute inflammatory bowel disease, diverticulitis, early intestinal obstruction or even (rarely) appendicitis may cause diarrhea. Chapter 3 discusses various aspects of acute diarrhea.

2. When constipation clearly precedes abdominal pain by a few or several days, disease of the colon or rectum is usually responsible, but any of the conditions noted in Table 11–1 should be considered. Failure to have a bowel movement during the course of abdominal pain is utterly nonspecific, unless that situation persists for several days, since intestinal ileus is a

TABLE 11–1. CAUSES OF ACUTE ABDOMINAL PAIN AND CONSTIPATION

Structural bowel obstruction	Possible iatrogenic causes
Fecal impaction	Laxative/cathartic abuse
Entrapped hernias	Analgesics
Adhesions	Antacids (aluminum)
Neoplasms	Antidepressants
Inflammatory strictures	Phenothiazines
Intussusception	Antiparkinsonism drugs
Subacute volvulus	Ganglionic blockers
	Clonidine
Proctocolitis	
	Possible metabolic causes
Anal fissure	Diabetes
	Uremia
Irritable bowel syndrome	Hypokalemia
	Hypercalcemia
Diverticulosis/diverticulitis	Hypothyroidism
Pregnancy	Rare causes
	Heavy metal poisoning
Neurologic disease	Porphyria
Spinal cord compression	Tabes dorsalis
Cauda equina syndrome	Scleroderma
Dysautonomia	Chagas' disease
Hirschsprung's disease	Amyloidosis
Myotonic dystrophy	
Dermatomyositis	

common *result* of many types of abdominal pain. Continuation of normal bowel movements during the course of acute abdominal pain is "soft" evidence against a primary lower intestinal cause of pain.

3. Most patients with urinary tract causes of abdominal pain will have associated urinary symptoms—dysuria, frequency, hesitancy, hematuria. Urinary infection is unlikely in the absence of such symptoms, especially if fever is also absent.

Ureteral calculi are not always associated with urinary symptoms.[9] Unilateral flank pain, sometimes radiating into the groin, associated with gross or microscopic hematuria, usually suggests the diagnosis, however.

4. Many women with pelvic origin of pain will describe associated vaginal discharge, dyspareunia, irregular menstruation, associated vaginal bleeding, or some association between pain and the menstrual cycle.

5. Vomiting is nonspecific and may accompany pain of any kind. In general, however, when vomiting precedes the onset of abdominal pain, "surgical disease" is very unlikely,[2] and gastroenteritis or some other non-surgical illness is more often responsible. Surgical disease more often causes pain followed by vomiting.

Table 11–2 indicates causes of acute abdominal pain in which vomiting is a common associated symptom. (Temporary) relief of pain by vomiting is common in peptic ulcer disease and in some instances of intestinal obstruction. Vomiting rarely relieves the pain of peritonitis, cholecystitis, or pancreatitis.

The absence of vomiting by no means excludes serious disease: Large-bowel obstruction, intra-abdominal hemorrhage, or acute vascular events are examples of potentially life-threatening illnesses that may present with abdominal pain without vomiting.

The odor of vomitus (especially if feculent), presence of frank blood (or "coffee grounds"), and the content of vomitus (for example, undigested

**TABLE 11–2. CAUSES OF ACUTE ABDOMINAL PAIN
ASSOCIATED WITH VOMITING**

Common
Small-bowel obstruction
Acute cholecystitis
Acute appendicitis
Complications of pregnancy
Gastroenteritis
Food poisoning
Alcoholic gastritis/hepatitis
Peptic ulcer disease
Acute (inferior) myocardial infarction
Acute pyelonephritis
Viral hepatitis

Uncommon
Acute pancreatitis
Diabetic ketoacidosis
Drug withdrawal
Uremia
Vasculitis
Psychogenic

Rare
Porphyria
Lead poisoning
Acute adrenal insufficiency
Hyperlipidemia
Abdominal epilepsy
Acute glaucoma

food) may suggest intestinal obstruction, gastrointestinal bleeding, or gastroesophageal obstruction, respectively.

Anorexia is nonspecific, but its absence makes serious disease less likely, i.e., the patient with acute abdominal pain who is hungry usually has either a peptic ulcer with hunger pain or no serious intra-abdominal disease.

6. The specific clinical setting is sometimes helpful. Table 11–3 lists various past or concurrent medical problems that may point to an otherwise unsuspected diagnosis.

7. High fever (temperature greater than 103° F) or rigors are unusual in "simple surgical" problems (Fig. 11–1). Pneumonia, pyelonephritis, bacterial

**TABLE 11–3. PAST OR CONCURRENT MEDICAL PROBLEMS THAT MAY INDICATE
CAUSE OF ACUTE ABDOMINAL PAIN**

MEDICAL PROBLEM	POSSIBLE CAUSE OF PAIN
Recurrence of documented prior disease?	Gallstones; kidney stones; peptic ulcer; intussusception; intra-abdominal adhesions; bowel neoplasms or strictures; pelvic disease; pancreatitis; volvulus
Diabetes?	Diabetic ketoacidosis; gastroparesis diabeticorum; pancreatitis; acute fatty liver; diabetic neuralgia
Alcoholism?	Gastritis; hepatitis; pancreatitis; ulcer disease
Ascites?	Spontaneous peritonitis[10]
Cardiac disease (valvular disease, cardiomyopathy, arrhythmias, prior emboli, congestive heart failure)?	Mesenteric infarction (embolism, thrombosis, "poor perfusion"); myocardial infarction
Prior surgery (appendectomy, cholecystectomy, total hysterectomy, bilateral salpingo-oophorectomy)?	Can we thus *exclude* appendicitis, cholecystitis, pelvic disease? Also consider: adhesions; stricture; postoperative pancreatitis/cholecystitis
Upper respiratory infection?	Mesenteric adenitis; gastroenteritis; pneumonia
Infectious mononucleosis?	Hepatitis; splenic rupture
Sickle cell disease?	Abdominal crisis; splenic infarction
Collagen vascular disease?	Abdominal vasculitis?[11]
Syncope/impaired mental status?	Abdominal epilepsy[12]
Menstrual cycle?	See page 563
Recurrent, localized edema?	C1 esterase deficiency

dysentery, ascending cholangitis, liver abscess, or intra-abdominal abscess (subphrenic, tubo-ovarian, pericolonic) should be suspected in such circumstances.

Physical examination reveals a healthy, but anxious, young woman who appears only mildly uncomfortable. Temperature is 37.8° C orally; other vital signs are normal—the pulse is 72.

The abdomen is flat, bowel sounds are present (or slightly diminished), and there is moderate tenderness and slight guarding on deep palpation of the right lower quadrant. There is no rigidity or rebound or percussion tenderness.

Physical Examination

The initial approach to the examination of the patient with acute abdominal pain is directed at quickly identifying those patients with serious (often, but not always, surgical) conditions. This can usually be done by answering three basic questions (see also Table 11–6, pages 544 and 545):

I. Is the patient "shocky"?

Obviously, vital signs must be carefully recorded. Blood pressure and pulse should be measured in supine and upright positions—orthostatic hypotension in the patient with acute abdominal pain usually implies either intra-abdominal hemorrhage or fluid loss ("third spacing").

A normal blood pressure by no means excludes "shock." The patient with cold, clammy extremities (and often the tip of the nose and the ears as well), tachycardia, impaired mentation, and oliguria is "shocky," even if not frankly hypotensive.

The patient in shock with acute abdominal pain may be suffering from one of many thoracic, intra-abdominal, or pelvic disorders. This subject is far beyond the scope of this text, but the location of pain and the remainder of the examination will usually greatly narrow the differential diagnosis (see Table 11–6).

When the abdominal examination is normal in such patients, it is crucial to remember that myocardial infarction, pulmonary embolism, pneumothorax, aortic dissection, intra-abdominal, gastrointestinal or retroperitoneal bleeding, mesenteric ischemia/infarction, and acute pancreatitis may cause acute abdominal pain, shock, and a surprisingly unimpressive abdominal examination.

More often, abdominal examination of the patient with acute abdominal pain who is shocky reveals evidence of either peritonitis or abdominal distention.

II. Are there peritoneal signs? (Table 11–4)

As noted previously, the patient with diffuse or focal peritonitis

TABLE 11–4. "PERITONEAL SIGNS" OF SERIOUS CONDITIONS ASSOCIATED WITH ACUTE ABDOMINAL PAIN

DIFFUSE PERITONITIS	LOCALIZED PERITONITIS
Very severe pain	Severe, focal pain
Patient lies motionless	Avoidance of movement, coughing
Bowel sounds absent	Bowel sounds diminished/absent
Diffuse percussion tenderness	Focal percussion tenderness
Palpable abdominal rigidity	Referred percussion tenderness
Diffuse tenderness and guarding with gentle palpation	Focal guarding and/or rigidity
	Referred guarding
	Rebound tenderness

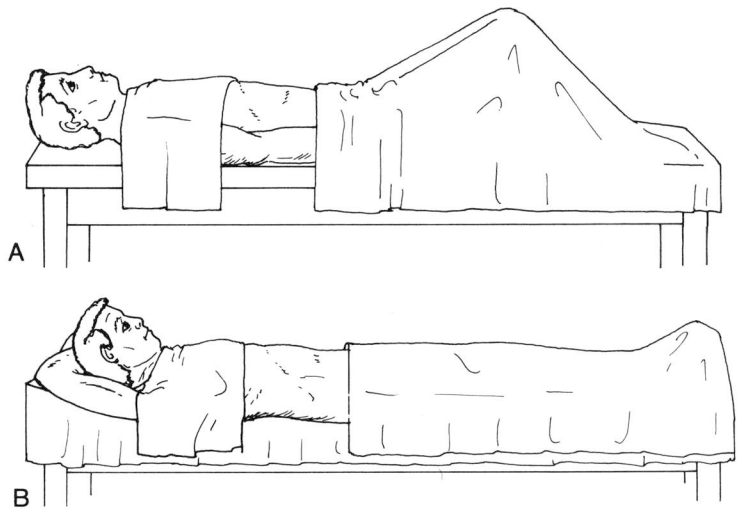

FIGURE 11–4. Positioning the patient. The patient should be well draped, lying supine, hands at the side, knees slightly flexed. *A,* Correct. *B,* Incorrect.

usually has severe pain that is worsened by movement or cough. Simple observation of the patient's posture is often a helpful clue. The patient with peritonitis usually lies still, often with both knees drawn up toward the chest, complaining bitterly when forced to move during the examination. Remember:

A. Before the abdomen is examined, the patient must be properly positioned.

   The patient's abdominal musculature should be fully relaxed: The patient should thus lie supine, head flat on the table, arms at the sides, knees slightly flexed (Fig. 11–4).

B. Auscultation of the abdomen should be performed before palpation.

   Three minutes of continuous auscultation should be allowed before bowel sounds are characterized as absent. Peritonitis and paralytic ileus are the common causes of true absence of bowel sounds. Dramatically hyperactive bowel sounds are often heard in the patient with hyperperistalsis due to gastroenteritis or intestinal bleeding. High-pitched rushes of bowel sounds that coincide with crampy abdominal pain but then resolve as cramping resolves is typical of partial bowel obstruction. (Characterizing bowel sounds as hyperactive or hypoactive is highly subjective, and such quantitative distinctions are more often helpful in following the patient: Subsequent examination that reveals definite increases or decreases in bowel sounds may point to important changes.)

C. The abdomen should be percussed before it is palpated.

   Percussion of the abdomen may identify areas of tympany (bowel gas), dullness (fluid, masses, feces, fat), or shifting dullness (ascites). Light percussion of all areas of the abdomen, beginning at a site distant from the area of most intense pain and ending over the painful area, will also identify local or generalized peritoneal irritation.

   Percussion tenderness (Fig. 11–5) refers to abdominal tenderness elicited by gently tapping the abdominal wall. Especially when this induces both pain and subjacent muscular guarding or when percussion of one area of the abdomen causes pain in a distant site (referred percussion tenderness, Fig. 11–5B), peritoneal irritation is likely. Deeper (more painful) palpation is unlikely to add helpful information when there is definite (localized or generalized) percussion tenderness with guarding.

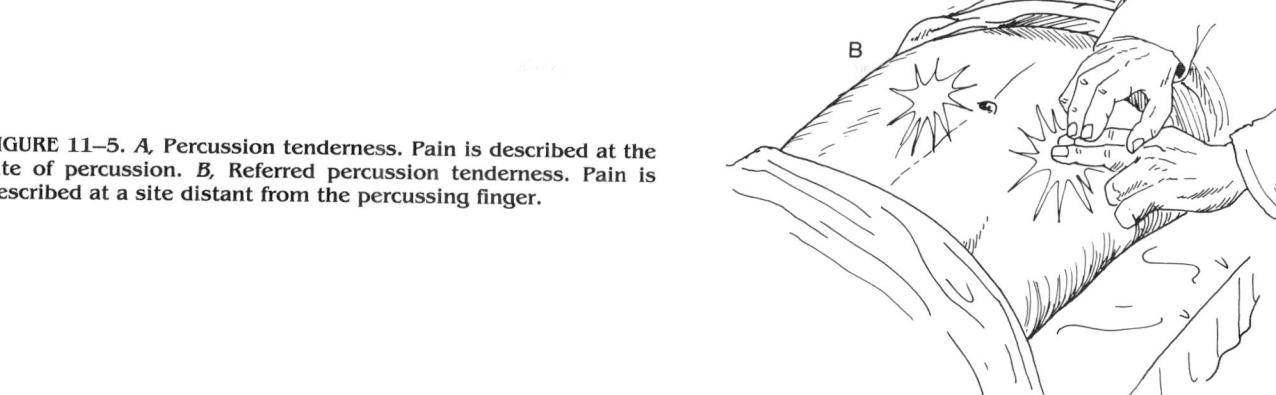

FIGURE 11–5. A, Percussion tenderness. Pain is described at the site of percussion. B, Referred percussion tenderness. Pain is described at a site distant from the percussing finger.

D. Following observation, auscultation, and percussion, gentle palpation of the abdomen will yield the most information.

By resting the palm and fingers of the examining hand on the abdomen while talking to the patient the physician will let the patient get used to palpation. It is remarkable how frequently tenderness to light palpation disappears or diminishes after the first moment of contact as the examiner's resting hand is accommodated by the anxious patient.

When even light palpation causes tensing of abdominal musculature, one of three situations is usually present.

First, the examiner's hands are too cold or are pressed too pointedly into the abdomen (Fig. 11–6B).

Second, the patient may be ticklish or guard involuntarily—here, compression of the patient's sternum with the examiner's left hand while the abdomen is palpated with the right hand may be helpful since the left hand thus forces abdominal breathing and at least intermittent abdominal relaxation.

Third, there may be "true guarding" because of a subjacent (usually inflammatory) disease process. In spite of all precautions, the abdomen then tenses as manual palpation elicits local tenderness. (Rigidity is unmistakable board-like hardness of the abdominal wall that overlies peritoneal irritation and that is constant and unyielding—this is usually seen only in advanced peritonitis.)

Palpation should begin, like percussion, at a site distant from the area of most intense pain. Rest your palm and fingers flat on the abdomen and then gently and repetitively flex the fingers, lightly kneading the abdomen as the fingers "crawl" from one quadrant to

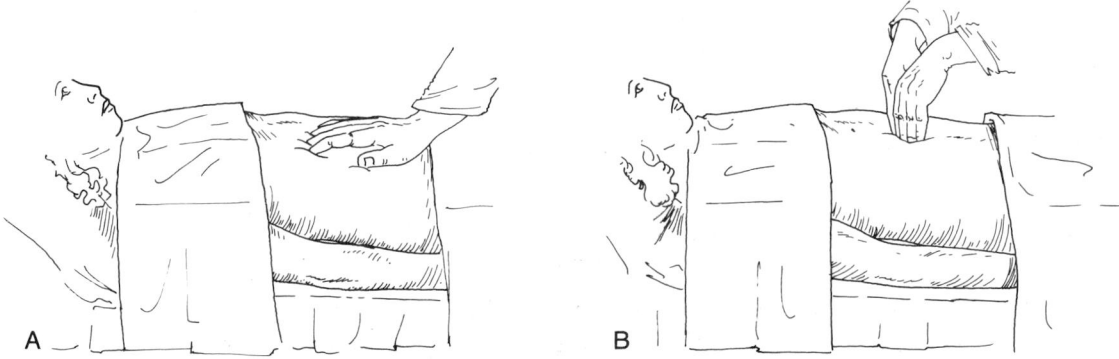

FIGURE 11–6. The examining hand should be flat on the abdomen, the tips of the fingers gently palpating. A, Correct. B, Incorrect.

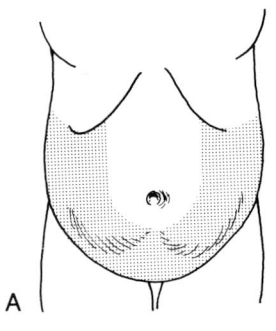
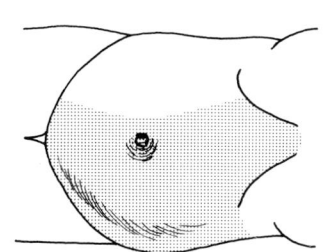

FIGURE 11–7. Abdominal distention: 5 Fs (fluid, feces, flatus, fetus, fat). A, Ascites (fluid). The dark area is dull to percussion. "Shifting dullness" is demonstrated with the patient in the decubitus position. B, Bowel distention (feces or flatus). In this condition, the abdomen is diffusely tympanitic on percussion, and bowel loops (with or without feces) may be palpable. C, A pelvic or other intra-abdominal mass (fetus) will either be discretely palpable or dull to percussion locally (dark area). D, The obese patient (fat) will have a large abdomen without shifting dullness, prominent tympany, palpable bowel or other masses, or localized dullness.

A

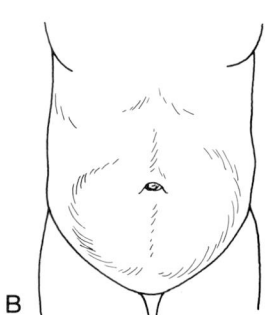
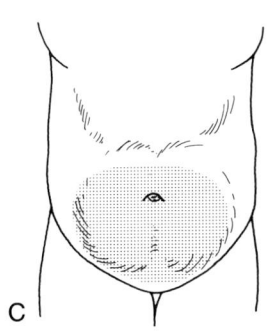
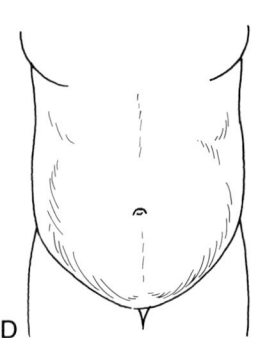

B   C   D

the next (Fig. 11–6). Deeper palpation is helpful when there is little or no tenderness on percussion or flat palpation, and areas of localized pain may then be more carefully examined for evidence of deep tenderness or masses. Rebound tenderness—worsening of pain with sudden release of the deeply palpating hand—is sometimes an indicator of early peritoneal irritation but is nonspecific.

III. Is the abdomen distended?

Increased abdominal girth is due to one of the five Fs: fat (obesity), feces or flatus (constipation or intestinal obstruction or both), fetus (pregnancy or other intra-abdominal masses), or fluid (ascites). Abdominal percussion and palpation will usually distinguish among intraperitoneal fluid, intra-abdominal masses, and excessive intestinal gas (Fig. 11–7). The patient with acute abdominal pain and a distended abdomen may then require paracentesis[10] (to diagnose infection or hemorrhage), further evaluation of palpable abdominal masses (see Tables 11–15 and 11–21) or abdominal x-rays to detect intestinal obstruction. (Occasionally, peritoneal lavage[13] will be diagnostically helpful, even when the abdomen is not distended. This is usually left to the surgeon and is most useful in the patient with post-traumatic abdominal pain.)

The absence of distention does not exclude early bowel obstruction, especially when the large intestine is obstructed or early in the course of distal small-bowel obstruction. Clinical differences between such low bowel obstruction and more proximal (high) obstruction are enumerated in Table 11–5, as are the most common causes of obstruction of the large and small intestine found in two large clinical series.[15, 16]

Table 11–6 indicates the usual differential diagnosis of acute abdominal pain according to the location of pain or tenderness, the severity and timing of pain, and the presence or absence of shock, peritoneal signs, or abdominal distention.

The independent significance of each of these clinical clues must be emphasized, i.e., whenever the patient with acute abdominal pain

TABLE 11–5A. CLINICAL DIFFERENCE BETWEEN LOW AND HIGH BOWEL OBSTRUCTION[14]

PROXIMAL BOWEL OBSTRUCTION	DISTAL BOWEL OBSTRUCTION
Acute onset	Less acute onset
Prominent vomiting	Less prominent vomiting
Nonfeculent vomitus	Vomitus may be feculent
Frequent intervals of pain	Less frequent intervals of pain
Minimal distention	Distention common

TABLE 11–5B. COMMON CAUSES OF INTESTINAL OBSTRUCTION[15, 16]

TYPE OF OBSTRUCTION	No.	%
Small intestinal obstruction (152 cases)[15]		
Postoperative adhesions	108	71.1
Carcinoma (primary or metastatic)	14	9.3
External hernia	8	5.3
Internal hernia	4	2.6
Crohn's disease	6	3.9
Inflammatory stricture	2	1.3
Gallstone ileus	2	1.3
Others	8	5.3
Large intestinal obstruction (554 cases)[16]		
Carcinoma	371	67
Sigmoid volvulus	49	9
Diverticulitis	39	7
Fecal impaction	26	4.7
Miscellaneous	44	8
Peritoneal carcinoma		
Cecal volvulus		
Toxic megacolon		
Undiagnosed	25	4.5

demonstrates any of these characteristics, serious disease must be excluded.

For example, the patient with a perforated peptic ulcer may describe very abrupt, severe abdominal pain and yet, during the first 6 to 12 hours of illness, may not have an impressive abdominal examination. Thereafter, such patients will develop peritonitis.

Any patient with acute abdominal pain who looks "shocky" requires emergency attention, whatever the remainder of the examination reveals. Intra-abdominal or retroperitoneal hemorrhage may be associated with a relatively benign abdominal examination, for example.

Definite peritoneal signs (Table 11–4) require surgical consultation, however atypical the history or however nontoxic the condition of the patient appears.

Abdominal distention may result from bowel obstruction without shock, peritonitis, or severe pain.

Thus, there can be no "cookbook approach"—Table 11–6 is merely a general outline of differential diagnosis. Nevertheless, most serious diseases that cause acute abdominal pain will be suspected early if the sequence of investigations outlined here is followed:

Where is the pain?
Did the pain begin (or worsen) abruptly?
Is the patient "shocky"?
Are there peritoneal signs?
Is the abdomen distended?

Unless the patient is in shock and requires immediate exploratory

TABLE 11–6. CRITICAL CLUES IN DIFFERENTIAL DIAGNOSIS OF ACUTE ABDOMINAL PAIN

	GENERALIZED ABDOMINAL PAIN	MIDLINE EPIGASTRIC PAIN	MIDLINE PERIUMBILICAL PAIN
1. Shocky? ↓ No	Perforated viscus Peritonitis Intra-abdominal hemorrhage Acute vascular event Pancreatitis	Myocardial infarction Pulmonary embolism Aortic dissection Pericardial tamponade Upper intestinal bleeding Perforated ulcer or gallbladder Acute pancreatitis	Myocardial infarction Mesenteric infarction Leaking abdominal aortic aneurysm Acute pancreatitis Small-bowel obstruction Ruptured ectopic pregnancy

2. Peritoneal signs?
↓ No
	Diffuse peritonitis
	Bowel infarction
	Bowel strangulation
		Perforated ulcer or gallbladder
		Acute cholecystitis
		Gallbladder empyema
		Severe pancreatitis
			Small-bowel strangulation/
			  infarction
			Meckel's diverticulitis
			Acute Crohn's disease
			  (perforation?)
			Acute appendicitis

3. Abdominal distention? ↓ No	Bowel obstruction Volvulus Paralytic ileus Intra-abdominal hemorrhage Bowel ischemia Ascites Constipation	Gastric outlet obstruction Gastric volvulus Pancreatitis with paralytic ileus Proximal bowel obstruction Constipation	Bowel obstruction Inflammatory bowel disease Toxic megacolon Mesenteric ischemia Constipation
4. Very abrupt severe pain? ↓	Perforated viscus Biliary/ureteral stones Acute vascular event Acute pancreatitis	Myocardial infarction Pulmonary embolism Aortic dissection Acute pancreatitis Biliary colic/acute cholecystitis Mesenteric ischemia	Volvulus Mesenteric infarction Leaking abdominal aortic aneurysm Early appendicitis
X-ray findings?	Free air Bowel obstruction Volvulus Stone Mass Stool	X-ray chest, abdomen ECG	X-ray chest, abdomen ECG

	MIDLINE HYPOGASTRIC PAIN	RIGHT UPPER QUADRANT PAIN*	LEFT UPPER QUADRANT PAIN*
1. Shocky? ↓ No	Ruptured ectopic pregnancy Perforated uterus Pelvic bleeding Lower intestinal bleeding Incomplete abortion Perforated duodenal ulcer Ruptured aneurysm	Pulmonary embolism Myocardial infarction Tension pneumothorax Pneumonia with sepsis Perforated gallbladder Ascending cholangitis Acute pancreatitis Perforated duodenal ulcer	Pulmonary embolism Myocardial infarction Tension pneumothorax Splenic rupture Leaking splenic artery Aneurysm Perforated gastric ulcer
2. Peritoneal signs? ↓ No	Pelvic abscess Bladder/uterine perforation	Acute cholecystitis Retrocecal appendicitis Ruptured ectopic pregnancy Ruptured tubal abscess Fitz-Hugh–Curtis syndrome Subphrenic abscess	Acute pancreatitis Perforated gastric ulcer Splenic rupture/bleeding Ruptured ectopic pregnancy Ruptured tubal abscess Subphrenic abscess

3. Abdominal distention?
↓ No
	Large bowel obstruction
	Constipation/impaction
	Toxic megacolon
	Ruptured ectopic pregnancy
	Intrauterine pregnancy
	Threatened abortion
	Distended bladder
		Hepatic flexure syndrome
		Hepatomegaly
		Constipation
		Upper abdominal mass (Table
		  11–21)
			Volvulus
			Toxic megacolon
			Sigmoid colon obstruction
			Splenomegaly/splenic bleeding
			Splenic flexure syndrome
			Upper abdominal mass (Table
			  11–21)

TABLE 11–6. CRITICAL CLUES IN DIFFERENTIAL DIAGNOSIS OF ACUTE ABDOMINAL PAIN *(Continued)*

	MIDLINE HYPOGASTRIC PAIN	RIGHT UPPER QUADRANT PAIN*	LEFT UPPER QUADRANT PAIN*
4. Very abrupt severe pain?	Volvulus Intra-abdominal bleeding Ruptured ectopic pregnancy Rupture of pelvic/colonic abscess	Pulmonary embolism Myocardial infarction Pneumothorax Ruptured esophagus Perforated duodenal ulcer Ruptured ectopic pregnancy Ruptured tubal abscess Ureteral stone Renal infarction	Pulmonary embolism Myocardial infarction Pneumothorax Ruptured esophagus Perforated ulcer Renal infarction Ruptured spleen Ectopic pregnancy Tubal abscess Ureteral stone
X-ray findings?	Pelvic ultrasound too	X-ray chest, abdomen ECG	X-ray chest, abdomen ECG

	RIGHT LOWER QUADRANT PAIN*	LEFT LOWER QUADRANT PAIN*
1. Shocky? No	Ruptured ectopic pregnancy Pelvic bleeding Perforated duodenal ulcer Aortoiliac dissection Perforated appendix Pyelonephritis/sepsis	Ruptured ectopic pregnancy Pelvic bleeding Aortoiliac dissection Perforated colon Pyelonephritis with sepsis Perforated ulcer Sigmoid diverticulitis with sepsis
2. Peritoneal signs? No	Acute appendicitis Perforated duodenal ulcer Acute cholecystitis Acute Crohn's disease Cecal diverticulitis Cecal carcinoma with perforation Tubo-ovarian abscess/acute PID Meckel's diverticulitis	Acute diverticulitis Left-sided appendicitis Colon carcinoma with pericolonic abscess Tubo-ovarian abscess/acute PID
3. Abdominal distention? No	Cecal volvulus Large bowel obstruction Pelvic-retroperitoneal hemorrhage Renal/colonic/pelvic mass (Table 11–15) Ectopic pregnancy Intrauterine pregnancy Constipation	Volvulus Pelvic/retroperitoneal hemorrhage Renal/colonic/pelvic mass (Table 11–15) Large bowel obstruction Ectopic pregnancy Intrauterine pregnancy Constipation Fecal impaction
4. Very abrupt severe pain?	Ruptured ectopic pregnancy Ruptured pelvic/colonic abscess Perforated duodenal ulcer Aortoiliac dissection Ureteral stone Spontaneous abortion Perforated pelvic appendix Renal/bowel infarction Hemorrhagic or ruptured ovarian cyst Ovarian torsion Strangulated hernia	Similar to right lower quadrant pain, except perforated duodenal ulcer rarely Perforated colon more often
X-ray findings?	Pelvic ultrasound too	Pelvic ultrasound too

*See also Figure 11–3.

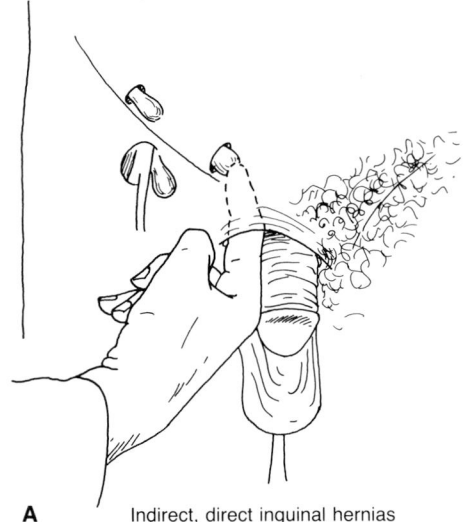

FIGURE 11–8. Hernias. *A*, In the male, indirect and direct inguinal hernias are most common. These are palpable above the inguinal ligament. The examiner's finger here palpates a direct inguinal hernia (extruding from the external inguinal ring) by invaginating the scrotal sac into the inguinal canal. An indirect hernia (extruding from the internal inguinal ring) lies lateral and superior to it. In the female, femoral hernias are more likely than inguinal hernias. The femoral hernia is palpable below the inguinal ligament, medial to the femoral artery and vein. Hernias of the abdominal wall are usually more obvious when the patient stands and/or strains the abdominal musculature. Umbilical (*C*) and postoperative (incisional) (*B*) hernias, as well as defects of the rectus abdominis muscle (*D*) and linea alba (*E*), are most common.

A   Indirect, direct inguinal hernias
Femoral hernia (arrow)

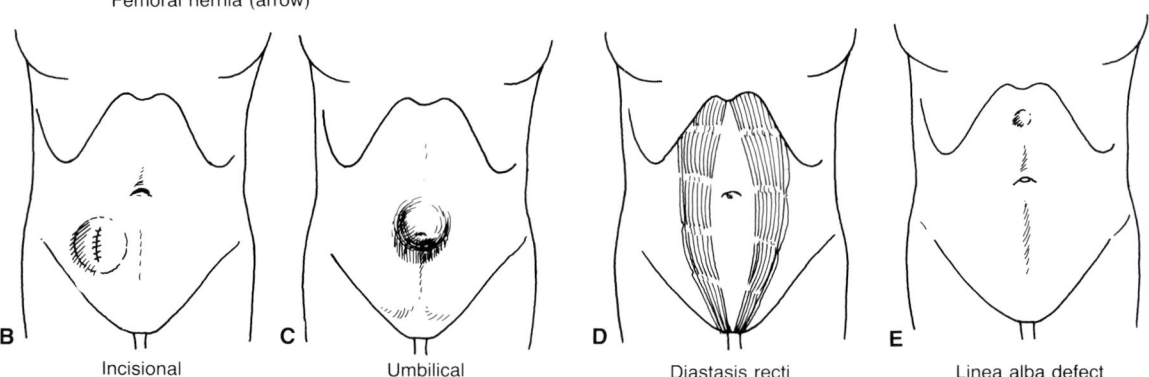

B   Incisional

C   Umbilical

D   Diastasis recti

E   Linea alba defect

surgery, *any* of the findings listed in Table 11–6—definite peritoneal signs, abdominal distention, or very severe pain and tenderness—mandate x-rays of the abdomen, a complete blood count, and urinalysis. Other tests (ECG, chest x-ray, serum amylase determination, abdominal/pelvic ultrasound, abdominal paracentesis, for example) may be indicated in specific situations. Such tests are briefly enumerated further in Table 11–10, page 556.

In Sally's case, there is no evidence of impending shock, peritoneal signs, or abdominal distention. Pain and tenderness are not very severe.

In addition to direct examination of the abdomen—observation, auscultation, percussion, and palpation—other indirect abdominal examinations are often very helpful. These include:

1. All potential hernia orifices should always be examined (Fig. 11–3). Inguinal hernias are most common in men; femoral hernias in women. Incisional hernias should be sought when pain overlies an operative scar; umbilical hernias usually bulge when the patient sits up, as does diastasis recti (a defect along the length of the rectus abdominis muscle).

Hernias are not uncommon causes of bowel obstruction (Table 11–5). Strangulation of a hernia—usually announced by severe local pain, inability to reduce the hernia, extreme focal tenderness often with peritoneal signs, with or without bowel obstruction and leukocytosis—is a surgical emergency. The nonobstructing hernia is usually asymptomatic or only mildly and intermittently uncomfortable, especially when the patient lifts or strains. Note that some hernias are internal (Table 11–5); these are not palpable.

The abdominal wall should also be examined for evidence of superficial muscular tenderness—localized pain and tenderness overlying some part of the rectus abdominis muscle is most common. Rectus abdominis contusion, tears, or hematomas usually present with highly localized tenderness or swelling, which are usually superficial, but which may be confused with local peritonitis, because pain and tenderness are localized and pain worsens with movement and may be associated with guarding or percussion tenderness.

In the patient with abdominal-wall pain, voluntary abdominal flexion or extension may exacerbate the pain. When a patient has highly localized abdominal pain and tenderness, but bowel sounds are active, the patient is not sick, and voluntary tensing of the abdominal muscles worsens the pain and the overlying tenderness, abdominal-wall disorders should be suspected.

> Palpation of inguinal and femoral canals bilaterally, while Sally stands and coughs, demonstrates that there are no hernias. There is no abdominal muscle tenderness while Sally sits up from the supine position—there are no umbilical hernias.

2. Examination of the back can be enlightening in some patients. Unilateral flank tenderness suggests renal/ureteral disease (stone, infection, infarct, tumor). Impaired back range of motion may implicate a thoracic or lumbar spine disorder that can occasionally cause primarily anterior (or radicular) abdominal pain. The elderly patient with osteoporotic kyphoscoliosis is a common victim. Hip disease may refer pain to the groin or lower abdomen—range of motion and palpation will help exclude degenerative joint disease, aseptic necrosis, and localized bursitis of the hips in such circumstances.

The obturator sign (Fig. 11–9A)—hypogastric abdominal pain during hip range of motion, especially flexion/internal rotation—may indicate either hip disease or irritation of the obturator internus muscle in the pelvis. Pelvic appendicitis, a pelvic abscess, or pelvic hemorrhage may be suggested by this maneuver. A rare obturator hernia may also be thus suspected.

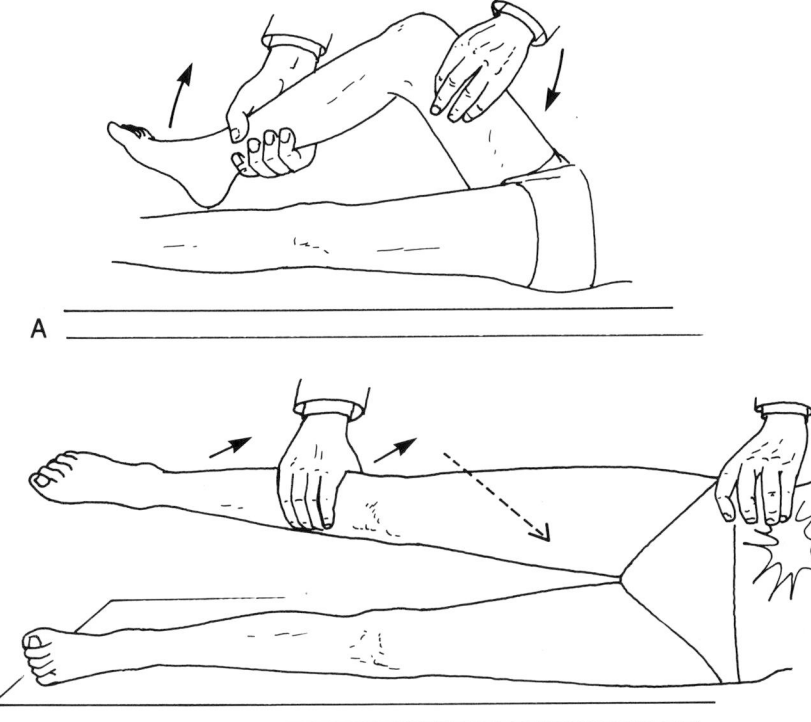

FIGURE 11–9. *A*, The obturator sign. Pain occurs when the hip is flexed and rotated. Internal rotation is most likely to cause pain due to pelvic or retroperitoneal disease or both. *B*, The psoas sign may be performed passively or actively. The hip is passively extended, thus stretching the psoas muscle (*solid arrow*). The hip is actively flexed, thus tensing the psoas muscle (*dotted arrow*).

The psoas sign (Fig. 11–9B) will elicit pain when an otherwise occult inflammatory process in the retroperitoneum or pelvis irritates the psoas muscle. Forceful hip flexion against resistance or passive hip extension stresses the psoas muscle—contiguous inflammation (classically with a psoas abscess) will induce pain with this maneuver.

> **The back and flanks are nontender. Hip range of motion is normal bilaterally, except that the obturator test on the right appears to slightly worsen Sally's discomfort. The psoas test is negative.**

3. Pelvic examination must be performed in all women with abdominal pain (especially those with lower abdominal pain, but even upper abdominal pain may have a pelvic source—Table 11–6). A variety of pelvic disorders comprise the majority of causes of lower abdominal pain in women— palpation (or absence) of localized tenderness or masses on pelvic examination is always crucial diagnostic information in such patients.

Bimanual palpation will be most revealing when the right hand is used internally to examine the right side of the pelvis and the left hand to examine the left (Fig. 11–10).

Genital and prostate examinations are crucial in all men with abdominal pain. Genital disorders are much less common causes of abdominal pain in men than are pelvic diseases in women, but testicular torsion, epididymitis, orchitis, and prostatitis should never be missed (see Chapter 8, "Male Genitourinary Infections"). Rarely, an undescended (intra-abdominal) testis will be discovered, or a testicular carcinoma will be palpated in a young male.

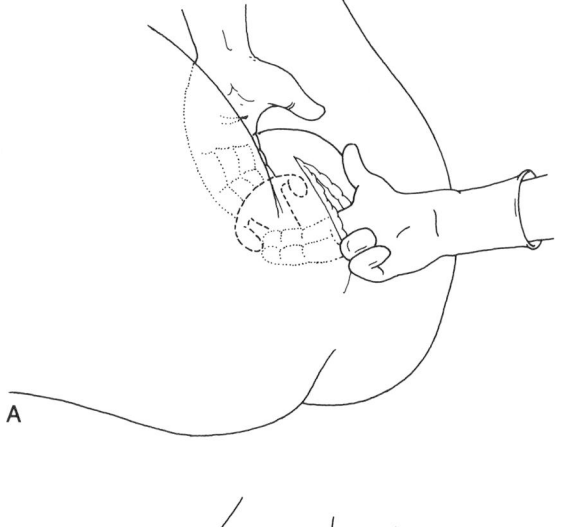

A

B

FIGURE 11–10. Bimanual pelvic examination. Pelvic organs will be adequately examined only by using both hands simultaneously, one internally, the other externally. Pelvic structures on the right are most easily examined with the examiner's right hand situated internally; structures on the left are easiest to feel with the left (internal) hand. A, Palpation of the right ovary and Fallopian tube. B, Palpation of the left tubo-ovarian structures.

**TABLE 11–7. CAUSES OF ABDOMINAL PAIN ASSOCIATED
WITH HEME-POSITIVE STOOL**

Esophagitis	Diverticulosis
Gastritis	Diverticulitis
Peptic ulcer	Meckel's diverticulum
Inflammatory bowel disease	Bacterial dysentery
Intestinal neoplasm	Amebiasis
Intestinal infarction or strangulation	Stercoral ulceration with constipation

4. Rectal examination is an essential part of the abdominal examination. The presence of blood in the stool always implicates the intestine as the site of disease (Table 11–7). Fecal impaction, rectal carcinoma, and inflammatory anorectal diseases can also be readily identified with the palpating finger. Rectal tenderness will be found when any localized perirectal inflammatory process is present (diverticular abscess, appendicitis, pelvic abscess, for example).

> Pelvic examination reveals normal external genitalia. The cervix appears normal but is moderately tender to manual palpation and manipulation. The uterus is normal in size and position, as are both ovaries and fallopian tubes, but there is moderate adnexal tenderness, more on the right than the left. Rectal examination is nontender. Stool is brown and Hematest negative.

5. Complete physical examination should be briefly reviewed in all patients with acute abdominal pain. Restricting the physical examination to the abdomen and pelvis will occasionally miss important clues that can suggest the cause of abdominal pain. As Table 11–8 suggests, a variety of extra-abdominal findings will occasionally suggest a specific diagnosis; most of these, importantly, are nonsurgical conditions.

> Examination of head, ears, eyes, nose, throat, lungs, and heart is normal. There is no lymphadenopathy. The aortic pulsation and all pulses are normal. There is no edema.

Thus the history and physical examination in Sally's case point to an inflammatory process of some intra-abdominal organ(s) in the right lower quadrant or pelvis. There is no physical evidence of peritoneal irritation, bowel obstruction, a localized (abdominal or pelvic) mass, intestinal bleeding, or extra-abdominal disease. These findings do narrow the differential diagnosis considerably, but a specific diagnosis cannot yet be made (see page 557 and Table 11–11, pages 560 and 561).

The results of a few simple laboratory tests can help to further narrow the differential diagnosis.

> Flat and upright x-rays of the abdomen and pelvis are normal. The urinalysis is completely normal. The white blood count is 10,200 with 80 per cent polymorphonuclears, 20 per cent lymphocytes.

What does this mean?

Tests

1. The plain abdominal x-ray (flat plate, KUB, scout film) is normal in the great majority of patients with abdominal pain. In one study (Table 11–9) of 1780 patients in whom abdominal pain was evaluated in an emergency

TABLE 11–8. EXTRA-ABDOMINAL PHYSICAL FINDINGS IN ACUTE ABDOMINAL PAIN

PHYSICAL FINDINGS	SUGGESTED DIAGNOSES
Very high temperature (> 103°F) and rigors	Cholangitis; pyelonephritis; peritonitis; intra-abdominal abscess; pneumonia; pelvic infection
Hypertension	Myocardial infarction; aortic dissection; abdominal aortic aneurysm; uremia. Rarely: acute glomerulonephritis; acute porphyria; renal infarction; vasculitis (SLE, polyarteritis)
Orthostatic hypotension	Blood loss or fluid loss; acute adrenal hemorrhage
Lymphadenopathy	Mononucleosis (spleen ruptured?); lymphoma; hepatitis
Pulse deficits	Aortic dissection; aortic aneurysm and/or thrombosis
Vascular bruits	Aortic dissection or aneurysm; dissection or aneurysm of splenic, renal, or iliac arteries; vascular tumor (hepatoma)
Friction rubs	Pericarditis; pleuritis; pulmonary embolism; subphrenic abscess; liver abscess/liver tumor; Fitz-Hugh–Curtis syndrome
Cardiac findings (atrial fibrillation, valvular disease, congestive heart failure)	Embolization to bowel, spleen, kidney?; mesenteric ischemia (arterial or venous) due to low cardiac output
Pleural effusion	Pneumonia; pulmonary embolism; subphrenic abscess; pancreatitis; esophageal rupture; ovarian tumor
Breast tenderness	Pregnancy (uterine or ectopic)
Flank tenderness	Pyelonephritis, kidney stone, renal infarct, renal vein thrombosis
Unilateral leg edema	Iliac phlebitis, pelvic neoplasm
Bilateral edema	Abdominal pain due to liver disease, congestive heart failure, renal disease, renal vein thrombosis
Ecchymoses	Henoch-Schönlein purpura; acute pancreatitis (Grey-Turner's sign); intra-abdominal bleeding; acute leukemia
Jaundice	Hepatobiliary disease; hemolytic crisis
Dark urine	Bile: hepatobiliary disease Blood: kidney stone; renal infarct; pyelonephritis; cystitis; acute glomerulonephritis; renal vein thrombosis; Henoch-Schönlein purpura; vasculitis Other: Possibly hemoglobinuria, myoglobinuria, porphyria?
Lipemia retinalis	Hyperlipidemic pancreatitis; diabetic ketoacidosis
Mental status deficit	Shock; abdominal epilepsy; multisystem disease (connective tissue disease or vasculitis)

TABLE 11–9. PLAIN ABDOMINAL X-RAYS IN EVALUATION OF ABDOMINAL PAIN IN 1780 PATIENTS

ABNORMALITY		No.
Renal calculi		46
Bowel obstruction		34
Gallstones		8
Free air		3
Thumbprinting		3
Pancreatic calcifications		3
Ileus		78
Generalized	50	
Localized	28	
Total		175 (10%)

Adapted from reference 17.

room, only 10 per cent of such x-rays were abnormal.[17] Many of the observed radiographic abnormalities were nonspecific (for example, ileus). Because of the low yield of these x-rays, the authors of this study suggest that the plain film of the abdomen is unlikely to alter diagnostic/therapeutic decisions except when physical examination reveals marked abdominal tenderness or when patients are clinically suspected of having bowel obstruction, renal/ureteral calculi, abdominal trauma, mesenteric ischemia, or gallbladder disease. Of note is the fact that most such cases will be detected (or suspected) by the brief scheme outlined in Table 11–6, i.e., the absence of peritoneal signs, abdominal distention, shock, or severe/abrupt onset of abdominal pain will usually predict a nondiagnostic x-ray.

It must be remembered, however, that the clinician may find abdominal x-rays helpful even if they are not specifically diagnostic.[18] Thus, the need for abdominal x-rays in the patient with acute abdominal pain must always be individualized. (In Sally's case, one can easily argue that an x-ray is superfluous.)

Figure 11–11 through 11–18 illustrate some of the abnormalities that may be diagnostically helpful when recognized on the plain abdominal x-ray.

When x-ray is performed, for whatever reason, what is the "reassurance value" of a normal x-ray?* In general, a normal plain abdominal x-ray excludes only free air (Fig. 11–11) (usually due to a perforated viscus) and bowel obstruction (Fig. 11–15) with or without volvulus (Figs. 11–16 and 11–18) (each of these is usually strongly suspected by the history and physical examination anyway). Gallstones (Fig. 11–13) are seen on the x-ray in only 10 to 15 per cent of cases. An appendiceal fecalith (Fig. 11–12) is seen in only 5 per cent of patients with acute appendicitis. Kidney stones (Fig. 11–14) are seen often on plain films—in perhaps 70 per cent of cases—but many stones are not radiopaque. Localized ileus is a common finding in acute pancreatitis and other focal inflammatory disorders, but such findings are usually nonspecific. The absence of thumbprinting (Fig. 11–17) by no means excludes mesenteric ischemia.

Thus the plain abdominal x-ray is only occasionally helpful (Table 11–9)—and usually when clinical findings are dramatic anyway.

2. Urinalysis is helpful in several ways and should, in general, be performed in all patients with acute abdominal pain. The following may be noted.

Microscopic hematuria (greater than 3 red cells per high-power field) will be found in perhaps 90 per cent of cases of acute ureteral calculus. The absence of red cells in the urine is usually strong evidence against a kidney stone, but a normal urinalysis must be disregarded when clinical evidence is compelling (for example, the patient with a past history of kidney stones and sudden onset of abdominal and flank pain). Hematuria is also common during urinary tract infections (cystitis or pyelonephritis), which are common causes of abdominal pain in females. Renal infarction, renal vein thrombosis, acute glomerulonephritis, and urorenal neoplasms will be rare causes of abdominal pain with hematuria.

Microscopic pyuria (greater than 5 white blood cells per high-power field) is virtually universal in patients with acute bacterial urinary infections (cystitis or pyelonephritis). The absence of white blood cells in the urine usually excludes urinary infections as the cause of abdominal pain. Many women will have *asymptomatic* bacteriuria or pyuria, however; thus these findings are never themselves diagnostic of the cause of abdominal pain.

---

*See also Chapter 4, Headache, pages 197 to 198, regarding "reassurance value."

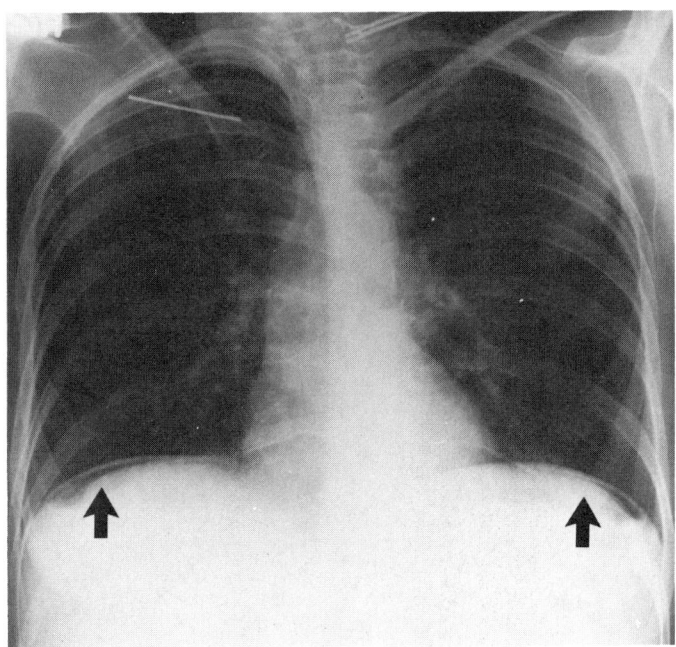

FIGURE 11–11. This 38-year-old woman presented with very abrupt onset of severe epigastric pain followed by a period of 6 to 8 hours during which her pain somewhat diminished. Pain then increased dramatically over the next 6 hours, and, on examination, she was in severe pain, with absent bowel sounds and diffuse peritoneal signs. The x-ray demonstrates free air under both diaphragms (arrows). A perforated duodenal ulcer was found at surgery.

FIGURE 11–12. This 26-year-old man described the gradual onset of anorexia, nausea, and vague periumbilical abdominal pain. Twenty-four hours later, the pain was much more severe in the right lower quadrant, where localized peritoneal signs were apparent. The flat plate reveals a huge calcified density in the right lower quadrant that proved to be an appendiceal fecalith at surgery.

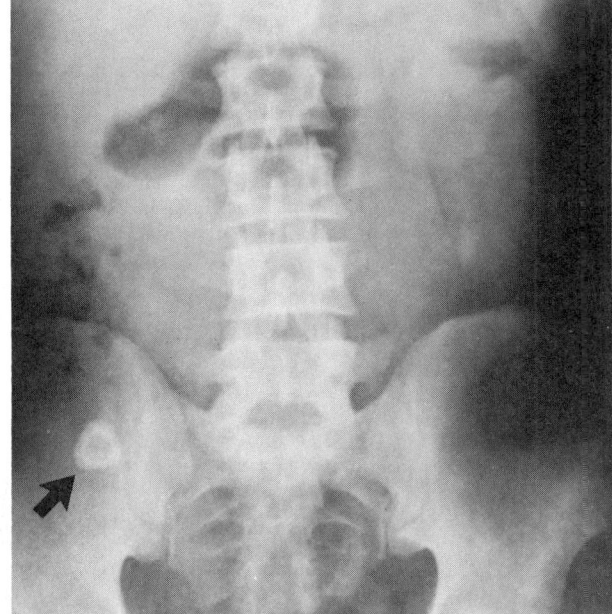

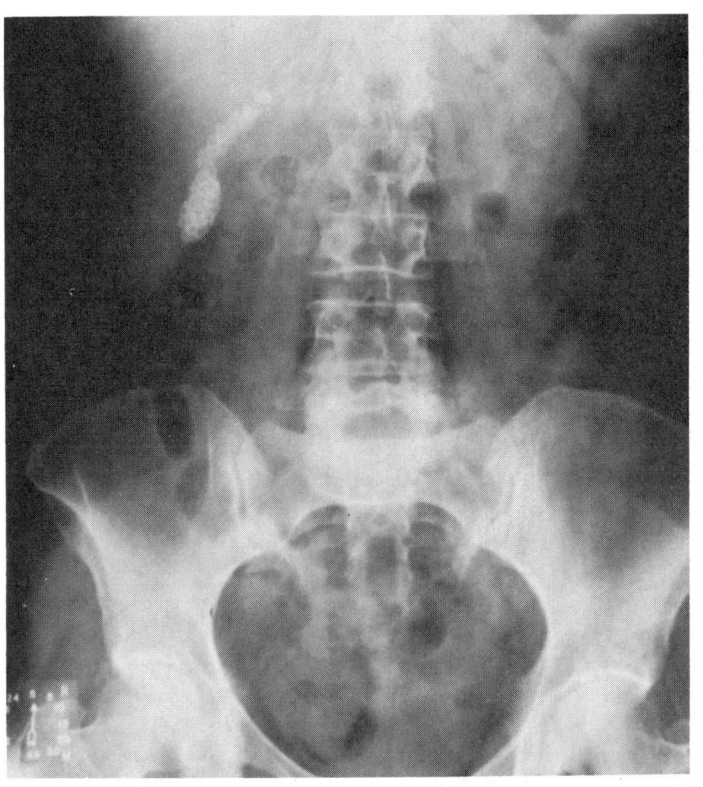

FIGURE 11–13. This 42-year-old obese woman described 4 hours of severe epigastric abdominal pain associated with nausea and vomiting. Examination of the abdomen was unremarkable. A flat plate demonstrates multiple gallstones outlying the gallbladder. The patient's pain resolved spontaneously after a total of 6 hours. This episode of biliary colic was the third such episode in the previous 18 months. Elective cholecystectomy was performed.

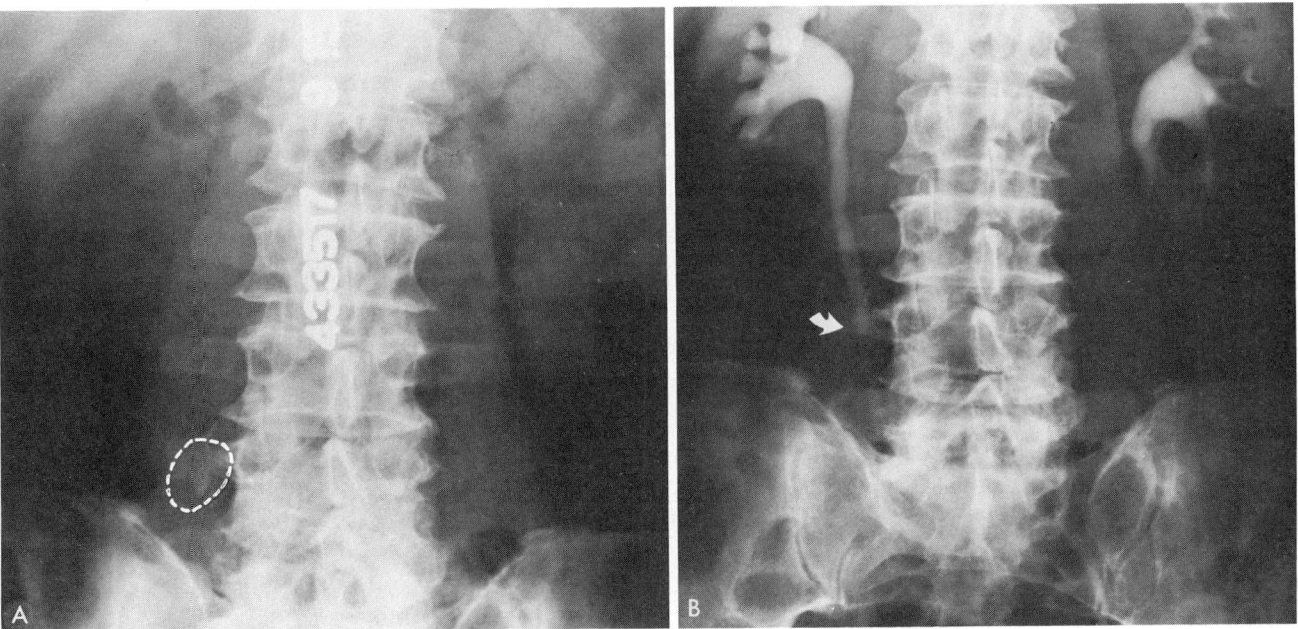

FIGURE 11-14. This 43-year-old man developed very severe right-sided abdominal pain radiating into the right groin. There was prominent nausea and vomiting but minimal back pain and no abdominal distention or peritoneal signs. There were no urinary complaints, but the urinalysis revealed microscopic hematuria. The abdominal flat plate (A) reveals a radiopaque calculus adjacent to the fourth lumbar vertebra on the right (circled). Intravenous pyelogram (B) demonstrates complete obstruction of the right ureter at that level (arrow). The patient was unable to pass the stone spontaneously. Retrograde retrieval of the stone was accomplished 24 hours later.

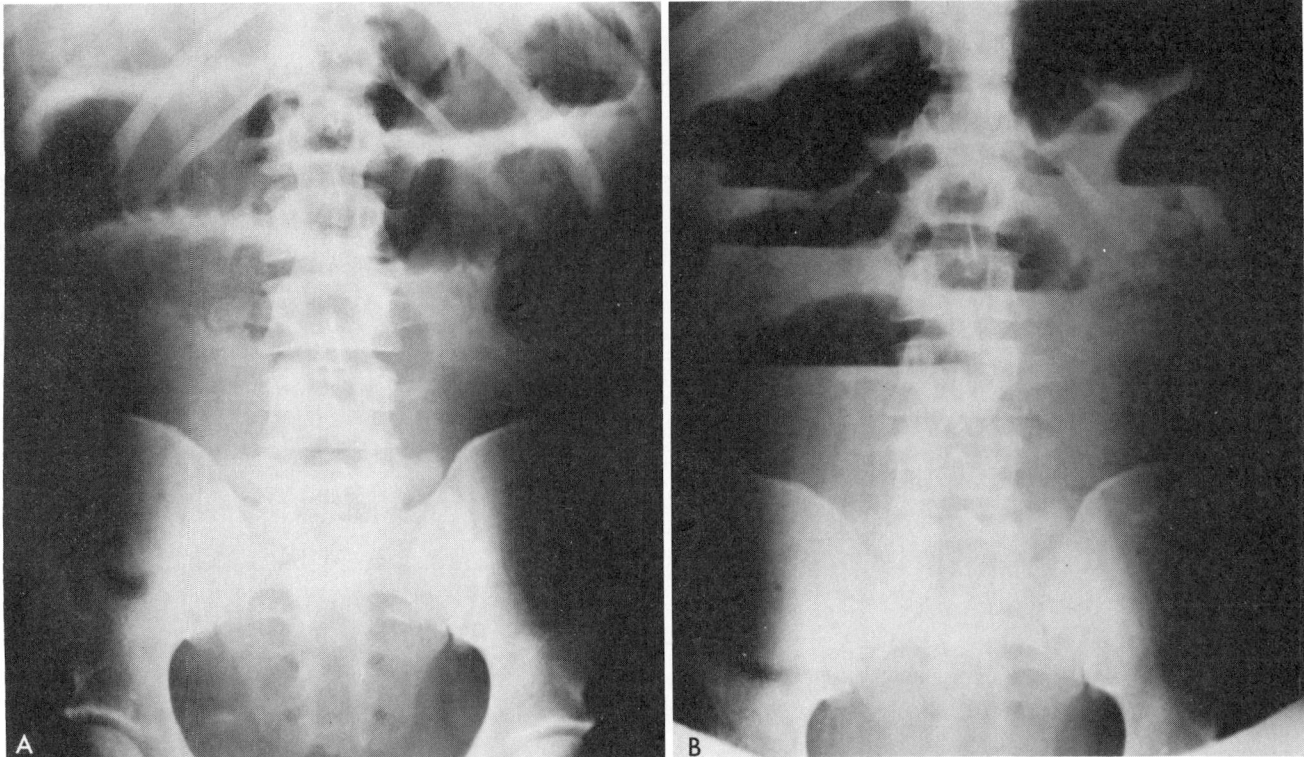

FIGURE 11-15. This 30-year-old man described progressively worsening periumbilical abdominal pain over the previous 24 hours. He described intermittent "waves" of crampy pain, lasting a few minutes, followed by pain-free intervals until the next "attack" of crampy pain. Repetitive vomiting then ensued. Examination revealed the abdomen to be moderately distended. High-pitched, hyperactive bowel sounds could be heard during the patient's attacks of intermittent pain. The abdominal flat plate (A) demonstrates dilated loops of small intestine that, on upright film (B), depict typical air-fluid levels in the small bowel. Laparotomy demonstrated obstruction of the distal small bowel due to postoperative adhesions (from a prior appendectomy).

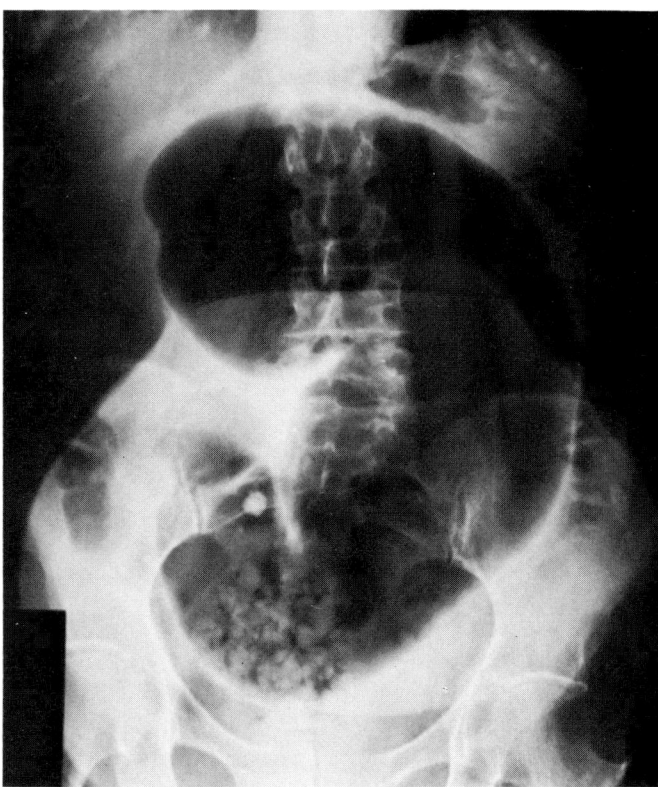

FIGURE 11–16. This 80-year-old woman described sudden onset of diffuse abdominal pain, initially worse in the lower abdomen. Examination revealed the abdomen to be distended and tympanitic. Bowel sounds were absent, but there were no peritoneal signs. The abdominal flat plate reveals the classic "reverse C loop" typical of cecal volvulus. Surgical decompression was required.

FIGURE 11–17. This 62-year-old man with longstanding rheumatic heart disease and atrial fibrillation developed very abrupt onset of excruciatingly severe central abdominal pain. Examination revealed mild abdominal distention and diffuse tenderness but no peritoneal signs. Abdominal flat plate reveals a greatly dilated loop of small intestine with "thumbprinting" (arrows) (due to edema of the bowel wall). An arteriogram demonstrated an embolus in the superior mesenteric artery. The patient did well after surgical embolectomy.

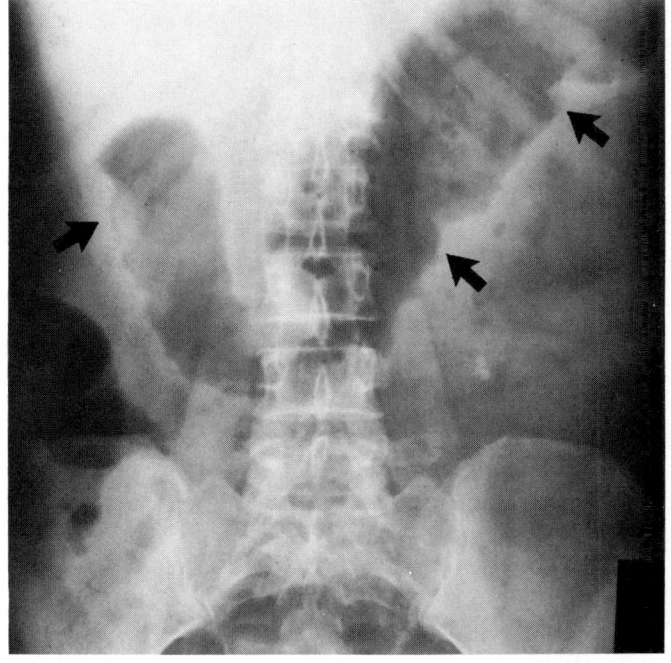

Glycosuria and ketonuria suggest diabetic ketoacidosis, which not infrequently presents with acute abdominal pain. Ketonuria without glycosuria usually reflects decreased food intake (starvation ketosis) and is nonspecific. Bilirubinuria implies a direct serum bilirubin value greater than 3 mg per 100 ml—this is a major clue to the presence of hepatobiliary disease (especially if visible jaundice is mild or equivocal). Proteinuria is nonspecific—it is commonly encountered in many types of acute illness, especially in patients with high fever, congestive heart failure, seizures, or pneumonia[19]—but heavy (4+) proteinuria should suggest intrinsic renal disease. Cellular (especially

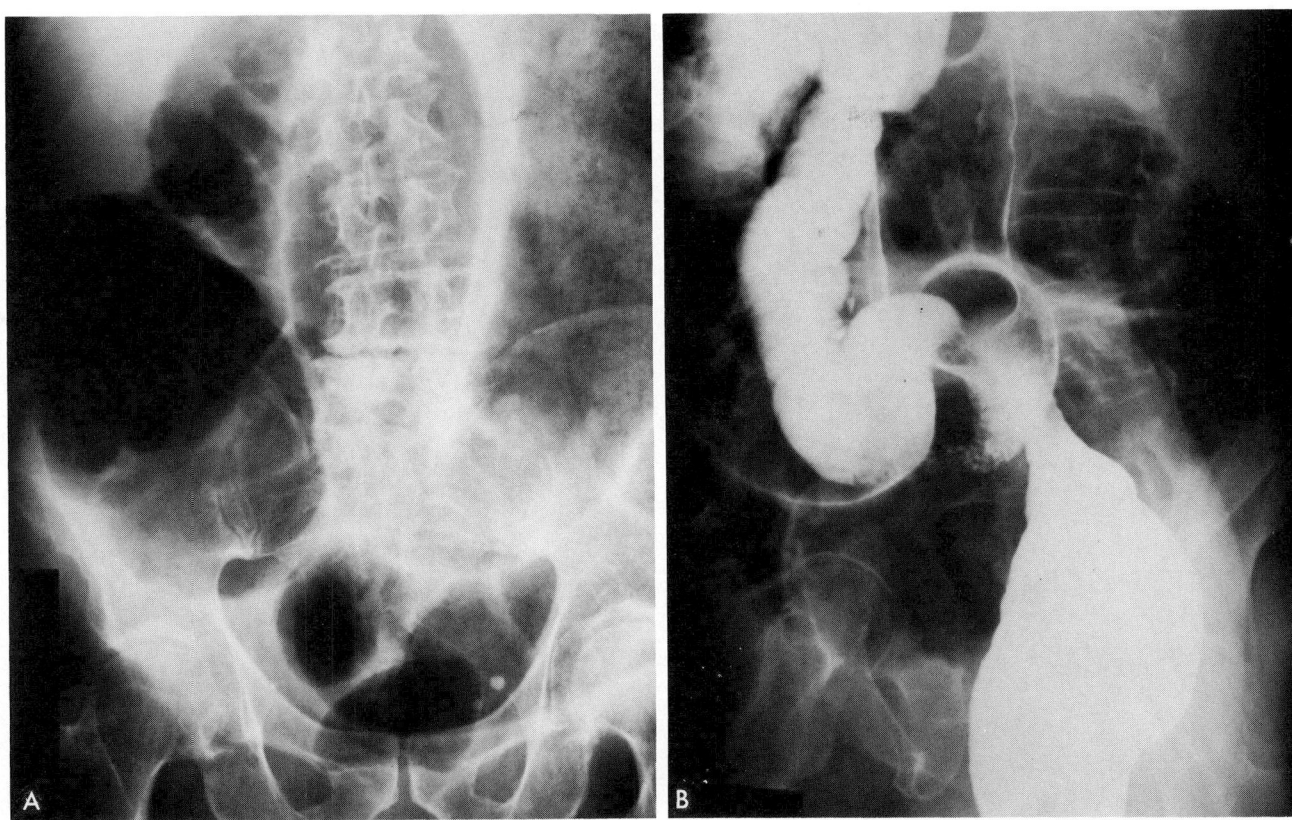

FIGURE 11–18. This 60-year-old woman described gradual onset of moderately severe lower abdominal pain over the previous 24 to 36 hours. Examination revealed a distended abdomen that was tympanitic but without peritoneal signs. A flat plate of the abdomen demonstrates marked dilatation of the large bowel (*A*). The barium enema (*B*) (lateral view) demonstrates torsion of the sigmoid colon that caused this large bowel obstruction—sigmoid volvulus. The barium enema relieved the obstruction. Surgery was not necessary.

red cell) casts should suggest acute glomerulonephritis, vasculitis (polyarteritis, systemic lupus erythematosus), Henoch-Schönlein disease—all of which may occasionally present with acute abdominal pain. Pigmented urine that contains no blood or bile should suggest at least the possibility of hemoglobinuria (which may be seen in acute hemolytic crises causing abdominal pain), acute myoglobinuria, or, even more rarely, acute intermittent porphyria.

3. The white blood cell count is often a routine component of the evaluation of acute abdominal pain, but its utility is sometimes misunderstood. In general, acute inflammatory disease causes leukocytosis, i.e., an elevation of the total white blood count (greater than 10,000 mm³) or a "left shift" (greater than 80 per cent polymorphonuclears), or both. Thus the great majority of patients with acute appendicitis (95 per cent)[5, 20, 21] or acute cholecystitis (90 per cent) will demonstrate leukocytosis. However, leukocytosis is nonspecific and may also be seen with a variety of nonsurgical diseases: pelvic inflammatory disease, gastroenteritis, alcoholic hepatitis, pyelonephritis, and mesenteric adenitis, for example. In addition, some patients with a surgical abdomen will have a normal white blood count—early bowel obstruction, ectopic pregnancy, abdominal aortic aneurysms, and rare cases of appendicitis and cholecystitis are among them.

Thus the white blood count is a helpful ancillary test that usually serves to confirm clinical impressions, but that should be disregarded when clinical findings are at variance with it. The patient with clinical acute appendicitis needs surgery, whatever the white blood count.[21, 22] The patient with clinical gastroenteritis should simply be observed, even if the white blood count is elevated.

Extreme leukocytosis (greater than 20,000) is much more specific for serious disease—especially localized peritonitis, bowel strangulation or infarction—but such extreme elevations are seen only uncommonly in patients with acute abdominal pain.

4. Other Tests. Many other tests can be useful in the diagnostic approach to the patient with acute abdominal pain. Table 11–10 enumerates some of these. There are usually specific indications for these tests, but each should be selected with a particular diagnosis or differential diagnosis in mind. Some of these examinations—especially barium studies and abdominal ultrasound examinations—are more helpful in the patient with chronic or recurrent abdominal pain (see page 577).

TABLE 11–10. TESTS IN ACUTE ABDOMINAL PAIN

Test	In Suspected Diagnosis of	Usually Excluded by Normal Study	Cost
Plain abdominal x-ray	Perforated viscus; bowel obstruction; volvulus; kidney stone; trauma; ischemia	Perforated viscus; bowel obstruction; volvulus	$47
Urinalysis	Kidney stone; urinary infection; pyelonephritis; diabetic ketoacidosis; intrinsic renal disease	Urinary infection; ketoacidosis; intrinsic acute renal disease	$8
CBC with differential count	Acute inflammatory disease; especially "surgical abdomen": acute appendicitis; acute cholecystitis; bowel strangulation	Intra-abdominal abscess; peritonitis; bowel strangulation/infarction; acute appendicitis (5 to 10% false negative); acute cholecystitis (10% false negative)	$13
Serum amylase	Pancreatitis (see also Table 11–23)	Acute pancreatitis	$21
Pregnancy test Urinary HCG	Intrauterine or	Gestation > 6 weeks	$10
Beta-subunit assay	Extrauterine pregnancy	Earlier pregnancy	$36
Abdominal ultrasound	Aortic aneurysm; gallstones; causes of jaundice?	Aortic aneurysm; gallstones; bile duct obstruction	$100–200*
Pelvic ultrasound	"Surgical pelvic disease": ectopic pregnancy, ovarian torsion, ovarian mass, ovarian hemorrhage, tubal abscess, threatened/incomplete abortion	"Surgical pelvic disease"	$80–160*
Biliary scan	Acute cholecystitis	Acute cholecystitis	$210
Upper GI series	Acute peptic ulcer disease	Gastric/duodenal ulcer (10–15% false negative)	$130
Barium enema†	Sigmoid volvulus (therapeutic)	Colon carcinoma (15% false negative); diverticulosis/diverticulitis	$130
Intravenous pyelography	Kidney/ureteral stone or obstruction	Stone/obstruction	$160
Visceral angiography	Dissecting aneurysm; leaking abdominal aortic aneurysm; mesenteric embolism/thrombosis; renal or splenic infarction; splenic rupture; severe gastrointestinal bleeding		$300–700*

*Cost depends on extent of examination.
†Single contrast study.

In Sally's case the normal urinalysis helps to exclude consideration of acute urinary disorders. The normal abdominal x-ray excludes the (clinically very unlikely) possibility of bowel obstruction or volvulus. The equivocal white blood count adds little to an equivocal physical examination.

> Cultures for gonorrhea are obtained from the cervix and rectum. Sally is told that her pain is probably due to mild inflammation of the pelvic organs, perhaps related to her recent menstrual period or perhaps due to an infection. Antibiotics are recommended, pending the results of the culture.
>
> Sally says that her menstrual pains bother her at the beginning of her period, not at the end. She says there is "no chance of venereal disease" since she and her husband have sexual relations only with each other. She refuses an antibiotic, saying, "I will wait until the tests are back. I just wanted to be sure that I did not have appendicitis."
>
> Sally is asked to return in 48 hours for a repeat examination, or before if she worsens.

NOTE

1. We have not made a specific diagnosis. As Figure 11–1 suggests, this is not an uncommon situation in the patient with abdominal pain. This does not mean that a rigorous attempt to achieve a specific diagnosis is unimportant. As Cope says,

> There are . . . occasions when, with some indefinite symptoms, there may be a tendency to wait for the development of clearer indications, to see if the condition will not improve spontaneously, and generally to temporize. (This) . . . course of conduct is the least justifiable, for it is a wise plan always to make a very thorough attempt to elucidate the problem when the patient is seen for the first time. Though in quite a number of cases it is impossible to be sure of the diagnosis, yet it is a good habit to come to a decision in each case; and it will be found that, after a short time, provided that no method of diagnosis be neglected, the percentage of correct diagnoses will rapidly increase.[23]

2. The most likely presumptive diagnosis here is pelvic inflammatory disease. (See below.) Figure 11–19 summarizes the clinical approach to acute (nontraumatic) abdominal pain.

3. Every patient with unexplained abdominal pain should be followed and reexamined. The logistics of follow-up depend on the specific clinical situation. As noted above and in Figure 11–19 when the patient is "sick," consultation with a surgeon or observation in the hospital usually makes sense.

In general, the longer the duration of pain, the less specific its location and the less localizing the physical examination, the less urgent is consultation or hospital observation. Thus the patient with vague abdominal pain of several days' (or longer) duration whose physical examination does not reveal localized tenderness, abdominal distention, or an abnormal mass can usually be followed as an outpatient.

Familiarity with the natural history of different disease processes is crucial here. For example, the patient with early appendicitis, incipient bowel obstruction, subacute mesenteric ischemia, or unruptured ectopic pregnancy may present with nonspecific midline visceral abdominal pain and an unimpressive physical examination. Repeat examination in the subsequent 12 to 24 hours will often be much more worrisome in such patients. Consider, for example, as in Sally's case, the following.

FIGURE 11–19. Acute (nontraumatic) abdominal pain.

1. Where is the pain?

Initially?
Now?   Midline "visceral" pain?   Epigastric?
Radiation?   Periumbilical? ⎫ Figure 11–2
                                               Hypogastric?   ⎭

              Lateralized "parietal" pain? ──→ Which quadrant? ──→ Figure 11–3

2. Timing of pain: Very abrupt onset → or suddenly much worse! → Viscus perforation?
                                                                  Viscus obstruction?
                                                                  Acute vascular event?

                  Gradual onset → progressively worsening? → Inflammatory process?
                                                             Intestinal obstruction?

                  Duration <24 hours: Observe!
                            >72 hours: "Surgical" abdomen less likely

   N.B. Acute abdominal pain in an elderly patient? ⎫ "Serious" disease common
        Pain that awakens the patient from sleep!   ⎭

3. Severity of pain   Very severe, abruptly! → Perforated viscus
                                                      Acute vascular event

4. Associated symptoms   Diarrhea: Gastroenteritis? (Chapter 3)
                             Constipation: Table 11–1
                             Urinary symptoms: UTI? Prostatitis? (Chapters 6 and 8)
                             Pelvic symptoms: PID? Pregnancy?
                             Vomiting: Worry! (Table 11–2)
                             Anorexia: Nonspecific but "worrisome"
                             High fever/chills: Pyelonephritis, cholangitis, abscess,
                                                     pneumonia?
                             Respiratory symptoms: Referred pain from thorax?
                                                   Pleurisy? Pneumonia?

   N.B. Vomiting that precedes onset of
        pain usually implies "nonsurgical"
        disease!

5. Clinical setting: Previous history of stones, adhesions, ulcer, neoplasm, pelvic disease, and so on?
                     Recurrence?

                     Diabetic?   ⎫
                     Alcoholic? ⎪ Table 11–3
                     Ascites?   ⎬
                     Cardiac disease? ⎭

6. Physical examination: Vital signs: Hypotensive or "shocky"?
Peritoneal findings?
Abdominal distention? } Table 11–6
Pelvic/rectal exam!
Extra-abdominal clues (Table 11–8)?

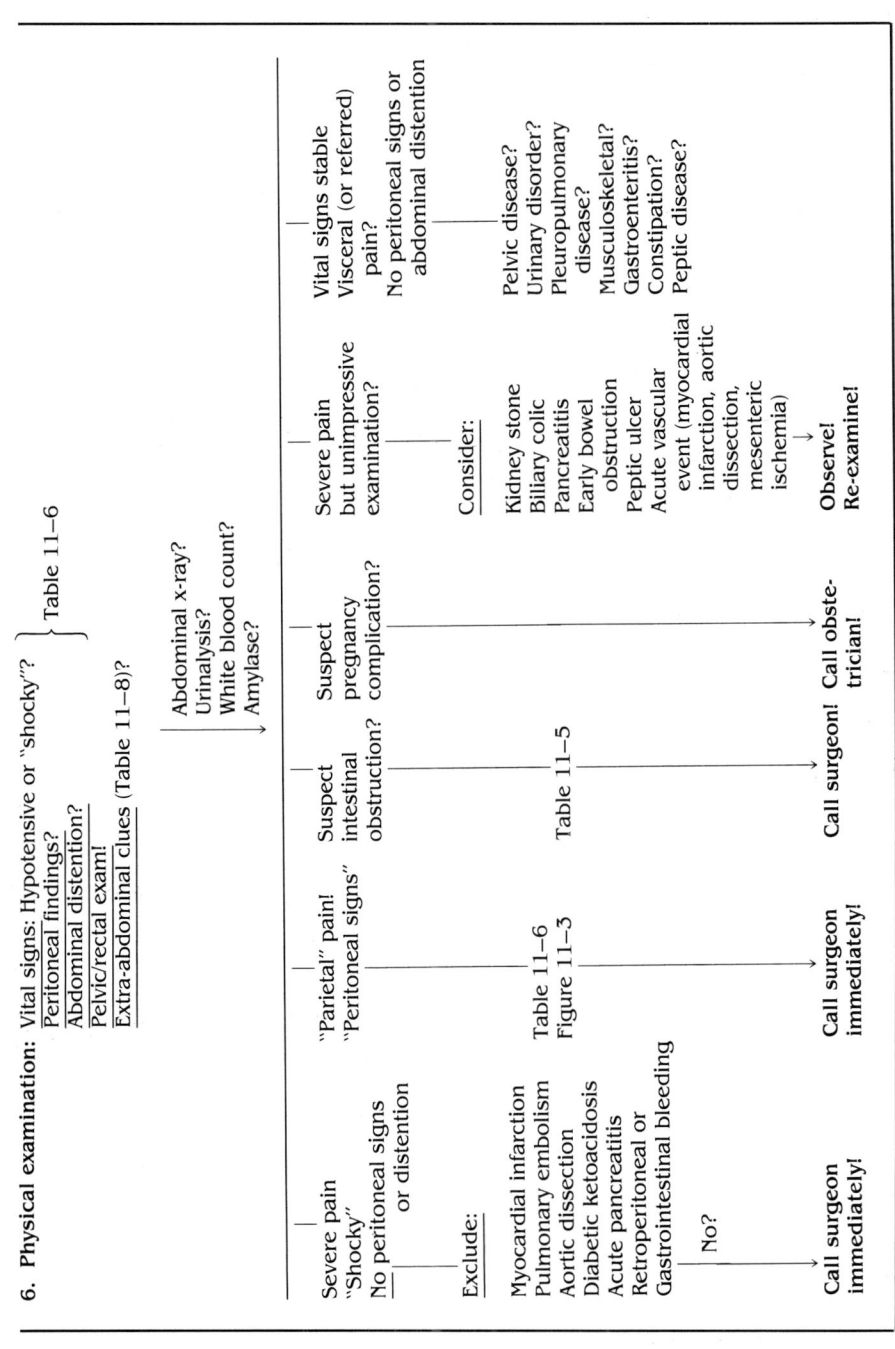

Abdominal x-ray?
Urinalysis?
White blood count?
Amylase?

Severe pain "Shocky" No peritoneal signs or distention	"Parietal" pain! "Peritoneal signs"	Suspect intestinal obstruction?	Suspect pregnancy complication?	Severe pain but unimpressive examination?	Vital signs stable Visceral (or referred) pain? No peritoneal signs or abdominal distention
Exclude:	Table 11–6 Figure 11–3	Table 11–5		Consider:	Pelvic disease? Urinary disorder? Pleuropulmonary disease? Musculoskeletal? Gastroenteritis? Constipation? Peptic disease?
Myocardial infarction Pulmonary embolism Aortic dissection Diabetic ketoacidosis Acute pancreatitis Retroperitoneal or Gastrointestinal bleeding				Kidney stone Biliary colic Pancreatitis Early bowel obstruction Peptic ulcer Acute vascular event (myocardial infarction, aortic dissection, mesenteric ischemia)	
No?					
Call surgeon immediately!	Call surgeon immediately!	Call surgeon!	Call obstetrician!	Observe! Re-examine!	

TABLE 11–11. DIFFERENTIAL DIAGNOSIS OF ACUTE RIGHT LOWER QUADRANT PAIN

DIAGNOSIS	SETTING	SYMPTOMS	SIGNS
Appendicitis*	Most often adolescents and young adults; any age (except infancy)	Midline abdominal pain (diffuse, periumbilical and/or epigastric), anorexia Nausea with or without vomiting Localized right lower quadrant pain	Early: may be normal examination After 12–24 hours: localized right lower quadrant tenderness, guarding Late: frank peritonitis and/or appendiceal/pelvic abscess
Ectopic pregnancy	Woman of childbearing age; history of PID, tubal pregnancy, or possibly tubal ligation	Menstrual period missed or late and/or vaginal spotting and/or pregnancy symptoms; nonspecific lower abdominal pain	Unruptured: extreme cervical tenderness and/or adnexal mass and/or cul-de-sac mass Ruptured: shock, abdominal distention, nonclotted blood at culdocentesis
Cecal volvulus[24]	More common in elderly	Acute, severe abdominal pain	Distention and/or localized tenderness; tympany
Strangulated hernia	Any age	Severe localized pain; generalized pain and distention with secondary bowel obstruction	Women: femoral; men: inguinal; distention if bowel obstruction coexists
Perforated duodenal ulcer[25]	Prior history of epigastric peptic symptoms and/or known ulcer	Abrupt onset; epigastric → right lower quadrant pain	Epigastric and right lower quadrant tenderness; possibly peritoneal signs, heme-positive stool
Ureteral calculus[9]	Any age; possibly past history of stones	Very severe pain with vomiting; usually flank pain, and/or testicular or groin radiation	Flank tenderness; vague abdominal tenderness; no peritoneal signs
Pyelonephritis; urinary infection (see Chap. 6)	Usually female	Dysuria, fever, flank pain	Flank tenderness; vague abdominal tenderness without peritoneal signs
Threatened abortion[26]	Young women	Period missed or late; vaginal spotting and/or pregnancy symptoms	Uterine tenderness; vaginal bleeding
Ovarian cyst: rupture/ hemorrhage	Usually young female often in latter half of menstrual cycle	Sudden onset unilateral pelvic pain (rarely shock due to extreme hemorrhage)	Adnexal tenderness and/or palpable ovarian mass
Pelvic inflammatory disease[27–31]	Young female, menses just completed Exposure to venereal disease?	Bilateral lower abdominal pain and/or fever, dyspareunia	Bilateral adnexal and cervical tenderness; possibly cervical discharge
Tubal abscess	Young female Exposure to venereal disease?	Bilateral lower abdominal pain and/or fever, dyspareunia	Unilateral tender adnexal mass
Mesenteric adenitis	Young patient with antecedent upper respiratory infection	Lower abdominal pain; appetite often normal; vomiting unusual; mimics appendicitis	Localized right lower quadrant tenderness; rarely, peritoneal findings
Others	**Mittelschmerz Dysmenorrhea Endometriosis Carcinoma of ovary or uterus**	**Meckel's diverticulum Crohn's disease Acute cholecystitis Cecal diverticulitis Cecal carcinoma and/or perforation Abdominal wall disorders (rectus hematoma, etc.)**	**Psoas bursitis Hip disease Iliac artery aneurysm/dissection Inguinal lymphadenitis Acute scrotal disease Iliofemoral thrombophlebitis**

*Retrocecal or pelvic appendicitis may be atypical; remember psoas test, obturator test, pelvic/rectal examination.

Acute Right Lower Quadrant Pain

Table 11–11 illustrates many of the disorders that should be considered in the patient with acute right lower quadrant pain. Usually the clinical setting, the severity and sequence of symptoms, careful examination, and routine tests will identify a specific diagnosis or at least greatly narrow the

DIAGNOSIS	X-RAY	WHITE BLOOD COUNT	URINALYSIS	DIAGNOSIS (dx) & TREATMENT (Rx)
Appendicitis*	Usually normal Fecalith rare (Fig. 11-12)	>10,000 and/or left shift in greater than 90% of adults	Usually normal	Laparotomy (dx and Rx)
Ectopic pregnancy	Usually normal	Variable	Normal	Pregnancy test and pelvic ultrasound and/or culdocentesis, laparoscopy, laparotomy. } (dx) Call gynecologist (Rx)
Cecal volvulus[24]	Diagnostic (Fig. 11-16)	Variable	Normal	X-ray (dx) Cecal decompression (Rx)
Strangulated hernia	Bowel obstruction? (Fig. 11-15)	Usually increased	Normal	Clinical examination (dx) Surgery (Rx)
Perforated duodenal ulcer[25]	Free air? (Fig. 11-11)	Usually increased	Normal	X-ray Upper GI series } (dx) Laparotomy Surgery, usually (Rx)
Ureteral calculus[9]	Opaque stone? (Fig. 11-14)	Variable; usually normal	Hematuria	IVP (dx) Retrieve stone versus spontaneous passage } (Rx)
Pyelonephritis; urinary infection (see Chap. 6)	Normal (unless stone)	Pyelonephritis: usually leukocytosis; cystitis: normal	Pyuria; bacteriuria; possibly white blood cell casts	Clinical findings and urinalysis } (dx) Urine culture Antibiotics (Rx)
Threatened abortion[26]	Normal or visible fetal parts	Normal	Normal	Positive pregnancy test } (dx) Pelvic ultrasound Call gynecologist (Rx)
Ovarian cyst: rupture/ hemorrhage	Normal	Normal	Normal	Negative pregnancy test } (dx) Pelvic ultrasound Laparoscopy
Pelvic inflammatory disease[27-31]	Normal	Variable	Normal or pyuria	Physical findings Cervical Gram's stain Gonococcal cultures } (dx) Normal pelvic ultrasound Antibiotic therapy (Rx)
Tubal abscess	Normal	Variable; usually increased	Normal or pyuria	Physical findings } (dx) Pelvic ultrasound Call gynecologist (Rx)
Mesenteric adenitis	Normal	Variable; usually normal	Normal	Improves with observation (dx and Rx)

*Retrocecal or pelvic appendicitis may be atypical; remember psoas test, obturator test, pelvic/rectal examination.

differential diagnosis. (In general, the differential diagnosis is much less extensive for males.)

Notice that in Sally's case several diagnoses can be dismissed as most unlikely:

There is no evidence of bowel obstruction on examination or x-ray. Cecal volvulus can be excluded in a patient with a normal x-ray. A strangulated external hernia can be excluded by careful physical examination (Fig. 11–8). A strangulated internal hernia cannot be so readily excluded, but the absence of peritoneal signs and bowel obstruction makes this unlikely.

The absence of hematuria, as well as the normal x-ray, makes a kidney stone highly unlikely, especially since the clinical suspicion is low in this case. The normal urinalysis and absence of fever and urinary symptoms virtually exclude the possibility of acute pyelonephritis and other urinary infections. As illustrated in Figure 11–3, duodenal ulcer may perforate and dissect into the right "gutter" of the abdomen, but a prior history of peptic symptoms and more localizing findings are almost always found in this unusual situation. Similarly, cecal diverticulitis or a pericolonic abscess with colon cancer will cause more localized tenderness (and almost always occur in an older patient population). Acute Crohn's disease cannot be excluded, but there is no specific reason to consider it here (in the absence of fever, diarrhea, heme-positive stool, or prior symptoms). Meckel's diverticulitis is a very rare condition whose clinical presentation usually mimics acute appendicitis. Acute cholecystitis can cause pain in the lower abdomen when the gallbladder is unusually low lying, but pelvic tenderness (in Sally's case) would not be expected in acute cholecystitis.

There is no evidence of an extra-abdominal (back, hips, thoracic) disorder.

In this case, then, as Table 11–11 suggests, the differential diagnosis must include a variety of acute pelvic disorders and acute appendicitis. The absence of a localized adnexal mass or prominent unilateral pelvic tenderness is usually evidence against ectopic pregnancy, a tubo-ovarian abscess, or torsion, rupture, or hemorrhage of an ovarian cyst or neoplasm. (The adequacy of the pelvic examination—Figure 11–10—is obviously the crucial issue here.) The absence of prior symptoms does not suggest endometriosis; the normal period makes pregnancy or its complications unlikely (but not impossible).

Virtually by exclusion, pelvic inflammatory disease is most likely. Nevertheless, because of their protean manifestations and potentially life-threatening consequences, acute appendicitis and ectopic pregnancy also deserve our closer attention. (Follow-up examination in this case is most important if these disorders are to be excluded with complete confidence.)

CONSIDER

Pelvic Inflammatory Disease. Pelvic inflammatory disease[27-31] (PID) is an acute infectious illness that afflicts (usually) young women of childbearing age, presenting most often as pelvic or low abdominal pain, with or without fever, usually with marked tenderness of the uterus and tubo-ovarian structures on bimanual pelvic examination. Manipulation of the cervix is usually very painful (chandelier sign). Gonococcal infection is the cause in one third to one half of cases. Various anaerobic bacteria and chlamydiae are the usual causes of the nongonococcal variety, which is *clinically* indistinguishable from gonococcal PID. (The endocervical Gram's stain will reveal intracellular gram-negative diplococci in two thirds of women with culture-proven gonorrhea. This is a helpful clue but is a nonspecific result, since nongonococcal *Neisseria* organisms are sometimes pelvic commensal organisms.)

The results of cervical cultures are used "operationally" to distinguish gonococcal (*Neisseria gonorrhoeae* isolated) from nongonococcal (*N. gonorrhoeae* not isolated) PID, although, strictly speaking, only isolation of the gonococcus from peritoneal fluid (during culdocentesis, laparoscopy, or laparotomy) is definitive proof of gonococcal PID. Treatment of uncomplicated PID usually involves tetracycline 500 mg qid for 10 days or ampicillin 3.5 gm orally followed by 500 mg qid for 10 days. Either of these regimens usually will be effective for gonococcal or culture-negative PID, but tetracycline is preferred for proven chlamydial infection. (Chlamydial cultures can be obtained but are not usually necessary and are not universally available.) Most women with PID become asymptomatic within the first week of therapy (the mean time to recovery in one study of 182 women was 3.8 days).[30]

Unfortunately the diagnosis of PID on clinical grounds alone is not always easy. Even when experienced gynecologists diagnose acute PID, laparoscopy will confirm that diagnosis in only about two thirds of cases.[31] One laparoscopic study of 814 women with clinical PID[31] revealed acute salpingitis in 532 (65 per cent), while 184 (23 per cent) patients were normal. More importantly, in 98 patients (12 percent) other diagnoses were made, several of which required very different and often urgent therapy: appendicitis (24), ectopic pregnancy (11), ovarian neoplasms (7), pelvic endometriosis (16), and corpus luteum hematomas (12).

On the other end of the spectrum are women with mild PID in whom pain is only mild or moderate, the uterus and adnexa are only slightly tender, or tenderness is elicited only on cervical manipulation—itself a nonspecific physical finding. Cultures should be obtained and antibiotics considered in such women, but PID is only sometimes proven among such patients, unless gonorrhea is diagnosed by culture.

Thus, while presumptive antibiotic therapy, pending cultures, often makes sense in the treatment of women with acute pelvic pain and tenderness, three generalizations about the woman with acute pelvic pain should be remembered:

1. A precise menstrual history must be elicited. Most cases of acute PID begin during or soon after menstruation. Simple dysmenorrhea will often be associated with pelvic tenderness, but this pain usually begins just before or at the onset of menstruation. Mittelschmerz (which usually causes unilateral pain—see below) occurs during ovulation. A ruptured or hemorrhagic corpus luteum cyst most often occurs in the latter half of the cycle.

If there is any suspicion of pregnancy (prior missed period, late period, breast tenderness, early morning nausea), a pregnancy test or pelvic ultrasound examination or both should be obtained. The latter study can be especially helpful in the early diagnosis of ectopic pregnancy, threatened or incomplete abortion, or intrauterine pregnancy with corpus luteum cyst hemorrhage.[32, 33]

2. When pelvic pain is primarily unilateral or when there is disproportionate unilateral adnexal tenderness or a palpable adnexal mass on pelvic examination, a pelvic ultrasound examination should be obtained immediately, when possible. This test will usually distinguish "surgical" pelvic pain—due to ectopic pregnancy, tubo-ovarian abscess, spontaneous (incomplete) abortion, adnexal neoplasms, or ovarian hemorrhagic cysts—from "medical" diagnoses—PID, small ovarian cysts with or without hemorrhage, normal intrauterine pregnancy, fibroids, endometritis, and so on.[32] When pelvic ultrasound examination is not available or (for whatever reason) is unreliable, a gynecologist should be consulted. Diagnostic laparoscopy is sometimes necessary in these circumstances.

3. When pelvic disorders cannot be confidently distinguished from other serious disease—especially appendicitis—the patient should be observed in the hospital. This is especially true when the patient is acutely ill and when

right lower quadrant pain is difficult to distinguish from pelvic pain. Exploratory laparotomy is not infrequently necessary to resolve this dilemma;[34] certainly careful observation and frequent reexamination over the next 12 to 24 hours are always indicated.

Appendicitis.[5, 34–38] A definitive diagnosis of acute appendicitis is made only in the operating room. In the vast majority of cases, however, a characteristic sequence of symptoms loudly announces the disease, and the physical examination (eventually) reveals highly localized tenderness in the right lower quadrant.

Usually acute (but not abrupt) onset of rather vague epigastric, periumbilical, or generalized abdominal pain is accompanied within several hours by anorexia, nausea or vomiting.* Sometimes pain *begins* in the right lower quadrant (perhaps most often with retrocecal appendicitis), but more often pain *moves into* the right lower quadrant within 12 to 24 hours after onset of the more diffuse or central pain. At this time, the patient often will point (with one finger) to McBurney's point† where, depending on the stage of disease, there may be highly localized tenderness, rebound, guarding, or percussion tenderness. (It is to be hoped that the diagnosis will be made before frank peritonitis with abdominal rigidity ensues.) Fever is low grade, if present at all, but leukocytosis is almost always present in adults;[20–22] the abdominal x-ray is rarely helpful.

It must be emphasized that this is the *usual* clinical presentation. Crucial to the early diagnosis of appendicitis is an appreciation of the typical sequence of events, as well as the variability of signs and symptoms, depending on the stage of disease and the anatomic location of the appendix:

1. As noted previously, any (especially young) patient with acute central abdominal pain who is anorectic or nauseated must be suspected of acute appendicitis, even when the examination is not localizing, especially when symptoms have been present for less than a day. Repeat examination several hours later will usually reveal localized parietal pain and (early) peritoneal inflammation when appendicitis is "brewing."

2. Figure 11–20 illustrates the iliac appendix, which is usually located anteriorly in the right lower quadrant, just beneath the parietal peritoneum. Inflammation of this appendix will result in the usual sequence of symptoms and signs noted above. Figure 11–20 also illustrates the retrocecal and the pelvic appendix. The retrocecal appendix is shielded from the parietal peritoneum by the overlying cecum; its location may be variable, depending on the mobility of the cecum (Fig. 11–20B). Thus the retrocecal appendix, when inflamed, may cause pain in the mid or upper right abdomen, and it may not be associated with such sharply delineated tenderness and peritoneal signs as the iliac appendix. Occasionally a positive psoas sign (Fig. 11–9) will suggest this process when other findings are equivocal. The pelvic appendix hangs over the pelvic brim and may thus be less accessible to abdominal palpation and less likely to incite highly localized peritoneal signs. Tenderness up high on rectal examination and a positive obturator sign (Fig. 11–9) may suggest this process. Pelvic appendicitis is often very difficult to distinguish

---

*As noted previously, experienced surgeons place much confidence in the notion that vomiting "never" precedes pain in acute appendicitis—vomiting before pain is more suggestive of a nonsurgical problem.

†McBurney's point is easy to locate by placing the little finger of one hand over the patient's umbilicus and the thumb of that hand over the patient's anterior superior iliac spine—then the index finger is extended perpendicularly to the abdominal wall—that is McBurney's point.[39]

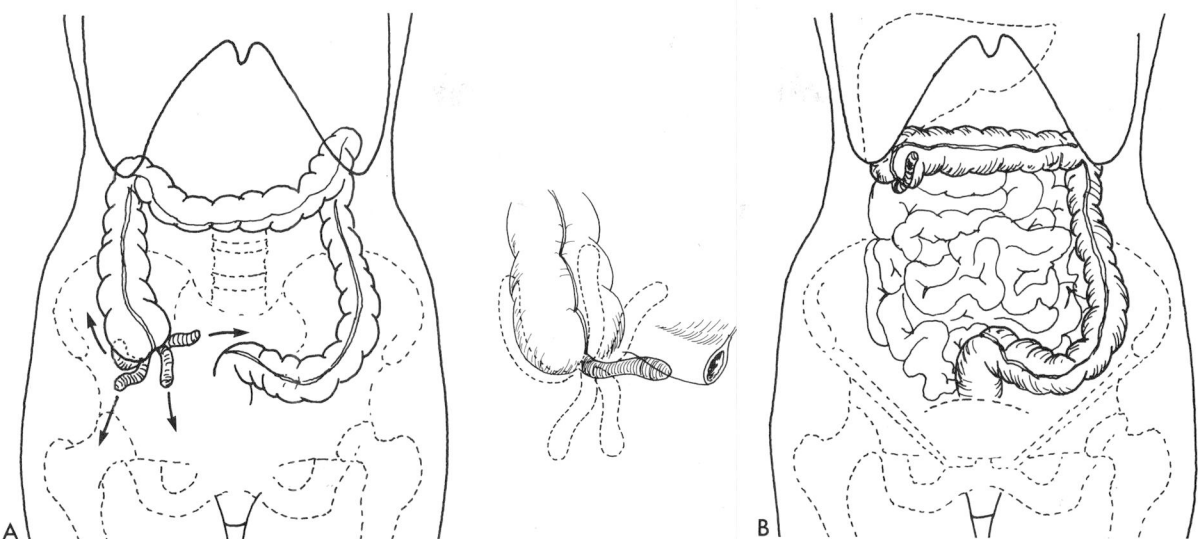

FIGURE 11–20. The Appendix. *A*, The appendix may be located anteriorly, medially, retrocecally, or in the pelvis. *B*, The location of the appendix obviously depends upon the location of the cecum in the abdomen. Because the bowel may be quite mobile in some patients, the appendix may be located in many different sites in the abdomen. In this figure, the appendix is in the right upper quadrant.

from a localized acute pelvic disorder—as discussed above, laparoscopy or laparotomy may be necessary to decide the issue in women.[34]

3. Clinical suspicions are always more important than laboratory tests in the patient with suspected appendicitis. A surgeon should be consulted immediately when the examination or symptoms suggests the diagnosis, even if physical findings are not classic.

Thus, in Sally's case, appendicitis is not likely, but it is a possibility. Sally's initial pain was in the midline, there is (mild) anorexia, and the pain

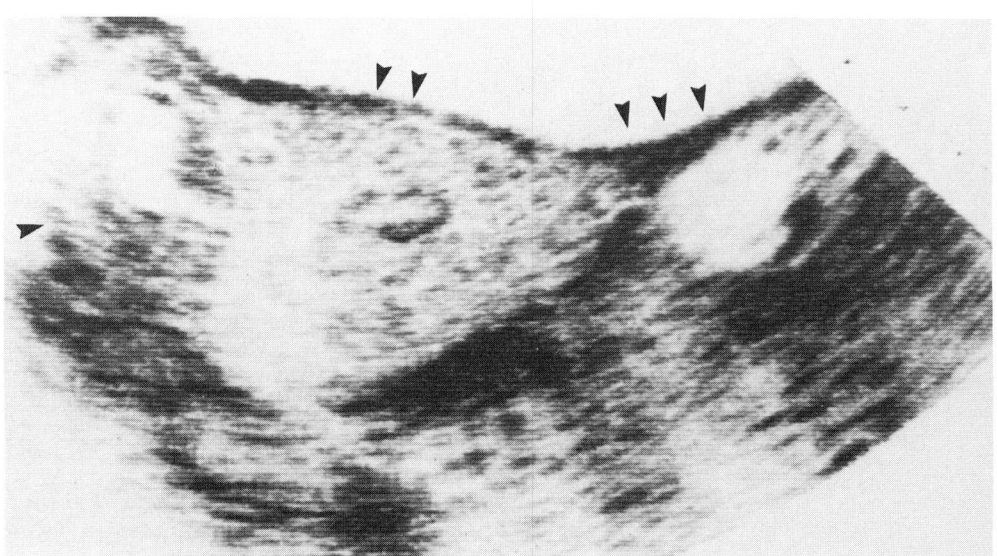

FIGURE 11–21. This 18-year-old woman described progressively worsening lower abdominal pain over the previous 3 days. Examination of the abdomen was unremarkable, but pelvic examination demonstrated marked tenderness on manipulation of the cervix, as well as fullness in the cul-de-sac and right adnexa. The ultrasound examination demonstrates an ectopic pregnancy in the right adnexa (*arrow*), a pseudogestational "sac" in the uterus (*two arrows*), and the corpus luteum of pregnancy on the left (*three arrows*). This patient admitted that she was a "week or two" late for her period but said, "That is not unusual for me." There had been no abnormal vaginal bleeding.

TABLE 11–12. SYMPTOMS AND SIGNS OF ECTOPIC PREGNANCY IN 654 PATIENTS*

SYMPTOMS	No.	(%)	SIGNS	No.	(%)
Pain	654	(100)	Shock	318	(49)
Amenorrhea	547	(84)	Abdominal tenderness	392	(60)
No missed period	76	(12)	Rebound tenderness	340	(52)
Vaginal bleeding	523	(80)	Rigidity	93	(14)
Nausea	114	(17)	Abdominal mass	36	(6)
			Abdominal distention	109	(15)
			Cervical tenderness	572	(87)
			Adnexal mass	310	(47)
			Cul-de-sac mass/fullness	568	(87)
			Fever	330	(50)

*Tubal, 639; abdominal, 9; uterine, 5; ovarian, 1.
Adapted from reference 42.

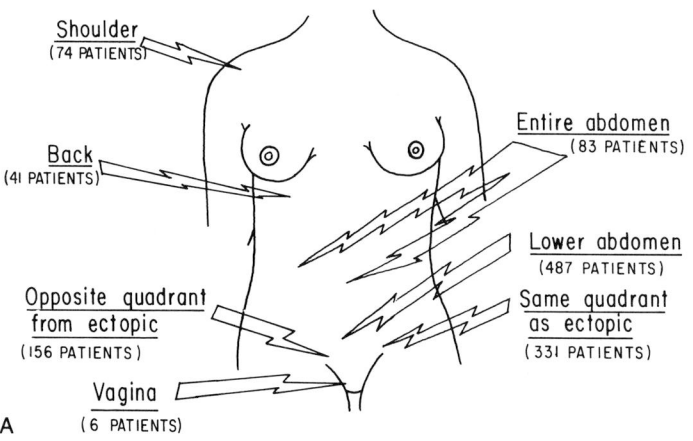

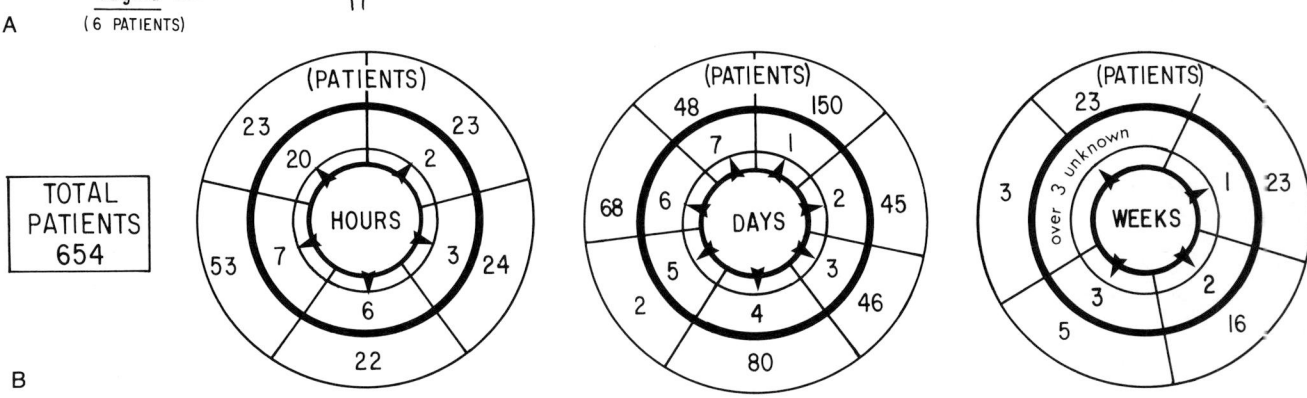

FIGURE 11–22. Ectopic pregnancy. *A,* Anatomic location of pain in 654 patients with ectopic pregnancy. *B,* Duration of abdominal pain before the diagnosis of ectopic pregnancy was confirmed among 654 patients. (Adapted from Breen, JL: A 21-year survey of 654 ectopic pregnancies. Am J Obstet Gynecol 106:1004–1019, 1970.)

and tenderness now involve the right lower quadrant. The x-ray and white blood count do not help here. Sally must be followed for the next day or two.

Ectopic Pregnancy.[40–44] Extrauterine pregnancies constitute about 1 per cent of all pregnancies; 95 per cent of these are in the fallopian tubes. As with acute appendicitis, there is a classic presentation that should never be missed: A woman of childbearing age misses a period (or two), develops lower abdominal, back, or pelvic pain and notices vaginal spotting or frank bleeding; physical examination reveals exquisite tenderness on cervical manipulation or a tender mass (or indistinct fullness) in the cul-de-sac or adnexa on bimanual examination. Breast tenderness, morning nausea or vomiting,

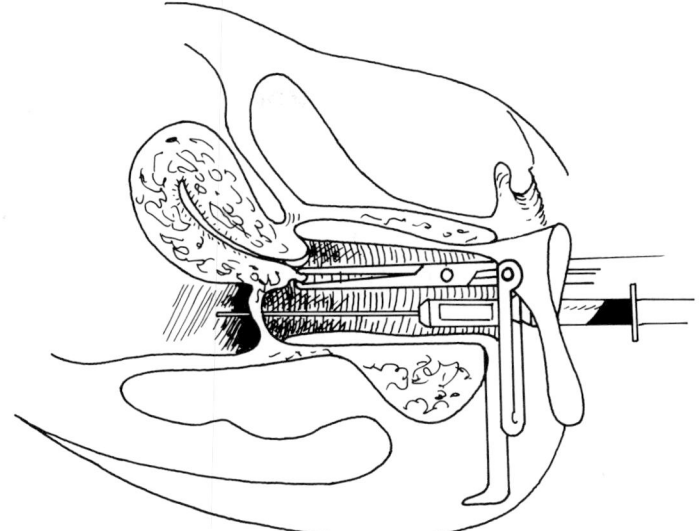

FIGURE 11–23. Culdocentesis. Aspiration of nonclotting blood from the posterior cul-de-sac provides presumptive evidence of pelvic bleeding. Such findings will be present in the vast majority of women with a leaking or ruptured ectopic pregnancy. Such findings may also be present in the patient with a hemorrhagic ovarian mass (neoplasm, cyst).

and other pregnancy symptoms may coexist. If the diagnosis is not made early, the ectopic pregnancy may eventually rupture into the peritoneal cavity—sudden acute abdominal pain, abdominal distention, with or without hypotension and syncope, then occur—a true medical/surgical emergency.

Before rupture, the diagnosis of ectopic pregnancy is usually confirmed by a positive pregnancy test and a pelvic ultrasound examination (Fig. 11–21), but laparoscopy or culdocentesis (see Fig. 11–23) may be necessary as well. (Pelvic ultrasound examination is extremely helpful since it will usually confirm the diagnosis, as well as exclude intrauterine pregnancy with threatened abortion.)

Unfortunately, as with acute appendicitis, the classic case is not the only possible presentation. Table 11–12 illustrates the spectrum of symptoms and signs among a group of 654 patients with surgically proven ectopic pregnancy. The great majority of these women were found to have a ruptured ectopic pregnancy: hence the impressive frequency of worrisome physical findings (shock) in this series. Physical examination will be much less impressive before rupture. Other factors deserve emphasis here:

1. Not all patients with ectopic pregnancy have acute abdominal pain. The duration of pain before diagnosis is usually brief (466 of 654 had pain for fewer than 4 days), but not always (Fig. 11–22).

2. A careful menstrual history is most important in the woman with lower abdominal pain, especially if there is marked cervical tenderness or a palpable pelvic mass. However, perhaps 10 to 15 per cent of women with ectopic pregnancy will *not* have missed a period, and thus symptoms may begin within 4 weeks of their prior menstruation. (In the majority, the prior period is 6 to 9 weeks previously.) Closer questioning will reveal that, in at least some, the prior period was abnormal—briefer in duration, scantier in flow, and the like.

3. Vaginal bleeding that coexists with abdominal pain may be mistaken for a normal menstrual period in some women. The examiner must be careful and do a thorough pelvic examination.

4. Pregnancy tests[45] may or may not be helpful. The usual urinary human chorionic gonadotropin (HCG) determination for pregnancy is sensitive to 2000 to 3000 IU—a level usually attained in the urine only after

4 to 6 weeks of gestation. A negative urine pregnancy test thus does not exclude early ectopic (or intrauterine) pregnancy. The serum B–subunit HCG assay is much more sensitive (detecting approximately 10 IU) and will be positive in more than 90 per cent of pregnancies even when an expected period is only a few days late (i.e., when the last period occurred approximately 1 month before). However, even this test may be negative in the woman with threatened abortion or early ectopic pregnancy.

    5. A gynecologist should be consulted immediately whenever this diagnosis is confirmed or strongly suspected. Culdocentesis (Fig. 11–23) or laparoscopy will usually make the diagnosis, even if pregnancy tests and pelvic ultrasound examinations are nondiagnostic.

> The next day, Sally returns saying, "I couldn't wait until tomorrow." Four hours ago, Sally developed the abrupt onset of a new, more severe "sharp" pain "under my right rib cage." Her previous lower abdominal pain persists but is overshadowed by this new pain. When asked to localized the pain, Sally places her palm across her right upper quadrant, below the costal margin. The pain does not radiate, and it cannot be localized with one finger. This pain perhaps hurts more when Sally takes a deep breath, but there is no dyspnea, cough, or hemoptysis. Sally denies diarrhea, rigors, or genitourinary symptoms. Sally has not vomited but is vaguely nauseated.

Acute Right Upper Quadrant Pain

NOTE

    The location, timing, and severity of Sally's pain tell us much about its possible origin(s).

    The general location of pain should suggest disease of the upper abdominal viscera—as Figure 11–2 illustrates, the esophagus, stomach, duodenum, pancreas, liver, or gallbladder—or the thorax. (The thorax is the most common locus of referred upper abdominal pain, just as the pelvis is the most common locus of referred lower abdominal pain.)

    The sharp lateralization of pain to one side should suggest either local irritation of parietal peritoneum overlying an upper intra-abdominal organ or disease of a unilaterally innervated, extraperitoneal structure, for example, the lung, diaphragm, kidney, or chest/abdominal wall. Physical examination will usually distinguish these two possibilities: The former will be associated with peritoneal signs, but the latter will not.

    The abrupt onset of pain should suggest perforation of an intra-abdominal viscus (especially esophagus, stomach, duodenum) or obstruction of a (non-intestinal) hollow viscus—gallbladder, bile duct, or ureter. As noted previously, acute pancreatitis and acute vascular events can also cause abrupt pain.*

    The severity of pain is subjective, but usually the pain of localized peritonitis, biliary or ureteral obstruction, or abdominal visceral perforation is very severe.

    The clinical setting—right upper quadrant pain following 2 days of lower abdominal pain in a young female—is also crucial here (see below).

    Physical examination, then, must assess how sick Sally is, whether pain

---

*These assumptions about abrupt abdominal pain depend on the supposition that the source of pain is, indeed, intra-abdominal: many thoracic disorders may begin abruptly and refer pain to the abdomen—myocardial infarction, pulmonary embolism or pneumonia, for example.

is intra-abdominal or referred from the thorax, and whether there is evidence of localized peritonitis.

> **Sally appears moderately ill but is not shocky. She is warm peripherally; blood pressure is 120/80, pulse 80, respirations 20, temperature 38.2°C rectally.**
>
> **Sally prefers to lie still during the examination—movement (involuntary coughing) seems to worsen her right upper quadrant pain. Physical examination is normal, except that of the abdomen and pelvis.**
>
> **The abdomen is flat, and bowel sounds are present (but are hypoactive). There is definite percussion tenderness in the right upper quadrant, but this is not well localized. In addition, percussion of the left upper quadrant "refers" tenderness to the right upper quadrant (see Fig. 11–5B). There are no palpable masses or organomegaly, but palpation of the right upper quadrant is difficult because of definite guarding (without frank rigidity) in this area with any attempt at deep palpation. Attempts to elicit rebound in the left upper quadrant cause pain in the right upper quadrant.**
>
> **Pelvic examination is unchanged from the previous day: There is moderate bilateral adnexal and cervical tenderness without palpable masses. Rectal examination is normal.**

What does this mean?

I. Physical examination clearly suggests localized peritoneal irritation in the right upper quadrant.

   As we have seen, localized percussion tenderness and, even more specifically, referred percussion tenderness and referred rebound (percussion and palpation on the left induce pain and guarding on the right) usually imply local peritoneal irritation. These physical findings have several pathoanatomic implications:

   A. Sally is sick—such peritoneal signs usually indicate a surgical abdomen.
   B. Localized intra-abdominal disease is documented.

      Referred pain from the thorax, back, or pelvis can cause poorly localized abdominal pain and tenderness, and rarely abdominal wall guarding during palpation, but pain and tenderness that localize to one area even during contralateral abdominal palpation are "never" due to extra-abdominal disease. (In other words, true peritoneal signs only rarely [if ever] are associated with referred abdominal pain. It is the terminology that is confusing here: Referred percussion tenderness or referred rebound tenderness is never associated with referred abdominal pain.)
   C. Moreover, intraperitoneal disease is most likely.

      It is rare for disease of extraperitoneal intra-abdominal structures to cause such localizing peritoneal signs. Disease of the kidneys, retroperitoneum, pelvis, and abdominal wall may cause localized pain and tenderness, but rarely with such definite evidence of peritoneal inflammation.

II. Table 11–13 indicates the common causes of acute right upper quadrant pain.

   Those that will (at least sometimes) present with true peritoneal signs include acute cholecystitis, perforated peptic ulcer, retrocecal appendicitis, colonic perforation with pericolonic abscess in the hepatic flexure, and gonococcal perihepatitis. Occasionally pleuritis or pneumonia will cause tenderness and splinting in the upper quadrant. A

TABLE 11–13. DIFFERENTIAL DIAGNOSIS OF ACUTE RIGHT UPPER QUADRANT PAIN

DISEASE	SETTING	SYMPTOMS	SIGNS	X-RAYS	WHITE CELL COUNT	URINALYSIS	DIAGNOSIS (dx)/ TREATMENT (Rx)
Biliary colic[6, 7, 46]	Fat, forty, fertile, female; 90%: age 30–80	Episodes (15 min to hours) of steady epigastric or right upper quadrant pain; anorexia; nausea. Self-limited. Rarely colicky	May be mild right upper quadrant tenderness; rarely palpable gallbladder, jaundice	Right upper quadrant calculi in 15 to 25% (Fig. 11–13). Ultrasound (Fig. 11–24) and/or oral cholecystogram: stones	Often normal	Normal	Clinical findings; HIDA scan (Fig. 11–25) or stones on ultrasound. Cholecystectomy (elective) (Rx) }(dx)
Acute cholecystitis[46-54]	Fat, forty, fertile female, age 30–80	Severe epigastric and/or right upper quadrant pain, prolonged (>6 hours); nausea/vomiting common; possibly past history of biliary colic. *Remember:* High fever, chills: ascending cholangitis. gallbladder empyema? Local or generalized peritonitis: gallbladder perforation? Jaundice: Common duct stone?	Epigastric and/or right upper quadrant tenderness; positive Murphy's sign and/or peritoneal signs	Ultrasound (Fig. 11–24): stones	Leukocytosis — Ultrasound! Surgery?	Normal; possibly bilirubinuria	Clinical findings and stones on ultrasound; HIDA scan. Cholecystectomy (Rx) }(dx)
Acute hepatitis viral[55-58]	Any age, usually young; drug addict? blood transfusion?	Usually subacute, indolent illness: malaise, anorexia, rash, arthralgias	Low-grade fever; hepatic tenderness and/or hepatomegaly; usually jaundiced	Normal	Leukocytosis uncommon; lymphocytosis about one-third	Possibly bilirubinuria	Abnormal liver enzymes. Find cause (hepatitis A?, hepatitis B?, etc.) }(dx)
Alcoholic hepatitis[59-60]	Usually age 30–65; heavy alcohol consumption	Usually subacute symptoms but may be fulminant with fever, right upper quadrant pain, toxicity	Liver enlarged, tender; fever; jaundice	Normal	Leukocytosis in about two-thirds	Possibly bilirubinuria	Clinical setting; abnormal liver enzymes; exclude biliary disease }(dx). Discontinue alcohol. Corticosteroids?[60] }(Rx)
Acute hepatic congestion	Usually elderly with congestive heart failure; rarely, Budd-Chiari syndrome. Massive pulmonary embolism. Pericardial disease	Right upper quadrant pain, symptoms of congestive heart failure	Liver enlarged, tender; congestive heart failure (increased jugular venous pressure, edema); ascites?	Normal abdomen and chest x-rays	Normal	Normal	Clinical setting; exclude other diseases }(dx). Resolves with diuresis/treatment of congestive heart failure }(Rx)
Fitz-Hugh–Curtis syndrome[61-63] (gonococcal perihepatitis)	Young sexually active female	Simultaneous or antecedent PID with (often severe) right upper quadrant pain	Right upper quadrant tenderness, sometimes with peritoneal signs. Rarely, hepatic rub. Pelvic tenderness (rule out tubal abscess)	Normal	Variable	Possibly pyuria	Clinical findings of PID plus upper quadrant pain; gonococcal (rarely chlamydial) cultures of the cervix, rectum, pharynx. Antibiotics (Rx) }(dx)

						(dx) (Rx) / (dx)
Subphrenic or subhepatic abscess[64]	Postoperative abdominal surgery; Perforated ulcer, gallbladder, appendix, colon?	Chest/right upper quadrant pain; possibly respirophasic pain; fever	Fever; tender right upper quadrant, usually without peritoneal signs; possibly absence of liver dullness	Elevated diaphragm; pleural effusion; rarely, gas fluid level	Leukocytosis	Normal	Clinical setting; echo/CT scan; Surgical drainage
Perforated peptic ulcer	Any age	Prior history of peptic disease; abrupt right upper quadrant pain	Tender epigastrium and/or right upper quadrant; peritoneal signs (usually); and/or fever	Free air (Fig. 11–11); localized ileus?	Leukocytosis	Normal	Clinical findings; Surgical exploration
Retrocecal appendicitis	Usually, adolescent or young adult	Pain in midline moving to right upper or lower quadrant; nausea; anorexia	Early: examination may be normal. After 12–24 hr: localized right upper or lower quadrant tenderness. Late: diffuse peritonitis and/or abscess	Fecalith rare	Leukocytosis	Normal	Laparotomy
Urorenal disease: acute pyelonephritis, kidney stone, renal infarct		Usually severe pain	"Never" peritoneal signs	IVP?	Variable	Abnormal	
Thoracic disease	Pneumonia, Pleuritis, Pulmonary embolism, Pneumothorax, Pericarditis, Myocardial infarction, Slipping rib	Usually cardiopulmonary symptoms (see Chap. 13)	"Never" peritoneal signs	Chest x-ray, lung scan?			
Others:	Hepatocellular adenoma; Hepatocellular carcinoma; Intrahepatic hemorrhage (cyst, neoplasm, abscess, trauma); Hepatic infarction or abscess	Ruptured ectopic pregnancy or tubal abscess	Pancreatitis (see Table 11–24); Pancreatic pseudocyst/abscess	Hepatic flexure (colon) syndrome; Chest wall disorder; Abdominal wall disorder			

variety of liver diseases will cause localized right upper quadrant pain and tenderness, but peritoneal signs are not found except in very unusual circumstances—for example, a ruptured hepatic abscess, intrahepatic bleeding. Rupture of a pelvic organ (e.g., ectopic pregnancy) can rarely cause localized peritonitis in the upper abdomen. Thus, localized peritonitis in the right upper quadrant usually has a limited differential diagnosis. Sometimes only surgical exploration will achieve a specific diagnosis.

On the other hand, localized right upper quadrant pain and tenderness without peritoneal signs have a much more lengthy differential diagnosis, as Table 11–13 suggests. A variety of hepatic disorders are most common. Usually hepatomegaly or tenderness clearly overlying the liver itself will be apparent in acute hepatitis, acute hepatic congestion, or when mass lesions (cysts, neoplasms, abscesses) involve the liver.

III. The clinical setting is of great importance.

There is no specific reason here to suggest a perforated peptic ulcer (prior ulcer symptoms) or carcinoma of the hepatic flexure of the colon (the patient is young and there is no family history of cancer).

Retrocecal appendicitis is possible, but, while appendicitis will (rarely) cause right upper quadrant peritoneal signs (when the cecum is highly placed and mobile (Fig. 11–20), the prior right lower quadrant pain and continuing pelvic tenderness would then be difficult to explain.

The prior history of possible PID makes the diagnosis of gonococcal perihepatitis (Fitz-Hugh–Curtis syndrome) a real possibility. A ruptured ectopic pregnancy or tubal abscess is also possible, since highly localized upper abdominal peritoneal signs may occasionally be seen in these circumstances.

Had the right upper quadrant pain and tenderness arisen de novo, the most likely diagnosis here would be acute cholecystitis. Rarely the pain of gallbladder disease will be felt in the lower abdomen, but pelvic tenderness is never part of this clinical syndrome.[46] Nevertheless, biliary tract disease is so often the cause of acute right upper quadrant pain that brief emphasis is worthwhile here.

The diagnosis of acute cholecystitis,[47–49] is largely clinical. As Table 11–13 suggests, most patients are middle-aged or older, usually female, and often obese; many patients, however, do not fit the "fat, forty, fertile female" stereotype. Often there is a prior history of recurrent dyspepsia or episodes of biliary colic[6, 46] (see page 598). Acute cholecystitis usually presents with acute epigastric or right upper quadrant pain that occasionally radiates to the subscapular area. Pain is usually deep, steady, and severe, but there is remarkable individual variation (and a few patients will have only mild pain). Nausea, anorexia, and vomiting occur frequently. The presence of jaundice or a palpable gallbladder is always a helpful clue but is found in only a minority of patients.

The findings on physical examination depend on the stage of disease: Cystic duct obstruction by gallstones (the cause of acute cholecystitis in greater than 90 per cent of cases) that does not resolve spontaneously (as does biliary colic) will progress to cause inflammation or infection or perforation of the gallbladder wall. In most patients with acute uncomplicated cholecystitis, there is localized tenderness in the right upper quadrant with a positive Murphy's sign (increased pain and tenderness on inspiration during palpation of the right upper quadrant). Frank peritoneal signs may be present in acute cholecystitis but should always suggest gallbladder empyema or perforation with a pericholecystic abscess. High fever and rigors are unusual in uncomplicated acute cholecystitis and should suggest ascending cholangitis, empyema of the gallbladder, or perforation with abscess. (These latter conditions almost always require emergency surgery,[50] unlike acute uncomplicated cholecystitis, which is often initially managed medically with elective cholecystectomy performed 4 to 6 weeks later.)

Since the diagnosis of acute cholecystitis may be confused with other disorders (Table 11–13), confirmation of the diagnosis preoperatively is always desirable (but is not always possible). A variety of imaging procedures are available—in most cases, only the abdominal ultrasound or nuclear scan is worthwhile. As noted previously, the abdominal flat plate reveals gallstones in only 15 to 25 per cent of cases. The oral cholecystogram is useful only in the diagnosis of chronic gallbladder disease (recurrent biliary colic or suspected cholelithiasis) and is not helpful in the patient with ongoing abdominal pain and suspected acute cholecystitis. The intravenous cholangiogram is useful only occasionally. Serum liver enzymes or amylase levels often rise transiently, but these results are nonspecific. Liver scans and CT scans of the abdomen are, in general, not helpful, unless intrahepatic disease (e.g., abscess, tumor) is also suspected.

The abdominal ultrasound examination (Fig. 11–24) is a very sensitive test for the presence of gallstones, but documentation of gallstones does not necessarily prove acute cholecystitis. (A normal gallbladder on ultrasound is very strong evidence against the diagnosis of acute cholecystitis, however.) When the patient is jaundiced or when ascending cholangitis is suspected, the ultrasound is often the procedure of choice to exclude common duct stones and to evaluate the site of biliary obstruction. Otherwise, radionuclide biliary imaging[53, 54] (Fig. 11–25) is currently the procedure of choice to confirm the diagnosis of acute cholecystitis. Failure to fill the gallbladder with radionuclide usually confirms the diagnosis of cystic duct obstruction (Fig. 11–25B), and this information can be available in less than an hour.

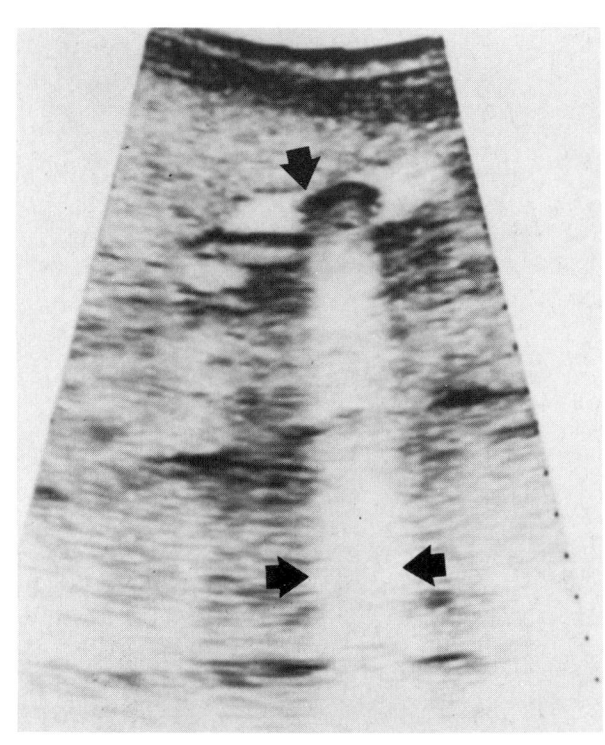

FIGURE 11–24. An abdominal ultrasound demonstrating a large gallstone within the gallbladder. The arrows point to the gallstone (*arrow*) and the "echo displacement" transmitted by the stone. This 44-year-old woman described recurrent attacks of epigastric and right upper quadrant abdominal pain, lasting several hours each and associated with nausea, but always resolving spontaneously—this is biliary colic.

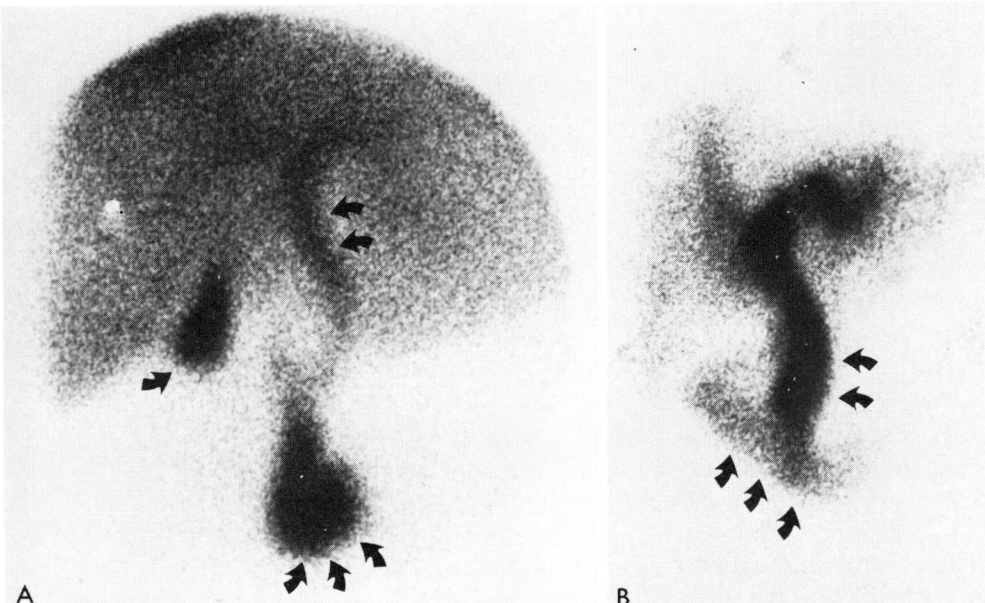

FIGURE 11–25. *A,* A normal nuclear biliary scan (HIDA scan). After 20 minutes, the gallbladder (*arrow*) is filled with isotope, and the common bile duct (*two arrows*) can be seen to be emptying into the duodenum (*three arrows*). *B,* This HIDA scan was obtained when the woman described in Figure 11–24 developed gradually worsening epigastric abdominal pain that persisted for 36 hours. Examination revealed marked tenderness in the right upper quadrant with a positive Murphy's sign. The nuclear scan reveals no filling of the gallbladder but prompt excretion of isotope in the common bile duct (*two arrows*) and into the duodenum (*three arrows*). As expected, cystic duct obstruction by an impacted gallstone was found at laparotomy, when the patient did not improve with intravenous fluids and antibiotics.

Biliary scans are not, however, universally available, nor are they perfectly sensitive or specific.

The clinical history and examination are the crucial diagnostic findings, whatever the results of biliary imaging procedures.

In Sally's case,

> Chest x-ray and abdominal flat plate are normal. The white blood count is 11,000 with a left shift; the urinalysis is normal.

> A surgical consultant is impressed by the right upper quadrant peritoneal signs, but finds that the percussion and referred tenderness are rather diffuse throughout the right upper quadrant and not sharply localized. This fact and the persistent pelvic tenderness raise the question of an intra-abdominal complication of pelvic disease. An abdominal and pelvic ultrasound examination is completely normal: There are no gallstones; pelvic structures are normal.

NOTE

1. The patient with localized peritoneal signs will usually have a surgical problem. The surgeon should always be consulted immediately in such cases.*

2. The normal ultrasound examination of the pelvis makes much less likely the diagnosis of a tubal abscess or an ectopic pregnancy. Similarly the normal gallbladder ultrasound examination excludes acute cholecystitis with a high degree of probability.

3. The clinical setting (prior PID?), as well as the persistent pelvic tenderness, strongly suggests ongoing PID with a relatively rare complication—the Fitz-Hugh–Curtis syndrome.

*Table 11–25 indicates general guidelines for surgical consultation in the patient with acute abdominal pain.

Cervical cultures from the day before are growing a few colonies of gram-negative diplococci, probably *Neisseria gonorrhoeae.*

Gonococcal perihepatitis[61-63] (Fitz-Hugh–Curtis syndrome) refers to a poorly understood inflammatory process involving the capsule of the liver, probably due to intraperitoneal infection complicating acute salpingitis, resulting ultimately in fibrous adhesions surrounding the liver. Gonococcal infection is almost always responsible, but chlamydial PID has been reported to cause a similar clinical picture. The illness is usually self-limited and will slowly resolve even if untreated, but it does respond dramatically to appropriate antibiotic therapy once recognized.

Hospitalization is recommended because of the severity of Sally's pain, but she refuses.

Procaine penicillin 4.8 million units intramuscularly with 1 gm of oral probenecid is administered. Sally is sent home with a prescription for ampicillin 500 mg qid for the next 10 days.

The next day Sally is "50 per cent better," and by week's end is completely asymptomatic. Her husband, who now admits to an extramarital liaison, is culture positive for urethral gonorrhea. Repeat cultures of Sally and her husband 10 days following treatment are sterile and serologic tests for syphilis are nonreactive.

NOTE

1. When gonococcal perihepatitis is well documented, hospitalization is often unnecessary. (Treatment of gonorrhea and PID is discussed on page 562 and in Chapter 8, "Male Genitourinary Infections.") When the patient initially presents with acute right upper quadrant pain, a presumptive diagnosis may be suspected, but the patient often requires hospitalization and observation pending the results of cultures and response to antibiotics.

2. Gonococcal perihepatitis is not a common cause of acute right upper quadrant pain. Nevertheless, this and other causes of right upper quadrant pain (Table 11–13) will often be readily identified after a careful, systematic analysis of clinical setting, symptoms, and physical findings.

Sally does well, but 3 months later she returns to the clinic complaining, "I'm having more stomach pain." For the past 6 weeks, Sally has experienced frequent episodes of lower abdominal pain, often several times per week. Sally admits to similar pains intermittently for the past 5 to 6 years, but "these are worse." These chronic/recurrent pains are "different" from her recent PID, which has resolved symptomatically.

CHRONIC/RECURRENT ABDOMINAL PAIN

While the general approach to the patient with chronic abdominal pain must emphasize the same basic approach as the approach to acute abdominal pain—the history and physical examination are the cornerstone—a somewhat distinctive mind set applies to the patient with nonacute pain. This is not simply a matter of degrees of urgency, although the initial question regarding the patient with acute pain—is this a surgical emergency?—is rarely uppermost when one is confronting the patient whose pain has persisted or recurred intermittently for many weeks, months, or years. Rather, that patient offers a distinctive differential diagnosis, i.e., the statistics illustrated in Figure 11–

1 do not apply well to patients with chronic/recurrent abdominal pain. There is, of course, some overlap here since chronic disorders must begin at some point (and hence may present acutely, initially). In addition, chronic disease processes can cause intermittent acute flares or complications as well as chronic, recurrent symptoms. (Peptic ulcer disease or diverticulosis, for example, usually causes chronic/recurrent symptoms, but perforation of an ulcer or development of acute diverticulitis will cause an "acute abdomen.") Nevertheless, a comparison of Figure 11–1 with Tables 11–14 and 11–19 indicates the very different spectrum of possibilities that apply to acute and chronic abdominal pain.

Tables 11–14 and 11–19 (page 594) are somewhat artificial because the distinction between upper abdominal pain and lower abdominal pain is not always obvious. Many patients with chronic/recurrent abdominal pain are vague or unreliable about the precise location of pain. Moreover, some so-called upper abdominal disorders (Table 11–19) will cause lower abdominal pain on occasion, and some so-called lower abdominal disorders (Table 11–14) can result in upper abdominal pain. (For example, duodenal ulcer disease may cause lower abdominal pain [Figure 11–30A, page 596]; irritable bowel syndrome may cause upper abdominal pain.) Even more confusing are patients with two or more simultaneous conditions (for example, esophagitis and irritable bowel syndrome). Such patients often cannot distinguish among different types of pain.

Obviously, then, the patient should not be forced to artificially label his or her pain as upper or lower abdominal pain; much more important is listening to the patient. Other characteristics of clinical symptoms—relation to meals, relieving factors, periodicity of symptoms, for example—are often

TABLE 11–14.   FREQUENCY OF CAUSES OF CHRONIC/RECURRENT LOWER ABDOMINAL PAIN*

GASTROINTESTINAL	PELVIC	GENITOURINARY	OTHER
	Common		
Irritable bowel syndrome	Dysmemorrhea	Recurrent urinary	Hernia
Diverticulosis	Endometriosis	infection	Abdominal wall pain
Constipation	Pelvic congestion	Chronic prostatitis	Hip disease (degenerative
Lactose intolerance	Mittelschmerz	Scrotal disorders	joint disease [DJD],
	Uterine fibroids		bursitis)
	Ovarian cyst(s)		
	Uncommon		
Carcinoma of colon	Chronic PID	Polycystic kidneys	Radiculitis
Abdominal aortic aneurysm	Adenomyosis uteri	Renal/ureteral neoplasm	Spinal disease
Upper GI diseases	Uterine cancer	Bladder neoplasm	Osteitis pubis
(e.g., duodenal ulcer)	Ovarian cancer	Chronic urolithiasis	Pelvic bone lesions
Inflammatory bowel disease	Cervical cancer		Sacroiliitis
			Aortoiliac claudication or
			aneurysm
	Rare		
Meckel's diverticulum	Many others†	Retroperitoneal tumors	Ilioinguinal neuritis
Intermittent large bowel			Vasculitis
obstruction			Abdominal epilepsy
Intestinal angina			Porphyria
Chronic abdominal abscess			Lead poisoning
(diverticular, appendiceal,			Sickle cell disease
pelvic)			Drug induced
			Uremia
			Diabetic enteropathy

*This refers to the frequency of these various diseases in all patients with lower abdominal pain, not necessarily the overall prevalence of the different diseases in the general population.

†See reference 65.

more important than the location of pain alone. Nevertheless, most patients with chronic/recurrent abdominal pain can localize, at least vaguely, their pain in either the upper or lower abdomen. This is very helpful because the diagnostic significance of the location of abdominal pain illustrated in Figure 11–2 does apply to both acute and chronic/recurrent pain. As we have seen, upper abdominal pain usually reflects disease of the upper abdominal organs or thorax; lower abdominal pain, disease of the pelvis, colon, or rectum. Midline periumbilical pain is not common in the patient with chronic abdominal pain, but that location must suggest disease of the small bowel, as well as "overlap" from organs above or below.

Sally localizes her current pain in the suprapubic and bilateral hypogastric regions—she places both hands across her lower abdomen when asked to point to the pain.

Sally's description is otherwise rather vague: Pains may be unilateral or bilateral, sometimes are mild, but may also be incapacitating (and require Sally to leave work and "lie down" occasionally); some last "a few minutes," others "all day."

Sally describes the pain as "sharp but aching," and says they are unpredictable—"Sometimes, they seem related to my periods, sometimes to bowel movements, I just don't know."

Chronic/Recurrent Lower Abdominal Pain

Most cases of chronic/recurrent lower abdominal pain are caused by disorders of the large bowel or pelvic organs. However, this usually reliable dictum can sometimes be responsible for diagnostic and therapeutic errors if relied upon too dogmatically. All too often, such patients are hastily examined and then subjected to diagnostic tests that are intended to exclude serious disease in the colon and pelvis, whether serious disease is clinically suspected or not. When these tests—usually a barium enema, proctoscopy, or pelvic ultrasound—are normal, the patient is often told "not to worry, it's nothing serious" or is subjected to additional tests (for example, gallbladder x-rays, upper gastrointestinal series) designed to exclude disease in organ systems that only uncommonly cause lower abdominal pain. That this stategy is inadequate is best emphasized not so much by diatribes about cost-efficient testing as by the clinical fact that the great majority of cases of chronic/ recurrent lower abdominal pain are due to diseases usually associated with normal laboratory tests and radiologic imaging procedures. The diagnosis of these disorders may sometimes require tests to exclude other possibilities, but the history and physical examination alone are very often sufficiently diagnostic of the most common causes of chronic lower abdominal pain.

Table 11–17 (pages 586 and 587) enumerates the common causes of chronic/recurrent lower abdominal pain. In many patients these disorders can be both diagnosed and treated presumptively, i.e., without testing. On the other hand, each of these disorders may be mimicked by much more serious diseases, some of which are enumerated in Table 11–18 (pages 592 and 593). Most of these serious disorders can be diagnosed (or excluded) only with a variety of tests. No wonder so many normal tests are performed in patients with chronic lower abdominal pain.

How, then, should we approach the patient with chronic/recurrent lower abdominal pain? Such patients can usually be best managed after first considering the answer(s) to four questions:

I. How long has the pain been a problem?

Sally admits to similar pains intermittently for the past 5 to 6 years. Usually these pains have been attributed to "my periods or my nerves" by other physicians. Sally is not certain that her present pains are the same as prior pains but she thinks so.

The patient who has had pain for more than a few years will almost never suffer from one of the serious disorders enumerated in Table 11–18. In this setting, neoplasms are most unlikely, although occasionally a slow-growing uterine, urologic, or retroperitoneal malignant tumor will be symptomatic for a few years before discovery. Chronic inflammatory disease of the bowels or pelvis will, at times, be very indolent in course, but there are almost always other clues (see below) in these cases.

The patient with lower abdominal pain for less than a year is more of a problem. None of the disorders in Table 11–18 can be neglected in such a patient, although the clinical setting, symptoms, and signs usually raise specific suspicions.

Thus, in Sally's case, the duration of pain is somewhat reassuring.

II. Are there clues that implicate a particular organ system?

A. Is the pain related to intestinal events?

Pain that is associated with gas, bloating, abdominal borborygmi, diarrhea, constipation, or rectal bleeding is usually gastrointestinal. This is even more likely when pain is fully or partly relieved by defecation, passing flatus, use of laxatives, or dietary alterations.

B. Is the pain related to gynecologic events?

Pelvic or gynecologic pain is usually associated with abnormal menstruation, vaginal bleeding, or dyspareunia or characteristically occurs at certain phases of the menstrual cycle.

C. Are there urinary symptoms?

Disorders of the prostate, bladder, or kidneys that may cause lower abdominal pain are almost always associated with urinary hesitancy, frequency, dysuria, hematuria, or some other perception of urinary dysfunction in association with abdominal pain. In the male, chronic prostatitis or prostatosis is the usual cause (Chapter 8, "Male Genitourinary Infections"); in the female, recurrent cystitis is much more common (Chapter 6, "Female Urinary Tract Infections").

D. Is the pain postural, exertional, or positional?

Lower abdominal pain may be caused by disease of the lumbosacral spine, hips, sacroiliac joints, and pelvic bones, as well as by disorders of the abdominal wall (muscle contusions, hernias). Pain that is precipitated by standing up, bending over, rolling over, walking, or other "mechanical factors" is often musculoskeletal (see also Chapter 1, "Low Back Pain"). Rarely, intermittent vascular claudication will cause lower abdominal pain (exertional groin, hip, or low back pain due to aortoiliac disease).

E. Is the pain postprandial?

Postprandial lower abdominal pain should suggest atypical location of upper abdominal disease (see Figs. 11–30 and 11–32, pages 596 and 599, respectively), food (especially lactose) intolerance (Chapter 3, "Diarrhea"), lower intestinal disease in which pain is affected by the gastrocolic reflex (colonic stimulation 15 to 30 minutes after eating),[66] or, rarely, intestinal angina due to meal-related mesenteric ischemia (see page 615).

On closer questioning it appears that Sally is describing two different types of abdominal pain:

One pain is clearly related to menstruation. Diffuse lower abdominal discomfort and cramping occur at the onset of menstruation and persists for 2 or 3 days. This pain is very similar to usual menstrual cramps, which have been present "ever since I began having periods" but, "they seem more bothersome now, the pain is worse, and I have to go to bed for a day or two."

The second pain is much less predictable. Here, pain occurs primarily in the left lower quadrant but may be felt throughout the hypogastrium and is episodic, lasting for several hours on most occasions. This pain occurs now at least twice a week. Sally denies any change in bowel habits but admits to chronic constipation for years and says that this pain is often associated with "bloating" and is somewhat relieved by "passing gas or having a bowel movement."

There is no history of rectal bleeding, tenesmus, diarrhea, weight loss, dyspareunia, abnormal vaginal bleeding, or urinary symptoms. Symptoms are unrelated to bodily position or eating but tend to feel better "lying down with a heating pad on my stomach."

Sally is not experiencing pain now. She is currently in the middle of her menstrual cycle.

Thus, in Sally's case, the history suggests both gynecologic and intestinal pain.

III. Are there any findings on history or physical examination that are specifically worrisome?

Lower abdominal pain that begins at an elderly age is worrisome. Most of the common benign causes of lower abdominal pain begin in young adulthood or early middle age. Exceptions include diverticular disease of the colon, musculoskeletal diseases of the hips and back (usually degenerative), and some prostatic disorders.

Associated weight loss is worrisome. The common tendency is to suspect neoplasm when weight loss is a prominent feature in the patient with chronic abdominal pain, but inflammatory disease of the bowel or pelvis may cause weight loss, as may intestinal angina (see below).

Abnormal vaginal bleeding in the perimenopausal or postmenopausal woman is worrisome. Any postmenopausal woman with vaginal bleeding (or spotting) and lower abdominal pain has a gynecologic (usually endometrial) malignant tumor until proven otherwise. Most ovarian and uterine cancers occur in middle-aged and elderly women (Table 11–18, pages 592 and 593).

A palpable pelvic or abdominal mass is always worrisome. Very large masses (which fill most of the abdomen) may originate anywhere, but most masses in the lower abdomen can be localized to the pelvic adnexa, cul-de-sac, or lower (midline or unilateral) abdomen. Table 11–15 indicates the most common causes of lower abdominal masses.

Recent changes in bowel habits in the middle-aged or elderly are worrisome. Stool that is positive for occult blood is always worrisome. Stool should be tested for occult blood in every patient with lower abdominal pain.

A family history of colorectal or gynecologic malignant neoplasms is worrisome. While these involve primarily the elderly and middle-aged, colorectal carcinoma and gynecologic malignant tumors certainly occur in younger patients. (Cervical carcinoma is largely a disease of young women, but this is an unusual cause of occult abdominal pain.) Even when there are no other worrisome findings, a family history of these malignant neoplasms always deserves attention.

TABLE 11–15.   CAUSES OF LOWER ABDOMINAL MASSES

ADNEXA				
CYSTIC*	**SOLID***	**CUL-DE-SAC**	**SUPRAPUBIC**	**MIDABDOMEN**
Benign or malignant ovarian cyst	Ovarian neoplasm	Ovarian cyst or neoplasm	Pregnant uterus	Bowel tumor
Tubo-ovarian abscess	Ectopic pregnancy	Ectopic pregnancy	Uterine neoplasm	Aortic aneurysm
Pyosalpinx	Fallopian tube neoplasm	Pyosalpinx	Distended bladder	Abdominal wall hematoma or abscess
Bowel gas	Pedunculated uterine myoma	Tubo-ovarian or pelvic abscess	Bladder neoplasm	Malignant peritoneal or omental tumor (metastatic)
Diverticular, appendiceal, or abdominal wall abscess	Colorectal cancer	Retroflexed uterus	Ovarian tumor	
	Diverticulitis	Uterine myoma	Bowel tumor	
	Appendicitis	Feces in bowel	Feces	
	Abdominal wall hematoma	Colon cancer	Abdominal wall hematoma or abscess	
		Diverticulitis		
		Appendicitis		
		Ectopic kidney		
		Retroperitoneal tumor		

*This designation refers usually to the ultrasound characteristics of the adnexal mass, although physical examination will sometimes distinguish solid from cystic masses.

There is no family history of malignant disease. Sally has not lost weight.

Physical examination is completely normal. There are no palpable abdominal or pelvic masses. Stool is brown and heme negative. Flanks, groin, hips, and back are normal.

The significance of a normal physical examination in the patient with chronic lower abdominal pain deserves brief emphasis. Many of the serious diseases listed in Table 11–18 will very often be associated with a normal examination:

The physical examination and Papanicolaou test are notoriously unreliable detectors of uterine carcinoma.[67]

Rectal examination will detect only a minority of colorectal carcinomas (Fig. 11–26),[68] and palpable abdominal masses are unusual in the

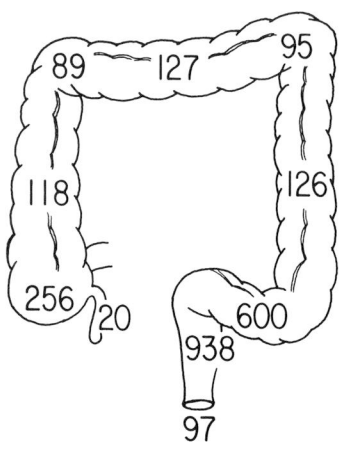

FIGURE 11–26. Common locations of colorectal carcinomas. There has been some change in the incidence of various locations over the past several decades. Previously, it was widely taught that most colorectal carcinomas were within reach of the palpating finger on rectal examination. This is no longer the case. The figure illustrates the review of Falterman et al. of location of 2313 colorectal carcinomas.[68]

majority of patients with colon cancer until very late in the course of the disease.[68] Hemoccult testing of the stool may be positive only intermittently.

Ovarian carcinoma usually is apparent on physical examination by the time symptoms of abdominal pain begin, but usually disease is far advanced at this time.[69, 70]

Renal, bladder, and retroperitoneal neoplasms are rarely palpable.

Abdominal aortic aneurysms will easily be missed in the obese patient.

Examination of the genitals, prostate, back, hips, groin, and femoral vessels is always helpful. For example, hip degenerative arthritis will cause groin or lower abdominal discomfort. Hip range of motion, especially internal rotation, will reproduce the pain.

Psoas bursitis presents with groin pain and sometimes tenderness, worsened by forced hip flexion or passive hip extension (Fig. 11–9). Vascular palpation may be the first clue to an iliac artery or femoral artery aneurysm. Ilioinguinal neuritis[71] is a rare entrapment neuropathy that causes peculiar pains in the groin (or inner proximal thigh); pressure at a point just medial to the anterior superior iliac spine reproduces pain or dysesthesias. The importance of inguinal and femoral hernias, scrotal disorders, and prostate disease has been mentioned previously.

IV. Finally, where there are no worrisome findings, are clinical findings typical of one of the common causes of chronic lower abdominal pain?

It is possible to make a presumptive diagnosis of the cause of chronic lower abdominal pain purely on the basis of the history and examination (see below and Fig. 11–27), especially:

A. When the patient is young, there are no worrisome findings on history or examination, and symptoms are typical of irritable bowel syndrome, primary dysmenorrhea, habitual constipation, or various benign menstrual cycle pains (due to mittelschmerz or pelvic congestion, for example.)

B. When there is a known history of diverticulosis or lactose intolerance and no reason to suspect another coexisting diagnosis.

C. When clinical findings document the presence of hernias, prostate disorders, abdominal wall disorders, or hip disease and there is no reason to doubt the relation between these findings and the patient's pain.

In Sally's case, clinical findings are typical of primary dysmenorrhea and the irritable bowel syndrome.

The premenstrual pelvic pain is longstanding and is typical of dysmenorrhea page 585). The only change is its apparent severity. (The severity of chronic/recurrent abdominal pain is always difficult to judge quantitatively—nevertheless, some superimposed cause of secondary dysmenorrhea [page 585] should also be considered.)

The second, intestinal, pain is highly suggestive of irritable bowel syndrome.

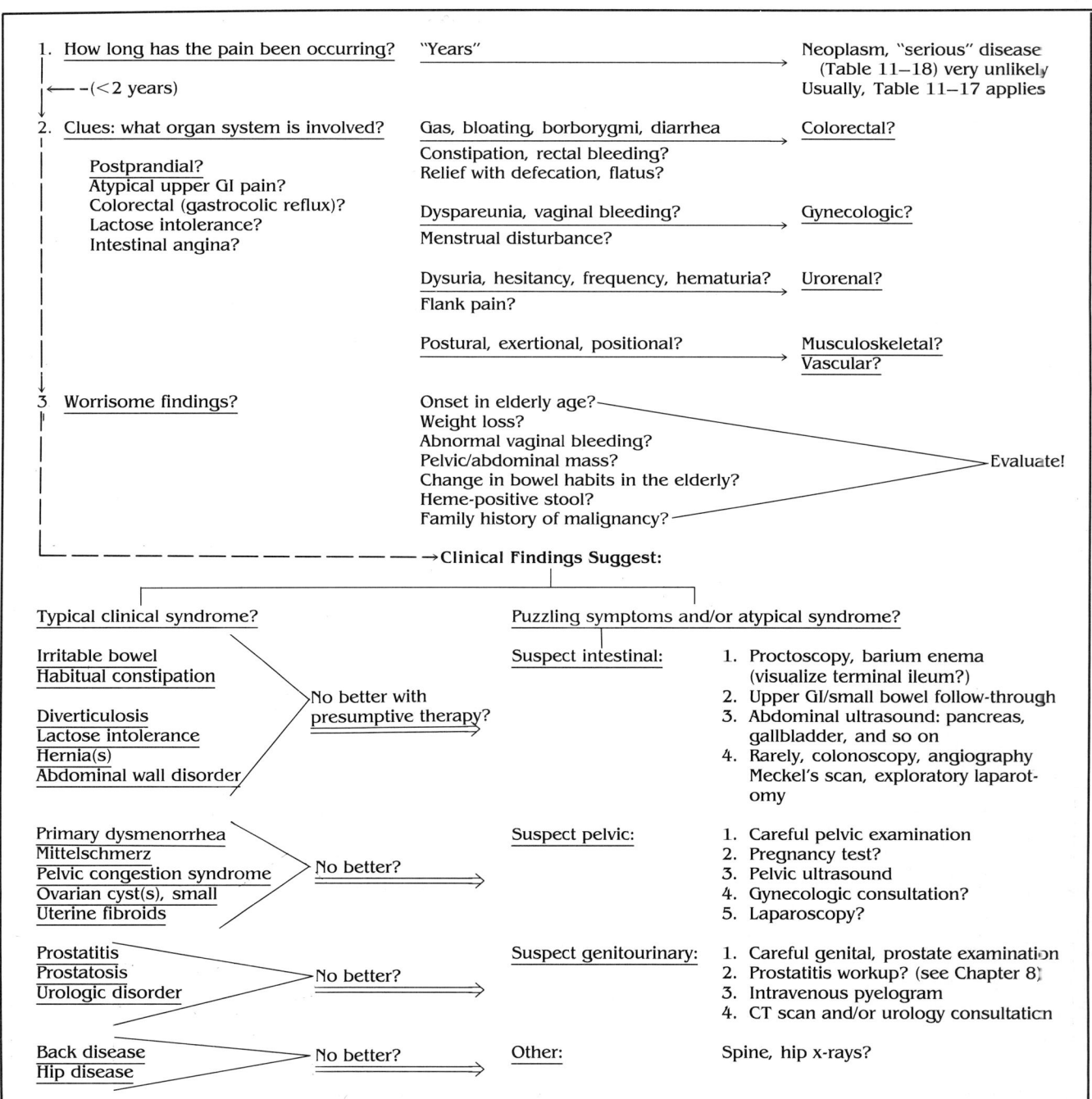

FIGURE 11–27. Chronic recurrent lower abdominal pain.

CONSIDER

Presumptive Diagnosis and Treatment of Chronic Lower Abdominal Pain

Whether diagnostic testing is performed in the patient with chronic lower abdominal pain depends on many factors. Certainly when pain is of fairly recent onset (months) or there are any worrisome clinical findings, investigation is necessary. Specific testing will depend upon whether the pain is suspected to be of intestinal, gynecologic, urorenal, musculoskeletal, or psychogenic origin (Fig. 11–27). In many patients, however, diagnosis can be presumptive and therapy initiated without testing (see Table 11–17, pages 586 and 587). Often such patients then require investigation only when they fail to respond to presumptive treatment. Just as the careful history and physical examination are the cornerstone of presumptive diagnosis, careful clinical follow-up is crucial whenever presumptive treatment is employed.

CONSIDER

Irritable Bowel Syndrome.[72-76] Sometimes called spastic colon, colitis, or mucous colitis, this disorder is surely the most common intestinal cause of lower abdominal pain in the Western world. Symptoms most often begin in adolescence or young adulthood (before the age of 30 years). Abdominal pain is usually hypogastric in location, crampy in nature, highly variable in frequency and duration, and often clearly associated with bowel function: associated borborygmi, gas, or bloating, abdominal distention, and partial or temporary relief of discomfort with passage of flatus or feces are common. Pain in the left lower quadrant is most common (but pain due to the irritable bowel may be remarkably varied in location).[72] Physical examination is normal, except that abdominal palpation may reveal a tender, palpable sigmoid colon, which becomes *less* tender with progressively (gentle but) deeper manual compression of that area. Rectal examination may indicate mild tenderness, and proctoscopy (if performed) may be difficult because of rectosigmoid spasm, especially during painful episodes.

A careful history will almost always reveal a history of coexistent or antecedent bowel dysfunction. Chronic constipation is most common, but periods of constipation (weeks) alternating with periods of small-volume diarrhea (see Chapter 3, "Diarrhea") are even more characteristic. Chronic or intermittent diarrhea without constipation is present in a minority. A very characteristic bowel pattern is seen in many: In the morning a constipated movement with passage of small, hard pellets of stool is followed in the next hour or two by one or more movements of small-volume diarrhea, often intermixed with visible mucus. Each morning, the sequence is repeated.

When recurrent episodes of such abdominal pain and bowel dysfunction can be correlated with various life stresses, the diagnosis is usually established. Almy's "life history" is time consuming but remarkably valuable in the approach to many patients.[77] Various personality types have been loosely correlated with different clinical manifestations[78, 79]—constipation in the hostile, "anal retentive"; diarrhea in the resentful or anxious patient. Diarrhea during school examinations or before a public appearance and constipation when frustrated, depressed, or unfulfilled are examples of behavioral bowel dysfunction common in irritable bowel syndrome. Remember however: Many patients with apparently well-adjusted personalities will develop the irritable bowel syndrome, sometimes in the absence of any demonstrable life stress.

Irritable bowel syndrome is never a presumptive diagnosis when symptoms begin at an elderly age, when stool is Hemoccult positive (or anemia is documented), or when there are associated systemic symptoms (weight loss, anorexia). In any of these circumstances, proctosigmoidoscopy and barium enema (at least) are mandatory. In the young patient, diseases often mistaken for irritable bowel syndrome include inflammatory bowel disease and lactose intolerance. In the older patient, diverticular disease and colorectal cancer are more common.

Presumptive treatment of irritable bowel syndrome includes:

1. Patient education—brief explanations about coordinated peristalsis, bowel spasm, gas buildup, and intestinal motility help most patients understand basic pathogenesis. The possible influence of life stresses on symptoms is usually illuminating for the patient, and brief description of the neural control of gut contractility helps the patient see the connection between stress and abdominal pain (see case, page 590). (The patient who denies an association between life stress and symptoms is occasionally correct, but here Almy's "life history"[77] will be valuable for patient and physician alike.) Physical exercise and promotion of general well-being help many.

2. Dietary modification—a high-fiber diet (see Appendix IV in Chapter 3, "Diarrhea"), sufficient liquids and taking a hydrophilic colloid preparation daily (for example, Metamucil) should be routine. The patient must understand that these measures must be followed for several weeks before improvement will occur. A brief trial of a lactose-free diet is sometimes worthwhile, since symptoms of the irritable bowel syndrome and lactose intolerance may overlap (and since each condition is so common).

3. Medication is only sometimes necessary. Antispasmodics (for example, chlordiazepoxide hydrochloride and clidinium bromide—Librax) are occasionally useful when bowel spasm is incompletely relieved with dietary modification and Metamucil. Antidiarrheal agents (for example, diphenoxylate hydrochloride and atropine—Lomotil) may be needed when recurrent diarrhea is the problem—interestingly, diet and Metamucil often relieve diarrhea as well as constipation; other causes of diarrhea (see Chapter 3, "Diarrhea") should be excluded when they do not. Laxatives and cathartics should be avoided when possible, as should all narcotic analgesics.

When the patient does not respond to these measures after a 6- to 8-week trial, laboratory and radiologic testing should be undertaken. The patient with a clinical diagnosis of irritable bowel syndrome who does not respond to such treatment *must* undergo proctoscopy and barium x-rays of the lower (and sometimes upper) bowel. Further investigation or consultation with a gastroenterologist (or psychiatrist) must then be individualized (Fig. 11–27).

Habitual constipation is, in some cases, a forme fruste of irritable bowel syndrome. Usually constipation in these patients is lifelong, probably engendered by sociocultural conditioning during early bowel training. Intermittent bouts of lower abdominal pain are relieved by defecation. Rarely, diarrhea will arise intermittently when fecal impaction occurs or, very rarely, severe constipation may cause a stercoral ulcer of the colon, and bleeding may ensue. Usually, however, the history of lifelong constipation in a young patient without "worrisome findings" is diagnostic. Laxative or cathartic

**TABLE 11–16. NONCATHARTIC PROPHYLAXIS OF
CHRONIC CONSTIPATION**

Daily
  6 prunes each morning; fresh fruits and vegetables
  each lunch and dinner; Metamucil, 1 tablespoonful in
  8 ounces of water before bedtime

Every 3 days
  Enema—1½ quarts warm tap water (no additives)

abuse is very common among such patients, and this is the reason treatment is so difficult in most refractory cases. An ongoing program of constipation prophylaxis (Table 11–16) is helpful for many. Search for rare causes of constipation (for example, Hirschsprung's disease, dysautonomia, scleroderma, myotonic dystrophy, intestinal pseudo-obstruction[80]) is important when such treatment is ineffective.[81]

Dysmenorrhea.[65, 82–84] Dysmenorrhea refers to lower abdominal cramping beginning a day or two before (or coincident with) the onset of menstrual flow, sometimes associated with nausea, headache, tension, irritability, and fatigue. Symptoms are usually most troublesome for the first 24 to 48 hours and they rapidly diminish as menses abate.

The majority of women develop some degree of dysmenorrhea. Most do not seek medical attention. For those who do, great care must be taken to distinguish primary dysmenorrhea from secondary dysmenorrhea.

Primary (natural) dysmenorrhea refers to symptoms that usually begin soon after menarche and gradually diminish with increasing age and parity; no structural disorder is likely in these circumstances, and symptoms are probably due to myometrial contractility (and local uterine ischemia) induced by prostaglandins released during normal menstruation.[83, 84]

Treatment of primary dysmenorrhea is pharmacologic. For some, mild analgesics suffice. When contraception is also desirable, oral contraceptives often achieve both goals. Nonsteroidal anti-inflammatory drugs (Table 1–4) that inhibit prostaglandins are most helpful—the best studied drugs are mefenamic acid (Ponstel), ibuprofen (Motrin), naproxen (Naprosyn), and indomethacin (Indocin). Medication is begun a day before anticipated symptoms and usually continued for 2 to 3 days. When one drug is ineffective, another should be tried.

A common misunderstanding among some young women with primary dysmenorrhea is the notion that "there must be something wrong with me." Latent concerns about cancer, sexual function, and future fertility are common. Brief patient education is always worthwhile. Careful pelvic examination is essential.

Secondary (acquired) dysmenorrhea refers to menstrual pain caused by some pelvic disease: most commonly uterine myomas, endometriosis, adenomyosis uteri, cervical stenosis, PID, or endometrial polyps, but many others are possible. Symptoms usually begin long after menarche (except for developmental disorders like cervical stenosis) and then worsen over time (as opposed to the usual resolution of primary dysmenorrhea as age increases). Thus, onset of dysmenorrhea long after menarche, worsening of symptoms in the late 20s or 30s or failure to respond to treatment of primary dysmenorrhea should certainly prompt investigation (gynecologic consultation, pelvic ultrasound).

Endometriosis.[85] Endometriosis is an important cause of dysmenorrhea that is often misdiagnosed. In this condition, endometrial tissue proliferates

TABLE 11–17. COMMON CAUSES OF CHRONIC/RECURRENT LOWER ABDOMINAL PAIN

DIAGNOSIS*	PRESUMPTIVE DIAGNOSIS WHEN	PRESUMPTIVE THERAPY	SUGGESTED TEST(S) AND THEIR TIMING
Irritable bowel syndrome[72–79] (spastic colon, mucous colitis)	Typical clinical symptoms beginning in early adulthood; associated bowel dysfunction "Normal" examination Hemetest-negative stool No family history of colorectal cancer or polyps	Diet: Bran, whole wheat bread, carrots, apples, oranges, salad greens (bulk) Medications: hydrophylic colloid (e.g., Metamucil) Antispasmodics: chlordiazepoxide HCl/ clidinium bromide (Librax) Patient education	Proctosigmoidoscopy and barium enema if: Onset of symptoms in middle-aged/elderly Heme-positive stool Family history of colorectal cancer or polyps Failure to improve after 6 to 8 weeks of presumptive therapy
Diverticular disease of colon[89–94]	Usually asymptomatic	See irritable bowel syndrome	
Painful diverticulosis (Fig. 11–29A)	Radiographic diverticulosis; no other source of pain	See irritable bowel syndrome	Barium enema (by definition)† Possibly proctoscopy and/or colonoscopy if rectal bleeding is a problem
Acute diverticulitis (Fig. 11–29B)	Localized (usually sigmoid) abdominal pain and tenderness Fever; elevated ESR; leukocytosis Known radiographic diverticulosis	Bowel rest (no oral intake) Usually hospitalize Broad-spectrum antibiotics (ampicillin, tetracycline, trimethoprim/ sulfamethoxazole)	After acute illness resolves (proctoscopy, barium enema, colonoscopy may perforate colon during acute illness)
Partial large bowel obstruction due to stricture (Fig. 11–29C)	Never	Surgery	Barium enema may suggest diagnosis, but colon carcinoma must be excluded (colonoscopy?)
Habitual constipation[95]	Life-long history Younger patient Normal examination Heme-negative stool	Withdraw cathartics, laxatives Exclude drug-induced constipation (Table 11–1) Bulk diet, liquids, hydrophilic colloid, tap water enemas (Table 11–16)	Proctoscopy, barium enema if: Metabolic or systemic cause suspected (Table 11–1) Heme-positive stool Onset in middle-age or beyond Failure to respond to treatment
Dysmenorrhea[65, 82–84] (menstrual cramps)	Typical premenstrual pain, onset soon after menarche, gradually diminishing with age Normal pelvic examination	Nonaddictive analgesics and/ or antiprostaglandin agents and/or oral contraceptives	Gynecologic consultation and/ or pelvic ultrasound or laparoscopy if secondary dysmenorrhea suspected because of pain onset years after menarche, increasing disability over time, abnormal pelvic examination, absence of response to presumptive therapy

*In addition to the diagnoses listed, chronic recurrent lower abdominal pain may be due to hip, back, urinary, prostate or genital disease or neuralgia as well as to atypical location of upper GI disease (e.g., peptic ulcer—see text).
†Only the barium enema confirms the diagnosis.

TABLE 11–17. COMMON CAUSES OF CHRONIC/RECURRENT LOWER ABDOMINAL PAIN (Continued)

DIAGNOSIS*	PRESUMPTIVE DIAGNOSIS WHEN	PRESUMPTIVE THERAPY	SUGGESTED TEST(S) AND THEIR TIMING
Uterine myomas[96] (fibroids)	Pain clearly related to menses, intercourse Palpable myomas No suspicion of other pelvic disorder (e.g., abnormal bleeding, unilateral adnexal mass)	Reassurance, mild analgesics Avoid estrogens Surgery: if disabled and beyond childbearing age Yearly examination	Pelvic ultrasound if ovarian, uterine neoplasm cannot be excluded Gynecologic consultation and/ or dilatation and curettage if abnormal bleeding, diagnosis uncertain, or severe symptoms
Premenstrual syndrome[97] (pelvic congestion)	Premenstrual (several days) abdominal and back pain; weight gain Irritability; headache Breast congestion	Reduce salt intake Regular exercise Pyridoxine Diuretics	Study if: Abnormal pelvic examination Failure to respond to presumptive therapy
Endometriosis[85]	Acquired (secondary) dysmenorrhea and palpable nodular implants in cul-de-sac, ovaries, and/or uterosacral ligaments in premenopausal female (usually age 30–40)	Rarely wise Hormonal therapy and/or surgery after documentation	Gynecologic consultation and/ or laparoscopy for documentation
Mittelschmerz[85] (ovulation pain)	Recurrent unilateral adnexal pain, always exactly at midcycle Otherwise asymptomatic and normal pelvic examination	Reassurance Mild analgesics	Gynecologic consultation and/ or pelvic ultrasound or laparoscopy if: Ovarian cyst, neoplasm cannot be excluded Secondary dysmenorrhea Abnormal bleeding
Hernia Males, inguinal Females, femoral	Physical examination documents hernia No other disorder suspected	Reassurance Truss Avoidance of strain	Proctoscopy, barium x-ray if strangulation or bowel obstruction suspected or if considering surgery
Ovarian cyst(s)	Young women; adnexal pain and palpable ovarian cyst(s), especially in late cycle (corpus luteum cysts)	Reassurance Mild analgesics	Pelvic ultrasound and/or laparoscopy if: There is infertility Severe recurrent pain Neoplasm cannot be excluded Patient is perimenopausal or postmenopausal
Abdominal Wall Disorder	History of trauma? Visible ecchymosis or swelling Palpable hernia Pain with rectus muscle tension or stress No GI/GU/systemic symptoms	Reassurance Local ice or heat Rest	Consider CT scan if: Internal disease cannot be excluded There is a local palpable mass
Lactose Intolerance	See Chap. 3		

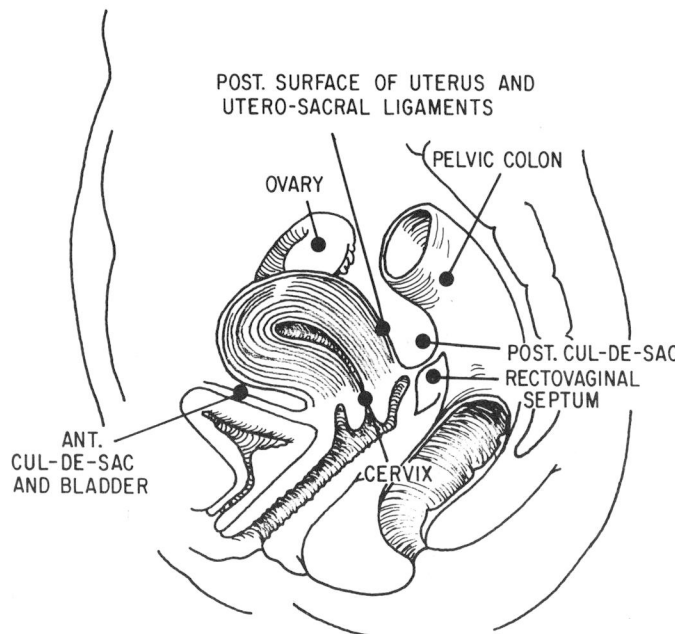

POST. SURFACE OF UTERUS AND
UTERO-SACRAL LIGAMENTS

PELVIC COLON

OVARY

POST. CUL-DE-SAC
RECTOVAGINAL
SEPTUM

ANT.
CUL-DE-SAC
AND BLADDER

CERVIX

FIGURE 11–28. The most common locations of ectopic endometrial tissue include the uterine surfaces, the cul-de-sac, the uterosacral ligaments, and the tubo-ovarian structures.

outside the uterine cavity (Fig. 11–28), most often in ovaries, rectovaginal cul-de-sac, uterosacral or broad ligaments, and on peritoneal surfaces of the uterus. (Endometrial "implants" may rarely be seen in extraordinarily diverse sites—pleura,[86] spinal cord,[87] bronchus[88]—giving rise to very bizarre presentations.) This ectopic endometrial tissue remains normally responsive to systemic hormonal events, and thus, while symptoms will vary with the location of the endometrial tissue, the usual symptoms are acquired dysmenorrhea, usually beginning in the 20s or 30s, with crampy lower abdominal pain during menstruation with or without abnormal vaginal bleeding or dyspareunia. Sometimes pain will be more constant—a vague fullness or bearing-down feeling in the pelvis or low back—or will be intermittently associated with bowel movements (when the colon is involved), cyclic hematuria (when the bladder is involved), or acute local peritonitis (when endometrial cysts rupture and bleed).

Thus the diagnosis may be difficult, either because symptoms are mistaken for primary dysmenorrhea in an overly reactive, complaining woman or because (rarely) symptoms are only sometimes related to menses. Pelvic examination, especially during a bout of pain, often reveals painful nodules in the characteristic locations—ovaries or tubes, cul-de-sac, or along the uterosacral ligaments (Fig. 11–28). X-rays and pelvic ultrasound are usually normal, except in unusual circumstances in which the bowel is involved or endometrial cysts ("endometriomas") are large. Laparoscopy or laparotomy is required for definitive diagnosis in most instances. Treatment usually involves various hormonal manipulations but is too specialized and individualized to be discussed here.[85]

As Table 11–17 shows, other common causes of pelvic pain are mittelschmerz—unilateral adnexal pain and tenderness occurring cyclically between periods (during ovulation); pelvic congestion syndrome[97]—premenstrual discomfort in association with weight gain, edema, bloating, headache, and irritability, sometimes for 7 to 10 days before menses, usually in the 30- to 40-year-old group; and intermittent adnexal pain due to ovarian cysts—resorption of a corpus luteum cyst late in the menstrual cycle causes recurrent late cycle pain in some women.

Diverticular Disease of the Colon.[89–94] Diverticulosis is a radiographic diagnosis (Fig. 11–29A). Perhaps one third of all elderly patients have colonic

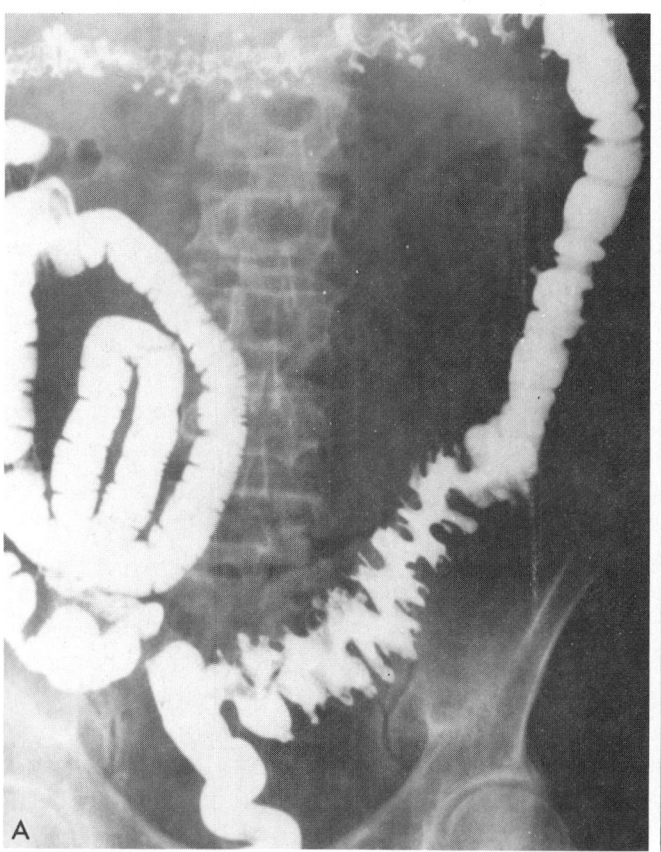

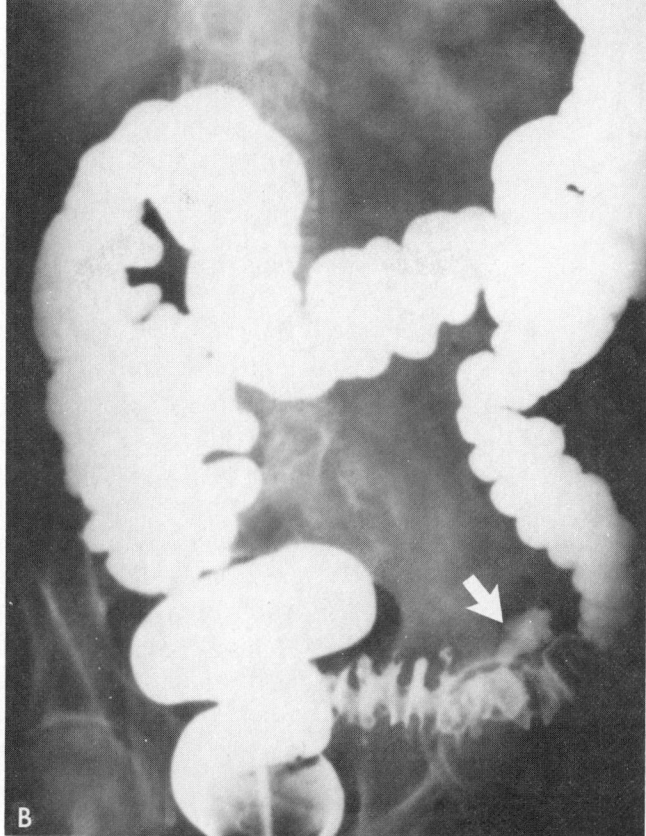

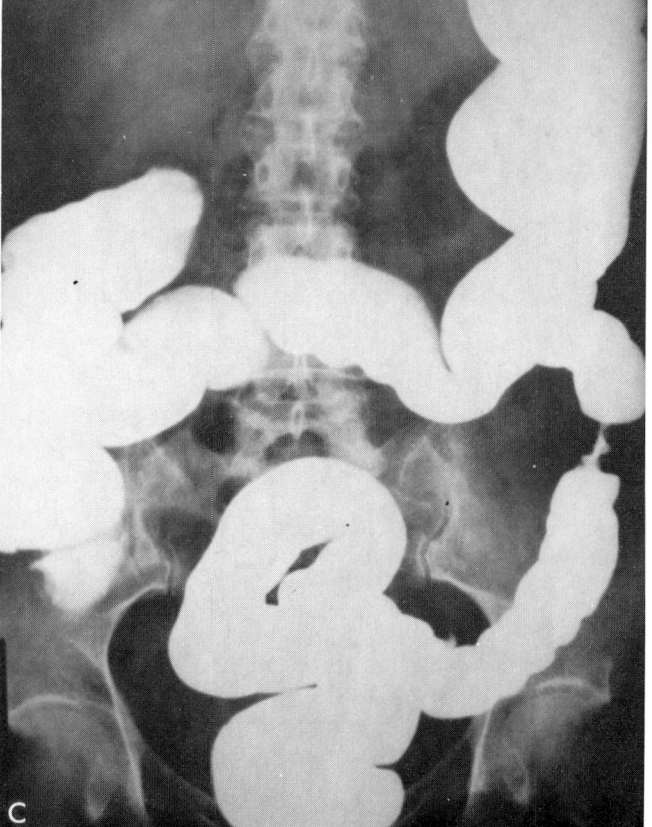

FIGURE 11–29. Diverticular disease. *A,* There is extensive diverticulosis of the colon, but the patient has no symptoms. *B,* A pericolonic abscess (*arrow*) is demonstrated on barium enema in this elderly patient with fever, left lower quadrant abdominal pain, and localized peritoneal signs. *C,* This barium enema is typical of the "napkin ring" obstruction of the colon so often seen in patients with colon carcinoma. Exploratory laparotomy revealed no carcinoma. This patient, whose symptoms were those of progressive distal bowel obstruction, was found to have a stricture due to prior diverticular disease. (Note the absence of prominent diverticulosis elsewhere in the colon—this is most unusual!)

diverticula—relatively few have any symptoms. Unlike the irritable bowel syndrome, however, diverticular disease can be serious: massive rectal bleeding, acute diverticulitis with pericolonic abscess formation (Fig. 11–29B), peritonitis after diverticular perforation, or bowel obstruction (sometimes mimicking colon cancer—Fig. 11–29C) may complicate diverticulosis.

Treatment usually involves a high-fiber diet, Metamucil, and (occasionally) antispasmodic drugs. Because diverticular disease is primarily a disease of the elderly, painful diverticulosis can never be presumptively diagnosed initially—colorectal carcinoma in particular must be excluded, and barium enema must be performed. When diverticulosis has been radiographically documented in the recent past, however, and when there are no new findings suggesting an additional diagnosis, treatment of recurrent diverticulosis *is* often presumptive.

Acute diverticulitis, on the other hand, often is treated presumptively, at least initially. Precise pathogenesis of acute diverticulitis remains somewhat controversial, but diverticular perforation with pericolonic abscess formation is usually responsible for the typical clinical findings: (usually) left lower quadrant abdominal pain, localized tenderness (often with local peritoneal signs), leukocytosis, and fever. The diagnosis can only be *proven* when a barium enema demonstrates extravasation of contrast material into a pericolonic abscess (Fig. 11–29B) (or, less often, at surgery). Other x-ray findings are often highly suspicious of acute diverticulitis but are nonspecific. Barium studies are, however, usually postponed until the patient improves symptomatically, since a barium enema performed during acute diverticulitis may do more harm than good (generalized barium peritonitis may result if a perforation is present). Thus the elderly patient (especially if prior diverticulosis is known) with clinical acute diverticulitis is often treated presumptively (usually in the hospital, with intravenous feedings and broad-spectrum antibiotics). After clinical improvement, studies must be undertaken to exclude colon carcinoma, which may present very similarly. Diagnostic studies are always indicated sooner if surgery[90] is contemplated or if the patient is seriously ill and does not respond to medical therapy.

Thus, in Sally's case, endometriosis involving the pelvis and colon is a remote possible unifying diagnosis, but it is much more likely that Sally suffers from primary dysmenorrhea as well as the irritable bowel syndrome.

> Sally is told that her pains are probably of two different origins. No laboratory or radiologic testing is performed.
>
> Sally is instructed in the use of Motrin 400 mg tid or qid, to be taken the day before and for the first few days of each menstrual period, to treat the menstrual pain. Sally is due to have her period in 10 days.
>
> The nonmenstrual pains are explained as spasms of the large intestine. Sally is told that the circumference of the large bowel contains layers of muscle and that sometimes these muscles become overreactive or uncoordinated, disrupting normal painless sequential peristalsis. Such spasms can then cause pain, gas buildup, and bowel dysfunction. A brief review of prior life events suggests flare of this problem during emotional circumstances—Sally specifically remembers difficulty during high school examinations and during the prolonged, ultimately fatal, illness of her mother.
>
> Sally is instructed in the use of a high-fiber diet and also to take 1 tablespoonful of Metamucil each night in 8 ounces of water. She is told this will help promote a softer, bulkier stool that can help avoid bowel spasm. Sally is told she will not see immediate benefit, but that after 4 to 6 weeks things will probably be better. A lactose-free diet is suggested for a week or two to see if it is helpful.
>
> Sally is then told that intestinal muscles are under the involuntary control of nerves that receive their instructions from the brain. The importance of

psychologic tension and upset as causes of bowel muscle spasm is re-viewed. Sally is asked whether she feels any emotional stress and answers simply, "We all have problems. There is nothing new or different." Sally is asked to think more about that and to return in 6 weeks.

NOTE

Figure 11–27 illustrates the general approach to the patient with chronic/recurrent abdominal pain. Note that in Sally's case symptoms are longstanding and quite typical of common benign disorders; thus "presumptive" diagnosis and treatment are reasonable, given her age and lack of worrisome findings. When such a strategy is employed, careful follow-up is essential.

When the patient demands abolute diagnostic certainty (or is requesting a second opinion), testing is necessary, but normal tests will sometimes be more reassuring to patients who are told beforehand, "Your tests will be normal—you have irritable bowel syndrome" (or whatever).

Table 11–18 illustrates some of the serious causes of chronic/recurrent lower abdominal pain. Most of these will be suspected on the basis of the clinical setting, symptoms, or signs. Usually there is some worrisome finding (page 579) among patients with these diseases. When diagnostic testing is performed because one or more of these serious disorders is suspected, remember: Those tests that usually diagnose these disorders are not neces-sarily the same as those tests that definitively exclude them! As suggested by Table 11–18, normal proctoscopy and barium enema usually, but *not always*, will exclude colon carcinoma; normal endometrial curettage does *not* neces-sarily exclude uterine carcinoma; Crohn's disease *may* be missed on barium x-rays; the normal pelvic ultrasound *almost* always excludes ovarian carci-noma. Each of these disorders cannot be discussed here in detail—in all patients, however, clinical suspicions based on the history and physical examination are most important; test results can be interpreted only in the light of these clinical findings.

Six weeks later, Sally returns for her follow-up appointment, saying, "I'm not much better." Closer questioning reveals that she has had two men-strual periods since her last visit, and that the premenstrual pain has been markedly relieved by the Motrin. However, the unpredictable lower abdom-inal cramping continues to recur, in spite of the high-fiber diet and daily Metamucil.

Sally admits that she is less constipated than previously but describes recurrent, usually left lower quadrant cramping, often associated with abdominal bloating and gas and partly relieved with the passage of feces or gas. She denies any other symptoms. Omission of lactose for 2 weeks did not appear to be helpful.

Physical examination is normal, except for mild, variable, fluctuating left lower quadrant tenderness.

The relations between life events and irritable bowel syndrome are again suggested. Sally is asked specifically about her job, marriage, home life, and future plans and whether there are any increasing anxieties, uncertain-ties, or frustrations about such matters. Sally says that she is happy in her job and that her career is quite satisfying. Her marriage and home life are another matter.

Sally's husband is not even apologetic about his previous fling that resulted in Sally's gonococcal PID. He continues to be "distant and uncaring," and Sally suspects that he is repeatedly unfaithful. When she is asked if they have sought counseling of any kind, Sally says it would not help because, "My grandfather is the real problem."

TABLE 11–18. SERIOUS CAUSES OF CHRONIC/RECURRENT LOWER ABDOMINAL PAIN

DISEASE	WHEN TO SUSPECT		
	SETTING	SYMPTOMS	SIGNS
Colorectal carcinoma[68]	Usually, middle-aged or elderly—less than 5% of colon cancers occur before age 40 (chronic ulcerative colitis and familial polyposis syndromes are exceptions)	Rectal: changes in bowel movement; rectal bleeding	Heme-positive stool; palpable rectal mass
		Left colon: changes in bowel movement; abdominal cramps	Heme-positive stool; physical examination often normal
		Right colon: weight loss; iron deficient anemia; possibly abdominal cramps	Heme-positive stool; possibly palpable cecal mass
Endometrial (uterine) carcinoma[67]	Usually perimenopausal or postmenopausal (80%) Premenopausal (20%)	Postmenopausal or otherwise abnormal vaginal bleeding Menstrual irregularity or decline in menses	Pelvic examination and Pap test often normal
Ovarian carcinoma[69]	Usually perimenopausal or postmenopausal	Rarely symptomatic until disease advanced; then ascites/abdominal pain, abdominal mass	Adnexal mass; ascites when disease is advanced
Inflammatory bowel disease (see Chap. 3)			
Crohn's disease	80% less than 40 years	Rarely abdominal pain alone; usually also diarrhea, GI bleeding, weight loss, fever, fatigue	Fever, right lower quadrant pain/mass; anemia; heme-positive stools
Ulcerative colitis	All ages		Heme-positive stool
Meckel's diverticulum[98]	Young	Intermittent pain, bleeding, or obstruction	Pseudoappendicitis; heme-positive stools; small-bowel obstruction (possibly intussusception)
Chronic abscess[64]	History of appendicitis, surgery, diverticulitis, PID, etc.	Fever, weight loss, indolent but progressive symptoms	Localized tenderness; fever; possibly enterocutaneous fistula
Chronic pelvic inflammatory disease	Premenopausal; history of acute PID, infertility?	Pelvic pain; dyspareunia; infertility; fever	Unilateral or bilateral tubo-ovarian swelling/tenderness (not as dramatic as acute PID)
Intestinal angina (see page 615; Table 11–22)	Usually elderly; diffuse vascular disease	Most often epigastric pain; postprandial abdominal pain; fear of eating; weight loss	Exam often normal Vascular bruits? Sometimes, heme + stool
Abdominal aortic aneurysm (see Table 11–22)	Usually elderly; diffuse vascular disease	Possibly claudication; "blue toe syndrome"; vague abdominal pain (usually asymptomatic)	Palpable aneurysm; bruit
Aortoiliac claudication	Usually beyond middle-aged, smoker, hypertension, etc.	Episodic exertional groin, hip, or back pain	Diminished pulses, cool feet, diminished toe hair
Remember:	**Neoplasm of pelvic bones, spine, or retroperitoneum** **Unsuspected uterine or ectopic pregnancy** **Polycystic kidneys**		

For the past 6 months, Sally has had her 72-year-old grandfather living with her. "He has nowhere else to go." He is losing weight, eats poorly, and is an increasing burden on Sally and her husband, who is adamantly opposed to caring for him at home. Sally admits that this is a major stress, but "What can I do about it? He can't take care of himself!"

Sally submits to urinalysis, proctoscopy, and barium enema. All studies are normal, except for visible sigmoid spasm on fluoroscopy during barium studies.

NOTE

The patient with irritable bowel syndrome very often is troubled by covert anxieties or unavoidable stresses. Denial of emotional precipitants is very common. Specific directed queries about the patient's current occupa-

TABLE 11–18. SERIOUS CAUSES OF CHRONIC/RECURRENT LOWER ABDOMINAL PAIN (*Continued*)

DISEASE	USUALLY DIAGNOSED BY	EXCLUDE IF	TREATMENT
Colorectal carcinoma[68]	Proctoscopy	Normal proctoscopy and rectal examination	Surgery
	Sigmoidoscopy and/or barium enema	Normal colonoscopy	Surgery
	Barium enema and/or colonoscopy	Normal colonoscopy (to terminal ileum)	Surgery
Endometrial (uterine) carcinoma[67]	Endometrial curettage and/or biopsy	Repeatedly normal biopsies and/or hysterectomy	Usually by hysterectomy Possibly radiation therapy, chemotherapy
Ovarian carcinoma[69]	Physical examination; ultrasound; exploration or laparoscopy	Normal laparoscopy and/or exploration	Surgery; possibly chemotherapy
Inflammatory bowel disease (see Chap. 3) Crohn's disease	Barium studies; rectal biopsy; colonoscopic biopsy	Normal laparotomy	Azulfidine, corticosteroids and/or surgery
Ulcerative colitis		Normal colonoscopy	
Meckel's diverticulum[98]	"Meckel's scan"	Laparotomy?	Surgery
Chronic abscess[64]	Ultrasound and/or CT scan, gallium scan	Normal laparotomy	Surgery and/or percutaneous drainage
Chronic pelvic inflammatory disease	Laparoscopy and/or hysterosalpingography, pelvic ultrasound	All studies normal	Antibiotics; sometimes surgery
Intestinal angina (see page 603; Table 11–22)	Clinical history and triple-vessel mesenteric disease on abdominal angiography	Normal angiography or less than multiple-vessel atherosclerosis	Revascularization
Abdominal aortic aneurysm (see Table 11–22)	Abdominal ultrasound	Normal aorta on ultrasound and arteriogram	Surgery, usually
Aortoiliac claudication	Clinical findings; Doppler and/or noninvasive vascular laboratory methods	Normal arteriography	Surgical bypass

tional, marital, sexual, family, and financial situation are always worthwhile when the irritable bowel syndrome is clinically very likely but when symptoms persist despite appropriate treatment.

(This by no means should imply that all painful episodes or flares of irritable bowel syndrome can be correlated with specific emotional stresses. Much more often, it is the ongoing, subliminal psychosocial stresses that form the substrate for symptomatic events. As noted previously, a substantial minority of patients with irritable bowel syndrome will have no demonstrable personality [or affective] disorder. Do not insist that the patient with irritable bowel syndrome must be stressed, anxious, frustrated, or depressed.)

Sally is given a prescription for Librax, is asked to speak to her husband about marital counseling, and is asked to bring her grandfather in for a medical examination.

Ichabod is a 72-year-old gentleman who has always been in good health except for longstanding borderline hypertension and a myocardial infarction 8 years previously. He is a thin, very alert, but somewhat depressed-looking man who complains, "My stomach hurts!" when asked what is bothering him. He places his hand over his epigastrium when localizing his pain.

Further questioning reveals that for the past 3 months (and perhaps longer than that), Ichabod has noticed intermittent epigastric pain that usually occurs after eating. This pain has increased in severity and frequency to the point that it occurs with almost every meal, and Ichabod has thus greatly decreased his food intake to try to avoid the pain. He thinks he "may have" lost weight, but, if so, this is because of inadequate food intake. Ichabod describes his pain as an "ache" that is sometimes associated with a "feeling of gas and bloating." Symptoms usually occur about half an hour after eating and last for 1 to 2 hours. "Tums don't help."

Chronic Recurrent Upper Abdominal Pain

Table 11–19 illustrates that the differential diagnosis of chronic/recurrent upper abdominal pain may be formidable, but most patients with recurrent or chronic upper abdominal pain suffer from one of a very few common gastrointestinal disorders. The overwhelming majority (96 per cent of one group of several hundred patients studied in England[99]) will be diagnosed as having esophagitis, duodenal ulcer, gastric ulcer, gastric carcinoma, biliary tract disease, or functional dyspepsia. Familiarity with typical clinical manifestations of these common disorders is thus crucial, especially since the history alone is sometimes classic and the (usually radiographic) documentation of these entities is then often simple and straightforward (Table 11–20).

CONSIDER

I. Esophagitis may coexist with duodenal ulcer disease, but more often esophagitis causes a distinctive symptom complex, discussed in Appendix II of Chapter 13, "Chest Pain." Retrosternal burning, sometimes associated with interscapular back discomfort, radiating up into the suprasternal area and associated with acid brash and eructation, is typical of

TABLE 11–19. CAUSES OF CHRONIC/RECURRENT UPPER ABDOMINAL PAIN

COMMON	UNCOMMON	RARE	RIGHT UPPER QUADRANT PAIN ONLY	LEFT UPPER QUADRANT PAIN ONLY
Esophagitis	Pancreatic carcinoma	Heavy metal poisoning	Biliary colic/cholelithiasis	Splenomegaly
Duodenal ulcer	Chronic pancreatitis	Porphyria	Gallbladder carcinoma	Splenic distention
Alcoholic gastritis	Pancreatic pseudocyst	Tabes dorsalis	Chronic hepatitis	Pancreatic disease
Gastric ulcer	Aortic aneurysm	Hyperlipidemia	Hepatocellular carcinoma	Splenic flexure syndrome
Gastric carcinoma	Intestinal angina	Familial Mediterranean	Hepatic distention (fat,	Renal/ureteral disease
Biliary colic	Superior mesenteric	fever	abscess, tumor,	Slipping rib
Functional dyspepsia	artery syndrome		congestive failure)	Radiculitis
	Celiac axis syndrome		Hepatic adenoma	
Lactose intolerance	Giardiasis		Hepatic flexure syndrome	
Angina pectoris	Gastroparesis		Renal/ureteral disease	
Rib cage disorders	diabeticorum		Slipping rib	
(xiphoidalgia,	Adrenal neoplasm		Radiculitis	
costochondritis)	Small-bowel disease			
Abdominal wall disorders	Colon disease			
(hernias, "scar" pain,	Vasculitis			
rectus muscle strains)	Psychogenic			
Irritable bowel syndrome				

TABLE 11–20. COMMON CAUSES OF CHRONIC/RECURRENT UPPER ABDOMINAL PAIN

DISEASE	WHEN TO SUSPECT	PRESUMPTIVE DIAGNOSIS	PROOF OF DIAGNOSIS	TREATMENT
Esophagitis	Heartburn, acid brash; usually retrosternal	History Dysphagia?	Barium swallow and/or endoscopy; (see Chap. 13)	See Chap. 13
Duodenal ulcer	Recurrent epigastric burning, discomfort; improves with antacids; usually related to meals	Upper GI series	Endoscopy (uncommonly necessary)	See Appendix
Duodenitis/gastritis	Aspirin; nonsteroidal anti-inflammatory drugs; alcoholic?	Ulcer symptoms; normal upper GI series; drug use	Endoscopy	Antacids; discontinuance of offending agents; see Appendix
Gastric ulcer		Upper GI series	Endoscopy and biopsy (often necessary)	See Appendix
Gastric carcinoma	Recurrent epigastric burning, discomfort; improves with antacids; usually related to meals Weight loss; possibly palpable mass; history of pernicious anemia; elderly patient	Upper GI series	Endoscopy and biopsy (always necessary)	Surgery and/or radiation therapy
Functional dyspepsia	Epigastric discomfort; dyspepsia less predictable in relation to meals/antacids	Normal upper GI series	Normal endoscopy (endoscopy rarely necessary)	Reassurance; antacids prn; follow-up
Biliary colic	Unpredictable *episodes* of more prolonged pain— asymptomatic between attacks (see Table 11–13)	History and gallstones on OCG or Echo	Resolution of symptoms after cholecystectomy	Surgery

Remember: Irritable bowel, angina pectoris, rib cage disorders, thoracic disease, abdominal wall disorders, lactose intolerance, giardiasis, and radiculopathy

esophagitis. Recumbency, bending forward, ingestion of large meals, and various dietary indiscretions often precipitate discomfort. Diagnosis and treatment are discussed further in Appendix II of Chapter 13.

II. Duodenal ulcer is classically announced by epigastric discomfort, often described as burning, gnawing, or hunger pains, which seem most prominent when the stomach is empty, i.e., during sleep or several hours after the last meal (or just prior to the next meal).

Ingestion of food or antacids often (at least temporarily) ameliorates symptoms. Thus, in many patients, the pain of duodenal ulcer is predictable. Such a symptom complex should strongly suggest duodenal ulcer disease, especially when the patient is young (peak incidence between 20 and 50 years) and when symptoms have recurred and remitted for a long time—many months to years (see Fig. 11–30).

It has long been known,[100] however, and more recently verified[101] that this classic presentation is not extremely common among patients with proven duodenal ulcer disease. In many patients, no definite relations among meals, hunger, and pain can be appreciated. In others, ingestion of food seems to cause pain rather than relieve it, and some patients will even purposely avoid eating to avoid pain. Several traditional adages about duodenal ulcers do seem to stand up well to careful scrutiny:[101] the location of pain is usually epigastric; symptoms tend to begin early in life (teenage and young adulthood) and to recur intermittently (with prolonged pain-free intervals); antacids usually (at least temporarily) help the patient's pain; and symptoms commonly awaken the patient from sleep.

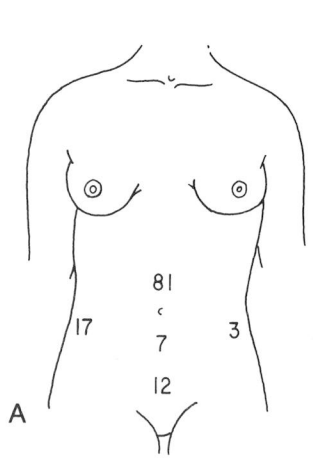

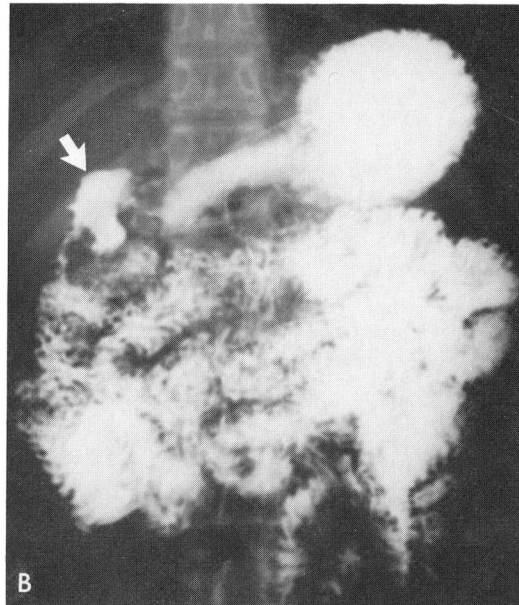

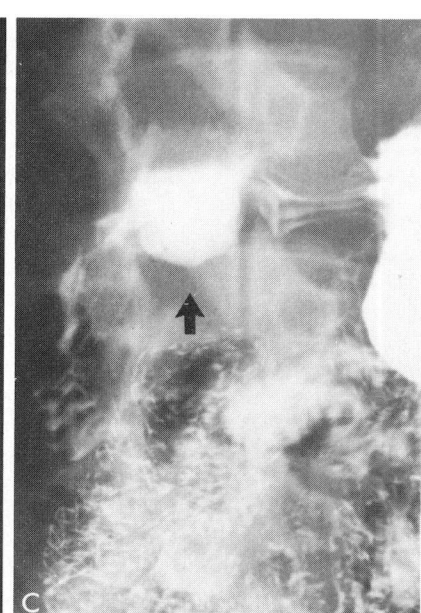

FIGURE 11–30. *A,* Primary site of pain among 120 patients with symptomatic duodenal ulcer disease. *B,C,* This 22-year-old man described epigastric discomfort intermittently over the previous 6 to 12 months. Pain was a "gnawing" hurt that was usually relieved by eating but returned a few hours after each meal. He was often awakened from sleep by the pain. Usually, antacids helped the pain but he sought medical attention when antacid tablets became less effective.

The UGI series reveals a very large duodenal ulcer (*arrow*). Cimetidine therapy resulted in initial cure, but there have been two recurrences since (see also Appendix). (*A* adapted from Branch, WT, and Trier, TS: Chronic dyspepsia and upper abdominal pain. *In* Branch, WT: Office Practice of Medicine. Philadelphia: W. B. Saunders Co., 1982.)

The upper gastrointestinal barium x-ray (Fig. 11–30*B* and *C*) will diagnose or exclude duodenal ulcer with about 90 per cent accuracy. Occasionally endoscopy is necessary to exclude false negative or false positive upper GI findings (see Appendix and page 606).[102] Gastritis or duodenitis (due to alcohol, aspirin, or nonsteroidal anti-inflammatory drugs) may cause symptoms indistinguishable from duodenal or gastric ulcer—only endoscopy will accurately diagnose these disorders.

III. <u>Gastric ulcer</u> tends to occur in an older age group (peak 40 to 60 years) than does duodenal ulcer.

Pain is usually epigastric and qualitatively similar to that of duodenal ulcer pain, but, for poorly understood reasons, pain location and quality are much more variable among patients with gastric ulcer. (For example, constant, aching pain in the mid lower abdomen will occasionally occur.) There is often some relation between eating and pain, but not always. Antacids sometimes are helpful, but this, too, is unpredictable.

Thus, in general, the pain of gastric ulcer disease is somewhat <u>less predictable</u> than that of duodenal ulcer disease.

The upper GI barium x-ray (Fig. 11–31) is highly accurate in demonstrating or excluding gastric ulcer (about 90 per cent). The 4- to 5-per cent incidence of gastric carcinoma among patients with gastric ulcer is a common rationale for more invasive diagnostic evaluation (endoscopy[103]) in such patients—this is discussed briefly in the appendix. However,

IV. <u>Gastric carcinoma</u>[103, 104] does not always present as gastric ulcer.

This neoplasm tends to occur in older patients (85 per cent of patients are older than 50 years) and appears to be diminishing in

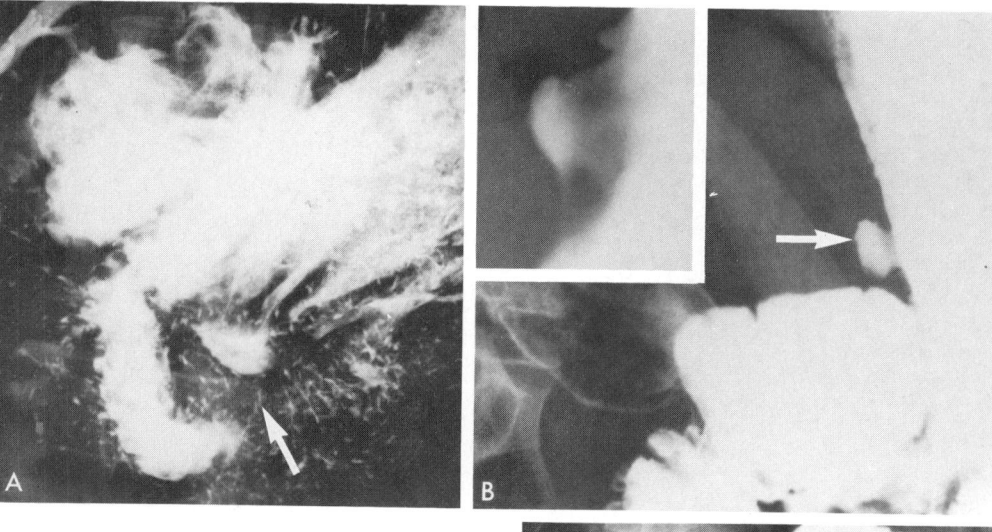

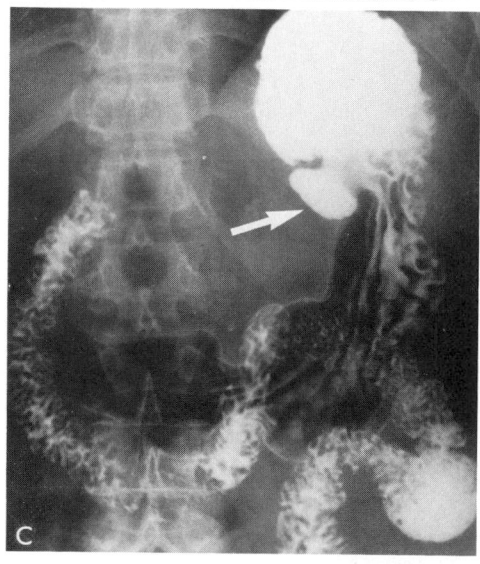

FIGURE 11–31. Gastric ulcers. Benign gastric ulcers are usually characterized radiographically by their smooth contours and the surrounding edema with radiating "folds"; they usually involve the lesser curvature of the stomach and project beyond the border of the gastric lumen as a "collar button" or a mushroom shape. Malignant gastric ulcers are more often irregular in outline, are surrounded by an irregular mass, and do not extend beyond the gastric lumen. A, A typical benign gastric ulcer of the greater curvature. Note the smooth, rounded contour of the ulcer and the "radiating folds" of edema. B, A typical benign ulcer of the lesser curvature. C, A "worrisome" gastric ulcer, proven at endoscopy to be malignant. The ulcer is irregular and does not extend beyond the gastric lumen. D, Certainly not all gastric cancers are ulcers. Infiltrating neoplasms, with or without partial gastric outlet obstruction, are also common. E, Similarly, it is not always possible to be sure about gastric ulcer purely on the basis of radiography. This lesion "looked benign" (radiographically) but failed to heal (see Appendix). Endoscopic biopsy revealed adenocarcinoma.

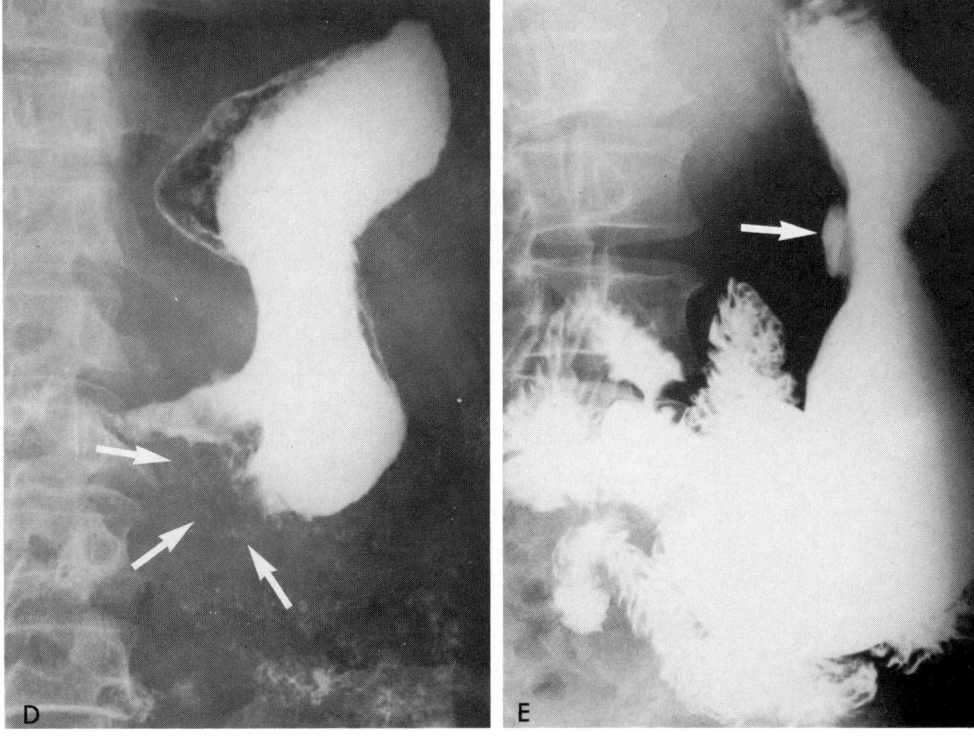

incidence, for obscure reasons. Epigastric discomfort, early satiety, postprandial vomiting, weight loss, anorexia, and occult gastrointestinal blood loss are common manifestations, but it is the extent (stage) of disease that usually dictates symptoms.[105, 106] Symptoms indistinguishable from gastric or duodenal ulcer symptoms are common early in the disease. The patient with previously documented achlorhydria or pernicious anemia is probably at greater risk of gastric carcinoma.

A barium upper GI series (Fig. 11–31D) will almost always suggest the diagnosis, but endoscopy, gastric cytologic studies, and/or surgery are required for definitive diagnosis.

V. <u>Biliary colic</u> is usually very different from the pain of esophagitis, duodenal or gastric ulcer, or gastric cancer.

The major difference is that biliary colic <u>is an infrequent (episodic) event, before and after which the patient is asymptomatic.</u> (The chronic dyspepsia, fatty food intolerance, and intermittent gas previously attributed to biliary disease in fact cannot be correlated with gallbladder disease.[107, 108]) Biliary colic is an attack,[6, 46] usually characterized by (often quite abrupt) onset of epigastric or right upper quadrant pain (Fig. 11–32) that is rarely colicky (it is usually steady) but is often quite severe.* Pain occasionally radiates to the shoulder or scapula, is often associated with nausea, anorexia, or vomiting, and typically lasts a few hours (range 15 minutes to several hours). Attacks of biliary colic are utterly *unpredictable*.

Unless frank acute cholecystitis (page 572) supervenes, the pain of biliary colic resolves spontaneously—the acute severe pain resolving in a few hours, while sometimes a residual ache slowly abates over the next day or so. The patient is then typically well until struck by the next unpredictable attack (which may be days, months or years thereafter).

VI. <u>Functional dyspepsia</u>[99, 109, 110] <u>is a term used to describe chronic/recurrent upper abdominal discomfort,</u> often associated with anorexia, eructation, bloating, or nausea <u>in patients whose diagnostic evaluation is normal</u> (hence, another diagnosis attributed to such patients is "x-ray–negative dyspepsia").

Depending upon how liberally one defines such symptoms, this is probably the most common cause of upper abdominal discomfort in the general population, i.e., if all patients with such intermittent discomfort were studied, most would be x-ray negative. (The fact is that most such patients do not seek medical attention at all.)

Whether there is a distinctive clinical entity here—an upper irritable bowel syndrome?[72]—is unclear. If there is, this group of patients tends to have symptoms that are vague, sporadic, or constant (rather than predictable, sterotyped, or unexpectedly episodic); symptoms are unconvincingly related to meals and are often unrelieved by antacids. There is never evidence of serious illness (weight loss, for example) in such patients unless major psychiatric disorders (depression, anorexia nervosa, for example) coexist.

<u>This concept of functional dyspepsia is of great importance for several reasons:</u>

---

*As with all diseases, there are occasions when symptoms are nonspecific and atypical. Cope's description of his own attacks of biliary colic[49]—characterized only by intermittent diaphoresis and tachycardia—is a case in point.

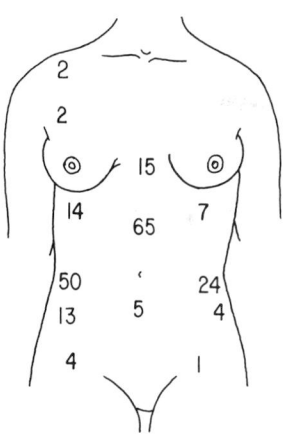
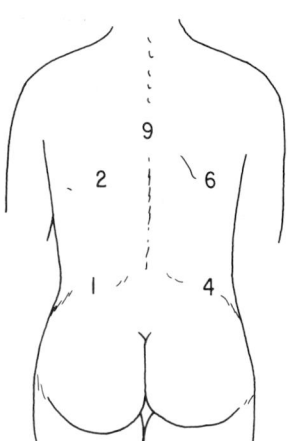

FIGURE 11–32. Primary site of pain among 227 patients with symptomatic gallbladder disease. (Adapted from Branch, WT, and Trier, JS: Chronic dyspepsia and upper abdominal pain. *In* Branch, WT: Office Practice of Medicine. Philadelphia: W. B. Saunders Co., 1982.)

A. This diagnosis may be used as a "wastebasket" for all patients whose symptoms and radiographic evaluation do not indicate esophagitis, duodenal or gastric ulcer, gastric carcinoma, or biliary tract disease.

   Since these diseases comprise such a large majority of the causes of upper abdominal pain and organic dyspepsia, there is a tendency to simply exclude these (usually with the upper GI series or endoscopy or gallbladder x-rays) and thereafter disregard rarer or more elusive diagnoses because an exclusionary diagnosis of functional dyspepsia is applied. In fact, the possible causes of chronic/recurrent upper abdominal pain are very numerous indeed (Table 11–19), and some uncommon causes are very serious (Table 11–22, pages 610 and 611).

B. Some patients with functional abdominal pain require psychiatric help.

   The problem of chronic psychogenic abdominal pain is beyond the scope of this text,[111, 112] but it is a major (and not rare) challenge. The borderline personality is most often afflicted (and help here is hard to come by). Evidence of depression, anxiety with hyperventilation/aerophagia (see Chapter 10, "Dizziness"), hysteria, hypochondriasis, or Munchausen's syndrome will be apparent in some, but the clinician must carefully exclude organic disease anyway: As Tables 11–19 and 11–22 and Figure 11–33 indicate, this may require very extensive investigation.

C. Most patients with functional dyspepsia have an excellent prognosis. Occasionally, symptomatic treatment with antacids, variations on the therapeutic regimen for irritable bowel (page 584), antigas (simethicone) or anticholinergic drugs may be helpful intermittently. The possibility of lactose intolerance or giardiasis should always be remembered in such patients, since these are common, curable problems (see Chapter 3, "Diarrhea").

How, then do we approach the patient with chronic/recurrent upper abdominal pain? Figure 11–33 illustrates the general strategy.

CONSIDER

Ichabod says his pain is "always" in the midline and epigastrium. There is no retrosternal, back, shoulder, or lower abdominal discomfort.

1. The pain is epigastric. Virtually all of the disorders listed in Table 11–19 may cause epigastric pain. As Figure 11–2 illustrates, disease of the

1. **Epigastric?**   No   ⟶ Retrosternal: esophageal, thoracic?
   Right upper quadrant only: liver, gallbladder, kidney, hepatic flexure, chest?
   Left upper quadrant only: spleen, pancreas, kidneys, splenic flexure, chest?

   Yes

2. **"Sounds" gastrointestinal?**   No   ⟶ Exertional: angina pectoris?
   Dyspepsia   Mechanical: chest wall disorders (see Chapter 13),
   Related to eating, hunger, defecation   abdominal wall disorders
   Associated "gas," bloating, borborygmi   Radicular: neuralgia, spine disease?

   Yes   Always postprandial?
                   Esophagitis? Ulcer? Lactose intolerance? Pancreatic disease? Intestinal ischemia?

3. **"Classic" clinical history?**   Esophagitis?   ⟶ Presumptive therapy (p. 767)
                                       Dysphagia? ⟶ **Barium swallow**

   Duodenal (gastric) ulcer?
   Prior ulcer history? ⟶ **UGI series** ⟨ Duodenal ulcer Treatment (Appendix)
                                        Gastric ulcer ⟩ **Endoscopy?**
                                        Nondiagnostic

   No

   or

   Equivocal   Biliary colic? ⟶ **Oral cholecystogram and/or ultrasound** ⟨ Normal
                                                   Gallstones ⟶ Surgery

   Associated borborygmi, diarrhea, relation to defecation? ⟶ Lactose intolerance?
                                          Giardiasis?
                                          Inflammatory bowel disease?
                                          Irritable colon?
                                          Atypical location of "lower" GI disorders (p. 577)?

   Epigastric and back pain? weight loss? ⟶ Pancreatic carcinoma? ⟶ Ultrasound ⟨ ERCP?
                                                           CT scan?

4. **Prior medical history: clues?** ⟶

                               Alcoholic ⟶ Gastritis, ulcer, hepatitis, pancreatitis?

   Rare multisystem diseases?
   Vasculitis:
     Polyarteritis
     SLE   Diabetic ⟶ Gastroparesis diabeticorum, fatty liver, neuritis?
   Neurologic: **Gallstones?**
     Porphyria
     Lead poisoning   Medication ⟶ Corticosteroids
     Tabes dorsalis   Aspirin   Ulcer, gastritis?
     Abdominal epilepsy   Nonsteroidal anti-inflammatory drugs
   Other: Contraceptives: esophagitis, hepatic adenoma
     Endometriosis?   Diffuse vascular disease
     Angioneurotic edema?   Bruits? ⟶ Angina? Aneurysm? Mesenteric ischemia?

                             Hematologic disease ⟶ Pernicious anemia: gastric cancer?
                                          Chronic leukemia/lymphoma: hepatosplenomegaly? coagulopathy? ischemia?
                                          Myeloproliferative disease: thrombocytosis? Polycythemia?
                                          Hemolytic disorders: gallstones? splenic disease? "crises?"

   No

FIGURE 11–33. Chronic or Recurrent Upper Abdominal Pain.

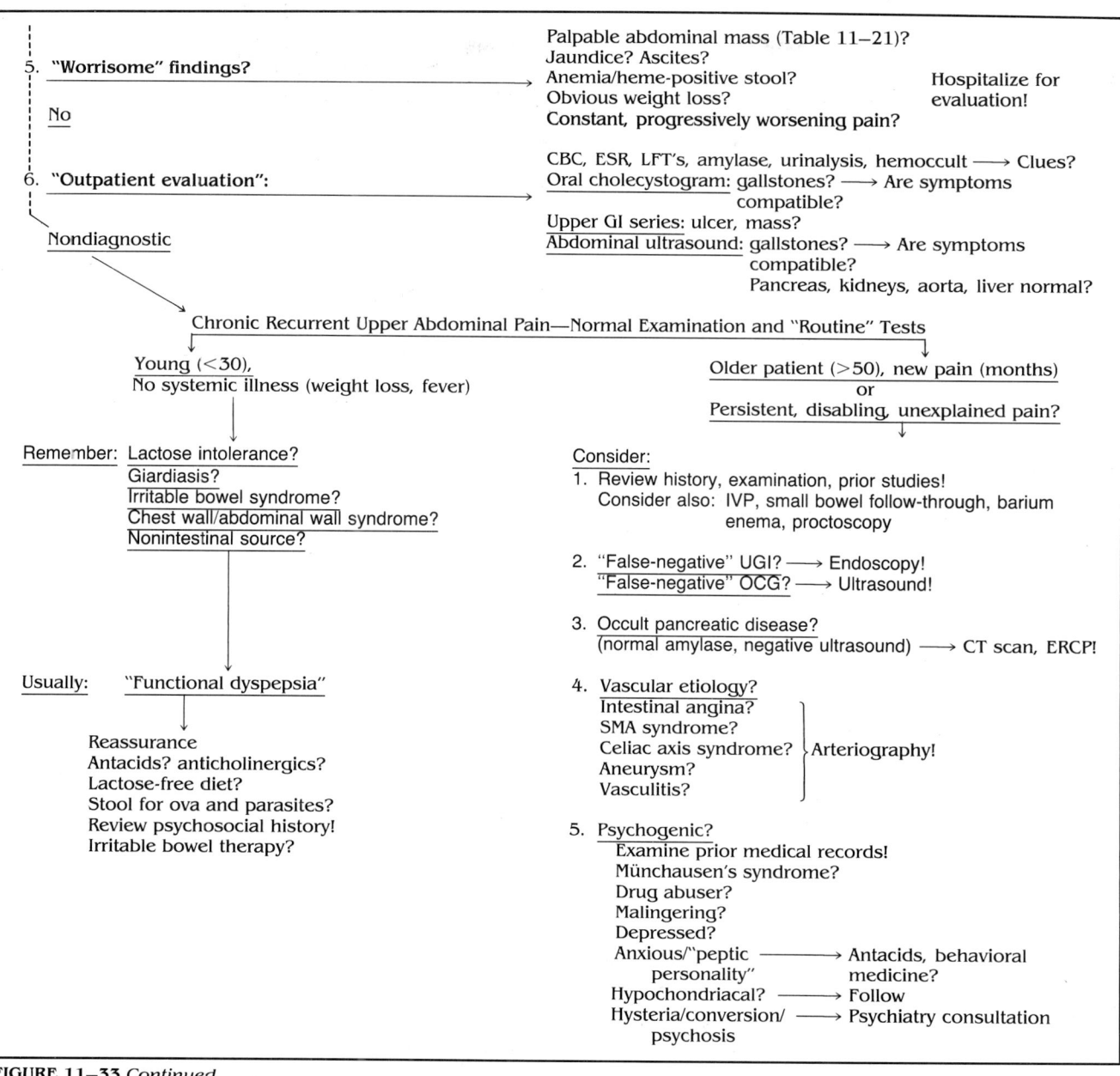

5. "Worrisome" findings? ———————————————→ Palpable abdominal mass (Table 11–21)?
   Jaundice? Ascites?
   Anemia/heme-positive stool?   Hospitalize for
   No   Obvious weight loss?   evaluation!
   Constant, progressively worsening pain?

6. "Outpatient evaluation": ———————————————→ CBC, ESR, LFT's, amylase, urinalysis, hemoccult ——→ Clues?
   Oral cholecystogram: gallstones? ——→ Are symptoms
                                                    compatible?
   Upper GI series: ulcer, mass?
   Nondiagnostic   Abdominal ultrasound: gallstones? ——→ Are symptoms
                                                    compatible?
   Pancreas, kidneys, aorta, liver normal?

Chronic Recurrent Upper Abdominal Pain—Normal Examination and "Routine" Tests

Young (<30),   Older patient (>50), new pain (months)
No systemic illness (weight loss, fever)   or
                                                  Persistent, disabling, unexplained pain?

Remember: Lactose intolerance?   Consider:
          Giardiasis?   1. Review history, examination, prior studies!
          Irritable bowel syndrome?   Consider also: IVP, small bowel follow-through, barium
          Chest wall/abdominal wall syndrome?   enema, proctoscopy
          Nonintestinal source?
                                                  2. "False-negative" UGI? ——→ Endoscopy!
                                                     "False-negative" OCG? ——→ Ultrasound!

                                                  3. Occult pancreatic disease?
                                                     (normal amylase, negative ultrasound) ——→ CT scan, ERCP!

Usually: "Functional dyspepsia"   4. Vascular etiology?
                                                     Intestinal angina?
          Reassurance   SMA syndrome?
          Antacids? anticholinergics?   Celiac axis syndrome? ⎬ Arteriography!
          Lactose-free diet?   Aneurysm?
          Stool for ova and parasites?   Vasculitis?
          Review psychosocial history!
          Irritable bowel therapy?   5. Psychogenic?
                                                     Examine prior medical records!
                                                     Münchausen's syndrome?
                                                     Drug abuser?
                                                     Malingering?
                                                     Depressed?
                                                     Anxious/"peptic ——————→ Antacids, behavioral
                                                        personality"   medicine?
                                                     Hypochondriacal? ——→ Follow
                                                     Hysteria/conversion/ ——→ Psychiatry consultation
                                                        psychosis

FIGURE 11–33 *Continued*

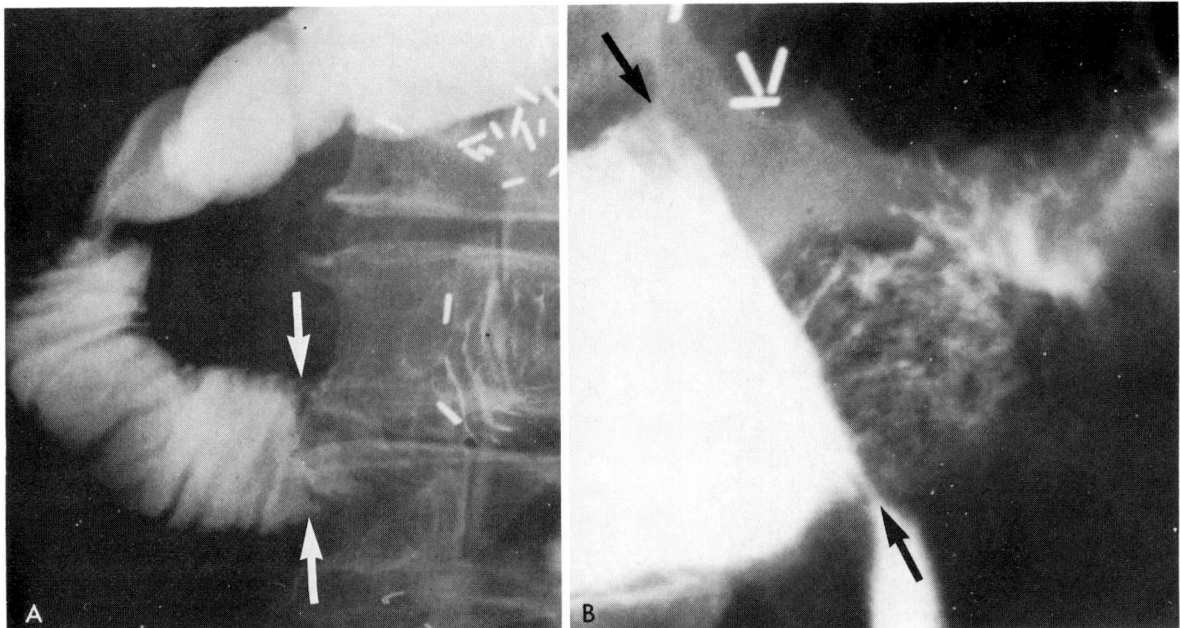

FIGURE 11–34. The superior mesenteric artery syndrome. Three months after resection of a benign retroperitoneal neoplasm (see surgical clips), this 36-year-old woman developed predictable postprandial abdominal pain and vomiting. She had lost 50 pounds. *A,* The upper GI series demonstrates abrupt cessation of barium flow in the area of the superior mesenteric artery. *B,* Shows abrupt, "linear" obstruction (*arrows*) to barium flow. Parenteral hyperalimentation with progressive weight gain resulted in complete amelioration of symptoms and a normal upper GI series 1 month later. This syndrome, caused by duodenal compression by the overlying superior mesenteric artery, is usually the *result* of weight loss and is most often seen in cachectic postperative or debilitated patients. Restoration of body weight alleviates the problem in most.

esophagus, stomach, duodenum, pancreas, liver, and gallbladder are the usual causes of epigastric pain.

When pain lateralizes primarily to the right or left upper quadrant, hepatobiliary disease, urorenal disorders, splenic disease, or disorders of the thorax or colonic flexures must be especially considered.

> Ichabod is convinced that his pain is somehow related to eating; he again confirms that "gas and bloating" are often associated with or follow the pain. Ichabod denies any relation of pain to physical exertion, bodily position, respiration, bowel movements, urination, or mechanical motion of the thorax and abdomen. The pain is "deep inside."

2. The pain sounds gastrointestinal. This is a crucial determination. It is not always possible to distinguish upper abdominal pain from lower chest pain (see also Chapter 13, "Chest Pain"). When pain is clearly related to or associated with other intestinal phenomena—for example, eating, defecation, belching, gas—one of the common disorders discussed above is most likely. When pain is not clearly "intestinal sounding," various gastrointestinal disorders may still be responsible, but the differential diagnosis must be expanded:

Angina pectoris is a common cause of epigastric pain. Rarely the pain is related only to eating (see Chapter 13, "Chest Pain"), but episodic constricting discomfort that occurs predictably with physical exertion or emotional tension is the rule.

Chest-wall disorders will often cause upper abdominal pain. The "slipping rib syndrome" and intercostal neuritis are usually unilateral; xiphodalgia and costochondritis are more often in the midline (see also "Chapter 13, "Chest Pain").

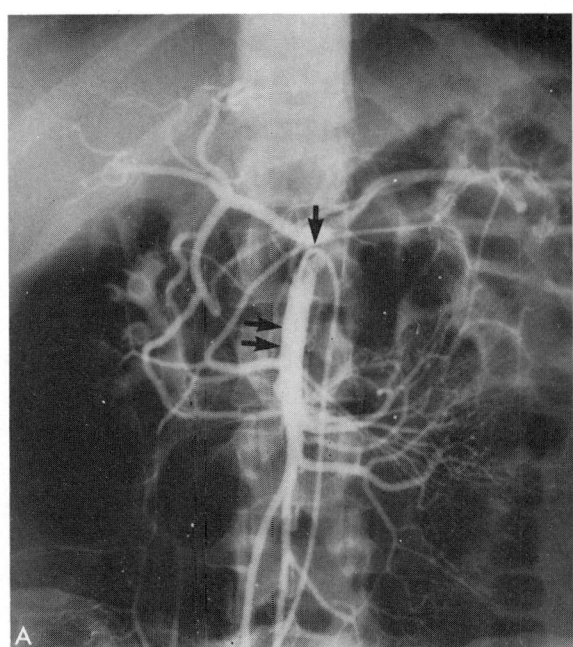 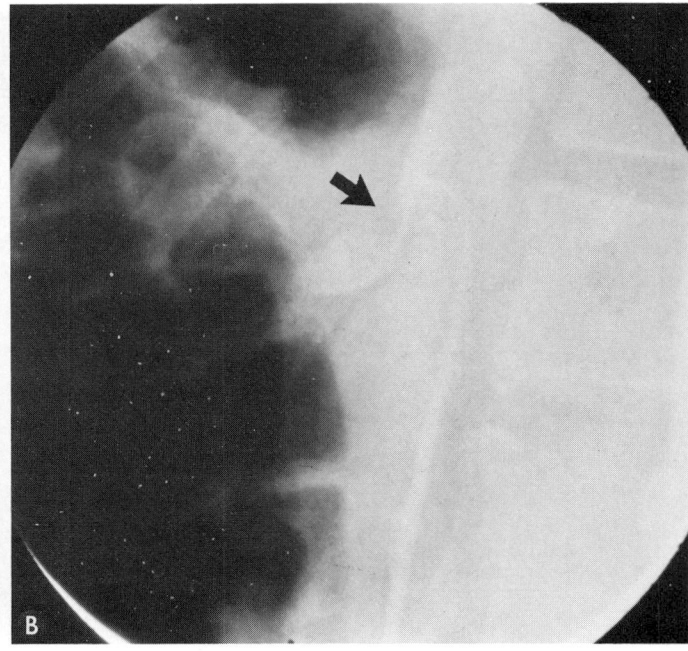

FIGURE 11–35. Celiac axis syndrome. This 24-year-old woman described predictable postprandial epigastric and periumbilical abdominal pain, usually after meals (within 15 to 45 minutes) and lasting for 1 to 2 hours. Physical examination was unremarkable, except for an epigastric systolic bruit. An extensive series of investigations was entirely normal. Finally, this arteriogram demonstrated the following: *A*, Retrograde filling of the celiac artery (*arrow*) after injection of the superior mesenteric artery (*double arrow*). *B*, On lateral view, high-grade stenosis (*arrow*) of the celiac artery soon after its origin from the aorta. At surgery, a hypertrophied median arcuate ligament was excised from around the celiac artery. The patient's symptoms completely resolved. This disorder is so rare that some authorities doubt its existence. This patient is a "believer."

Radicular abdominal pain may superficially resemble visceral abdominal disease. Usually, however, pain is unilateral and/or is associated with back pain. Postherpetic neuralgia, diabetic mononeuritis, rare abdominal entrapment neuropathies, and thoracic spine disease affecting T4–10 (osteoporosis with compression fractures, degenerative arthritis, (rare) discs or spinal cord diseases) will occasionally so present.

When pain is predictably postprandial, several disorders must be suspected: Esophagitis, duodenal or gastric ulcer, and functional dyspepsia are most common. Further history may reveal that only certain foods elicit symptoms, as in the patient with lactose intolerance; associated flatulence, borborygmi, and diarrhea should suggest this diagnosis, as well as that of giardiasis, while atypical presentations of inflammatory bowel disease, the irritable bowel syndrome, or diverticular disease are also possible.

Postprandial vomiting with pain may imply gastric outlet obstruction (due to carcinoma or ulcer), diabetic gastroparesis, or recurrent pancreatitis, pancreatic carcinoma, pancreatic pseudocysts, or the superior mesenteric artery syndrome (Fig. 11–34). The timing of postprandial pain sometimes helps: rare cases of intestinal ischemia (intestinal angina[113–116] in the elderly [see Fig. 11–37, page 612], celiac axis syndrome [Fig. 11–35] in the young[117]) usually cause pain within 15 to 30 minutes after eating—fear of eating is then often a more prominent symptom than pain. Esophageal or ulcer disease more often causes pain an hour or more after eating (but, as noted above, such a history may be unreliable).

Ichabod is not sure how long after eating his pain usually occurs (perhaps an hour). Pain does not occur after every meal, and perhaps small feedings are better tolerated. There has been no vomiting.

> Symptoms are definitely intermittent—Ichabod is pain free most of the day, but symptoms do occur "almost every day now." Symptoms seem always related to meals.

> There is no "heartburn." Antacids do not relieve the pain. The pain resolves slowly but spontaneously each time. Average duration of pain is (perhaps) an hour or two. Pain does not awaken Ichabod at night "unless I eat before I go to bed."

3. Symptoms are not classic for any of the common causes of dyspepsia and upper abdominal pain. Ichabod's symptoms are not typical of esophagitis.

Pain due to gallbladder disease is most unlikely. Ichabod's pain is not unpredictably episodic, prolonged, or associated with nausea and vomiting. Biliary colic rarely occurs every day or in such a predictable postprandial fashion. (This, of course, does not mean that gallstones—so commonly asymptomatic—are not present.[118])

Ichabod's age, negative past history, absence of nocturnal pain, and failure of symptomatic antacid therapy are atypical of duodenal ulcer disease. Gastric ulcer (or gastric carcinoma) is certainly a possibility, given the location of pain, the relation to meals, and the associated weight loss.

When a careful history is obtained, many patients with one of the common causes of upper abdominal pain will describe a classic history (Table 11–20). The absence of such a history by no means excludes any of these diseases, but its presence often allows selective testing and prompt diagnosis (see Fig. 11–33, 3).

> Ichabod denies any prior history of "stomach trouble." There is no history of ulcers, diabetes, alcoholism, aspirin ingestion (he takes hydrochlorothiazide 50 mg per day), pernicious anemia, or gastrointestinal bleeding or family history of cancer.

4. Past medical history is not very helpful in Ichabod's case. On the other hand:

The chronic alcoholic is susceptible to alcoholic gastritis, duodenal or gastric ulcer disease, painful alcoholic hepatitis, and acute, chronic relapsing, or chronic pancreatitis.

The diabetic patient, especially the longstanding insulin-dependent diabetic, may develop gastroparesis owing to visceral neuropathy, painful fatty liver, or radicular mononeuritis of thoracic spinal nerves. Gallbladder disease in diabetics[119] is often very atypical in presentation. Rarely, chronic pancreatitis will be the *cause* of diabetes.

The patient taking corticosteroids, aspirin, or other nonsteroidal anti-inflammatory agents may develop gastritis, esophagitis, or ulcer. Oral contraceptives may worsen esophagitis or, rarely, induce painful hepatic adenomas.[120, 121]

The elderly patient with diffuse vascular disease must be suspected of angina pectoris, abdominal aortic aneurysms (which only rarely cause chronic pain), or recurrent mesenteric ischemia (see below).

Various hematologic disorders may be associated with or cause recurrent abdominal pain. Pernicious anemia probably predisposes to gastric carcinoma. Myeloproliferative disorders (chronic leukemias, polycythemia vera, myeloid metaplasia) and lymphomas will cause hepatosplenomegaly (distention of liver or spleen may be symptomatic) or coagulopathies (thrombocytosis, polycythemia) that predispose to vascular occlusion. Hemolytic diseases may cause intermittent abdominal crises, gallstones, or splenic infarction.

The patient with recurrent abdominal pain and evidence of multisystem disease (renal, rheumatologic, pulmonary, neurologic, cardiac) may have systemic lupus erythematosus, polyarteritis nodosa,[11] porphyria, lead poisoning, or other rare entities.

> Physical examination is normal, except for questionable appearance of weight loss.
>
> Ichabod is anicteric, in no distress, and has normal vital signs. There are no palpable abdominal masses or organomegaly. There is no ascites. Rectal examination reveals heme-negative stool.
>
> Examination of the lungs, heart, back, chest, and abdominal wall is unremarkable. There is no abdominal tenderness. There are no vascular bruits.

5. There are no unequivocally worrisome findings in Ichabod's case. Objective physical findings that are invariably worrisome include: jaundice, palpable abdominal mass(es) (Table 11–21), pallor (anemia), heme-positive stool, ascites, and obvious weight loss. Such findings always require investigation, usually in the hospital.

Historical findings that are always worrisome are a history of weight loss or a description of constant, unrelenting, progressively worsening upper abdominal pain. The last pain pattern, especially when associated with weight loss, must always raise the suspicion of pancreatic carcinoma, chronic pancreatitis,[123–125] or gastric carcinoma. Such disorders often present with pain that is present day and night, anorexia, or back pain.

Occasionally the patient with "functional" abdominal pain or depressive illness will describe constant pain. The younger patient who does not look ill and whose weight is stable despite very prolonged duration of pain (months to years) can often be suspected early of "nonorganic" disease. Nevertheless, full evaluation is always necessary.

TABLE 11–21. PALPABLE UPPER ABDOMINAL MASSES

EPIGASTRIC	RIGHT UPPER QUADRANT	LEFT UPPER QUADRANT
Neoplasm	Hepatomegaly	Splenomegaly
Stomach	Abscess	*Sequestration (hemolytic
Colon	Neoplasm	disease)
Pancreas	Adenoma	Proliferation (chronic
Peritoneal	Infiltrative disease	infection)
(metastatic)	(e.g., fat, iron,	Lipid (storage disorders)
	copper, amyloid)	Engorgement (portal
Organomegaly	Congestion	hypertension,
Liver		hemoglobinopathies)
Gallbladder	Neoplasm	Endowment (congenital)
Spleen	Liver	INvasion
	Colon	Neoplasm
Pancreatic pseudocyst	Gallbladder	Lymphoma
	Kidney	Leukemia
Abdominal aortic	Adrenal	Granulomatous disease
aneurysm		
	Enlarged gallbladder	Neoplasm
Abdominal wall		Spleen
hernia	Polycystic kidneys	Pancreas
		Kidney
		Adrenal
		Stomach
		Colon
		Polycystic kidneys

*This mnemonic adapted from reference 122.

Complete blood count, urinalysis, sedimentation rate, liver enzymes, and amylase are normal. A barium swallow with upper GI series is normal.

Two days later an abdominal ultrasound examination is normal. The gallbladder, pancreas, liver, kidneys, and aorta are all well visualized; all are normal.

6. In Ichabod's case, outpatient testing is nondiagnostic. What does this mean?

a. The normal upper GI series excludes duodenal and gastric ulcer with about 80 to 90 per cent accuracy. Like any test, the upper GI series is only as accurate as its performance is expert: double-contrast barium upper GI series performed by experienced radiologists compare favorably with endoscopy in overall diagnostic accuracy of ulcers and neoplasms.[126] Under these circumstances, the symptomatic patient with "x-ray negative dyspepsia" is unlikely to harbor an endoscopically visible ulcer: One study demonstrated three benign ulcers—two duodenal, one gastric—among 140 such patients.[127]

Nevertheless, when clinical suspicion of ulcer disease is strong but barium studies are nondiagnostic (the patient with prior ulcer disease and duodenal "scarring" is a common example), esophagogastroduodenoscopy is the "gold standard" in diagnosis.[128–130] Whether missing the occasional ulcer on barium studies is sufficient reason to routinely perform endoscopy in patients with "x-ray negative dyspepsia" is highly questionable. That strategy is certainly expensive. The cost of endoscopy just in patients with radiographically documented gastric ulcers is staggering.[131] Such strategies in the treatment of documented ulcer disease are discussed briefly in the Appendix.

(The decision to perform the upper GI series in the first place deserves brief comment. One study demonstrated inappropriate abuse of this test in a large number of ambulatory patients.[132] In general, patients in older age groups [over 50], those with a history of prior ulcer disease, and those whose symptoms are clearly postprandial or relieved with food/milk are most likely to have a "diagnostic" upper GI series. The decision to perform such tests must, of course, be individualized.)

b. When biliary colic or cholelithiasis is suspected, the oral cholecystogram is usually a highly reliable test. A completely normal oral cholecystogram makes gallstones very unlikely (greater than 90 per cent accuracy). Conversely, failure to visualize the gallbladder after a "double-dose oral cholecystogram" is very strong presumptive evidence favoring gallbladder disease[133] (assuming, of course, that cholecystectomy has not been performed and that the patient does not have severe liver disease). Gallbladder ultrasound is always the preferred diagnostic method in the patient who is pregnant, jaundiced, or allergic to the radiographic dye. (It is also occasionally useful in the patient strongly suspected of gallbladder disease whose oral cholecystogram is normal.) In many centers now, ultrasound is the initial procedure of choice. (The cost of ultrasound limited to the gallbladder is $100 [Table 11–10]: the oral cholecystogram costs about the same.)

A normal abdominal ultrasound examination excludes: biliary tract disease with about 95 per cent accuracy,[51, 52] pancreatic disease[134–136] with about 75 per cent accuracy, and most neoplasms of the kidney and liver. (A normal abdominal ultrasound examination may mean one of two things: All organs were visualized and all were normal, or all visualized organs were normal but not all organs were visualized. The radiologist's exact conclusions must be obtained.)

In Ichabod's case, gallbladder disease is clinically most unlikely. The abdominal ultrasound examination is performed not so much to evaluate the

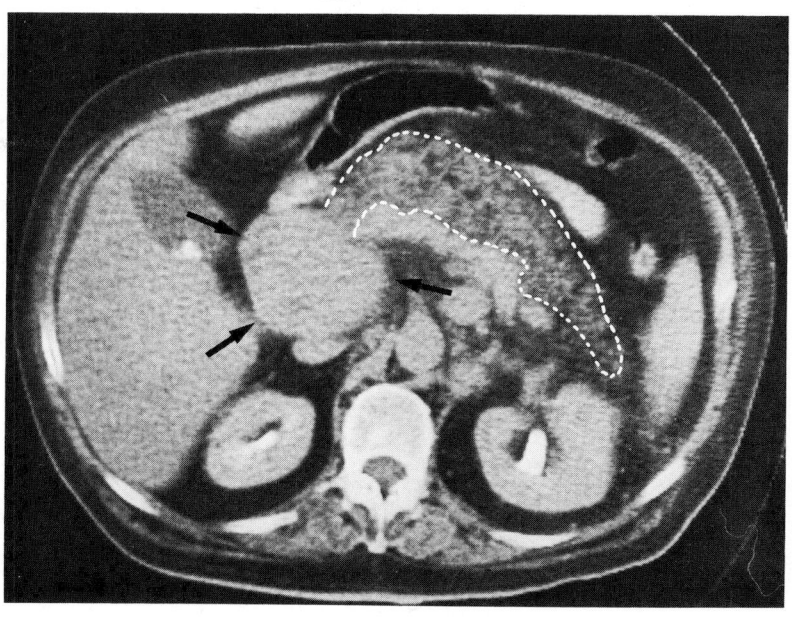

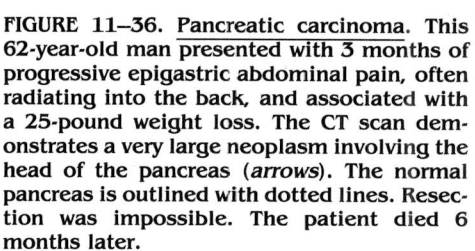

FIGURE 11–36. Pancreatic carcinoma. This 62-year-old man presented with 3 months of progressive epigastric abdominal pain, often radiating into the back, and associated with a 25-pound weight loss. The CT scan demonstrates a very large neoplasm involving the head of the pancreas (*arrows*). The normal pancreas is outlined with dotted lines. Resection was impossible. The patient died 6 months later.

gallbladder as to visualize the pancreas. Negative information about liver, gallbladder, kidneys, and aorta is reassuring as well. Any elderly patient with chronic upper abdominal pain (especially if associated with jaundice, a palpable gallbladder, weight loss, or back pain) must be suspected of pancreatic carcinoma (Fig. 11–36) (or, rarely, gallbladder carcinoma).[137] A normal pancreas on ultrasound examination is good evidence that pancreatic carcinoma is not the problem, but CT scans or ERCP will be necessary to diagnose or exclude that disease in some patients.[136] A normal pancreatic ultrasound examination almost always excludes a pancreatic pseudocyst.

c. Chronic pancreatitis[123–125] may closely mimic pancreatic carcinoma. Persistent, severe epigastric/back pain, often exacerbated by eating, develops in the chronic alcoholic or, less often, in the nonalcoholic patient who has had recurrent prior episodes of acute pancreatitis. The alcoholic variety is easily the most common. Weight loss may be prominent, either when malabsorption results from exocrine pancreatic insufficiency or when eating precipitates pain so predictably that food intake diminishes. Pancreatic calcifications (Fig. 3–13) will be seen on abdominal flat plate in only a minority. In their absence, ERCP is often needed to document the disease. Treatment of painful chronic pancreatitis is very difficult; surgery is usually a last resort and thus narcotic abuse is a common complication in the medically managed patient with chronic pancreatitis.

d. Normal liver enzymes are helpful in that most hepatic causes of chronic/recurrent upper abdominal pain (alcoholic hepatitis, chronic active hepatitis, fatty liver, hepatic congestion, and hepatocellular carcinoma are probably most common) are usually associated with some increase of liver enzymes. One (very uncommon) exception is the hepatic adenoma usually related to oral contraceptive drug use[121]—when this is suspected, a liver scan will be needed even when liver function tests are normal.[120]

e. A normal serum amylase value is not very helpful in the patient with chronic abdominal pain. Neither pancreatic carcinoma nor chronic pancreatitis is often associated with increased serum amylase.[138] (Acute pancreatitis or episodic, recurrent/relapsing acute pancreatitis—see page 614—almost always is.)

Ichabod is told that all his tests are normal and that an "acid stomach" might be causing his trouble. A dose of Mylanta II (See Appendix) 1 and 3 hours after each meal is prescribed. Stool is collected for tests for ova and parasites. A lactose-free diet is suggested.

Ichabod admits that he is depressed, "but I'm depressed because my stomach hurts. Wouldn't you be depressed if you couldn't eat?"

Again, Figure 11–33 illustrates the general approach to the patient with chronic/recurrent upper abdominal pain.

NOTE

Were Ichabod a young, otherwise healthy patient, the diagnosis of functional dyspepsia with or without some underlying psychologic disability might be the most likely diagnosis at this point. In such a patient, watchful waiting, perhaps in tandem with various symptomatic treatments (antacids, anticholinergic agents, high-fiber diet), is often indicated rather that further extensive testing. A trial of a lactose-free diet or collections of stool for ova and parasites will occasionally yield surprising results in such patients.

Ichabod, however, is elderly and is significantly disabled by his symptoms. This by no means proves serious disease, and depression with somatic symptoms is still a real possibility here, but a variety of uncommon disorders must be suspected (Table 11–22) in such patients.

Especially in the elderly patient, the diagnosis of psychosomatic abdominal pain should never be made before the gamut of organic disease is excluded.

Getting to know the patient with chronic abdominal pain will usually distinguish psychogenic from organic disease. All prior medical records must be obtained. Malingering, drug abuse, or Munchausen's syndrome will often thus come to light. The depressed patient must be studied carefully: organic disease must always be excluded before depression is labeled primary rather than secondary to the cause of pain. The anxious, hypochondriacal patient or the patient with a "peptic personality" (the compulsive, introspective, or angry overachiever) may be much helped with behavioral modification therapy, an "open office-door policy," and occasional antacids or anticholinergics. The patient with psychosis, hysteria,[150] or suspected conversion symptoms must be referred to a psychiatrist.

The patient's response to a brief trial of presumptive therapy is often a helpful clue. Functional dyspepsia usually resolves with reassurance and time.

SEVERE CENTRAL ABDOMINAL PAIN

Admission to the hospital is tentatively scheduled for 2 weeks hence, if symptoms do not resolve with antacids and a change of diet. Hospital procedures that are anticipated include observation (especially after eating), small-bowel and colon barium studies, esophagogastroscopy, and perhaps ECRP or CT scan—roughly in that order.

Ten days later, Sally calls to say that Ichabod has had severe, constant abdominal pain for the past 3 to 4 hours.

Ichabod says his pain is a very severe, deep ache, "The worst I ever had," in the periumbilical area. It began abruptly, soon after he arose from sleep this morning. It has been progressively worsening over the past 3 hours. Ichabod denies vomiting or pulmonary or urinary symptoms. He did feel a sudden urge to move his bowels at the onset of pain but has had no diarrhea. Ichabod says that there had been no change in his prior pattern of postprandial abdominal pain; neither antacids nor the lactose-free diet seem to have helped. This "feels like the same pain, but much worse."

NOTE

1. The location of pain is periumbilical. As Figure 11–2 illustrates, this should raise specific questions about disease of the small bowel, cecum, or appendix. As Table 11–6 suggests, disease of the heart, aorta, and pancreas must also be remembered in the patient with central abdominal pain.

As we have seen, however, a variety of disorders may begin as central abdominal pain, only to move thereafter into a more localized (and diagnostically localizing) area of the abdomen, as Figure 11–38 illustrates. When severe central abdominal pain persists without secondary localization, consider bowel obstruction, pancreatitis, peptic ulcer disease, aortic aneurysm, myocardial infarction, mesenteric ischemia, intra-abdominal bleeding, or visceral perforation with (impending) generalized peritonitis. Prior history and physical examination will often distinguish among these possibilities (page 614). For example,

2. The (allegedly) abrupt onset of pain is worrisome—visceral perforation or obstruction, as well as acute vascular events, must be considered.

3. Ichabod's age is also cause for concern—acute abdominal pain in the elderly is more often serious.[1]

4. The prior history of postprandial upper abdominal pain may or may not be pertinent here. If it is, major considerations include a perforated peptic ulcer (missed on the previous upper GI series), acute cholecystitis or pancreatitis (false-negative ultrasound examination of the gallbladder and pancreas previously?), or mesenteric ischemia following progressive intestinal angina (Fig. 11–37, page 612).

> On examination, Ichabod is clearly in pain and places both hands around the umbilicus when describing its location. The pain does not radiate but is "all over" the abdomen. Blood pressure is normal without orthostatic changes. The pulse is 100. Ichabod is slightly diaphoretic, but his color is good and his extremities are warm. Physical examination is otherwise completely normal, except for the abdomen: bowel sounds are greatly diminished and there is (perhaps) slight abdominal distention. There is no percussion tenderness, guarding, or rebound tenderness, but there is moderate generalized abdominal tenderness, especially in the central abdomen. There are no palpable hernias. All pulses are normal. Examination of the back, hips, genitals, chest, flanks, and rectum is normal. Psoas and obturator signs are unremarkable. The stool is Hematest negative.

NOTE

I. Ichabod is not "shocky."

The patient with acute abdominal pain who is in shock usually requires surgical attention. The location of pain is often the best guide to diagnosis in such patients (see Table 11–6). Usually such patients have generalized peritonitis, intra-abdominal hemorrhage (due, for example, to a ruptured ectopic pregnancy, spleen, or aorta) or third spacing due to pancreatitis, bowel obstruction, or bowel infarction.

Remember: Myocardial infarction, pulmonary embolism, sepsis, diabetic ketoacidosis, gastrointestinal bleeding, or aortic dissection may all present with shock and acute abdominal pain—exploratory laparotomy in such patients could be disastrous.

II. There is no evidence of peritonitis.

Acute central abdominal pain associated with diffuse abdominal

TABLE 11–22. UNCOMMON CAUSES OF CHRONIC/RECURRENT UPPER ABDOMINAL PAIN

DISEASE*	WHEN TO SUSPECT		
	SETTING	SYMPTOMS	SIGNS
Pancreatic carcinoma[136]	95% older than 40	Epigastric pain; back pain; weight loss	Possibly jaundice; weight loss; palpable gallbladder or mass
Chronic pancreatitis*[123–125]	Chronic alcoholic (usually)	As in pancreatic carcinoma	Possibly malabsorption; weight loss
Pancreatic pseudocyst[140]	Persistent pain and hyperamylasemia after acute pancreatitis	May be asymptomatic; possibly persistent epigastric pain	Large pseudocyst may be palpable
Intestinal angina[113–116]	Usually elderly patient with diffuse vascular disease	Postprandial (15–30 min) pain lasting 1–2 hours; fear of eating	Weight loss common; diffuse vascular disease; bruits
Superior mesenteric artery syndrome[142]	Asthenic patient or following extreme weight loss (from another cause); often young	Postprandial pain, vomiting; weight loss; relief with eating in prone or knee/chest position	Weight loss
Celiac axis syndrome[117]	Usually young female	Epigastric (often postprandial), abdominal pain	Epigastric bruit
Abdominal aortic aneurysm[143–146]	Middle-aged or elderly patient (with or without other vascular disease)	Often absent; sometimes persistent vague, midline abdominal, back, flank pain	Palpable aneurysm in thin patient; normal examination in obese and/or muscular patient
Gastroparesis diabeticorum[147] (or postvagotomy gastroparesis)	Insulin-dependent diabetic, usually more than 10 years' duration or Postvagotomy	Postprandial pain, gas, nausea, vomiting	Diabetics often with nephropathy, autonomic neuropathy
Hepatic flexure syndrome		Symptoms of irritable bowel syndrome with pain localized to right upper quadrant	
Splenic flexure syndrome		Symptoms of irritable bowel syndrome with pain localized to left upper quadrant	
Carcinoma of gallbladder[137]	Elderly patient; gallstones in 85%	Acute or chronic cholelithiasis; palpable mass in two-thirds; weight loss common	
Hepatocellular adenoma[120, 121]	Young female taking oral contraceptives	Right upper quadrant pain, often acute; may be subacute	Right upper quadrant tenderness, hepatomegaly?
Hepatocellular carcinoma[148]	Usually males with cirrhosis, hemochromatosis, chronic active hepatitis	Right upper quadrant pain; hepatomegaly; weight loss	Jaundice? Fever? Ascites? Bruit/rub over liver?
Remember:	**Small bowel colon disease** **Connective tissue disease; vasculitis**[11] **Psychogenic** **"Rare" medical disease: familial Mediterranean fever, lead poisoning, porphyria, tabes dorsalis** **Chronic active hepatitis**[149] **Renal/ureteral disease, neoplasm** **Symptomatic hepatosplenomegaly** **Congestive heart failure with hepatic congestion** **Hepatic abscess** **Splenic disease**		

*A different disease from acute or relapsing pancreatitis.

TABLE 11–22. UNCOMMON CAUSES OF CHRONIC/RECURRENT UPPER ABDOMINAL PAIN *(Continued)*

DISEASE*	USUALLY DIAGNOSED BY	EXCLUDE IF	TREATMENT
Pancreatic carcinoma[136]	Ultrasound, CT scan, ERCP, with percutaneous biopsy[139]; surgical exploration	Normal ultrasound and CT scan	Surgery and/or radiation therapy
Chronic pancreatitis†[123–125]	Steatorrhea and pain in chronic alcoholic; calcified pancreas on x-ray (around 30%); no mass on ultrasound or CT scan; ERCP	Normal ERCP	Pain control Treat steatorrhea Resect pseudocyst, if present Explore if cannot exclude carcinoma
Pancreatic pseudocyst[140]	Ultrasound; CT scan	Normal ultrasound and CT scan	Resect large, painful pseudocyst Watch and wait with smaller, asymptomatic pseudocysts
Intestinal angina[113–116]	Clinical syndrome *and* no evidence of other intra-abdominal disease *and* arteriography: *more than* two-vessel mesenteric vascular obstruction	Arteriography normal or insignificant vessel obstruction (less than 50% occlusion of fewer than three vessels)	Vascular bypass
Superior mesenteric artery syndrome[142]	Postprandial duodenal distention on upper GI series: compression of third portion of duodenum between superior mesenteric artery anteriorly and retroperitoneum posteriorly	No weight loss; upper GI normal	Gain weight; eat in prone position; possibly hyperalimentation
Celiac axis syndrome[117]	Celiac artery compression on arteriography (compressed usually by median arcuate ligament of the diaphragm)	Normal arteriography	Wait; rarely requires surgery ("positive" arteriogram not uncommon in asymptomatic patients)
Abdominal aortic aneurysm[143–146]	Abdominal ultrasound	Normal aortography and ultrasound	Surgery if symptomatic; if asymptomatic; surgery when increasing in size and/or exceeds 5 cm in diameter
Gastroparesis diabeticorum[147] (or postvagotomy gastroparesis)	Upper GI series (exclude other obstructive process)	Not diabetic; other cause for symptoms found	Metoclopramide; soft foods; possibly cholinergic drugs, surgery (gastroenterostomy)
Hepatic flexure syndrome **Splenic flexure syndrome**	Clinical history; normal proctoscopy, barium enema (exclude colon cancer)	No features of irritable bowel syndrome and another diagnosis found	High-fiber diet; Metamucil
Carcinoma of gallbladder[137]	Surgery	Negative exploration	Resection
Hepatocellular adenoma[120, 121]	"Cold" spot(s) on liver scan; (liver function tests may be normal)	Normal liver scan and hepatic angiography	Surgery versus wait: stop oral contraceptives
Hepatocellular carcinoma[148]	"Cold" liver scan defect(s); hypervascular mass on angiogram; positive cytologic findings in ascites	Normal liver scan and angiography	Surgery and/or radiation therapy, chemosurgery

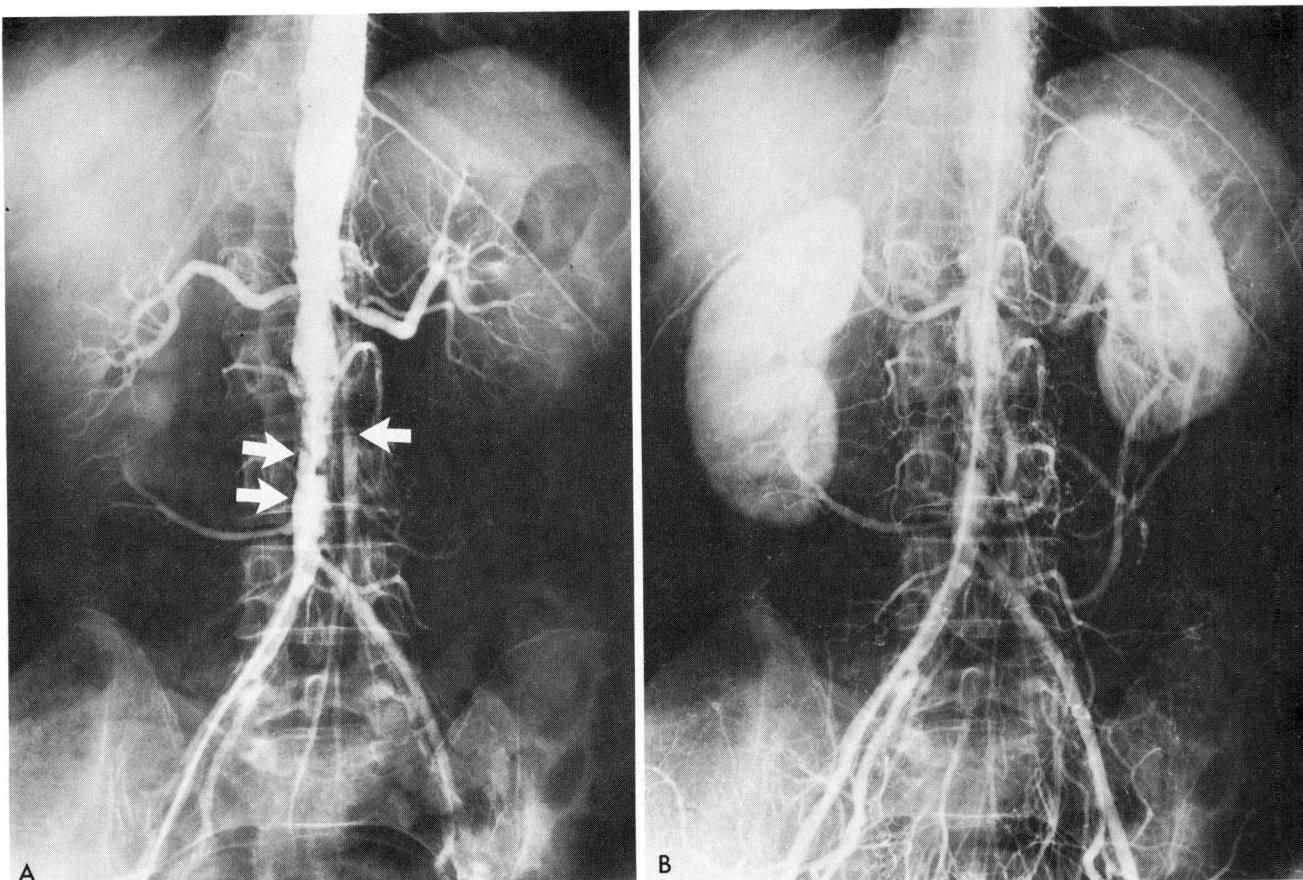

FIGURE 11-37. This 73-year-old diabetic, hypertensive woman with diffuse atherosclerotic vascular disease lost 20 pounds over a 6-week period because of severe postprandial abdominal pain that caused her to limit her food intake greatly. After normal barium x-rays of the upper and lower intestine, abdominal ultrasound, and CT scan, this mesenteric arteriogram, performed after injection into the proximal aorta (see catheter in *B*), demonstrates the following: *A*, Minimal visualization of the upper abdominal vessels—there is virtually complete occlusion of the celiac and superior mesenteric arteries. There is severe stenosis of the inferior mesenteric artery (*arrow*) and extensive aortic atherosclerosis (*two arrows*). The kidneys perfuse. *B*, A later film shows delayed perfusion in the distribution of all major mesenteric vessels via collateral pathways. Mesenteric bypass grafting was decided upon. Massive myocardial infarction prevented surgery. The patient died.

rigidity is almost always due to a perforated viscus—peptic ulcer, colonic diverticula, appendicitis, or bowel neoplasm is the cause in most. Less dramatic peritoneal signs (guarding, percussion, or rebound tenderness) will be seen early in such patients. More localized pain and peritonitis raise other possibilities (see Table 11–6). Remember:

A. Some patients who are elderly, uremic, neurologically impaired, or previously receiving corticosteroids or potent analgesics may not demonstrate remarkable abdominal findings even in the presence of frank peritonitis.

B. The absence of peritoneal signs in the patient who is obviously ill with severe central abdominal pain must raise suspicion that pain is referred (from the thorax or spine) or that an intra-abdominal, extraperitoneal organ is the source of symptoms. Thus, disease of the pancreas, aorta, great vessels, pelvic organs, and retroperitoneal structures must be considered. Diseases of intra-abdominal/intraperitoneal organs that typically do not cause peritoneal signs (until very late, if at all) are intestinal obstruction and acute mesenteric ischemia.

C. The development of peritoneal signs takes time, at least in some cases.

As noted previously, a perforated peptic ulcer may cause abrupt, severe abdominal pain followed by an interval of several hours during which pain and tenderness are unimpressive; 6 to 12 hours later more dramatic physical findings and recurrence of severe pain then develop. As we have seen, peritoneal signs do not usually develop immediately in the patient with acute appendicitis or acute cholecystitis, either.

III. There is mild (early?) abdominal distention.

As noted previously, the distended abdomen may be due to a variety of different problems, not all of which are serious. In the setting of severe acute abdominal pain, however, bowel obstruction (the abdomen should be tympanitic), intra-abdominal bleeding (the abdomen rapidly enlarges and is dull to percussion), and ascites (with bacterial peritonitis) must be especially considered. Abdominal paracentesis or peritoneal lavage[13] (following the flat plate to rule out intestinal obstruction) will distinguish intraperitoneal infection from intra-abdominal hemorrhage.

Abdominal flat plate is normal.

A chest x-ray and ECG are unremarkable.

The white blood count is 14,000 with a left shift. The hemoglobin is unchanged from previously (15 gm/per 100 ml). The urinalysis is normal.

Serum amylase is 560 (normal up to 200).

What does this mean?

1. There is no radiographic evidence of intestinal obstruction or of a perforated intra-abdominal viscus (free air). Cardiopulmonary causes of referred pain (myocardial infarction, aortic dissection, for example) seem unlikely, given the normal ECG and normal chest x-ray (see Chapter 13, "Chest Pain").

2. Leukocytosis is worrisome but is nonspecific.

A normal hemoglobin does not exclude bleeding (since intravascular equilibration might not yet have occurred), but this is less likely. An *elevated* hemoglobin level may point to significant "third spacing" of fluid.

TABLE 11–23. HYPERAMYLASEMIA IN ASSOCIATION WITH CAUSES OF ABDOMINAL PAIN*†

Pancreatic disease	Perforated peptic ulcer
Acute pancreatitis	Intestinal obstruction
Chronic pancreatitis	
Pancreatic pseudocyst	Ruptured ectopic pregnancy
Pancreatic abscess	Mesenteric infarction
Pancreatic carcinoma	
	Aortic dissection
Biliary tract disease	Peritonitis
Cholecystitis	
Cholelithiasis	Acute appendicitis
Choledocholithiasis	Diabetic ketoacidosis
Ruptured gallbladder	
Fulminant hepatitis	

*Adapted from reference 138.
†Hyperamylasemia may occur in the absence of intra-abdominal disease as a result of macroamylasemia, renal insufficiency, salivary gland lesion, pregnancy, burns, lung cancer.

3. Hyperamylasemia must raise the question of acute pancreatitis, but, as Table 11–23 suggests, hyperamylasemia in the patient with acute abdominal pain may have many other causes.

> **Ichabod's pain persists 2 hours later and is, if anything, worse. Physical examination is unchanged. The abdomen is diffusely tender without peritoneal signs and remains mildly distended.**

What does this mean?

Ichabod has severe central abdominal pain and abdominal tenderness. In the absence of shock, definite peritoneal signs, or radiographic intestinal obstruction—all indications for immediate surgical consultation—there are several diagnostic possibilities:

1. Acute pancreatitis.[151, 152]

The pain of acute pancreatitis may be generalized but is more often epigastric, periumbilical, or referred to the back. Nausea and vomiting are usually prominent symptoms, and abdominal tenderness (if present) is usually epigastric or in the left upper quadrant. The serum amylase is "always" elevated in acute pancreatitis. Alcoholism and gallstones are the causes of acute pancreatitis in at least 90 per cent of cases. Table 11–24 illustrates other much less common causes.

If Ichabod's current acute pain is related to his prior postprandial pain, pancreatitis is not an attractive unifying diagnosis, given the previously normal ultrasound examination of the gallbladder (excluding gallstones with 90 per cent accuracy) and the absence of chronic alcoholism by history. A peptic ulcer may penetrate posteriorly into the pancreas, resulting in clinical acute pancreatitis, but, again, the prior normal upper GI series makes this unlikely as well. Some cases of acute pancreatitis are idiopathic, and thus

TABLE 11–24. CAUSES OF PANCREATITIS

Alcohol	Drug induced
	Analgesics (morphine, codeine, Demerol)
Cholelithiasis	Steroids
	Oral contraceptives
Metabolic	Antibiotics (isoniazid, tetracycline)
Uremia	Diuretics (chlorothiazide, furosemide,
Hyperlipidemia (Types I, IV)	chlorthalidone)
Hypercalcemia	Salicylates, indomethacin
Diabetic ketoacidosis	6-Mercaptopurine, L-aparaginase
Hemochromatosis	
Cystinuria	Idiopathic
Trauma	Malignant
	Lymphoma
Infectious	Pancreatic carcinoma
Mumps, mononucleosis, viral	
hepatitis	Others
Gram-negative sepsis	Penetrating duodenal ulcer
Typhoid fever	Pregnancy
Scarlet fever	Post partum
Other viral infections	Cystic fibrosis
	Nutritional
Vascular	
Polyarteritis nodosa	
Systemic lupus erythematosus	
Atherosclerotic embolization	

the absence of gallstones, peptic ulcers, or alcoholism certainly does not exclude acute pancreatitis. Interestingly, Ichabod does take one drug (hydrochlorothiazide) that has been reported to cause pancreatitis.

(The pancreas is an intra-abdominal extraperitoneal organ—so are the kidneys, the aorta, pelvic organs, retroperitoneal space, and great vessels. The absence of peritoneal signs is never evidence against disorders involving these structures.)

2. Aortic dissection[153] or leaking aortic aneurysm must be considered, especially in an elderly, hypertensive patient. Nevertheless, the normal chest x-ray and previously normal ultrasound examination of the aorta are strong evidence against these diagnoses, and the prior bouts of pain would be unexplained by these very acute disorders. (Occasionally an abdominal aortic aneurysm may cause insidious intermittent pain before frank rupture.)

3. Mesenteric ischemia[141] must be strongly considered here. Acute severe abdominal pain in an elderly patient, with or without known cardiac or vascular disease, must always suggest this possibility. After frank bowel infarction occurs as a result of impaired mesenteric blood supply, abdominal distention, diffuse peritonitis, increasing leukocytosis, shock, and intestinal bleeding are common, but, early in the clinical course, physical examination of the patient with mesenteric ischemia/infarction may be remarkably unremarkable. In fact, a vaunted clinical hallmark of (impending) mesenteric infarction is the disproportionate severity of pain (usually in an elderly patient) when compared with a relatively benign physical examination. Early diagnosis is crucial, since mortality is extremely high, and only early diagnosis and aggressive (medical and surgical) management can improve the usually dismal prognosis.

Most instances of intestinal ischemia or infarction are due to nonocclusive vascular insufficiency of the bowel due to "low-flow states"—prolonged hypotension, myocardial infarction, for example—or to acute embolic occlusion of a major mesenteric vessel in patients with congestive heart failure, cardiac arrhythmias, or valvular heart disease. The diagnosis is thus usually suspected because of the clinical setting. A minority, however, is due to atherosclerotic mesenteric vascular thrombosis—the prior history of post-prandial abdominal pain, perhaps due to intestinal angina, makes this an especially attractive possibility in Ichabod's case. (Note that hyperamylasemia will occur in this setting—Table 11–23.)

4. As noted previously, the initial pain of acute appendicitis, acute cholecystitis, or other inflammatory processes may be visceral and poorly localized, as in this case. Subsequent examination over the next several hours will then reveal evidence of localization to the appropriate abdominal quadrant as localized peritonitis ensues (or when acute perforation results). Figure 11–38 illustrates some of these events.

5. A variety of benign abdominal disorders—gastroenteritis, for example—may cause acute generalized abdominal pain. Hyperamylasemia does not occur in the patient with gastroenteritis, but remember: A variety of extra-abdominal disorders may cause (especially mild) hyperamylasemia, i.e., the serum amylase may be a "red herring" and unrelated to the cause of abdominal pain (Table 11–23).

Serial examinations will usually distinguish gastroenteritis from more severe disease when the pain migrates into various locales in the abdomen and diarrhea develops.

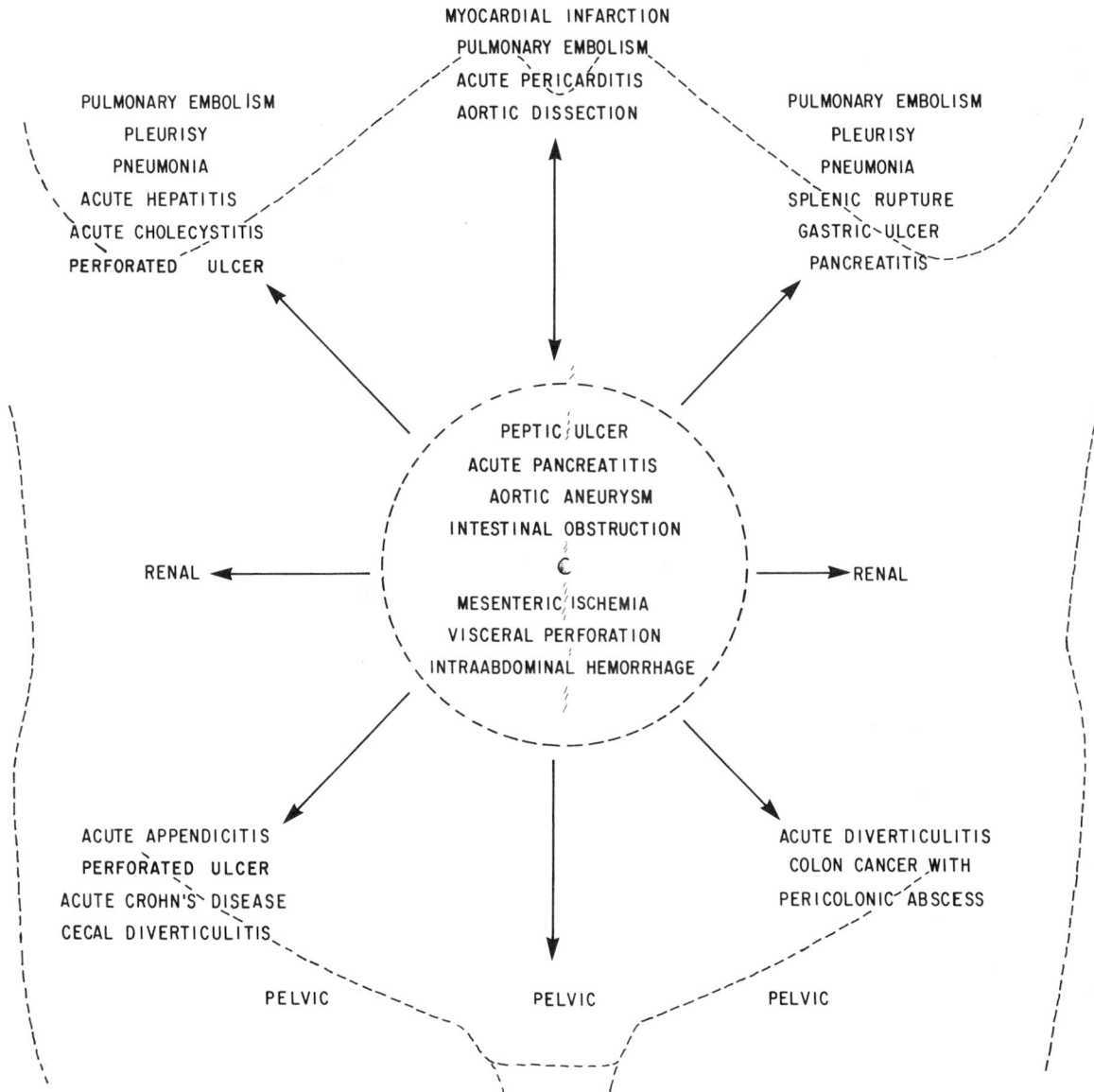

FIGURE 11–38. Central abdominal pain. Many causes of abdominal pain will begin in the central abdomen, only to "migrate" subsequently into a more "localizing" position in the abdomen. When severe abdominal pain persists without localization to one specific quadrant, those entities grouped in the periumbilical area of the figure must be especially considered.

Thus a variety of serious conditions may be responsible for Ichabod's pain. The most likely diagnoses at this time, however, are acute pancreatitis, mesenteric ischemia/infarction, or early acute appendicitis.

The patient with severe abdominal pain of acute onset that has been present for several hours must be reexamined or hospitalized for observation, even in the absence of definite peritoneal signs, abdominal distention, or shock. Normal x-rays, white blood count, or serum amylase does not alter this caveat. While it is always desirable to attempt a specific diagnosis at initial presentation, such tentative diagnoses will often be invalidated or confirmed only by serial observations and physical examination.

Ichabod is hospitalized. A nasogastric tube is placed—there is no blood in the drainage. Intravenous fluids are begun. Urea nitrogen, electrolytes, and glucose are normal.

A surgical consultant who examines Ichabod is impressed by the severity of his pain and also by the relatively unimpressive abdominal findings.

Acute pancreatitis is deemed most likely, but the prior abdominal pain history is considered suggestive of mesenteric ischemia.

Four hours later, Ichabod is worse. His pain is even more severe, and his abdomen is now more distended, despite nasogastric suction. Repeat white blood count is 20,000 with a left shift. Repeat x-rays of the abdomen show nonspecific bowel gas but a question of early thumbprinting of the small bowel (Fig. 11–17).

Emergency visceral angiography reveals complete occlusion of the superior mesenteric artery without adequate collateral circulation to the small bowel. Laparotomy reveals impending infarction of the small bowel with thrombosis of the origin of the superior mesenteric artery. Bypass grafting of the superior mesenteric artery does not reverse the dusky, cyanotic appearance of the small bowel. Extensive small-bowel resection is performed.

A stormy postoperative course ensues—a "second-look" operation 24 hours later reveals further infarction of the remaining small bowel; additional resection is performed. Multiple postoperative complications follow—Ichabod dies on the 26th hospital day.

The management of suspected acute mesenteric ischemia or infarction is far beyond the scope of this text.[141] Of more importance here is emphasis on the fact that a surgeon must be consulted in a variety of situations, as suggested in Table 11–25. Most often, a specific surgical illness is suspected, and the need for the surgeon is obvious. Even when this is not the case, however, the patient with severe acute abdominal pain should be examined by the surgeon and carefully observed for at least the next several hours.

TABLE 11–25. CONSULTATION WITH SURGEON FOR PATIENTS WITH ACUTE ABDOMINAL PAIN

ALL POST-TRAUMATIC ABDOMINAL PAIN*

DOCUMENTED:

Shock and abdominal pain (always remember myocardial infarction, pulmonary embolism, sepsis, diabetic ketoacidosis, gastrointestinal bleeding, aortic dissection)

Peritonitis, diffuse or localized

Free air on x-ray: perforated viscus

Volvulus

Bowel obstruction?

SUSPECTED:

Acute appendicitis

Acute cholecystitis

Gynecologic emergency (ruptured ectopic pregnancy, pelvic hemorrhage, perforated uterus, threatened abortion)

Intra-abdominal hemorrhage

Abdominal aortic aneurysm

Mesenteric ischemia/infarction

PERHAPS:

Severe abdominal pain, cause unknown

Moderate to severe abdominal tenderness, cause unknown

*Except obvious superficial abdominal wall injury.

Repeated careful observation will usually then separate serious (often surgical) disease from self-limited causes of acute abdominal pain.

> Sally ultimately requires psychiatric consultation because of her remorse and guilt about the death of her grandfather. Her dysmenorrhea and irritable bowel symptoms improve with the medical management previously described but then wax and wane with her emotional state.
>
> A year later, Sally's abdominal complaints worsen, coincident with preparations for divorce proceedings. Repeat diagnostic investigations are not performed. Since resolution of these personal crises, Sally has done well, except for intermittent flares easily managed with Metamucil and antispasmodic drugs.

Ambulatory Treatment of Peptic Ulcer Disease

When duodenal ulcer is documented radiographically or endoscopically, initial treatment is usually straightforward. In the absence of bleeding, perforation, obstruction, or posterior penetration (with pancreatitis), the great majority of patients will do well when treated as outpatients.

Placebo treatment alone may result in healing of as many as half of all duodenal ulcers,[154-156] but if patients comply with a simple treatment regimen for 4 to 6 weeks, more than 90 per cent will achieve (at least temporary) cure:

1. Diet: Coffee[157] (caffeinated and decaffeinated), tea, cola drinks, and alcohol should be avoided. Excessive milk and cream[158] should be avoided. Many patients report that avoidance of spicy or acid food (citrus fruits, for example) is also symptomatically helpful, but there is little statistical evidence to support that dietary modification.

2. Smoking[159, 160] should be discontinued.

3. All medications containing aspirin and all nonsteroidal anti-inflammatory drugs should be stopped (when possible).[161]

4. The patient should attempt a relaxing life style. For some, this means staying out of work. For others, avoiding work is more stressful (and is thus counterproductive). All patients should eat at least three nutritious meals a day, reserve at least 8 hours a night for sleep, and generally "go easy."

5. Cimetidine* is the current drug of choice for treatment of duodenal ulcer.[162, 163] When it is taken with each meal and at bedtime in 300-mg doses (1.2 gm qd), ulcer healing rates approximate 90 per cent. While the drug is expensive (Table 11–26), it is no more costly than the alternative treatment: antacids (which are probably equally effective but are more cumbersome to administer) and sucralfate (which may be as effective but is less well studied). Cimetidine side effects—rash, diarrhea, dizziness, somnolence—are unusual (less than 5 per cent). Drug interactions are occasionally of great importance. (Dosage of coumarin, phenytoin, propranolol, diazepam, chlordiazepoxide, and theophylline may have to be reduced if they are given concomitantly with cimetidine.)

Antacids[164, 165, 167] are available in an extraordinary variety of commercial preparations. Table 11–26 lists some of the more commonly prescribed antacids and their relative cost, salt content, and acid-neutralizing capability as determined by two studies. (Neutralization of 140 mEq of acid is considered the standard by which to judge antacid dose effectiveness, although careful studies of the precise amount of acid neutralization that correlates with ulcer

---

*Ranitidine is a similar drug, recently released. It may replace cimetidine as the drug of choice, but further experience with ranitidine is needed.

TABLE 11–26A. ANTACIDS IN TREATMENT OF DUODENAL ULCER[164, 165]

ANTACID (LIQUID)*†	DOSE (ML) TO NEUTRALIZE 140 mEQ ACID	SODIUM (MG) PER 30 ML	COST PER MONTH
Maalox TC (aluminum hydroxide, magnesium hydroxide)	33	7.2	$44
Delcid (aluminum hydroxide, magnesium hydroxide)	17–34‡	9	$31–57‡
Mylanta-II (aluminum hydroxide, magnesium hydroxide, simethicone)	39	6.6	$63
Gelusil-II (aluminum hydroxide, magnesium hydroxide, simethicone)	32–47‡	7.8	$48–74‡
Maalox Plus (aluminum hydroxide, magnesium hydroxide, simethicone)	60	15	$68
Gelusil (aluminum hydroxide, magnesium hydroxide, simethicone)	65	4.2	$80
Riopan Plus (aluminum hydroxide, magnesium hydroxide, simethicone)	78	4.2	$78
ALternaGEL (aluminum hydroxide)	63	4	$75
Amphojel (aluminum hydroxide)	100	42	$114

*Omitted from this table are the many antacids that contain either calcium or carbonate, each of which is at least theoretically contraindicated in the treatment of peptic ulcer disease.[166]

†Magnesium-containing antacids often cause diarrhea. Antacids that contain only aluminum are more often constipating.

‡The variations in neutralizing capacity and thus monthly cost are a result of variable findings in the two cited studies.[164, 165]

TABLE 11–26B. AGENTS OTHER THAN ANTACIDS IN TREATMENT OF DUODENAL ULCER

PRODUCT	USUAL DOSE	SIDE EFFECTS	COST PER MONTH
Cimetidine	300 mg q6h with meals and at bedtime; 1.2 gm qd	Uncommon (less than 5%); diarrhea; nausea; vomiting; rash; dizziness; epigastric pain; gynecomastia; constipation; drowsiness; muscular pain	$42/120 tablets
Ranitidine*	150 mg bid	(Allegedly) few	$55/60 tablets
Sucralfate	1 gm 1 hour before meals and at bedtime; 4 gm qd	Uncommon; constipation; dry mouth	$36/120 tablets

*Recently released.

healing are not available. Surely there is individual variation among different patients in this regard.) Cost-efficacy analysis suggests that Maalox TC, Delcid, Mylanta-II, and Gelusil are preferred. ALternaGEL is necessary for some patients (or one can alternate ALternaGEL with one of the above antacids) when diarrhea is caused by the magnesium-containing antacids. Liquid preparations, taken 1 hour and 3 hours after each meal and at bedtime (seven doses per day), are recommended.

Sucralfate[168] is a newer agent that may be equally as effective as antacids or cimetidine. Taken 1 hour before meals and at bedtime, in dosages of 1 gm (4 gm qd), sucralfate binds to the ulcer and may thus promote healing by a different mechanism than either antacids or cimetidine.

After 6 to 8 weeks of initial treatment, the condition of the patient is reassessed (Fig. 11–39). If the patient is now completely asymptomatic, repeat upper GI x-rays and endoscopy are usually not necessary. Recurrence of duodenal ulcer is, however, very common,[169] and absence of symptoms does not guarantee cure. For this reason, some physicians routinely repeat x-rays or endoscopy to document healing.

Indefinite continuation of dietary, smoking, and medicinal restrictions makes sense, but is of unproven efficacy. Cimetidine maintenance therapy, 400 mg each night (for up to 1 year) has been found to be effective in reducing the incidence of recurrent ulcer.

When, after 4 to 6 weeks' therapy, symptoms persist, repeat upper GI series or endoscopy is necessary. When healing of the ulcer is documented (by endoscopy), persistent symptoms usually indicate persistent dyspepsia or "acid symptoms," and occasional antacids or nightly cimetidine may be helpful. (Associated pathologic states—in the gallbladder or pancreas, for example—must also be considered.)

When a duodenal ulcer persists (radiographically or endoscopically) after 4 to 6 weeks' initial therapy, consider:

1. Patient compliance—failure to stop smoking, avoid alcohol or aspirin, and to use faithfully the prescribed antiulcer regimen are currently the most common noncompliance causes of treatment failure.

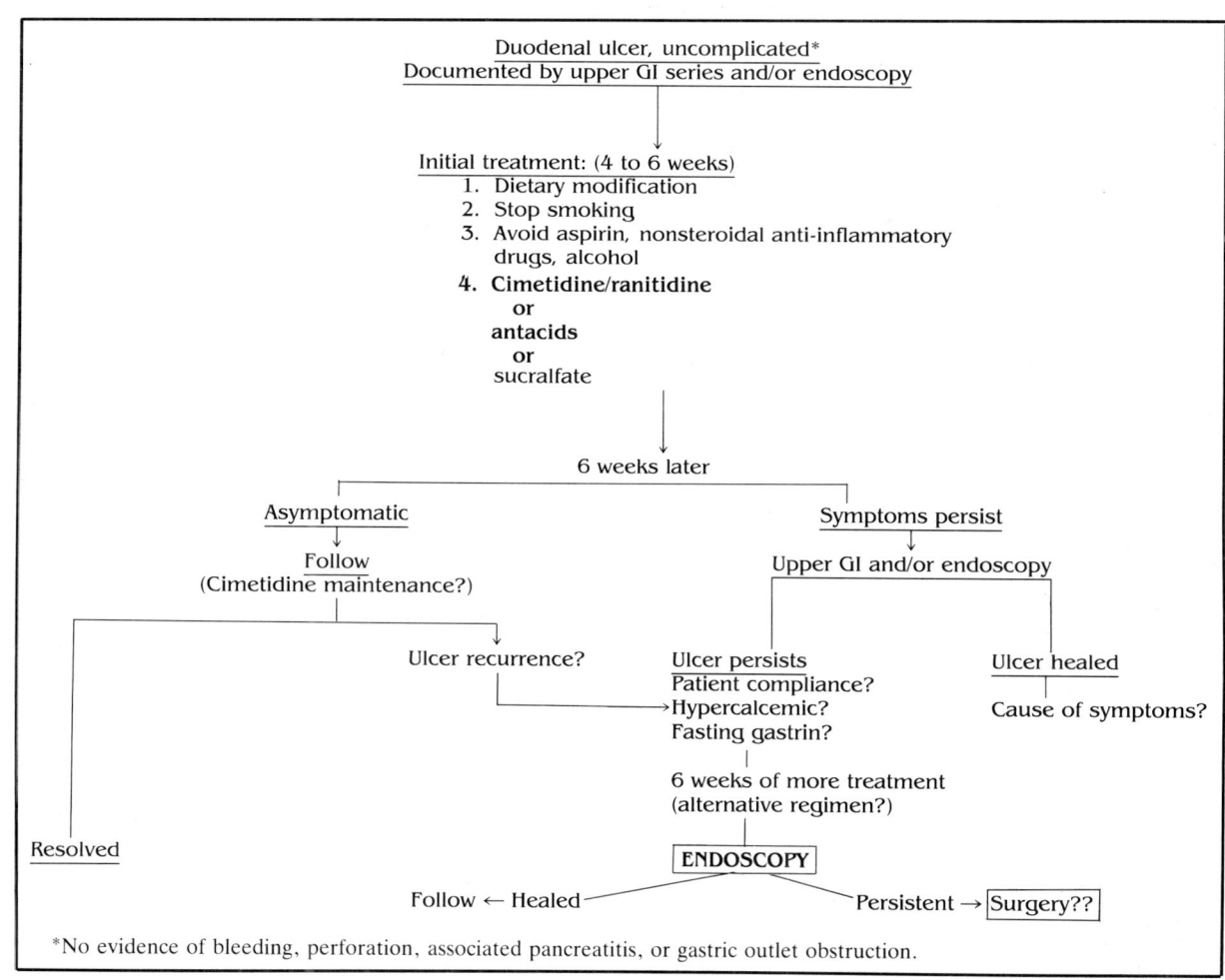

FIGURE 11–39.

TABLE 11–27. CAUSES OF ELEVATED SERUM GASTRIN LEVEL

Normal or Decreased Gastric Acid Secretion	Increased Gastric Acid Secretion
Pernicious anemia	Zollinger-Ellison syndrome
Chronic gastritis	Retained gastric antrum
Gastric cancer	Gastric outlet obstruction
Vagotomy	Renal failure
Pheochromocytoma	Antral G-cell hyperfunction
	Antral G-cell hyperplasia
	Short-bowel syndrome

Adapted from reference 170.

2. Hypercalcemia should be excluded, as should the Zollinger-Ellison syndrome[170] (the fasting serum gastrin level is the best screening test for the latter, but an elevated serum gastrin level may have many other causes—Table 11–27).

3. Surgery may be necessary but is rarely indicated before more prolonged medical therapy is attempted. Higher doses of cimetidine (for example, 600 mg qid), an alternative regimen (for example, sucralfate), or combined treatment (antacids plus sucralfate, for example) for at least another 1 to 2 months are usually indicated. Documentation of acid neutralization is often worthwhile in this setting—a pH probe or nasogastric tube for pH analysis during the first few days of treatment may reveal inadequate acid neutralization (gastric pH less than 5) in spite of treatment—treatment changes should then be made accordingly, since some patients will require higher doses or more frequent administration of antacids or Cimetidine.

Surgical treatment of ulcer disease is beyond the scope of this text.[171–173] Table 11–28 illustrates one author's compilation of surgical results and complications after several of the many available surgical procedures. Obviously, before surgery is recommended, persistent ulcer disease must be proven endoscopically, patient compliance with medical treatment must be reconsidered, and (sometimes) hospitalization is warranted for optimal medical treatment.

Grossman et al.,[174] and McCarthy[175] have reviewed many of the recent developments in the diagnosis and treatment of duodenal ulcer disease.

When gastric ulcer[176–178] is documented radiographically, initial treatment is generally identical to that of duodenal ulcer, with the following exception (Fig. 11–40):

1. While duodenal ulcer is "never" malignant, 4 to 5 per cent of gastric ulcers are malignant. When the ulcer is radiographically benign, and the

TABLE 11–28. SURGICAL TREATMENT OF PEPTIC ULCER*

PROCEDURE	INCIDENCE OF RECURRENT ULCER (%)	POSTPRANDIAL SYMPTOMS (%)	WEIGHT LOSS	DIARRHEA (%)
Subtotal gastrectomy	2–5	38–40	+ +	7
Truncal vagotomy and antrectomy	0–3	34–39	+ +	20–23
Truncal vagotomy and drainage	7–15	21–40	+	25–26
Proximal gastric vagotomy	1–22	0–14	+	0–14

*Adapted from reference 173.
+ = mild weight loss
+ + = more pronounced weight loss

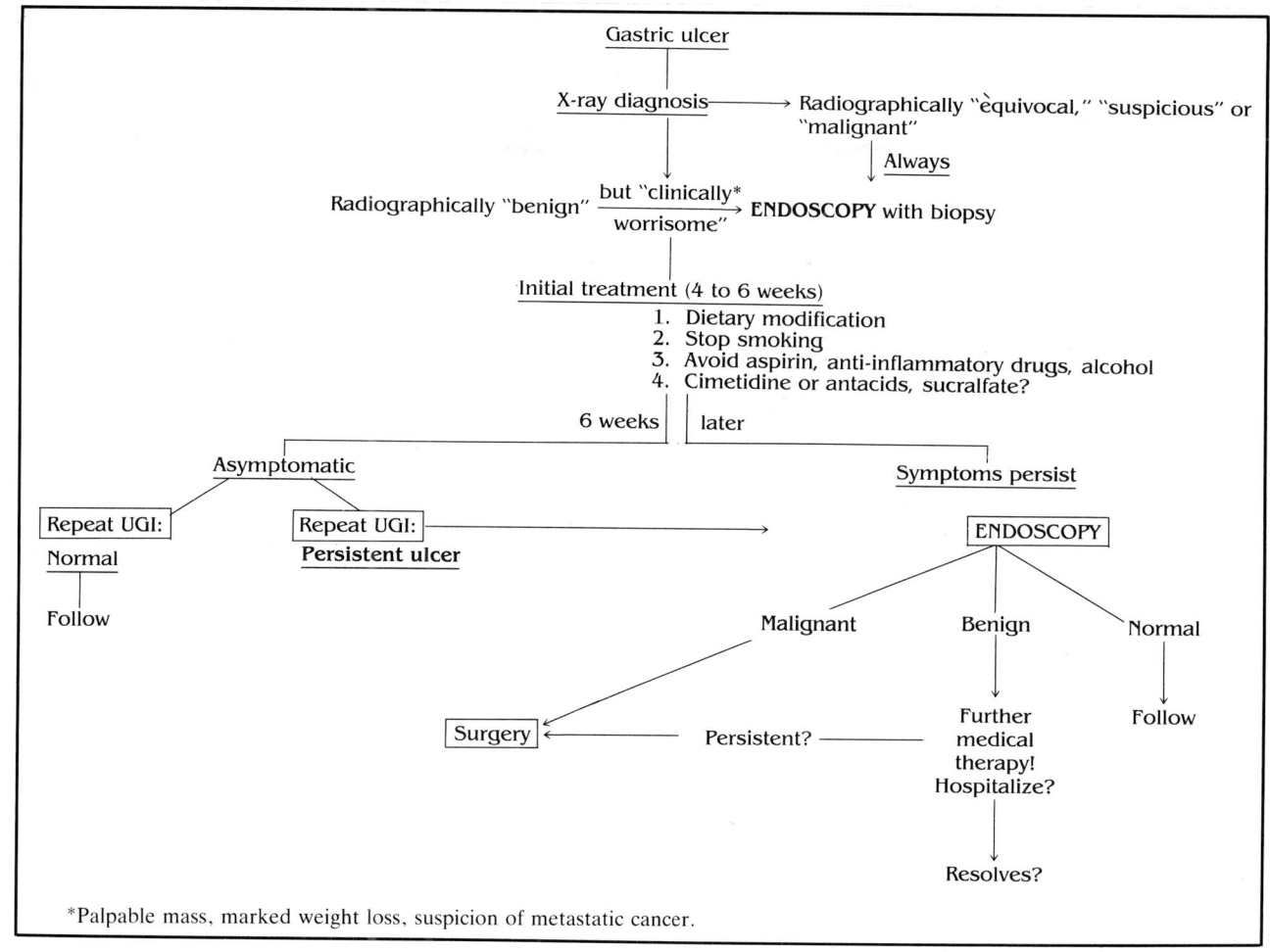

FIGURE 11–40.

patient is not clinically worrisome (no palpable mass, weight loss, history of pernicious anemia, or family history of gastric carcinoma), endoscopy is usually unnecessary (Fig. 11–31).

Some authorities prefer endoscopy in all patients with gastric ulcer because "radiographic benignity" is not invariably reliable.[105, 106, 179] and, rarely, even malignant ulcers may heal (temporarily) with medical treatment.[170] Routine endoscopy of all patients with gastric ulcer is extremely expensive when one considers the frequency of gastric ulcers and the relative rarity of a healing malignant ulcer. Nevertheless, whenever a gastric ulcer is not a typical benign ulcer radiographically or the patient is worrisome, endoscopy is essential.

2. Antacids or cimetidine is the preferred treatment of gastric ulcer. Sucralfate may be effective for gastric ulcer, but this remains uncertain.[168]

3. Documentation of healing is essential in all patients with gastric ulcer. All patients with gastric ulcer need either an upper GI series or endoscopy after completion of therapy, even when they are asymptomatic. The best approach to documentation of healing remains controversial. Endoscopy is the most reliable method, but a radiographically benign ulcer that is healed completely on repeat upper GI series usually does not require confirmatory endoscopy.

4. Hospitalization has long been thought to be more often necessary in the patient with gastric ulcer. This is probably not the case.[177] Most patients with an otherwise uncomplicated gastric ulcer can be treated as outpatients.

REFERENCES

1. Brewer, RJ, et al.: Abdominal pain. An analysis of 1,000 consecutive cases in a university hospital emergency room. Am J Surg 131:219–223, 1976.
2. Botsford, T, Wilson, RE: The Acute Abdomen: An Approach to Diagnosis and Management, 2nd ed. Philadelphia: W. B. Saunders, 1977.
3. Way, LW: Abdominal pain and the acute abdomen. In Sleisenger, MH, Fordtran, JS (eds.): Gastrointestinal Diseases, 2nd ed. Philadelphia: W. B. Saunders, 1978, pp. 394–410.
4. Jones, CM: Digestive Tract Pain. New York: MacMillan, 1938.
5. Ferrier, PK: Acute appendicitis in university students: A twenty-year study of 1,028 cases. J Am Coll Health Assoc 20:287–290, 1972.
6. French EG, Robb, WAT: Biliary and renal colic. Br Med J 3:121, 1963.
7. Glenn, F: Pain in biliary tract disease. Surg Gynecol Obstet 122:495, 1966.
8. Morton, JJ: Diverticulitis of the colon. Ann Surg 124:725–745, 1946.
9. Wax, SH, Frank, IN: A retrospective study of upper urinary tract calculi. J Urol 94:28–32, 1965.
10. Weinstein, M, et al.: Spontaneous bacterial peritonitis. Am J Med 64:592–598, 1978.
11. Zizic, TM, et al.: Acute abdominal complications of systemic lupus erythematosus and polyarteritis nodosa. Am J Med 73:525–531, 1982.
12. Peppercorn, MA, et al.: Abdominal epilepsy. A cause of abdominal pain in adults. JAMA 240:2450–2451, 1978.
13. Fischer, RP, et al.: Diagnostic peritoneal lavage: 14 years and 2,586 patients later. Am J Surg 136:701–704, 1978.
14. Jones, RS: Intestinal obstruction, pseudo-obstruction and ileus. In Sleisenger, MH, Fordtran, JS (eds.): Gastrointestinal Diseases, 2nd ed, Philadelphia: W. B. Saunders, pp. 425–436.
15. Davis, SE, Sperling, L.: Obstruction of the small intestine. Arch Surg 99:424–426, 1969.
16. Carden, ABG: Acute large bowel obstruction: Etiology and mortality. Med J Aust 1:662–663, 1966.
17. Eisenberg, RL, et al.: Evaluation of plain abdominal radiographs in the diagnosis of abdominal pain. Ann Intern Med 97:257–261, 1982.
18. Lee, PWR: The plain x-ray in the acute abdomen: A surgeon's evaluation. Br J Surg 63:763–766, 1976.
19. Reuben, DB, et al.: Transient proteinuria in emergency medical admissions. N Engl J Med 306:1031–1033, 1982.
20. Raftery, AT: The value of the leukocyte count in the diagnosis of acute appendicitis. Br J Surg 63:143–144, 1976.
21. Sasso, RD, et al.: Leukocyte and neutrophil counts in acute appendicitis. Am J Surg 120:563–566, 1970.
22. Bolton, JP, et al.: An assessment of the value of the white cell count in the management of suspected acute appendicitis. Br J Surg 62:906–908, 1975.
23. Cope, Z: The Early Diagnosis of the Acute Abdomen, 14th ed. London: Oxford University Press, 1972, p. 1.
24. Hendrick, JW: Treatment of volvulus of the cecum and right colon: A report of six acute and thirteen recurrent cases. Arch Surg 88:364–374, 1964.
25. Cope, Z: The Early Diagnosis of the Acute Abdomen, 14th ed. London: Oxford University Press, 1972, pp. 79–90.
26. Andersen, SG: Management of threatened abortion with real-time sonography. Obstet Gynecol 55:259–262, 1980.
27. Eschenbach, DA, Holmes, KK: Acute pelvic inflammatory disease: Current concepts of pathogenesis, etiology and management. Clin Obstet Gynecol 18:35–56, 1975.
28. Chow, AW, et al.: The bacteriology of acute pelvic inflammatory disease. Am J Obstet Gynecol 122:876–879, 1975.
29. Eschenbach, DA, et al.: Polymicrobial etiology of acute pelvic inflammatory disease. N Engl J Med 293:166–171, 1975.
30. Cunningham, FG, et al.: Evaluation of tetracycline or penicillin and ampicillin for treatment of acute pelvic inflammatory disease. N Engl J Med 296:1380–1383, 1977.
31. Jacobson, L, Westron, L: Objective diagnosis of acute pelvic inflammatory disease. Diagnostic and prognostic value of routine laparoscopy. Am J Obstet Gynecol 105:1088–1098, 1969.
32. Vine, HS, Birnholz, JC: Ultrasound evaluation of pelvic pain. JAMA 244:2540–2542, 1980.
33. Abrahams, J: Ultrasonography. When it is and isn't indicated for OB/GYN patients. Consultant 55–64, (Sept) 1982.
34. Girardet, R, Enquist, I: Differential diagnosis between appendicitis and acute pelvic inflammatory disease. Surg Gynecol Obstet 116:212–216, 1963.
35. Cope, Z: The Early Diagnosis of the Acute Abdomen, 14th ed. London: Oxford University Press, 1972, pp. 48–78.
36. Mittelpunkt, A, Nora, PF: Current features in the treatment of acute appendicitis: An analysis of 1,000 consecutive cases. Surgery 60:971–975, 1966.
37. Peltokallio, P, Janhainen, K: Acute appendicitis in the aged patient. Study of 300 cases after the age of 60. Arch Surg 100:140–143, 1970.
38. Lewis, FR, et al.: Appendicitis. A critical review of diagnosis and treatment in 1,000 cases. Arch Surg 110:677–684, 1975.
39. Manning, RT: Signs that point to appendicitis. Diagnosis pp 88–90, (Feb) 1982.
40. Fitzgerald, JE, Brewer, JI: Extrauterine pregnancy: A clinical study of 500 cases. Am J Obstet Gynecol 30:264–269, 1935.
41. Webster, HD, et al.: Ectopic pregnancy. A 17-year review. Am J Obstet Gynecol 92:23–34, 1965.
42. Breen, JL: A 21-year survey of 654 ectopic pregnancies. Am J Obstet Gynecol 106:1004–1019, 1970.
43. Kitchin, JD, et al.: Ectopic pregnancy: Current clinical trends. Am J Obstet Gynecol 134:47–476, 1979.
44. Hsu Wu, DI, Langer, A: Ectopic pregnancy. Am Fam Physician 26:161–166, 1982.

45. Lorenz, RP, et al.: A radioreceptor assay for human chorionic gonadotropin in normal and abnormal pregnancies. A clinical evaluation. Am J Obstet Gynecol 134:471–475, 1979.
46. Gunn, A, Keddie, N: Some clinical observations on patients with gallstones. Lancet 2:239, 1972.
47. Byrne, JJ: Acute cholecystitis. Am J Surg 97:156–172, 1959.
48. Raine, PAM, Gunn, AA: Acute cholecystitis. Br J Surg 62:697–700, 1975.
49. Cope, Z: The Early Diagnosis of the Acute Abdomen, 14th ed. London: Oxford University Press, 1972, pp. 152–160.
50. Gardner, B, et al.: Factors influencing the timing of the surgery and acute cholecystitis. Am J Surg 125:730–733, 1973.
51. Bartrum, R, et al.: Ultrasonic and radiographic cholecystography. N Engl J Med 296:538, 1977.
52. Lee, JKT, et al.: Cholecystosonography: Accuracy, pitfalls and unusual findings. Am J Surg 139:223, 1980.
53. Weissman, HS, et al.: Rapid and accurate diagnosis of acute cholecystitis with 99m-Tc HIDA cholescintigraphy. AJR 135:523, 1979.
54. Freitas, JE: Cholescintigraphy in acute and chronic cholecystitis. Sem Nucl Med 18:26, 1982.
55. Zimmerman, HJ, et al.: Infectious hepatitis: Clinical and laboratory features of 295 cases. Am J Med Sci 213:395–409, 1947.
56. Lewis, JH, et al.: Hepatitis B. A study of 200 cases positive for the hepatitis B antigen. Am J Dig Dis 18:921–929, 1973.
57. Petersen, P, et al.: Acute viral hepatitis: A survey of 500 patients. Scand J Gastroenterol 9:607–613, 1974.
58. Gitnick, GL: Viral hepatitis. West J Med 128:117–126, 1978.
59. Green, J, et al.: Acute alcoholic hepatitis. Arch Intern Med 112:113–124, 1963.
60. Conn, HO: Steroid treatment of alcoholic hepatitis. The yeas and the nays. Gastroenterology 74:319–326, 1978.
61. Curtis, AH: Adhesions of the anterior surface of the liver. JAMA 99:2010–2012, 1932.
62. Fitzhugh, T, Jr: Acute gonococcic peritonitis of the right upper quadrant in women. JAMA 102:2094–2096, 1934.
63. Stanley, MM: Gonococcic peritonitis of the upper part of the abdomen in young women. Arch Intern Med 78:1–13, 1946.
64. Miller, WT, Talman, EA: Subphrenic abscess. Am J Roentgenol 101:961–969, 1967.
65. Romney, SL, et al. (eds.): Obstetrics and Gynecology: Health Care for Women, 2nd ed. New York: McGraw-Hill, 1981, pp. 489, 889–891.
66. Duthrie, HL: Colonic response to eating. Gastroenterology 75:527–528, 1978.
67. Perez, CA, et al.: Carcinoma of the endometrium. In DeVita, VT, et al. (eds.): Cancer: Principles and Practice of Oncology. Philadelphia: J. B. Lippincott, 1982, pp. 849–860.
68. Falterman, KW, et al.: Cancer of the colon, rectum and anus. A review of 2,313 cases. Cancer 34:951–959, 1974.
69. Kent, SW, McKay, DG: Primary cancer of the ovary. Am J Obstet Gynecol 80:430–438, 1960.
70. Young, TC, et al.: Cancer of the ovary. In DeVita, VT, et al. (eds.): Cancer: Principles and Practice of Oncology. Philadelphia: J. B. Lippincott, 1982, pp. 884–913.
71. Kopell, H, Thompson, WAL: Peripheral Entrapment Neuropathies. Baltimore: Williams and Wilkins, 1963.
72. Swarbrick, ET, et al.: Site of pain from the irritable bowel. Lancet 2: 443–446, 1980.
73. Drossman, DA, et al.: The irritable bowel syndrome. Gastroenterology 73:811–822, 1977.
74. Manning, AP, et al.: Towards a positive diagnosis of the irritable bowel. Br Med J 2:653–654, 1978.
75. Prout, BJ: The irritable colon syndrome—very common but often missed. Mod Med 36–40, (July) 1977.
76. Whitehead, WE, Schuster, MM: Psychological management of the irritable bowel syndrome. Pract Gastroenterol 3:32–36, 1979.
77. Almy, TP: Diagnostic Approaches to Presenting Syndromes. Baltimore: Williams and Wilkins, 1971, pp. 167–196.
78. Almy, TP: Experimental studies on the irritable colon. Am J Med 10:60–67, 1951.
79. Almy, TP, et al.: Alterations in colonic function in man under stress. IV. Hypomotility of the sigmoid colon, and its relationship to the mechanics of functional diarrhea. Gastroenterology 15:95–103, 1950.
80. Schuffler, MD, et al.: Chronic intestinal pseudo-obstruction: A report of 27 cases and a review of the literature. Medicine 60:173–196, 1981.
81. Haddad, H, Devroede-Bertrand, G: Large bowel motility disorders. Med Clin North Am 65:1377–1396, 1981.
82. Ylikorkala, O, Dawood, MY: New concepts in dysmenorrhea. Am J Obstet Gynecol 130:833, 1978.
83. Chan, WY, et al.: Prostaglandins in primary dysmenorrhea. Comparison of prophylactic and nonprophylactic treatment with ibuprofen and use of all contraceptives. Am J Med 70:535–541, 1981.
84. Swartz, A, et al.: Primary dysmenorrhea: Alleviation by an inhibitor of prostaglandin synthesis and action. Obstet Gynecol 44:709, 1974.
85. Merrill, JA: Endometriosis. In Romney, SL, et al. (eds.): Obstetrics and Gynecology: Health Care for Women, 2nd ed. McGraw-Hill, 1981, pp. 931–945.
86. Kovarik, JL, Toll, GD: Thoracic endometriosis with recurrent spontaneous pneumothorax. JAMA 196:595, 1966.
87. Lombardo, L, et al.: Subarachnoid hemorrhage due to endometriosis of the spinal canal. Neurology 19:423, 1968.
88. Rodman, MH, Jones, CW: Catamenial hemoptysis due to bronchial endometriosis. N Engl J Med 266:805, 1962.
89. Morton, JJ: Diverticulitis of the colon. Ann Surg 124:725–745, 1946.
90. Botsford, TW, Curtis, LE: Diverticulitis coli. Criteria of management for the physician and the surgeon. N Engl J Med 265:618–623, 1961.

91. Morton, DL, Goldman, L: Differential diagnosis of diverticulitis and carcinoma of the sigmoid colon. Am J Surg 103:55–61, 1962.
92. Roth, JLA: Diagnosis and differential diagnosis of colonic diverticulitis. Postgrad Med 60:85–90, 1976.
93. Almy, TP, Howell, DA: Diverticular disease of the colon. N Engl J Med 302:324–330, 1980.
94. Renny, A, Snape, WJ: Diverticular disease: A common disorder, a common mimic. Diagnosis 28–37, (Mar) 1982.
95. Devroede, G: Constipation: Mechanisms and management. In Sleisenger, MH, Fordtran, JS (eds.): Gastrointestinal Diseases, 2nd ed. Philadelphia: W. B. Saunders, 1978, pp. 368–386.
96. Romney, SL, et al. (eds.): Obstetrics and Gynecology: Health Care for Women, 2nd ed. New York: McGraw-Hill, 1981, pp. 1983–1985.
97. Jessop, C: Women's curse: A general internist's approach to common menstrual problems. West J Med 138:76–82, 1983.
98. Aubrey, DA: Meckel's diverticulum. A review of 66 emergency Meckel's diverticulectomies. Arch Surg 100:144–146, 1970.
99. Horrocks, JC, deDombal, FT: Clinical presentation of patients with dyspepsia. Detailed symptomatic study of 360 patients. Gut 19:19–26, 1978.
100. Friedenwald, J: A clinical study of a thousand cases of ulcer of the stomach and duodenum. Am J Med Sci 144:157–170, 1912.
101. Earlam, R: A computerized questionnaire analysis of duodeal ulcer symptoms. Gastroenterology 71:314–317, 1976.
102. Belber, JP: Endoscopic examination of the duodenal bulb: A comparison with x-ray. Gastroenterology 61:55, 1979.
103. Decker, W, Tytgat, GW: Diagnostic accuracy of fiberendoscopy in detection of upper GI malignancy: A follow-up analysis. Gastroenterology 73:710, 1977.
104. Rubin, P, et al.: Cancer of the GI tract. C. Gastric cancer diagnosis. JAMA 228:883–896, 1974.
105. Green, PHR, et al.: Early gastric cancer. Gastroenterology 81:247–256, 1981.
106. Green, PHR, O'Toole, KM: Early gastric cancer. Ann Intern Med 97:272–273, 1982.
107. Price, WH: Gallbladder dyspepsia. Br Med J 2:138–141, 1963.
108. Koch, JP, Donaldson, RM: A survey of food intolerance in hospitalized patients. N Engl J Med 271:657–660, 1964.
109. Gregory, DW, et al.: Natural history of patients with x-ray negative dyspepsia in general practice. Br Med J 4:519–522, 1972.
110. Horrocks, JC, deDombal, FT: Computer aided diagnosis of "dyspepsia." Am J Dig Dis 20:397–406, 1975.
111. Weddington, WW: Psychiatric aspects of chronic abdominal pain. Drug Ther 97–111, (Feb) 1982.
112. Winans, CS: The challenge of chronic abdominal pain. Drug Ther 48–50, (Mar) 1982.
113. Morris, GC, et al.: Abdominal angina. Surg Clin North Am 46:919–930, 1966.
114. Willian, LF: Vascular insufficiency of the intestines. Gastroenterology 61:757–777, 1971.
115. Watt, JK, et al.: Chronic intestinal ischemia. Br Med J 3:199–202, 1967.
116. Hansen, HJB: Abdominal angina. Results of arterial reconstruction in 12 patients. Acta Chir Scand 142:319–325, 1976.
117. Watson, WC, Sadikali, F: Celiac axis compression. Experience with 20 patients, and a critical appraisal of the syndrome. Ann Intern Med 86:278–284, 1977.
118. Gracie, WA, Ransohoff, DF: The natural history of silent gallstones. The innocent gallstone is not a myth. N Engl J Med 307:798–800, 1982.
119. Grodski, M, et al.: Diabetic cholecystopathy. Diabetologia 4:345, 1968.
120. Knowles, DM, et al.: Clinical, radiologic and pathologic characterization of benign hepatic neoplasm. Alleged association with oral contraceptives. Medicine 57:223, 1978.
121. Edmonson, H, et al.: Liver cell adenoma associated with use of oral contraceptives. N Engl J Med 294:470, 1976.
122. Gottlieb, AJ, et al. (eds.): The Whole Internist Catalog. Philadelphia: W. B. Saunders, 1980, p. 10.
123. Mackie, CR, et al.: Nonoperative differentiation between pancreatic cancer and chronic pancreatitis. Ann Surg 189:480, 1979.
124. Sarles, H: Chronic calcifying pancreatitis—chronic alcoholic pancreatitis. Gastroenterology 66:604, 1974.
125. Strum, WS, Spiro, HM: Chronic pancreatitis. Ann Intern Med 74:264–277, 1971.
126. Herlinger, H, et al.: An evaluation of the double contrast barium meal (DCBM) against endoscopy. Clin Radio 28:307–314, 1977.
127. Salter, RH: X-ray negative dyspepsia. Br Med J 2:235–236, 1977.
128. Laufer, I, et al.: The diagnostic accuracy of barium studies of the stomach and duodenum—correlation with endoscopy. Radiology 115:569–573, 1975.
129. Cotton, PB: Fiberoptic endoscopy and the barium meal—results and implications. Br Med J 2:161–165, 1973.
130. Gore, RM, Goldberg, HI: Current indications for radiology and endoscopy in the evaluation of upper gastrointestinal tract disease. Intern Med 3:77–85, 1982.
131. Isenberg JI: Peptic ulcer disease. In Beeson, PB, McDermott, W, Wyngaarden, JB (eds.): Cecil's Textbook of Medicine, 16th ed. Philadelphia: W. B. Saunders, 1982, pp. 642–646.
132. Marton, KI, et al.: The clinical value of the upper gastrointestinal tract roentgenogram series. Arch Intern Med 140:191–195, 1980.
133. Mujahed, Z, et al.: The nonopacified gallbladder on oral cholecystography. Radiology 112:1, 1974.
134. Lawson, T: Sensitivity of pancreatic ultrasonography in the detection of pancreatic disease. Radiology 128:733, 1978.
135. Simeone, JF, et al.: Modern concepts of imaging of the pancreas. Invest Radiol 15:6, 1980.
136. Moss, AA, et al.: The combined use of CT and ERCP in the assessment of suspected pancreatic neoplasm: A blind clinical evaluation. Radiology 134:159, 1980.

137. Piehler, JM, Crichlow, RW: Primary carcinoma of the gallbladder. Surg Gynecol Obstet 147:929, 1978.
138. Salt, WB, Schenker, S: Amylase—its clinical significance: A review of the literature. Medicine 55:269–289, 1976.
139. Goldstein, HM, et al.: Percutaneous fine needle aspiration of pancreatic and other abdominal masses. Radiology 123:319, 1977.
140. Winship, D, et al.: Pancreatitis: Pancreatic pseudocysts and their complications. Gastroenterology 73:593, 1977.
141. Boley, SJ, et al.: Ischemic disease of the intestine. Curr Probl Surg 15:1, 1978.
142. Superior mesenteric artery syndrome. In Beeson, PB, McDermott, W, Wyngaarden, JB (eds.): Cecil's Textbook of Medicine, 16th ed. Philadelphia: W. B. Saunders, 1982, pp. 722–723.
143. Bergan, JJ, Yao, JST: Modern concepts of abdominal aortic aneurysms. Surg Clin North Am 54:175, 1974.
144. Darling, RC, et al.: Autopsy studies of unoperated abdominal aortic aneurysms: The case for early resection. Circulation 56 (suppl. 2):161, 1977.
145. Gardner, RJ, et al.: The surgical experience and a 1-to-16 year follow-up of 272 abdominal aortic aneurysms. Am J Surg 135:226, 1978.
146. Collins, JJ, et al.: Common aortic aneurysms: When to intervene. J Cardiovasc Med 8:245–254, (Feb) 1983.
147. Malagelada, JR, et al.: Gastric motor abnormalities in diabetic and post-gastrectomy gastroparesis: Effective metoclopramide and bethanechol. Gastroenterology 78:286, 1980.
148. Ihde, DC, et al.: Clinical manifestations of hepatoma. A review of 6 years' experience at a cancer hospital. Am J Med 56:83, 1974.
149. Czaja, AJ: Current problems in the diagnosis and management of chronic active hepatitis. Mayo Clin Proc 56:311–323, 1981.
150. Murphy, GE: The clinical management of hysteria. JAMA 247:2559–2564, 1982.
151. Brandborg, LL: Acute pancreatitis. In Sleisenger, MH, Fordtran, JS (eds.): Gastrointestinal Diseases, 2nd ed. Philadelphia: W. B. Saunders, 1978, pp. 1409–1439.
152. Paloyan, D, Simonowitz, D: Diagnostic considerations in acute alcoholic and gallstone pancreatitis. Am J Surg 132:329, 1976.
153. Slater, EE, DeSanctis, RW: Clinical recognition of dissecting aortic aneurysm. Am J Med 60:625, 1976.
154. Binder, HJ, et al.: Cimetidine in the treatment of duodenal ulcer: A multivariate double-blind study. Gastroenterology 74:380–388, 1978.
155. Hetzel, DJ, et al.: Cimetidine treatment of duodenal ulceration. Short-term clinical trial and maintenance study. Gastroenterology 74:389–392, 1978.
156. Hollander, D, Harlan, J: Antacids versus placebos in peptic ulcer therapy: A controlled double-blind investigation. JAMA 226:1181–1185, 1973.
157. Cohen, S, Barth, GH: Gastric acid secretion and lower esophageal sphincter pressure in response to coffee and caffeine. N Engl J Med 293:897, 1975.
158. Ippoliti, AF, et al.: The effect of various forms of milk on gastric acid secretion. Ann Intern Med 84:296–289, 1976.
159. Korman, MG, et al.: Influence of smoking on healing rate of duodenal ulcer in response to cimetidine or high dose antacids. Gastroenterology 80:1451–1453, 1981.
160. Ross, AHM, et al.: Late mortality after surgery for peptic ulcer. N Engl J Med 307:519–522, 1982.
161. Caruso, I, Bianchi Perro, G: Gastroscopic evaluation of anti-inflammatory agents. Br Med 1:75–78, 1980.
162. Freston, JW: Cimetidine. I. Developments, pharmacology, and efficacy. Ann Intern Med 97:573–580, 1982.
163. Freston, JW: Cimetidine. II. Adverse reactions and pattern of use. Ann Intern Med 97:728–734, 1982.
164. Drake, D, Hollander, D: Neutralizing capacity and cost effectiveness of antacids. Ann Intern Med 94:215–217, 1981.
165. Dutro, MP, Amerson, AB: Comparison of liquid antacids (Letter). N Engl J Med 302:1967, 1980.
166. Barreras, RF: Acid secretion after calcium carbonate in patients with duodenal ulcer. N Engl J Med 282:1402–1405, 1970.
167. Graham, DY, Smith, JL: Antacids—where they stand in clinical medicine. Consultant:33–41, (Apr) 1982.
168. Richardson, CT: Sucralfate (Editorial). Ann Intern Med 97:272, 1982.
169. Korman, MG, et al.: Relapse rate of duodenal ulcer after cessation of long-term cimetidine treatment. Dig Dis Sci 25:88–91, 1980.
170. Jensen, RT, et al.: Zollinger-Ellison syndrome: Current concepts in management. Ann Intern Med 98:59–75, 1983.
171. Symposium on duodenal peptic ulceration—1980. Mayo Clin Proc 55:3, 1980.
172. Thompson, JC: The role of surgery in peptic ulcer. N Engl J Med 307:550–551, 1982.
173. Meyer, JH: Peptic ulcer: Complications and surgical treatment. In Beeson, PB, McDermott, W, Wyngaarden, JB (eds.): Cecil's Textbook of Medicine, 16th ed. Philadelphia: W. B. Saunders, 1982, p. 652.
174. Grossman, MI, et al.: Peptic ulcer: New therapies, new diseases. Ann Intern Med 95:609–627, 1981.
175. McCarthy, DM: Peptic ulcer heterogeneity and clinical implications. Ann Intern Med 95:507–508, 1981.
176. Veterans Administration cooperative study of gastric ulcer. Gastroenterology 61:567–641, 1971.
177. Englert, E, et al.: Cimetidine, antacids, and hospitalization in the treatment of benign gastric ulcer. Gastroenterology 74:416–425, 1978.
178. Fordtran, JS, et al.: Round table discussion on gastric ulcer. Gastroenterology 74:431–434, 1978.
179. Sakita, T, et al.: Observation on the healing of ulceration in early gastric cancer. Gastroenterology 60:835–844, 1971.

12
COUGH

ACUTE COUGH................................... 629
   Initial Approach 629
   Bronchitis versus Pneumonia 631
   Treatment of Acute Bronchitis 638
      When the Patient Does Not Improve.......... 640
   Hemoptysis..................................... 642
   Diagnosis of Pneumonia 643
   Treatment of Pneumonia....................... 657
      Follow-up................................... 664

CHRONIC COUGH................................ 667

APPENDIX: THE WORRIED WELL 672

REFERENCES...................................... 674

Most cough is involuntary and is initiated through a complex reflex arc.[1] The afferent arm of that reflex is served by many different nerves (primarily the vagus, trigeminal, glossopharyngeal, and phrenic), which may be stimulated by a remarkable variety of receptors in many different organ systems (Fig. 12–1). This partly explains the lengthy differential diagnosis of cough (Table 12–1) since pathologic and physiologic events both within and outside the laryngotracheobronchial tree can cause coughing. After synapse in cough centers in the medulla of the brain stem, the efferent arm of the cough reflex, modulated by vagus, phrenic, and spinal motor nerves, then initiates cough.

The motor mechanism of cough involves three successive phases. The inspiratory phase consists of the characteristic deep inspiration that precedes cough, whereby high lung volumes are achieved. During this phase, the

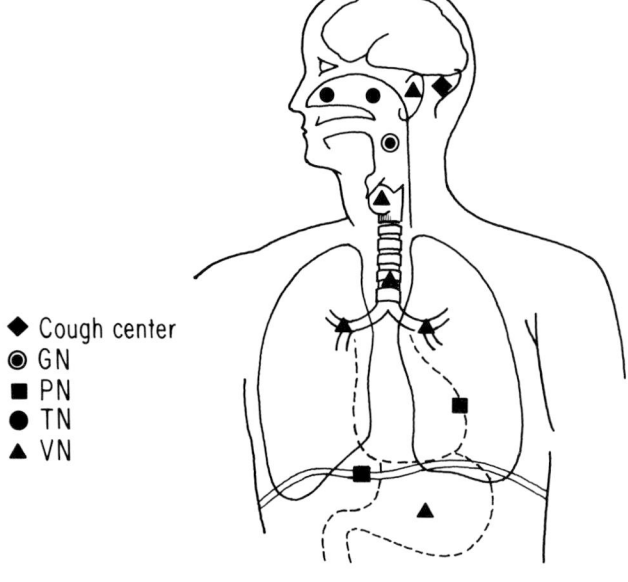

♦ Cough center
◉ GN
■ PN
● TN
▲ VN

FIGURE 12–1. The cough reflex arc. GN = Glossopharyngeal nerve innervates pharynx. PN = Phrenic nerve innervates pericardium and diaphragm. TN = Trigeminal nerve innervates nose and sinuses. VN = Vagus nerve innervates ear canals, tympanic membrane, larynx, trachea, bronchi, pleura, esophagus, and stomach.

TABLE 12–1. CAUSES OF COUGH

Upper Respiratory	Lower Respiratory	Others
Common		
Allergic rhinitis	Acute bronchitis	Subphrenic abscess
Sinusitis	Chronic bronchitis	Ruptured spleen
Nasal polyps	Asthma	Aortic aneurysm
Pharyngitis	Obstructive lung disease	Pericardial disease
Tracheolaryngitis	Bronchiectasis	Mediastinal neoplasm
Tonsillar hypertrophy	Pneumonia	Reflux esophagitis
	Tuberculosis	Angina pectoris
	Lung cancer	Glossopharyngeal neuralgia
	Congestive heart failure	Vagus nerve tumors
	Pneumothorax	Psychogenic
	Pleural effusion	Cervical spine osteophytosis
	Bronchial irritants	(phrenic nerve)
		Aortic dissection
Uncommon		Pneumomediastinum
Uvular enlargement	Tracheobronchial foreign	Esophageal rupture
Nasopharyngeal	body	Anaphylaxis
neoplasm	Aspiration	
Laryngeal polyps	Pulmonary embolism	
External otitis	Interstitial lung disease	
Hair/wax in ear canal	Pulmonary vasculitis	
	Bronchial adenoma	
	Lung contusion	

glottis opens, the chest expands, and the bronchial tree enlarges. Deep inspiration facilitates subsequent high-velocity air flow by increasing static elastic recoil of the lungs and decreasing airway resistance. At the height of inspiration, the second phase of cough, the compressive phase, occurs—the glottis closes and expiratory chest muscles contract, thus raising intrathoracic pressures to generate high flow rates during the cough itself. Sudden opening of the glottis then initiates the third phase, the expiratory phase—compressed intrabronchial air releases as the cough explosion occurs. Early in the expiratory phase, when lung volumes are high, pleural pressures are sufficient to compress large airways. At lower lung volumes (as progressive cough follows a single inspiration), smaller airways are compressed. This sequence of successive coughs with decreasing lung volumes thus allows initial clearance of large proximal airways followed by clearance of the smaller distal airways. Repetition of these three phases then permits progressive clearing of airways of all sizes, as secretions are mobilized from distal to proximal airways and then expelled.

ACUTE COUGH

Initial Approach

As Table 12–1 suggests, the causes of cough are many. The great majority of patients with cough have one of the common upper or lower respiratory disorders. The clinical approach to the patient with acute cough depends on a careful history and examination.

CONSIDER

> Brenda Bronchitis, a healthy 35-year-old divorced schoolteacher, enters the clinic complaining of 5 days of gradually increasing cough. One week before, Brenda noted the onset of rhinorrhea, hoarseness, and low-grade fever. These symptoms have largely resolved, but spasmodic coughing, occasionally productive of small amounts of yellow sputum, persists. There is no history of chills, chest pain, or dyspnea, or any prior history of asthma or heart disease.
>
> Brenda has been a pack-a-day smoker for the past 15 years, but denies chronic cough. Brenda's father, who lives with her, has had similar symptoms for the past 2 weeks.

In the patient with cough, the <u>history</u> will answer several important questions:

I. <u>Is the cough acute or chronic?</u>

Chronic or recurrent cough requires a different approach entirely (see page 667). Most acute cough (present for a few days or a week) is caused by upper or lower respiratory tract infections. Hence, the importance of the following question:

II. <u>Does the cough "sound" infectious or noninfectious?</u>

Fever, associated upper respiratory infection symptoms (rhinitis, myalgias, hoarseness, headache), or a highly likely epidemiologic source of infection (a "community bug," a sick family member) suggests infectious cough.

<u>When acute cough is not associated with these "infectious clues," several possibilities should come to mind:</u>

A. Asthma.

Cough without clinically apparent bronchospasm (audible wheezing) is not uncommon among asthmatics. Many patients with mild asthma are unaware of their problem, but most admit to a prior history of similar (often seasonal) symptoms, repeated bouts of "bronchitis," other manifestations of atopy (eczema, allergic rhinitis), or intermittent (especially exertional) wheezing or dyspnea. When a careful history is obtained, only rarely is cough the solitary manifestation of asthma.[2] Pulmonary function testing may reveal "reactive airways disease," and especially when extrinsic (allergic) asthma is suspected, a <u>Wright's stain of sputum for eosinophils</u> will be a helpful clue.

B. Aspiration.

Foreign body aspiration should be suspected in the very young or the very old, but especially in patients with known disorders that predispose to aspiration. Neuromuscular diseases (e.g., myasthenia gravis, bulbar palsies, polymyositis), esophageal disorders (esophageal stricture, Zenker's diverticulum, motility disorders), alcoholism or sedative use, seizure disorders, or a recent history of stupor or loss of consciousness (drug addicts) must always raise suspicion of aspiration, since the history of actual aspiration is often elusive.[3]

C. Other upper respiratory disorders.

As noted in Table 12–1, some ear, nose, and throat disorders may cause cough, even when the tracheobronchial tree is normal. Careful examination of ears, throat, nose, and neck is always crucial here.

D. Bronchial irritants.

A wide variety of industrial and environmental substances are known to cause bronchitis and asthma, both in normal patients and in those with underlying airway disease. *Bacillus subtilis*[4] enzymes in detergent manufacture and toluene diisocyanate[5, 6] in polyurethane are examples of dust- and chemical-induced asthma, respectively. Fumes, tobacco smoke, woodstove emissions, and many other substances may cause acute cough. A brief environmental and occupational history is worthwhile when cough is puzzling.

E. Congestive heart failure, pulmonary embolism, and angina pectoris may present as acute cough.

Very sudden onset of acute cough should also suggest (early) anaphylaxis, pneumothorax, pneumomediastinum, aortic dissection, or esophageal rupture, but there are usually other clues to each of these diagnoses (see Chapter 13, Chest Pain).

III. Is the patient with acute infectious cough a normal or abnormal host?

In the otherwise healthy patient with acute infectious cough, the history and physical examination are usually reliable in distinguishing acute bronchitis from pneumonia, and thus subsequent strategies can usually be formulated purely on the basis of these clinical findings (see below).

In the abnormal host, however, such clinical findings are much less reliable. The chronically ill patient who is uremic, alcoholic, or malnourished or who suffers from chronic cardiopulmonary disease will often present with atypical clinical symptoms or signs. The immunosuppressed patient not only may present atypically but will also be susceptible to a variety of serious diseases rarely encountered in the healthy patient (see page 652).

Bronchitis versus Pneumonia

When the patient is otherwise healthy, however, consider:

IV. In the patient with "infectious cough," do symptoms suggest bronchitis or pneumonia?

Several symptoms are common in both bronchitis and pneumonia:

Fever almost always accompanies pneumonia in the normal host, and its absence is strong evidence against pneumonia (assuming antipyretic medications have not obscured the picture). Many patients with bronchitis as part of a "viral syndrome" will also have fever, however. Thus the presence of fever is nonspecific, but its absence is a helpful finding.

Chills are nonspecific. Many patients with viral bronchitis will describe "chills," i.e., intermittent "hot and cold feelings." Only rarely will such patients experience true rigors (teeth chattering, visible shaking). Sudden onset of a single rigor is typical of pneumococcal pneumonia but may also be seen with other types of pneumonia. Thus, true rigors should suggest pneumonia. The absence of chills or rigors is nonspecific.

Chest pain may occur in bronchitis or pneumonia, but certain characteristics of the chest pain are often helpful in diagnosis. Many patients with bronchitis will complain of vague substernal and bilateral chest discomfort, usually described as "tight" or "congested," often worsened with coughing. Classic pleuritic chest pain, i.e., sharp, knifelike unilateral respirophasic pain, always must suggest pneumonia (with or without pleuritis or empyema—see also Chapter 13, "Chest Pain").

Dyspnea is uncommon in acute bronchitis unless there is superimposed bronchospasm (see below), underlying cardiopulmonary disease, or excessive anxiety. True shortness of breath in the patient with acute infectious cough is much more common in pneumonia. The patient with pleuritic chest pain often cannot distinguish between dyspnea (air hunger) and painful breathing, but either symptom should suggest pneumonia.

Sputum is much misunderstood. Thick, discolored sputum is often erroneously believed to be synonymous with purulent (bacterial) infection. In fact, the thickness, i.e., viscosity, of the sputum is determined by its content of relative amounts of mucus, fibrin, and water—all thick sputum is not pus. The presence of sputum, then, is nonspecific. Both bronchitis and pneumonia may cause sputum production.

Similarly, (yellow or green) discoloration of sputum may result from prolonged bronchial stasis of secretions and does not necessarily imply purulence (inflammatory cells). The purulence of sputum is determined with a microscope, not the naked eye. The sputum Gram's stain is most important (see below). When blood is present in sputum (hemoptysis), other considerations arise (see page 642).

In Brenda's case the history suggests acute infectious bronchitis in a normal host.

Physical examination reveals a healthy-looking female who coughs frequently during the examination. Oral temperature is 37.5° C, pulse is 70, respiratory rate 16. Examination of the eyes, ears, nose, and throat is normal, except for mild nasal congestion and slight hoarseness. The lungs are clear to auscultation, except for occasional scattered early inspiratory rhonchi that diminish after coughing. Cardiac examination is normal. Brenda is unable to produce any sputum.

Examination does not, then, suggest pneumonia.

Why?

1. The patient is not very "sick." Most patients with (especially bacterial) pneumonia are clearly quite ill. These patients are usually febrile, tachycardic, tachypneic, diaphoretic, i.e., their condition is "toxic." When present, pleuritic chest pain just makes matters worse. While many patients with nonbacterial pneumonia are not so toxic (see below), the general appearance and vital signs of the patient are often the best physical clue to the presence of pneumonia. High fever, tachycardia, and increased respiratory rate (greater than 16 to 20 breaths per minute) are most unusual in uncomplicated bronchitis. Conversely, an occasional patient with nonbacterial pneumonia may have normal vital signs (see page 644).

2. Lung auscultation does not demonstrate consolidation. The classic physical findings in the patient with bacterial pneumonia include localized (lobar) tubular breathing, dullness to percussion, egophony, increased tactile and vocal fremitus, and inspiratory crackles (or rales). The presence of such findings is virtually diagnostic of bacterial pneumonia in the patient with appropriate symptoms—subsequent efforts are then devoted to identifying the specific pathogen (see below).

Auscultatory consolidation, however, is today somewhat uncommon among patients with pneumonia—it is rare in patients with nonbacterial pneumonia and may be a late finding (only appearing after several days of illness) in patients with bacterial pneumonia. More often, only slight dullness to percussion, localized crackles (see below), and diminished breath sounds or equivocal tubular breathing will be found in the patient with early pneumonia. The localization of abnormal auscultatory findings to one lobe of the lung is a very helpful diagnostic clue—most bacterial and nonbacterial pneumonias are localized to one lobe. The "auscultatory anatomy" of the lungs must be remembered here (Fig. 12–2). Notice that abnormalities of both upper lobes will be missed if the axillae are not examined, as will findings in the right middle lobe, left lower lobe, and lingula if the lateral and lower anterior chest are ignored. (Especially the right middle lobe, a common locale for pneumonia, is often ignored when auscultation does not proceed in a sequential lobar orientation.)

3. Adventitious lung sounds usually, but not always, should suggest pneumonia. Most patients with bronchitis have a normal lung examination. Some will demonstrate rhonchi—coarse snoring or rattling sounds that usually are prominent early in inspiration and tend to diminish or disappear after a vigorous cough. Rhonchi are caused by secretions in the large airways—especially when such sounds are heard in scattered locations or over the upper anterior chest in the midline (over the trachea), parenchymal lung disease (pneumonia) need not be assumed.

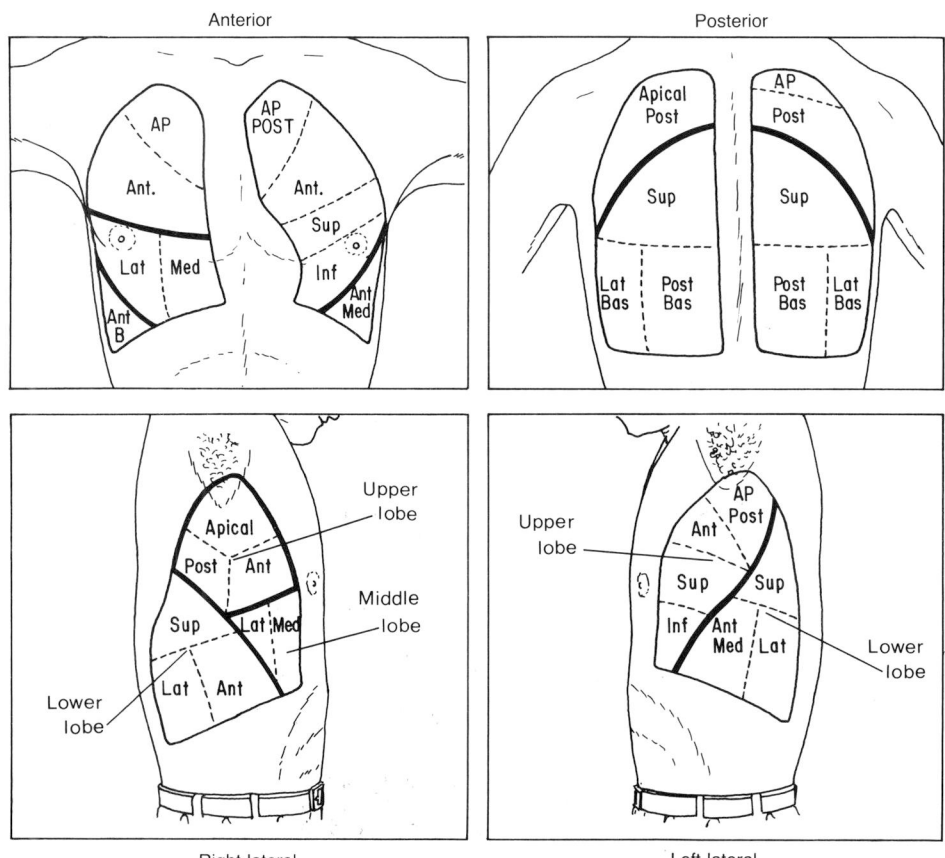

FIGURE 12–2. The topography of the five lung lobes and their major segments as viewed from anterior, posterior, right lateral, and left lateral orientations. The solid lines demarcate lobes; the dotted lines, separate segments. Note that the upper lobes are primarily anterior, the lower lobes are primarily posterior, and the right middle lobe is located in the lower lateral and anterior right chest.

Some patients with bronchitis will demonstrate crackles (rales), which are finer, higher-pitched sounds produced by sudden opening of small bronchioles and alveoli. Crackles in bronchitis tend to occur early in inspiration, to clear with coughing, and to be heard in more than one lobar location simultaneously. On the other hand, crackles in pneumonia tend to occur late in inspiration, to not clear with coughing, and to be focal (lobar). In some patients with pneumonia, crackles will not be heard at all if the infected segment of lung is poorly ventilated. In such patients, several deep breaths or a quick cough at the end of expiration will often reveal transitory crackles during the next inspiration.

Precise description and recording of abnormal lung sounds are often ignored today, since chest x-rays are so routinely performed. Our approach here, however, will attempt to minimize the use of unnecessary chest x-rays (see below). The distinction between *early inspiratory* crackles (bronchial) and *late inspiratory* crackles (lung parenchyma)[7, 8] has not been studied in the clinical evaluation of *acute* cough. Nevertheless, "fine tuning" our lung examination[9] can be helpful in the practical management of patients. The characteristics listed in Figure 12–3 are by no means highly discriminating per se, but when considered in the context of other symptoms and signs—see below—can be useful.

> In Brenda's case, physical examination supports the diagnosis of infectious bronchitis. There is no specific reason to suspect pneumonia.

Figure 12–4 illustrates the general clinical approach to acute cough.

NOTE

1. The history and the physical examination are of *equal* importance in deciding who needs a chest x-ray. Wood, et al.,[10] studied 947 consecutive

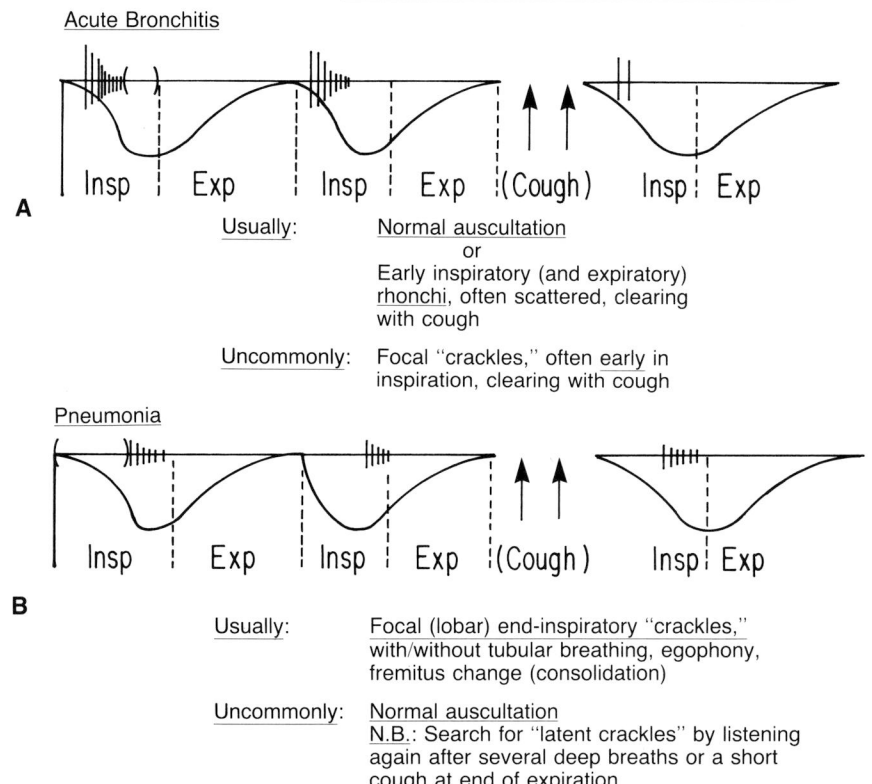

FIGURE 12–3. Auscultatory findings in *(A)* bronchitis and *(B)* pneumonia.

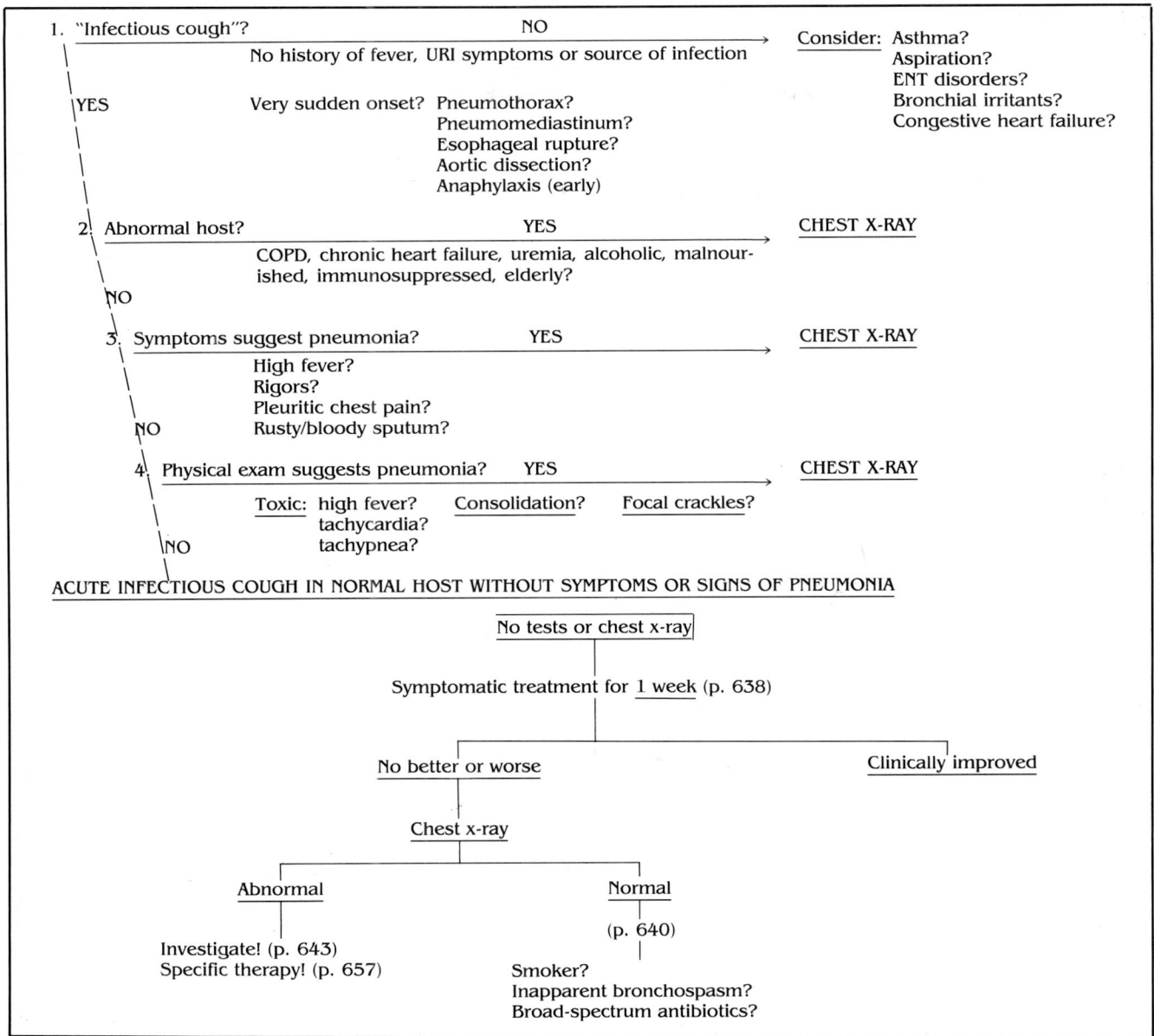

FIGURE 12—4. The general approach to acute cough.

adults with acute infectious cough, of whom 57 (6 per cent) had pneumonia; 52 of these 57 patients had an oral temperature greater than 38.3°C, an abnormal chest examination, or a history of shaking chills (rigors), or some combination of these. Among the other (5) patients with pneumonia who had none of these "pneumonia clues," 4 were elderly, and 1 had classic pleuritic chest pain (Fig. 12–5).

The importance of the history and the overall "look" of the patient are emphasized by studies that reveal the relative insensitivity of chest auscultation in the diagnosis of pneumonia in some patients. In one such study, 200 young men with radiographic pneumonia, sick enough to be hospitalized, underwent careful clinical chest examination.[11] (Microbial causes were not specified—the patients' ages and clinical findings suggest nonbacterial pneumonia was common.) Fifty (25 per cent) had completely normal lungs on examination. In only one half of all patients were crackles heard in any portion of the lungs, and in even fewer (83 of 200) were any abnormal lung

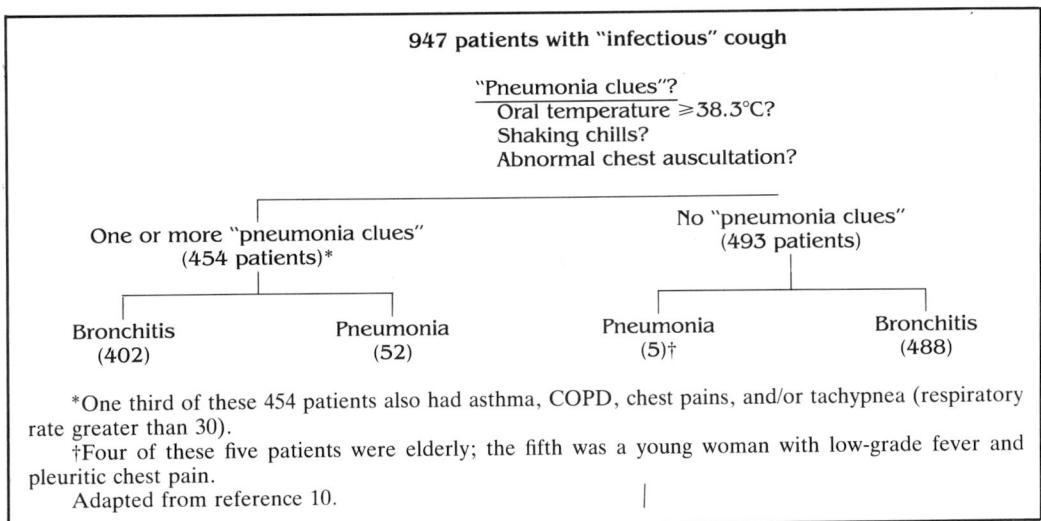

947 patients with "infectious" cough

"Pneumonia clues"?
Oral temperature ⩾38.3°C?
Shaking chills?
Abnormal chest auscultation?

One or more "pneumonia clues"
(454 patients)*

No "pneumonia clues"
(493 patients)

Bronchitis
(402)

Pneumonia
(52)

Pneumonia
(5)†

Bronchitis
(488)

*One third of these 454 patients also had asthma, COPD, chest pains, and/or tachypnea (respiratory rate greater than 30).
†Four of these five patients were elderly; the fifth was a young woman with low-grade fever and pleuritic chest pain.
Adapted from reference 10.

FIGURE 12–5.

sounds described in the area of radiographic pneumonia. The authors of this study "do not suggest that the stethoscope should be hung in the closet,"[11] but, even in the normal host, physical examination of the lungs may be unimpressive in the presence of pneumonia. This is especially true of nonbacterial pneumonia. Almost all patients with bacterial pneumonia will have abnormal auscultatory findings, but very early in their clinical course (the first 24 to 48 hours), or when all of the bronchial anatomy is not carefully examined (Fig. 12–2), the chest may be "clear."

Hence, the history and physical examination are *complementary*: The coughing patient with high fever, rigors, and/or pleuritic chest pain needs a chest x-ray, whatever the auscultatory findings on examination. On the other hand,

2. Many patients with acute cough do not need chest x-rays. In the study by Wood and associates,[10] 488 patients (51 per cent of the group) had no clinical features that suggested pneumonia (Fig. 12–5). Chest x-rays are not necessary in such patients. The economic implications here are significant.*

Whether it is possible to be even more selective among patients with cough in determining the need for x-rays requires further study. Certainly, there is room for improvement: Of the 454 patients in the study of Wood and co-workers who did have high fever, rigors, or abnormal chest examinations, only 52 had pneumonia. Thus, even among such selected patients, only 1 in 9 will have radiographic pneumonia.

Interest in improved test selection is all the more important if one believes that:

3. Antibiotics are not indicated in otherwise healthy patients with acute bronchitis. Some physicians treat all infectious cough with broad-spectrum antibiotics (e.g., tetracycline, erythromycin). There are several reasons to object to this strategy:

First, as we have seen, very few such patients have pneumonia.[10]

Second, while there are surprisingly few data available on this subject, the small number of pertinent studies suggest that antibiotics do not help the patient with acute bronchitis.[12, 13]

---

*If more than half of the many millions of Americans with respiratory infections can be spared the cost of a chest x-ray ($30 to $50), the annual impact on the "health dollar" is impressive.

Finally, casual "shotgun therapy" may condone a less rigorous diagnostic approach to the patient with acute cough—sometimes this is a serious mistake (see Table 12–1).

Acute bronchitis is usually a viral infection[14–16] in which cough is often but one of several symptoms—fever, rhinitis, hoarseness, headache, and myalgias often coexist. Specific manifestations and clinical courses will vary with the specific infectious agent, but so much overlap occurs among these different syndromes that differential diagnosis is impossible without serologic studies or viral cultures (which are currently only of academic or epidemiologic interest). Table 12–2 illustrates clinical features of some of the common causes of acute bronchitis.

Mycoplasma infections may be a frequent cause of acute bronchitis (without pneumonia) in some populations[19, 20]—primarily the young—but there is little evidence that documents efficacy of antibiotic therapy in mycoplasmal bronchitis (unlike mycoplasma pneumonia, which can be ameliorated with antibiotics—see page 661). Nevertheless, the possibility of mycoplasma infection in the patient with acute bronchitis is a common (unproven) rationale for antibiotic therapy in the minds of many clinicians.* It is likely that bacterial infection rarely, if ever, causes acute bronchitis in normal adults.

4. Once the diagnosis of acute bronchitis is established (with or without chest x-rays), no further diagnostic testing is useful.

Sputum Gram's stains and sputum cultures are sometimes obtained in this setting as a guide to antibiotic therapy. Such studies are spurious. As noted above, a Wright's stain of sputum may be helpful when allergic cough is suspected—eosinophilia in sputum will support that suspicion. Otherwise, attempts at bacteriologic diagnosis of acute bronchitis are useful only in research studies and (perhaps) in the patient with chronic lung disease. (The patient with severe obstructive lung disease who develops an infectious flare without radiographic pneumonia may benefit from antibiotic therapy.[24])

---

*Whether prevalence of treatable chlamydial respiratory infections[21–23] will buttress the rationale for broad-spectrum antibiotic therapy of bronchitis remains to be seen—in normal adults, probably not.

TABLE 12–2. CLINICAL FEATURES OF ACUTE INFECTIOUS BRONCHITIS[17]

Causative Organism	Setting	Typical Syndrome
Rhinovirus	Universal	Common cold, rhinitis, malaise
Parainfluenza	Universal	Hoarseness prominent
Influenza virus, A and B	Epidemic, pandemic	Abrupt-onset headache, fever, myalgias
Adenovirus	Young, military population	Fever, prominent pharyngitis, rhinitis
Coxsackievirus	Young, military population	Fever, prominent headache, rhinitis
Respiratory syncytial virus	Children, elderly/COPD[18]	Myalgias, headache
Mycoplasma	Young adults	Insidious-onset headache, cough, malaise

Brenda is told that she most likely has acute viral bronchitis and that antibiotics will not help her, but that her illness will run its own self-limited course. Brenda is told that symptomatic therapy may help relieve her discomfort, and she is treated with a cough suppressant (elixir of terpin hydrate with codeine) and told to call if she has not improved in 1 week. The symptoms of bacterial pneumonia are briefly explained (fever, rigors, pleurisy), and she is warned that very occasionally this may follow viral bronchitis and that she must be seen again and have a chest x-ray should this occur. Brenda is told that stopping smoking will help her to improve more quickly.

Treatment of Acute Bronchitis

Most patients with acute bronchitis improve gradually without any treatment and are well within 1 to 3 weeks. Many types of symptomatic therapy may be helpful. None is essential. Antibiotics are not recommended here, except in unusual circumstances (the patient with severe chronic obstructive lung disease and perhaps the patient who does not improve—page 641).

Cough suppression may be theoretically undesirable since cough is a valuable defense mechanism that clears bronchial debris, thus preventing mucus plugging, atelectasis, and (perhaps) parenchymal lung infection. However, cough itself may be disabling, especially when frequent and prolonged or when associated with other medical problems that it may exacerbate. The patient with symptomatic intervertebral disc disease, headache, urinary stress incontinence, hemorrhoids, or a hernia will be grateful for effective cough suppression, as will the patient with other common or uncommon complications of cough (Table 12–3).

Most effective cough suppressants act by raising the cough threshold of the central nervous system rather than by any peripheral bronchial mechanism.[25] Many antitussive drugs are marketed in combination with other drugs (usually antihistamines, decongestants, alcohol, or expectorants) whose pharmacologic actions are separate. While these substances are often helpful in relieving coexisting symptoms—rhinorrhea, congestion, sore throat[26]—antitussive potency depends simply on the dose of codeine, hydrocodone, or dextromethorphan that reaches the cough center in the brain stem.

Codeine and hydrocodone are the most effective cough suppressants. Most preparations containing codeine are marketed as liquids containing 10

TABLE 12–3. COMPLICATIONS OF COUGH

COMMON	UNCOMMON BUT SERIOUS	EXACERBATION OF PRIOR PROBLEM
Chest-wall pain	Rib fracture	Herniated disc
Fatigue	Ruptured rectus abdominis	Ventral hernia
Insomnia	Pneumothorax	Inguinal hernia
Mild hemoptysis	Pneumomediastinum	Urinary incontinence
Nosebleed	Syncope	Hemorrhoidal bleeding
Conjunctival hemorrhage	Bradyarrhythmias	Headache

TABLE 12–4. COUGH SUPPRESSANTS CONTAINING CODEINE OR HYDROCODONE

BRAND OR GENERIC NAME	ANTITUSSIVE CODEINE	ANTITUSSIVE HYDROCODONE	ALSO CONTAINS:*	ALCOHOL %	DOSE	COST/ AMOUNT
Codeine	15, 30, or 60 mg/tablet				15–30 mg q4h	$4.00/15 (30 mg tablets)
Hydrocodone		5, 10 mg/tablet			5–10 mg q4h	$3.00/15 (10 mg tablets)
Terpin hydrate with codeine	10 mg/tsp		E	40	1–2 tsp q4h	$3.00/4 oz
Hycodan		5 mg/tablet, tsp	Ac		1–2 tab q4h; 1–2 tsp q4h	$8.00/30; $7.00/4 oz
Robitussin A-C	10 mg/tsp		E	3.5	1–2 tsp q4h	$5.50/4 oz
Hycomine		5 mg/tsp	D		1–2 tsp q4h	$7.50/4 oz
Robitussin-DAC	10 mg/tsp		D, E	1.4	1–2 tsp q4h	$5.50/4 oz
Tussionex		5 mg/tablet, tsp	Ah		1–2 tab q8–12h; 1–2 tsp q8–12h	$8.00/15; $4.50/2 oz
Novahistine DH	10 mg/tsp		D, Ah	5	1–2 tsp q4h	$6.00/4 oz
Tussend		5 mg/tablet, tsp	D	5 (liquid)	1–2 tab q4h; 1–2 tsp q4h	$9.50/30; $4.50/4 oz
Triaminic expectorant with codeine	10 mg/tsp		D, Ah, E	5	1–2 tsp q4h	$6.50/4 oz
Actifed-C expectorant	10 mg/tsp		D, Ah, E		1–2 tsp q4h	$5.00/4 oz
Dimetane expectorant-DC	10 mg/tsp		D, Ah, E	3.5	1–2 tsp q4h	$5.00/4 oz
Omni-Tuss	10 mg/tsp		Ah, E		1–2 tsp q8–12h	$4.50/2 oz
Phenergan expectorant with codeine	10 mg/tsp		Ah, E	7	1–2 tsp q4h	$5.00/4 oz
Nucofed	20 mg/cap		D		1 cap q4–6h	$6.00/30
	20 mg/tsp		D		1–2 tsp q4h	$7.00/4 oz

*Other pharmacologic agents beside antitussive and alcohol: D, decongestant; Ah, antihistamine; Ac, anticholinergic; E, expectorant.

mg of codeine per 5 cc, often in combination with other drugs. Codeine tablets (15, 30, or 60 mg) are just as effective, but the higher dose is more likely to cause constipation or drowsiness. Hydrocodone is a narcotic, like codeine. Most hydrocodone preparations contain 5 mg per 5 cc, in various combinations with other preparations. Dextromethorphan (the d-isomer of the codeine analog of levorphanol) is commonly marketed in over-the-counter preparations. Dextromethorphan is not a narcotic (like codeine and hydrocodone), and it is much less potent as a cough suppressant.

In general, cough suppressants should be used at night, to allow restful sleep. During the day, mild cough should be encouraged as a defense mechanism except when the cough is itself disabling (Table 12–3). The abuse potential of narcotic cough suppressants must be remembered in the patient who demands frequent refills or excessive amounts of these drugs, and the alcohol content of various preparations is worthy of note as well.

Table 12–4 lists some of the commonly prescribed cough suppressants that contain either codeine or hydrocodone.

Expectorants[27] are designed to liquefy those components of sputum that contribute to its viscosity: mucus, pus, and fibrin. The ideal expectorant or mucolytic agent would liquefy all of these substances and induce minimal side effects. No presently formulated preparation meets these needs. Acetylcysteine (Mucomyst) and iodides are used by some physicians, but their efficacy is unproven, and side effects may be a problem (gastrointestinal symptoms or parotitis with iodides, for example). Humidification is an age-old, simple, nontoxic therapy that often helps "loosen" secretions. Oral fluids, a vaporizer in the bedroom at night, a steam tent, or simply standing in a hot, steaming shower or inhaling the steam vapor from a sink or a pot of boiling water will help many.

Many expectorants are combined with cough suppressants (Table 12–4). (The combination of cough suppressants and expectorants in a single preparation *is* confusing.) There is no firm evidence that these expectorants are helpful, but they probably do not counteract the antitussive properties of codeine or hydrocodone.

Bronchodilators (see below) may be very useful as expectorants in some patients. Table 12–5 lists some of the commonly used bronchodilators.

> One week later, Brenda calls to say she is worse. Her fever and rhinitis have subsided, but she is coughing more frequently and has difficulty sleeping because of the annoying cough. Brenda has also noticed a few "flecks of blood" in her (infrequent) sputum, which worries her greatly. There is no dyspnea, pleuritic chest pain, chills, or other new symptoms.
>
> On repeat examination, Brenda is afebrile, looks fatigued, and coughs spasmodically. No hemoptysis or sputum is observed. Examination of the chest is unremarkable, except for a few coarse rhonchi at the base of each lung. Auscultation while Brenda performs repeated forced expiratory maneuvers induces more coughing and elicits mild diffuse expiratory wheezing.
>
> Chest x-ray is normal.

When the Patient Does Not Improve. When the patient with acute bronchitis does not improve as expected, several things should be considered:

1. Is the patient a smoker? Recent evidence documents that cigarette smokers (without chronic lung disease) are not only more likely to develop acute infectious bronchitis but will often experience symptoms for a longer duration than nonsmokers.[28, 29] In one small study, symptoms lasted twice as long in smokers.[30] This "extended natural history" of acute bronchitis should be remembered when persistent symptoms raise the question of further diagnostic evaluation in patients with cough (see below, "Chronic Cough").

TABLE 12–5. BRONCHODILATORS

GENERIC NAME	TRADE NAME	DOSE	INSTRUCTIONS	COST/AMOUNT
Metered-dose inhalers				
Metaproterenol sulfate	Alupent	0.65 mg/inhalation	2 inhalations q4h	$8.00/15 cc
	Metaprel	0.65 mg/inhalation	2 inhalations q4h	$8.00/15 cc
Albuterol	Proventil	90 μg/inhalation	2 inhalations q4h	$10.00/17 gm
	Ventolin	90 μg/inhalation	2 inhalations q4h	$10.00/17 gm
Isoetharine	Bronkometer	340 μg/inhalation	1–2 inhalations q4h	$10.00/20 cc
Isoproterenol	Isuprel	131 μg/inhalation	1–2 inhalations q4h	$8.00/15 cc
Oral preparations				
Theophylline, regular	Bronkodyl	100, 200 mg capsules	100–200 mg q6h*	$6.00/30 (100 mg)
	Elixophyllin	100, 200 mg capsules		$6.00/30
	Slo-Phyllin	100, 200 mg tablets		$4.00/30
	Theolair	125, 250 mg tablets	125–250 mg q6h*	$6.00/30 (125 mg)
	Theoclear	100, 200 mg tablets	100–200 mg q6h*	$4.00/30 (100 mg)
Theophylline, sustained release†	Theo-Dur	100, 200, 300 mg tablets	q12h*	$4.00/20 (200 mg)
	Elixophyllin SR	125, 250 mg capsules	q12h*	$4.00/20 (125 mg)
	Slo-Phyllin	60, 125, 250 mg capsules	q12h*	$5.00/20 (125 mg)
	Theolair	250, 500 mg tablets	q12h*	$6.00/20 (200 mg)
Metaproterenol	Alupent	10, 20 mg	10–20 mg qid	$7.00/30
	Metaprel	10, 20 mg	10–20 mg qid	$7.00/30
Terbutaline	Brethine	2.5, 5 mg	2.5–5 mg tid	$7.00/30
	Bricanyl	2.5, 5 mg	2.5–5 mg tid	$6.00/30
Albuterol	Proventil	2, 4 mg	2–4 mg qid	$8.50/30
	Ventolin	2, 4 mg	2–4 mg qid	$8.50/30

*Recommended average dose of theophylline, 16 mg/kg body weight/24 h. This applies primarily to patients with asthma who require maintenance dose of bronchodilators. Most patients with acute bronchitis complicated by mild bronchospasm require lower doses, and these guidelines need not be so strictly observed.

†These are but a few of very many sustained-release preparations currently marketed. Costs are very similar for most.

This observation might also be used to bolster the patient's resolve to stop smoking.

Perhaps the smoker's persistent cough is related to subclinical airways disease,[29] and this may have relevance to the more general problem (in smokers and nonsmokers) of "postbronchitic bronchospasm."

2. Postbronchitic bronchospasm is common. A small but definite minority of patients with apparently uncomplicated acute infectious bronchitis will develop persistent (longer than 3 to 4 weeks) cough with or without clinical evidence of bronchospasm (audible wheezing, dyspnea, abnormal pulmonary function tests), even in the absence of any prior history of smoking, atopy, or other lung disease. The etiology of this problem is unclear, but postinfectious bronchospasm may be one contributing factor.[30, 31] Reversible self-limited bronchospasm may be demonstrated by pulmonary function testing during otherwise uncomplicated infectious bronchitis.[31] Asking the patient to perform forced expiratory maneuvers ("Deep breath in, then deep breath out, hard, until all the air is gone from your lungs") during auscultation will reveal audible wheezing in some such patients.

A brief course of oral bronchodilators[32] is often helpful in these patients. Aerosolized bronchodilators are especially effective, since inhalation of the drug will often induce coughing and allow mobilization of secretions. A second inhalation then allows better deposition of the drug into the more peripheral airways. Hence, prescription orders are written: two inhalations 1 to 2 minutes apart, four times per day. The aerosolized drugs are only slightly more expensive than oral theophylline preparations. Table 12–5 illustrates the most useful bronchodilators. (Notice that "combination drugs" and epinephrine preparations are not included here. These may be useful in some patients, but the current generation of bronchodilator drugs makes most of these obsolete.) Unless the patient has chronic asthma or chronic obstructive pulmonary disease (COPD), 1- to 2-week courses of therapy are usually sufficient for the patient with acute bronchitis who fails to improve.

3. Is the diagnosis correct? Pneumonia, tuberculosis, and lung cancer are among the literally hundreds of respiratory diseases that may present with poorly resolving acute cough. Especially when the selective approach to testing and x-rays is advocated (see above) and the chest x-ray is initially omitted, all patients who do not improve do require posteroanterior and lateral chest x-rays. The need for additional studies (pulmonary function tests, bronchoscopy) depends on the x-ray results as well as the subsequent clinical course.

4. Should antibiotics be prescribed? Patients who do not improve with symptomatic therapy, especially those who continue to produce purulent sputum (in the absence of pneumonia or any other explanation) are often treated with broad-spectrum antibiotics. Considering the relative benignity and low cost of such drugs (tetracycline, erythromycin, ampicillin) and our limited understanding of the etiology of this problem, it is difficult to argue with this approach. (There are no prospective clinical studies that address this issue, and it is not at all a rare problem.) Nevertheless, virtually all patients with acute bronchitis do eventually improve with or without antibiotics. The few who do not improve (after 4 to 6 weeks) have chronic cough—this requires investigation (page 667).

Brenda is told that she has "only" bronchitis and that her chest x-ray is normal, but that she is not improving as quickly as she might because of

her continued smoking. She is told to stop smoking and to continue using the codeine at night, but to add tetracycline 500 mg qid × 7 days and a metaproterenol inhaler, two inhalations 1 to 2 minutes apart, four times a day.

Brenda is told that the normal chest x-ray implies that she need not worry about the hemoptysis since repetitive coughing can sometimes "break small blood vessels" in the bronchial tubes. She is instructed that, if cough or hemoptysis persists, further investigation will be needed.

Hemoptysis

Coughing up blood is a frightening symptom that deserves special emphasis. The differential diagnosis is lengthy and includes disorders of the entire respiratory system (including the nose and throat) as well as various systemic disorders.[33, 34] Table 12–6 lists various common and uncommon causes of hemoptysis.

Massive hemoptysis obviously requires emergency attention[34]—usually rigid bronchoscopy followed by thoracotomy. Most hemoptysis is mild and subacute; however, all patients with even minimal hemoptysis must undergo:

1. Chest x-ray. Some of the common causes of hemoptysis may be associated with a normal chest x-ray (Table 12–6). Often, however, the x-ray will reveal a likely source (pneumonia, cancer, tuberculosis).

When the x-ray is normal, several considerations are especially important:

2. The history must include consideration of the patient's age and smoking history. All patients over the age of 40 years with *unexplained* hemoptysis (however brief) should be considered for bronchoscopy to exclude endobronchial carcinoma,[35] even if the chest x-ray is normal.

The younger nonsmoker with hemoptysis should be questioned about associated symptoms—nasal or oropharyngeal bleeding, hematuria (systemic lupus erythematosus, Goodpasture's syndrome, Wegener's granulomatosis), bleeding diathesis, symptoms of bronchiectasis, for example. Often specific clinical settings will suggest the correct diagnosis immediately (pulmonary

TABLE 12–6. CAUSES OF HEMOPTYSIS

COMMON

Acute bronchitis*	Lung cancer
Chronic bronchitis*	Pulmonary embolism*
Pneumonia	Congestive heart failure
Trauma/contusion	Congenital heart disease
Gum bleeding* (gingivitis)	Bronchiectasis
Nosebleeds*	Tuberculosis

UNCOMMON

Bleeding diathesis*	Broncholithiasis
Bronchial adenoma*	Bronchopleural fistula
Arteriovenous aneurysm*	Granulomatous lung disease
Bronchial endometriosis*	Cystic fibrosis
Pneumoconiosis	Foreign body*
Polyarteritis nodosa	Lung abscess
Goodpasture's syndrome	Pulmonary hemosiderosis
Pulmonary hypertension*	Mycetoma
Systemic lupus erythematosus	Transtracheal aspiration
Wegener's granulomatosis	Lung biopsy

*Causes of hemoptysis often associated with "normal" chest x-rays.

embolism, mitral stenosis, known pulmonary hypertension, recent transtracheal aspiration or lung biopsy, or the like).

3. Complete physical examination is crucial. Chest and heart examination must not preclude ear, nose, and throat examination or evaluation for lymphadenopathy, polyarthritis, evidence of other bleeding disorders, and other systemic clues. A complete blood count, coagulation studies, urinalysis, and various other studies may then be indicated, depending upon the specific setting (Table 12–6).

One group has suggested that when hemoptysis is brief (less than 1 week in duration) in a patient under the age of 40 years (even if a smoker) with a normal chest x-ray, further, i.e., invasive, testing (bronchoscopy) is highly unlikely to yield significant results.[36] Foregoing bronchoscopy in this setting makes sense when there is a reason for hemoptysis (for example, acute bronchitis with prolonged and vigorous coughing, as in Brenda's case) but, even here, a repeat chest x-ray should be obtained a few months later to exclude initially inapparent but serious disease. Unfortunately, young patients do develop lung cancer.[37]

Thus, not all patients with (any) hemoptysis require bronchoscopy.[36, 38] In the low-risk patient (the young nonsmoker, for example) who has mild, brief hemoptysis in the setting of prolonged and vigorous coughing and a normal chest x-ray, careful follow-up rather than immediate exhaustive testing is recommended. The need for further studies should be individualized in the patient with hemoptysis.

Sometimes a cause for hemoptysis cannot be found in spite of extensive investigation. In such a situation (idiopathic hemoptysis) the long-term prognosis is good;[39] the hemoptysis is probably most often the result of acute or chronic bronchitis.[33]

> Brenda now reveals that she has "dragged in" her father, Norman P. Neumonia, who continues to cough and feel bad.
>
> Norman is a 69-year-old man with longstanding chronic bronchitis and emphysema. He describes 3 weeks of increasingly severe cough, productive of thick yellow sputum. He has experienced such symptoms many times in the past, but, for the past 3 days, he has felt "feverish" and has noted a new pain in the right lower "rib cage" that hurts with coughing and respiration. There is no history of shaking chills or hemoptysis.
>
> On examination, Norman appears chronically ill, is mildly cyanotic, and has a temperature of 38.8° C orally. His respiratory rate is 28 per minute, pulse is 90 and regular, blood pressure 140/80. The chest is greatly expanded, and accessory muscles of respiration are prominent in the neck. Breath sounds are diminished throughout the lung fields, but there are diffuse expiratory rhonchi, as well as a few inspiratory crackles localized over the right posterior and lateral chest areas.
>
> Chest x-ray reveals "partial" consolidation of the right lower lobe and blunting of the right costophrenic angle on the lateral film, with a question of a pleural effusion in that location. The white blood count is 10,200 with a left shift.

Diagnosis of Pneumonia

Table 12–7 gives clinical clues in the differential diagnosis of community-acquired pneumonia in adults and adolescents. No one clinical finding at the time of *initial* evaluation of such patients will be reliably diagnostic of a specific form of pneumonia. Among patients with various types of bacterial and nonbacterial pneumonia, there is considerable overlap in clinical findings, chest x-ray patterns, peripheral white blood count, and sputum examinations.[44] *Proof* of diagnosis depends on isolation of the pathogenic organism from blood, pleural fluid, or lung tissue in bacterial pneumonia and definitive serial serologic evidence in nonbacterial pneumonias. Such proof is rarely available when the patient is initially seen (and is frequently never available, even if all reasonable diagnostic efforts are attempted).

Often, then, the diagnosis of a specific type of pneumonia is presumptive and is based on an analysis of several pieces of information:

I. The history and physical examination usually will suggest whether the pneumonia is bacterial or nonbacterial.

As we have seen, bacterial pneumonia often presents with sudden onset of fever and shaking chills (often in the setting of an antecedent upper respiratory infection), pleuritic chest pain, tachypnea, copious purulent or "rusty" sputum, and (sometimes) consolidation on auscul-

TABLE 12–7. DIFFERENTIAL DIAGNOSIS OF COMMUNITY-ACQUIRED PNEUMONIA IN ADULTS AND ADOLESCENTS

	BACTERIAL[40, 41]	NONBACTERIAL[42, 43]
Age	Any age	Usually young
Symptoms and signs	Antecedent URI Onset sudden Shaking chills Pleuritic chest pain Tachycardia/tachypnea Purulent sputum Consolidation on auscultation	Headache, malaise, URI symptoms Onset more gradual Rigors uncommon Pleuritic pain uncommon Condition less toxic Sputum scant, mucoid, or absent Localized crackles without consolidation
Sputum Gram's stain	Many polymorphonuclears; one predominant organism	Variable number of polymorphonuclear or mononuclear cells; no predominant organism
Chest x-ray	Lobar/segmental consolidation; may be patchy "bronchopneumonia"	Unilateral or bilateral interstitial, patchy infiltrates
White blood count	Usually 15,000–25,000, left shift; occasionally normal	Usually normal (less than 10,000)
Cause		
Common	*Streptococcus pneumoniae*	*Mycoplasma pneumoniae*
Uncommon	*Hemophilus influenzae; Klebsiella; Legionella pneumophila;* aspiration	Influenza A and B; adenovirus; varicella; chlamydial?
Rare	*Staphylococcus aureus;* gram-negative bacilli; *Streptococcus pyogenes; Neisseria meningitidis;* tuberculosis; plague; anthrax; leptospirosis; melioidosis; *Nocardia;* tularemia; *Listeria; Branhamella*	Measles; Q fever; ornithosis; pneumocystosis; histoplasmosis; coccidioidomycosis; blastomycosis; cryptococcosis
Definitive diagnosis	Blood culture; pleural fluid culture; lung tissue culture	Lung biopsy; serologic titers over time

tation of the involved lung(s). Nonbacterial pneumonias are more often gradual in onset, the condition of the patient is usually less toxic, pleuritic pain and rigors are decidedly uncommon, sputum is often scanty or absent, and auscultation of the lungs is commonly unimpressive, especially when compared with the chest x-ray findings.

As Tables 12–7, 12–8, and 12–9 suggest, however, none of these clinical findings is at all specific. Some patients with bacterial pneumonia will present with more indolent symptoms, do not appear to be in a toxic state, and may not produce any sputum. The elderly and the patient with chronic lung disease are often among these atypical patients. A few patients with nonbacterial pneumonia may be very ill, with high fever, chest pain, rigors, and sputum.

In general, however, distinctions in Table 12–7 are helpful in beginning to formulate a likely presumptive diagnosis. The clinical setting is always helpful. Various types of pneumonia are common in some situations and very rare in others. In general, nonbacterial pneumonias are probably most common among young, healthy patients; bacterial pneumonia is far more likely in the elderly patient or the patient with underlying cardiopulmonary disease.*

Mycoplasma pneumoniae is probably the most common cause of all pneumonias in young, healthy adults. Viral pneumonia is rare in the normal adult, except during (influenza) epidemics, in military recruits (where adenovirus pneumonia occurs), or when systemic viral illness is obvious (measles or varicella). In certain geographic areas, primary fungal pneumonias are not rare—histoplasmosis in the Midwest, coccidioidomycosis in the Southwest, for example. Rarely, Q fever or ornithosis (psittacosis) will be suspected when there has been documented exposure to sick livestock or birds respectively. Some male homosexuals are now at risk for *Pneumocystis carinii* and/or cytomegalovirus pneumonia.[116, 117] *Chlamydia trachomatis* infection may be associated with pneumonia in adults, but this requires further study.[21]

Community-acquired bacterial pneumonia in healthy adults is usually pneumococcal.[91–94] Patients with COPD are likely to develop *Hemophilus influenzae* pneumonia as well. Gram-negative bacillary pneumonias are rare, except in immunosuppressed patients, alcoholics, diabetics, the very elderly (especially those living in nursing homes),[94] or patients recently hospitalized or receiving antibiotic therapy.[95, 96] Staphylococcal pneumonia is rarely community acquired, except in debilitated or immunosuppressed hosts or during influenza epidemics. *Legionella* pneumonia usually occurs in the elderly or immunosuppressed patient. Aspiration pneumonia[75–78] should be suspected in the patient who has impaired mental status, esophageal, or neuromuscular diseases—usually these patients are elderly or hospitalized or both. Rarely, *Streptococcus pyogenes*,[97] *Neisseria meningitidis*,[98] or *Branhamella catarrhalis*[141] will cause community-acquired bacterial pneumonia.

The approach to the patient with hospital-acquired pneumonia or the immunocompromised patient with pneumonia is far beyond the scope of this text. There are now, however, many ambulatory patients undergoing chemotherapy for cancer, leukemia, or lymphoma, or re-

---

*It is not possible to be precise about the quantitative frequency of various types of pneumonia in ambulatory patients.[88–91] Most clinical studies of pneumonia deal with chronically ill or hospitalized patients or both.[92, 93] Even in such populations, a specific pathogen is often not *proven*, i.e., by blood, pleural fluid, or lung tissue cultures.[21, 70]

TABLE 12–8. NONBACTERIAL PNEUMONIAS IN ADULTS AND ADOLESCENTS

	Mycoplasma pneumoniae[45–48]	INFLUENZA[40, 49–53]	ADENOVIRUS[49, 54, 55]
When to suspect	Most common in young adults; rare in elderly patients; gradual onset; headaches, myalgias, sore throat; bullous myringitis (rare)	Very rare except during influenza epidemic; usually severely ill	Usually in closed populations (military recruits); young adults/adolescents; clinical findings similar to *Mycoplasma* pneumonia; pharyngitis often prominent
Diagnosis	Young adult with clinical nonbacterial pneumonia Chest x-ray: patchy lower lobe infiltrate(s) (Fig. 12–6A) Serology: Cold agglutinins 1:64 mycoplasma complement fixation Sputum: few polys; no bacteria	Clinical influenza and relentless cough, tachypnea Chest x-ray: diffuse interstitial infiltrates (Fig. 12–6C) Serology: complement fixation Sputum: rarely present	Often epidemic Chest x-ray: patchy (usually unilateral) infiltrate(s) Serology: complement fixation Sputum: rarely present
Treatment	Tetracycline 500 mg qid × 10–14 days or erythromycin 250 mg qid × 10–14 days	None	None
Complications	Many, but all uncommon:[46] hemolytic anemia; anorexia; arthritis; cardiac involvement; aseptic meningitis; Guillain-Barré syndrome	Bacterial (especially staphylococcal) pneumonia; respiratory failure common	Rare
Usual course	Gradual resolution over 1–3 wk	Variable, but morbidity high	Usually mild and self-limited over 1–3 wk

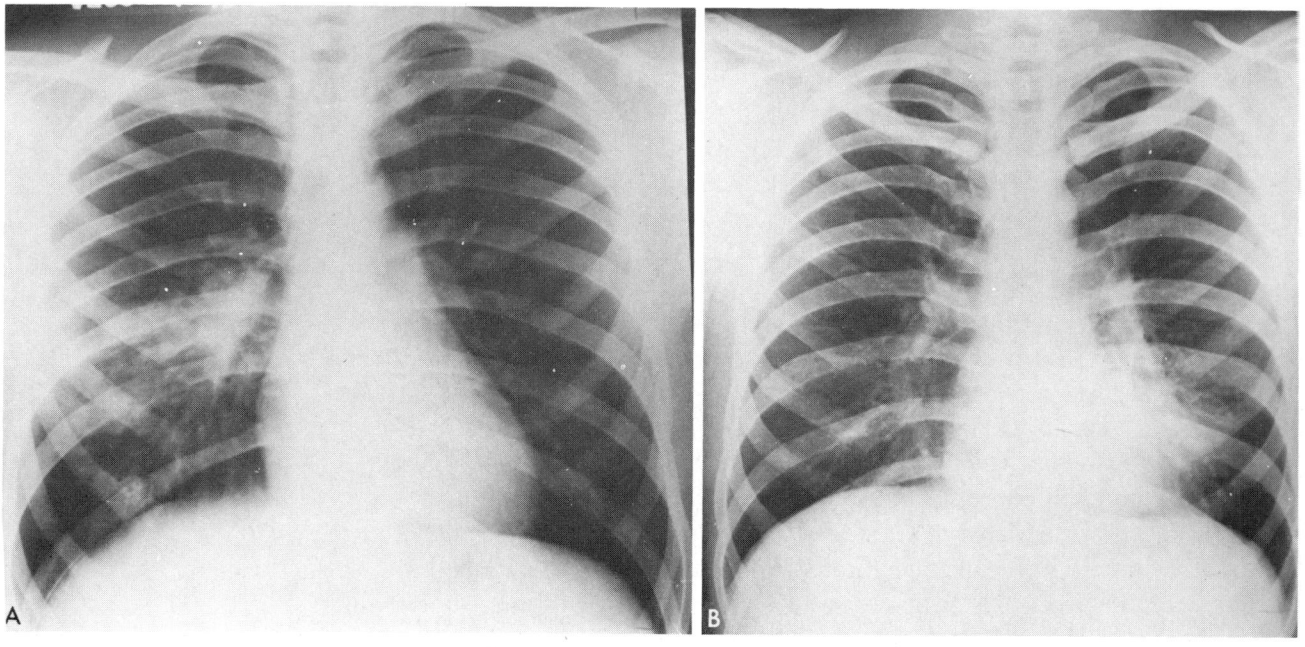

FIGURE 12–6 *See legend on opposite page.*

TABLE 12–8. NONBACTERIAL PNEUMONIAS IN ADULTS AND ADOLESCENTS *(Continued)*

MEASLES[56, 57]	VARICELLA[57, 58]	PSITTACOSIS (ORNITHOSIS)[42, 43, 59, 60] *(Chlamydia psittaci)*	Q FEVER[42, 43, 61, 62] *(Coxiella burnetti)*
Extremely rare in adults, unless immunosuppressed	Respiratory symptoms during clinical chickenpox infection	Known contact with psittacine birds (parrots, parakeets); recent contact with atypical pneumonia patient	Documented exposure to sick livestock; abattoir workers
Diagnose systemic illness (rash always present)	Diagnose systemic illness (rash always present)	Clinical nonbacterial pneumonia in appropriate setting Occasionally may mimic bacterial pneumonia: abrupt onset, rigors, pleurisy, high fever, acutely ill Sputum: few mononuclear cells without predominant organism Serology: complement fixation Chest x-ray: lobar and/or bronchopneumonia	Clinical nonbacterial pneumonia in appropriate setting Occasionally may mimic bacterial pneumonia: abrupt onset, rigors, pleurisy, high fever, acutely ill Sputum: few mononuclear cells without predominant organisms Serology: complement fixation Chest x-ray: usual interstitial patchy infiltrate(s)
None	None	Tetracycline 500 mg qid × 3 wk (alternative drug: chloramphenicol)	Tetracycline 500 mg qid × 2–3 wk (alternative drug: chloramphenicol)
Superimposed bacterial pneumonia common	Rarely, superimposed bacterial pneumonia	Myocarditis; encephalitis; splenomegaly; hepatitis; acute renal failure	Hepatitis; uveitis; thrombophlebitis/arteritis; cardiac involvement; meningitis
May be very ill, but usually self-limited illness	Often quite ill, but usually resolves without treatment	May be fulminant and fatal, but usually slow, gradual recovery; relapse not uncommon	Usually benign and often improves spontaneously in 1–2 wk; occasionally may be prolonged and relapsing

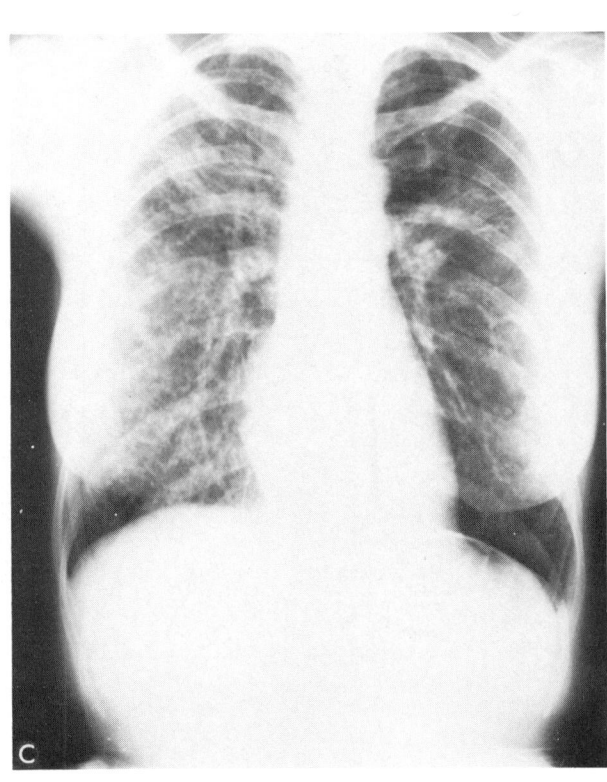

FIGURE 12–6. Nonbacterial pneumonias. *A*, This 31-year-old man presented with 1 week of malaise, headache, sore throat, low-grade fever, and nonproductive cough. Physical examination demonstrated a temperature of 38.6° C and late inspiratory crackles located only over the right lower lobe. The x-ray demonstrated a mixed alveolar-interstitial bronchopneumonia of the right lower lobe. The WBC count was 9000. Sputum was scant: a few polys and no organisms could be seen on Gram's stain. The patient improved dramatically with oral erythromycin. Serum cold agglutinin titers reached 1:256 10 days later. This is a typical example of mycoplasma pneumonia.

B, This 35-year-old woman presented with rather abrupt onset of high fever, rigors, and nonproductive cough. Examination was unremarkable except for fever and focal inspiratory crackles over the left lateral and lower chest. Chest x-ray demonstrates a patchy infiltrate in the lingula of the left lung. Sputum Gram's stain demonstrated moderate numbers of white blood cells but no microorganisms. The WBC count was 8000. The patient then volunteered the history that 12 of her cows had had "pneumonia" 4 weeks previously and 1 had died. (Subsequent complement fixation tests on the patient's serum were diagnostic of Q fever.) The patient improved over the next 10 days with oral tetracycline.

C, This 19-year-old woman developed an upper respiratory infection characterized by the abrupt onset of severe headache, myalgias, and shaking chills. Five days later, the patient developed severe dyspnea, tachypnea, and a relentless but dry cough. Sputum Gram's stain from a transtracheal aspirate (Fig. 12–17) revealed a few inflammatory cells and no microorganisms. The WBC count was 12,000. The patient ultimately recovered from serologically diagnosed influenza pneumonia. The x-ray demonstrates diffuse interstitial bilateral pulmonary infiltrates.

TABLE 12–9.   BACTERIAL PNEUMONIAS IN ADULTS AND ADOLESCENTS

	Streptococcus pneumoniae[40, 41, 63-70] (FIG. 12–18)	*Staphylococcus aureus*[40, 41, 69, 71] (FIG. 12–10)	*Klebsiella Pneumoniae*[40, 41, 72, 73] (FIG. 12–7)
When to suspect	Most community-acquired bacterial pneumonias are pneumococcal	Rarely community-acquired in normal host; common in influenza epidemic; debilitated or immunosuppressed host	Alcoholic; elderly (nursing home resident); debilitated, immunosuppressed
Diagnosis	Sputum Gram's stain: lancet-shaped gram-positive diplococci Sputum culture: positive 50% Blood culture: positive 5–30% Chest x-ray: lobar consolidation (but may be "bronchopneumonia"); necrotizing, rarely	Sputum Gram's stain: gram-positive cocci in clusters Sputum culture: usually positive Blood culture: positive 10% Chest x-ray: diffuse bronchopneumonia with cavitation/pneumatoceles	Sputum Gram's stain: gram-negative encapsulated rods Sputum culture: usually positive Blood culture: positive 20% Chest x-ray: lobar consolidation with necrosis; commonly affects upper lobes
Treatment	Penicillin 1.2–2.4 million units/24 hr parenterally; or penicillin 250 mg po qid × 10 days; or erythromycin 250 mg po qid × 10 days; or cephalosporin	Nafcillin, methicillin, oxacillin 6–12 gm/24 hr parenterally × 2–3 wk; or vancomycin 500 mg q6h IV (preferred if methicillin-resistant staphylococcus); or cephalosporin	Cephalosporin 6–12 gm/day plus aminoglycoside 3–5 mg/kg/day parenterally × 3–4 weeks
Complications	Parapneumonic effusion 20–40%; empyema rare; meningitis, endocarditis, pericarditis, lung abscess very rare	Usually very sick; respiratory failure common; lung abscess, empyema not uncommon; if bacteremia: possibly endocarditis, osteomyelitis, "metastatic infection"	Empyema common, lung abscess not rare
Usual course	Crisis (defervescence in 24–48 hr) or lysis (7–10 days)	Mortality high; often fulminant respiratory failure; slow recovery the rule	Slow recovery; mortality high

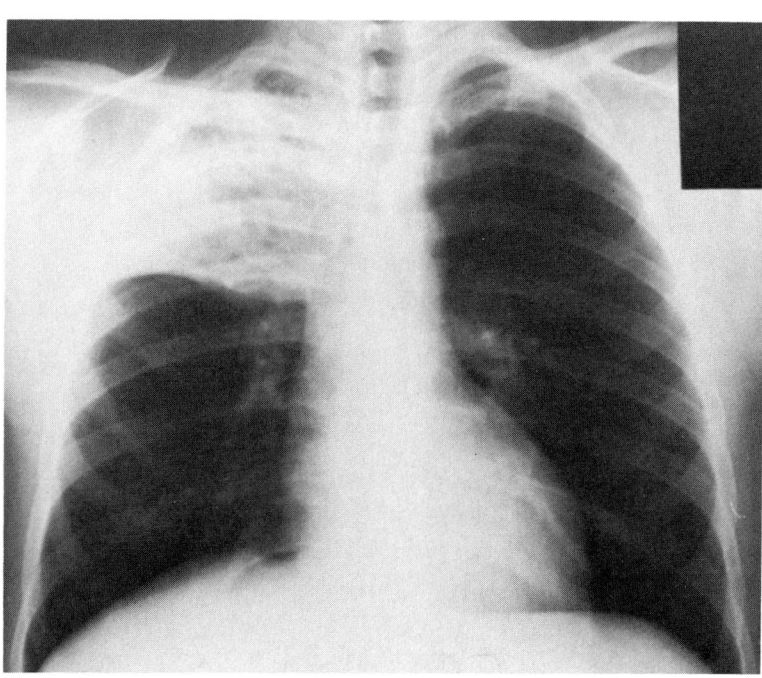

FIGURE 12–7. This 49-year-old male chronic alcoholic developed high fevers, rigors, and cough productive of thick, tenacious sputum. On examination, the patient was febrile but not extremely toxic, and examination revealed crackles and tubular breath sounds over the anterior right upper lobe. The WBC count was 16,000. The chest x-ray demonstrates necrotizing lobar consolidation of the right upper lobe (with a "bulging fissure"). Sputum and blood grew *Klebsiella pneumoniae*. The patient improved slowly but required hospitalization for 4 weeks.

TABLE 12–9. BACTERIAL PNEUMONIAS IN ADULTS AND ADOLESCENTS (Continued)

	ASPIRATION PNEUMONIA[28, 74–78] (MIXED ANAEROBIC INFECTION) (FIG. 12–9)	Hemophilus Influenzae[40, 41, 72, 73, 79, 80] (FIG. 12–19)	LEGIONNAIRES' DISEASE[81–86] Legionella pneumophila (FIG. 12–8)
When to suspect	History of vomiting, coma, seizures; neuromuscular disease, esophageal disease; elderly patient	COPD; alcoholic, debilitated; may occur in normal host	Usually middle-aged or older and/or immunosuppressed; rarely, epidemic; multiple recurrent rigors, headache, diarrhea, obtundation; proteinuria, hyponatremia, abnormal liver enzymes
Diagnosis	Sputum Gram's stain: mixed oral flora, many polymorphonuclears Sputum foul, fetid Sputum culture: mixed flora and/or Bacteroides and/or anaerobic streptococci Blood culture: usually negative Chest x-ray: Lower lobes, usually; may be necrotizing	Sputum Gram's stain: gram-negative pleomorphic, slender, small, coccobacilli Sputum culture: positive 50% Blood culture: often positive (in type B infection) Chest x-ray: Lobar or bronchopneumonia; may be necrotizing	Sputum Gram's stain: many polymorphonuclears, no organisms Sputum culture: negative Blood culture: negative Chest x-ray: lobar pneumonia, rapidly progressive Diagnosis by direct immunofluorescent stain of sputum and/or lung biopsy and/or pleural fluid OR indirect fluorescent antibody titers in serum
Treatment	Parenteral penicillin 6 million units/24 hr × 2 wk; or clindamycin 600–2400 mg/24 hr × 2 weeks parenterally; or chloramphenicol 3–4 gm/24 hr × 2 weeks	Ampicillin 4–12 gm/24 hr × 1–2 wk and/or chloramphenicol; or cefamandole 2–12 gm/24 hr	Erythromycin 1 gm q6h IV, then erythromycin 500 mg po qid × 3 weeks or rifampin or trimethoprim-sulfamethoxazole
Complications	Lung abscess, empyema not rare; repeated aspiration	Non-type B: complications rare; type B: bacteremia, empyema, abscess common	Multisystem failure; respiratory failure very common
Usual course	Depends on underlying condition; slow recovery the rule	Usually slow recovery; mortality higher with type B	Mortality high; often rapid progression to multilobar disease; usually slow difficult recovery

ceiving high-dose corticosteroid therapy for various reasons, or who are leukopenic or uremic. Table 12–10 (page 652) indicates the extraordinary spectrum of pulmonary infectious processes that must be suspected in such patients, according to the specific immune dysfunction categorized by Matthay and Greene.[99] Thus, the clinical setting—the status of the host—is crucial.

II. The chest x-ray[100] is helpful when it reveals classic lobar or segmental consolidation.

Such a finding is unusual in nonbacterial pneumonia and is more typical of various types of bacterial pneumonia—especially pneumococcal (Fig. 12–18, page 660), *Hemophilus influenzae* (Fig. 12–19, page 661) and *Klebsiella* pneumonia (Fig. 12–7). Involvement of multiple lobes or segments in one or both lungs is more commonly seen with fulminant bacterial pneumonia—staphylococcal (Fig. 12–10), gram-negative bacillary, and *Legionella* pneumonia (Fig. 12–8) often so present.

Many bacterial pneumonias do not present with classic lobar pneumonia on chest x-ray, however. Bronchopneumonia—a patchy infiltrate confined to a single segment or lobe—is very common in patients with various types of bacterial pneumonia. The patient with underlying chronic lung disease, especially emphysema, will very often present with patchy consolidation when afflicted with bacterial pneumonia.[101]

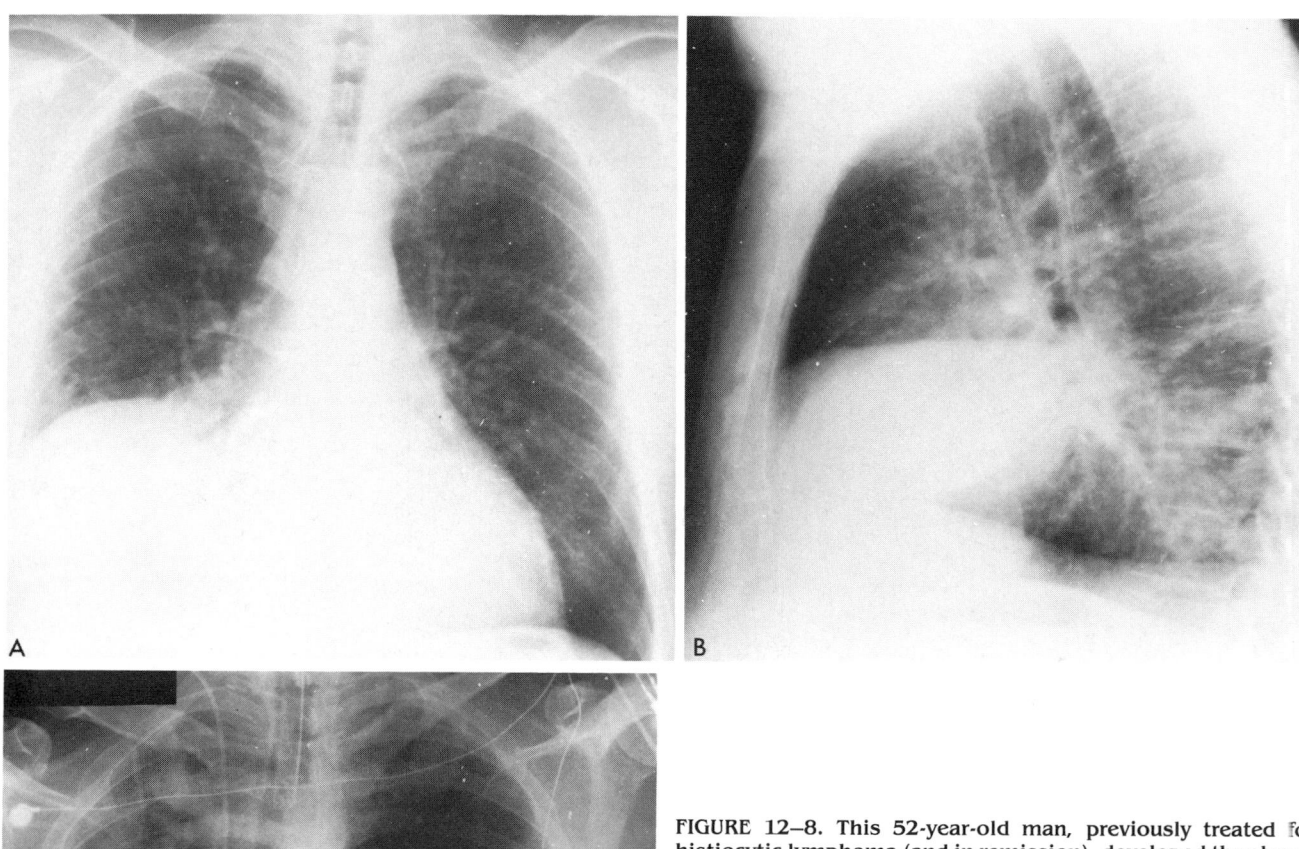

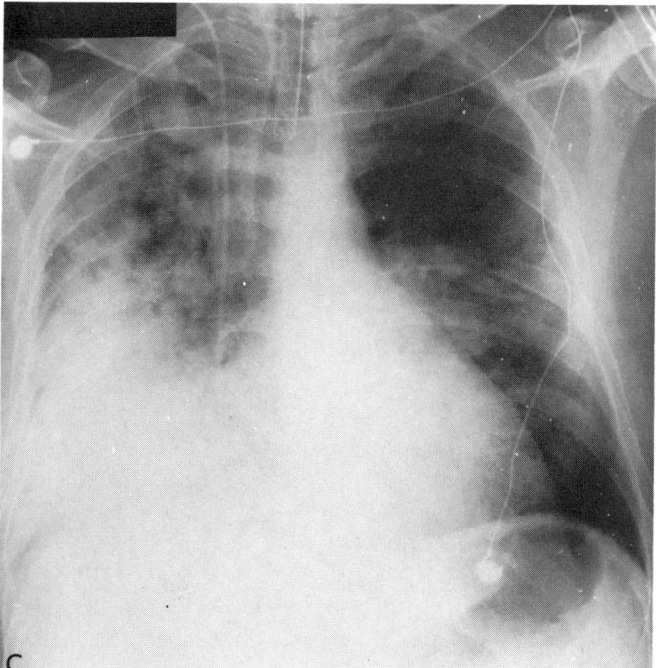

FIGURE 12–8. This 52-year-old man, previously treated for histiocytic lymphoma (and in remission), developed the abrupt onset of severe headache, diarrhea, high fever, and recurrent severe rigors. The patient did not complain of cough. Physical examination demonstrated crackles and tubular breathing over the right middle lobe. Initial chest x-ray (A and B) demonstrates lobar consolidation in the right middle lobe. Sputum Gram's stain demonstrated many leukocytes but no microorganisms. The WBC count was 6000. The patient was hospitalized and treated initially with intravenous erythromycin but 24 hours later was in respiratory failure, with pneumonia involving four lobes of the lung (C). Serologic studies ultimately confirmed *Legionella* pneumonia. The patient recovered from this illness but died during the same hospitalization of a nosocomial gram-negative bacillary pneumonia. Autopsy demonstrated no evidence of recurrent lymphoma.

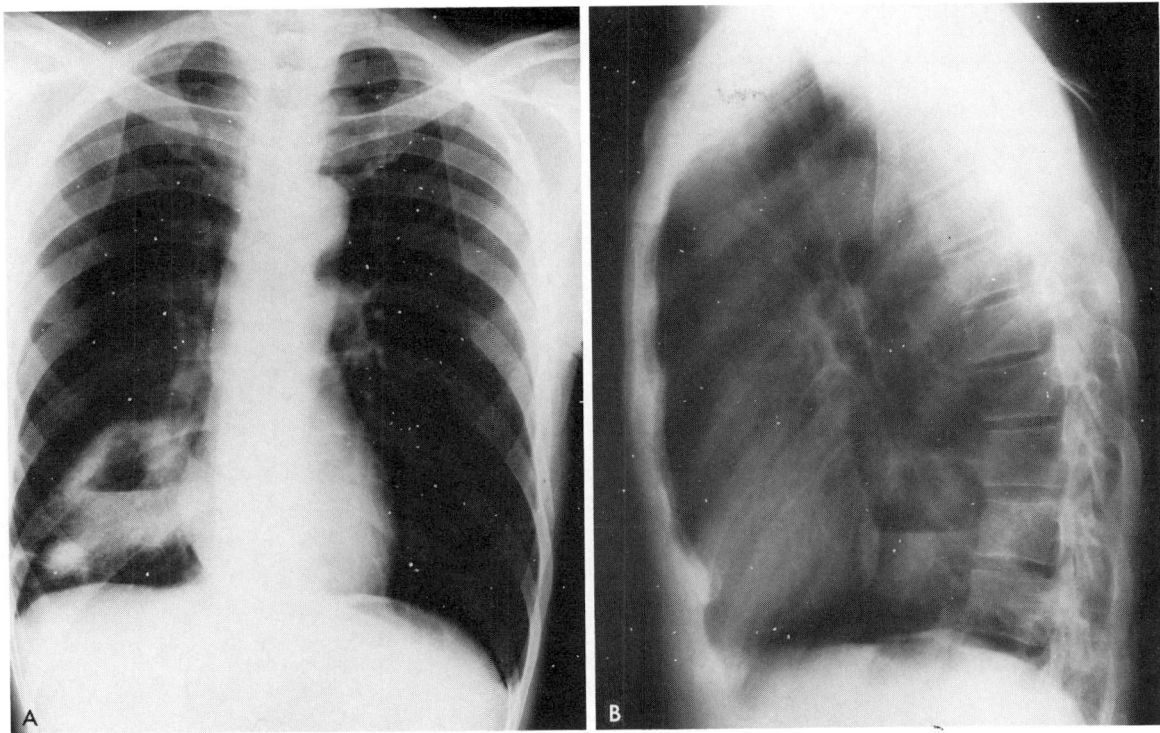

FIGURE 12–9. *A* and *B,* This 27-year-old heroin addict complained of insidious onset of low-grade fever, productive cough, and foul-smelling sputum. Chest x-ray demonstrates an abscess in the right lower lung. Sputum Gram's stain demonstrated many inflammatory cells with a mixture of oral flora. Culture of this extremely foul sputum ultimately grew four different anaerobic bacteria. Prolonged intravenous antibiotic therapy was successful without surgical resection. This anaerobic lung abscess was presumed to be due to aspiration.

FIGURE 12–10. This 26-year-old man receiving immunosuppressive drugs for chronic active hepatitis developed high fevers, recurrent rigors, and productive cough. On physical examination, he was extremely toxic, hypotensive, and hypoxemic and was coughing sputum that demonstrated many leukocytes and gram-positive cocci in clusters. Sputum cultures grew pure isolates of *Staphylococcus aureus.* The patient ultimately required intubation but did survive after a stormy hospital course. The chest x-ray demonstrates extensive cavitating consolidation in both lungs.

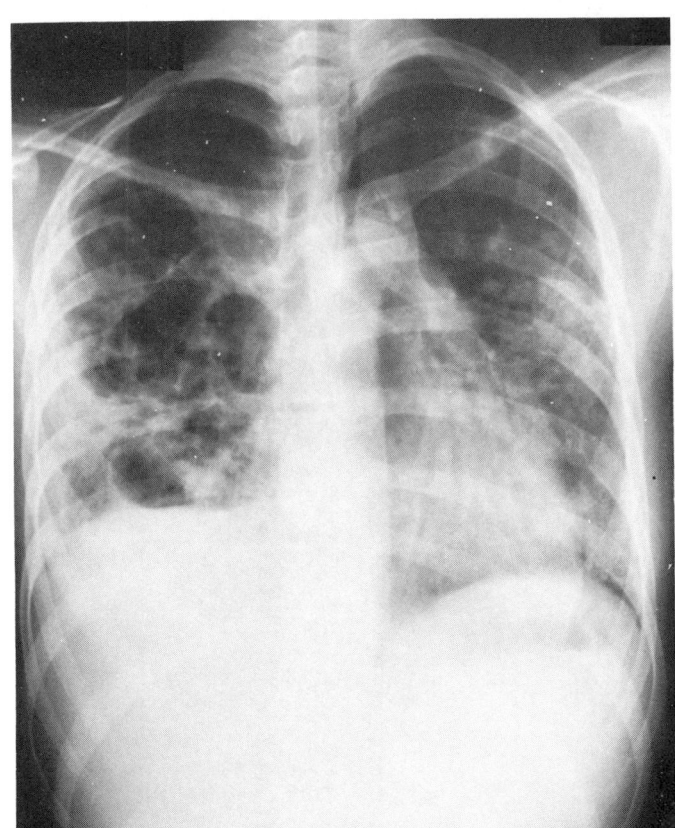

TABLE 12–10. RESPIRATORY INFECTIONS IN THE IMMUNOCOMPROMISED HOST*

HOST DEFENSE IMPAIRMENT	TYPICAL SETTINGS	OPPORTUNISTIC PATHOGENS
Leukocyte dysfunction	Myelocytic leukemia; chronic granulomatous disease; leukopenia; corticosteroid therapy	*Pseudomonas; Serratia;* Staphylococcus; *Nocardia; Candida; Aspergillus*
Impaired humoral immunity	Lymphoma; myeloma; lymphatic leukemia; cancer; cytotoxic therapy; hypogammaglobulinemia; splenectomy	Pneumococcus; *Hemophilus; Pseudomonas; Pneumocystis*
Impaired cellular immunity	Hodgkin's disease; corticosteroid therapy; uremia; cancer; cytotoxic therapy; homosexual males†	Tuberculosis; *Listeria; Candida;* herpesvirus; cytomegalovirus; *Toxoplasma; Pneumocystis; Strongyloides*
Disrupted infection "boundary"	Intubated; indwelling catheter; skin breakdown; altered normal flora (debilitated, on antibiotic regimen)	*Escherichia coli; Staphylococcus; Klebsiella; Pseudomonas;* anaerobes; *Candida*

*Adapted from Reference 99.
†Those with AIDS (acquired immune deficiency syndrome).

Unilateral (less often, bilateral) interstitial or patchy infiltrates are more typical of nonbacterial pneumonias (Fig. 12–6). *Mycoplasma* pneumonia usually presents with a patchy unilateral lower lobe infiltrate. Influenza or adenoviral pneumonia usually results in diffuse interstitial infiltrates, but this same picture may be seen with *Mycoplasma*, Q fever, or ornithosis.

III. <u>The white blood count may or may not help.</u>

In bacterial pneumonias, the white blood count *usually* ranges between 15,000 and 25,000 with a marked left shift, but normal (or even low) white blood counts are not at all rare. Leukopenia associated with proven bacterial pneumonia is often a poor prognostic sign.

Most patients with nonbacterial pneumonia have a normal white blood count, but a few may have extreme leukocytosis.

IV. <u>Sputum Gram's stain is the most important single piece of clinical information.</u>

Several aspects of the sputum Gram's stain should be emphasized:

A. <u>Unless the patient has radiographic pneumonitis, the sputum examination is rarely worthwhile.</u> The patient with acute bronchitis may produce sputum that contains white blood cells and various (usually multiple) microorganisms. Except in the patient with severe chronic lung disease, sputum in acute bronchitis need not be studied.

(Ampicillin is usually chosen for the patient with chronic obstructive lung disease and acute bronchitis because *Hemophilus influenzae* or pneumococcus is most often implicated in infectious flares, but a sputum Gram's stain may be worthwhile if the patient is penicillin allergic or if there is a high incidence of ampicillin-resistant *Hemophilus influenzae* in a certain locale. Antibiotics can then be chosen according to sputum appearance on Gram's stain [see Table 12–13, page 662].)

B. The sputum specimen must be deep.

Oropharyngeal flora contaminate expectorated sputum specimens. The presence of numerous squamous epithelial cells on Gram's stain indicates that microorgansims on or around these cells must be presumed to be oropharyngeal in origin. A deep sputum specimen contains few (or no) squamous cells—only under these circumstances is the analysis of cellular and bacterial forms worthwhile (Fig. 12–11).

C. The Gram's stain must be carefully prepared.

Variations in staining, timing, and decoloration of the Gram's stain can create very misleading information. For example, gramnegative organisms like *Hemophilus* or *Neisseria meningitidis* or even *Klebsiella* can sometimes be mistaken for gram-positive diplococci if the stain is "overdecolorized." Important therapeutic errors then result. In doubtful cases, the quellung reaction is a quick and simple

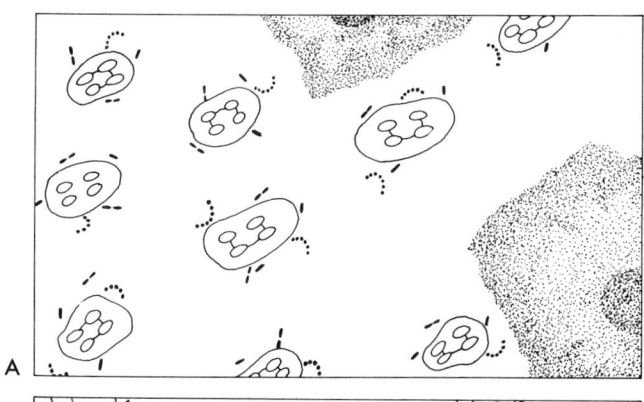

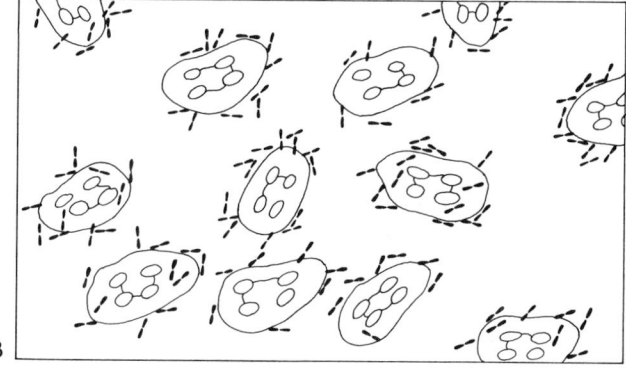

FIGURE 12–11. Common results of the sputum Gram's stain in patients with cough, fever, and pulmonary infiltrates. *A,* The top panel demonstrates inflammatory cells, large squamous (oropharyngeal) epithelial cells, and a variety of microorganisms that are primarily extracellular. Such a specimen almost always reflects oropharyngeal flora rather than a deep respiratory pathogen. *B,* The middle panel demonstrates many inflammatory cells, a preponderance of intracellular and extracellular grampositive diplococci, and no visible squamous epithelial cells. This is a typical Gram's stain in a patient with pneumococcal pneumonia. *C,* The bottom panel demonstrates many inflammatory cells without squamous epithelial cells or visible microorganisms. This may reflect a variety of conditions, but Legionella pneumonia, mycoplasma pneumonia, tuberculosis, partially treated bacterial pneumonia, and noninfectious inflammatory lung diseases are among the many.

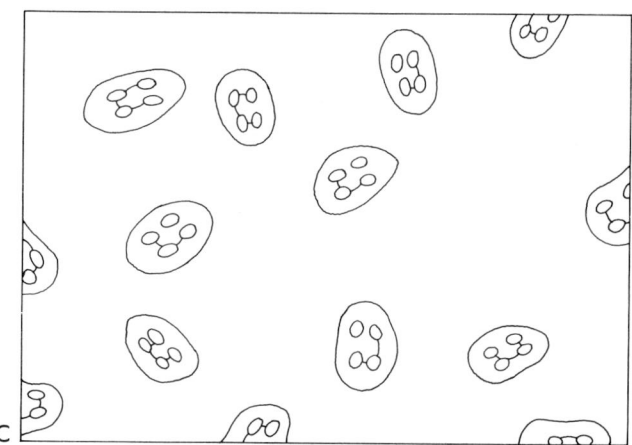

procedure that will highlight the capsule of the pneumococcus, and diagnosis may then be more confident.[102]

D. **The Gram's stain must be interpreted in the light of other clinical findings.**

The expectorated sputum specimen does not necessarily reflect the pathology of lung parenchyma in the patient with cough and pulmonary infiltrates. This is especially a problem in the patient with chronic obstructive lung disease in whom purulent sputum (containing pneumococci or *Hemophilus* organisms) may be a common finding whether or not pneumonia is present. Thus, the patient with chronic bronchitis who develops tuberculosis or lung cancer or pulmonary infarction will be a diagnostic and therapeutic problem if too much reliance is placed on the sputum Gram's stain alone.

E. **The Gram's stain is never "negative."**

The sputum specimen may be unacceptable (Fig. 12–11A) or the Gram's stain may be nondiagnostic, but a "negative" Gram's stain of deep, well-prepared sputum is often very helpful diagnostically. For example:

A deep sputum specimen that reveals little inflammation (white blood cells) and no predominant organism should suggest the possibility that infection may not be the problem at all (Figs. 12–12, 12–13, and 12–14). Cough, fever, and pulmonary infiltrates may be the presenting manifestation of many noninfectious illnesses:[103] congestive heart failure, pulmonary emboli, lung cancer (especially alveolar cell carcinoma), vasculitis (systemic lupus, Wegener's granulomatosis, polyarteritis), interstitial lung disease (sarcoidosis, pneumoconiosis), pulmonary hemorrhage or contusion, bronchiectasis, or drug/toxin-induced pneumonitis (hypersensitivity pneumonitis, for example).

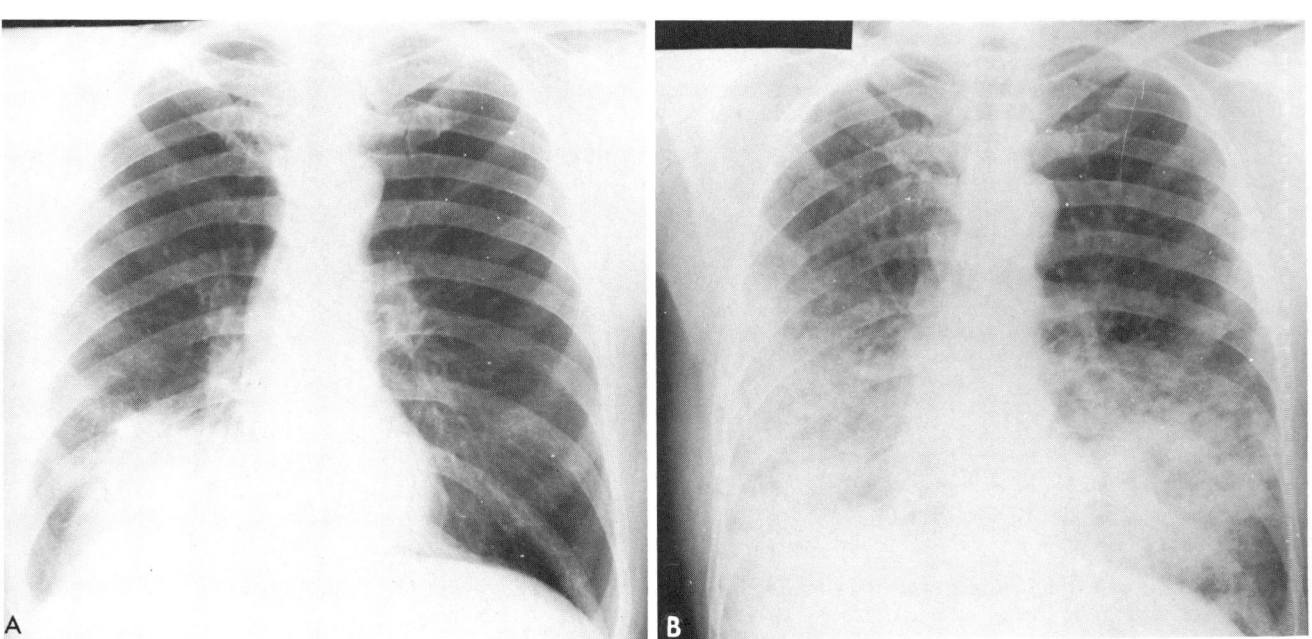

FIGURE 12–12. This 67-year-old nonsmoking man developed a productive cough and low-grade fever that persisted for the next 5 weeks. Physical examination was normal except for a few crackles in the right lower lobe. Chest x-ray shows an infiltrate in the right middle and lower lobes (A). The patient did not appear ill but had an almost continuous cough productive of thin, watery secretions. Sputum Gram's stain revealed neither inflammatory cells nor microorganisms. Alveolar cell carcinoma was diagnosed on sputum cytology. Three months later the patient died of rapid progression of his carcinoma (B).

FIGURE 12–13 *(right)*. This 62-year-old man described 4 weeks of low-grade fever, dry cough, and diffuse arthralgias. Physical examination was unremarkable except for diffuse end-inspiratory crackles in both lung fields. Chest x-ray demonstrates extensive interstitial infiltrates in both lung fields. Lung biopsy ultimately revealed severe, inflammatory, <u>fibrosing alveolitis</u>.

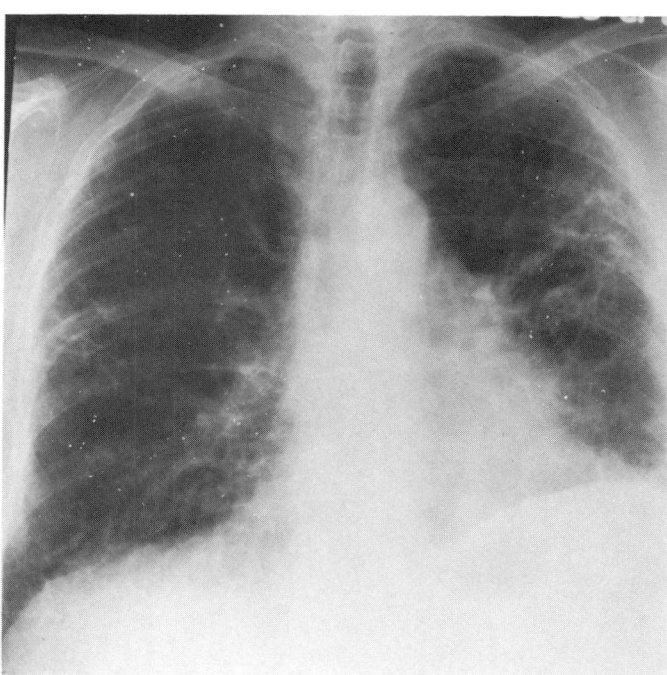

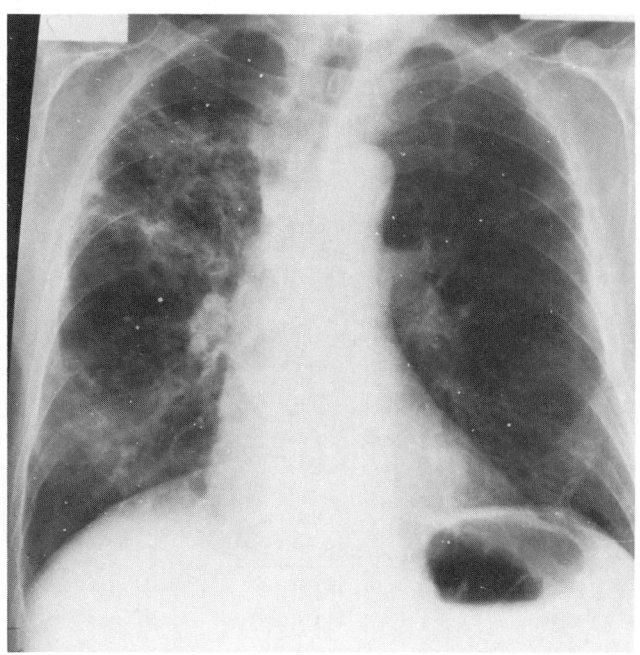

FIGURE 12–14 *(left)*. This 52-year-old farmer developed sudden onset of shortness of breath, high fever, wheezing, and productive cough. Examination was unremarkable except for low-grade fever and diffuse end-inspiratory crackles in both lung fields, much more prominent on the right. Sputum Gram's stain revealed a few inflammatory cells and no microorganisms. Broad-spectrum antibiotic therapy resulted in apparent cure. Three weeks later, the patient returned with an identical clinical syndrome. Further study demonstrated <u>hypersensitivity pneumonitis</u> caused by thermophilic actinomycetes in the patient's hay bin.

When deep sputum reveals <u>many leukocytes but no bacteria</u>, bacterial pneumonia cannot be excluded, but special consideration should then be given to the possibility of *Legionella* (Fig. 12–8),[81–85] *Mycoplasma* and other nonbacterial pneumonias (Table 12–8 and Fig. 12–6), primary tuberculosis (Fig. 12–15),[104, 105] partially treated bacterial pneumonia, and other noninfectious inflammatory lung diseases. Depending upon other aspects of the clinical picture, <u>sputum AFB smears</u>[106] (which are very helpful in the diagnosis of tuberculosis when expertly prepared), and serum titers for <u>cold agglutinins</u> (a nonspecific test for *Mycoplasma pneumoniae*—positive in titers greater than 1:32 in only about 50 per cent of such patients) may be helpful.*

In Norman's case the clinical presentation (see page 643) <u>suggests bacterial pneumonia, and the chest x-ray is compatible with that diagnosis. Community-acquired bacterial pneumonia in the patient with chronic obstructive lung disease is usually due to pneumococcal or *Hemophilus* infection.</u>

A sample of expectorated sputum that is thick and yellow is cultured for bacterial pathogens after performance of the Gram's stain, which reveals only rare squamous epithelial cells, sheets of polymorphonuclear leukocytes, and many intracellular and extracellular gram-positive lancet-shaped diplococci.

---

*"Bedside" cold agglutinin testing is a simple, quick procedure that may correlate with serologic positivity in *Mycoplasma pneumoniae* infection, but this test is positive in only about 10 per cent of cases.[107]

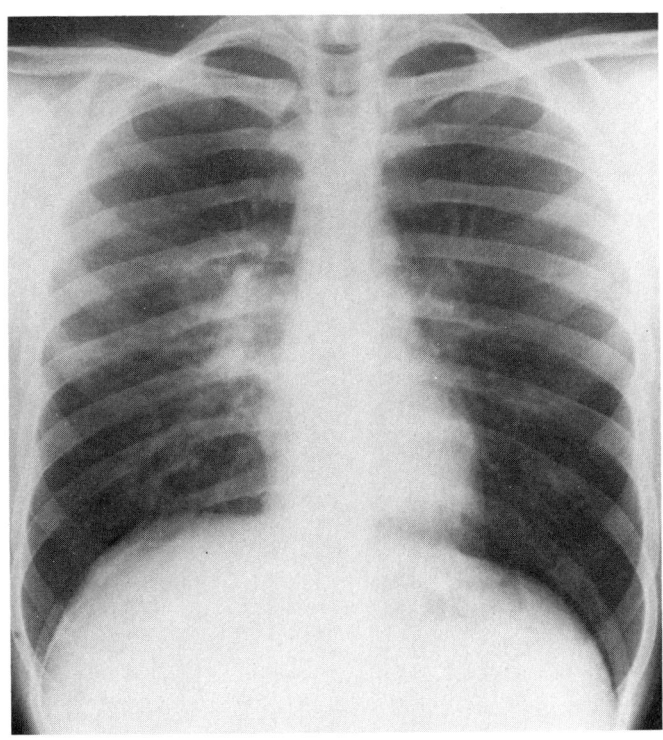

FIGURE 12–15. This 29-year-old male nurse developed insidious onset of nonproductive cough, low-grade fever, and night sweats. Physical examination was completely normal. Chest x-ray demonstrates a poorly defined infiltrate in the right midlung field. Sputum Gram's stain revealed a few inflammatory cells and no microorganisms. Acid-fast smear of the sputum demonstrated tubercle bacilli. Six weeks later, sputum cultures grew *Mycobacterium tuberculosis*.

NOTE

1. The diagnosis of pneumococcal pneumonia is very likely. The sputum Gram's stain demonstrates typical pneumococci from a sputum specimen which appears adequate for diagnosis. The fact that Norman has chronic obstructive lung disease should be remembered, since such a sputum specimen does not necessarily reflect the pathologic findings of the pulmonary infiltrate (see above). In addition, remember that the Gram's stain is not a bacteriologic test—morphology of stained organisms is often very helpful in identifying specific organisms, but sometimes pneumococci, staphylococci, and other streptococci cannot be differentiated by morphologic means alone. That problem is even more formidable when gram-negative organisms are seen. Nevertheless, when the pneumococcus is suspected clinically and is the only organism identified on sputum Gram's stain, one can usually assume that pneumococcal pneumonia is the problem.

2. A sputum culture is obtained. Growth of a pure culture of a single organism from a deep sputum specimen is often very helpful in confirming the diagnosis of a specific bacterial pneumonia, but sputum cultures are sometimes not so helpful as one might hope. For example, in proven (bacteremic) pneumococcal pneumonia, the sputum culture may grow pneumococci in only 50 per cent of cases.[108] While different culture techniques might improve the sensitivity of the sputum culture,[109] the fact remains that many patients with typical bacterial pneumonia will have nondiagnostic sputum cultures. Conversely, as noted above, some patients carry various organisms in the oropharynx or tracheobronchial tree—a positive culture sometimes reflects carriage rather than pulmonary infection, especially in the patient with chronic lung disease.

Thus, both positive and negative sputum cultures must be interpreted with caution. Frequently the sputum Gram's stain provides the only clue to bacteriologic diagnosis in patients with pneumonia.

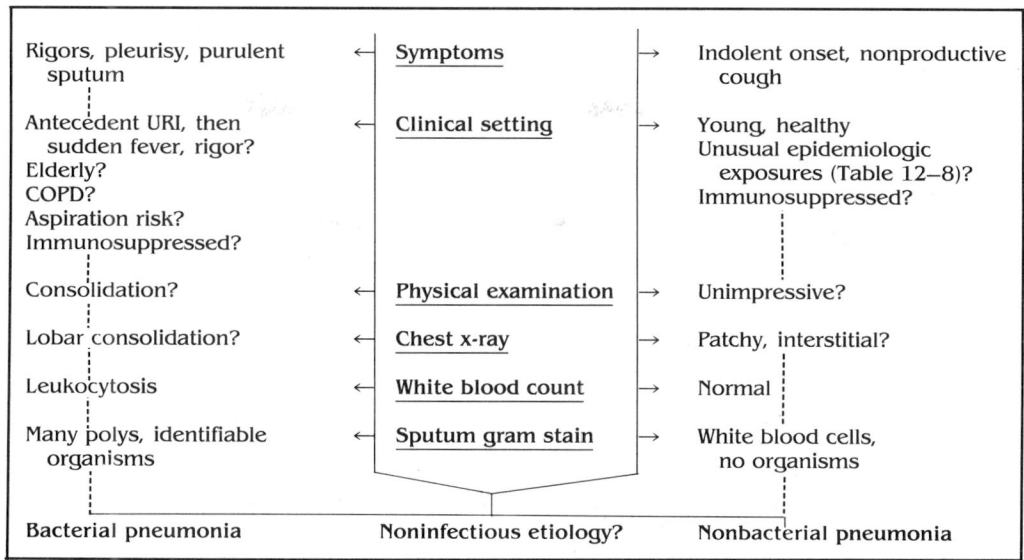

	Symptoms	
Rigors, pleurisy, purulent ← sputum		→ Indolent onset, nonproductive cough
	Clinical setting	
Antecedent URI, then ← sudden fever, rigor? Elderly? COPD? Aspiration risk? Immunosuppressed?		→ Young, healthy Unusual epidemiologic exposures (Table 12–8)? Immunosuppressed?
	Physical examination	
Consolidation? ←		→ Unimpressive?
	Chest x-ray	
Lobar consolidation? ←		→ Patchy, interstitial?
	White blood count	
Leukocytosis ←		→ Normal
	Sputum gram stain	
Many polys, identifiable ← organisms		→ White blood cells, no organisms
Bacterial pneumonia	Noninfectious etiology?	Nonbacterial pneumonia

FIGURE 12–16. The patient with cough, fever, and pulmonary infiltrate(s).

3. Sometimes the patient cannot produce sputum. When this is the case, respiratory therapy (inhaled nebulized aerosols, "cupping and coughing," stimulation of cough with postural drainage) may help induce production of sputum. Transtracheal aspiration (Fig. 12–17) is a safe procedure only when the physician is very experienced in its performance. While this procedure should always be considered in the acutely ill patient who cannot produce sputum and in whom a rapid specific presumptive diagnosis is important, this situation applies primarily to patients requiring hospitalization. Transtracheal aspiration is rarely, if ever, indicated in the patient whose condition is not toxic and who does not require hospitalization. In those patients with "outpatient pneumonia," antibiotic therapy is often prescribed to cover the various likely possibilities (see below), without resorting to this invasive procedure.

Arterial blood gases demonstrate a pH of 7.45 P_{CO_2} of 36, P_{O_2} of 51.

Norman is told that he should be admitted to the hospital for treatment of his pneumonia. Despite a prolonged explanation of the need for hospitalization in his case, Norman adamantly refuses.

Treatment of Pneumonia

I. Nonbacterial (especially mycoplasmal) pneumonia can often be treated with oral antibiotics.

Young, healthy adults with pneumococcal pneumonia can also often be treated with oral antibiotics at home.[66]

Most patients with pneumonia, however, should be hospitalized, especially: (Table 12–11)

A. When the patient is acutely ill, i.e., in a toxic state, with high fever, severe pleuritic pain, dehydration, hypotension, obtundation, hypoxemia, or tachypnea/tachycardia.

Many patients of all ages with acute bacterial pneumonia will fit this description. The patient with leukopenia and involvement of more than one lobe of the lung is especially worrisome.

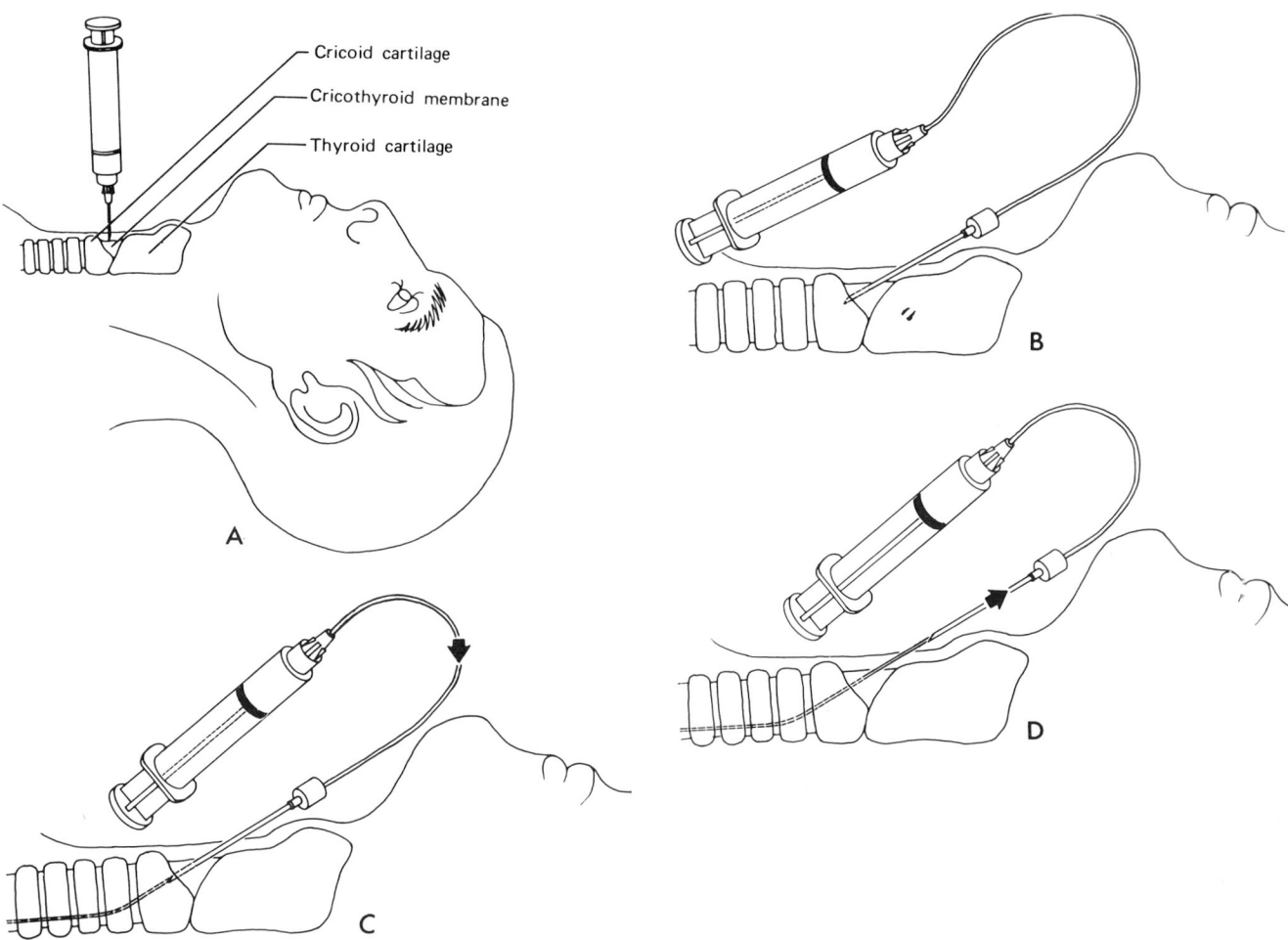

FIGURE 12–17. Transtracheal aspiration. *A,* Local anesthesia is applied to the skin over the cricothyroid membrane. The patient's neck is hyperextended. *B,* A larger bore needle with an indwelling catheter is then inserted through the cricothyroid membrane into the trachea. *C,* The catheter is then advanced into the trachea through the catheter. *D,* The needle is withdrawn, leaving the catheter in place. Secretions are then obtained by aspiration through the catheter. (Reproduced with permission from Mandell, GL, et al. (ed.): Principles and Practices of Infectious Disease. New York: John Wiley, 1979, p. 494.)

B. When the known or suspected pathogen(s) requires parenteral antibiotic therapy.

    Pneumonia due to *Staphylococcus aureus, Klebsiella,* other gram-negative bacilli, aspiration with mixed anaerobic infection, or *Legionella* should always be treated with parenteral antibiotics. This is also true of the patient with known or suspected lung abscess. Most such patients are acutely ill (see above).

TABLE 12–11. HOSPITALIZE THE PATIENT WITH PNEUMONIA WHEN:

Acutely ill	Underlying severe cardiopulmonary disease
Hypoxemia significant (Po_2 less than 60)	Alcoholic
Leukopenic and/or immunosuppressed	Malnourished
Multilobar involvement	Pregnant
Parenteral antibiotics mandatory	Empyema suspected/proven

C. When the patient is an abnormal host.

Observation in the hospital, parenteral antibiotic therapy for presumed pathogens (based on clinical findings and culture results) or invasive diagnostic testing (bronchoscopy, open lung biopsy) will be necessary in different circumstances in the immunocompromised patient (Table 12–10).

The patient with chronic cardiopulmonary disease is an abnormal host in a different sense. Impaired respiratory mechanics result in poor mobilization of infected secretions. i.e., cough is inadequate. Bronchial plugging or reactive bronchospasm will worsen ventilation-perfusion relationships, resulting in hypoxemia and pulmonary hypertension. Impaired cardiac reserve, susceptibility to ischemic myocardial damage and cardiac arrhythmias, the risk of venous thrombosis and superimposed pulmonary embolism during convalescence, as well as the generalized debilitation of severe infection all conspire to place such patients at great risk. (There is no such thing as a "little pneumonia" in the patient with severe COPD or chronic congestive heart failure.) The physiologic burden of pneumonia—hypoxemia, bronchial plugging, dehydration, cardiac stress—is as important in these patients as are the impaired host defenses in the immunocompromised patient (Table 12–10).

Patients who are alcoholic, malnourished, or pregnant are also abnormal hosts. The elderly patient with pneumonia, even if not "toxic," is usually best taken care of in the hospital.

D. When tube thoracostomy drainage of pleural fluid is necessary.

Infection of pleural fluid rarely, if ever, complicates nonbacterial pneumonias, but empyema (Table 12–12) is not uncommon among patients with bacterial pneumonia. Most pleural infections occur in the context of pneumonia that requires hospitalization anyway—staphylococcal pneumonia, gram-negative pneumonias, and aspiration pneumonias, most often.

When the chest x-ray suggests a pleural effusion in the patient with pneumonia, obtain a lateral decubitus x-ray with the involved side down (Figs 12–18 and 12–19). Most parapneumonic (noninfected) effusions are small—less than 10 mm in "thickness" (measure the distance from the fluid level to the inside of the chest wall on the decubitus x-ray).[110] Such effusions are very common in patients with bacterial pneumonia, but almost always resolve with routine antibiotic therapy. When the effusion is larger (greater than 10 mm in thickness), thoracentesis should be performed. The need for tube drainage of the pleural space can then usually be predicted by pleural fluid analysis.[110-112] When the pleural fluid Gram's stain reveals microorganisms or when the fluid is grossly purulent or has a glucose level less than 40 mg per 100 ml or a pH less than 7.00, immediate

TABLE 12–12. SUSPECT EMPYEMA

Decubitus chest film!

Tap all large effusions!

Thoracostomy drainage if:
  Fluid grossly purulent!
  Gram's stain identifies organism!
  pH less than 7.00!
  Glucose less than 40 mg/100 ml!

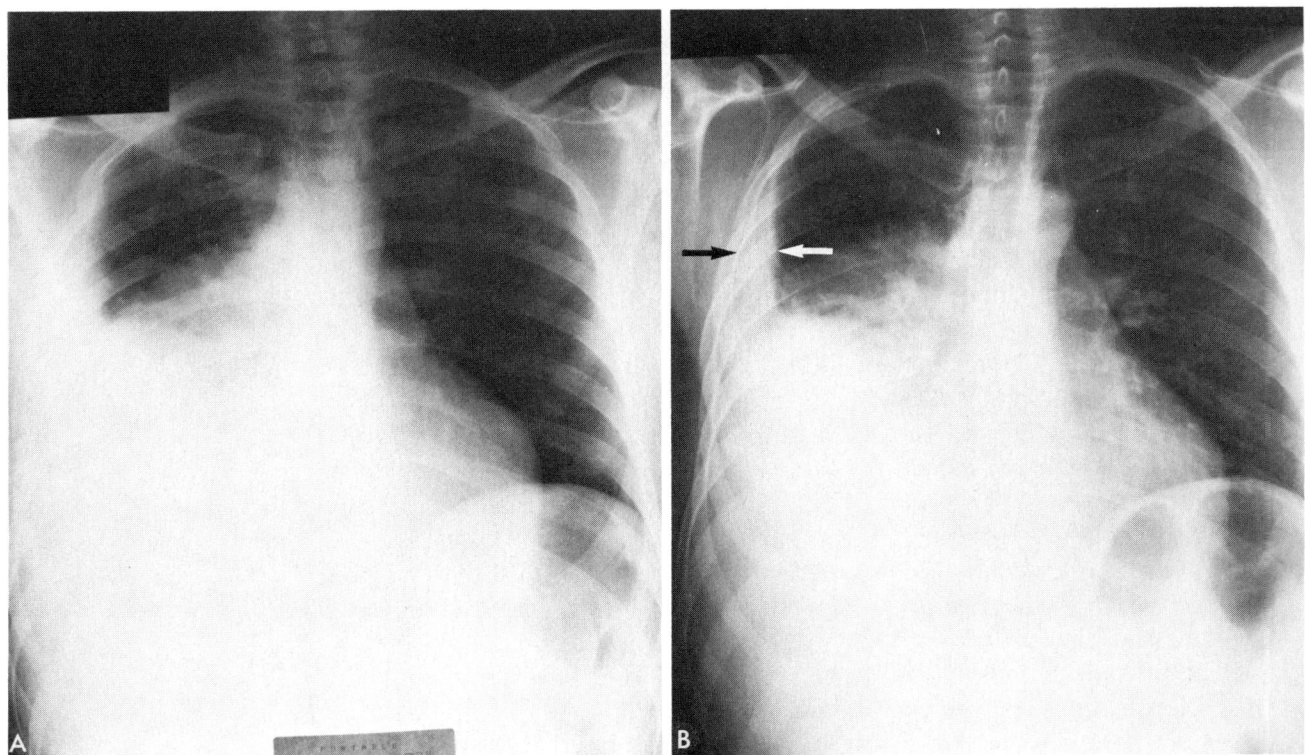

FIGURE 12–18. Empyema. This healthy 32-year-old man developed an upper respiratory infection, followed 4 days later by the abrupt onset of a single rigor, high fever, and cough productive of purulent sputum. Gram's stain demonstrated many white blood cells and gram-positive diplococci. The x-ray (A) demonstrates extensive consolidation of the right lower and right middle lobes. The decubitus chest film (B) demonstrates a large pleural effusion (arrow). Thoracentesis revealed purulent fluid, with a pH of 6.94, and gram-positive diplococci on Gram's stain. After a prolonged hospital course, complicated by purulent pericarditis and bilateral empyema, the patient recovered completely.

Most pneumococcal pneumonia is not nearly so severe, nor accompanied by such complications. Nevertheless, pneumococcal pneumonia can be a devastating and fatal illness.

thoracostomy is indicated. (The pleural fluid white blood count and protein are not helpful here. The pleural fluid lactic dehydrogenase [LDH] value may be useful in equivocal situations; for example, when the pleural fluid pH is between 7.00 and 7.20, and LDH level is greater than 1000, a repeat thoracentesis in a day or two should be considered if empyema is not proven initially.)

Early recognition of empyema is very important to ultimate prognosis. Failure to recognize this complication often leads to loculation of pleural fluid, which may then be a diagnostic[113] and therapeutic problem.[114, 115] Surgical decortication of a pleural "peel" is sometimes necessary in the patient with inadequately treated empyema.

II. Whether the patient is hospitalized or not, antibiotic therapy should be as specific as possible.

Three clinical situations are most common:

A. When a specific pathogenic organism is considered highly likely on the basis of the clinical findings, x-ray, and sputum examination.

When pneumococcal pneumonia is the presumptive diagnosis, penicillin is the preferred treatment. The hospitalized patient will be treated with intravenous penicillin G 200,000 to 400,000 units q4h or intramuscular procaine penicillin 600,000 to 1.2 million units

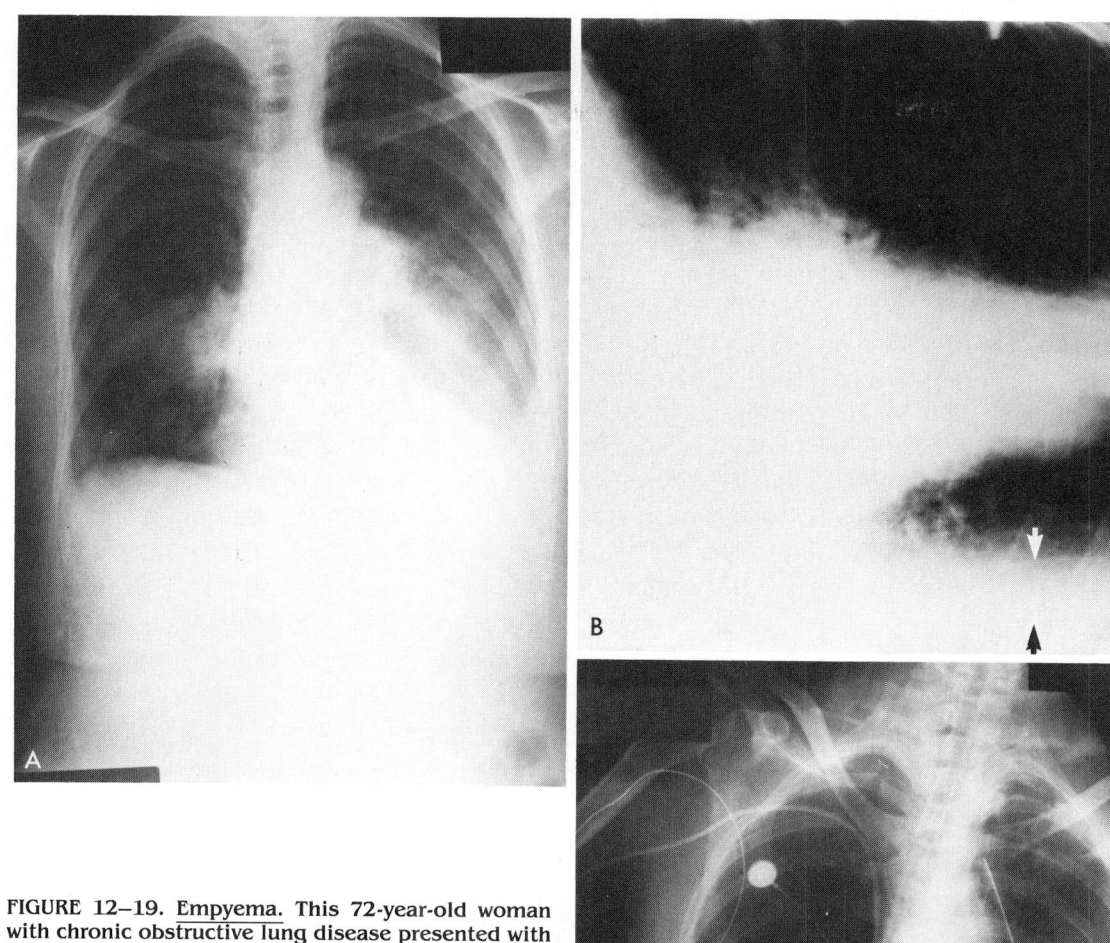

FIGURE 12–19. Empyema. This 72-year-old woman with chronic obstructive lung disease presented with a 1-week history of fever, productive cough, and 2 days of severe left pleuritic chest pain. Examination revealed diminished breath sounds at the left base. Sputum Gram's stain demonstrated many inflammatory cells and microorganisms typical of *Hemophilus influenzae*. The chest x-ray *(A)* demonstrates haziness in the left lower lung field and a suspicion of a pleural effusion. Decubitus chest x-ray *(B)* reveals that the pleural effusion *(arrow)* is very large (it measured 30 mm between arrows). Sputum, blood, and pleural fluid cultures grew *Hemophilus influenzae*, type B. After immediate, thoracostomy drainage *(C)* and prolonged intravenous antibiotic therapy, the patient did well.

bid. The patient in a less toxic condition who can be treated at home is often given a single intramuscular injection of 1.2 million units of procaine penicillin followed by 10 days of oral penicillin 250 mg qid.

When mycoplasma pneumonia is most likely, tetracycline is the drug of choice, 500 mg qid orally for 10 to 14 days. Erythromycin in similar doses is probably equally effective but is less well tolerated because of more frequent gastrointestinal upset (nausea, borborygmi, diarrhea). Antibiotic treatment of mycoplasma pneumonia is probably effective only when instituted early in the clinical course (within the first week).

Tables 12–8 and 12–9 describe recommended treatment in various other types of bacterial and nonbacterial pneumonia.

B. When bacterial pneumonia is the likely clinical diagnosis, but the sputum Gram's stain is either inadequate or unavailable.

In this setting, definitive diagnosis will depend on subsequent results of sputum, blood, or pleural fluid cultures (which may or may not be helpful). Presumptive therapy is then indicated, based on the specific clinical setting.

When the patient is only mildly ill and there are no specific indications for hospitalization, erythromycin 250 mg qid × 10 days is preferred. This regimen will "cover" pneumococcal pneumonia and is acceptable for *Mycoplasma* pneumonia, which can, at times, mimic bacterial pneumonia. (*Legionella* pneumonia may at times cause only mild infection, and erythromycin will be helpful here as well.) In certain such patients who are only mildly ill, alternatives should be considered: ampicillin (in the patient with chronic lung disease to cover hemophilus organisms and pneumococci) or oral cephalosporins (cephalexin, cefaclor) in the elderly, debilitated, alcoholic, or nursing home patient (Table 12–13).

When the patient is more severely ill, hospitalization and more vigorous diagnostic attempts are always important. Transtracheal aspiration, bronchoscopy, or lung biopsy may be needed. Therapy is then based on the results of those procedures.

TABLE 12–13. ANTIBIOTIC THERAPY FOR NONHOSPITALIZED PATIENTS WITH PNEUMONIA

DRUG/DOSE (10–14 DAYS USUAL DURATION OF THERAPY)	TREATMENT OF CHOICE IN	ALSO CONSIDER IN	COST/NO. TABLETS
Tetracycline 500 mg qid	*Mycoplasma* pneumonia	*Hemophilus influenzae* pneumonia in ampicillin-allergic patient; suspected Q fever, psittacosis	$6/40
Erythromycin† 250 mg qid	*Mycoplasma* pneumonia	Pneumococcal pneumonia, penicillin-allergic patient Suspect *Legionella*?*	$8/40
Penicillin V 250 mg qid 500 mg qid	Pneumococcal pneumonia	Suspected aspiration?*	$6/40 $9/40
Ampicillin 250 mg qid	*Hemophilus influenzae* pneumonia	COPD; unidentified organism*	$7/40
Chloramphenicol 500 mg qid	*Hemophilus influenzae* pneumonia, ampicillin-resistant, or in penicillin-allergic patient	Q fever or psittacosis suspected (and tetracycline contraindicated)	$22/80 (250 mg)
Trimethoprim-sulfamethoxazole 160/800 mg bid		*Hemophilus influenzae* pneumonia in penicillin-allergic patient	$7/20
Cephalexin 250 mg qid	Pneumococcal pneumonia in penicillin-allergic patient	Suspected gram-negative infection* (nursing home resident?)	$25/40
Cefaclor 250 mg tid		*Hemophilus influenzae* pneumonia in ampicillin-allergic patient; suspected gram-negative infection*	$28/30
Clindamycin 300 mg q6h		Pneumococcal pneumonia in penicillin-allergic patient; suspected aspiration pneumonia*	$70–80/100 (150 mg)

*Under these circumstances, hospitalization and precise documentation of cause (usually followed by parenteral antibiotics) is most often indicated. In circumstances in which this is *impossible*, these oral medications can be tried.

†Erythromycin, 500 mg qid, is preferred to the smaller dose (250 mg), but many patients cannot tolerate 2 gm of erythromycin each day.

C. When nonbacterial pneumonia is clinically likely.

Many such patients require no treatment at all when illness is mild or appears to be improving spontaneously. Tetracycline 500 mg qid is effective therapy for most treatable nonbacterial pneumonias (Table 12–8) that might be encountered under various circumstances (mycoplasma, chlamydiae (?),[21] psittacosis, Q fever).

The homosexual male with nonbacterial pneumonia must be suspected of cytomegalovirus and pneumocystis infection.[116, 117] Invasive studies are often required.

Geographic variables may suggest histoplasmosis,[118, 119] coccidioidomycosis,[120] or blastomycosis.[118]

A tuberculin skin test, sputum AFB smears, and TB cultures should always be considered in the pneumonia patient following recent third-world travel or other tuberculosis exposure, or in the patient with atypical pulmonary infiltrates (especially in the apex of the lung).

Norman's decubitus chest film reveals little, if any, pleural effusion. A blood culture is obtained.

An intramuscular injection of 1.2 million units of procaine penicillin G is administered to Norman, and a prescription is provided for oral penicillin (Pen-Vee K) 250 mg qid × 14 days. Theophylline 100 mg tid and a metaproterenol inhaler are provided as well. Arrangements are made for oxygen delivery at home—to be set at 1 to 2 liters per minute—and Brenda is briefly instructed about oxygen therapy and chest physical therapy. Brenda is very upset with her father who remains adamant about going home.

NOTE

1. Again, ideally, Norman should be hospitalized (Table 12–11).

2. Penicillin is the antibiotic of choice here because all clinical findings and the sputum Gram's stain suggest pneumococcal pneumonia. Were Normal penicillin allergic, erythromycin or clindamycin would be acceptable alternatives, as would an oral cephalosporin (unless there were a history of penicillin anaphylaxis).

If an acceptable sputum sample could not be obtained, ampicillin would be a logical choice to cover the most common organisms in this setting—pneumococcus and *Hemophilus influenzae* in the patient with chronic lung disease. Table 12–13 enumerates antibiotics commonly used in the treatment of outpatients with pneumonia.

3. Blood cultures should be obtained from all patients with pneumonia. The published frequency of positive blood cultures varies with the different bacterial pneumonias (Table 12–9), but such data are unreliable since bacteremia may be the criterion that defines the disease in some clinical studies (thus greatly overestimating its incidence), or the diagnosis in such studies may be based on much less specific criteria (thus underestimating the incidence of bacteremia). Even though blood cultures are only rarely positive in patients with "outpatient pneumonia," documentation of bacteremia assures a specific diagnosis and guides future antibiotic therapy.

4. Adjuvant therapy of pneumonia in outpatients may include: cough suppressants (to allow restful sleep); oral hydration; oral or aerosolized bronchodilators (especially for the patient with asthma or chronic lung

disease); chest physical therapy (cupping and coughing, "mobilizing secretions" are of unproven efficacy,[45] but are widely recommended); and oxygen therapy at home (when hypoxemia is a significant problem).[91] The need for daily chest physical therapy, oxygen, and hydration is usually sufficient reason for hospitalization, but, as in Norman's case, this is not always feasible.

> **Two days later, blood and sputum cultures are negative. (See page 656 concerning sensitivity of sputum cultures.) Brenda reports by telephone that Norman is "about the same," remains febrile (38.5° C orally), but appears less short of breath with oxygen therapy and is coughing up much thick sputum without difficulty. Norman has not changed his mind about hospitalization.**
>
> **(Brenda herself is very anxious about her father, but she feels "a little better," coughs less, has had no further hemoptysis, and is continuing use of the bronchodilators and intermittent cough suppressants.)**

Follow-up. Many patients with pneumonia are unnecessarily subjected to frequently repeated examinations, sputum cultures, and chest x-rays. While careful follow-up is important, the practical logistics depend on several considerations:

I. The natural history of specific types of pneumonia varies.

Different types of pneumonia resolve in different patterns—failure to respond to treatment must be defined with this in mind.

Pneumococcal pneumonia[40, 67] typically improves dramatically and rapidly after institution of antibiotics—the "crisis" (and fever) passes in 12 to 48 hours in many patients. Occasionally, pneumococcal pneumonia resolves more gradually; "lysis" of fever occurs over 7 to 10 days. Thus, continuing low-grade fever for 1 week is not necessarily a harbinger of complications (or mistaken diagnosis) in the patient with (presumed) pneumococcal pneumonia treated with penicillin. On the other hand, such a patient who responds rapidly to penicillin only to become febrile *again* several days after initial defervescence must be suspected of complications:

A. Local or systemic infectious complications—for example, empyema, pericarditis, endocarditis, meningitis.
B. Microbial superinfection with penicillin-resistant organisms.
C. Penicillin drug reaction.
D. An inaccurate original diagnosis.

Mycoplasma pneumonia, on the other hand, typically follows a more gradual resolution,[54, 121] over the course of 1 to 3 weeks. Most nonbacterial pneumonias will follow a similar course. (Occasionally, common nonbacterial pneumonias will progressively worsen, but this is unusual.)

Staphylococcal, *Klebsiella,* and (other) gram-negative pneumonias usually cause severe, fulminant disease followed by slow, difficult, and prolonged (many weeks) recovery in hospital.

Aspiration pneumonia and Legionnaires' disease follow highly variable courses, and generalizations are meaningless here.

Clinical improvement is the index to follow during the first 1 to 2 weeks in outpatients with pneumonia. Repeated cultures and chest x-rays are unnecessary during this time, as long as the patient is doing well.

II. The incidence of complications and the clinical course of pneumonia depend on the status of the infected host as well as the specific pathogen involved.

As noted in Tables 12–8 and 12–9, specific complications vary with the specific type of pneumonia. For example, although parapneumonic effusions are common in pneumococcal pneumonia, empyema is rare.[40, 41] On the other hand, empyema *is* common in pneumonia due to *Hemophilus influenzae, Staphylococcus aureus,* or *Streptococcus pyogenes. Mycoplasma* pneumonia has been associated with a plethora of systemic, hematologic, and neurologic complications,[46] but these are rare. Other nonbacterial pneumonias may be associated with multisystem disease as well. Specific microbial diagnosis helps anticipate specific complications.

The host is also important. In addition to the immunosuppressed patient or the patient with chronic heart or lung disease, the patient who is pregnant, alcoholic, uremic, very elderly, malnourished, diabetic, or neurologically impaired is always more of a problem. Such patients in general have a worse prognosis and/or improve more slowly.

III. The timing of repeat chest x-rays must be individualized.

Nonbacterial pneumonia (especially *Mycoplasma*) tends to resolve radiographically in tandem with clinical resolution.[54, 122, 123] While clinical improvement usually occurs over 1 to 3 weeks, and auscultation of the lungs is often abnormal throughout this time, the chest x-ray returns to normal within 4 weeks in most. Perhaps 20 per cent, but certainly only a minority, will require 6 to 8 weeks before complete radiographic resolution occurs.

Pneumococcal pneumonia is much more variable.[68] In the normal host (young and otherwise healthy), chest x-rays will return to normal within 6 weeks. (Abnormal physical findings often persist for 1 to 2 weeks beyond defervescence but will usually clear before the x-ray does.) Among abnormal hosts (especially elderly patients with chronic obstructive lung disease), many patients will have persistently abnormal chest x-rays beyond 6 weeks, and radiographic resolution may not be complete for 3 months or longer, even when clinical resolution is complete and no other underlying problem (for example, lung cancer) can be identified.[68]

While mycoplasma, other nonbacterial, and pneumococcal pneumonias usually resolve *completely* radiographically, other bacterial pneumonias may not. Especially the necrotizing pneumonias (staphylococcal, gram-negative bacillary, aspiration) may result in permanent lung tissue destruction and persistently abnormal chest x-rays because of scarring (Fig. 12–10). The patient with inadequately treated empyema will often develop extensive pleural scarring.

Thus, when "outpatient pneumonia" is being treated, the chest x-ray should be repeated when the clinician expects it to be normal. An interval of 6 weeks between the initial diagnostic x-ray and the first follow-up x-ray is usually reasonable, as long as the patient has done well clinically and there is no reason to suspect an underlying neoplasm (Fig. 12–20). A final x-ray another 2 months later is then necessary in those patients whose x-ray is not normal after 6 weeks.

To our surprise, Norman does well at home. Over the next 10 days, he becomes afebrile, coughs less, and is "close to normal."

Six weeks later, a repeat chest x-ray reveals only partial clearing of the right lower lobe infiltrate. Norman feels well, is afebrile, and auscultation of the lungs reveals a few persistent crackles in the right lower lobe. There is no suggestion of mediastinal widening or a hilar mass on chest x-ray. There has been no hemoptysis.

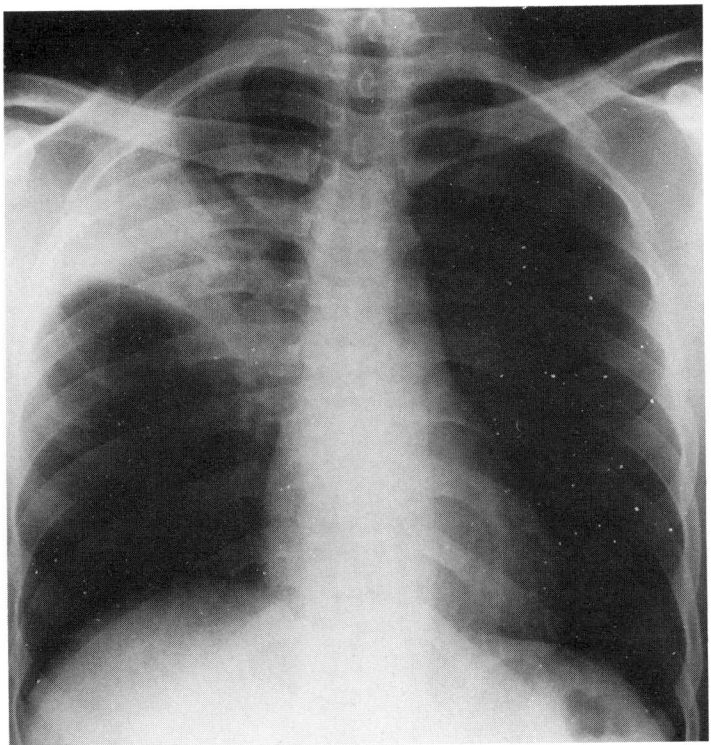

FIGURE 12–20. This 67-year-old smoker described 1 week of low-grade fever, night sweats, and an increasingly productive cough. Physical examination revealed low-grade fever and diminished breath sounds over the anterior right upper lobe. Sputum was purulent and suggested pneumococcal pneumonia. Chest x-ray demonstrated consolidation and partial atelectasis of the right upper lobe. The patient then admitted to four *months* of new cough, with several episodes of hemoptysis. Antibiotic treatment of presumed pneumococcal pneumonia resulted in rapid improvement of fever, cough, and night sweats but bronchoscopy demonstrated a squamous cell carcinoma at the orifice of the right upper lobe.

One interesting study of "poorly resolving pneumonia" (Table 12–14) included patients with (presumably infectious) pulmonary infiltrates "who continued to show roentgenographic densities after 30 days or failed to show clinical improvement after 7 days of antimicrobial therapy."[103] As we have seen, <u>failure to improve clinically is always a cause for concern</u> about the accuracy of the original diagnosis or as a clue to the development of complications. <u>Failure to resolve radiographically is another matter entirely.</u> While tuberculosis, lung cancer, pulmonary infarction, and a variety of other infectious and noninfectious diseases

TABLE 12–14. CAUSES OF POORLY RESOLVING "PNEUMONIA" IN 209 PATIENTS

INFECTIOUS PNEUMONIA		NONINFECTIOUS CAUSE		UNKNOWN CAUSE
Pneumococcal	41	Pulmonary infarction	12	Total 31
Tuberculosis	18	Bronchogenic carcinoma	10	
Aspiration	15	Other neoplasms‡	5	
Staphylococcal	14	Sarcoidosis	1	
Gram-negative bacilli	14	SLE	1	
Histoplasmosis	9	Hypersensitivity pneumonitis	1	
Psittacosis	5	Middle lobe atelectasis	1	
Tularemia	5	Silicosis	1	
Blastomycosis	5	Others§	4	
Mycoplasma	4	Total	36	
Nocardia	4			
Others†	8			
Total	142			

*Adapted from Reference 103. Data derived from Infectious Disease Consultation Service at Vanderbilt Hospital, 1961–1967.
†Cryptococcus, atypical mycobacteria, aspergillus, candida, cytomegalovirus infections.
‡Bronchial adenoma, alveolar cell carcinoma, lymphoma, leukemia, metastatic carcinoma.
§Pulmonary edema, pulmonary hemosiderosis, rheumatic disease, Hamman-Rich disease.

may initially mimic uncomplicated pneumonia but then fail to improve radiographically, uncomplicated pneumococcal pneumonia is the most common cause of poorly resolving pneumonia, radiographically defined.[103]

Thus, the natural history of radiographic resolution of pneumonia must be understood before the physician considers exhaustive diagnostic investigations (sputum cytology, pulmonary function tests, bronchoscopy, lung biopsy) in the patient whose pneumonia does not clear radiographically several weeks later.

Over the next 3 months, Norman remains well (for him) and his chest x-ray returns to normal, now 4 months after his acute pneumonia. No further studies are undertaken.

Throughout Norman's illness, however, Brenda Bronchitis has continued to cough. Her cough is now dry, infrequent, and occurs mostly during the day. The cough is clearly less severe than at the onset of her own illness and now "feels more like I have trouble clearing my throat." Brenda has stopped smoking. A physical examination is entirely normal. A repeat chest x-ray is normal, and pulmonary function tests are also completely normal. There has been no further hemoptysis since the first week of illness. Bronchodilators are no longer helpful, but Brenda has continued to use the codeine cough syrup.

Antihistamines, decongestants, two different trials of broad-spectrum antibiotics, and even a 1-week course of oral corticosteroids have not been helpful.

CHRONIC COUGH

The patient with chronic cough can be a perplexing challenge, but a systematic approach will almost always rise to the occasion.

The most important considerations in the evaluation of the patient with chronic cough are:

1. Is the patient a smoker? Chronic bronchitis, defined as daily production of sputum for at least 3 months per year for 2 consecutive years, is the cause of chronic cough in most smokers. The role of infection in chronic bronchitis continues to generate controversy,[124] and, while there is some evidence that antibiotics are useful in patients with acute bronchitis superimposed on chronic lung disease,[24] there are few data to support the use of daily antibiotics for chronic infection in this population. Only stopping smoking will help.

Chronic bronchitis or a history of repeated "acute bronchitis" in the *nonsmoker* should at least suggest the possibility of rarer phenomena: cystic fibrosis (yes, even in adults),[125, 126] alpha$_1$-antitrypsin deficiency,[127, 128] bronchiectasis (Fig. 12–21), atypical asthma,[2] or various host deficiency states (immunoglobulin deficiences,[129] immotile cilia syndrome,[130, 131] for example).

2. Does the patient perceive the cough to be high (oropharyngeal or "throat clearing"), or low (bronchial) in origin?[91]

Postnasal drip is the mundane but difficult problem that may be the most common cause of chronic cough in nonsmokers. Most often related to allergic rhinitis, chronic sinusitis, or structural nasopharyngeal abnormalities (nasal polyps, enlarged uvula, hypertrophied adenoids, or chronic tonsillitis), postnasal drip induces cough that is usually perceived by the patient as "high" or "throat clearing." Other suggestive clues include the presence of

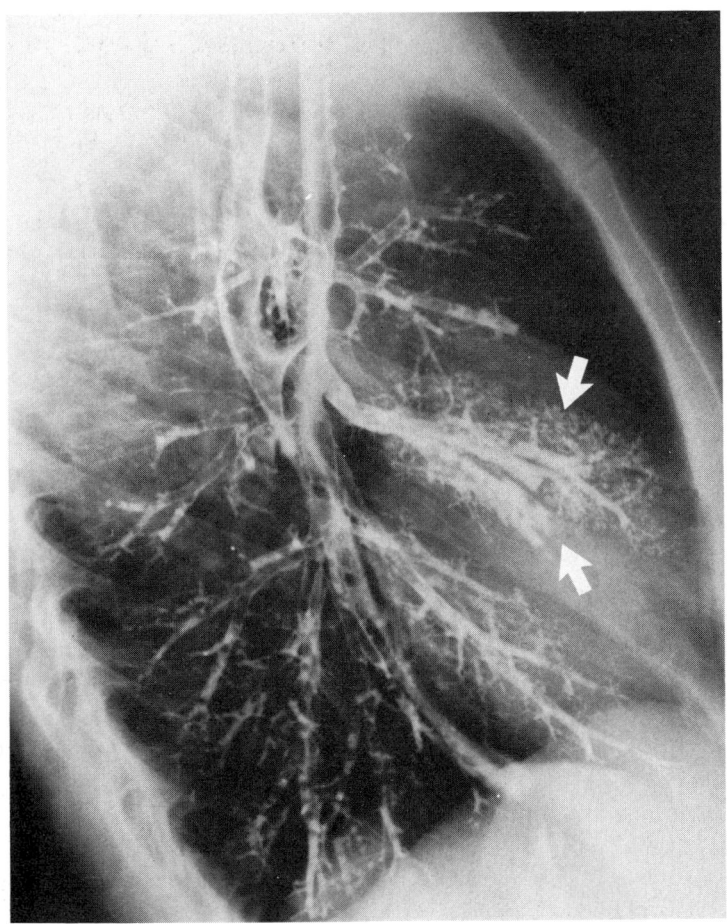

FIGURE 12–21. This 26-year-old man described a 3-year history of "frequent colds." On numerous occasions, the patient developed a productive cough without fever, which usually responded temporarily to broad-spectrum antibiotics. Chest x-rays were normal. Continuing recurrence of these episodes prompted investigation—the x-rays demonstrate bronchiectasis of the right middle lobe on bronchography (arrows). Right middle lobectomy resulted in permanent cure.

associated nasal or sinus symptoms (nasal voice or obstruction, head fullness, documented sinusitis), seasonal variation in cough (especially with allergic rhinitis), a response in the past to decongestant-antihistamine therapy, symptomatic fluctuations with weather (especially humidity), and prominence of symptoms early in the day (secretions pool in the hypopharynx during sleep and cause symptoms upon arising from bed) with improvement later in the day.

Treatment of postnasal drip is difficult but obviously depends on establishing a specific diagnosis. Intermittent use of antihistamine-decongestant preparations helps most patients with mild allergic rhinitis or sinusitis. (Many preparations can be bought over the counter— for example, 4 mg chlorpheniramine [Chlor-Trimeton—antihistamine] and 30 mg of pseudoephedrine [decongestant]. Antihistamines often produce drowsiness and are poorly tolerated by some patients.) Nasal sprays or drops should be avoided, except when used for no more than 2 to 3 consecutive days (rhinitis medicamentosus is a common complication of chronic nasal spray use). Topical nasal corticosteroid preparations (for example, nasal beclomethasone) are very helpful in patients with transient allergic rhinitis or during withdrawal from nasal spray-induced rhinitis medicamentosus, but these substances should not be used over a long term except on the advice of an allergist. Allergy evaluation, with skin testing and hyposensitization injection therapy, is important in many patients, both young and old.

Careful ear, nose, and throat examination and x-rays of the sinuses will also be useful in some patients whose symptoms point to the nose and sinuses as the cause of cough.

Always question the patient about symptoms of reflux esophagitis (Chapter 13, Appendix II)—this is not a rare cause of chronic unexplained cough, especially in the middle-aged and elderly.

3. Physical examination should always, then, include careful ear, nose, and throat examination, auscultation of the chest during forced expiration (to detect inapparent bronchospasm), cardiac examination for evidence of congestive heart failure or valvular disease (mitral stenosis, for example, can cause cough), and evaluation of physical findings that may herald lung cancer—unilateral immobility of the diagragm (phrenic nerve paralysis), Horner's syndrome, supraclavicular lymphadenopathy, localized wheezing, or hoarseness due to unilateral vocal cord paralysis (recurrent laryngeal nerve injury).

REMEMBER ALSO:

4. A normal chest x-ray does not exclude serious lung disease as a source of chronic cough. Carcinoma of the lung can present with cough and a normal chest x-ray when the cancer is entirely endobronchial.[35, 132]

Obstructive lung disease is diagnosed by history, physical examination, and pulmonary function test. The chest x-ray is often normal.

Various interstitial lung diseases may be associated with a normal chest x-ray—perhaps 10 per cent of the time.[133]

Occasionally, repeating the chest x-ray weeks or months later will yield surprising results (Figs. 12–22 and 12–23).

5. Pulmonary function tests may be very helpful in the patient with chronic cough. In the nonsmoker, documentation of reversible obstructive

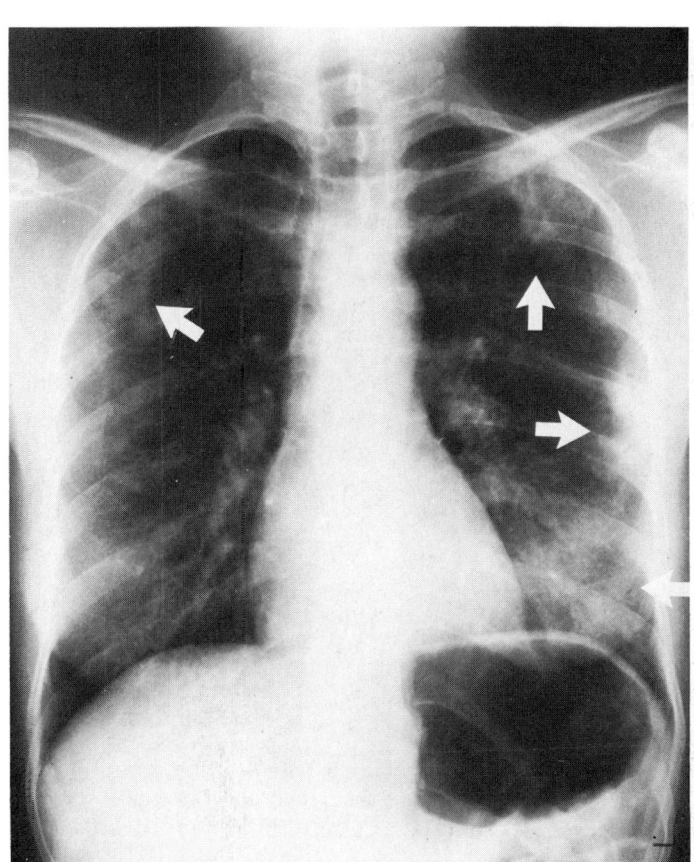

FIGURE 12–22. This 31-year-old woman with allergic rhinitis described chronic, recurrent, nonproductive cough. Sinus x-rays suggested chronic sinusitis, but decongestants and antibiotics did not help. An initial chest x-ray was completely normal. Three months later, the patient complained of persistent dry cough. Chest x-ray then demonstrated fluffy bilateral peripheral infiltrates (arrows), and the patient developed necrotizing glomerulonephritis. Cytotoxic therapy has resulted in dramatic improvement in this patient with Wegener's granulomatosis.

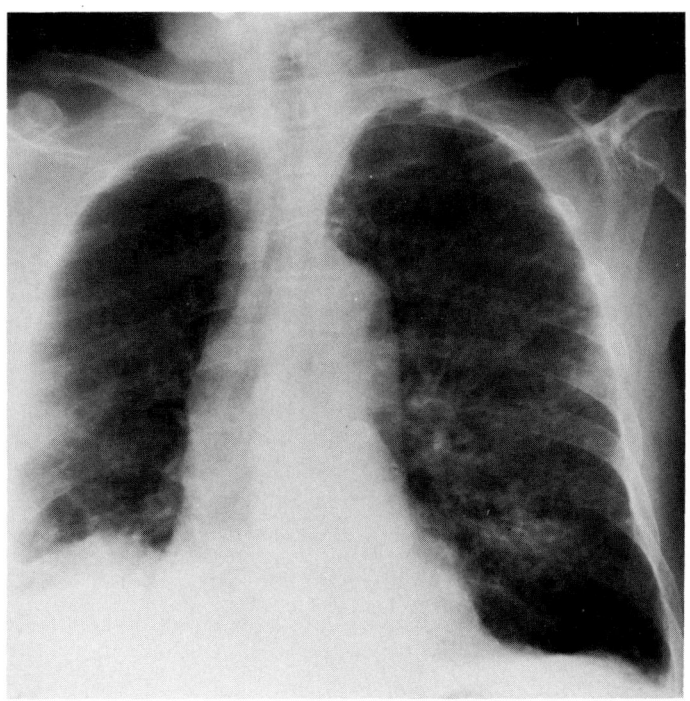

FIGURE 12–23. This 78-year-old man presented with low-grade fever, mild cough, night sweats, and weight loss over the previous 6 weeks. His initial chest x-ray was completely normal. An extensive workup in hospital for fever of unknown origin was completely normal. Two weeks after discharge from hospital, he returned with persistence of low-grade fever and cough. Chest x-ray now demonstrated diffuse miliary infiltrates in both lung fields. The patient improved dramatically with antibiotic therapy of culture-proven miliary tuberculosis.

deficits (decreased FEV_1/vital capacity, increased residual volume, decreased flow rates) may point to inapparent asthma. Bronchodilator therapy or short-term corticosteroids will then often be helpful.

In the smoker with chronic bronchitis,[134–137] documentation of obstructive deficits is useful in assessing prognosis and response to medical therapy and may also be a productive educational device for the physician trying to convince the chronic bronchitic to stop smoking.[136]

Virtually all patients with interstitial lung disease will demonstrate either abnormal pulmonary function tests (decreased vital capacity, decreased total lung volumes, decreased diffusing capacity) or an abnormal chest x-ray. Thus, in the unusual patient whose interstitial lung disease is not evident on chest x-ray, pulmonary function testing may provide the clue. (The great majority of patients with interstitial lung disease will have *both* abnormal x-rays and abnormal pulmonary function tests.)

6. Bronchoscopy is now widely available and in experienced hands is a benign procedure for most patients.

A patient whose chronic cough remains unexplained in spite of careful clinical examination, chest x-ray, and pulmonary function tests (and perhaps various therapeutic trials) should undergo bronchoscopy, especially if the patient is a smoker, over 40 years of age, or has a history of hemoptysis or progressively worsening cough.

At times, bronchoscopy is performed primarily for reassurance. As noted previously, normal fiberoptic bronchoscopy in the patient with a normal chest x-ray is almost always reason for optimism that occult carcinoma is not present.

After prolonged and ongoing discussion about her recurrent symptoms, Brenda admits that she is "deathly afraid" of lung cancer and emphysema, especially following her father's illness. Brenda is reassured that she does not have emphysema and vows to continue to avoid smoking. She asks if we can be absolutely certain that she does not have cancer. With this in mind, fiberoptic bronchoscopy and careful ear, nose, and throat examination are performed and are entirely normal.

Over the next 2 weeks, the cough resolves entirely, and Brenda feels completely well.

Psychogenic cough is an uncommon but real entity that may be a major therapeutic problem. The diagnosis is extremely difficult to document. It should be suspected when careful repeated evaluation is normal; when cough recurs and abates in association with stress, and relief of stress, respectively; when cough is prominent while the patient is among company but inapparent when the patient is observed during sleep or when the patient (thinks) he or she is alone; when obvious "secondary gain" is achieved by persistent cough; and when other manifestations of anxiety or depression coexist. None of these features is diagnostic, and psychogenic cough must always be a diagnosis of exclusion.

Psychogenic cough often begins during a legitimate bout of bronchitis or pneumonia, and the distinction between refractory (or slowly resolving) bronchitis and psychogenic cough can be very fine indeed. In a minority, overt psychiatric illness will be obvious, and psychiatric consultation will be helpful. In most, however, persistent cough, like many other persistent somatic symptoms, reflects a variety of unspoken fears, expectations, and needs that are not recognized or communicated by the patient. Our success with such patients, or lack thereof, says something about how we practice medicine today (see Appendix).

APPENDIX

The Worried Well

Most adults with acute cough have infectious bronchitis, while most with chronic cough have tobacco-related chronic bronchitis. The former is a benign, ubiquitous entity that is almost always self-limited; the latter is rarely a diagnostic challenge, even to the unsophisticated patient who so often complains of a "smoker's cough." Most patients with cough, then, know what is the matter with them and usually know what will make them better—for acute bronchitis—time; for chronic bronchitis—stopping smoking. The great majority of patients so afflicted never seek medical attention at all. Nevertheless, acute and chronic cough are extremely common complaints in ambulatory medical practices.[138] Why do some people seek advice while others do not?

In all ambulatory medical practices, the "worried well" are now legion. Among such people minor illness precipitates anxieties and concerns that are disproportionately intense. All experienced practitioners must be struck by the dramatic variation among patients in their "threshold" for seeking medical advice. Surely this is a complicated matter, and variables of socioeconomic status, cultural conditioning, and accessibility of medical care play major roles. But if the individual physician is to help such patients, if busy clinics are to smoothly orchestrate the care of both the worried well and the more seriously ill, if indeed society is to defeat its most devastating illnesses,[139] we health practitioners must begin to *educate* our patients.

Consider the patient with cough. He or she consults a physician for many reasons:

1. Fear. Well-intentioned media propaganda fill the airwaves with warnings about emphysema and lung cancer. Unfortunately, as Lewis Thomas has said,

> There is no discernible counter-propaganda. Nothing has changed so much in the past 25 years as the public's perception of its own health. The change amounts to a loss of confidence in the human form. The general belief these days seems to be that the body is fundamentally flawed, subject to disintegration at any moment, always on the verge of mortal disease, always in need of continual monitoring and support by health care professionals. . . . Left alone, unadvised by professionals, the tendency of the human body is perceived as prone to steady failure.[139]

2. Excessive expectations. The public at large attributes to modern medicine an omnipotence it does not begin to deserve. Moreover, much of patients' expectations are conditioned by previous contact with physicians who falsely imply value to the treatments we commonly prescribe. Any physician who has tried to downplay the need for antibiotics in the patient with acute bronchitis (who "knows" that penicillin "cures me"—the classic uncontrolled clinical trial) can attest to the counterproductive impact of uncommunicative "pill-pushing" practitioners.

3. The need for reassurance and nonspecific symptomatic therapy. These are the primary goals of the physician in so much of acute ambulatory illness—in this case, to temporarily suppress an annoying cough that prevents restful sleep and to bolster the patient's confidence in his or her own general good health.

Finding out why the patient consults us, then, is often as important in the management of minor illness as is making a specific clinical diagnosis. Viewing the patient as a customer[140] may be a useful model when considering patients' needs. Especially in the patient who does not appear acutely ill, the simple question, What worries you about your illness? may evoke surprising and insightful remarks that reveal the patient's deepest concerns and fears. In the neurotic and anxious patient, this can also open Pandora's box (listen and ye shall find—more than ye want). But the general principle is valid: Allowing the patient a simple but more active role in his or her interaction with the physician defuses the common disgruntlement at "being treated like a piece of meat" and allows the physician to negotiate the patient's real demands and concerns to a mutual settlement. Similarly, asking the patient at the end of the interview, Do you have any questions? or, Did you have in mind some other treatment that has helped you in the past? concludes the negotiations by allowing the physician a brief opportunity to educate the patient about an illness that is so common that it will probably recur again. (It may also, on occasion, suggest to the physician a type of therapy that he had not considered and that could be useful.) The physician can then briefly take the initiative even when the patient expresses no particular concern. For example,

> I ask you these questions because different doctors treat different problems in different ways, and, as time passes, we learn more about what is the best treatment for this problem. We now know that penicillin does not help the common cold, but we also know that stopping your smoking will both help make you better faster and stop you from getting emphysema. Some patients with your problem are also worried about lung cancer. I'm glad to say that there is no sign of cancer in your case, but I wish you would stop smoking so that I can say the same thing 5 or 10 years from now.

Many physicians will object that this process takes too much time. In fact, most patients can succinctly express their fears and expectations. Those few minutes can be as valuable to the physician as to the patient. The extraordinarily broad range of human response to illness is the heart of the matter: surely, if we are to help the worried well, we must understand why people worry.

It may be that this extra effort will not be rewarded. It may be that such a response on the part of health practitioners to the worried well will have little impact, in the larger view, on our society's health care system. But listen again to Lewis Thomas:

> The system is being overused, swamped by expectant overdemands for services that are frequently trivial or unproductive. . . . The health care system should be designed for use when it is really needed and when it has something of genuine value to offer. If designed, or redesigned, in this way the system would function far more effectively, and would probably cost very much less.[139]

But surely our system operates in response to patients' demands. The prospects of changing an entire society's demand for health care are negligible if individual health practitioners do not attempt to educate their patients. What can I offer this patient that is of genuine value? It may often be nothing more than explaining <u>why</u> I have nothing to offer.

If health care is to be made available to all citizens in a society in which costs can no longer be ignored, physicians and patients must educate each other—physicians educing from patients worries and fears as well as symptoms, and patients educing from physicians honesty and insight as well as prescriptions. So long as patients' abuse of the system is encouraged by physicians' indifference to that abuse, cost efficiency in the health care system will remain a dream, and more of us who are well will worry.

REFERENCES

1. Irwin, RS, et al.: Cough. A comprehensive review. Arch Intern Med 137:1186, 1977.
2. Corrao, WM, et al.: Chronic cough as the sole presenting manifestation of bronchial asthma. N Engl J Med 300:633, 1979.
3. Wolkove, N, et al.: Occult foreign body aspiration in adults. JAMA 248:1350–1352, 1982.
4. Biological effects of proteolytic enzyme detergents (Report of a symposium). Thorax 31:621, 1977.
5. Peters, JM, Murphy, RLH: Pulmonary toxicity of isocyanates. Ann Intern Med 73:654, 1970.
6. Butcher, BT, et al.: Longitudinal study of workers employed in the manufacture of toluene-diisocyanate. Am Rev Respir Dis 116:411, 1977.
7. Forgacs, P: Crackles and wheezes. Lancet 2:203, 1967.
8. Nath, AR, Capel, LH: Inspiratory crackles—early and late. Thorax 29:223, 1974.
9. Murphy, R, Holford, SK: Lung sounds. Basics of Respiratory Disease. American Thoracic Society, 1980, vol. 8 (#4), pp 1–6.
10. Wood, RW, et al.: An efficient strategy for managing acute respiratory illnesses in adults. Ann Intern Med 93:757, 1980.
11. Osmer, JC, Cole, BK: The stethoscope and roentgenogram in acute pneumonia. South Med J 59:75, 1966.
12. Stott, NCH, West, RR: Randomized controlled trial of antibiotics in patients with cough and purulent sputum. Br Med J 2:556, 1976.
13. Taylor, B, et al: Amoxicillin and co-trimoxazole in presumed viral respiratory infection of childhood: Placebo-controlled trial. Br Med J 2:552, 1977.
14. Howie, JGR: A new look at respiratory illness in general practice. J R Coll Gen Pract 23:895, 1973.
15. Edwards, G: Acute bronchitis—etiology, diagnosis, and management. Br Med J 1:963, 1966.
16. Monto, AS, Ullman, BM: Acute respiratory illness in an American community. The Tecumseh Study. JAMA 227:164, 1974.
17. Knight, V: Viral and Mycoplasmal Infections of the Respiratory Tract. Philadelphia: Lea & Febiger, 1973.
18. Franson, H, et al.: Acute lower respiratory illness in elderly patients with respiratory syncytial virus infection. Acta Med Scand 182:323, 1967.
19. Evans, AS, et al: Mycoplasma pneumoniae infections in University of Wisconsin students. Am Rev Respir Dis 96:237, 1967.
20. Mogabgab, WJ: Mycoplasma pneumoniae and adenovirus respiratory illnesses in military and university personnel. Am Rev Respir Dis 97:345, 1968.
21. Komaroff, A, et al: Chlamydia trachomatis infection in adults with community-acquired pneumonia. JAMA 245:1319–1322, 1981.
22. Harrison, HR, et al.: Chlamydia trachomatis infant pneumonitis. N Engl J Med 298:702–708, 1978.
23. Ito, JI, et al.: Pneumonia due to Chlamydia trachomatis in an immunocompromised adult. N Engl J Med 307:95–98, 1982.
24. Pines, IC, et al.: Antibiotic regimens in moderately ill patients with purulent exacerbations of chronic bronchitis. Br J Dis Chest 66:107, 1972.
25. Chakravarty, NK, et al.: Central effects of antitussive drugs on cough and respiration. J Pharmacol Exp Ther 117:127, 1956.
26. Howard, JC, et al.: Effectiveness of antihistamines in the symptomatic management of the common cold. JAMA 242:2414, 1979.
27. Watts, RW: New mucolytic agent for sputum liquefaction. Postgrad Med 36:449, 1964.
28. Aronson, MD, et al.: Association between cigarette smoking and acute respiratory tract illness in young adults. JAMA 248:181–183, 1982.
29. Niewoehner, DE, et al.: Pathologic changes in peripheral airways of young cigarette smokers. N Engl J Med 291:755–758, 1974.
30. Fridy, WW, et al.: Airways function during mild viral respiratory illness. Ann Intern Med 80:150, 1974.
31. Empey, DW, et al.: Mechanisms of bronchial hyperreactivity in normal subjects after upper respiratory infection. Am Rev Respir Dis 113:131, 1976.
32. Webb-Johnson, DC, Andrews, JL: Bronchodilator therapy. N Engl J Med 297:476, 758, 1977.
33. Wolfe, JD, Simmons, DH: Hemoptysis: Diagnosis and management. West J Med 127:383, 1977.
34. Boren, HG, et al.: The management of hemoptysis. Am Rev Respir Dis 93:471, 1966.
35. Schneider, L: Bronchogenic carcinoma heralded by hemoptysis and ignored because of negative chest x-ray results. NY State J Med 59:637, 1959.
36. Weaver, LJ, et al.: Selection of patients with hemoptysis for fiberoptic bronchoscopy. Chest 76:7, 1979.
37. Ganz, PA, et al.: Lung cancer in young patients. West J Med 133:373, 1980.
38. Snider, GL: When not to use the bronchoscope for hemoptysis. Chest 76:1, 1979.
39. Douglass, BE, Carr, DT: Prognosis in idiopathic hemoptysis. JAMA 150:764, 1952.
40. Hook, EW: Acute inflammatory diseases of the lung. In Barondess, J (ed.): Diagnostic Approaches to Presenting Syndromes. Baltimore: Williams and Wilkins, 1971, pp 333–402.
41. Lerner, AM, Jankauskas, K: The classical bacterial pneumonias. Disease-A-Month, February 1975.
42. Cunha, BA, Quintiliani, R: The atypical pneumonias. A diagnostic and therapeutic approach. Postgrad Med 66:95, 1979.
43. Murray, HW, Tuazon, C: Atypical pneumonias. Med Clin North Am, 64:507, 1980.
44. Shulman, JA, et al.: Errors and hazards in the diagnosis and treatment of bacterial pneumonias. Ann Intern Med 62:41, 1965.
45. Graham, WGB, Bradley, DA: Efficacy of chest physiotherapy and intermittent positive pressure breathing in the resolution of pneumonia. N Engl J Med 299:624, 1978.
46. Murray, HW, et al.: The protean manifestations of Mycoplasma pneumoniae infection in adults. Am J Med 58:229, 1975.

47. Cassell, GH, et al.: Mycoplasmas as agents of human disease. N Engl J Med 304:80, 1981.
48. Denny, FW, et al.: Mycoplasma pneumoniae disease: Clinical spectrum, pathophysiology, epidemiology, and control. J Infect Dis 123:74, 1971.
49. Mufson, MA, Zollar, LM: Nonbacterial respiratory infections. Disease-A-Month, November, 1975.
50. Knight, V: Influenza. Disease-A-Month, August 1976.
51. Kaye, D, et al.: Endemic influenza. II. The nature of the disease in the post-pandemic period. Am Rev Respir Dis 84:9, 1962.
52. Louria, DB, et al.: Studies of influenza in the pandemic of 1957–1958. II. Pulmonary complications of influenza. J Clin Invest 38:213, 1959.
53. Douglas, R: Influenza: The disease and its complications. Hosp Pract 11(12):43, 1976.
54. Mufson, MA, et al.: Eaton agent pneumonia—Clinical features. JAMA 178:369, 1961.
55. Bryant, RE, Rhoades, ER: Clinical features of adenoviral pneumonia in Air Force recruits. Am Rev Respir Dis 96:717, 1967.
56. Olson, RW, Hodges, GR: Measles pneumonia. Bacterial suprainfection as a complicating factor. JAMA 232:363, 1975.
57. Reichman, RC, Dolin, R: Viral pneumonias. Med Clin North Am, 64:491, 1980.
58. Treibwasser, JH et al.: Varicella pneumonia in adults. Medicine 46:409, 1967.
59. Schaffner, W, et al.: The clinical spectrum of endemic psittacosis. Arch Intern Med 119:433, 1967.
60. Covelli, HD, et al.: Psittacosis. Clinical presentation and therapeutic observations. West J Med 132:242, 1980.
61. Hueber, RJ, et al.: Q fever: A review. Ann Intern Med 30:495, 1949.
62. Denlinger, RB: Clinical aspects of Q fever in southern California. A study of 80 hospitalized cases. Ann Intern Med 30:510, 1949.
63. Van Metre, TE: Pneumococcal pneumonia treated with antibiotics: The prognostic significance of certain clinical findings. N Engl J Med 251:1048, 1954.
64. Austrian, R, Gold, J: Pneumococcal bacteremia with especial reference to bacteremic pneumococcal pneumonia. Ann Intern Med 60:759, 1964.
65. Brewin, A, et al.: High dose penicillin therapy and pneumococcal pneumonia. JAMA 230:409, 1974.
66. Reeves, JT, et al.: The treatment of moderate and severe pneumococcal pneumonia with oral phenoxymethyl penicillin. Arch Intern Med 103:184, 1958.
67. Hook, EW: Pneumococcal pneumonia. In Beeson, PB, McDermott, W, Wyngaarden, JB: Cecil's Textbook of Medicine, 15th ed. Philadelphia: WB Saunders, 1979, pp 347–357.
68. Jay, SJ et al.: The radiographic resolution of Streptococcus pneumoniae pneumonia. N Engl J Med 293:798, 1975.
69. Tuazon, CU: Gram-positive pneumonias. Med Clin North Am 64:343, 1980.
70. Smith, FE, Mann, JM: Pneumococcal pneumonia: Experience in a community hospital. West J Med 136:1–5, 1982.
71. Chickering, HT, Park, JH: Staphylococcus aureus pneumonia. JAMA 72:681, 1919.
72. Reyes, MP: The aerobic gram-negative bacillary pneumonias. Med Clin North Am 64:363, 1980.
73. Pierce, AK, Sanford, JP: Aerobic gram-negative bacillary pneumonias. Am Rev Respir Dis 110:647, 1974.
74. Bartlett, JG, Finegold, SN: Anaerobic infection of the lung and pleural space. Am Rev Respir Dis 110:56, 1974.
75. Johanson, WG, Harris, GD: Aspiration pneumonia, anaerobic infection, and lung abscess. Med Clin North Am 64:385, 1980.
76. Bartlett, JG, Finegold, SN: Anaerobic pleuropulmonary infections. Medicine 51:413–450, 1972.
77. Bartlett, JG, Finegold, SN: Anaerobic infections of the lung and pleural space. Am Rev Respir Dis 110:56–77, 1974.
78. Bartlett, JG, et al.: The bacteriology of aspiration pneumonia. Am J Med 56:202–207, 1974.
79. Tillotson, JR, Lerner, AM: Hemophilus influenzae bronchopneumonia in adults. Arch Intern Med 121:428, 1968.
80. Levin, DC, et al.: Bacteremic Hemophilus influenzae pneumonia in adults. Am J Med 62:219, 1977.
81. Sanford, JP: Legionnaire's disease—The first thousand days. N Engl J Med 300:654, 1979.
82. Beaty, HN, et al.: Legionnaire's disease in Vermont, May to October 1977. JAMA 240:127, 1978.
83. Balows, A, Fraser, DW (eds.): International Symposium on Legionnaire's Disease. Ann Intern Med 90:489, 1979.
84. Cordes, LG, Fraser, DW: Legionellosis: Legionnaire's disease; Pontiac fever. Med Clin North Am 64:395, 1980.
85. Kirby, BD, et al.: Legionnaire's disease: Report of 65 nosocomially acquired cases and review of the literature. Medicine 59:188, 1980.
86. Broome, CV, et al.: Rapid diagnosis of Legionnaire's disease by direct immunofluorescent staining. Ann Intern Med 90:1–4, 1979.
87. Rein, MF, et al.: Accuracy of Gram's stain in identifying pneumococci in sputum. JAMA 239:2671–2673, 1978.
88. Mufson, MA, et al.: The role of viruses, mycoplasmas, and bacteria in acute pneumonia in civilian adults. Am J Epidemiol 86:526, 1967.
89. Fiala, MA: Study of the combined role of viruses, mycoplasmas, and bacteria in adult pneumonia. Am J Med Sci 257:44, 1969.
90. Foy, HM, et al.: Viral and mycoplasmal pneumonia in a prepaid medical care group during an eight-year period. Am J Epidemiol 97:93, 1973.
91. Mostow, SR: Pneumonias acquired outside the hospital. Recognition and treatment. Med Clin North Am 58:555, 1974.
92. Sullivan, RJ, et al.: Adult pneumonia in a general hospital. Arch Intern Med 129:935, 1972.
93. Dorff, GJ, et al.: Etiologies and characteristic features of pneumonia in a municipal hospital. Am J Med Sci 266:349, 1973.
94. Garb, JL, et al.: Differences in etiology of pneumonia in nursing home and community patients. JAMA 240:2169, 1978.

95. McHenry, MC, et al.: Hospital-acquired pneumonia. Med Clin North Am 58:565, 1974.
96. Crane, LR, Lerner, AM: Gram-negative pneumonia in hospitalized patients. Postgrad Med 58:35, 1975.
97. Basiliere, JL, et al.: Steptococcal pneumonia. Am J Med 44:580, 1968.
98. Rose, HD, et al.: Meningococcal pneumonia. A source of nosocomial infection. Arch Intern Med 141:575–577, 1981.
99. Matthay, RA, Greene, WH: Pulmonary infections in the immunocompromised patient. Med Clin North Am 64:529, 1980.
100. Goodman, LR, et al.: The radiographic evaluation of pulmonary infection. Med Clin North Am 64:553, 1980.
101. Ziskind, MM, et al.: Incomplete consolidation in pneumococcal lobar pneumonia complicating pulmonary emphysema. Ann Intern Med 72:835, 1970.
102. Merrill, CW, et al.: Rapid identification of pneumococci. Gram's stain versus the quellung reaction. N Engl J Med 288:510, 1973.
103. Goodman, JS, Rogers, DE: Poorly resolving pneumonia. In Barondess, J (ed.): Diagnostic Approaches to Presenting Syndromes. Baltimore: Williams and Wilkins, 1971, pp 403–441.
104. Berger, HW, Granada, MG: Lower lung field tuberculosis. Chest 65:522, 1974.
105. Khan, MA, et al.: Clinical and roentgenographic spectrum of pulmonary tuberculosis in the adult. Am J Med 62:31, 1977.
106. Murray, RP, et al.: The acid-fast stain: A specific and predictive test for mycobacterial disease. Ann Intern Med 92:512, 1980.
107. Griffin, JP: Bedside cold agglutinins in the diagnosis of mycoplasma pneumonia. Ann Intern Med 70:701, 1969.
108. Barrett-Connor, E: The non-value of sputum culture in the diagnosis of pneumococcal pneumonia. Am Rev Respir Dis 103:845, 1971.
109. Drew, WL: Value of sputum culture in diagnosis of pneumococcal pneumonia. J Clin Microbiol 6:62, 1977.
110. Light, RW: Management of parapneumonic effusion. Arch Int Med 141:1339–1341, 1981.
111. Light, RW, et al.: Parapneumonic effusion. Am J Med 69:507–512, 1980.
112. Light, RW, et al.: Diagnostic significance of pleural fluid pH and PCO_2. Chest 64:591, 1973.
113. Sandweiss, DA, et al.: Ultrasound for diagnosis, localization and treatment of loculated pleural empyema. Ann Intern Med 82:50–53, 1975.
114. Morin, JE, et al.: Early thoracotomy for empyema. J Thorac Cardiovasc Surg 44:530–534, 1972
115. Bergh, NP, et al.: Intrapleural streptokinase in the treatment of hemothorax and empyema. Scand J Thorac Cardiovasc Surg 11:265–268, 1977.
116. Gottlieb, MS, et al.: Pneumocystis carinii pneumonia and mucosal candidiasis in previously healthy homosexual men. N Engl J Med 305:1425–1431, 1981.
117. Masur, H, et al.: An outbreak of community-acquired Pneumocystis carinii pneumonia. N Engl J Med 305:1431–1438, 1981.
118. Macher, A: Histoplasmosis and blastomycosis. Med Clin North Am 64:447–460, 1980.
119. Goodman, R, DesPrez, R: Histoplasmosis. Am Rev Respir Dis 117:929, 1978.
120. Cantanzaro, A: Pulmonary coccidioidomycosis. Med Clin North Am 64(3):461–474, 1980.
121. Foy, HM, et al.: Mycoplasma pneumoniae pneumonia in an urban area. JAMA 214:1606, 1970
122. Foy, HM, et al.: Radiographic study of Mycoplasma pneumoniae pneumonia. Am Rev Respir Dis 108:469, 1973.
123. Putman, CE, et al.: Mycoplasma pneumonia, clinical and roentgenographic patterns. Am J Roentgenol 124:417, 1975.
124. Tager, I, Speizer, FE: Role of infection in chronic bronchitis. N Engl J Med 292:563, 1975.
125. Shwachman, H, et al.: Cystic fibrosis: A new outlook. Medicine 56:129, 1977.
126. Rosenstein, BJ, et al.: Cystic fibrosis. Problems encountered with sweat testing. JAMA 240:1987, 1978.
127. Morse, JO: Alpha₁ antitrypsin deficiency. N Engl J Med 299:1045, 1099, 1978.
128. Kueppers, F, Black, LF: Alpha₁ antitrypsin and its deficiency. Am Rev Respir Dis 110:176, 1974.
129. Hermans, PE, et al.: Idiopathic late-onset immunoglobulin deficiency. Clinical observations in 50 patients. Am J Med 61:221, 1976.
130. Eliasson, R, et al.: The immotile cilia syndrome. A congenital ciliary abnormality as an etiologic factor in chronic airways infection and male sterility. N Engl J Med 297:1, 1977.
131. Sturgess, JM, et al.: Cilia with defective radial spokes. A cause of human respiratory disease. N Engl J Med 300:53, 1979.
132. Richardson, RH, et al.: The use of fiberoptic bronchoscopy and brush biopsy in the diagnosis of suspected pulmonary malignancy. Am Rev Respir Dis 109:63, 1974.
133. Epler, GR, et al.: Normal chest roentgenogram in chronic diffuse infiltrative lung disease. N Engl J Med 298:934, 1978.
134. Lertzman, MM, Cherniack, RM: Rehabilitation of patients with chronic obstructive pulmonary disease. Am Rev Respir Dis 114:1145, 1976.
135. Burrows, B, Earle, RH: Course and prognosis of chronic obstructive lung disease. A prospective study of 200 patients. N Engl J Med 280:397, 1969.
136. McCarthy, DS, et al.: Effect of modification of the smoking habit on lung function. Am Rev Respir Dis 114:113, 1976.
137. Bates, DV: The fate of the chronic bronchitic: A report of the ten-year followup in the Canadian Department of Veterans' Affairs Coordinated Study of Chronic Bronchitis. Am Rev Respir Dis 108:1043, 1973.
138. Moffett, HL: Common infections in ambulatory patients. Ann Intern Med 89(part 2):743, 1978.
139. Thomas, L.: On the science and technology of medicine. In Knowles, J (ed.): Doing Better and Feeling Worse. New York: WW Norton, 1977, pp 35–46.
140. Lazare, A, et al.: The customer approach to patienthood. Arch Gen Psychiatry, 32:553, 1975.
141. Louie, MH, et al.: Branhamella catarrhalis pneumonia. West J Med 138: 47–49, 1983.

13

CHEST PAIN

EPISODIC (RECURRENT) CHEST PAIN.............. 678

Typical Angina Pectoris........................ 682
Nonangina...................................... 687
"Compatible" Chest Pain....................... 693
Physical Examination........................... 694
Chest-Wall Syndromes 698
Tests and Chest Pain.......................... 705

MANAGEMENT OF ANGINA PECTORIS.............. 713

Drug Therapy................................... 713
Coronary Artery Surgery....................... 718
Patient Education.............................. 720
When to Worry, When to Refer, When to
Hospitalize.................................... 725

ACUTE SEVERE CHEST PAIN 727

ACUTE PLEURITIC CHEST PAIN 741

APPENDIX I: EXERCISE TESTING AND
CHEST PAIN: POPULATIONS AND PERSONS 754

APPENDIX II: ESOPHAGEAL CHEST PAIN 766

APPENDIX III: PSYCHOSOMATIC CHEST PAIN...... 770

APPENDIX IV: LUNG SCANS AND PULMONARY
EMBOLISM 772

REFERENCES..................................... 780

Chest pain may be caused by so many different clinical entities that any general overview of the problem tends to be either too superficial or too encyclopedic to be practically useful. Each of the individual diseases that may cause chest pain can be touched upon only briefly and inadequately here. Such disclaimers aside, the experienced clinician does usually follow a systematic (if often subconscious) practical strategy when confronted by the patient with chest pain, and it is this strategy that is our subject here.

In general, the specific clinical strategy useful in a given patient will vary according to which of three common situations pertains: (1) the patient with episodic, recurrent chest pain; (2) the patient with acute pleuritic chest pain; (3) the patient with acute nonpleuritic chest pain. As Table 13–1 suggests, the diagnostic emphasis varies for each of these different clinical situations, even though there is considerable overlap among them in differential diagnosis. Thus these clinical presentations are considered separately here but not because the diagnostic possibilities for each subset are mutually exclusive. They are not. A single disease entity (for example, coronary artery disease or a chest-wall disorder or esophageal disease) may result in any or all of these three clinical presentations over the course of its own natural history. Moreover, many patients have more than one type of chest pain simultane-

TABLE 13–1. DIAGNOSTIC EMPHASIS ACCORDING TO CLINICAL
PRESENTATION OF CHEST PAIN

ACUTE NONPLEURITIC CHEST PAIN	EPISODIC RECURRENT CHEST PAIN	ACUTE PLEURITIC CHEST PAIN
Myocardial infarction	Angina pectoris	Pleurisy
Pericarditis	Chest-wall disorder	Pneumonia
Aortic dissection	Hyperventilation/anxiety	Pericarditis
Pulmonary embolism	Esophageal disease	Pulmonary embolism
Cholecystitis	Others (see Table 13–2)	Chest-wall disorders
Others (see Table 13–14)		Others (see Table 13–16)

ously—two typical clinical syndromes that coexist may produce a combined presentation that is puzzlingly atypical.

Nevertheless, the practical diagnostic approach to each of these three subsets of chest pain does tend to follow a distinctive pattern or flow. For each subset, the emphasis on specific aspects of the history and physical examination and the need for (and timing of) various diagnostic tests, consultations, or hospitalization will be somewhat different.

CONSIDER

> Angela Angina, a 53-year-old secretary, enters the clinic asking for advice about recurrent chest pain. For the past 6 months, Angela has experienced episodic anterior chest pains that have recently occurred almost every day, although, "Naturally, I don't have it when I come to the doctor." Angela has always been healthy in the past but has been told that "I am overweight and my blood pressure is on the border line." One month ago, Angela's younger brother died suddenly of myocardial infarction and "so I am worried about my heart."

> When asked to describe her chest pain, Angela says, "It catches me around my heart (she points to the left submammary area) or sometimes inside my breast bone (she points to the lower sternum). It feels like getting stabbed with a knife, and then it will ache like someone keeps twisting the knife inside me. It doesn't usually last very long—a few minutes, maybe—but a few times it has lasted much longer, and I just can't figure out what is doing it, so here I am."

EPISODIC (RECURRENT) CHEST PAIN

Causes of episodic chest pain are listed in Table 13–2. The breadth of this differential diagnosis can be intimidating. Nevertheless, a careful clinical history and examination will usually distinguish among these many different entities. Sometimes the history will be unmistakably typical of a specific disorder: This is common among patients with angina pectoris, esophagitis, anxiety or hyperventilation, as well as some of the specific chest-wall disorders (see page 698). At other times, the history is less specific but at least strongly suggests one general type of chest pain, for example, chest-wall pain. While there will always be patients with chest pain who would tax even Osler's clinical skills, it is unusual to be just as confused about the cause of a particular patient's chest pain after taking a careful history as before. We shall see that the clinical history is always the most important diagnostic information—subsequent evaluation depends utterly on the history elicited.

Nevertheless, the degree of diagnostic confidence the clinician can derive from the history depends upon more than just the skill and patience with

TABLE 13–2. CAUSES OF EPISODIC CHEST PAIN

CHEST WALL	GASTROINTESTINAL	PSYCHOGENIC	OTHER CARDIOPULMONARY DISEASE	ANGINA PECTORIS
Costochondritis	Esophagitis	Hyperventilation	Mitral valve prolapse	Typical angina
Cervical/thoracic spine disease	Esophageal spasm	Anxiety	Pulmonary embolism	Atypical angina
Tietze's syndrome	Peptic ulcer disease	Hypochondriasis	Pleuritis	
Rib fractures	Cholecystitis/biliary colic	Depression	Bronchitis/asthma	
Xiphoidalgia	Pancreatitis	Malingering	Pericarditis	
Myodynia	Colonic flexure syndrome	Cardiac neurosis		
Fibrositis				
Breast disorders				
Mondor's disease				
Herpes zoster				
Slipping rib				
Pectoral muscle syndromes				
Thoracic outlet syndromes				
Sternoclavicular disease				

which the history is obtained. Several issues often conspire to muddle the diagnostic value of the clinical history in patients with chest pain. Constant reminds us of these issues when he warns of a common clinical misperception, pointing out that some think

> there are only two types of chest pain, typical angina and atypical angina. There is a reluctance to add a third category—nonangina. Patients with peculiar chest pain who are found to have significant coronary disease tend to be classified as having atypical angina. Thus, the idea of nonanginal pain is thrust increasingly into limbo as a most unlikely and rare cause of chest pain.[1]

This reminder illustrates three important generalizations about episodic chest pain:

1. Coronary artery disease is not the most common cause of episodic chest pain. The problem of ischemic heart disease is, understandably, so preeminent in the minds (and hearts?) of patients and physicians that the diagnosis or exclusion of coronary artery disease (CAD) often becomes the clinician's obsessive concern, regardless of the history. Sometimes this concern can be counterproductive. Because of our preoccupation with CAD, clinicians will often pursue various tests to diagnose or exclude CAD even when the patient's chest pain is clearly not angina pectoris by history. While such a strategy is usually well intentioned, it often leads to the abuse (and even misinterpretation) of diagnostic tests. The importance of the concept of "nonangina" lies in its allowing the clinician to avoid such tests and to concentrate on a differential diagnosis that does not include angina pectoris.

Table 13–3 contrasts the characteristics of episodic chest pain that are *typical* of angina pectoris with those pain characteristics that *exclude* angina pectoris. These symptoms will be discussed in greater detail below. Notice, however, that the symptoms of nonangina do not simply reflect the absence of typical anginal symptoms—the symptoms of nonangina serve as specific *positive* identifying characteristics whose presence *excludes* angina pectoris from consideration. Recognition of nonangina is only a first step, since the clinician must, of course, still distinguish among the other cardiopulmonary, gastrointestinal, chest-wall, and psychogenic syndromes that may cause nonangina (Table 13–2). Nevertheless, early recognition of chest pain as definite nonangina is very helpful in orienting subsequent clinical strategies. (Notice also that many patients with episodic chest pain do not readily fit into either category in Table 13–3. Such patients thus have neither typical angina pectoris nor definite nonangina—here the differential diagnosis cannot be so readily narrowed—see pages 693 and 695, Figure 13–5.)

2. Diagnostic tests in the evaluation of chest pain may be either helpful or misleading, depending on the patient's clinical history. In general, the usefulness of a test depends on the diagnostic information it *adds* to the clinical impression derived from the patient's history and physical examination. This seems obvious enough, but Constant's warning reminds us that the clinician sometimes allows the test results to interpret the history, rather than vice versa.

The use of exercise testing in the diagnosis of coronary artery disease—discussed briefly in Appendix I—exemplifies some of these interrelations. For example, a positive exercise test in a patient whose chest pain is definitely not angina (by history) is usually a false positive. As such, the rationale for performing the test in the first place is questionable. The actual interpretation of the test often depends as much on the patient tested as on the test result itself. Similarly, a negative exercise test in the patient with typical angina pectoris is often falsely negative and does not necessarily argue against the diagnosis of coronary artery disease.

The temptation to attribute more diagnostic importance to objective test results than to a subjective (but careful) clinical history and examination is understandable but will often be misleading.

TABLE 13–3. CHARACTERISTICS OF TYPICAL ANGINA PECTORIS AND DEFINITE NONANGINA

CHARACTERISTIC	TYPICAL ANGINA	DEFINITE NONANGINA
Onset and precipitating factor	Usually sudden onset during physical exertion (especially climbing, after meals, in cold or wind; hurrying) and/or emotional stress Sometimes only at rest, during sexual intercourse, after meals, when upset	Induced by: Bending forward Local chest-wall pressure Respiration Sudden single motion of torso or arm(s)
Duration	Usually 1–15 min subjectively; when actually timed ≤ 5 min	"A second" or constant (hours, days) > 1 hr, as a rule
Predictable relief	Rest; nitroglycerin	Immediately upon lying down
Location	Usually restrosternal; sometimes epigastric, neck, throat, jaw, arms, or interscapular area	Not helpful
Quality	Heavy, constricting, choking, tight Levine's sign (Fig. 13–2)	Not helpful

3. The designation "atypical chest pain" is more a camouflage than a diagnosis. Occasionally, when even a probing history and careful physical examination do not narrow the differential diagnosis, the tentative diagnosis of atypical chest pain may be applied. In such circumstances, there is a common tendency to "rule out" serious diseases by extensive testing for disorders that could uncommonly present atypically and that are detectable by objective tests. Unfortunately, when such tests are positive, this often results in misdiagnosis—the patient's atypical pain is "explained away" by angiographically proven (but in fact asymptomatic) coronary artery disease, for example. Unnecessary treatment is thus begun. More often, the tests are negative, and this too may result in misinformation—the patient is told that the tests are normal: thus, the pain is "not serious" or is "probably psychosomatic."

Sometimes this "rule-out approach" is unavoidable. Indeed, some causes of chest pain may produce symptoms that are unpredictable, qualitatively peculiar, and difficult to pin down even after a very careful interview and examination. "Rule-out testing" may then be necessary. (Mitral valve prolapse, anxiety disorders, and unusual cases of esophageal spasm or variant angina will cause atypical chest pain.) As a general strategy, however, every attempt should be made to minimize the number of patients with chest pain approached in this way. Too often, atypical chest pain is a meaningless label applied to symptoms that are not deemed typical of any of the disorders listed in Table 13–2 precisely because the history and examination are too hurried or too inattentive to be more discriminating.

How then does the clinician precisely diagnose the cause of episodic chest pain in a thorough but practical and cost-conscious manner?

The most important initial step is to discriminate among the three general historical types of episodic chest pain:

1. Typical angina pectoris. As Table 13–3 notes, typical angina refers to brief episodic discomfort in the chest, neck, or arms that is precipitated by physical exertion or emotional stress and is quickly relieved by rest (or nitroglycerin). Most patients with typical angina pectoris will describe a symptom complex that is itself virtually diagnostic (see below).

2. Definite nonangina. As noted above, identifying this subset of patients allows the clinician to forgo consideration of (symptomatic) coronary artery disease and to concentrate on a distinctive differential diagnosis. In fact, specific nonanginal symptoms (Table 13–3) often point to specific diagnoses. For example, pain readily induced by bending forward is often due to esophagitis or chest-wall disorders. Chest pain that is fleetingly transient (a "second" or a "quick stab") is usually psychogenic or musculoskeletal in origin. Respirophasic chest pain has its own differential diagnosis (see "Pleuritic Chest Pain," page 741).

3. Compatible chest pain. This subset includes patients whose chest pain is not typical of angina pectoris but who do not describe definite nonanginal symptoms either. As such, the chest pain is "compatible with" any or all of the disorders listed in Table 13–2 except typical angina. When this is the case, specific characteristics of the history and physical examination usually point to a specific diagnosis (see Fig. 13–5, page 695). Nevertheless, this is the group in whom diagnostic testing is most often necessary.

It may not be at all obvious that this subclassification of episodic chest pain is helpful. Often it is superfluous; for example, when the patient

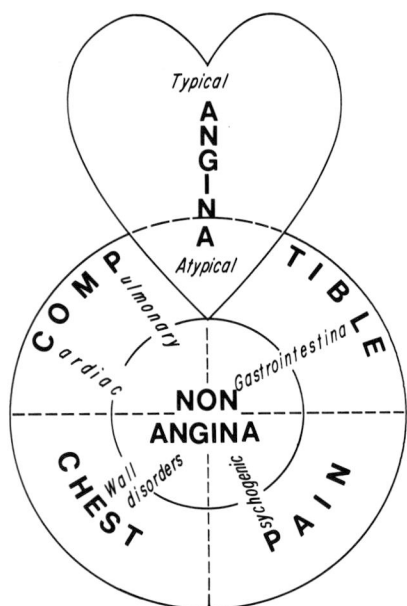

FIGURE 13–1. The three clinical subsets of episodic chest pain: typical angina, nonangina, and compatible chest pain.

describes a symptom complex that readily identifies the problem as one of the specific entities listed in Table 13–2. However, even the experienced clinician commonly encounters patients whose chest pain cannot be so confidently pigeon-holed. In such circumstances, this initial subclassification can be very useful.

The interrelationships among these three clinical types or subsets of episodic chest pain are schematized in Figure 13–1. The large circle represents all causes of episodic chest pain listed in Table 13–2 except for typical angina pectoris. The "heart" represents angina pectoris, in its typical and atypical presentations.

Most of the time, angina pectoris is typical—when this is so, the diagnosis is not usually confused with other types of episodic chest pain; hence, most of the heart does not overlap the circle in Figure 13–1. Sometimes, however, angina pectoris is atypical or is difficult to distinguish from other causes of episodic chest pain—here the circle and the heart intersect.

The clinical value of recognizing definite nonangina is illustrated by the small circle (the hole in the doughnut). The differential diagnosis of definite nonangina includes many causes of episodic chest pain but not (typical or atypical) angina.

The subset of "compatible chest pain" is represented by the doughnut itself. Here, symptoms are compatible with all types of chest pain listed in Table 13–2, but symptoms are neither typical of angina pectoris nor are they definitely nonanginal. A few such patients have atypical angina, but most do not.

As we shall see, it is only the persistent and inquisitive clinical historian who can use this scheme to good advantage; such an approach can greatly reduce the number of patients whose chest pain remains so puzzling or atypical that extensive "rule-out testing" must be employed. Thus, greater familiarity with each of these clinical subsets is crucial. Consider, in more detail, the problem of:

Typical Angina Pectoris

There is a common impression that angina pectoris may have such diverse clinical manifestations that reliance on the clinical history alone often leads to diagnostic errors. It is true that atypical angina is not rare, especially when one considers the spectrum of patients' reliability as historians as well as the popularization of different anginal syndromes—variant (Prinzmetal's) angina,[2] unstable angina,[3, 4] coronary insufficiency,[5] and angina equivalents.[6] Increased awareness of the role of coronary artery spasm[7, 8] and the syndrome of angina pectoris with normal coronary arteries[9-11] threatens to confuse matters even more. Nevertheless, most patients with angina pectoris have typical or classic angina (Table 13–3). Conversely, atypical angina is a common problem only if one too narrowly restricts the definition of typical angina or disregards the changing clinical characteristics of typical angina pectoris as its natural history evolves over time.

William Herberden recognized much of this over 200 years ago, and his description of *pectoris dolor* remains vividly instructive today:

> There is a disorder of the breast marked with strong and peculiar symptoms . . . the seat of it, and sense of strangling, and anxiety with which it is attended, may make it not improperly be called angina pectoris.
>
> They who are afflicted with it are seized while they are walking (more especially if it be uphill, and soon after eating) with a painful and most disagreeable sensation in the breast, which seems as if it would extinguish life, if it were to increase or continue; but the moment they stand still, all the uneasiness vanishes.
>
> In all other respects, the patients are, at the beginning of this disorder, perfectly well . . . the pain is sometimes situated in the upper part, sometimes in the middle, sometimes at the bottom of the os sterni, and often more inclined to the left than to the right side. It likewise very frequently extends from the breast to the middle of the left arm . . .
>
> After it has continued a year or more, it will not cease so instantaneously upon standing still; and it will come on not only when the persons are walking, but when they are lying down . . . and oblige them to rise up out of their beds. In some inveterate cases, it has been brought on by the motion of a horse, or a carriage, and even by swallowing, coughing, going to stool, or speaking, or any disturbance of mind.[12]

NOTE

1. The patient is "seized" suddenly and episodically. The patient with typical angina is asymptomatic between episodes.

2. The location of angina pectoris is usually retrosternal, i.e., behind the sternum, but it may be highly variable in different patients. Angina may appear anywhere in the anterior chest, neck, throat, or jaw or in either (or both) shoulder or arm. Epigastric or posterior chest (especially interscapular) locations are not at all rare. Each *individual* patient, however, usually develops symptoms of his or her angina in a predictable, unvarying location.

3. The symptom of angina (Table 13–4) is "disagreeable" but "peculiar"—angina is often not easy to describe qualitatively. Even the most articulate patients may use "Levine's sign" (Fig. 13–2) to explain themselves—a clenched fist placed over the sternum to elaborate on the verbal inadequacy of the commonly used descriptives—"pressing," "tightness," "constriction," "a vise around my chest." Such sensations are often not described as "pain." Many patients with classic angina pectoris will deny chest "pain" of any kind.*

4. Physical exertion is the usual, but not the only, precipitating factor. Physical exercise that causes a sustained increase in myocardial oxygen

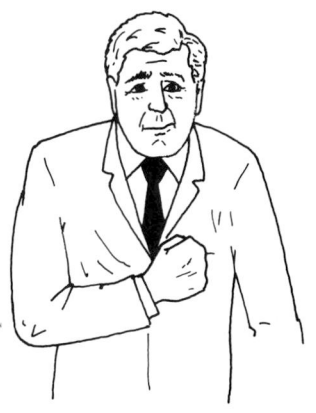

FIGURE 13–2. Levine's sign.

---

*While our concern here is the patient with episodic chest pain, some patients with angina pectoris manifest their symptoms in the form of angina equivalents. Such symptoms include dyspnea on exertion, paroxysmal cough on exertion, exertional syncope or presyncope, palpitations, or episodic exertional sweating.[6]

TABLE 13–4. SYMPTOMS OF ANGINA PECTORIS

Always *episodic*	
Often not a "pain" at all	
Exertional, usually	Remember the *pace* of exercise, associated emotional *stress,* and environmental conditions affect the anginal threshold
Occurs at rest?	May be unstable/progressive angina, variant angina (coronary spasm), or *not angina at all*
Duration *brief*	
Location highly variable among different patients, but usually stereotyped in individual patients	

demand—by increasing the pulse, blood pressure, and myocardial contractility—is the usual precipitant of angina pectoris. In fact, typical angina is often called "exertional" angina. Thus, as Heberden says, "walking, more especially if it be uphill" is a typical provocation, but sustained use of the arms—for example, washing windows—may be just as strenuous.* Under controlled circumstances, i.e., in the cardiac exercise laboratory, angina tends to be a predictable, reproducible phenomenon at certain levels of energy expenditure—thus, in an individual patient, typical angina is expected at a certain heart rate after a certain level of cardiac work ("aerobic capacity") is achieved. (This predictability can be helpful in the management of angina pectoris—see page 720—since patients can then be counseled to exercise within limits.)

However, daily life is hardly a controlled environment. Many different precipitating factors commonly add up to induce angina pectoris at lower than predicted levels of cardiac exercise. Thus, sometimes, chest pain may seem unlike typical angina pectoris if symptoms do not *always* correlate well with the degree or predictability of physical exertion that causes discomfort. In fact, it is not at all unusual for patients with typical angina pectoris to note that on some days they can "climb that hill without any trouble," and yet on other days just climbing a few stairs brings on their pain. Such a pain pattern should not be dismissed as atypical of angina pectoris, since the emotional energy expended during a given amount of physical work may determine whether that level of physical work induces angina pectoris. The carefree, unhurried angina patient can often achieve exercise levels that exceed his or her "aerobic capacity" when frustrated, tense, angry, worried, or impatient.

Thus the pace and familiarity of physical exertion may be as important as the quantitative myocardial oxygen demand imposed by such exercise. The patient who hurries to a destination will often experience angina early (for example, after the first block of a mile walk) but after a brief rest will endure more prolonged exercise (for example, the rest of the mile walk) without any symptoms. Mild exercise in an emotionally charged setting may induce angina in the patient with otherwise excellent exercise tolerance— sexual intercourse, for example, may be more exciting than strenuous, but it is the combined influence of emotion and exertion that often matters here.

---

*Probably the best "screening test" for angina is the question, "How do you feel when you walk a long way up a hill?"

Thus, various "nonaerobic" factors can influence the "anginal threshold." Different types of emotional stress are the most prevalent of these. Mild physical exertion immediately after a heavy meal or in very cold or windy weather is another common example.[13]

Typical angina then may occur at rest, during sleep, after eating, or during emotional stress, as well as during physical exertion. It is, however, unusual for angina to develop in an individual *only* during emotional stresses or after meals or during sleep, and yet *not* occur during vigorous physical exercise.[13] When this is the case, as Heberden himself recognized, it often reflects progression of symptomatic coronary artery disease from typical exertional angina to a more advanced and "unstable" pattern (see page 725).

Remember that sometimes, the patient who presents with nonexertional chest pain has so self-restricted physical exertion (*because of* progressive angina) that the change from typical exertional angina to (unstable) "rest angina" is inapparent. Such a history may be especially elusive in the anxious or sedentary patient who is a vague historian. In such patients, progressive unstable angina (page 725) may be mistaken for nonischemic chest pain—a potentially disastrous oversight. Thus, chest pain that occurs only at rest is not necessarily atypical of angina—such patients must be carefully questioned about previous precipitating factors. Always ask the patient with episodic chest pain what the pain used to be like when it first began.

Rest angina due to coronary artery spasm is *usually* typical of angina pectoris in all respects except that it occurs at rest. Such pain may recur at predictable times of day (commonly in the middle of the night).

5. The duration of angina is usually brief, but the "anxiety with which it is attended" often distorts the patient's subjective sense of time. In one study,[13] objective measurement of duration of typical angina showed that most attacks actually lasted only 2 or 3 minutes; many of these patients, however, subjectively described durations up to, and sometimes beyond, 15 minutes.

Since the clinician only rarely has the opportunity to observe an actual episode of angina, it is the patient's subjective description that usually matters: Typical angina rarely lasts more than "20 or 30 minutes." When episodic chest pain is *usually* more prolonged than this, it is not typical angina, but the patient's reliability as "timer" must be questioned. (Asking the patient to "clock" his symptoms is always informative—to the patient and the clinician.)

Occasionally the patient with typical angina purposefully challenges himself or herself by continuing painful exercise: Under these circumstances, typical angina may be atypically prolonged. Otherwise, prolonged chest pain is either not due to angina pectoris or represents a more serious complication of coronary artery disease—acute coronary insufficiency, impending myocardial infarction, or unstable angina (see below).

6. Angina does not always "cease instantaneously upon standing still," but, in general, exertional angina is relieved by rest within a few minutes. This does not mean that rest is a necessary requirement for the relief of pain—some patients can "walk through" their angina by subtly slowing the pace of exercise without actually stopping.

These variables in timing help us understand some of the difficulties in deciding whether nitroglycerin relieves the patient's pain—an important historical clue in the diagnosis of angina pectoris. Angina may be so brief in duration, or so poorly timed by the patient, or so quickly relieved by other factors (for example, rest) that subsidence of pain after the administration of nitroglycerin may not be necessarily related to the nitroglycerin. In general, it takes nitroglycerin 1 to 2 minutes to take effect pharmacologically—truly *immediate* relief or relief only after "15 to 20 minutes" is not typical of angina pectoris.[14] (An occasional patient with definite angina will demonstrate a delayed response to nitroglycerin—in such patients relief may not occur until 10 to 15 minutes have passed.)

Figure 13–3 illustrates the general approach to the patient with symptoms typical of angina pectoris. It must be remembered that angina pectoris is a clinical syndrome and not a specific diagnosis. In other words, while angina pectoris usually reflects coronary artery disease, a variety of other cardiac diseases may cause otherwise typical angina—valvular aortic stenosis, asymmetric septal hypertrophy, and severe pulmonary arterial hypertension are examples. Similarly, a variety of noncardiac syndromes may seem to exactly mimic typical angina pectoris—esophageal disease (see Appendix II), various chest-wall syndromes (page 698), and hyperventilation with or without anxiety (see Appendix III) are most common.

These qualifiers do not devalue the importance of recognizing typical angina. The diagnostic (Figure 13–3) and therapeutic (page 713) orientation such a history provides is very different from that which is necessary in patients with less specific "compatible" chest pain (see page 693) or those with:

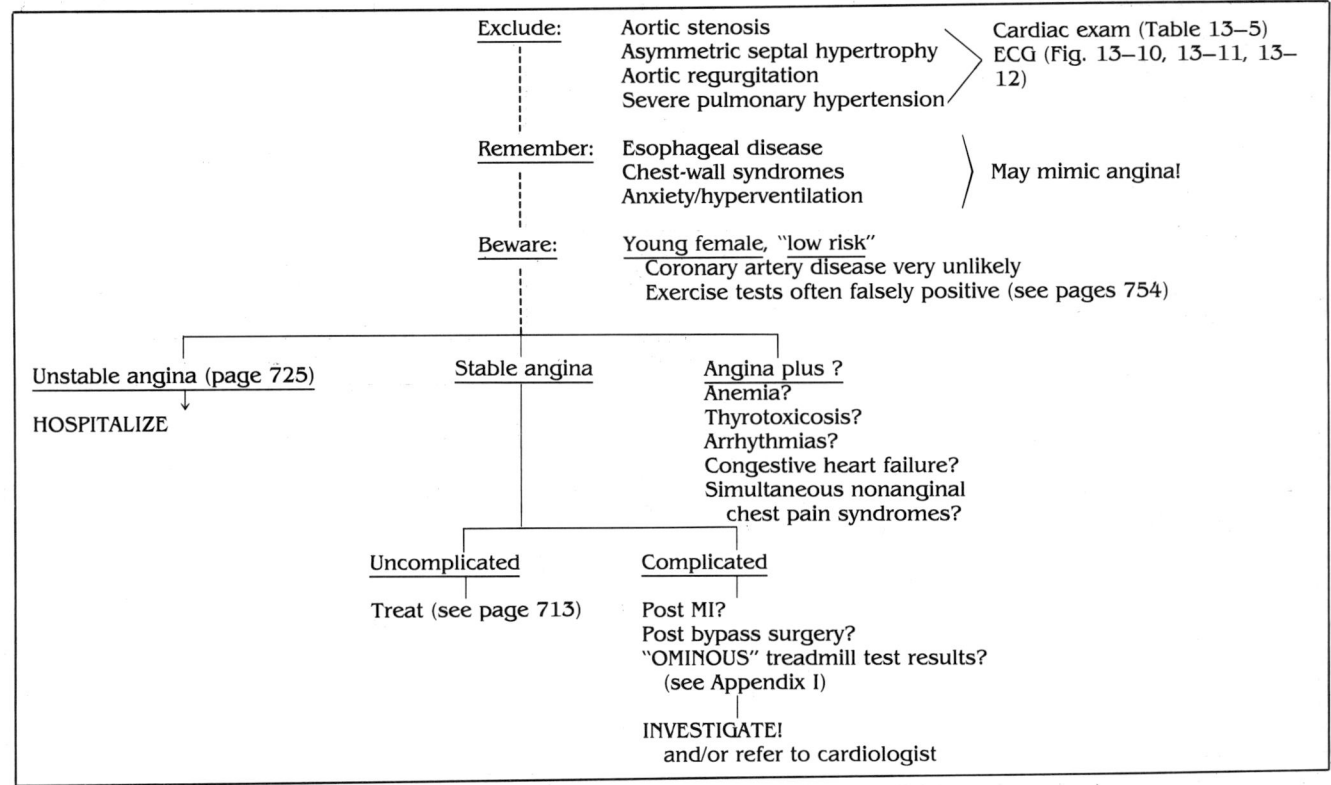

FIGURE 13–3. Typical angina pectoris.

Nonangina[1, 14, 15]

Table 13-2 lists symptom characteristics of episodic chest pain that can exclude angina pectoris from further consideration (remember that such symptoms by no means exclude *asymptomatic* coronary artery disease)—the clinician must be careful here because some patients will have more than one type of chest pain simultaneously. It is at least fair to say that nonanginal symptoms imply that chest pain is not *only* due to angina. Again, such symptoms may be very helpful diagnostically, because as Constant says,

> If a patient has a classic history of typical angina but has one nonanginal symptom, then that symptom cancels out all the typical anginal symptoms. This is because such thoracic origins of pain as esophageal spasm can mimic angina *almost* completely but there will *almost* always be one nonanginal symptom to help discount all the others (emphasis added).[1]

As with typical angina pectoris, the most telling symptom characteristics are timing, duration, and precipitating and relieving factors. The quality and location of pain are not so helpful.

NOTE

1. The timing and duration of pain.

Episodic chest pain that is constantly present for days, weeks, or longer is not angina. Such pain is usually psychogenic or originates in the chest wall (pages 698 and 770).

Chest pain that comes and goes in a "second" is not angina. The most common causes of such symptoms are psychogenic or chest-wall syndromes. Occasionally, mitral valve prolapse will be discovered in such patients. Remember that some patients with chronic, typical stable angina can recognize its onset so early that immediate rest from exercise will make the symptoms go away in "just a second."

Episodically recurrent chest pain that *usually* lasts more than 1 hour is not angina. Gastrointestinal disorders (especially biliary colic or peptic ulcer disease), chest-wall syndromes, and anxiety are more common causes of such prolonged chest pain.

Remember that patients with myocardial infarction or other prolonged ischemic events (for example, due to cardiac tachyarrhythmia) do experience prolonged chest pain. Certainly, then, one episode of prolonged pain (see page 692) by no means excludes symptomatic coronary artery disease, but repetitive episodes of such prolonged pain recurring over many months or years—especially when more typical previous angina is denied—will almost never be angina. *Very recent onset* (days or weeks) of recurrent, prolonged "anginal" pain must raise suspicion of "crescendo" or unstable angina (see page 725).

2. Precipitating factors.

Chest pain induced by or exacerbated by respiration is not angina. Angina may be accompanied by dyspnea or tachypnea (but it often is not), but angina is never respirophasic (pleuritic). Respirophasic chest pain has a distinctive differential diagnosis (see page 741).

Chest pain that is precipitated by bending forward is not angina. Such a story should suggest esophagitis, chest-wall syndromes, or psychogenic factors. (Remember that a precise history is always important: bending over—to tie a shoe?—during a long walk uphill may seem to "cause" the angina.

Chest pain that is reproduced or precipitated by local pressure on the chest is not angina. Such symptoms usually implicate one of several chest-wall syndromes (see page 698).

Chest pain brought on by a sudden, single movement of the torso or arm is not angina. Exertional chest pain must be carefully analyzed: Pain brought on by exercise that, in fact, involves a single brief movement to reach overhead, rotate the neck or chest, lean forward, push forward with the arms, or lift a light object (once) is not angina, as a rule. (Certainly the cumulative toll of such movements repeated again and again—during vacuuming, for example, or stocking a cabinet or a truck—may well induce angina.)

3. Relieving factors.

Chest pain that is always immediately relieved by lying down is not angina. If anything, the supine position lowers the "anginal threshold" (perhaps by increasing myocardial preload)—one form of unstable angina is angina decubitus where lying, especially on the left side, seems to induce angina.

Similarly, relief of those factors that typically precipitate nonangina does not relieve angina. For example, holding one's breath, standing upright (after bending), avoiding the local painful area on the chest wall, or holding the arms and chest motionless after a sudden painful twist or movement does not relieve angina pectoris.

(The pitfalls here are obvious: the patient experiencing angina may well stand still, try to relax the breathing, and hold the arms and chest motionless, and may even eventually lie down to rest.)

4. The quality and location of pain are not so helpful.

Angina may be so qualitatively imprecise and so diverse in location that there are few descriptions or locations that will exclude angina. It is, however, very rare for patients with angina to describe their chest symptoms as "tingling" or as "electric shocks" (although such symptoms in the arms or hands will sometimes coexist with typical angina). Chest pain located with one finger "over the heart" (the submammary area) is rarely angina. Similarly, associated lower abdominal, lower back, or leg symptoms are not due to angina. (However, anxiety induced by angina may be sufficient to distort perceptions such that secondary "functional" symptoms—aches all over—will occasionally produce peculiar pain radiation.)

It is then the other characteristics of pain that are most important—the timing and duration as well as the precipitating and relieving factors. "Tingling" pain in the right shoulder is most unlikely to be angina, but it certainly is suspicious if such symptoms occur only during physical exertion, last a few minutes, and are always relieved by rest or nitroglycerin.

Thus it can be seen that the history must be very carefully recorded if reliable distinctions between typical angina pectoris and definite nonangina are to be made. When the history (for whatever reason) does not allow such clear distinctions, the episodic chest pain is initially categorized as "compatible" chest pain (see page 693). Distinctions among these three historical types of chest pain will perhaps be more clear after considering again Angela Angina, our patient with episodic chest pain (who has been waiting anxiously on page 678):

"Angela, you say these pains have been happening to you for the past 6 months?"

"Yes."

"Before 6 months ago, did you ever experience chest pain?"

"No."

"And these pains now occur every day?"

"Yes, now almost every day. At first, I only got a pain once in a while, maybe once a week or so, but now I get them more often."

"What seems to you to cause the pain?"

"I don't know. That's why I'm here."

"Well, do you relate the pain to anything in particular?"

"I've tried to, but I can't."

"For instance, are you just as likely to get this pain when you are sitting down and resting as when you are up and around, working or exercising?"

"Oh, it usually happens when I'm busy doing something. Like if I vacuum the house, that gives me the pain sometimes. Or after I get out of bed in the morning and do a few chores before work, I might get it then, too." [ANGINA?]

"What kind of chores?"

"Oh, bringing up the laundry from the basement maybe, or putting wood on the fire. Things like that."

"What if you walk a long way up a hill?"

"I don't know. I don't walk up hills. I do walk three blocks from the bus to work every day—that doesn't bother me."

"What is the most strenuous physical exercise you do?"

"Not much. Vacuuming, maybe."

"What if you hurry while walking?"

"I don't usually hurry."

"You get the chest pain when you vacuum?"

"Sometimes. Not always."

"How much vacuuming do you do before it comes on?"

"It varies. Sometimes it comes on right when I start to vacuum."

"Do you ever get the pain just sitting still, doing nothing?"

"No, I guess not."

"When you get a pain—let's say when you're vacuuming—what do you do?"

"I just rest a minute or two and then it gets better." [ANGINA?]

"After it gets better, will it come back if you resume vacuuming?"

"Sometimes."

"If you don't stop vacuuming, what happens to the pain?"

"I don't know. I always stop."

"You say the pain lasts 'a minute or two.' A minute is a long time. Do you mean seconds or minutes?"

"I guess the average is 2 or 3 minutes." [ANGINA?]

"What would you say is the longest it lasts?"

"I'm not sure. Sometimes it will last longer—a half hour maybe. I did have one bad spell a few weeks back when I had a pain that lasted most of the day, and I got real sick and threw up, but I'm not sure that was the same thing. I think I ate something bad that day." [NONANGINA?]

"Where was that pain?"

"Same place (points to subxiphoid area). That only happened that one time, and it was different. I never throw up with this pain. That one was real bad, though."

"And it lasted how long?"

"All day. Six hours at least. I was just about to come to the hospital, but it went away." [NONANGINA? MYOCARDIAL INFARCTION?]

"How were you after that?"

"Tired, but okay."

"Your usual chest pain—is it ever shorter than 2 or 3 minutes?"

"Maybe. I'm not sure."

"Is it every very quick—just a second or two and then gone?"

"No."

"Have you ever taken medicine for this pain?"

"No. Oh, I've tried Rolaids a couple of times, but that doesn't help, and it usually goes away quickly anyway."

"Have you ever taken nitroglycerin?"

"No! So it is my heart, is that it?"

"We'll see. When you have the pain, does it hurt more to breathe?"

"Well, I feel like my breath is a little short, but I wouldn't say it hurts to breathe, no."

"Is there any place that is tender to touch on your chest—now, or when you have the pain?"

"No."

"Does bending over, or twisting your chest, or moving your arms seem to bring on the pain?"

"Well, vacuuming and carrying things do make you bend and lift, don't they? So, I guess so, maybe."

NOTE

1. When one is analyzing the history of episodic recurrent chest pain, it is always helpful to first elicit a general overview—What is the pain usually like?—regarding the quality, location, onset, and duration of pain, as well as its precipitating and relieving factors.

2. In this case, it seems fair to conclude that the composite picture is that of recurrent anterior chest pain that is usually brief in duration, associated with various types of physical exertion, and apparently relieved by rest.

Such a pattern is suspicious for angina pectoris, but there are a few peculiar features. For example, while there are no definite nonanginal symptoms, most of the precipitating activities (bending and lifting, for example) do stress the chest muscles and skeleton as much as the coronary circulation. Similarly, the pain is quite unpredictable: It may or may not occur during vacuuming; sometimes it occurs as soon as the vacuuming is begun, at other times not; and it does not seem to occur during walking. Finally, there appear to be (at least) two different kinds of chest pain—one of these (the severe pain that lasted for 6 hours) is definitely not angina (although it could still be due to coronary artery disease, as noted above).

3. When the "usual" history is confusing, as in this case, it always helps to analyze in detail one typical episode of chest pain that is fresh in the patient's mind—usually, the most recent one.

"Can you tell me about the last time you had chest pain?"

"Last night after supper. I was working in the kitchen and the pain started. I tried to ignore it for a few minutes, but it kept up, and so I sat down and rested a while. I was all right after that."

"It would help if we could go through that step by step. How did you feel before supper?"

"A little tired. I worked all day, but I hadn't had any chest pain."

"And during supper, did you feel well?"

"Fine."

"Did you have a heavy meal?"

"No. Just salad and chicken. I'm on a diet."

"And did you go in to work in the kitchen right after supper?"

"Oh no. My husband did the dishes, and I took my walk. I always try to take a walk after supper. It's good exercise, and it helps my digestion."

"Did you have any chest pain during your walk?"

"No, I felt fine."

"How far do you walk?"

"Just around the block—it takes about 10 minutes."

"Do you ever get your chest pain during your walk after supper?"

"Not that I can remember. Like I said, sometimes I get a little indigestion, that's all."

"Do you mean you get indigestion when you walk after supper?"

"Sometimes. Hardly ever now. I used to get it more often before I went on my diet and before we moved."

"Moved?"

"Yes, we moved last year. Our old neighborhood was kind of hilly, and walking up and down hills wasn't very relaxing. Now we live on a nice, flat street."

"Do you mean that you would get indigestion more when walking up and down hills than when walking on level ground?" [ANGINA?]

"Well, I never thought of it that way. I think it's just my diet. I don't know."

"What does this indigestion feel like?"

"Well, you know, I get this heavy kind of feeling (she points to the lower sternum and throat) and so I just stop for a minute and try to get up the gas, and then I'm fine." [ANGINA?]

"So this indigestion pain is different from your other chest pain?"

"Oh sure. I wouldn't call indigestion a 'pain,' would you?"

"Maybe not. Pain means different things to different people. Do you get this indigestion only when you walk or at other times, too?"

"Like I said, I hardly ever get it now. I'm not here about my indigestion."

"Okay. Back to last night. Did you get any pain—or indigestion—during your walk?"

"No."

"What did you do after your walk?"

"I came inside and began to tidy up the kitchen—put the dishes away and everything. You know, men never do it right, but I am grateful for the help. Anyway, I had been at it for a few minutes when I noticed the chest pain starting."

"Do you remember exactly what you were doing when the pain started?"

"I think I was putting the dishes away."

"Were you annoyed with your husband or upset about anything at the time?"

"No."

"Had you been mopping, or sweeping, or working hard at anything before that?"

"No, just cleaned out the sink, that's all."

"Is putting the dishes away hard to do?"

"No, of course not. I have to reach up high for a few and bend down to the floor cabinets a couple of times, but I wouldn't call that hard."

"Were you bending or reaching when you got your pain?"

"I guess so. I don't know. It just started, and I rested a minute, and that was it."

"So it lasted how long?"

"A minute or two—not seconds, minutes. Then I was fine the rest of the night. That wasn't a very bad one."

"Some are worse than others?"

"Well, like I said, sometimes it can last longer—a half-hour or more." [NONANGINA?]

"Can you tell when that will happen?"

"Not really. Maybe if I keep on working—vacuuming, for instance—even with the pain. Then I may have it for quite a while longer, even after I stop." [ANGINA?]

"Was the pain last night a typical pain?"

"Yes, I guess so. Now that you mention it, maybe there is more than one kind of pain. I don't know."

NOTE

1. When one is taking the history, it is essential to be as precise as possible. Listen to the patient, pick up cues, and follow them (even maddeningly) to their conclusion. Only in this way will the clinical history provide the crucial diagnostic data. We can draw a few tentative conclusions:

2. Angela's pain is compatible with, but not typical of, angina pectoris. The incident described reveals the pain was exertional in onset, but the type and degree of exertion involved (putting away dishes) was at least seemingly less stressful than a type of exertion more typically associated with classic angina—walking after eating—and yet this activity was tolerated without symptoms. Again, typical angina pectoris occurs *during* exertion—while it could be argued that putting dishes away after walking was the "last straw," this is not at all typical of angina pectoris.

Similarly, two features vaguely suggest nonangina, but these are indefinite: The duration of pain is sometimes atypically long for angina (a half-hour or more), and the usual precipitating events seem more often to involve bending and reaching (chest wall and arm use) than classic "cardiac exertion."

Thus, Angela's pain cannot be categorized clearly as either typical angina pectoris or as definite nonangina.

3. Angela does complain of more than one type of chest discomfort. The one prolonged episode of chest pain may or may not be related to these episodic chest pains. If Angela has angina, was this event a myocardial

infarction? Or is there another unrelated occult process (gallbladder disease, for example)? The diagnosis of acute, prolonged chest pain is discussed more fully on page 727.

Certainly, Angela's "indigestion" deserves further attention.

4. Angela's chest pain should thus be categorized initially as "compatible" chest pain.

"Compatible" Chest Pain

Because most angina pectoris is typical angina, most patients with compatible chest pain do not have angina. Thus, most patients with compatible chest pain should be first suspected of one or more of the gastrointestinal, cardiopulmonary, psychogenic, or chest-wall disorders noted in Table 13–2.

As is pointed out by Figure 13–5 (page 695), the approach to patients with compatible chest pain obviously varies with individual circumstances:

1. Usually the history alone will be suggestive of the various causes of psychogenic chest pain (see Appendix III).

2. Similarly, most of the gastrointestinal causes of chest pain will be suspected on the basis of the history. Esophagitis or esophageal spasm is certainly the most common cause of gastrointestinal chest pain. Usually, the history alone is diagnostic. Nevertheless, a definitive diagnosis of esophageal spasm or proof that esophagitis is the cause of a patient's pain is not always easy to establish. Appendix II briefly discusses the approach to these problems.

As Figure 13–4 illustrates, the patient with symptomatic gallstones commonly experiences pain whose localization is intermediate between lower chest and upper abdomen.[16] Episodic chest/epigastric pain due to biliary colic is usually suggested by the duration of pain and the prominence of nausea, vomiting, or anorexia during the attacks. "Biliary colic" is a misnomer[16] for usually steady (noncolicky) pain resulting from transient obstruction of the cystic duct by an impacted gallstone. Pain *may* be brief (15 to 20 minutes), but usually lasts 2 to 6 hours, and is most often associated with some anorexia, nausea, or vomiting during the attack. Symptoms of biliary colic overlap somewhat with the manifestations of actual acute cholecystitis,[16–18] but the latter entity usually causes more severe, more prolonged pain that requires medical attention. (See Chapter 11, "Abdominal Pain".) Radiation of epigastric/chest pain to the back or shoulder blade is a helpful clue in the diagnosis of biliary disease, but this pain pattern is not common.[16–18]

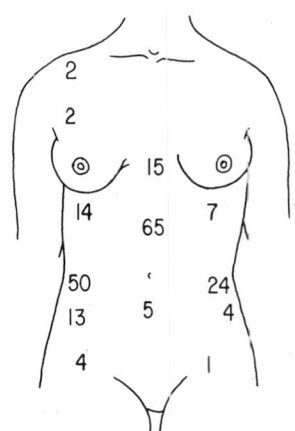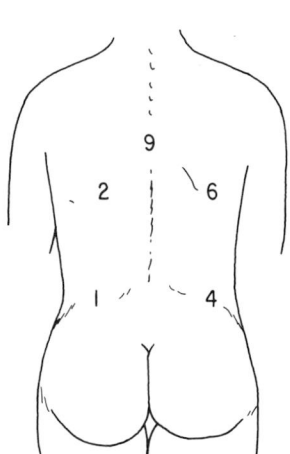

FIGURE 13–4. The location of pain among patients with biliary colic.

The pain of peptic ulcer disease can sometimes be puzzling, but this pain is usually clearly epigastric (unless associated with heartburn—see Appendix II). Ulcer pain and various disorders of the liver, spleen, pancreas, stomach, and colon (colonic flexure syndrome[19]) will occasionally be confused with other causes of episodic chest pain—these are discussed further in Chapter 11.

3. As we shall see, the physical examination is most helpful in the diagnosis of chest-wall syndromes.

4. Cardiopulmonary disease other than coronary artery disease that may either cause compatible chest pain or precisely mimic typical angina will usually be detected by physical examination (see below).

When the history and physical examination do not achieve a presumptive diagnosis, observation of the patient during an episode of pain may be very helpful. Transient ECG ischemic changes during pain, for example, may document otherwise atypical angina. A Holter monitor may be useful for this purpose as well.

Finally, in the patient with compatible chest pain, atypical angina must be considered as strongly as any other diagnosis when the initial approach in Figure 13–5 does not point to a specific disease entity. As is emphasized by Figure 13–5 and Appendix I, exercise testing or more invasive studies may then be indicated to exclude ischemic cardiac symptoms. Herein lies the crucial importance of first distinguishing definite nonangina from compatible chest pain whenever possible—when pain is definitely nonanginal, cardiac testing is rarely necessary.

Physical Examination

In patients with episodic chest pain, the physical examination is only sometimes revealing. Most patients with angina pectoris or gastrointestinal or psychogenic causes of chest pain will have normal physical examinations. Patients with other cardiopulmonary causes (see below) and patients with various chest-wall syndromes will usually demonstrate important physical findings. Note:

I. The patient with typical or suspected angina.

When (uncommonly) an episode of chest pain occurs in the presence of the clinician, certain findings strongly support the diagnosis of angina. These include transient physical findings (absent before and after pain, but present during pain): tachycardia, hypertension, and especially a cardiac gallop (S_4 or S_3), apical systolic murmur (due to papillary muscle dysfunction), or paradoxically split S_2.
More often, the patient's episodic pain is not observed. Here, physical examination should exclude valvular aortic stenosis (or insufficiency), asymmetric septal hypertrophy, pulmonic stenosis, and pulmonary hypertension—all of which may cause angina pectoris without coronary artery disease. It is always wise to look for evidence of congestive heart failure, anemia, hyperthyroidism, or cardiac arrhythmias that may precipitate or worsen angina pectoris. (Finally, in the patient with angina pectoris other coronary artery disease risk factors should be evaluated whose amelioration might help in overall patient management—hypertension, obesity, hyperlipidemias—see page 721.)

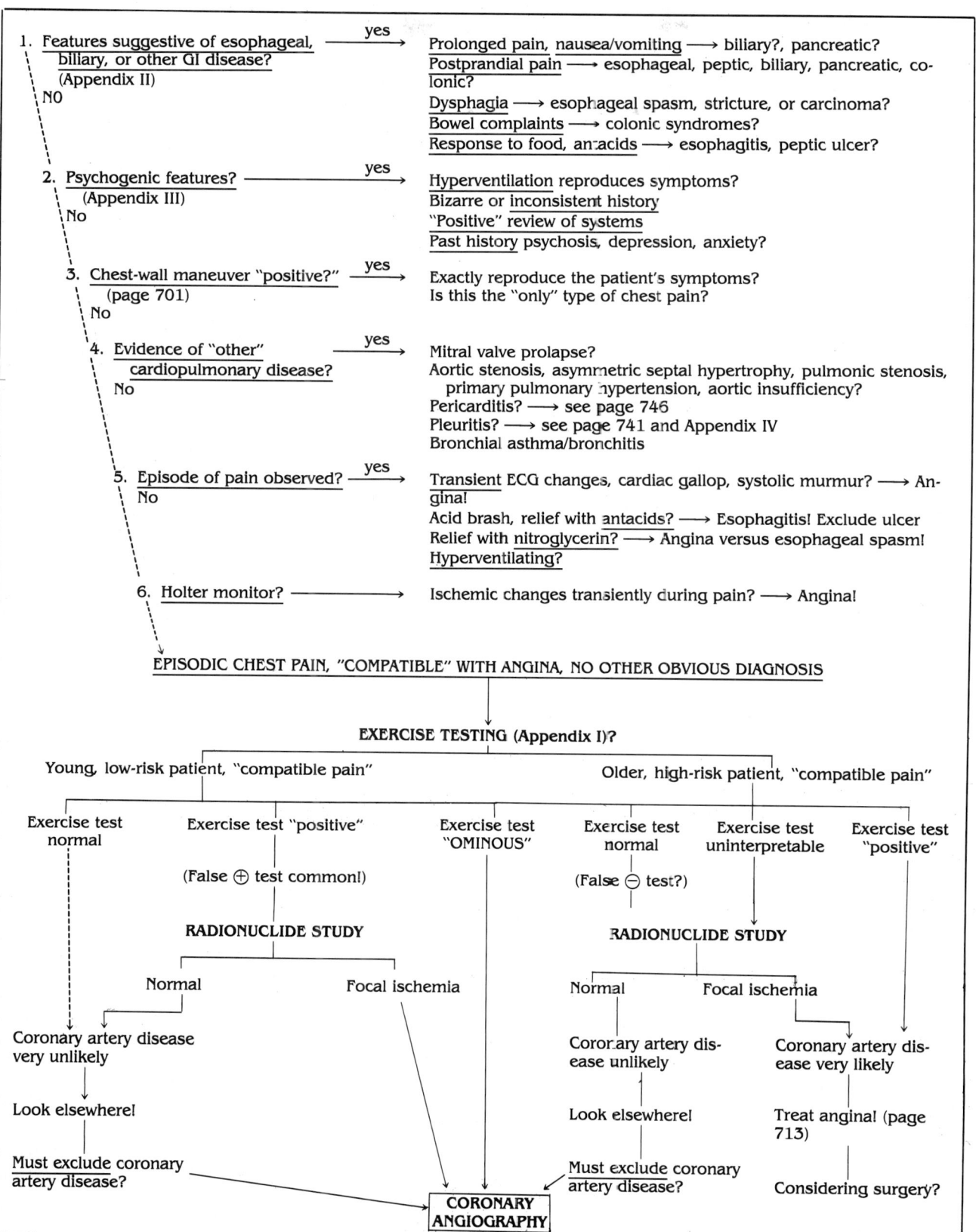

1. Features suggestive of esophageal, ——yes——→ Prolonged pain, nausea/vomiting ——→ biliary?, pancreatic?
   biliary, or other GI disease?
   (Appendix II)

   NO

   Postprandial pain ——→ esophageal, peptic, biliary, pancreatic, colonic?

   Dysphagia ——→ esophageal spasm, stricture, or carcinoma?
   Bowel complaints ——→ colonic syndromes?
   Response to food, antacids ——→ esophagitis, peptic ulcer?

2. Psychogenic features? ——yes——→ Hyperventilation reproduces symptoms?
   (Appendix III)

   No

   Bizarre or inconsistent history
   "Positive" review of systems
   Past history psychosis, depression, anxiety?

3. Chest-wall maneuver "positive?" ——yes——→ Exactly reproduce the patient's symptoms?
   (page 701)

   No

   Is this the "only" type of chest pain?

4. Evidence of "other" ——yes——→ Mitral valve prolapse?
   cardiopulmonary disease?

   No

   Aortic stenosis, asymmetric septal hypertrophy, pulmonic stenosis,
      primary pulmonary hypertension, aortic insufficiency?
   Pericarditis? ——→ see page 746
   Pleuritis? ——→ see page 741 and Appendix IV
   Bronchial asthma/bronchitis

5. Episode of pain observed? ——yes——→ Transient ECG changes, cardiac gallop, systolic murmur? ——→ Angina!

   No

   Acid brash, relief with antacids? ——→ Esophagitis! Exclude ulcer
   Relief with nitroglycerin? ——→ Angina versus esophageal spasm!
   Hyperventilating?

6. Holter monitor? ——————→ Ischemic changes transiently during pain? ——→ Angina!

EPISODIC CHEST PAIN, "COMPATIBLE" WITH ANGINA, NO OTHER OBVIOUS DIAGNOSIS

EXERCISE TESTING (Appendix I)?

Young, low-risk patient, "compatible pain"   Older, high-risk patient, "compatible pain"

Exercise test normal | Exercise test "positive" | Exercise test "OMINOUS" | Exercise test normal | Exercise test uninterpretable | Exercise test "positive"

(False ⊕ test common!)   (False ⊖ test?)

RADIONUCLIDE STUDY   RADIONUCLIDE STUDY

Normal   Focal ischemia   Normal   Focal ischemia

Coronary artery disease very unlikely

Look elsewhere!

Must exclude coronary artery disease?

Coronary artery disease unlikely

Look elsewhere!

Must exclude coronary artery disease?

Coronary artery disease very likely

Treat angina! (page 713)

Considering surgery?

CORONARY ANGIOGRAPHY

FIGURE 13–5. "Compatible" chest pain (neither typical angina pectoris nor definite nonangina).

Most patients with angina pectoris have a normal physical examination.

II. Most gastrointestinal causes of episodic chest pain are suspected purely on the basis of the clinical history.

The physical examination helps little unless an episode of pain is observed—in such cases, examination of the abdomen for evidence of cholecystitis, pancreatitis, or a colonic flexure syndrome is always important. A beneficial response to antacids during an episode of pain may suggest peptic ulcer disease or esophagitis.

Subsequent testing, however, usually depends on the specific history. Appendix II discusses briefly esophageal causes of episodic chest pain—the most common gastrointestinal source of chest pain.

III. Psychogenic chest pain is easy to diagnosis when it is caused by hyperventilation.

This is a very important cause of episodic chest pain,[20, 21] and voluntary hyperventilation for 2 to 3 minutes should be a routine part of the examination (see Chapter 10, "Dizziness"). However, anxiety (without hyperventilation), depression, hysteria, and cardiac neurosis are also common causes of episodic chest pain, and the physical examination is usually normal here (see Appendix III).

IV. Other cardiopulmonary causes of chest pain will usually present with a distinctive history—for example, *pleuritic* chest pain (see page 741)—that distinguishes it from angina and other entities discussed here, or will demonstrate certain typical physical findings.

Mitral valve prolapse is very common in healthy young women and is usually associated with a systolic click and/or a mid to late systolic murmur, best heard along the left sternal border with the patient sitting forward and exhaling. Chest pain in such patients is usually "compatible" with many other diagnoses—it may be exertional and simulate angina, but more often it is nonexertional, brief, and unpredictable.

Pericarditis may cause nonpleuritic chest pain but is almost always associated with either a pericardial friction rub or ECG changes (see page 746) and only uncommonly causes episodic, intermittent, nonpleuritic chest pain.

Recurrent pulmonary emboli may rarely cause episodic chest pain that simulates coronary insufficiency,[22] but pleuritic pain and other clues to this diagnosis (see page 744) are usually present.

Bronchial asthma or emphysema may cause vague recurrent chest pains, but usually the relationship to labored respiration and the abnormal lung examination is obvious. Acute bronchitis, viral syndromes, or prolonged coughing of any cause can result in episodic chest pain, but this is usually of the "chest-wall" variety (see below).

V. Otherwise, physical examination is most helpful in the diagnosis of chest-wall causes of episodic chest pain.

It must be remembered that the physical examination may be normal in such patients, but this is less common the more carefully one examines the patient.

The chest wall is examined in two ways:

A. Palpation for local tenderness, swelling, or masses.[23]

Figure 13–6 illustrates some palpable or visible abnormalities of the chest wall associated with various common causes of chest-wall pain (see below). Even when visible or palpable swelling is not apparent, gentle manual pressure over the sternum, xiphoid process, costochondral junctions, intercostal spaces, ribs, and insertions of sternocleidomastoid, pectoralis major and minor muscles, and rectus abdominis muscles should always be quickly applied. The breasts, sternoclavicular joints, and posterior chest wall (see also Chapter 9, "Shoulder Pain") should be examined.

B. Mechanical manipulation of the thorax.

The most puzzling chest-wall syndromes are those in which there is no palpable chest-wall tenderness or visible abnormality. All patients with puzzling chest pain should be subjected to several maneuvers that stress musculoskeletal structures of the thorax and the cervicothoracic spine. These include:

Bending forward at the waist
Lateral rotation of the torso (Fig. 1–3E)
Full expansion of the chest; active retraction of the chest
The scissors maneuver (Fig. 13–7A and B)
The hedge clipper maneuver (Fig. 13–7C)
The racing dive maneuver (Fig. 13–7D)
The crowing rooster maneuver (Fig. 13–7E)
The hooking maneuver (Fig. 13–7F)
The high ten maneuver (Fig. 13–7G)
Neck range of motion (Fig. 9–2)
Thoracic outlet maneuvers (Fig. 9–46)

The examiner should be creative here. As Allison[24] notes, "The simplest test is to get the patient to raise the arms and then press forward against resistance applied with the hands. In some cases, it is only turning the trunk, or some sudden and unexpected movement, that will reproduce the pain." A few clinical descriptions of these different maneuvers are available,[24-28] but these common problems are inadequately studied.

Further questioning of Angela reveals no gastrointestinal complaints except the "indigestion," and Angela remains vague about that complaint. There are no obvious psychosocial stresses, other than the recent death of Angela's brother and Angela's concern about her own health. She is a nonsmoker.

Angela is obese (5 feet 4 inches, 170 pounds), slightly anxious, but in no distress (and is not experiencing any pain at this time).

Blood pressure is 162/94 in both arms, pulse 88 and regular. Physical examination is otherwise normal except for mild retinal arteriolar narrowing and a II/VI midsystolic murmur heard at the lower left sternal border. The heart is not enlarged, and there are no gallops or clicks.

Voluntary hyperventilation is unremarkable.

There is mild tenderness to palpation along the lower left parasternal area but this is "nothing like" Angela's pain. Bending forward, chest expansion and retraction, the scissors maneuver, shoulder and neck range of motion, pectoralis major and pectoralis minor testing, and the hooking maneuver are accomplished painlessly. However, when Angela raises both her arms overhead and forcefully pushes her hands forward against the examiner's resistance, the "high ten" maneuver, (Fig. 13–7G), she experiences severe sternal chest pain that forces her to grab her chest and exclaim, "That's my pain." The pain resolves over 2 to 3 minutes and is reproduced when that maneuver is repeated. The "crowing rooster" maneuver (Fig. 13–7E) precipitates similar, but less severe, pain.

What does this mean?

Angela's frequent episodic chest pains are exactly reproduced by mechanical manipulation of the thorax. Chest-wall pain is thus highly likely, especially since the clinical history is compatible with that diagnosis.

Chest-Wall Syndromes

There are two general categories of chest-wall syndromes:

I. Syndromes usually characterized by visible/palpable swellings or localized tenderness.

    Many of these are illustrated in Figure 13–6.

    A. Disorders of the breast are usually easy to separate from other chest-pain syndromes.

        Tender intramammary masses in the female may be carcinomatous, fibroadenomatous, or inflammatory (or, in the male, due to gynecomastia). Pregnancy, caffeine use, and hormonal flux during the menstrual cycle may be responsible for more diffuse breast pain and tenderness. Occasionally the woman with large or pendulous breasts who does not wear properly supportive undergarments will complain of more vague discomfort where the breast tissue joins the chest wall—proper bra support often alleviates the discomfort. At times there is an element of panniculitis in such patients.

    B. Rib fractures are usually traumatic but may also follow prolonged or vigorous coughing; they are occasionally "pathologic" (due to a local neoplasm or metabolic bone disease, for example). There is usually sharply localized tenderness over the fracture site, often with palpable crepitus as the examiner's fingers straddle either side of the fracture and alternately depress each side of the rib. Treatment

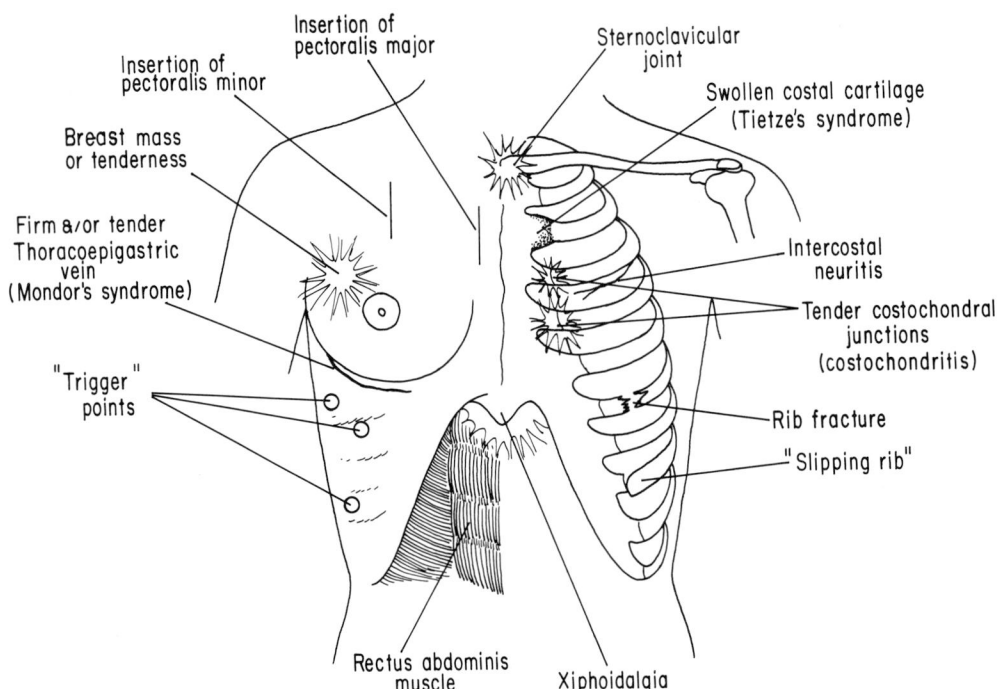

FIGURE 13–6. Palpable and/or visible abnormalities of the chest wall that may be found in different "chest-wall syndromes."

usually involves reassurance, analgesics, and sometimes use of a rib binder.

C. Xiphoidalgia refers to pain and tenderness of the xiphoid process at the lower end of the sternum.

This may be post-traumatic, but pathogenesis is often unknown; reassurance alone is usually successful in treatment, but rarely resection may be necessary for intractable pain. This pain is often worsened with bending, lifting, or twisting the torso.

Very rarely, tenderness of the sternum itself will be the result of serious hematologic disease (e.g., myelofibrosis, leukemia).

D. Costochondritis is a "wastebasket term" used to describe tenderness of the costochondral junction, usually without swelling, heat, or erythema.

Sometimes this is due to specific disorders of the costochondral junction itself—traumatic costochondral separations, rheumatoid arthritis (usually seen only in very extensive polyarticular disease), or local traumatic/inflammatory processes; much more often, there is no definable cause. Treatment usually involves local heat, anti-inflammatory medications, and reassurance.

E. Myodynia refers to localized tenderness of chest-wall muscles, usually the intercostal muscles, but occasionally the pectoralis major or pectoralis minor muscle can be specifically implicated (see below).

F. Fibrositis (see also Chapters 1, "Low Back Pain," and 9, "Shoulder Pain") refers to highly localized point tenderness, usually in the parasternal or intercostal areas, sometimes with a palpable nodular swelling whose palpation triggers local chest pain.

Local anesthetic infiltration is often curative, while anti-inflammatory drugs may be helpful as well. Diffuse fibrositis often requires tricyclic antidepressant medication.

G. Herpes zoster is usually obvious when its typical vesicular rash appears over a unilateral dermatome.

Other causes of intercostal neuritis (post-traumatic or postoperative) may induce a similar syndrome but without the characteristic dermatitis.

H. Tietze's syndrome[29] is commonly diagnosed but is, in fact, quite rare.

Properly defined, this syndrome refers to painful, tender (bulbous or fusiform) swelling of one or more (usually upper) costal cartilages, without overlying heat or erythema. This syndrome does not refer simply to costochondral tenderness—a local mass is palpable.

Pain usually worsens with chest-wall motion or fatigue. Tietze's syndrome tends to follow a self-limited course in which the costal swelling persists, but pain diminishes gradually over time. Occasionally, other specific lesions (rheumatoid arthritis, osteomyelitis, local tumors, callous formation after fracture or costochondral separation) can be confused with Tietze's syndrome, but rib biopsy (rarely necessary) reveals normal cartilage in Tietze's syndrome. Usually no extensive diagnostic testing is necessary.

I. Mondor's syndrome[23] refers to painful, tender, superficial thrombophlebitis of a superficial vein of the chest or upper abdominal wall.

The thoracoepigastric vein (over the lateral chest wall) is said to be most commonly involved, but similar findings within breast tissue itself may also occur. The involved area is easy to recognize since the vein stands out beneath the skin as a tender cord "attached" to the overlying skin. Spontaneous resolution of pain and tenderness (often leaving a residual painless venous cord) is the rule.

Localized chest-wall syndromes entirely confined to the posterior chest—due to scapular disorders or cervicothoracic arthritis, for example—are discussed briefly in Chapter 9, "Shoulder Pain."

Poorly localized, diffuse, or equivocal chest-wall tenderness is nonspecific and is never sufficient evidence to diagnose a chest-wall disorder and to exclude other diseases that might cause chest pain.

II. Syndromes in which chest-wall tenderness may be mild or absent but in which pain is reproduced by specific mechanical manipulation of the thorax.

These include:

A. Cervical or thoracic spine disease.[30]

Disorders of the cervical spine may cause pain limited to the anterior (usually upper) chest, shoulder, or arm but usually involve the posterior chest as well. Range of motion of the cervical spine (see Fig. 9–2), downward vertical pressure on the top of the head, or the "crowing rooster" maneuver (Fig. 13–7E) will usually elicit such pain and help localize the problem to the neck. Degenerative arthritis of the cervical spine is the most common cause of such symptoms. Anti-inflammatory drugs, neck traction, and other forms of physical therapy will be helpful.

Thoracic spine disease, especially kyphoscoliosis with or without osteoporosis or degenerative arthritis, will also cause chest pain—again, movement of the torso (torsion, bending), the "scissors" manuever, chest expansion/retraction, or the "high ten" maneuver will often reproduce this pain (see Fig. 13–7).

B. The slipping rib syndrome.[28, 31]

This probably results from recurrent subluxation of a costal cartilage (usually the eighth, ninth, or tenth rib), which then causes lower thoracic and/or upper abdominal pain.

Sometimes symptoms are described as a characteristic "grating" in the rib cage, but often the symptoms are much more puzzling. Bending over, rolling over in bed, or sudden use of the arms or torso are common precipitants of pain. The precise cause of pain is unclear, but traction on the subjacent intercostal nerve by the "subluxed" rib is one possible mechanism. Some observers insist that localized tenderness or swelling is often present or that abduction of the ipsilateral arm can reproduce the pain, but these findings are variable; hence, the value of the "hooking" maneuver (Fig. 13–7F).

Treatment involves reassurance and perhaps a chest-wall binder. Intercostal nerve blocks rarely help. Surgical resection of the involved rib is occasionally necessary.

Whether the precordial catch syndrome[32] is one form of the slipping rib syndrome is unclear. The former syndrome usually refers to the sudden onset of very brief pleuritic chest pain seen in patients with a slouched posture and often related in onset to bending over. Sometimes this benign syndrome will enter into the differential diagnosis of acute pleuritic chest pain (see page 741), but rarely is it a diagnostic problem.

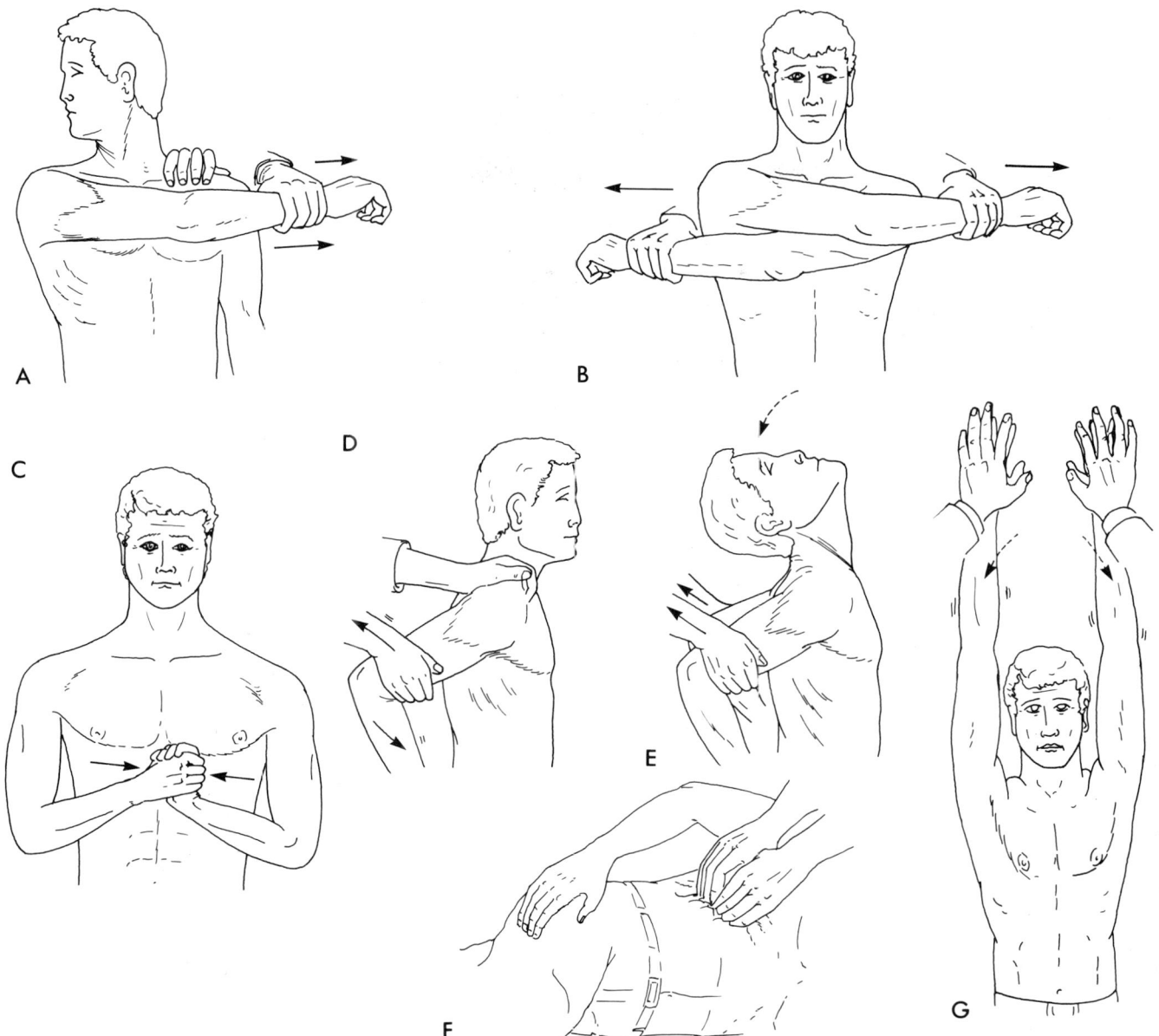

FIGURE 13–7. Chest-wall maneuvers.

A, B, "Scissors" maneuver. The patient's arm is adducted across the anterior chest, and the examiner pulls the patient's hand beyond the contralateral shoulder *(A)*. When both arms are tested together, traction is applied to both *(B)*, and the patient turns the head to either side—the arms form a "scissors." Pain originating in the scapula, thoracic spine, pectoral muscles, or ribs and intercostal structures will often be precipitated by the "scissors" maneuver.

C, The "hedge clipper" maneuver. The pectoralis major muscles are stressed by asking the patient to "press" the palms forcefully together with the elbows flexed anterior to the chest. The pectorals are thus more clearly defined, and pain will often be appreciated within the muscles or at their insertion in the upper parasternal area (Fig. 13–6).

D, The "racing dive" maneuver. The pectoralis minor muscles[26] are stressed by forcefully resisting the patient's attempt to throw forward the shoulder and upper arm from an initial position behind (dorsal to) the chest wall. The attempted arm motion is that of flinging the arm and hand forward, as a swim racer would when beginning a racing dive. The examiner resists this forward arm and shoulder motion.

E, The "crowing rooster" maneuver.[27] The patient hyperextends the neck while the examiner lifts both of the patient's arms backward and superiorly. Pain originating in the cervical spine or anterior chest wall or both will often thus be reproduced.

F, The "hooking" maneuver. With the patient supine, the examiner stands at the patient's side, facing the patient's feet. The examiner than "hooks" his or her fingers around the lower costal margin of the rib cage and pulls anteriorly (ventrally) and superiorly (cephalad). This maneuver may elicit pain when costochondritis or traumatic rib injuries involve the lower rib cage, when the upper rectus abdominis muscle is torn, or when a "slipping rib" is the problem.[28, 31]

G, The "high ten" maneuver. The patient raises both hands overhead, elbows extended, and then presses forward with the hands against resistance offered by the examiner. Pain originating in the anterior rib cage, thoracic spine, or pectoral muscles may be elicited here.

701

C. Pectoralis major syndrome.

Chest pain usually involves the upper anterior chest or shoulder. Usually some type of exertional overuse is responsible—such as unaccustomed calisthenics or lifting—but such a history may be inapparent. There may be tenderness along the upper parasternal area (where the pectoralis major inserts), or pain will be reproduced with the "hedge clipper" maneuver.

Usually, rest of the arm and shoulder, anti-inflammatory drugs, and local heat are sufficient therapy. Only rarely is surgical repair or further evaluation required.

D. Pectoralis minor syndrome.[26]

There may be vague tenderness in the upper midclavicular line (at the level of the third through fifth ribs) where the pectoralis minor muscle inserts, and specific stress of the pectoralis minor muscle will reproduce the pain (the "racing dive" maneuver).

E. Sternoclavicular disorders.

Sternoclavicular separation and degenerative (or inflammatory) arthritis are usually easily localized to the sternoclavicular joint but may initially present with vague upper anterior chest pain. Manipulation of the sternoclavicular joint by full ipsilateral shoulder abduction to 180 degrees with simultaneous palpation of the sternoclavicular joint will demonstrate the problem (see also Fig. 9–11).

F. Thoracic outlet syndromes.

These should be especially considered when pain or dysesthesias involve the upper (usually inner) arm and forearm or hand. Isolated anterior upper chest pain without pain radiation will sometimes result from one of these conditions, and thus the thoracic outlet maneuvers can be helpful. (The three common thoracic outlet disorders are discussed further in Chapter 9, "Shoulder Pain," Appendix III.)

Sometimes a specific thoracic outlet syndrome cannot be documented by palpation of the pulse and elicitation of neurologic symptoms during the various thoracic outlet maneuvers. These maneuvers, however—hyperabduction, the Adson maneuver, and the costoclavicular maneuver—are also very helpful nonspecific chest-wall maneuvers that may reveal that chest pain is in fact originating from the chest wall (even when a more specific diagnosis cannot be made).

Treatment of chest-wall disorders most often involves avoidance of typical precipitating factors, short courses of anti-inflammatory medications, changes in posture, muscular conditioning, local anesthetic infiltrations, or a combination of these treatments. Often it is helpful for patients to initiate daily chest-wall exercises that include pectoral muscle strengthening, as well as the shoulder and thoracic outlet exercise discussed in Chapter 9. Very often, simple reassurance that there is no more serious cause of chest pain is sufficient therapy.

Thoracic palpation and manipulation can be adequately performed in just a minute or two. Often it will be possible to make a specific diagnosis (e.g., xiphoidalgia, pectoral muscle strain). Equally often, however, it is not possible to identify a specific syndrome—sometimes the best we can do is to diagnose "chest-wall pain." This is so in Angela's case. When considering the diagnosis of such nonspecific chest-wall pain, remember:

1. Not all patients with chest-wall pain will demonstrate chest-wall

tenderness or positive maneuvers. Sometimes only the history (definite intermittent precipitation of pain by chest torsion, for example) and careful exclusion of other problems will suggest the diagnosis.

2. Unless this careful thoracic examination is performed routinely in patients with chest pain, mistakes will be inevitable. Often chest-wall pain very closely mimics the pain of more serious disease, for example, angina pectoris. It is likely that a number of patients with nonanginal chest pain but angiographically demonstrable coronary artery disease in fact suffer from chest-wall syndromes. Attributing pain to the coronary artery disease may lead to gross mismanagement of the patient (for example, unnecessary surgery). Similarly, at least some patients with the syndrome of angina with normal coronary arteries do not have angina at all, but have chest-wall disorders instead.[25]

3. Attribute the patient's chest pain to one of these chest-wall disorders only when the examination exactly and reproducibly elicits the patient's pain and when there are no clinical suspicions that another type of chest pain coexists. It is not rare, for example, to see patients with definite angina pectoris *and* chest-wall pain.[33] Failure to recognize combined disorders can be disastrous—the patient with stable angina who develops chest-wall pain may be mistakenly diagnosed as having unstable angina (page 725), for example.

> Angela is told that her chest pains are caused by a "strain" of the chest-wall muscles. She is told that avoidance of precipitating movements—reaching overhead, vacuuming, and the like—will be helpful, as will daily exercises for the chest wall, neck, and upper arms (see Chapter 9). Angela is instructed about such exercises and is visibly greatly relieved.
>
> Angela is told, however, of her risk factors for coronary artery disease and the need for dieting, exercise, and possibly antihypertensive therapy. She is also told that the symptoms of coronary artery disease may be quite subtle—that severe chest pain is not so common as is "tightness" or "pressure" in the chest, but that usually it is physical exertion that brings on such symptoms—e.g., walking, climbing a hill. Angela is surprised but does admit that on at least several occasions her "indigestion" did appear related to such physical exercise.
>
> The ECG is completely normal.

NOTE

1. Whatever the cause of Angela's various pains (and there appears to be more than one type), Angela is at high risk for coronary artery disease. She is obese, sedentary, mildly hypertensive, and has a positive family history for (early) coronary artery disease. Coronary risk factor identification and modification (page 721) are important in all patients with or without episodic chest pain, but these factors make all the more important further inquiry into Angela's other vague pain and "indigestion" (see below).

2. A systolic murmur is heard. In the patient with episodic chest pain, it is always important to distinguish benign systolic murmurs from those due to asymmetric septal hypertrophy, valvular aortic stenosis, and mitral valve prolapse (Table 13–5).

> Angela is placed on a diet and is given a prescription for sublingual nitroglycerin and is instructed in its use. She is asked to avoid exercises that stress the chest wall but is told to walk every day, sometimes uphill,

TABLE 13–5. IMPORTANCE OF SYSTOLIC MURMURS IN PATIENTS WITH EPISODIC CHEST PAIN

Disorder	Physical Examination	"Bedside" Maneuvers	ECG	Remember
Innocent ejection murmur	Murmur heard best along left sternal border and at base; 1/6 to 3/6 intensity; peaks early in systole; carotid upstroke normal; no click, gallop, thrill, heave, or diastolic murmur	Murmur diminishes with standing or Valsalva maneuver	Normal	Fever; anemia; thyrotoxicosis; pregnancy; consider: mild aortic stenosis, mild pulmonic stenosis, atrial septal defect
Valvular aortic stenosis[34] Mild	Similar to innocent murmur but possible ejection click		Normal	In elderly patients[34] may be difficult to distinguish mild from severe aortic stenosis Echocardiogram *usually* diagnostic
Severe	Murmur heard best at second right intercostal space, peaks late in systole; delayed carotid upstroke; palpable thrill at second right intercostal space; left ventricular heave; audible S₄ gallop; possible aortic insufficiency murmur too		Left ventricular hypertrophy (Fig. 13–10)	
Asymmetric septal hypertrophy	Murmur heard best at left sternal border, peaks in midsystole; carotid upstroke brisk and/or bisferiens; no aortic insufficiency murmur	Murmur increases with standing or Valsalva maneuver; decreases on squatting	Left ventricular hypertrophy; deep septal Q waves (Fig. 13–11)	Echocardiogram diagnostic
Pulmonic stenosis Mild	Similar to innocent murmur but possible ejection click		Normal	
Severe	Murmur heard best second left intercostal space, loud, prolonged; widely split S₂; palpable thrill at second left intercostal space; right ventricular heave; ejection click at second left intercostal space	Murmur and/or click may increase with inspiration	Right ventricular hypertrophy (Fig. 13–12)	On chest x-ray post-stenotic dilatation of pulmonary artery Echocardiogram *usually* diagnostic
Atrial septal defect	"Innocent" murmur but wide, fixed splitting of S₂		rSR' in V₁ and/or right bundle-branch block	On echocardiogram paradoxical septal motion common
Mitral valve prolapse	Murmur best heard at left sternal border and apex; mid to late systolic murmur; click(s) precede murmur	Murmur often increases with patient sitting forward, during expiration	Normal	Echocardiogram diagnostic

not necessarily just after meals, and is asked to keep track of any symptoms that occur during such exercise. Angela is told to take nitroglycerin if chest pain or indigestion occurs during such exercise and is asked to assess whether she thinks nitroglycerin helps to relieve her symptoms.

Angela is asked to return in a few weeks, at which time her "experiments" with exercise and nitroglycerin will be discussed further. An echocardiogram will be obtained to assess her heart murmur, which is "most likely not anything to be concerned about."

A chest x-ray is normal, as are a blood count and blood chemistry studies, except for a (fasting) cholesterol value of 295 mg per 100 ml. A lipid profile reveals an elevated cholesterol/HDL ratio.

Tests and Chest Pain

The most important "test" in the patient with episodic chest pain is the history and physical examination. When the history and examination do not strongly suggest a specific cause of chest pain, several tests are commonly performed (Table 13–6). As noted previously, many of these tests are much abused—they are ordered for the wrong reasons, or routinely, or are

TABLE 13–6. TESTS AND CHEST PAIN

Test	Cost	Possible Indications
Electrocardiography	$45	During episode of chest pain (Fig. 13–8) Suspected prior myocardial infarction (Fig. 13–9) Angina pectoris: Exclude left ventricular hypertrophy, right ventricular hypertrophy (Figs. 13–10 through 13–12)
Chest x-ray	$50	Pleuritic chest pain Acute severe chest pain

Echocardiography	$170 (M-mode)
	$230 (two-dimensional)
		Suspect
		  Valvular heart disease
		  Asymmetric septal hypertrophy (ASH)
		  Mitral valve prolapse
		  Atrial septal defect

Holter monitor (24 hour)	$130	Episodic chest pain: angina? arrhythmia?
Lipid profile (cholesterol/HDL)	$40	Coronary artery disease risk factors
Stress test		
ECG	$175	See Appendix I
Thallium (nuclear)	$300	
Nuclear ("gated") blood pool scan	$300	Noninvasive assessment of left ventricular function; rarely necessary in patient with undifferentiated chest pain
Coronary arteriography	$1500	Contemplated coronary artery bypass surgery (see Appendix I and page 754)
Oral cholecystography	$100	Gallstones?
Abdominal ultrasound		
Gallbladder only	$100	Gallstones?
Full abdomen	$200	Pancreatic disease?
Barium swallow/upper GI series	$100	Ulcers? esophageal reflux?
Esophageal manometry	$300	Esophageal spasm? Achalasia? Hypertensive lower esophageal sphincter? (see Appendix III)
Ventilation/perfusion lung scan	$185/130 ($315)	Pulmonary embolism? (see Appendix IV)

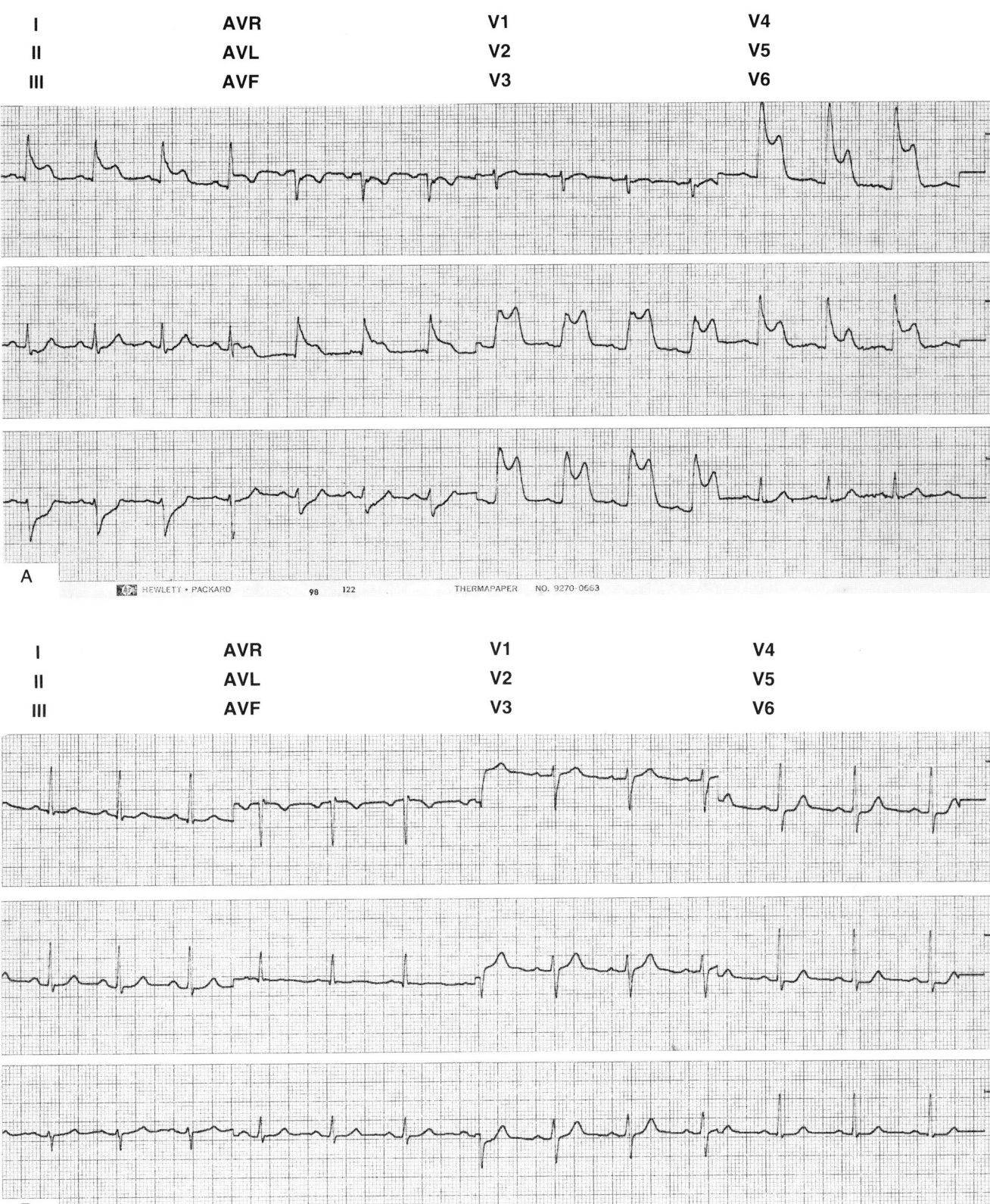

I	AVR	V1	V4
II	AVL	V2	V5
III	AVF	V3	V6

A

HEWLETT • PACKARD   98   122   THERMAPAPER   NO. 9270-0663

I	AVR	V1	V4
II	AVL	V2	V5
III	AVF	V3	V6

B

HEWLETT • PACKARD   98   122   THERMAPAPER   NO. 9270-0663

FIGURE 13–8. This 48-year-old man described episodic substernal chest pain very typical of angina pectoris (positive Levine's sign and prompt relief with sublingual nitroglycerin) but never related to physical exertion. An ECG exercise test was unremarkable. Observation in hospital documented dramatic anterolateral ST elevations on ECG *(A)* during a bout of spontaneous chest pain, relieved promptly by nitroglycerin. An electrocardiogram taken 18 minutes later (after subsidence of pain) is completely normal *(B)*. The coronary arteries were normal except for marked spasm of the left anterior descendng coronary artery after ergonovine administration during coronary arteriography. Nifedipine therapy (p. 717) prevented future pain. This is a relatively unusual ECG. Much more common is transient ST depression during a bout of angina pectoris due to atherosclerosis (see also Fig. 13–31, Appendix I).

misinterpreted because of failure to correlate the test result with the patient's clinical situation. Consider the tests selected for Angela:

I. The ECG.

The resting ECG is usually normal in patients with angina pectoris (and other types of episodic chest pain as well). Electrocardiography is not a routine examination in every patient with chest pain but should always be performed in the patient with acute severe chest pain (page 727). Obtaining an ECG during an episode of pain[35] may be very helpful (Fig. 13–8), but this is not usually possible. The usefulness of the resting ECG can be illustrated by its indications in Angela's case:

A. To recognize prior myocardial infarction.

Angela's recent, severe, prolonged bout of chest pain could have been due to myocardial infarction. It must be remembered that a normal ECG by no means excludes previous infarction, but often the telltale changes are found (Fig. 13–9).

B. To recognize other important cardiac problems.

The absence of ECG left ventricular hypertrophy (Fig. 13–10) is helpful regarding the duration and severity of Angela's (now borderline) hypertension, since both hypertension and left ventricular hypertrophy are significant risk factors for coronary artery disease (see page 720). Occasionally the resting ECG will suggest other important entities: asymmetric septal hypertrophy (Fig. 13–11), pul-

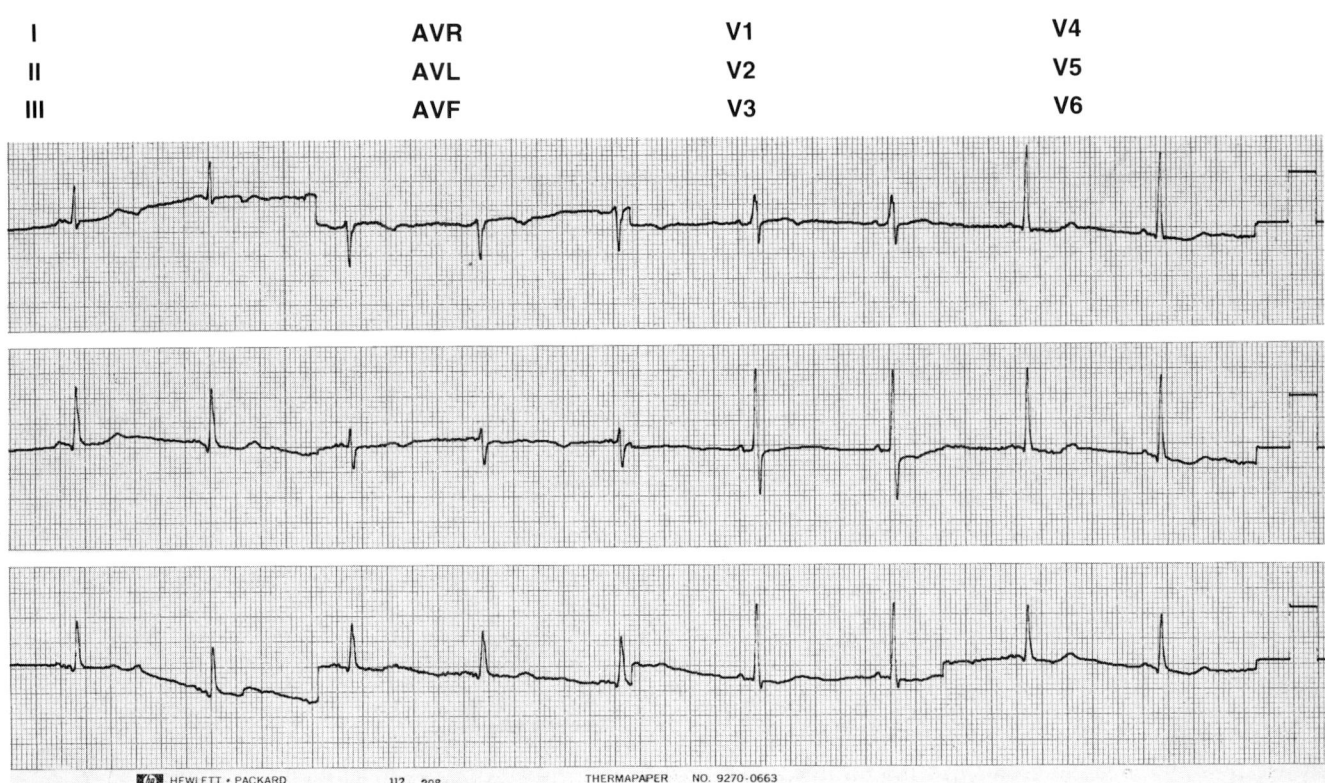

FIGURE 13–9. Prior myocardial infarction. This 63-year-old woman presented with episodic chest pain that was very difficult to analyze because she was such a vague historian. This electrocardiogram (obtained when the patient was asymptomatic) demonstrates an old posterior infarction (large R wave in lead V1), confirmed by radionuclide imaging. Subsequent evaluation revealed severe three-vessel coronary artery disease that required bypass surgery.

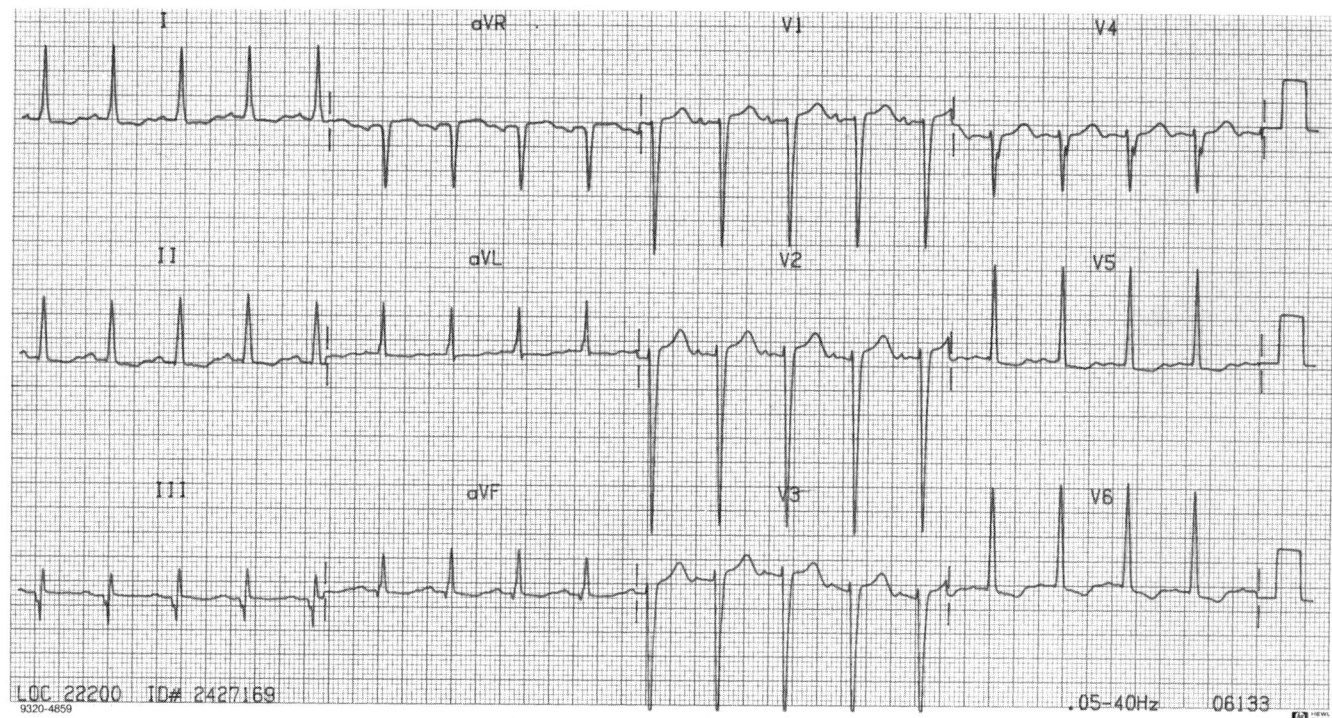

FIGURE 13–10. Left ventricular hypertrophy. This 70-year-old woman presented with typical exertional angina. Examination revealed a basal systolic murmur that radiated to the carotids, peaked late in systole, and was associated with a palpable thrill over the second right intercostal space. The carotid upstroke was delayed and diminished. The electrocardiogram reveals left ventricular hypertrophy with strain. Cardiac catheterization revealed severe valvular aortic stenosis with normal coronary arteries. The patient became completely asymptomatic after valve replacement surgery.

I	AVR	V1	V4
II	AVL	V2	V5
III	AVF	V3	V6

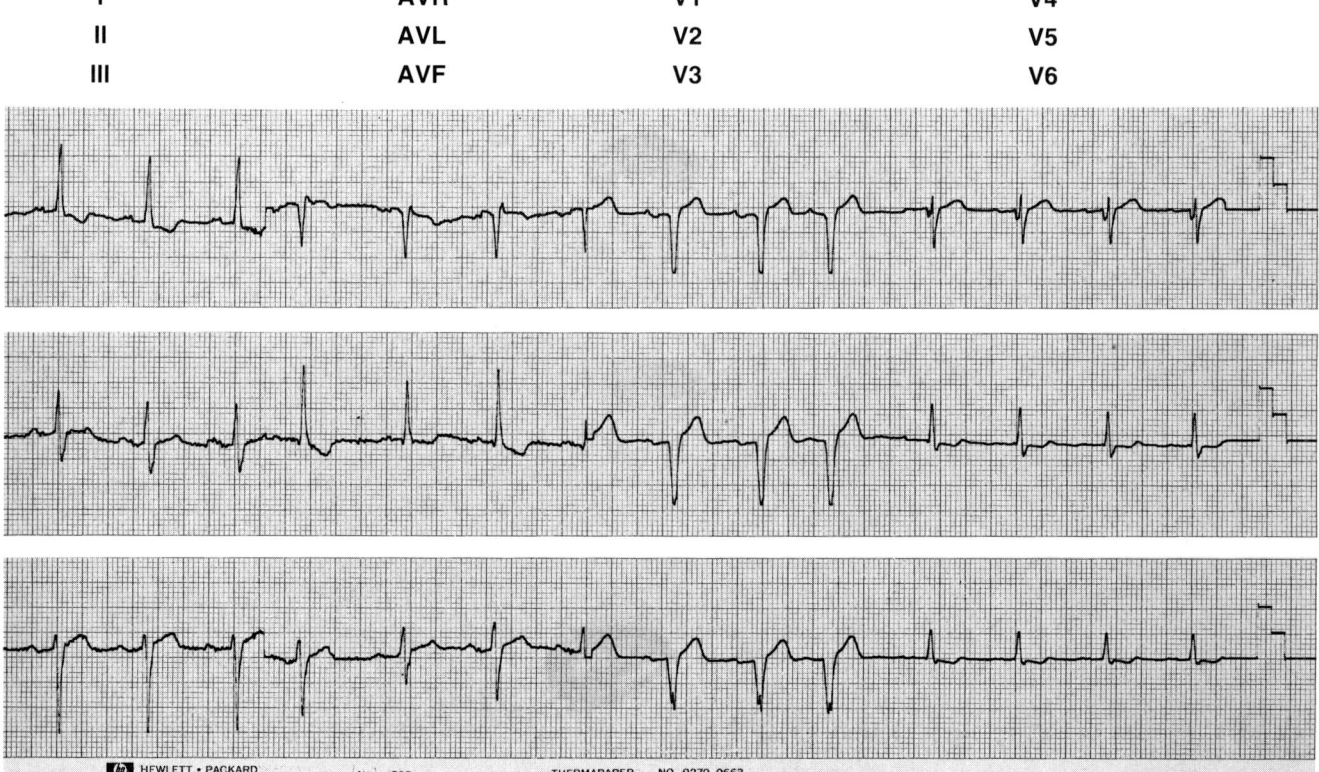

FIGURE 13–11. Asymmetric septal hypertrophy. This 42-year-old man described typical exertional angina. Examination was unremarkable except for a midsystolic murmur best heard along the left sternal border that increased on Valsalva maneuver. Echocardiogram demonstrated severe asymmetric septal hypertrophy. Electrocardiogram demonstrates deep septal Q waves and excessive left ventricular voltage (the leads are *half-standardized*). There was no evidence of prior myocardial infarction (the ECG is also consistent with a prior anterior infarct—see Fig. 13–17C). Coronary arteriography was normal.

monary hypertension (Fig. 13–12), or predisposition to arrhythmias (e.g., short PR interval).

C. As a baseline examination.

   The routine or annual ECG is wasteful in most patients. On the other hand, a resting ECG is essential when exercise testing is contemplated: Certain baseline ECG abnormalities will render ECG stress testing difficult to interpret (see Appendix I). Such findings (left bundle branch block or left ventricular hypertrophy, for example) usually require that exercise testing utilize radionuclide imaging rather than the ECG.

II. Chest x-rays are only rarely helpful in patients with episodic, nonpleuritic chest pain, and in general are unnecessary (but the chest x-ray *is* crucial in patients with pleuritic chest pain—see page 741).

   In Angela's case the specific cause of her chest-wall pain cannot be defined clinically, and only very rarely are bony abnormalities of the thorax (metastatic bony lesions or pathologic fractures, for example) or intrathoracic (especially mediastinal) masses found in such circumstances (Fig. 13–13). In general, chest x-rays are not helpful in evaluating chest-wall pain.

III. Echocardiography is very valuable in the assessment of heart murmurs, but not so much in the evaluation of episodic chest pain.

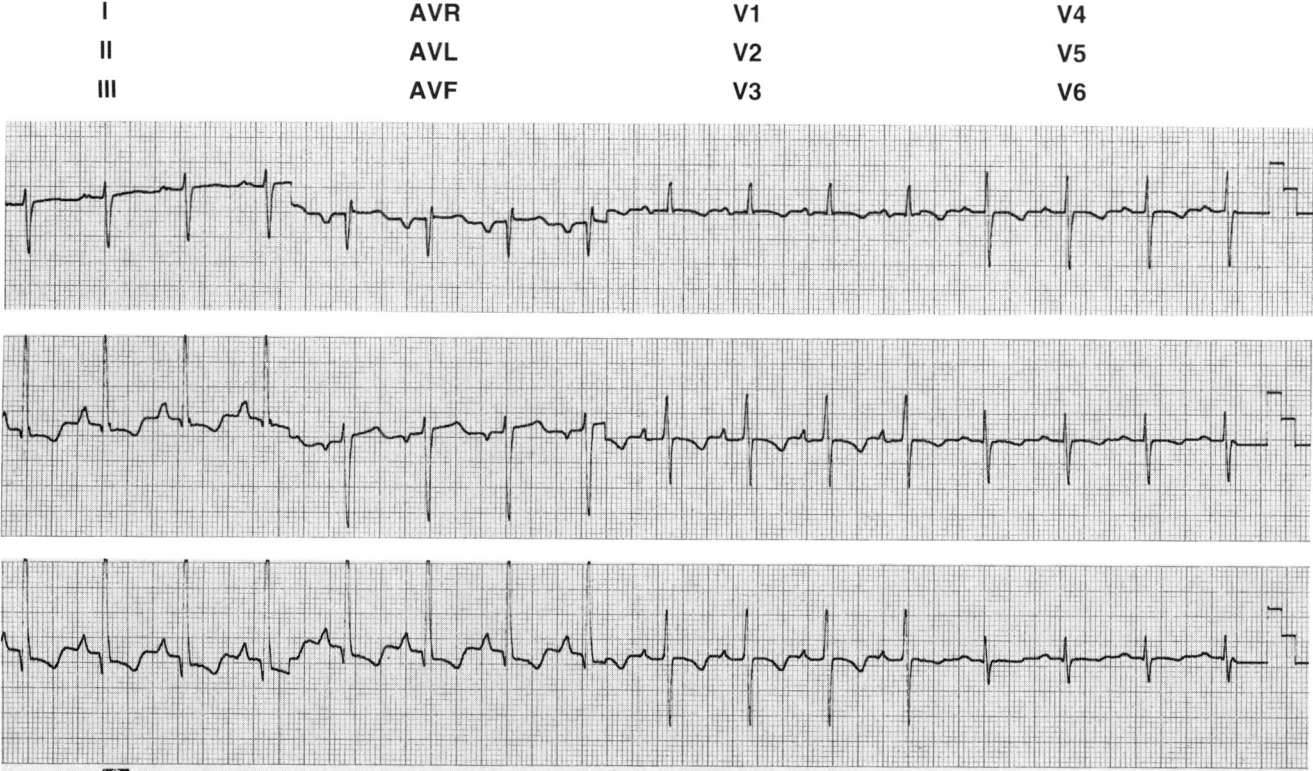

FIGURE 13–12. Right ventricular hypertrophy. This 26-year-old woman presented with classic exertional angina. Physical examination was unremarkable except for a palpable right ventricular heave. The electrocardiogram demonstrates abnormal voltage in the inferior and right precordial leads (the voltage is half-standardized), with "right ventricular strain." Cardiac catheterization demonstrated findings compatible with severe primary pulmonary hypertension. The coronary arteries were normal.

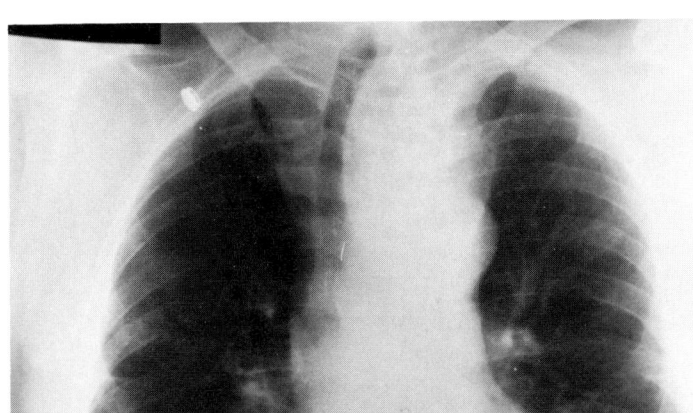

FIGURE 13–13. This 65-year-old man described peculiar episodic substernal chest pains that were never exertional and that were difficult to analyze on the basis of the history. Chest x-ray demonstrates a superior mediastinal mass deviating the trachea to the right. Subsequent exploration revealed a large substernal goiter with multiple areas of (presumably spontaneous) hemorrhage. The patient's chest pains resolved after removal of the goiter.

In Angela's case the echocardiogram is obtained to distinguish mitral valve prolapse and asymmetric septal hypertrophy from benign systolic murmur. Significant valvular aortic stenosis is usually easy to distinguish from a benign murmur, but in the elderly patient this may be more of a problem.[34]

This does not mean that echocardiography should be performed whenever a systolic murmur is heard. Physical examination—with special attention to quality and timing of the murmur; presence of click, gallop, diastolic murmur, thrills, or heaves; quality of the S_2 and carotid pulse; and response of the murmur to "bedside" maneuvers (Table 13–5)—and (sometimes) an ECG or chest x-ray are usually sufficient. In children with systolic murmurs, echocardiography only occasionally adds significant information to a sophisticated cardiac examination[36]—similar comparative studies should be performed in adults.

IV. Coronary artery disease risk-factor analysis is probably worthwhile in all patients.

While reversibility of coronary artery disease by therapeutic modification of risk factors remains a controversial subject, documentation of diabetes mellitus or hypercholesterolemia is helpful in overall patient management (see page 721). As above, smoking, family history, and blood pressure must also be noted.

V. As noted above, routine use of gallbladder and bowel x-rays should be avoided; the history will almost always suggest the need for such tests.

Documentation of a hiatal hernia on upper GI series by no means diagnoses the cause of a patient's chest pain (Appendix II): the value of demonstrating asymptomatic gallstones is similarly questionable.[37]

VI. Exercise testing.

As Figure 13–3 illustrates, when no other cause of episodic chest pain can be diagnosed by the history and physical examination, one is often left with the problem: Is this chest pain (atypical) angina? In such circumstances, exercise testing may be very helpful. (Appendix II briefly outlines the utility and interpretation of exercise testing.) Figure 13–3 illustrates just two ends of a very broad spectrum: Every patient is different. Exercise testing is no more than a winnowing process when used as a diagnostic test in patients with puzzling chest pain. For example, the young, low-risk patient with pain very atypical of angina pectoris will usually have a negative test: This can be useful information. Indiscriminate use of exercise testing in such a setting, however, will result in many false-positive tests, and one is then usually obliged to pursue that positive test with further studies, most of which are expensive, time consuming (and usually normal in that particular subset of patients). In the older high-risk patient with probable (mildly atypical) angina pectoris, positive exercise tests usually imply coronary artery disease, but negative tests are often falsely negative. Between these two ends of the spectrum are patients at intermediate risk in whom exercise testing is both less sensitive and less specific, but, paradoxically, these are the patients in whom exercise testing is often most helpful (see Appendix I).

In Angela's case it makes sense to first acquire more clinical information before resorting to exercise testing, especially since most of her chest pain appears to be "benign" chest-wall pain, and because, if she has angina, it is infrequent. A chest-pain diary will often be helpful, as will an analysis of the patient's response to nitroglycerin.

(Had we reached no other reliable explanation for Angela's frequent and unpredictable chest pains, immediate exercise testing or even hospitalization might have been necessary. If *all* of Angela's chest pains were thought due to angina, the situation would be "unstable" (page 725) and would require immediate attention.)

> Three weeks later, Angela returns and seems upset. Her previous chest pains now occur only infrequently, and she is convinced that these are related to chest-wall and arm use. She has begun daily neck, chest, and arm exercises (Chapter 9, Appendix III).
>
> Angela's "indigestion" does, however, appear to be exertional and does appear to respond to nitroglycerin. Angela develops her typical vague substernal discomfort, which feels "heavy and gassy," when she walks quickly up an incline, and this appears unrelated to meals or time of day. Sublingual nitroglycerin relieves her discomfort within 2 minutes, while rest alone allows the discomfort to continue for about 5 minutes. On several occasions she has taken nitroglycerin before climbing a hill and has not experienced any discomfort.
>
> Walking briskly up an incline appears to be the only activity that precipitates such discomfort, however, and Angela has walked over 1 mile on a flat surface at a brisk pace without any symptoms at all.
>
> Angela's blood pressure is 165/95 and pulse is 80 and regular. The echocardiogram is normal.

NOTE

1. This history is typical of angina pectoris. Discomfort is qualitatively suggestive of angina, is clearly related to cardiac exertion, is brief in duration, relieved by rest, and can be prevented or relieved by sublingual nitroglycerin. In a patient of this age with known risk factors, such a history is virtually diagnostic.

2. Angela's angina occurs only with rather vigorous physical exertion

TABLE 13–7. NEW YORK HEART ASSOCIATION CLASSIFICATION OF ANGINA

Class I	Proven coronary artery disease but asymptomatic
Class II	Angina pectoris only after unusually strenuous physical exertion
Class III	Angina pectoris with routine physical activity
Class IV	Angina with minimal activity or at rest

and does not compromise her usual daily activities (New York Heart Association Class II). As we shall see below, the specific treatment of angina pectoris depends as much on the patient's subjective disability as on any other factor. Table 13–7 is the New York Heart Association's classification of angina.

3. The importance of documenting exertional angina by exercise testing depends on the clinical setting (Appendix I):

Under usual circumstances, typical angina pectoris is diagnosed entirely by the history, and the exercise test is then not necessarily helpful *as a diagnostic test.*

When, however, symptoms seem to occur at very low levels of exercise (Class III or Class IV), documentation with exercise testing may be very important.

When chest pain is unpredictable or is intermingled with other chest pains the patient finds hard to distinguish from angina, an exercise test may be educational.

When the patient or physician is uncertain or fearful about how much exercise can be performed before angina develops, an exercise tolerance test will document exercise tolerance and the patient can then be better instructed about a "custom-made" exercise program (see page 724).

> Angela is told that her indigestion is angina pectoris. It is explained that this results when the blood supply to a part of the heart muscle fails to meet its need—in her case, during rather vigorous exercise. Angela is told that weight reduction, daily exercise, and blood pressure reduction will help to strengthen her heart and that angina can improve over time.
>
> Angela asks, "Will I have a heart attack?" The difference between angina pectoris and myocardial infarction is explained, as is the variable natural history of angina and the usefulness of medications in its treatment. Angela is told that her angina is quite mild, and while she should take nitroglycerin when symptoms occur (or before they are likely to develop), there is no danger of a heart attack now. The importance of "understanding her own angina" is emphasized—she must become aware of what she can and cannot do, so that she may exercise painlessly and also so that she will recognize any change in her angina that should be discussed with her physician—for example, if it begins to occur more frequently or with less exercise, lasts longer, or does not respond as quickly to nitroglycerin.
>
> Angela is provided with "angina literature" from the American Heart Association and is given a prescription for hydrochlorothiazide 50 mg per day for her hypertension. Angela is told to walk one-half to one mile every day on flat ground unless this causes chest pain. She is asked to return in 1 month. An ECG exercise tolerance test is scheduled for that time.

NOTE

Patient education is crucial in the management of angina pectoris (see page 720).

A general approach to the management of angina pectoris is outlined below, but these are general guidelines only. Every patient is different.

MANAGEMENT OF ANGINA PECTORIS

Unfortunately, atherosclerotic coronary artery disease is an incurable, usually progressive, condition for which all current pharmacologic and surgical interventions are palliative only. As noted above, a relatively few patients with angina pectoris will be found to have curable, noncoronary disease (for example, aortic stenosis) or other treatable complicating conditions (anemia, thyrotoxicosis, arrhythmias) that may temporarily precipitate symptoms of otherwise asymptomatic coronary artery disease. For the great majority of patients, however, angina must be "managed," i.e., manipulated and (it is hoped) controlled, rather than treated with the expectation of permanent cure.

The physician's role here must be broadly and creatively defined because the quality of life for many angina patients will be directly proportional to their physician's interest and attention to detail in helping them to cope with both the physical limitations and the psychologic burdens angina may impose. In a very real sense, the patient must manage his or her *own* angina. The generalist physician who limits his or her role to simply dispensing medications and "triaging" for cardiologists and cardiac surgeons has more to offer patients. There are four areas with which the generalist should be familiar:

1. Drug therapy—How to use which drug, when?

2. Surgical therapy—What is the role of coronary artery bypass surgery in the management of stable angina?

3. Patient education—How does one explain angina and its treatment so as to improve the patient's understanding, ensure compliance, and attend to the patient's sense of well-being?

4. When to worry—What are the indications for hospitalization, invasive studies, referral to a cardiologist or cardiac surgeon?

DRUG THERAPY. All patients with angina require drug therapy of some kind. Nitroglycerin, long-acting nitrates, and beta blockers are the mainstays of treatment.

Nitrates. All patients with angina pectoris should carry with them a supply of sublingual nitroglycerin. Sublingual nitroglycerin is available in several different dosages (Table 13–8). For each patient, dose is titrated according to efficacy, side effects, and individual needs. Tablets are now packaged in quantities of 25 or 100. To prevent loss of potency, it helps to refrigerate some of the total number and to carry the rest in an airtight amber glass vial that is easy to open (any "child-proof" bottle caps should be avoided and any cumbersome cotton plugs removed). The patient should be told to take the nitroglycerin at the first sign of chest pain, even when the patient is not certain whether the pain is anginal or not. If pain persists beyond 15 minutes despite three nitroglycerin pills taken 5 minutes apart, medical attention should be sought immediately. When the patient knows that angina will likely occur during a specific activity or event (a walk uphill, sexual intercourse, or a tension-charged encounter), nitroglycerin can be taken a few minutes *before*hand to help prevent the occurence of angina.

All patients should be given a test dose of nitroglycerin, preferably in the physician's office. (One tablet of 0.3 mg (1/200 grains) nitroglycerin should be administered sublingually in the presence of the physician.) Why? For one thing, the drug name sounds like an explosive, and a few patients are quite simply afraid to take it; this mistaken impression may be reinforced if the patient experiences a pulsating vascular headache and flushing of the skin after an initial dose of nitroglycerin. While transient flushing and briefly pronounced cranial pulsations (without severe headache) are common side effects, these effects tend to subside with regular usage and are rarely so disabling that even low doses of sublingual nitroglycerin cannot be tolerated. When such side effects occur in the physician's presence, their benignity can be emphasized and the therapeutic value of nitroglycerin's vasodilating action can be explained. Occasionally, nitroglycerin will cause dizziness and ortho-static hypotension. This may be especially common in the elderly or those with left ventricular dysfunction who cannot sufficiently increase cardiac output to compensate for the peripheral vasodilatation produced by nitroglyc-erin. (The patient whose angina pectoris results from severe valvular aortic stenosis is a typical example—all the more reason to remember that not all angina is due to coronary artery disease!)

It should be explained to the patient that nitroglycerin is not addictive—many patients are afraid of becoming dependent on nitroglycerin or think that the drug will lose its effectiveness if used too frequently over time.

Some patients believe that the more often they take nitroglycerin, the worse off they are. Many physicians lend credence to this belief by "meas-uring" the patient's angina according to the number of nitroglycerin tablets consumed per week (or unit time). Certainly the clinician should pay attention to the patient's quantitative use of nitroglycerin, since that consideration often is the best way to decide whether additional drug therapy is worthwhile (see below). Nevertheless, the patient should understand that nitroglycerin works by improving the heart's blood supply during exercise or stress; hence the drug should be used as a helpful means of doing more, rather than as a crutch.

In general, when the patient experiences angina more often than rarely, long-acting nitrates[38] or beta blockers[39] are indicated. As always, benefits must be balanced against risks and costs. For some patients, brief episodes of angina several times per week are not enough reason to use daily prophylactic medication, because of side effects, cost, nuisance value, or personality foibles; for other patients, one anginal episode per month is too much, and daily drug therapy is gratefully accepted.

Long-acting nitrates are often the clinician's first choice as a prophylactic antianginal agent. These drugs are highly effective, relatively inexpensive, usually well tolerated, and are available in several different forms (Table 13–8). Oral isosorbide dinitrate is the most commonly used: Administration every 6 hours is usually sufficient, and the dose is gradually increased, "titrating" therapeutic effects and side effects. Headache is the most common side effect but is usually transient, or the patient will develop tolerance to headache when dosage is temporarily decreased and then gradually increased again a week or two later. (The patient who is troubled by headaches from intermittent sublingual nitroglycerin will often develop similar problems with the long-acting nitrates. Occasionally, substitution of another nitrate will be helpful when headache is unavoidable. Usually, dose titration will avoid this

TABLE 13–8. NITRATES

Drug	Usual Dosage	Side Effects	Amount/Monthly Cost
Nitroglycerin Sublingual (Nitrostat)	0.15 mg (1/400 grain) ⎫ 0.30 mg (1/200 grain) ⎬ prn 0.60 mg (1/100 grain) ⎭	Headache, flushing, tachycardia, orthostatic hypotension	100 (0.3 mg) /$2.50
Oral capsules (Nitro-Bid, Nitrospan)	2.5–9 mg bid-qid	Same	5 mg qid/$38
Topical Ointment (2%) (Nitro-Bid, Nitrol, Nitrong)	½–5 in. q3–4h	Same; rarely, dermatitis	2 in. q4h/$30
Transdermal dressing (Nitro-Disc, Nitro-Dur, Transderm-Nitro)	5–10 mg pad(s) applied to skin once a day	Same	10 mg pad qd/$35
Isosorbide dinitrate (Isordil, Sorbitrate)			
Sublingual	2.5–20 mg q2–3h	Same	10 mg q6h oral/$12
Chewable	5–20 mg q2–3h		
Oral	5–60 mg q4–6h		
Erythrityl tetranitrate (Cardilate)			
Sublingual	5–20 mg q2–3h	Same	10 mg q6h oral/$12
Chewable	5–20 mg q2–3h		
Oral tablets	5–60 mg q4–6h		
Pentaerythritol tetranitrate (Peritrate)			
Tablets	5–60 mg q4–6h	Same	10 mg q6h/$9

problem, but such patients are often more easily treated with beta blockers—see below.)

The most common error in the use of nitrates is failure to prescribe adequate therapeutic dosage. Isosorbide dinitrate is often begun as 5 or 10 mg every 6 hours, but doses as high as 360 mg per day may be needed (and well tolerated). (Many patients are incorrectly deemed "refractory" to medical management when in fact nitrates can still be used to good advantage at higher doses.) In addition, the availability of many different nitrate preparations is sometimes forgotten in particular situations: Topical nitroglycerin ointment is especially helpful for the patient with nocturnal angina; transdermal nitroglycerin can be applied just once a day and should be considered when the patient with angina is temporarily unable to take pills (perioperatively, for example).

Beta Blockers[39, 40] (Table 13–9). For at least two reasons, it makes sense to use beta blockers in patients whose angina is more frequent than rare. First, these drugs reduce myocardial oxygen consumption by pharmacologic blockade of beta adrenergic receptors in the heart and circulation. As such, the myocardial hemodynamic effects of beta blockers complement those of the nitrates—the latter reduce preload, increase contractility, and cause reflex tachycardia with peripheral vasodilatation, while beta blockers do the opposite. For this reason (and because the symptomatic side effects of each class of drugs tend to offset those of the other), the combination of beta blockers and nitrates is especially appealing. Second, there is considerable evidence that the recent decline in mortality from ischemic heart disease is at least partly related to widespread use of beta blockers.[41] In patients who have already suffered myocardial infarction(s), there is now substantial evidence that beta blockade reduces the incidence of subsequent myocardial infarction or sudden death.[42, 43]

Especially good candidates for beta blockade are patients who are

TABLE 13–9. BETA BLOCKERS

DRUG	DOSAGE	SIDE EFFECTS	ADVANTAGES	AMOUNT/ MONTHLY COST
Propranolol hydrochloride (Inderal)	10–120 mg q6–8h	Bronchospasm, congestive heart failure, heart block, bradycardia, impotence, fatigue, depression, vasospasm (Raynaud's), worsening claudication, nasal congestion	Time-tested gold standard	40 mg qid/$17
Metoprolol tartrate (Lopressor)	25–100 mg q6h	Same	Cardioselective at low doses	25 mg qid/$16
Atenolol (Tenormin)	25–100 mg qd	Same	Cardioselective at low doses; once daily dosage	50 mg qd/$13
Timolol (Blocadren)	10–20 mg bid	Same	Twice daily dosage	10 mg bid/$18
Nadolol (Corgard)	40–240 mg qd	Same	Once daily dosage	160 mg qd/$25
Pindolol (Visken)	5 mg–30 mg bid	Same	ISA*	10 mg bid/$18

*Pindolol is the first available beta blocker with "intrinsic sympathomimetic activity" (ISA). This drug *may* cause less bradycardia and less depression of cardiac output. Nevertheless, heart failure and heart block remain contraindications.

hypertensive, susceptible to ventricular ectopy or supraventricular tachycardias, those with "hyperdynamic" circulation,* or those who are susceptible to nitrate-induced headache (some migraineurs, for example).

Congestive heart failure and advanced degrees of heart block are the only absolute contraindications to beta blockade. The recent availability of cardioselective beta blockers has allowed cautious use of low doses of metoprolol or atenolol in the patient with obstructive lung disease or asthma, but as can be noted from Table 13–9, these drugs lose their cardioselectivity at higher doses and preexistent bronchospasm is a strong, if not absolute, contraindication to these drugs. Relative contraindications include Raynaud's phenomenon, peripheral vascular disease, or known coronary artery spasm (which may be exacerbated by beta blockade); severe chronic nasal congestion; and the brittle insulin-dependent diabetic whose hypoglycemic symptoms (tachycardia, sweating, anxiety) may be masked by beta blockers.

Doses of beta blocker are titrated according to frequency of incidence of angina, severity of side effects, and the effect on pulse rate. The average effective dose of propranolol is 40 mg qid, but there is wide individual variation, and, as with nitrates, many practitioners do not prescribe sufficient amounts (over 500 mg per day may be needed). The pulse rate, at rest and during mild exercise, is a helpful indicator of the adequacy of beta blockade. When the resting pulse is greater than 70 per minute, or a brief walk induces tachycardia, beta blockade is incomplete and the dose may be increased. Conversely, when angina persists at unacceptable levels in spite of apparently adequate beta blockade (i.e., the patient remains bradycardic with exercise), additional therapeutic measures will be necessary, since further increasing the dose of beta blocker often will not then produce further salutary effects. (Remember that occurrence of bradycardia does not mean that the dose must be reduced: An ECG should be obtained to be certain that the bradycardia is not due to heart block—a rare complication of beta blockers—but asymptomatic sinus bradycardia is not only acceptable but is *desirable* in most patients as a therapeutic end point.)

Serious side effects of beta blockers—congestive heart failure, heart

*A small subset of patients with resting tachycardia, increased myocardial contractility, and other signs of "epinephrine excess" of uncertain cause. (These patients do not have pheochromocytomas or hyperthyroidism.)

block, and bronchospasm—are uncommon but are usually obvious when they occur. (An occasional exception is the patient with intermittent coughing, the result of beta blockade–induced bronchospasm, in whom audible wheezing cannot be heard.)

More frequent, however, are the minor side effects that may be critically important in the overall management of the angina patient. These include fatigue, depression, and sexual impotence (in the male). These symptoms may be so subtle, and are so commonly psychogenic in origin otherwise, that only the physician who knows the patient well will manage this dilemma skillfully. Some attempt at a brief psychologic profile and sexual history before the administration of beta blockers will be useful. In general, it helps not to warn the patient prospectively about such "minor" side effects (since the power of suggestion is mighty), but rather to periodically ask a few probing questions as treatment continues. Impotence usually occurs early in the course of treatment, but fatigue and depression may be much more insidious in onset.

When beta blockers are withdrawn (for whatever reason), they should be withdrawn gradually (over the course of several days) because of the small but definite risk of the propranolol withdrawal rebound phenomenon[44, 45] precipitating unstable angina or even myocardial infarction.

Calcium Channel Blockers. [46–53] These newer agents—nifedipine, verapamil, and diltiazem (the only ones available at the time of printing—there will almost certainly be more)—should be considered in the patient with angina pectoris under certain circumstances. These include:

1. When coronary artery spasm is known (by angiography or documented transient ST elevations during angina;* Fig. 13–8). Nifedipine has clearly been shown to be highly effective in this situation.[46]

2. When coronary artery spasm is suspected.[160] There are no completely reliable clinical indicators of coronary spasm, but otherwise typical angina that is especially prominent at rest[53] or in cold weather or that occurs at predictable and reproducible times of the day or night is suspicious for coronary spasm. Sudden *worsening* of angina after beginning beta blocker therapy should also raise this question.

Often coronary artery spasm is superimposed on otherwise fixed atherosclerotic coronary stenoses. (Only one third of patients with coronary spasm will not also have angiographic coronary atherosclerosis; in these, spasm alone is responsible for pain.) Remember: Calcium channel agents are effective in management of chronic, stable exertional angina pectoris (without spasm) as well.[47] Thus, calcium agents should be considered as a therapeutic trial even when spasm has not been angiographically documented, especially:

3. When maximal doses of beta blockers and nitrates are ineffective. As noted above, many physicians do not push adequate amounts of traditional drugs, especially the nitrates. There is, however, evidence that combining calcium agents with beta blockers can improve treatment results.[48]

While it is in general advisable to use as simple a drug regimen as possible, combining calcium channel agents with low-dose beta blockers or nitrates should also be considered, especially:

4. When therapeutic doses of beta blockers or nitrates cannot be tolerated.

---

*Transient ST elevation during angina does not *prove* spasm, but it is suggestive.

TABLE 13–10.   CALCIUM CHANNEL BLOCKERS

DRUG	DOSAGE	SIDE EFFECTS	AMOUNT/MONTHLY COST
Nifedipine (Procardia)	10–30 mg q6–8h	Hypotension, dizziness, headache, flushing, diarrhea, constipation, pedal edema, tachycardia, paresthesias	10 mg q8h/$25
Verapamil (Calan, Isoptin)	40–120 mg q6–8h	Same plus atrioventricular block	40 mg q8h/$25
Diltiazem (Cardizem)	30–120 mg q6–8h	Same	30 mg q8h/$25

5. When angina becomes unstable (see also page 725).[49, 50]

The calcium channel agents have many effects other than their influence on coronary artery disease. They are useful as antiarrhythmic drugs and as antihypertensives. Thus a variety of side effects are possible (Table 13–10). Verapamil and diltiazem are especially useful as antiarrhythmic drugs for tachyarrhythmias, and, because they may prolong atrioventricular conduction time, these should be used with great caution (if at all) in the patient also taking beta blockers or other antiarrhythmic drugs that slow conduction through the atrioventricular node. The most common side effects of these agents are dizziness, flushing, headache, pedal edema, and a variety of bowel complaints. As can be seen in Table 13–10, these drugs can be expensive.

Coronary Artery Surgery

Decisions about coronary artery bypass procedures (and other promising nonsurgical procedures like transluminal coronary angioplasty) are made by cardiologists and cardiac surgeons, not by the generalist physician. The number of variables that may enter into such decisions are many, and this complex and controversial subject cannot possibly be reviewed here. Several reviews may be helpful.[54-62] Nevertheless, when one considers the paucity of data about the long-term risk/benefit analysis of bypass surgery, as well as the improving efficacy of pharmacologic therapy of angina pectoris, it is probably fair to say that too many surgical bypass procedures are performed currently in the United States. There are many reasons for this, but the generalist physician should at least remember a few basic facts before referring patients for consideration of surgical procedures:

1. Except for the small minority of patients who have significant narrowing of the left main coronary artery—in these patients (perhaps 5 per cent of the angina population) bypass surgery will definitely improve long-term survival—coronary artery bypass surgery is undertaken primarily to relieve the patient of symptomatic angina.*[163] Under most circumstances, then, surgical therapy is advisable when medical therapy is unsuccessful, for whatever reasons. There are exceptions to this general rule,[60] but certainly prospective surgical candidates must understand that coronary artery surgery may cure angina, but it does not cure coronary artery disease.

More than one opinion is always desirable when surgery is contemplated in the patient with chronic stable angina.

*Our understanding of the relative benefits of surgical vs. medical therapy on long-term morbidity and mortality continues to evolve. All the answers are not known.[59]

2. In some medical centers, coronary arteriography is performed routinely in patients with even mild stable angina.[63] Such practices are often justified by the fact that long-term prognosis in the patient with angina depends ultimately on the extent and anatomy of that individual's coronary artery disease (Table 13–11). For example, patients with single-vessel (not main left) coronary artery disease and good left ventricular function have a good prognosis without surgery. However, further prospective studies are needed to determine the role of coronary artery surgery in altering long-term prognosis among different subsets of patients with coronary artery disease. Such studies must categorize patients according to coronary anatomy, hemodynamic function, and symptomatic status—for each subset, medical and surgical therapy must then be compared.*

Thus, while surgery will improve statistical long-term survival in some selected patients (those with "left main disease" and perhaps "left main equivalent disease"[62]), this does not mean that all patients with known or suspected coronary artery disease should be studied by arteriography[63] to find these relative few (perhaps 10 per cent of all patients with angina). Unfortunately there are currently no noninvasive (and inexpensive) studies that accurately predict the presence of left main coronary artery disease.[64]

In general, referral for arteriography is indicated only under certain worrisome conditions (see page 725) or when the patient's angina remains symptomatically unacceptable in spite of appropriate medical therapy.

3. Every patient is different. Some patients are unwilling or unable to comply with the pharmacologic and behavioral measures so important to the medical management of angina pectoris. Other patients prefer the "one-shot" surgical approach. Still others will do almost anything to avoid the knife. While the patient's own wishes and attitudes should never be the sole determining factor, decisions for or against surgery must always be individualized.

---

*The recent Coronary Artery Surgery Study is an excellent beginning.[164, 165]

TABLE 13–11. MORTALITY AFTER NONSURGICAL TREATMENT OF CORONARY ARTERY DISEASE

	% Mortality per Year	% Mortality per 5 Years
Normal arteriogram	0	0
Single vessel		
LAD*	2–4	10–20
RCA†	1–2	2–8
Circumflex	0–1	0–2
Two vessel		
LAD plus RCA or circumflex	7–10	35–50
Before first septal perforator		12
After first septal perforator		12
RCA plus circumflex	3–6	15–30
Three vessel	10–12	50–60
Left main‡	15–25	70

(Reproduced with permission from Humphries, JO: Expected course of patients with coronary artery disease. In Rahimtoola, SH (ed.): Coronary Bypass Surgery. Philadelphia: F. A. Davis Co., 1977, p. 48.)
*LAD, left anterior descending coronary artery.
†RCA, right coronary artery.
‡Left main: stenosis of the proximal "take off" of the left coronary artery.

TABLE 13–12. PROBABILITY OF DEVELOPING CORONARY HEART DISEASE IN 8 YEARS*

45-YEAR-OLD MAN†

DOES NOT SMOKE CIGARETTES | SMOKE CIGARETTES

LVH-ECG Negative

	Chol	SBP 105	120	135	150	165	180		Chol	SBP 105	120	135	150	165	180
Glucose intolerance absent	185	20	24	29	35	42	51		185	32	39	46	56	67	81
	210	25	30	36	44	53	64		210	40	48	58	69	83	99
	235	31	38	45	55	66	79		235	50	60	72	86	103	122
	260	39	47	56	68	81	97		260	62	74	89	106	126	149
	285	48	58	70	84	100	119		285	76	92	109	130	153	181
	310	60	72	87	104	123	146		310	94	113	134	158	186	217

	Chol	SBP 105	120	135	150	165	180		Chol	SBP 105	120	135	150	165	180
Glucose intolerance present	185	25	30	36	44	53	64		185	40	48	58	69	83	99
	210	31	38	45	55	66	79		210	50	60	72	86	102	122
	235	39	47	56	68	81	97		235	62	74	89	106	126	149
	260	48	58	70	84	100	119		260	76	91	109	130	153	181
	285	60	72	87	103	123	146		285	94	112	134	158	186	217
	310	75	89	107	127	150	177		310	116	138	163	191	223	259

LVH-ECG Positive

	Chol	SBP 105	120	135	150	165	180		Chol	SBP 105	120	135	150	165	180
Glucose intolerance absent	185	41	50	60	72	86	102		185	65	78	93	111	132	157
	210	51	62	74	89	106	126		210	81	96	115	136	161	189
	235	64	76	91	109	130	153		235	100	118	141	166	195	227
	260	79	94	112	134	158	186		260	122	145	171	200	234	270
	285	97	116	138	163	191	223		285	149	176	206	240	277	318
	310	120	142	167	196	229	266		310	181	212	246	284	326	370

	Chol	SBP 105	120	135	150	165	180		Chol	SBP 105	120	135	150	165	180
Glucose intolerance absent	185	51	62	74	88	105	126		185	81	96	115	136	161	189
	210	64	76	91	109	129	153		210	99	118	140	166	195	227
	235	79	94	112	133	158	186		235	122	145	171	200	233	270
	260	97	116	137	162	191	223		260	149	176	206	240	277	318
	285	119	142	167	196	229	265		285	181	211	246	284	325	370
	310	146	172	202	235	272	313		310	217	252	291	333	378	425

(From Gordon, T, Sorlie, P, Kannel, WB: Coronary heart disease, atherothrombotic brain infarction, intermittent claudication—A multivariate analysis of some factors related to their incidence. Framingham Study, 16-year follow-up. In Kannel, WB, Gordon, T (eds.): The Framingham Study. An Epidemiological Investigation of Cardiovascular Disease. Section 27, 1971.)

*Sixteen-year follow-up of the Framingham Study. Probability is shown in thousandths.

†Men aged 45 years have an average systolic blood pressure (SBP) of 131 mm Hg and an average serum cholesterol (Chol) of 235 mg per 100 ml; 67 per cent smoke cigarettes, 1.3 per cent have definite left ventricular hypertrophy (LVH) according to ECG findings, and 3.8 per cent have glucose intolerance. At these average values, the probability of developing coronary heart disease in 8 years is 60/1000.

Patient Education

Fundamental to the management of angina pectoris is the notion that the patient should understand its basic pathophysiology. The degree to which this is feasible will depend on the individual patient's interest and capability, but most patients comprehend the simplified supply-and-demand concept of coronary artery disease: Cardiac muscle can perform painlessly the effort demanded of it only when it is provided with adequate blood supply; angina occurs when the heart muscle demands more blood than can be supplied; the treatment of angina must then either improve the blood supply or lessen the demand for it. This concept emphasizes the difference between coronary artery disease and its symptoms, since some components of treatment are aimed at angina (drugs, exercise) and others are directed at coronary artery disease itself (risk factor modification). The supply-and-demand theory, however simplistic, will make more obvious to the patient the rationale for pharmacologic therapy, surgical intervention, exercise, and other necessary alterations in life style. It is hoped that this improved understanding will improve patient compliance. Consider especially:

TABLE 13–12. PROBABILITY OF DEVELOPING CORONARY HEART DISEASE IN 8 YEARS* (Continued)

65-YEAR-OLD MAN‡

		DOES NOT SMOKE CIGARETTES								SMOKE CIGARETTES					

LVH-ECG Negative

	SBP	105	120	135	150	165	180	SBP	105	120	135	150	165	180
Chol								**Chol**						
Glucose intolerance absent — 185		67	80	96	115	136	161	185	105	124	147	174	204	237
210		69	83	99	118	140	165	210	107	128	151	178	209	243
235		71	85	102	121	143	169	235	111	131	155	183	214	249
260		73	88	104	124	147	174	260	114	135	159	187	219	254
285		75	90	107	128	151	178	285	117	139	164	192	224	260
310		77	93	110	131	155	183	310	120	142	168	197	230	266

	SBP	105	120	135	150	165	180	SBP	105	120	135	150	165	180
Chol								**Chol**						
Glucose intolerance absent — 185		83	99	1118	140	165	194	185	128	152	179	209	243	281
210		85	102	121	144	169	199	210	132	156	183	214	249	287
235		88	105	125	148	174	204	235	135	160	188	220	255	294
260		90	108	128	151	178	209	260	139	164	193	225	261	300
285		93	111	131	155	183	214	285	143	168	197	230	267	307
310		95	114	135	160	188	219	310	146	173	202	236	273	314

LVH-ECG Positive

	SBP	105	120	135	150	165	180	SBP	105	120	135	150	165	180
Chol								**Chol**						
Glucose intolerance absent — 185		132	156	184	215	250	288	185	198	231	268	308	351	397
210		136	160	188	220	256	295	210	203	237	274	314	358	404
235		139	164	193	226	262	301	235	208	242	280	321	365	412
260		143	169	198	231	268	308	260	213	248	286	328	373	419
285		147	173	203	237	274	314	285	219	254	293	335	380	427
310		151	178	208	242	280	321	310	224	260	299	342	387	435

	SBP	105	120	135	150	165	180	SBP	105	120	135	150	165	180
Chol								**Chol**						
Glucose intolerance absent — 185		161	189	221	256	295	337	185	237	274	315	359	405	453
210		165	193	226	262	302	344	210	243	281	322	366	412	461
235		169	198	231	268	308	351	235	248	287	329	373	420	468
260		173	203	237	274	315	359	260	254	293	335	380	428	476
285		178	208	243	280	322	366	285	260	300	342	388	435	484
310		183	214	248	287	328	373	310	266	306	349	395	443	491

(From Gordon, T, Sorlie, P, and Kannel, WB: Coronary heart disease, atherothrombotic brain infarction, intermittent claudication— A multivariate analysis of some factors related to their incidence. Framingham Study, 16-year follow-up. In Kannel, WB, Gordon, T (eds): The Framingham Study. An Epidemiological Investigation of Cardiovascular Disease. Section 27, 1971.)

*Sixteen-year follow-up of the Framingham Study. Probability is shown in thousandths.

‡Men aged 65 years have an average systolic blood pressure (SBP) of 143 mm Hg and an average serum cholesterol (Chol) of 236 mg per 100 ml; 45 per cent smoke cigarettes, 7.9 per cent have definite left ventricular hypertrophy (LVH) according to ECG findings, and 9.6 per cent have glucose intolerance. At these average values, the probability of developing coronary heart disease in 8 years is 145/1000.

I. Risk factor modification.

Whether the modification of various coronary risk factors—especially hypertension, hypercholesterolemia, smoking, obesity, glucose intolerance, and sedentary life styles—will alter the ultimate progression of established coronary artery disease in an individual patient is unknown. Surely, attempted prevention of these risk factors before development of coronary artery disease makes more sense. Nevertheless, patients can be told (albeit simplistically) that smoking and hypercholesterolemia and glucose intolerance reduce myocardial blood supply by accelerating atherosclerosis while hypertension, obesity, and poor physical conditioning place excessive demands on the heart muscle. Thus, altering these factors may change the balance of supply and demand so that angina pectoris will improve. Two concepts deserve emphasis here:

A. The cumulative impact of the various risk factors should be emphasized.

Actually showing patients the dramatic data from the Framingham study will raise more than a few eyebrows (Table 13–12)

HOW TO COUNT YOUR PULSE

1. Locate your pulse in either the carotid artery in the neck (left) or the radial artery at the wrist (right).

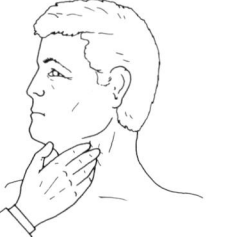 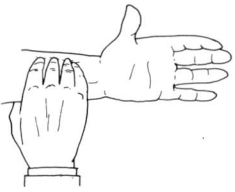

2. Count the number of pulse beats in ten seconds, using a timepiece with a second hand. Note if your pulse is regular or irregular ("skipping").

3. Calculate your pulse per minute from the table, and record!

Beats in Ten Seconds	Pulse Per minute	Beats in Ten Seconds	Pulse Per Minute
7	42	19	114
8	48	20	120
9	54	21	126
10	60	22	132
11	66	23	138
12	72	24	144
13	78	25	150
14	84	26	156
15	90	27	162
16	96	28	168
17	102	29	174
18	108	30	180

A

WALK PROGRAM

Conditions: Loose, comfortable clothing and comfortable shoes should be worn for the walks. If you have been instructed to walk indoors, be sure you are walking in a comfortable "in-door" temperature (60 to 75 degrees Fahrenheit). Remember to relax as you walk, particularly back, shoulders, and arms.

Frequency: Exercises should be done _every other day_ . Take pulse and record before exercise begins.

Warm-up: _Walk slowly for 10 minutes_ .

Routine: Walk for _1 mile_ at a rate of _2 miles / hour_ . Stop, sit down, and immediately record pulse. Allow pulse to return to resting pulse (at least 3 minutes).

Complete second walk for _½ mile_ at a rate of _2 miles / hour_ .

Cool-down: _Walk slowly for 10 minutes_ .

If at any time you experience chest pain or discomfort, shortness of breath, sweating, or undue fatigue, you should stop.

Remember: Wait 1½ hours after meals, skip exercise on "bad" days.

B   Maximum pulse _120_ .

FIGURE 13–14. *A,* How to count your pulse. *B,* Walk program and heart rate profile.

HEART RATE PROFILE

Instructions: Count your heart rate for only 10 seconds, beginning one second or less after you start palpating your pulse. Multiply each value by 6 to obtain the heart rate per minute.

Week	Rest	Warmup	Stimulus Period						Cooldown Period	
	Resting Rate	After Warmup	After 5 min.	10 min.	15 min.	20 min.	25 min.	30 min.	After 2 min.	After 10 min.
1										
2										
3										
4										
5										
6										
7										
8										
9										
10										
11										
12										
13										
14										
15										

FIGURE 13–14. Continued.

and will underline the importance of cumulative risk factors. For the patient with hypertension and angina, for example, it should be made plain that taking antihypertensive medication is not enough if the patient continues to smoke. Other practical issues may thus be clarified for different patients: for example, even borderline hypertension should be treated, all the more so in the sedentary smoker with hypercholesterolemia.

B. Patients should understand that risk factor modification is largely up to them.

Diet, exercise, stopping smoking, and complying with antihypertensive therapy all depend ultimately on patient complicance. None of these major alterations in habit and life style is easy, but all are under the patient's own control—this is an important psychologic plus for many patients. The monolithic myth of angina pectoris should be specifically debunked: Angina pectoris is not necessarily a death sentence, nor does every patient with angina pectoris suffer myocardial infarction. The notion that patients can do something about it themselves is always worth emphasis.

II. Exercise should be scientific, specific, and sometimes supervised.

Many people do not know how to exercise. Explaining the concept of aerobic exercise (walking, jogging, bicycling), which conditions the heart without straining it, will help many patients understand that a gradual, controlled exercise program can ultimately allow the heart to perform more work despite a fixed coronary blood supply.

Figure 13–14 illustrates a walking program designed for a relatively sedentary patient with mild exertional angina (NYHA Class II or III). Similar programs for bicycling, swimming, or jogging can be easily prescribed. Whatever exercise is to be used, careful prescriptions of frequency, duration, and rate of exercise should be tailored to the individual patient—gradual modification can then follow in the subsequent weeks and months. In general, 30 minutes per day of aerobic exercise is the goal. Patients should be instructed how to take their own pulse and to follow their progress over time with a heart rate profile.

Exercise testing may be especially helpful as an educational device—both initially, to document exercise tolerance and to set a maximum pulse, and serially, to demonstrate (to the physician and the patient) the value of progressive exercise training (see Appendix I).[65]

It is never advisable to simply tell the patient to "get some exercise." Specifically, nonaerobic exercise—weight lifting, push-ups, and the like—should be deemphasized in the patient with angina.

III. Alterations in life style.

While the supply/demand balance may tip in the patient's favor when earnest attempts are made to exercise, diet, stop smoking, and take appropriate medications, such efforts require major life style changes for many patients. Some will be able to conform, but many will not. Whatever the results of their own efforts, patients will often be grateful to the physician who takes the time to explain and to listen. Patients must understand, for example, that what we demand of our heart is rooted deeply in what we demand of ourselves. It is not just *what* we demand, but *how* we demand it, that may tip the balance favorably or unfavorably. The impact of emotional stresses and the liability of certain personality types in the precipitation and treatment

TABLE 13–13. TREATMENT OF ANGINA

STEP 1

Exclude treatable causes (e.g., aortic stenosis) and precipitating factors
(anemia, thyrotoxicosis, arrhythmias, hypertension)
Hospitalize, investigate, and/or refer the patient with unstable angina,
"ominous" exercise tests, or angina after myocardial infarction or
bypass surgery

STEP 2

Instruct in use of sublingual nitroglycerin
Explain angina
Risk factor modification: stop smoking; treat hypertension, diet
Graduated "cardiac exercise" program
Evaluate life style, stress: modulate "demands"

STEP 3 (Step 2 plus)

Long-acting nitrates (Table 13–8)
      and/or
Beta blockers (Table 13–9)
      and/or
Calcium channel antagonists (Table 13–10)
  (Suspect coronary spasm)

STEP 4

Maximize dosage of nitrates, beta blockers, and calcium channel agents
If refractory to optimal therapy, consider surgery
Consider arteriography → surgery?

---

of angina must be made clear to individual patients. Above all, this requires that the physician get to know the patient, often with attention to seemingly unimportant details, as Graboys and Lown explain:

> For example, consider the patient who awakens late each morning, is in a mad rush to shower, shave, dress, and have breakfast before racing down to the automobile, and then experiences angina while reaching for the ignition key. Counseling such a patient to arise 5 to 10 minutes earlier may eliminate this pattern of angina. Simply slowing the tempo of activity still allows the patient to reach the planned destination but prevents chest discomfort.
>
> If the patient exercises on an empty stomach, angina will be prevented and there will be no need to give up a favored activity . . . the imaginative, caring physician can find ingenious but nontaxing solutions to a myriad of other similar problems.[66]

Absolute restrictions on physical activity and life style are sometimes not so necessary as are a sensitization to self-expectations and modulation of the tempo of life. The "imaginative, caring physician" can be very helpful here. The value of stress management training in this setting deserves further study.[67]

The goal of antianginal therapy is total elimination of angina. This is possible only sometimes. The general approach summarized in Table 13–13 will usually help.

When to Worry, When to Refer, When to Hospitalize

There are several situations in which worry is appropriate when treating the angina patient. These are also the usual reasons to either hospitalize the patient or immediately seek a specialist's help.

1. The patient with unstable angina. Stable angina means that angina is chronic and predictable—i.e., induced by the same degree of physical or psychic stress, relieved reproducibly with rest or nitroglycerin, and requiring relatively stable doses of nitrates, beta blockers, or other drugs. Unstable angina thus refers to angina that is new or accelerating or recently unpredictable. For example, the patient with no prior history of angina who develops frequent, severe, and prolonged anginal episodes over the preceding

several days or weeks has unstable angina. So does the patient with chronic, exertional angina whose pain is now provoked by much less activity than previously, which now occurs at rest or during sleep, or which is now not so reliably relieved with the usual pause for rest or nitroglycerin. Even more unstable is angina in the patient with severe, prolonged chest pain associated with transient ECG changes (preinfarction angina[3]), especially when such symptoms occur at rest or with little provocation.[68]

It is always important to remember that unstable angina may be mistaken for stable angina complicated by other remediable problems (anemia, hyperthyroidism, congestive heart failure, arrhythmias), as mentioned previously. New nocturnal angina, for example, often prompts concern about unstable coronary artery disease or impending myocardial infarction, but such symptoms may also at times simply reflect stressful dreams, reflux esophagitis, paroxysmal noctural dyspnea due to congestive heart failure, hypoglycemia in the diabetic, or nocturnal cardiac arrhythmias—each of these obviously requires a very different therapeutic approach than does unstable angina.

In general, hospitalization and intensive medical therapy are indicated for the patient with unstable angina.[69] Immediate arteriography or coronary surgery is not usually necessary or beneficial (an exception is the patient already refractory to optimal medical therapy—urgent arteriography and surgery may be necessary here). Arteriography after stabilization in the hospital is usually worthwhile to detect the minority with main left coronary artery stenoses (in whom surgery must be considered), those few with normal coronary arteries, and those whose coronary anatomy or ventricular function proves them noncandidates for surgery anyway.

2. The patient with "ominous" exercise tolerance test results. Various "ominous" findings on stress testing sometimes indicate dangerous coronary artery disease—i.e., main left disease or multiple-vessel disease. This does not mean that surgery is indicated in all patients with such stress test results, since medical therapy may be very effective in many such patients,[70] but often patients in this group should at least be subjected to coronary arteriography (see Appendix I).

3. The patient who develops angina pectoris following myocardial infarction. Especially when the patient develops angina and ischemic changes (on resting ECG or stress test) in an area of myocardium distant from the previous infarction (for example, anterior ischemia in the patient after inferior myocardial infarction), one must always be concerned about the prognostic implications of jeopardizing "critical myocardial mass."[71] The patient who develops angina soon after documented myocardial infarction is probably at especially high risk.[72]

4. The patient who develops angina after coronary artery surgery. Early postoperative angina may reflect graft closure, while later development of angina usually implies progression of underlying coronary artery disease. Nevertheless, such patients usually require referral and study.

5. Obviously, the patient in whom myocardial infarction is suspected. Thus:

Three days later, Angela arrives in the clinic unannounced, complaining of severe lower retrosternal chest pain of 2 hours' duration which has not responded to nitroglycerin times four doses. Angela is slightly pale and diaphoretic, and is obviously in pain. Blood pressure is 160/105, pulse 100 and regular, temperature 38°C rectally, respiratory rate 16 per minute.

Angela explains that the pain began while sitting at her desk, working. She had felt well for the previous 3 days. The pain began "sort of" suddenly, but became gradually worse over the next hour. She became nauseated and has vomited twice since. The pain is constant, deep, and aching, is unrelated to body position, and is not respirophasic. When asked to point to the pain, she placed her open hand over her upper epigastrium and lower sternum. The pain does not radiate. The pain is similar to one prior episode of prolonged pain mentioned during her previous visit.

Angela is anxious and seems restless, preferring to frequently shift position rather than to lie still. Physical examination of the head, eyes, ears, nose, throat, chest, heart, pulses, and abdomen is normal except for vague, mild discomfort on deep palpation of the subxiphoid area. Deep breaths do not worsen the pain, nor do chest-wall maneuvers.

The ECG is normal except for sinus tachycardia of 100 per minute. The chest x-ray is normal. The white blood count is 10,000 with 80 per cent polymorphonuclears.

Pain persists 1 hour after arrival. Angela vomits again.

ACUTE SEVERE CHEST PAIN

While any of the causes of episodic chest pain (discussed above) may cause acute severe chest pain, patients who are obviously acutely ill with severe chest pain usually will have one of the serious illnesses in Table 13–14. While the differential diagnosis is very broad—it includes cardiac, pulmonary, vascular, mediastinal, spinal, and gastrointestinal disease—it is usually possible to make the correct diagnosis (and exclude others) after careful clinical examination and a few simple tests.

I. History.

Several factors are important in the history:

A. The location or radiation of pain may or may not help (Fig. 13–15).
Subxiphoid or epigastric pain suggests gastrointestinal causes (especially biliary, pancreatic, esophageal, and gastroduodenal), but

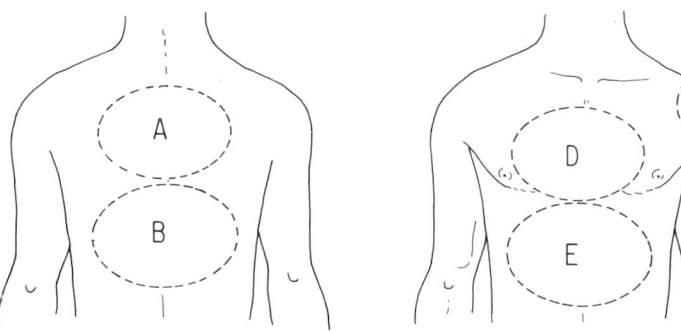

A. Upper posterior chest
Myocardial infarction?
Aortic dissection?
Esophageal disease?
Cervical/thoracic spine disease

B. Lower posterior chest
Pancreatic disease?
Aortic dissection/aneurysm?
(Penetrating) peptic ulcer?
Acute cholecystitis?
Spinal disease?
Renal/retroperitoneal disease?

C. Shoulder
Local shoulder disorder?
Cervical spine disease?
Cardiac disease?
Esophageal/mediastinal disease?
Pleuropulmonary disease?

D. Upper anterior chest
Myocardial infarction?
Pericarditis?
Aortic dissection?
Esophageal disease?
Cholecystitis?
Pulmonary embolism?

E. Lower anterior chest
Myocardial infarction?
Aortic dissection/aneurysm?
Peptic ulcer?
Cholecystitis?
Pancreatitis?

FIGURE 13–15. Common locations of chest pain.

TABLE 13–14. CAUSES OF ACUTE NONPLEURITIC CHEST PAIN

DISEASE	USUAL SYMPTOMS	HELPFUL CLUES	USUALLY EXCLUDE BY	DEFINITIVELY CONFIRMED BY
Myocardial infarction[73]	Severe, oppressive, constricting retrosternal pain; onset usually at rest, lasting more than 30 min; often anxious, restless, diaphoretic, dyspneic	Prior history of angina or myocardial infarction; ischemic ECG (Fig. 13–17); Levine's sign; associated arrhythmias and/or congestive heart failure	Normal ECG and/or observation in hospital and normal cardiac enzymes	ECG evolution (usually); cardiac enzymes increase[74, 75]; nuclear scan (sometimes)[76, 158]
Aortic dissection[77, 78]	Very abrupt, tearing pain in anterior or posterior chest, migrating to arms, abdomen, legs	Pulse deficits; shocky but hypertensive; neurologic findings; aortic insufficiency murmur; history of hypertension (especially with "distal dissection")[77]; normal ECG/abnormal chest x-ray (Fig. 13–19)	Normal mediastinum on chest x-ray and no "helpful clues", but only angiography definitively excludes	Angiography
Pericarditis[79, 80]	Pleuritic chest pain or nonpleuritic myocardial infarction type of chest pain; pain often worse supine, better sitting up; referral to trapezius ridge	Underlying disease (viral infection, connective tissue disease, uremia—Table 13–15); typical ECG evolution (Fig. 13–26); pericardial friction rub	Normal ECG and absence of pericardial friction rub	Typical ECG evolution; pericardial rub
Acute coronary insufficiency[5, 68]	Severe, oppressive, constricting retrosternal pain; onset usually at rest; lasting more than 30 min; often anxious, restless, diaphoretic, dyspneic	Prior history of angina or myocardial infarction; ischemic ECG; Levine's sign; associated arrhythmias and/or congestive heart failure	Normal ECG; observation in hospital—normal stress tests and/or arteriography when stable	Clinical findings with transient ECG ischemic changes without infarction per enzymes or ECG; stress test and/or arteriography
Pulmonary embolism[95, 96]	Pleuritic chest pain and/or sudden dyspnea, apprehension, palpitations; occasionally, acute nonpleuritic chest "pressure"	Factors predisposing to venous thrombosis—postoperative, post partum, birth control pills, prolonged bedrest or immobilization, cancer, congestive heart failure; hemoptysis; clinical deep vein thrombosis (legs)	Normal perfusion lung scan	Ventilation perfusion lung scans and/or pulmonary angiography (see Appendix IV)
Pneumothorax[159]	Sudden dyspnea, cough, chest pain	Diminished breath sounds; mediastinal shift?	Normal chest x-ray	Chest x-ray (Fig. 13–20)
Pneumomediastinum[81]	Sudden retrosternal pain and dyspnea	Bronchial asthma; chest trauma; suspected esophageal or tracheal perforation; subcutaneous emphysema/"crunch"	Normal chest x-ray (PA and lateral film); look carefully at lateral!	Chest x-ray (Fig. 13–21)

Esophageal rupture[82,83]	Sudden substernal (usually) left chest pain (sometimes pleuritic); dyspnea; sometimes fever	Onset immediately after vomiting and/or esophageal instrumentation; unexplained left pleural effusion and/or mediastinitis	Normal chest x-ray and unlikely clinical setting	Gastrografin barium swallow (Fig. 13–22); endoscopy (find cause)
Pneumonia	Usually pleuritic chest pain with cough and fever	History, chest x-ray	Normal chest x-ray (after 24 hours of symptoms)	Chest x-ray; sputum analysis
Esophageal spasm[84,85]	Substernal constricting chest pain, often at time of swallowing	History of dysphagia; relation of pain to cold/carbonated beverages or foods	Normal esophageal manometry with or without ergonovine "challenge"[86]	Barium swallow, endoscopy, and/or esophageal manometry (see Appendix II)
Esophagitis*	Heartburn	Acid brash; worse bending over, supine; better with antacids	Endoscopy and biopsy	Endoscopy; biopsy; acid perfusion test (see Appendix II)
Biliary colic*	15 min to 6 hr epigastric/right upper quadrant constant pain with nausea and vomiting—self-limited	Examination often normal; recurrent attacks; fat, forty, fertile female	Absence of gallstones radiographically (oral cholecystography, abdominal ultrasound)	Clinical history; oral cholecystography, abdominal ultrasound, and/or radionuclide biliary scan
Acute cholecystitis*	Prolonged, (hours—days) epigastric and/or right upper quadrant pain with nausea and vomiting; fever/chills → cholangitis	Murphy's sign and/or tender epigastrium/right upper quadrant; prior history biliary colic	Absence of gallstones radiographically (oral cholecystography, ultrasound)	Abdominal ultrasound, radionuclide scan, and/or surgical exploration
Pancreatitis, acute*	Severe epigastric/periumbilical pain radiating to the back with nausea and vomiting; "sick"	Tender epigastrium; history of alcohol or gallstones; increased serum amylase	Normal amylase and lipase	Clinical picture; increased serum amylase and lipase
Hepatic congestion*	Vague right upper quadrant and/or epigastric discomfort	Tender, enlarged liver; congestive heart failure	Absence of hepatomegaly, right upper quadrant tenderness, and congestive heart failure	Improvement with treatment of underlying condition (usually congestive heart failure)
Peptic ulcer disease*	Epigastric postprandial discomfort, usually relieved with antacids and/or food	History; antacid trial	Endoscopy	Upper GI series and/or endoscopy
Perforated ulcer*	"Acute abdomen" and/or pancreatitis	Increased amylase (posterior penetration of duodenal ulcer); "acute abdomen;" air under diaphragm (p. 552); Fig. 11–11	Normal abdominal examination, normal amylase, and normal abdominal x-ray	Endoscopy
Cervical/thoracic spine disease: degenerative spondylosis, osteoporosis, thoracic disc, metastatic neoplasm	Usually posterior chest pain, exacerbated by spinal range of motion; sometimes, radicular pain increased with Valsalva maneuver	Increased pain with neck/torso range of motion; increased pain with Valsalva maneuver; radicular pain	Clinical findings; normal spine films; sometimes bone scan, myelography	Clinical findings; spine x-rays; sometimes myelography, bone scan

*See Chapter 11, "Abdominal Pain."

the pain of myocardial infarction, aortic dissection, or pericarditis may also be located in the epigastrium.

Upper anterior chest pain is not usually associated with gastrointestinal diseases, except those of esophageal origin.

Pain involving the left arm is utterly nonspecific, despite the "left arm–cardiac pain" myth.

Pain in the upper midback (interscapular area) should suggest either disease of the spine or of the mediastinum—especially the aorta, esophagus, or heart.

Pain in the midback (lower thoracic spine) should suggest pancreatic or spinal disease but aortic, biliary, or peptic ulcer disease may so present as well.

B. The quality of pain sometimes helps.

Pleuritic chest pain—sharp, "sticking," lateralized, respirophasic pain—involves a differential diagnosis discussed on page 741, but since some of the common causes of pleuritic pain—especially pulmonary embolism and pericarditis—will occasionally cause nonpleuritic chest pain, these disorders must be considered here as well.

Severe pain described as ripping or tearing, especially when such pain migrates up the chest, into the neck or arms or down the back, should suggest aortic dissection. Conversely, the pain of myocardial infarction is usually an oppressive, constricting, suffocating discomfort that is usually quite severe. (Remember, however, that as many as 10 to 20 per cent of patients suffering myocardial infarction may not have chest discomfort at all.)

Pain that is radicular, i.e., encircles the chest unilaterally from back to front and is qualitatively electric, shooting, or prickly suggests neuritis of some form—for example, incipient herpes zoster (before the rash appears), diabetic neuritis, or thoracic spine disease.

Burning pain is nonspecific. This is a common descriptor for esophageal or peptic ulcer pain, but a few patients will describe myocardial infarction in the same way.

Pain at the left breast border that is synchronous with the heart beat is a rare manifestation of pericarditis.

Pain that is very brief ("a second") but intermittently recurrent and severe is usually of psychogenic or chest-wall origin, but intercostal neuralgia may also be so described (as may, very rarely, coronary artery spasm).

C. Precise timing of the onset and the severity of pain helps.

Acute chest pain that is very severe and at its worst from the moment of onset is typical of aortic dissection, spontaneous pneumothorax, esophageal rupture, pneumomediastinum, and perforation of an intra-abdominal viscus. Many other diseases may cause sudden chest pain—pulmonary embolism, pericarditis, biliary colic, esophageal spasm—but these usually are not of maximal intensity quite so immediately. The pain of myocardial infarction, acute cholecystitis, pericarditis, and peptic ulcer disease can begin suddenly but is usually more gradual in onset and then worsens over time.

D. Occasionally, specific events will seem to have triggered the pain.

When pain immediately follows vomiting—consider esophageal rupture; swallowing—consider esophageal spasm; coughing—consider pneumothorax, pneumomediastinum, or rib fracture; Valsalva maneuvers (straining at stool, for example)—consider pulmonary embolism, herniated thoracic disc, aortic dissection, or pneumo-thorax/pneumomediastinum.

E. Associated or antecedent symptoms usually help.

Nausea and vomiting are nonspecific since they may occur with severe pain of any kind, but they are typical of biliary disease, pancreatitis, and (inferior) myocardial infarction.

Acute dyspnea should suggest myocardial infarction, pulmonary embolism, pneumothorax, or pneumonia. Subdiaphragmatic disease (especially acute cholecystitis or subdiaphragmatic abscess) or disease associated with a sudden pleural effusion (esophageal rupture or aortic dissection) may also cause acute shortness of breath.

Dysphagia suggests esophageal disease but may be seen with other mediastinal disorders as well.

Many patients with myocardial infarction give a history of preceding angina pectoris.

Many patients with acute cholecystitis give a history of prior biliary colic (page 693). Most patients with pulmonary embolism have some underlying predisposition to venous thrombosis (page 744).

Most patients with severe peptic disease (or a perforated ulcer) give a prior history of typical postprandial abdominal discomfort (page 595).

In Angela's case, pain is epigastric and substernal, is constant and severe but is not pleuritic, has worsened gradually over 2 hours' time, and is associated with nausea and vomiting. Pain continues.

Thus, Angela's symptoms are not diagnostic of any one disorder, but they are most suggestive of myocardial infarction or acute gastrointestinal disease, especially biliary disease or pancreatitis. Nonpleuritic pericarditis or pulmonary emboli are possible, and no one cause of pain listed in Table 13–14 could be summarily excluded on the basis of the history alone.

II. Physical Examination.

Vital signs and general appearance are crucial.

Most of the disorders listed in Table 13–14 can be associated with shock. (Esophagitis, esophageal spasm, biliary colic, and thoracic spine disease do not cause shock.) This designation usually refers to the presence of hypotension, but not always—the patient with severe chest pain who is shocky (pale, clammy, disoriented, restless, and diaphoretic) but hypertensive should suggest aortic dissection (or myocardial infarction).

Hypotension in the patient with severe chest pain may be the result of: cardiac compromise—due to myocardial infarction, pulmonary embolism, pericardial tamponade, massive pneumothorax or pneumomediastinum, or aortic dissection with congestive heart failure and aortic insufficiency; sepsis—pneumonia, cholangitis, purulent pericarditis, perforated abdominal viscus, or subdiaphragmatic abscess should be remembered; or "occult" causes—acute pancreatitis or rupture of the esophagus, aorta, or an intra-abdominal viscus.

Blood pressure should be taken in both arms and all peripheral pulses recorded—discrepancies (for example, absence of left carotid, left branchial, or femoral pulses) should suggest acute aortic dissection.

Restlessness may reflect incipient shock but may also be a characteristic response to certain types of pain. For example, biliary colic, pulmonary embolism, and esophageal spasm commonly cause fright and an impulse to move about. Conversely, acute cholecystitis, myocardial infarction, and acute pancreatitis usually cause the patient to remain motionless, passively awaiting relief or doom.

Fever is nonspecific, since it may be associated with pulmonary emboli, aortic dissection, and pancreatitis as well as with the infectious or inflammatory processes listed in Table 13–14. High fever and rigors should suggest bacterial infection (in the biliary tract, lung, or pericardium, for example).

Examination of the thorax and lungs will usually diagnose (or suggest) pneumonia—consolidation or focal crackles—as well as pneumothorax—unilateral diminished breath sounds.

Cardiac examination will often diagnose pericarditis—pericardial friction rub; proximal aortic dissection—a new aortic insufficiency murmur; or various complications of myocardial infarction—papillary muscle dysfunction or congestive heart failure.

Abdominal examination will usually be revealing during acute cholecystitis or pancreatitis; after a ruptured abdominal viscus; or when hepatic congestion is the problem, but is often unimpressive during biliary colic or esophageal disorders.

Tenderness of the chest or abdominal wall during acute chest pain is nonspecific: It is not unusual for patients with all varieties of severe "internal" chest pain to admit to vague tenderness of the overlying chest or abdominal surface.

In Angela's case, physical examination is normal except for mild hypertension, tachycardia, (perhaps) low-grade fever, restlessness, and (perhaps) mild subxiphoid tenderness.

Thus, physical examination is rather unrevealing and does not add much to the differential diagnosis suggested by Angela's symptoms. There is, however, no physical finding that suggests pericarditis, pneumonia, pneumothorax, hepatic congestion, or a perforated intra-abdominal viscus.

III. Tests.

The ECG and chest x-ray are always helpful in the patient with acute severe chest pain. In Angela's case, both are normal.

A. The electrocardiogram is usually diagnostic of acute transmural myocardial infarction, but this is not always so (Figs. 13–16 through 13–18).

As Table 13–14 suggests, myocardial infarction can be excluded only by serial ECGs and cardiac enzyme determinations over the course of 24 hours, and it is often the history and physical findings, rather than the ECG that determine the need for hospitalization for suspected myocardial infarction. The distinction among acute coronary insufficiency,[5, 68] subendocardial infarction,[88] and transmural myocardial infarction[89] has blurred, not just because the clinical symptoms of each may be identical, but because the ultimate prognosis of each may be similar. Thus, while in most instances threatened or actual myocardial infarction produces an abnormal ECG, nonspecific ECG changes (or even a normal ECG) in such settings are not at all uncommon. The initial absence of "classic" ECG abnormalities is the most common reason for failure to diagnose acute myocardial infarction.[159]

Pericarditis cannot be diagnosed in the absence of a pericardial friction rub when the ECG is also normal (see page 746).

B. A normal chest x-ray *usually* excludes aortic dissection, pneumothorax, pneumonia, pneumomediastinum, and esophageal rupture.

Caution is advised here. For example, 90 per cent of aortic dissections will be associated with an abnormal aortic knob or widening of the mediastinum (Fig. 13–19, page 736).[77, 78] These changes may be very subtle, however, and when other clinical findings are suggestive, a normal chest x-ray by no means excludes the diagnosis (and ultrasound and/or arteriography is necessary). A small or loculated pneumothorax may be missed;[160] a large one is usually obvious (Fig. 13–20, page 737). Pneumomediastinum may be very subtle (but a lateral chest film usually helps) (Fig. 13–21, page 737). Pneumonia will occasionally not appear radiographically until symptoms have been present for 24 to 48 hours (page 634). Esophageal rupture usually causes at least some change in the chest x-ray (almost always on the left), but these changes may be hidden by the heart shadow (Fig. 13–22, page 738).

C. Other tests will occasionally help.

Leukocytosis, like fever, is relatively nonspecific, but extreme white count elevations (greater than 20,000) normally suggest infection—pneumonia, esophageal or abdominal visceral rupture, chole-

I	AVR	V1	V4
II	AVL	V2	V5
III	AVF	V3	V6

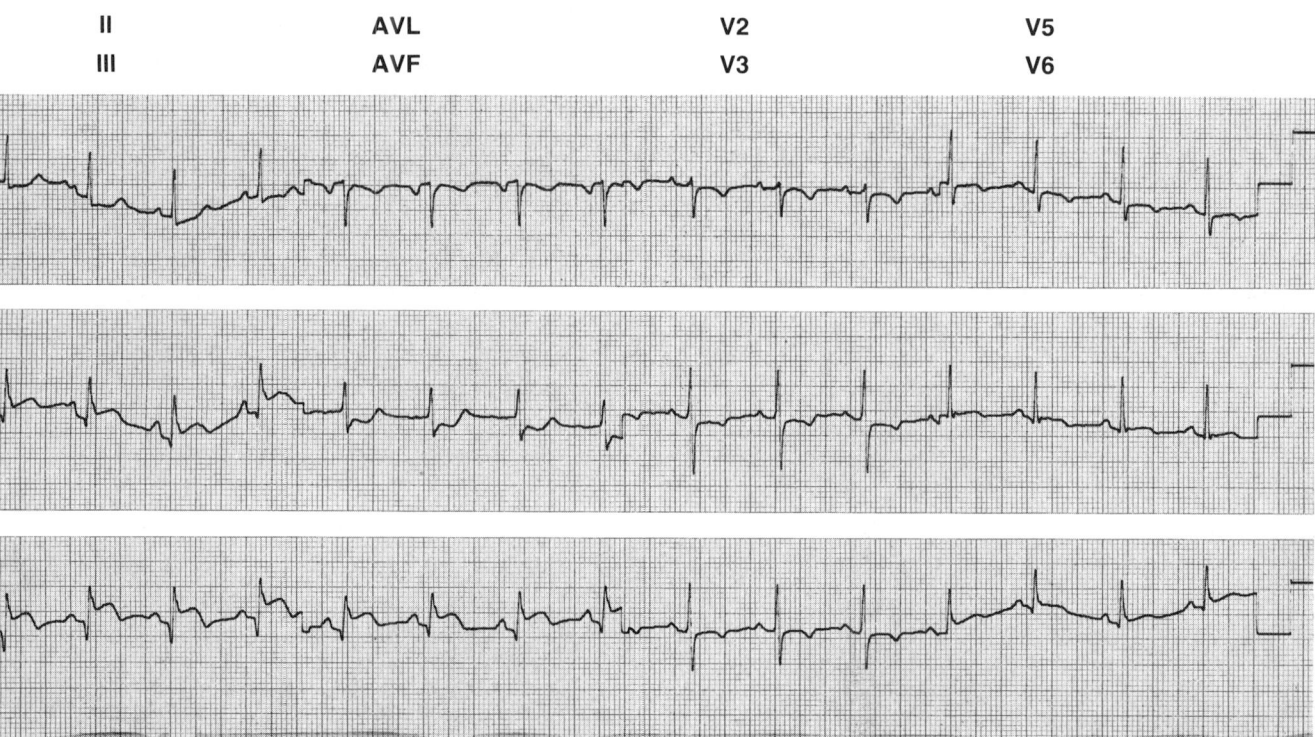

HEWLETT • PACKARD   112 308   THERMAPAPER   NO. 9270-0663

FIGURE 13–16. Inferior myocardial infarction. This 32-year-old hypertensive diabetic female described severe oppressive substernal constriction and shortness of breath over the previous 3 hours. The electrocardiogram demonstrates ST elevations in the inferior leads as well as nondiagnostic anterolateral T wave changes. Transmural inferior myocardial infarction was subsequently documented.

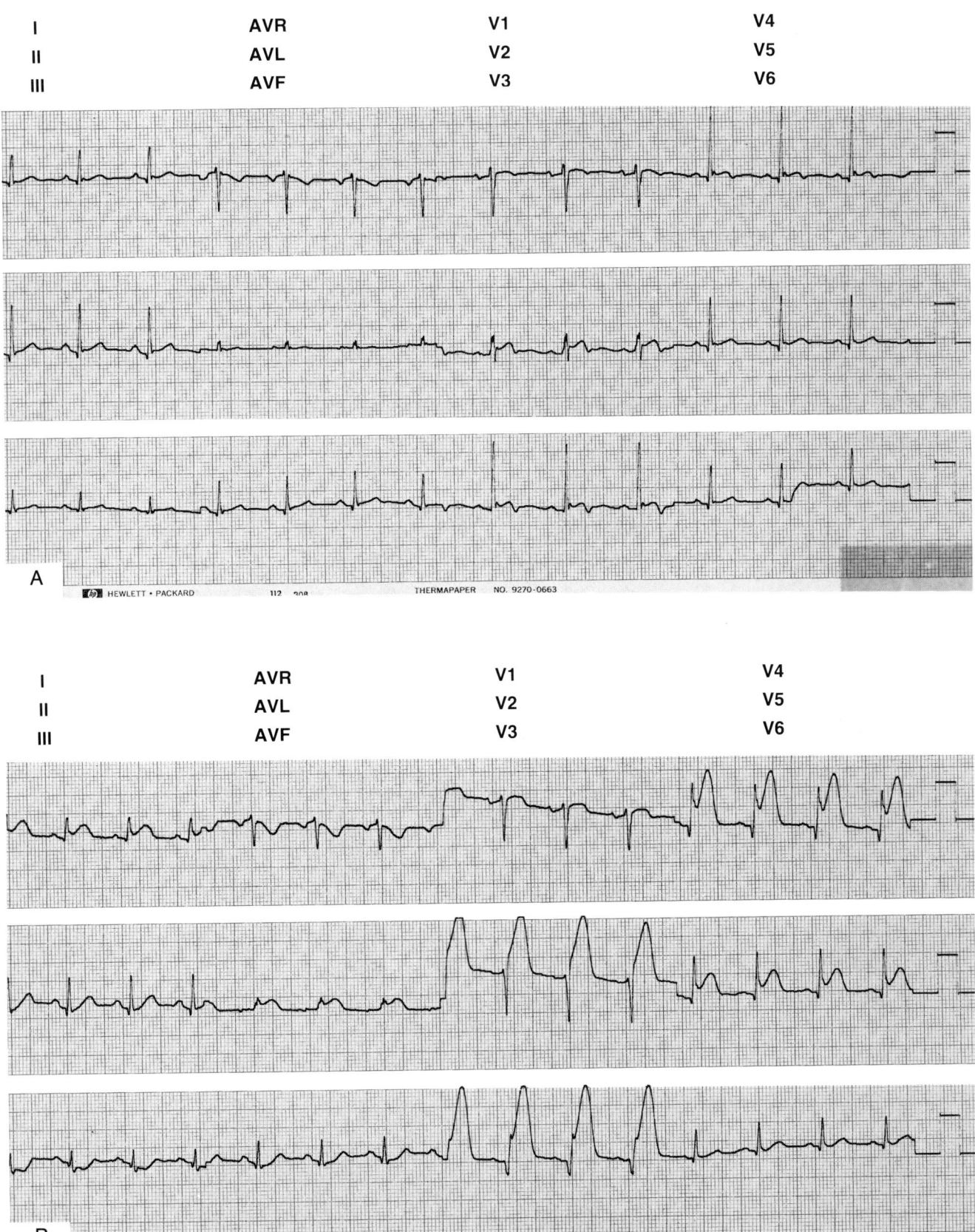

I	AVR	V1	V4
II	AVL	V2	V5
III	AVF	V3	V6

A

I	AVR	V1	V4
II	AVL	V2	V5
III	AVF	V3	V6

B

FIGURE 13—17 *See legend on opposite page*

I	AVR	V1	V4
II	AVL	V2	V5
III	AVF	V3	V6

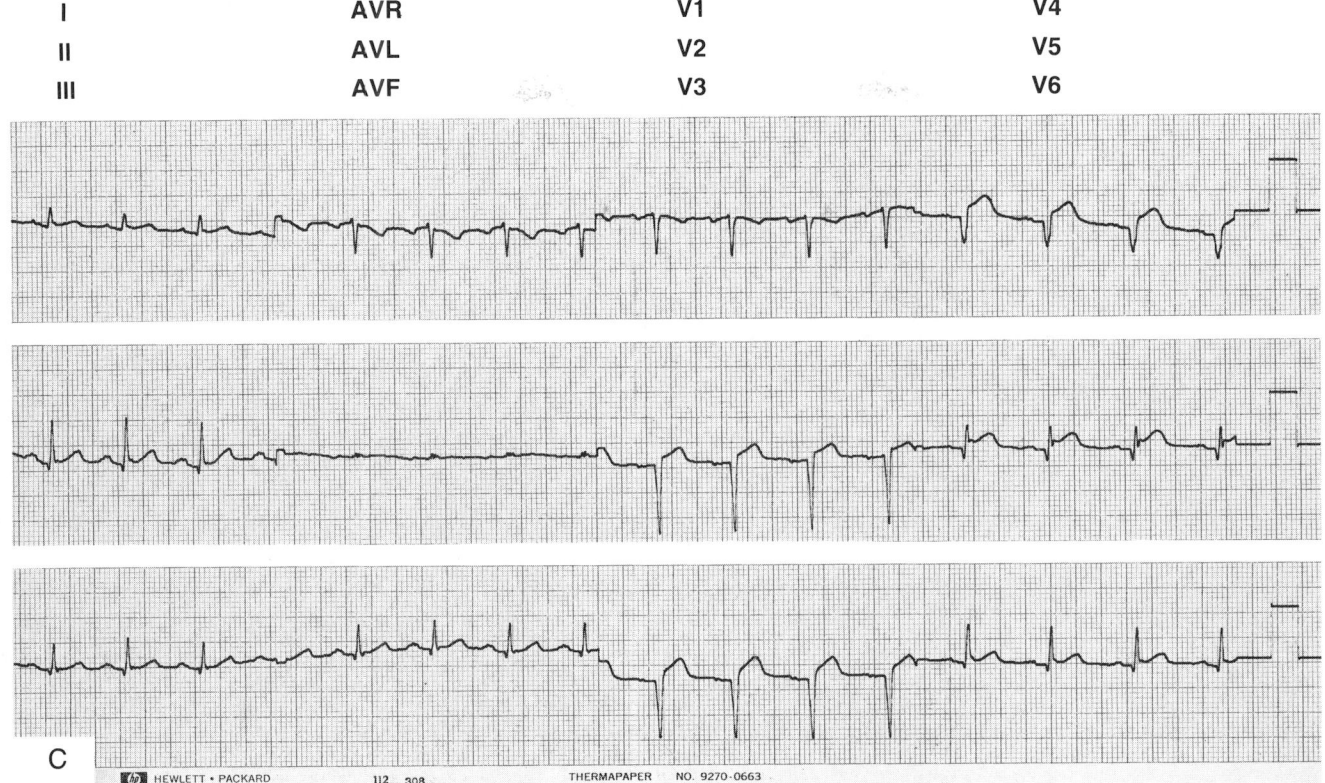

HEWLETT · PACKARD   112 308   THERMAPAPER   NO. 9270-0663

C

FIGURE 13–17. Anterior myocardial infarction. This 49-year-old man described mild but persistent "tightness" in the upper chest and throat for the previous 7 hours. The electrocardiogram (A) demonstrates 1- to 2-mm ST elevations in the anterior precordial leads. The patient's previous electrocardiogram demonstrated "early repolarization" (see Fig. 13–26) in these same leads, and initially it was unclear whether this electrocardiogram represented a change or not. After admission to the coronary care unit, a repeat electrocardiogram 12 hours later (B) demonstrates marked anterolateral ST elevations, "hyperacute T waves," and new anterolateral Q waves. Two days later, the electrocardiogram demonstrates extensive loss of voltage and Q waves in the anterolateral leads with resolving ST-T wave changes (C). Cardiac enzyme determinations documented a large anterolateral transmural myocardial infarction.

cystitis (with cholangitis), or pancreatitis. Cardiac enzymes, serum amylase and lipase, ventilation perfusion lung scans, abdominal x-rays, and abdominal ultrasound or nuclear scans will be helpful in different circumstances (Table 13–14).

After a careful history, examination, chest x-ray, and ECG, the patient with acute severe chest pain will fall into one of several categories (Fig. 13–23, page 739).

1. The patient with acute pleuritic chest pain. Such patients are discussed on page 741. In most instances the differential diagnosis is brief, but it can be very extensive (see Table 13–16, page 747).

2. The patient with suspected subdiaphragmatic/intra-abdominal disease. Usually the history and physical examination will strongly suggest acute cholecystitis, biliary colic, pancreatitis, (complications of) peptic ulcer disease, or other causes of acute upper abdominal pain (see Chapter 11, "Abdominal Pain").

3. The patient whose examination, chest x-ray, or ECG strongly suggests or documents a specific diagnosis. This is usually the case in patients with myocardial infarction, pericarditis, pneumothorax, pneumomediastinum, and aortic dissection.

I	AVR	V1	V4
II	AVL	V2	V5
III	AVF	V3	V6

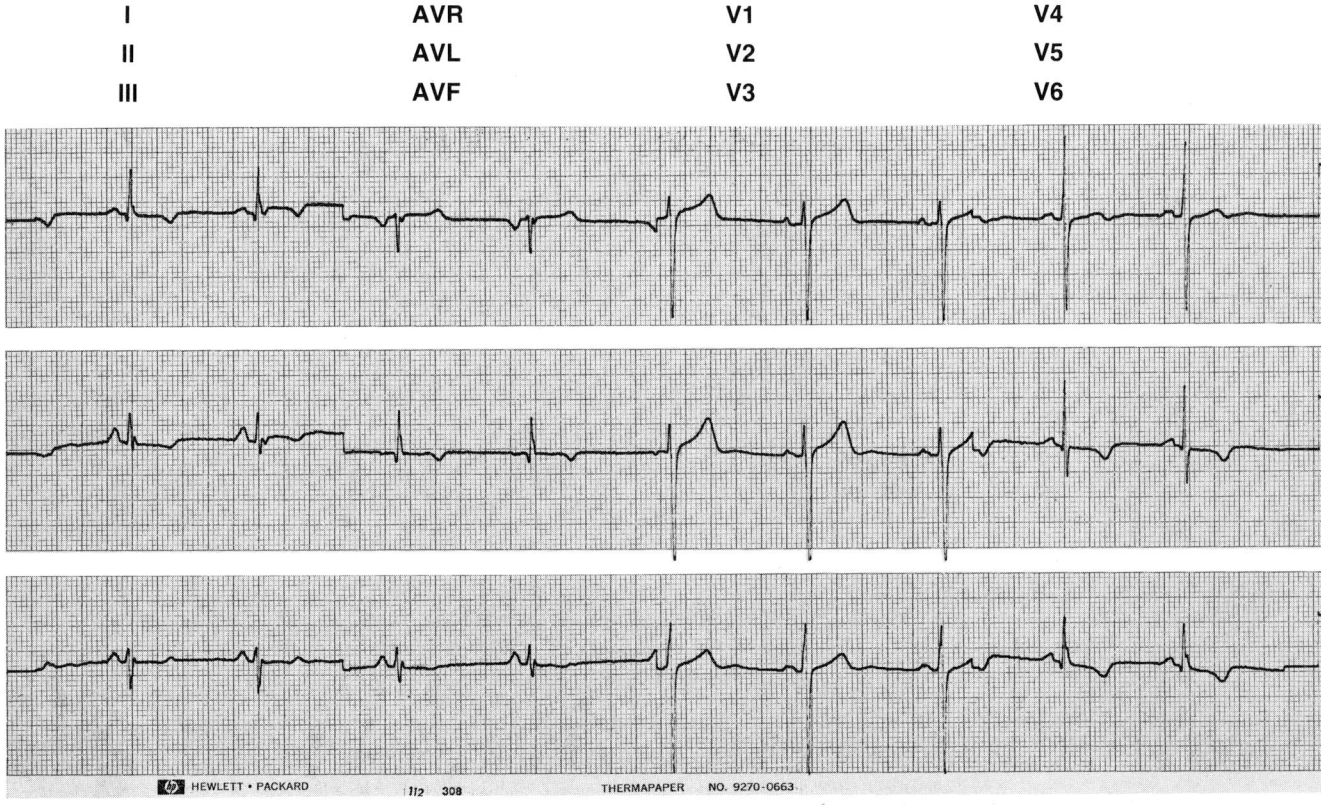

HEWLETT · PACKARD   112 308   THERMAPAPER   NO. 9270-0663

FIGURE 13–18. This 47-year-old man with known asymmetric septal hypertrophy treated with propranolol described 5 hours of severe interscapular and bilateral arm pain. The electrocardiogram demonstrates "nonspecific" lateral T wave inversions. Observation in the coronary care unit and serum cardiac enzymes documented myocardial infarction ("subendocardial"). Coronary arteriography revealed extensive three-vessel disease, which ultimately required bypass surgery.

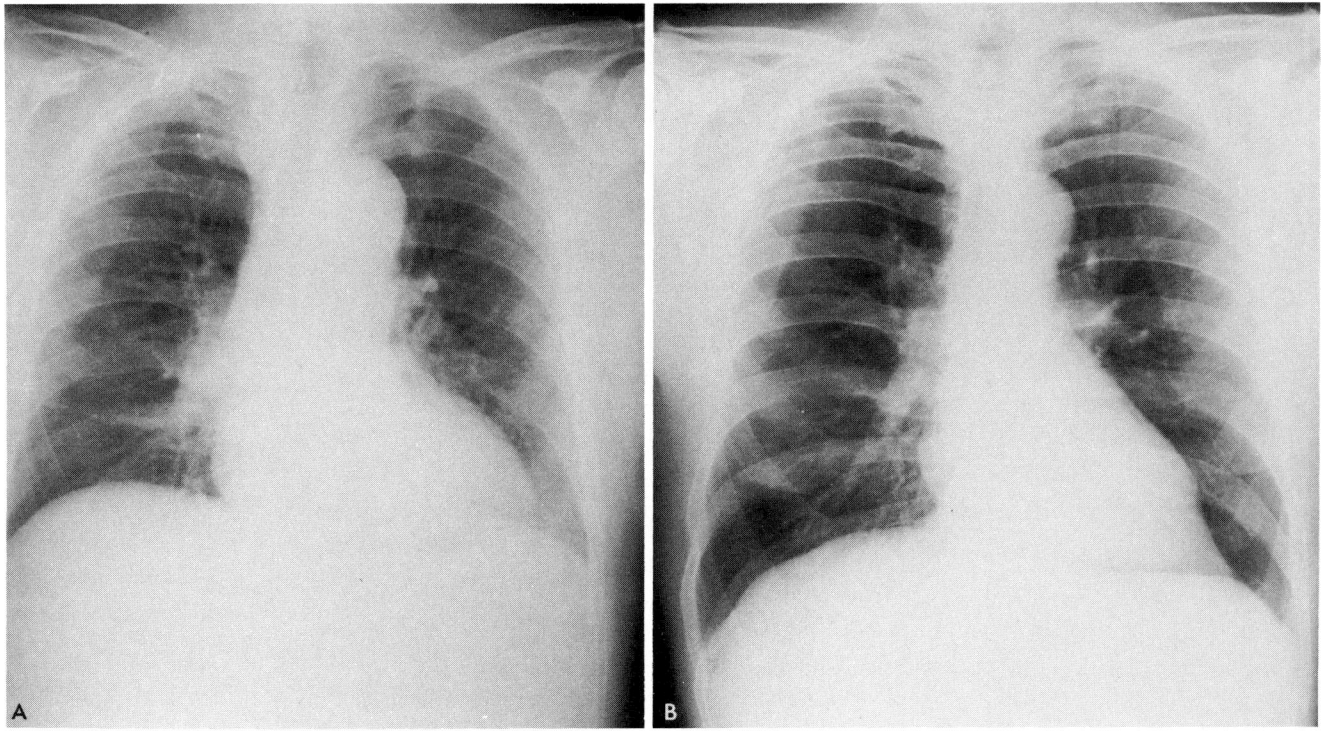

FIGURE 13–19. This 72-year-old hypertensive man described the sudden onset of severe, "ripping" pain in the upper anterior and posterior (interscapular) chest, radiating down into the lower back. The ECG was normal. All peripheral pulses were normal. The x-ray (A) might have been interpreted as unremarkable, had it not been compared with the patient's previous (B) chest x-ray (performed two years before). There is now definite widening of the thoracic aorta and mediastinum. Arteriography demonstrated an aortic dissection beginning just proximal to the left subclavian artery. (Repeat physical examination revealed a diminished left axillary, brachial, and radial pulsation.) Surgery was successful.

736

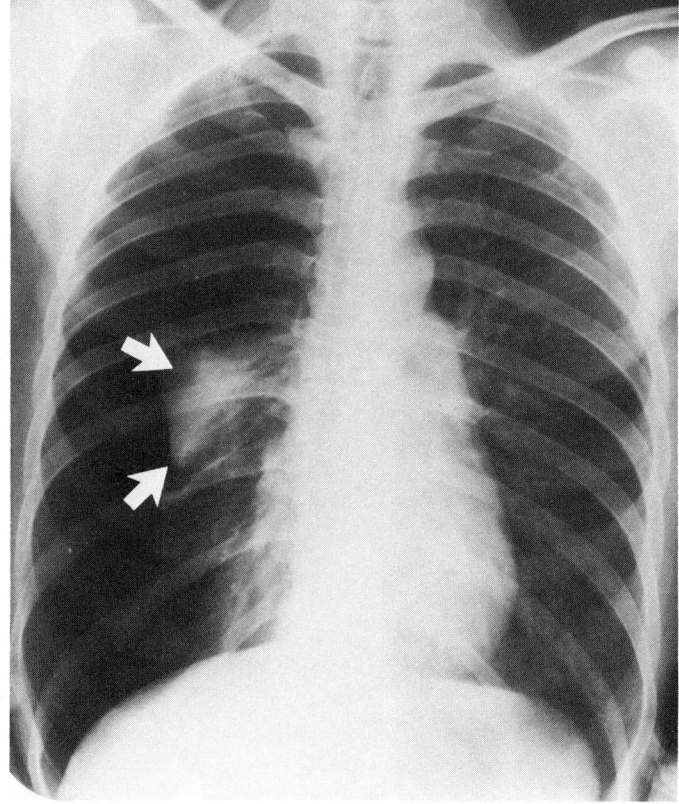

FIGURE 13–20. This 19-year-old man described the very abrupt onset of severe right chest pain and dyspnea. There is a large right pneumothorax with collapse of the entire right lung (*arrows*).

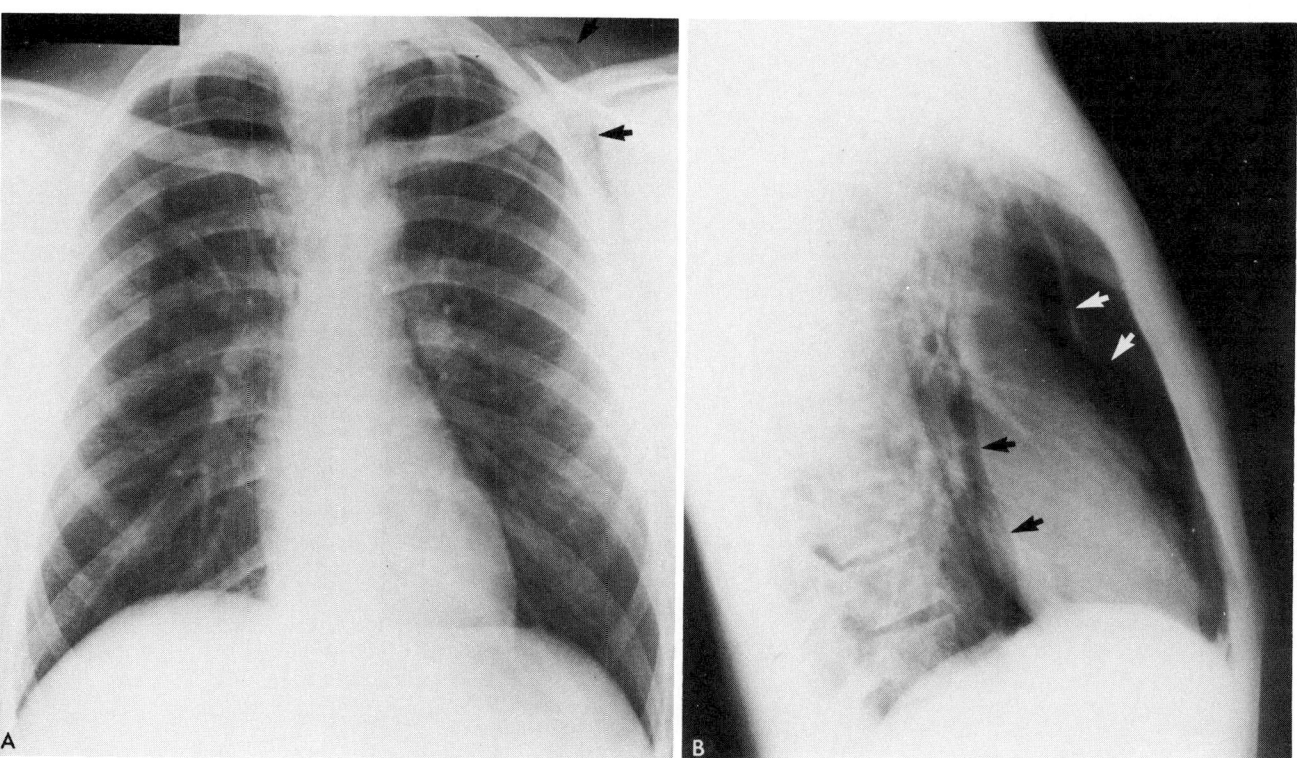

FIGURE 13–21. This 47-year-old male asthmatic described the abrupt onset of very severe substernal chest pain after a bout of prolonged coughing. Careful examination revealed palpable crepitance in the suprasternal and left supraclavicular area (note free air above the clavicle on the left [*arrows*]). The posteroanterior chest film (*A*) does demonstrate unusually clear delineation of the left heart border, but the lateral film (*B*) illustrates best the extensive pneumomediastinum (*arrows*) outlining the anterior and posterior cardiac silhouette. The patient recovered spontaneously.

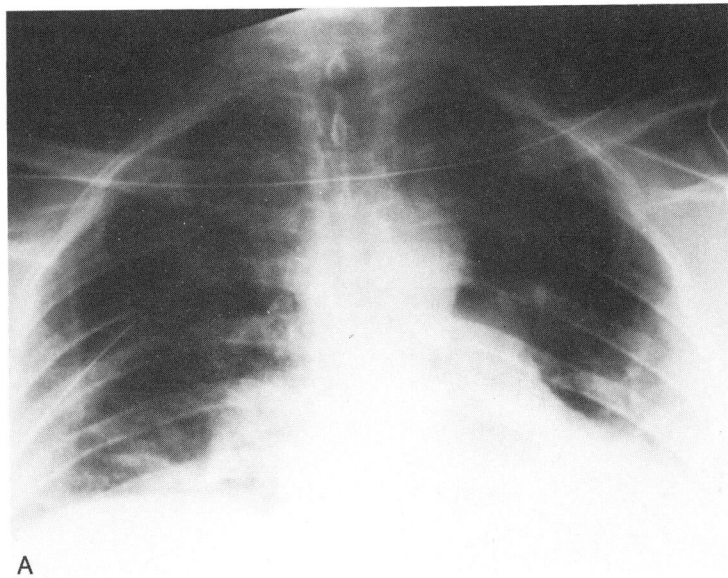
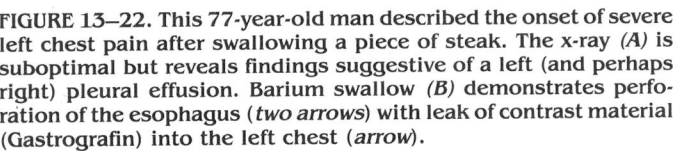
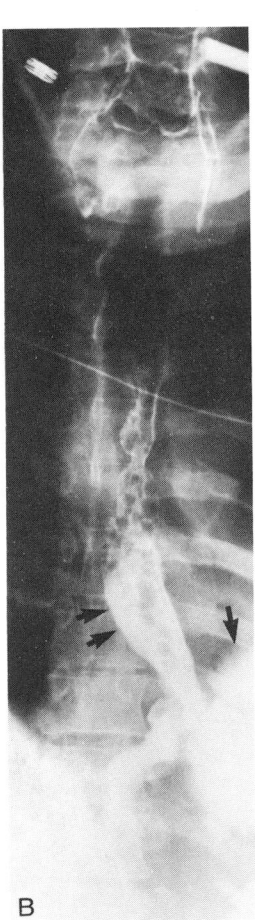

FIGURE 13–22. This 77-year-old man described the onset of severe left chest pain after swallowing a piece of steak. The x-ray *(A)* is suboptimal but reveals findings suggestive of a left (and perhaps right) pleural effusion. Barium swallow *(B)* demonstrates perforation of the esophagus (*two arrows*) with leak of contrast material (Gastrografin) into the left chest (*arrow*).

4. The patient with nonpleuritic chest pain whose physical examination, ECG, and chest x-ray are normal; and intra-abdominal disease is not suspected. As Figure 13–23 suggests, such patients should be suspected of esophageal, chest-wall/spinal, or psychogenic pain, but it is often impossible to exclude more serious disease in an outpatient setting. As discussed previously, myocardial infarction, pulmonary embolism, aortic dissection, and other serious diseases must still be considered when the patient is sick and pain is severe, even when the ECG and chest x-ray are not diagnostic.

Further history, voluntary hyperventilation, and the various chest-wall maneuvers (page 701) will sometimes be helpful in this setting, but observation in the hospital is often necessary in such patients.

In Angela's case, pain is severe but nonpleuritic. Physical examination, chest x-ray, and ECG do not readily point to a specific diagnosis. The location of pain, persistent vomiting, and (equivocal) epigastric tenderness suggest the possibility of an intra-abdominal cause of "chest" pain—especially biliary colic, pancreatitis, or peptic ulcer disease. Despite the normal ECG and chest x-ray, myocardial infarction and pulmonary embolism cannot be excluded. An esophageal source of pain is also possible. Thus,

1. The diagnosis is unclear.

2. Angela is "sick."

3. Pain persists.

4. Angela should be hospitalized, preferably in an intensive or coronary care unit. Admission to the latter is debatable, but studies that attempt to

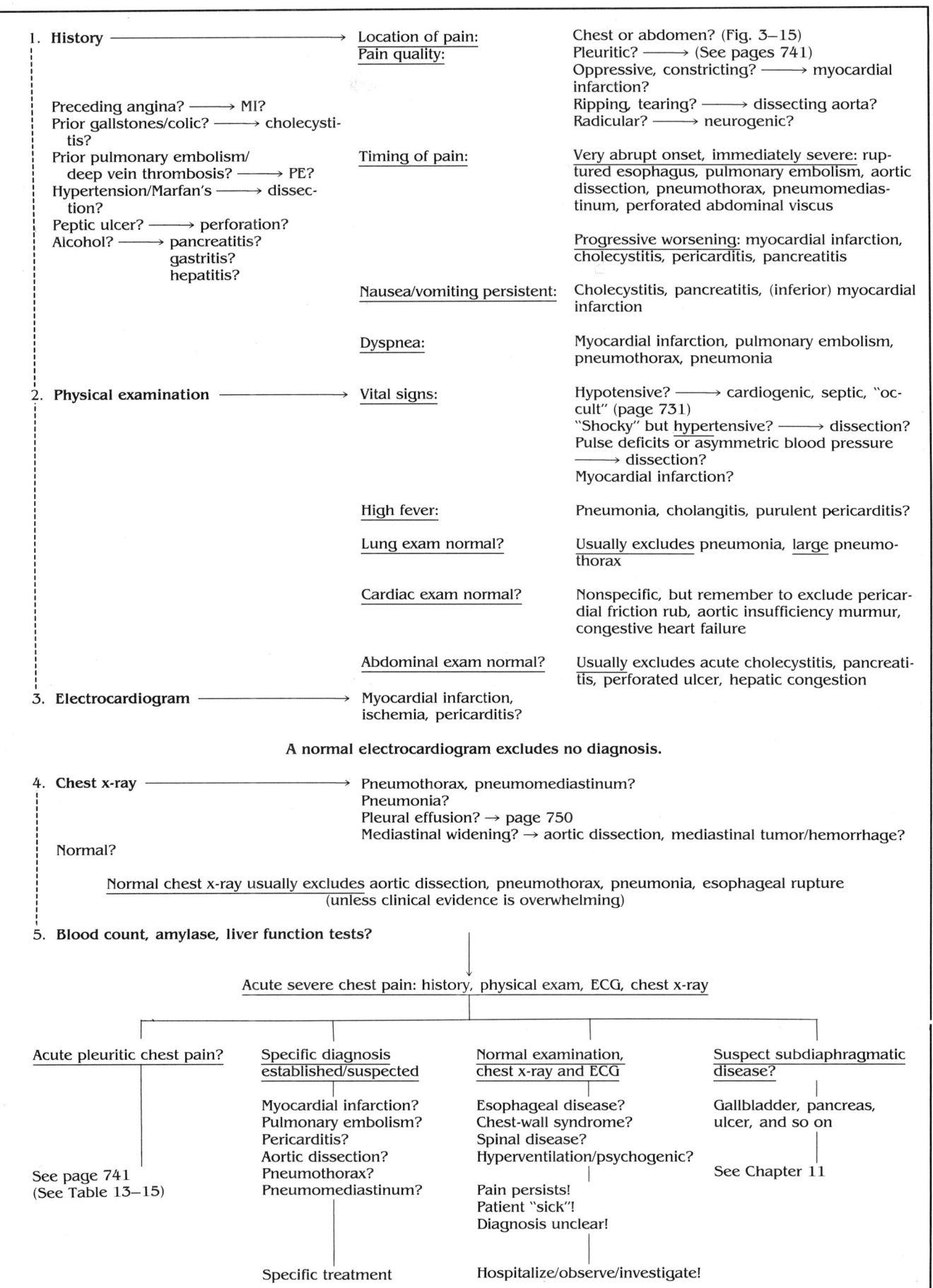

1. History ──────────────→ Location of pain: Chest or abdomen? (Fig. 3–15)
          Pain quality: Pleuritic? ──────→ (See pages 741)
           Oppressive, constricting? ──────→ myocardial infarction?

Preceding angina? ──────→ MI?
Prior gallstones/colic? ──────→ cholecystitis?
          Ripping, tearing? ──────→ dissecting aorta?
          Radicular? ──────→ neurogenic?

Prior pulmonary embolism/
   deep vein thrombosis? ──────→ PE?
Hypertension/Marfan's ──────→ dissec-
   tion?
Peptic ulcer? ──────→ perforation?
Alcohol? ──────→ pancreatitis?
         gastritis?
         hepatitis?

          Timing of pain: Very abrupt onset, immediately severe: rup-
           tured esophagus, pulmonary embolism, aortic
           dissection, pneumothorax, pneumomedias-
           tinum, perforated abdominal viscus

           Progressive worsening: myocardial infarction,
           cholecystitis, pericarditis, pancreatitis

          Nausea/vomiting persistent: Cholecystitis, pancreatitis, (inferior) myocardial
           infarction

          Dyspnea: Myocardial infarction, pulmonary embolism,
           pneumothorax, pneumonia

2. Physical examination ──────────→ Vital signs: Hypotensive? ──────→ cardiogenic, septic, "oc-
           cult" (page 731)
           "Shocky" but hypertensive? ──────→ dissection?
           Pulse deficits or asymmetric blood pressure
           ──────→ dissection?
           Myocardial infarction?

          High fever: Pneumonia, cholangitis, purulent pericarditis?

          Lung exam normal?   Usually excludes pneumonia, large pneumo-
           thorax

          Cardiac exam normal?   Nonspecific, but remember to exclude pericar-
           dial friction rub, aortic insufficiency murmur,
           congestive heart failure

          Abdominal exam normal?   Usually excludes acute cholecystitis, pancreati-
           tis, perforated ulcer, hepatic congestion

3. Electrocardiogram ──────────→ Myocardial infarction,
          ischemia, pericarditis?

A normal electrocardiogram excludes no diagnosis.

4. Chest x-ray ──────────→ Pneumothorax, pneumomediastinum?
          Pneumonia?
          Pleural effusion? → page 750
          Mediastinal widening? → aortic dissection, mediastinal tumor/hemorrhage?

Normal?

    Normal chest x-ray usually excludes aortic dissection, pneumothorax, pneumonia, esophageal rupture
               (unless clinical evidence is overwhelming)

5. **Blood count, amylase, liver function tests?**

Acute severe chest pain: history, physical exam, ECG, chest x-ray

Acute pleuritic chest pain?	Specific diagnosis established/suspected	Normal examination, chest x-ray and ECG	Suspect subdiaphragmatic disease?
	Myocardial infarction?	Esophageal disease?	Gallbladder, pancreas,
	Pulmonary embolism?	Chest-wall syndrome?	ulcer, and so on
	Pericarditis?	Spinal disease?	
	Aortic dissection?	Hyperventilation/psychogenic?	
	Pneumothorax?		See Chapter 11
See page 741	Pneumomediastinum?	Pain persists!	
(See Table 13–15)		Patient "sick"!	
		Diagnosis unclear!	
	Specific treatment	Hospitalize/observe/investigate!	

FIGURE 13–23. Acute severe chest pain.

delineate improved criteria for admission to cardiac care units[90] suggest that ongoing chest pain suspected to be myocardial in origin is one such criterion (as is congestive heart failure, arrhythmias, or hypotension). A nondiagnostic ECG does not alter this decision[158] (although a completely normal ECG certainly lessens the probability of myocardial infarction).

> Angela is admitted to the coronary care unit. Antiemetics and antacids provide no relief. The pain gradually subsides over the next 4 hours. Serum amylase is normal, as are serial ECGs, cardiac enzymes, and physical examination.
>
> Angela is up and walking 48 hours later, afebrile, with normal vital signs and no pain. A barium swallow and upper GI series are normal, except for a hiatal hernia without definite gastroesophageal reflux. An oral cholecystogram reveals multiple gallstones; abdominal ultrasound confirms gallstones but is otherwise normal; there is no abnormality of the pancreas or biliary ducts. Angela admits that this episode of severe pain was identical to that which occurred a few months before. A Bernstein test is normal (see Appendix II).
>
> A diagnosis of recurrent biliary colic is made. Preoperatively Angela undergoes an exercise tolerance test—at a heart rate of 150 per minute and 10 METS exercise level, she develops her typical exertional transient "indigestion," which is associated with 1.5-mm downsloping ST depressions in the inferior limb leads (see Appendix I).
>
> An elective cholecystectomy is performed. Common duct exploration is unrevealing, but the gallbladder is inflamed and contains several stones. There are no postoperative complications except for low-grade fever and incisional chest pain. Seven days later, Angela is discharged from the hospital with a prescription for nitroglycerin prn.

NOTE

1. Again, myocardial infarction can be excluded only by serial ECGs and cardiac enzymes (CPK and LDH isoenzymes) determinations under observation in the hospital. These serial observations will usually distinguish acute transmural myocardial infarction from "subendocardial infarction" (slight enzyme increases without new Q waves on ECG) and from "coronary insufficiency" or unstable, prolonged angina (transient ischemic ST-T wave changes, no enzyme changes).*

The absence of any ECG or enzyme changes usually* excludes cardiac pain from consideration, but stress testing is sometimes thereafter performed in such circumstances to more definitively exclude coronary artery disease—see also Appendix I.

2. The exercise tolerance test is helpful here in several ways. It documents good exercise tolerance without "ominous" findings (see Appendix I). It establishes that Angela's "indigestion" is clearly ischemic cardiac pain. It supports the clinical conclusion that Angela's angina is mild and associated only with vigorous exertion. Elective abdominal surgery is thus likely to be relatively well tolerated[91] despite the presence of coronary artery disease.

3. As noted in Chapter 11, "Abdominal Pain," demonstration of gallstones radiographically or by ultrasound no more definitively diagnoses biliary colic or acute cholecystitis than does x-ray visualization of a hiatus hernia or

---

*Pathologic studies at autopsy[158] suggest that even serial ECG and isoenzyme determinations will "miss" some myocardial infarctions. Radionuclide "infarct scans" should be considered in such cases.

gastroesophageal reflux definitely prove that reflux esophagitis is the cause of chest pain. Here the clinical symptoms, together with a normal acid perfusion test (Bernstein test) make symptomatic esophagitis most unlikely as the cause of Angela's symptoms—see Appendix II. In this case, however, the history *is* strongly suggestive of biliary colic. Given the radiographic documentation of gallstones and the absence of any other likely diagnosis it can be assumed that gallstones are the problem.

4. Preoperative, intraoperative, and postoperative management of angina patients is a complicated subject. Rose and associates' review is instructive.[91]

> Ten days after hospital discharge, Angela calls complaining of new right pleuritic chest pain. She says she has been recovering slowly at home with minor right upper quadrant discomfort "from my incision," but yesterday noted the onset of sharp, "sticking" respirophasic chest pain, more at the end of inspiration, located at the right lateral lower chest and costal margin. The pain is worse today and "it bothers my breathing."
>
> On examination, Angela is in obvious pain, holding her right lower rib cage and breathing shallowly. Blood pressure is 140/90, pulse 90 and regular, temperature 38.7°C rectally (101.6°F), and respiratory rate 22. Physical examination is unremarkable otherwise, except for diminished breath sounds in the right posterior lung field and tenderness of palpation over the right lower rib cage. The heart and abdominal examinations are normal except for vague equivocal right upper quadrant tenderness. The incision is well healed. The extremities are normal without edema. There is no calf or leg tenderness or swelling.
>
> White blood count is 12,800 with 88 per cent polymorphonuclears. Chest x-ray shows a small right pleural effusion without parenchymal infiltrates. The ECG is normal.
>
> Angela denies upper respiratory infection symptoms, myalgias, arthralgias, cough, hemoptysis, or dyspnea, but "it does hurt to breathe." The chest pain is not positional.

ACUTE PLEURITIC CHEST PAIN

Pleuritic chest pain refers to pain which is clearly induced or exacerbated by respiration—perhaps a better description is respirophasic. Usually, pleuritic pain is unilateral, sharp, "sticking" or "stabbing" and accompanied by brief, shallow respirations to avoid more severe pain.

Most patients with acute pleuritic chest pain suffer from one of several common disorders, but the differential diagnosis can be wide-ranged. (Table 13–15 lists most of the common, uncommon, and rare causes.) Precise diagnosis sometimes requires extensive invasive testing (e.g., pulmonary angiography or pleural biopsy), but usually the clinical setting, examination of the patient, and careful review of the chest x-ray will strongly suggest the correct diagnosis. Familiarity with the clinical disorders that most commonly cause acute pleuritic chest pain will allow judicious use of further testing when the diagnosis is unclear. The most common causes of acute pleuritic chest pain include:

Viral or Idiopathic Pleuritis. This problem is especially common in healthy young adults and may occur in either endemic[92] or epidemic[93] forms; often Coxsackie B viruses are responsible for this "pleurodynia" (sometimes

TABLE 13–15. ACUTE PLEURITIC CHEST PAIN

	TYPICAL CLINICAL PICTURE	TYPICAL CHEST X-RAY	THINK OTHERWISE IF	USUAL DIFFERENTIAL DIAGNOSIS	CONFIRM DIAGNOSIS BY
COMMON CAUSES					
Viral or idiopathic pleurisy[92, 93]	Young, healthy adult; symptoms of upper respiratory infection; low-grade fever; sudden onset	Normal	Predisposition to pulmonary embolism Chest x-ray: parenchymal infiltrate; pleural effusion	Pulmonary embolism; chest-wall causes; pneumonia	Normal lung scan; clinical follow-up; viral serologic tests?
Pericarditis[79, 80, 102, 104]	Pain worse when recumbent, better sitting up; radiation to trapezius ridge; pericardial friction rub; abnormal ECG (Fig. 13–26)	Normal	No pericardial rub and normal ECG	Pulmonary embolism; myocardial infarction	Pericardial friction rub and ECG evolution; find specific cause
Pulmonary embolism[94-98]	Sudden dyspnea and acute apprehension (hemoptysis uncommon); obvious predisposing factors (Table 13–14)	Normal or small pleural effusion or peripheral infiltrate/atelectasis (Figs. 13–24, 13–25)	No predisposing factors, dyspnea, or pleural effusion; normal perfusion lung scan excludes diagnosis	Pleurisy; pneumonia; pericarditis; chest-wall causes	Lung scan and/or pulmonary angiography (see Appendix IV)
Pneumonia	Fever/chills; productive cough; symptoms of upper respiratory infection	Parenchymal infiltrate(s) with or without pleural effusion	No fever or cough; normal chest x-ray	Pulmonary embolism; tuberculosis; empyema	Typical clinical picture and chest x-ray; isolate microorganism
Chest-wall pain	Pain with chest movement; chest-wall tenderness; positive "chest-wall maneuvers"; normal cardiac and lung examination	Normal	Abnormal lung examination and chest x-ray; systemic symptoms	Pleurisy; pneumonia; pulmonary embolism	Clinical status; normal chest x-ray; reproduce all symptoms with chest-wall maneuvers
Nonpenetrating chest trauma[113]	Obvious chest trauma	Pneumothorax? Rib fracture? Hemothorax? Contusion?	No trauma or chest-wall tenderness	When chest x-ray normal—other chest-wall syndromes. When chest x-ray reveals pleural effusion—aortic dissection, hemothorax, esophageal rupture, bronchopleural fistula	Clinical picture
Post-thoracotomy pain[113]	Incisional pain and/or recurrent "pleurisy" with upper respiratory infection, weather changes, fatigue, etc.	Normal or postoperative changes	Chest x-ray abnormality resolves after surgery but then recurs	Pulmonary embolism; empyema	Exclude other diagnoses
UNCOMMON CAUSES					
Tuberculosis[114]	Cough, fever	Pleural effusion, often large (with or without associated infiltrate)	Repeatedly negative PPD over 2 months' time; failure to grow organism	Pneumonia/empyema; neoplasm	Positive PPD; pleural fluid culture; pleural biopsy

Pleuritis due to connective tissue diseases (especially systemic lupus erythematosus)[109, 110]	Acute pleuritic pain rarely only manifestation; usually rash, Raynaud's, arthritis, renal disease	Small effusion(s) usually with parenchymal infiltrate(s); often bilateral (or alternating)	No other SLE symptoms; ANA negative	Pleurisy; pneumonia; pulmonary embolism; pericarditis	Clinical course; positive ANA
Neoplasm	Usually insidious onset; other evidence of cancer (pleural involvement usually metastatic)	Large pleural effusion with or without primary lesion	Resolves spontaneously	Tuberculosis; empyema; many others[115]	Pleural fluid cytologic tests, pleural biopsy, and/or surgical exploration[116]
Empyema[117-120]	Often insidious onset; fever, dyspnea, cough; usually associated pulmonary infection and/or postsurgical complication. Sometimes post-traumatic, post-thoracentesis, esophageal fistula, subdiaphragmatic disease	Usually associated pneumona, elevated diaphragm and pleural effusion	Small pleural effusion without infiltrate or predisposing cause; no fever or leukocytosis	Pneumonia with parapneumonic effusion[121-122]; pulmonary embolism; tuberculosis; neoplasm	Thoracentesis—pH less than 7; positive Gram stain; positive culture; low glucose level; gross purulent fluid (see Chapter 12)
Subphrenic abscess[106, 107]	Fever; sometimes only minimal abdominal findings; usually associated hepatic, biliary or pancreatic disease or postoperative abdominal surgery	Small pleural effusion, atelectasis, and/or elevated hemidiaphragm	No known associated disease or prior surgery; no fever	Many of above	Possibly liver/lung scan, gallium scan, CT scan; surgical drainage
Intrahepatic abscess[123-125]	Fever; chills; hepatomegaly; bacteremia	Elevated hemidiaphragm, pleural effusion, or normal	No fever; normal liver scan	Subphrenic abscess; pneumonia; empyema	Liver scan; possibly angiography; needle aspiration and/or surgical exploration
Dressler's syndrome[108] or postpericardiotomy syndrome	After myocardial infarction, cardiac surgery, cardiac trauma (usually within 6 wk)	Pleural effusion(s) (often bilateral), with or without pulmonary infiltrates	No prior event; normal chest x-ray	Pericarditis; SLE; congestive heart failure; pulmonary emboli	Clinical picture; exclude other diagnoses; prompt response to anti-inflammatory drugs
Drug induced[126]	Procainamide- and/or hydralazine-induced SLE*. Nitrofurantoin- and/or methysergide-induced pleural reaction	SLE-like picture. SLE-like picture or diffuse infiltrates with or without effusions	No drugs	SLE; other hypersensitivity diseases; pneumonia	Clinical picture; positive ANA; resolving with drug withdrawal

RARE CAUSES

Uremia	**Rheumatoid arthritis**
Aortic dissection	**Myxedema**
Esophageal rupture	**Asbestosis**
Bronchopleural fistula	**Whipple's disease**
Sickle-cell disease	**Sarcoidosis**
Mesothelioma	**Pancreatitis**
Fungal disease	**Hypersensitivity**
Parasitic disease	**pneumonitis**

*SLE = Systemic lupus erythematosus.

called devil's grip or Bornholm's disease). Sudden, very severe pleuritic chest pain usually occurs in association with other viral symptoms—headache, myalgias, cough, chills—and may be associated with a pleural friction rub and chest-wall or upper abdominal tenderness on the involved side. Temperature ranges from 99°F to 104°F but fever is usually low grade (101°F). The chest x-ray is typically normal; rarely, a small pleural effusion or nondescript parenchymal infiltrate will be seen. The illness is usually self-limited, lasting an average of 1 week (rarely, symptoms may persist for several weeks or recur after apparent remission).

The usual differential diagnosis includes the common disorders in Table 13–15. The normal chest x-ray will (usually) exclude pneumonia; the prominence of systemic or pulmonary symptoms (fever, dyspnea, cough) will usually exclude chest-wall syndromes (although chest-wall tenderness may be seen with either); a normal cardiac examination and ECG will exclude pericarditis (see below). The most problematic differential diagnosis is usually that between idiopathic pleuritis and

Pulmonary Embolism.[94–97] In most patients with pulmonary embolism there are one or more features that specifically suggest the possibility of embolic disease or that are atypical of idiopathic pleuritis. These include:

1. Predisposing factors—pulmonary embolism should be suspected when there is a history of prolonged bedrest or immobilization, congestive heart

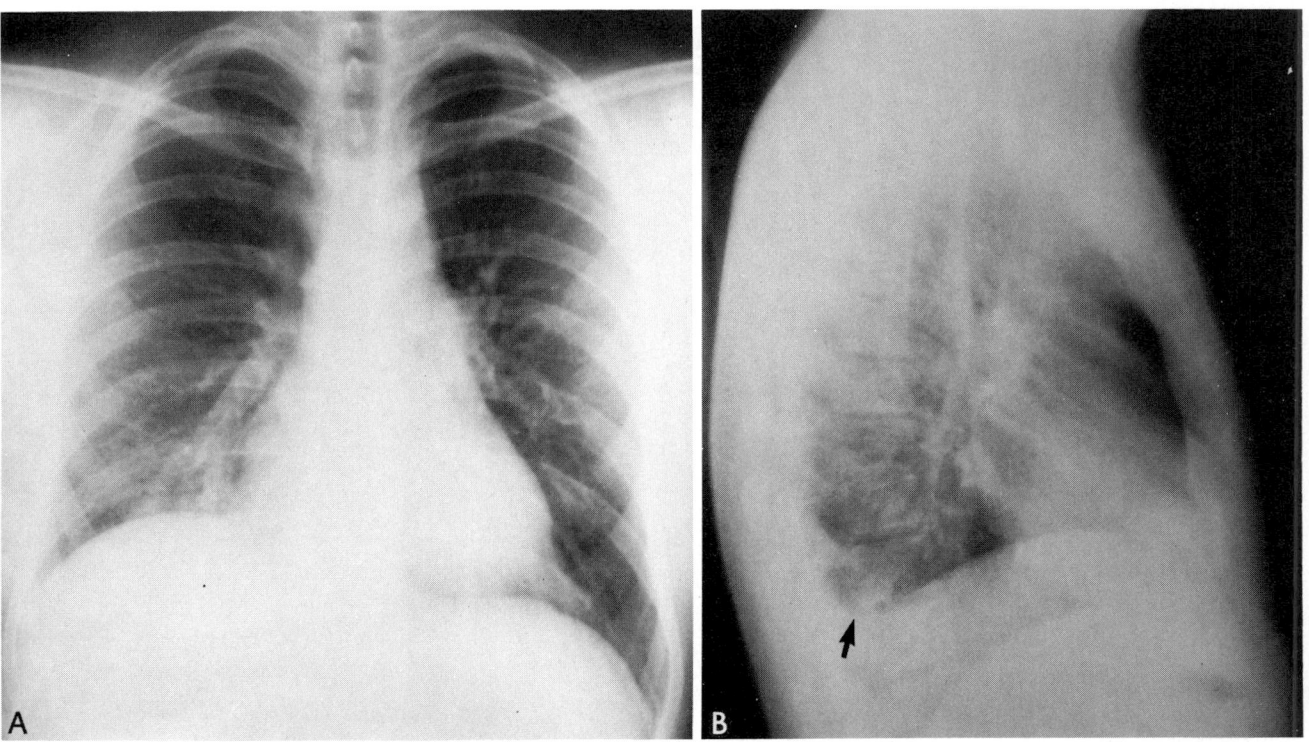

FIGURE 13–24. A, B, This healthy 35-year-old lawyer described low-grade temperature, myalgias, and mild right pleuritic chest pain over the previous 48 hours. Physical examination was unremarkable. The chest x-ray is unimpressive except for a small right pleural effusion best demonstrated on the lateral film (*arrow*). The diagnosis of idiopathic pleuritis was considered most likely. Six hours later, the patient returned complaining of more severe pain, having coughed up a moderate amount of blood. A lung scan was "indeterminate" (see Fig. 13–39, Appendix IV), but subsequent arteriography documented pulmonary embolism.

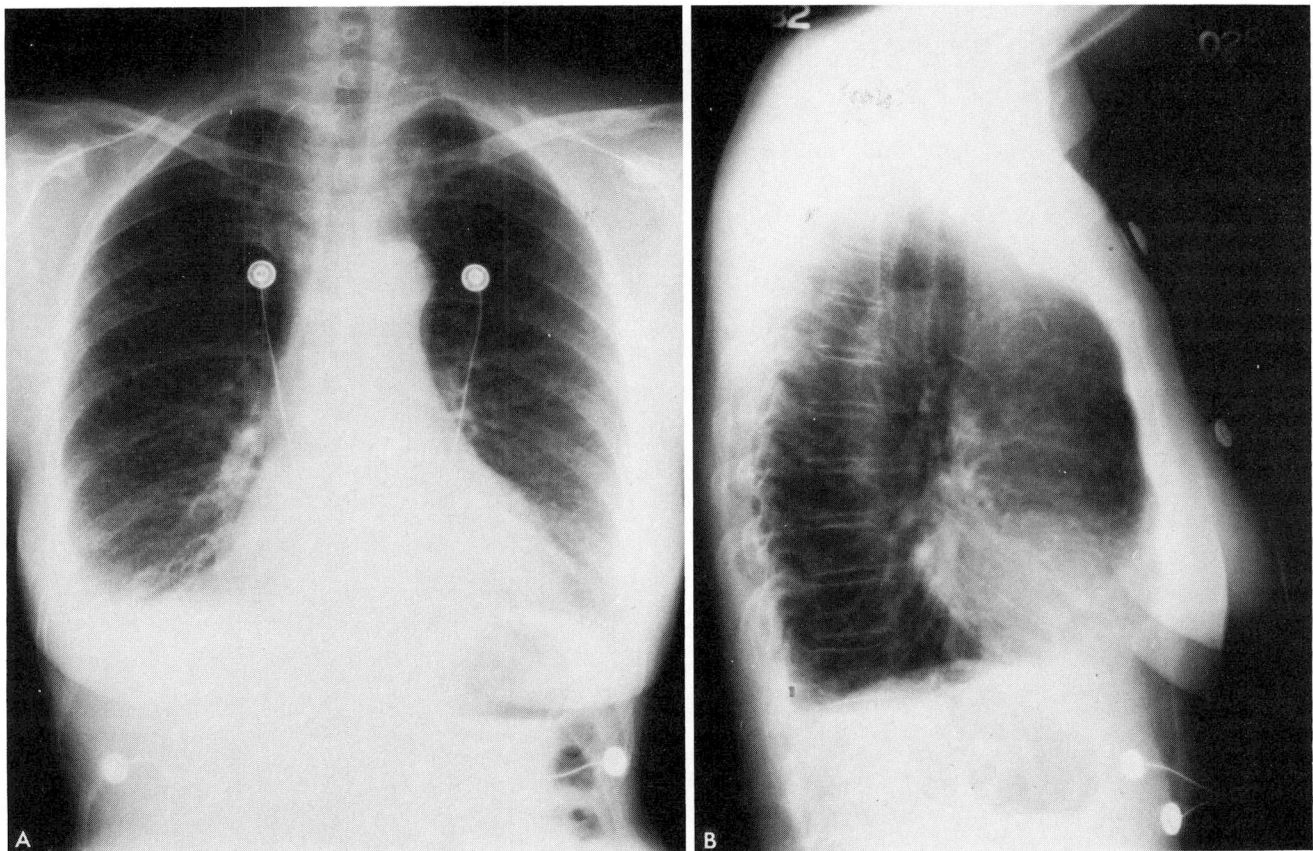

FIGURE 13–25. *A, B,* This 63-year-old woman described the sudden onset of severe right pleuritic chest pain without hemoptysis or dyspnea. Examination revealed diminished breath sounds in the right lung posteriorly. X-ray reveals a hazy, "wedge-shaped" infiltrate in the right lower lobe and a small pleural effusion. Examination of the legs disclosed a 2-cm difference in calf diameter without edema or discomfort in the legs. Subsequent venography and lung scanning documented deep vein thrombosis with pulmonary embolism.

failure, cancer, prior or current deep vein thrombosis, prolonged travel (e.g., in cars and trains), oral contraceptive use, or when the patient is postoperative or post partum (within the past month).

2. An abnormal chest x-ray (Figs. 13–24 and 13–25), especially a small pleural effusion or peripheral, nondescript, or wedge-shaped pulmonary infiltrate, is distinctly unusual in viral pleuritis and should always suggest pulmonary embolism (among other possibilities). The chest x-ray is often normal in pulmonary embolism, however.

3. Hemoptysis and severe dyspnea are not typical of viral pleuritis and should always suggest another diagnosis. (True dyspnea may, however, be difficult to distinguish from the splinting often associated with any pleuritic chest pain.)

When any of these clinical features is present, acute pulmonary embolism must be considered strongly. In healthy young adults (who are the usual victims of viral pleuritis), a perfusion lung scan will usually answer the question since a normal scan is expected in pleuritis and *excludes* pulmonary embolism.[98] When the clinical situation is more complicated (in an older patient, a smoker, or a patient with cardiopulmonary disease), however, the lung scan may or may not help (see Appendix IV), and only pulmonary angiography will definitively prove (or exclude) the diagnosis.

(It should be emphasized that determinations of the values of arterial blood gases, serum enzymes, and fibrin split products, the ECG, and other "tests" are entirely nonspecific for pulmonary embolism. The diagnosis of pulmonary embolism is suspected on clinical grounds and is then either proven or excluded by lung scanning or angiography—see Appendix IV.)

Pericarditis. Pericarditis usually causes pleuritic chest pain—often the pain is worse when the patient lies supine and seems to improve with sitting forward. Shoulder pain over the trapezius ridge is a common site of pain radiation.[79, 80] While the diagnosis should be suspected when these pain patterns are present (or when specific causes of pericarditis are known to be present in the individual patient—Table 13–16), the diagnosis of pericarditis depends on auscultation of a pericardial friction rub and/or documentation of ECG changes typical of pericarditis (Fig. 13–26):

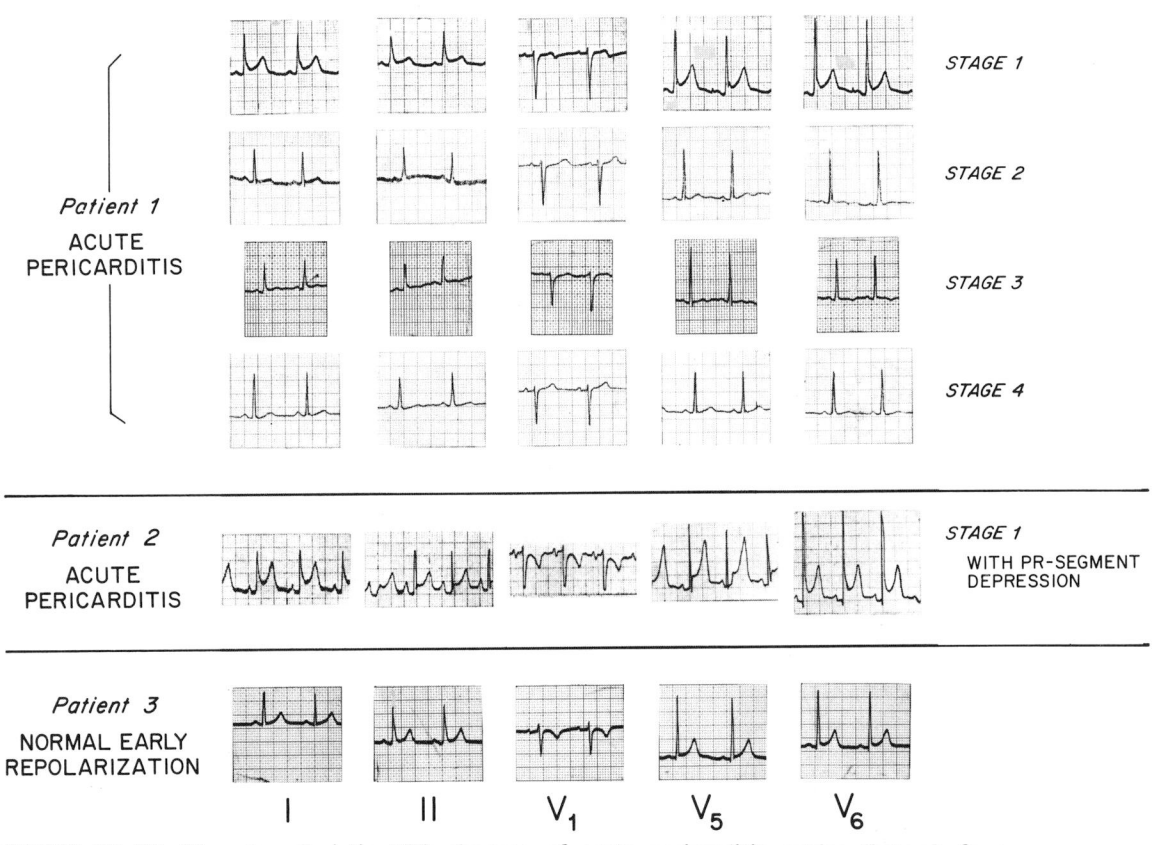

FIGURE 13–26. The characteristic ECG changes of acute pericarditis evolve through four stages.[99, 100] Evolution through these various stages may proceed slowly (days to weeks) or rapidly (hours). Thus, the electrocardiographic manifestations of acute pericarditis vary, depending upon the stage of illness in each individual patient. Stage I involves acute ST segment elevations, which are usually present diffusely throughout the precordial and limb leads. These ST elevations tend to be concave upward, and are associated with upright T waves, and depressed PR segments, as well as with ST depressions in leads AVR and V1. In Stage II, the ST segments become isoelectric, and the T waves are flattened. PR segments may remain depressed during this stage. In Stage III the T waves invert. Q waves do not develop. In Stage IV the electrocardiogram reverts to normal. (Patients 1 and 3 reproduced with permission from Johnson, RA, et al. (ed.): The Practice of Cardiology. Boston: Little, Brown and Co., © 1980, p. 668; Patient 2 reproduced with permission from the American Heart Association, Inc., from Spodick, DH: Diagnostic electrocardiographic sequences in acute pericarditis. Circulation 48:575, 1973.)

1. Most pericardial fricton rubs (82 per cent in Spodick's series[101]) are either *triphasic* (during atrial systole, ventricular systole, and ventricular diastole) or *biphasic*—the rub is characteristically scratchy, grating, high pitched, and "superficial sounding." Usually, then, the absence of a rub, combined with a normal ECG, excludes the diagnosis of pericarditis.

TABLE 13–16. CAUSES OF ACUTE PERICARDITIS

INFECTIOUS
Viral*
  Coxsackievirus (A or B)
  Echovirus
  Influenza
  Infectious mononucleosis
  Mumps
  Varicella
  Lymphogranuloma venereum
  Q fever
  Boutonneuse fever
  Typhus (*R. prowazeki)*
Tuberculous
Bacterial
  Staphylococcus
  Hemophilus influenzae
  Meningococcus
  Salmonella typhosa
  Salmonella, other
  Shigella
  Plague
  Tularemia
  Mycoplasma pneumoniae
  Gram-negative coliform bacteria
  Anaerobic bacteria
  Pneumococcus
  Gonococcus
  Streptococcus (hemolytic)
  Neisseria mucosus
  Brucellosis
  Melioidosis
  Yaws
  Listeria
Spread from contiguous source
  Intrathoracic infection
  Infective endocarditis
  Esophageal perforation
Mycotic
  Actinomycosis
  Histoplasmosis
  Coccidioidomycosis
  Nocardiosis
  Aspergillosis
  Blastomycosis
Parasitic
  Toxoplasmosis
  Amebiasis
  Chagas' disease
  Echinococcosis
  Filariasis
NEOPLASTIC*
Contiguous spread from local neoplasm
Metastatic spread
Primary pericardial tumor

UREMIA*
RHEUMATOLOGIC DISEASE* with pericarditis
A major or frequent feature
  Rheumatoid arthritis
  Systemic lupus erythematosus
  Mixed connective tissue disease
  Sjögren's syndrome
  Whipple's disease
  Scleroderma
An occasional feature
  Reiter's syndrome
  Ankylosing spondylitis
  Inflammatory bowel disease
  Serum sickness
  Wegener's granulomatosis
A rare feature
  Other vasculitis syndromes
  Polymyositis
  Behçet's disease
  Familial Mediterranean fever
  Amyloidosis
  Gout
Other systemic diseases
  Sarcoidosis
  Hemochromatosis
  Syndrome of pulmonary infiltrates with eosinophilia
  Gaucher's disease
  Polyserositis
  Diabetic ketoacidosis
  Degos' disease
AFTER TRANSMURAL MYOCARDIAL INFARCTION* (1–4 days)
AFTER CARDIAC INJURY
  Postpericardiotomy syndrome
  After blunt chest trauma
  Dressler's syndrome
RADIATION INJURY
DRUG-INDUCED*
  Procainamide
  Hydralazine
  Quinidine
  Phenylbutazone
  Isoniazid
  Penicillin
  Streptomycin
  Methysergide
  Daunorubicin
CONTIGUOUS PLEURITIS

Adapted from Reference 71.
*Most common causes of acute pericarditis.

However, the clinician must be careful here.

Some pericardial friction rubs (18 per cent in Spodick's series[101]) are only *monophasic*—these may easily be confused with benign murmurs (especially when systolic).

Some pericardial friction rubs are audible only intermittently (and thus may be missed if the clinician listens at just one point in time). Auscultation should be performed with the patient in several different positions (supine, sitting up). There is no one best position. Auscultation while the patient leans forward during held expiration is especially recommended by some authorities.[102] Finally, some pericardial friction rubs have a respirophasic accentuation and may easily be confused with pleural friction rubs.

2. The ECG changes of pericarditis may also be confused with other benign (early repolarization) and serious (myocardial infarction, ventricular aneurysm) conditions: It is often the *evolution over time* that is the most specific ECG evidence for acute pericarditis[103] (Fig. 13–26).

Despite the lengthy differential diagnosis listed in Table 13–16, the most common cause of acute pericarditis is idiopathic or viral[104] (especially when there is no history of myocardial infarction, neoplasm, cardiac surgery, connective tissue disease, uremia, or drug ingestion—the other common causes[102]). Treatment usually includes nonsteroidal anti-inflammatory drugs for 4 to 6 weeks. Systemic corticosteroids are usually reserved for cases unresponsive to those more benign medications. The clinical course of most patients is uneventful. Nevertheless, establishing a specific diagnosis (when possible) is always important.

Pneumonia. Pneumonia commonly causes acute pleuritic chest pain, but usually clinical symptoms (productive cough, fever), focal abnormalities on lung auscultation (inspiratory crackles or consolidation), and pulmonary infiltrate on chest x-ray will make this diagnosis. Bacterial pneumonias are the usual cause, but viral or mycoplasmal pneumonia may occasionally produce a similar picture[105] (Chapter 12, "Cough").

Chest-Wall Pain. Chest-wall pain may be "pleuritic." However, usually such pain is also related to thoracic motions (e.g., twisting, lifting) or is clearly related to various chest-wall maneuvers (see page 701). The absence of systemic or pulmonary symptoms, a normal cardiac and lung examination, and a normal chest x-ray and ECG are expected when chest-wall pain is the cause of pleuritic pain.

For several weeks or months after thoracotomy or upper quadrant abdominal surgery the patient may develop intermittent "pleuritic" pain, sometimes precipitated by fatigue, weather changes, or other poorly understood phenomena.

The patient with nonpenetrating chest trauma and pleuritic chest pain deserves careful attention, even when the chest x-ray is normal, since the devastating effects of lung contusion are occasionally delayed—the chest x-ray may be normal during the first 24 hours.

Bronchial Asthma. Bronchial asthma or severe, prolonged infectious bronchitis may cause a forme fruste of pleuritic chest pain. This pain is clearly related to respiration but is more often caused by chest-wall fatigue or other undefined factors associated with prolonged coughing, wheezing, or respiratory distress. Often, the pain is central (sternal) rather than sharply unilateral, tends to worsen with cough or chest motion as well as respiration, and is typically associated with other obvious findings of asthma or an upper respiratory infection (and usually a normal chest x-ray).

After consideration of typical features of these common causes of acute pleuritic chest pain, several generalizations emerge (Fig. 13–27):

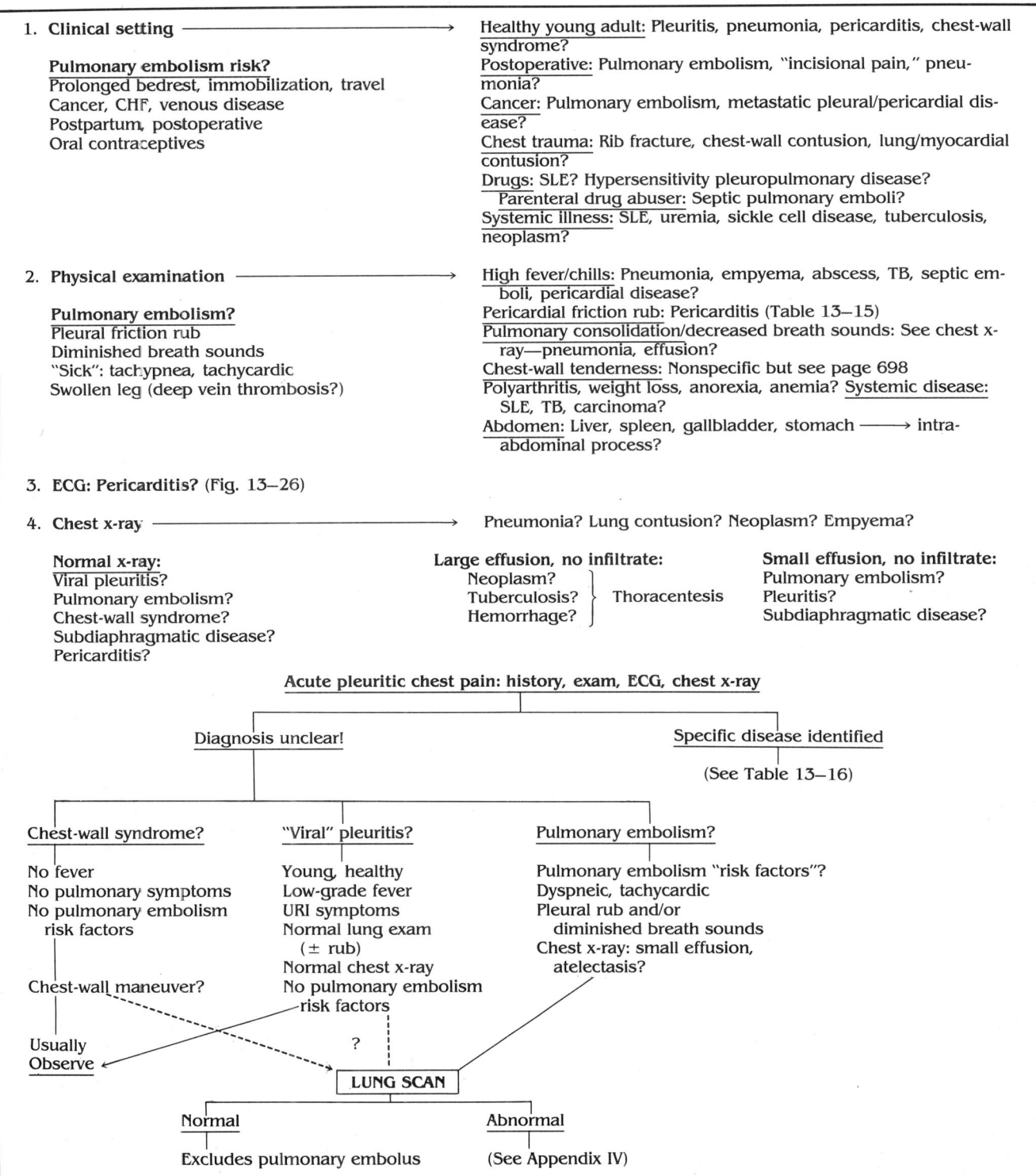

FIGURE 13–27. Acute pleuritic chest pain.

1. Clinical setting is all-important. Most healthy young adults with acute pleuritic chest pain will have viral pleuritis, pneumonia, pericarditis, or acute chest-wall pain. Usually a careful history, physical examination, chest x-ray and ECG will settle the question, but a lung scan is sometimes needed to distinguish pleuritis from pulmonary embolism (see below and Appendix IV).

The postoperative patient is, in general, at risk for pulmonary embolism, atelectasis with pneumonia, or incisional (chest-wall) pain. The post-thoracotomy patient may be susceptible to mild incisional pain (as noted above), but may also rarely develop postoperative empyema or bronchopleural fistula. After abdominal surgery, patients are at risk of postoperative pancreatitis or cholecystitis, intra-abdominal (subdiaphragmatic) abscesses,[106, 107] flares of systemic lupus erythematosus, or empyema (when surgery involves the upper quadrant). Dressler's syndrome[108] (post–cardiac injury syndrome) may follow pericardial or cardiac surgery (or myocardial infarction).

Specific questions arise in the patient with known or suspected cancer: To be remembered are metastatic pleural or pericardial disease, pulmonary emboli, bizarre pneumonias (in the immunosuppressed patient), bronchopleural fistulas due to primary lung carcinoma, or esophageal rupture due to esophageal carcinoma.

Other systemic symptoms or diseases raise different questions: systemic lupus erythematosus (SLE),[109, 110] uremia, sickle cell disease, and rheumatoid arthritis are among those systemic illnesses that can produce acute pleuritic chest pain. Various medications may induce SLE (procainamide or hydralazine, for example) or hypersensitivity pneumonitis/pleuritis (nitrofurantoin or methysergide, for example).

2. Physical examination may or may not help. Examination of the heart and lungs will be normal in most patients with viral pleuritis and chest wall pain and often in the patient with pulmonary embolism. Examination may occasionally be normal in patients with pericarditis (when the rub is not heard) or pneumonia (especially in nonbacterial pneumonia or during the first 24 hours of bacterial pneumonia).

Remember that subdiaphragmatic disease (especially subphrenic abscess[106, 107]) may present with acute pleuritic chest pain without prominent abdominal symptoms and signs (Fig. 13–28).

The presence of fever is nonspecific—virtually all entities in Table 13–15 may cause fever (except the chest-wall disorders). Very high fever, especially with shaking chills, would be unusual except in the "septic" processes—pneumonia, empyema, subphrenic abscess, tuberculosis, purulent pericarditis, septic pulmonary emboli. The absence of fever usually (but not always) exclude these entities.

3. The chest x-ray always helps. A normal chest x-ray in a patient with acute pleuritic pain should suggest viral pleuritis, pulmonary emboli, pericarditis, or chest-wall pain (or, very rarely, such entities as SLE, sickle cell disease, or pancreatitis). Note that the definition of a "normal" chest x-ray must be strict—a good quality posteroanterior and lateral film that is completely normal. Minor changes are often important (see Figure 13–24, for example): elevation of a hemidiaphragm may suggest subpulmonic effusion, subdiaphragmatic abscess, or pulmonary embolism.

Radiographic pleural effusions without pulmonary infiltrate usually exclude pneumonia, SLE, and empyema. (SLE usually causes infiltrates *and*

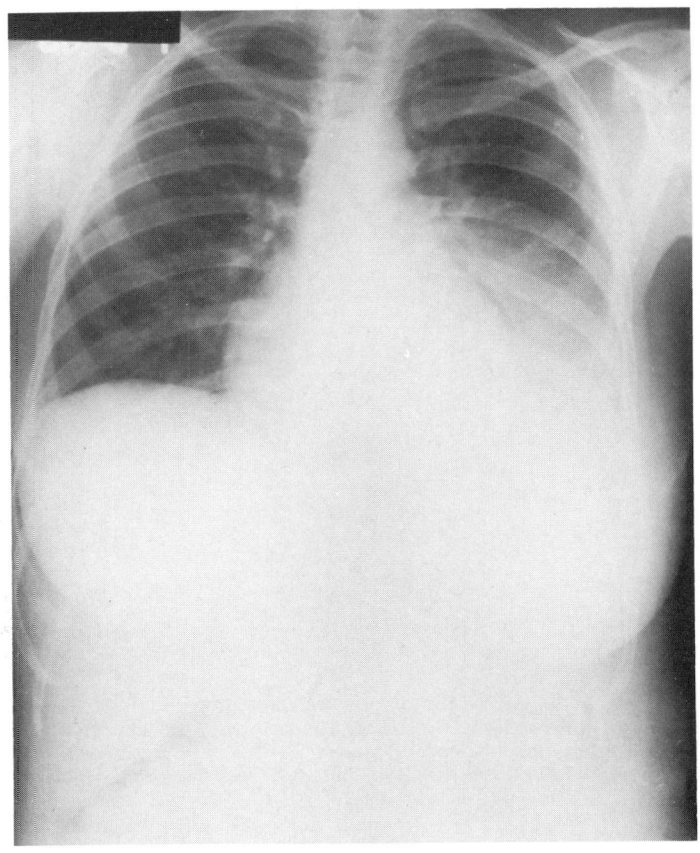

FIGURE 13–28. This 48-year-old woman complained of progressive left lower chest pain 3 weeks after splenectomy for staging of lymphoma. Abdominal examination was benign. X-rays reveal findings suggestive of a left pleural effusion. A large left subphrenic abscess was subsequently drained.

effusions. Empyema occasionally is a late, unrecognized complication of a prior pneumonia or is due to thoracentesis, thoracic surgery, trauma, esophageal rupture, or subdiaphragmatic disease—here, *only* an effusion may be present.)

A large pleural effusion without an infiltrate (Fig. 13–29) would be most unusual in viral pleurisy, pulmonary embolism, connective tissue disease, Dressler's syndrome, or drug-induced disease: Such an x-ray should always suggest neoplasm or tuberculosis (or, rarely, inapparent trauma, aortic dissection, esophageal rupture, or asbestosis).

A small pleural effusion (Figs. 13–24 and 13–25) without an infiltrate should especially suggest pulmonary embolism, pleuritis, or a subdiaphragmatic process.

Bilateral pleural effusions should suggest pulmonary emboli, SLE, Dressler's syndrome, drug-induced disease, or rarely tuberculosis.

(Note that these "x-ray clues" apply here to patients whose presenting complaint is acute pleuritic chest pain—there are scores of other causes of pleural effusions in which differential diagnosis depends on thoracentesis,[111] pleural biopsy, or surgical exploration[112] as well as the overall clinical setting.)

4. The subsequent clinical course may or may not help.

Notice, for example, that most of the common and uncommon disorders listed in Table 13–15 may resolve or remit spontaneously. Viral pleuritis, nonbacterial pneumonia, benign "viral" pericarditis, chest-wall syndromes, and post-traumatic and post-thoracotomy syndromes *usually* resolve spontaneously. Pulmonary embolism, tuberculous pleuritis, and systemic lupus erythematosus often will resolve without treatment (but may then recur). Drug-induced syndromes may "mysteriously" improve after unwitting dis-

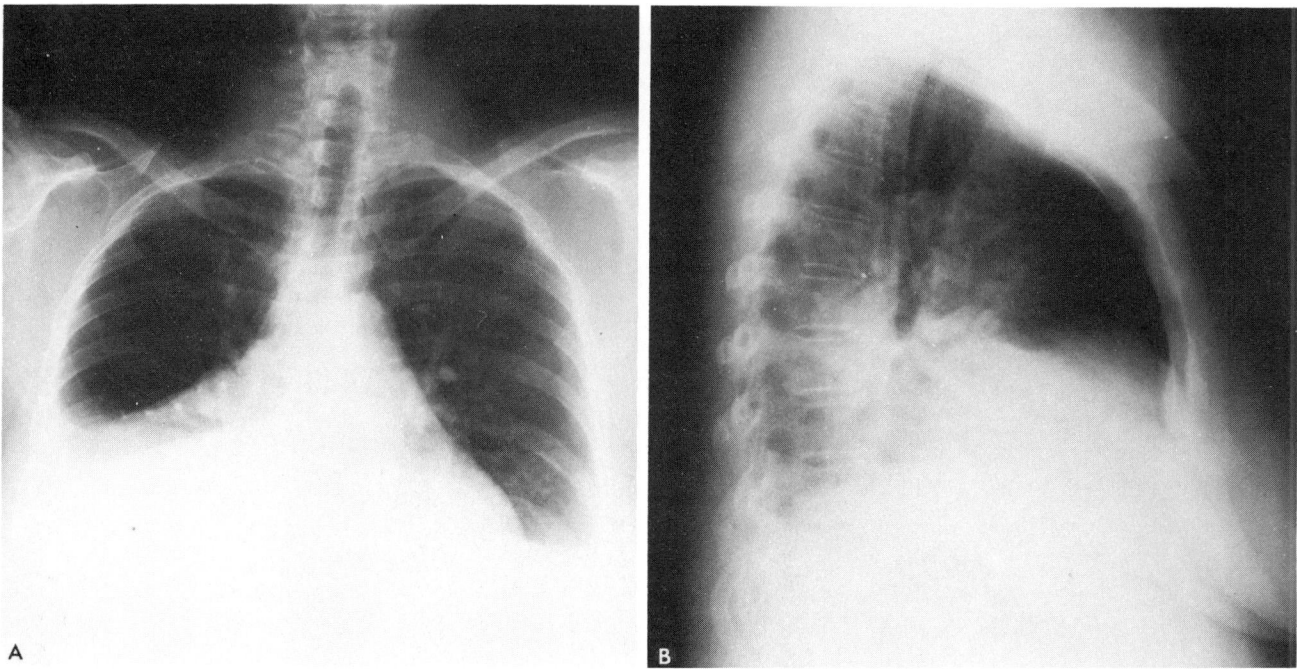

FIGURE 13–29. *A, B,* This 50-year-old previously healthy woman described the subacute onset of mild right pleuritic chest pain, associated with increasing shortness of breath. Chest x-ray reveals a large right pleural effusion (2 liters of fluid were removed from the right pleural cavity) and a small left pleural effusion. Metastatic ovarian carcinoma was ultimately proven and treated.

continuation of the offending agent. Even bacterial pneumonia can resolve without treatment.

Thus, spontaneous improvement of acute pleuritic chest pain does not always exclude serious disease. A specific diagnosis should always be sought in such patients.

Conversely, processes in Table 13–15 that typically persist or worsen over time include neoplasms, empyema, subdiaphragmatic abscesses, and (sometimes) pleural tuberculosis. Thus, acute pleuritic pain syndromes that persist, worsen, or are associated with progressively enlarging pleural effusions should suggest one of these possibilities.

In Angela's case, several conclusions are reasonable:

1. Acute pleuritic chest pain with low-grade fever, a (relatively) normal physical examination and ECG, and a chest x-ray that reveals a new, small pleural effusion without pulmonary infiltrates is most suggestive of viral pleuritis, pulmonary embolism, or a subdiaphragmatic process. The last two are especially suspect because Angela has recently had intra-abdominal surgery (in the right upper quadrant). Much less likely, but possible, are tuberculosis, empyema, or "postoperative" SLE. We can reasonably exclude pericarditis, pneumonia, chest-wall pain, trauma, neoplasm, drug-induced disease, and most of the rare diseases listed in Table 13–15.

2. A lung scan should be performed. The *clinical* probability of pulmonary embolism is very high in this setting. Appendix IV discusses the interpretation and utility of lung scanning in this and other situations.

3. One can argue that hospitalization is indicated whatever the results of tests. If, however, the lung scan is normal (Appendix IV), one might

decide to follow Angela as an outpatient. The subsequent course would then distinguish between a subdiaphragmatic process and viral pleuritis—the other likely possibilities. Thoracentesis might be helpful, but small effusions may be difficult to tap.

> Angela is admitted to the hospital.
>
> A perfusion lung scan reveals a single, segmental defect in the posterobasal segment of the right lower lobe, in the same area as the pleural effusion on chest x-ray. The perfusion defect is of approximately the same size as the effusion. (A ventilation scan is thus not obtained; see Appendix IV.) Pulmonary arteriography is performed and is normal.
>
> Over the next 3 days, the pleural effusion increases slightly in size, and right upper quadrant abdominal tenderness increases. The white blood count rises to 18,000 with a marked left shift. Serum amylase, tuberculin skin tests, and antinuclear antibodies (ANA) are negative. Thoracentesis reveals exudative fluid with a low white cell count and normal glucose, Gram stain, AFB smear, and bacterial cultures. One blood culture grows gram-negative bacilli.
>
> Surgical exploration and drainage of a suprahepatic abscess are accomplished without complications, and Angela is discharged 2 weeks later, feeling well.

NOTE

1. While the clinical probability of pulmonary embolism was high in this case, the lung scan result was indeterminate (see Appendix IV), and the differential diagnosis in this case included disease (for example, an intra-abdominal abscess) that might worsen during therapeutic anticoagulation—thus, arteriography was absolutely essential to rule out (or diagnose) pulmonary embolism in this setting (see Appendix IV).

2. Most causes of pleuritic chest pain are thoracic in origin, but subdiaphragmatic processes must always be remembered, especially in certain suspicious clinical settings.

> Angela resumes her gradual daily exercise program and tolerates exercise with a heart rate of 130 without symptoms. She loses weight, continues antihypertensive therapy, and becomes angina free except during unusually vigorous exercise.

APPENDIX I

Exercise Testing and Chest Pain: Populations and Persons

Exercise (stress) testing is a valuable clinical tool in a variety of clinical circumstances. Table 13–17 indicates some of these clinical situations (while Table 13–18 enumerates some contraindications to stress testing). It can be seen that exercise testing may be useful diagnostically or therapeutically—its broad role in the overall management of patients with known or suspected ischemic heart disease is far beyond the scope of this text. Ellestad and associates' review[127] is recommended.

Here we will focus on the *diagnostic* utility of the exercise test in the patient with chest pain. As we shall see, exercise testing may or may not be helpful in the diagnosis of episodic chest pain,[128] and it is the clinical setting that helps determine this.

TABLE 13–17. POSSIBLE INDICATIONS FOR STRESS TESTING

Evaluation of patient with symptoms suggestive of coronary artery disease.
Determination of patient's physical work capacity and aerobic capacity.
Determination of patient's physical limitations after infarction and as aid in design of rehabilitation exercise program.
Evaluation of status of patient after bypass to aid in rehabilitation exercise program and to detect residual ischemia.
Evaluation of status of asymptomatic patient over age 40 with risk factors for coronary artery disease.
Evaluation of arrhythmias.
Evaluation of therapeutic drug regimens for arrhythmias, angina, or ischemia.
Stimulation of patients to conform to risk factor modification.

(Adapted with permission from Ellestad, MH, et al.: Stress testing: Clinical application and predictive capacity. Prog Cardiovasc Dis 21:431–460, 1979.)

TABLE 13–18. POSSIBLE CONTRAINDICATIONS TO STRESS TESTING

1. Acute myocardial infarction.*
2. Acute myocarditis or pericarditis.
3. Symptomatology suggestive of unstable angina.
4. Rapid atrial arrhythmias.
5. Advanced atrioventricular block (second or third degree).
6. Uncompensated congestive heart failure.
7. Acute noncardiac illnesses (e.g., hyperthyroidism, infection, pulmonary disease).
8. Aortic stenosis (relative contraindication).
9. Known left main coronary artery disease (relative contraindication).
10. False-positive or false-negative test very likely.

(Adapted with permission from Ellestad, MH, et al.: Stress testing: Clinical application and predictive capacity. Prog Cardiovasc Dis 21:431–460, 1979.)
*However, many centers are routinely subjecting patients to a submaximal (70 per cent) symptom-limited test prior to discharge.

EXERCISE TESTING AND
THE PREVALENCE OF DISEASE IN A POPULATION

Table 13–19 indicates the results of ECG exercise testing and coronary arteriography among 1703 symptomatic patients divided into subsets according to sex and clinical classification of chest pain as definite angina, probable angina, and nonischemic chest pain.[129] (Notice that these subsets are not exactly identical with those subsets discussed in the text—"probable angina" in Table 13–19 would, however, be one type of "compatible chest pain" according to our scheme.)

NOTE

1. <u>As expected, the prevalence of coronary artery disease (CAD) among patients with chest pain varies directly with the patient's sex and clinical history.</u> It will also vary with the patient's age and coronary risk factors—see page 721.

CAD is more common in men than women. For each sex, CAD is much more common when chest pain is clearly anginal than when it is clearly nonanginal; prevalence of disease in patients with "probable angina" is intermediate between those two extremes. (As discussed in the text proper, prevalence of CAD in "probable angina" will vary with *how* probable or *how* atypical is the history of pain.)

2. <u>When the prevalence of CAD is either very high or very low, exercise testing is not very helpful as a *diagnostic* test for CAD.</u>[128, 130] For example, a history of definite angina among men was itself so highly predictive of CAD (88 per cent) that a positive exercise test in such patients did not add much diagnostic information to the history alone (95 per cent predictive value of a positive test versus 88 per cent prevalence of disease). Similarly, a negative exercise test would often be falsely reassuring because 62 per cent of such patients did have CAD in spite of the negative test.

At the other end of the spectrum, a history of nonischemic pain among women was so unlikely to be associated with CAD (5 per cent) that a negative exercise test was no more reassuring (95 per cent true negative) than the history alone, while a positive exercise test in such patients was usually misleading, since it was almost always (94 per cent) falsely positive.

3. <u>When the prevalence of CAD is intermediate between these two extremes, the results of exercise testing can heighten or lessen the probability of CAD, but probability is not certainty.</u> Consider, for example, the results of exercise testing among men with probable angina and among women with either definite angina or probable angina. The respective prevalence of CAD in these groups was 67, 58, and 35 per cent. Note that the higher the prevalence of CAD, the fewer tests are false-positive, but false-negative tests are more frequent. Thus in men with probable angina, a positive exercise test strongly implied CAD, but a negative test was not reassuring (because false-negatives were so common); in women with probable angina, a negative test was more reassuring than in the men, but a positive test did not help very much (because it was almost as likely to be falsely positive as truly positive).

Thus, when prevalence of CAD is intermediate, exercise tests may or may not help. The higher the prevalence of CAD, the more predictive is a

TABLE 13–19. CORRELATIONS AMONG CLINICAL HISTORY OF CHEST PAIN, ECG EXERCISE TEST RESULTS, AND CORONARY ARTERIOGRAPHY IN MEN AND WOMEN

	PREVALENCE OF CORONARY ARTERY DISEASE (DEFINED ARTERIOGRAPHICALLY)†			EXERCISE TEST POSITIVE*			EXERCISE TEST NEGATIVE			EXERCISE TEST SENSITIVITY %/ SPECIFICITY %
Males	Total	CAD +	CAD −	Total	CAD +	CAD −	Total	CAD +	CAD −	
Definite angina	487	428	59	377	360	17	110	68	42	
	Prevalence coronary artery disease = 88% (428/487)			Predictive value of positive test = 95% (360/377) False positive = 5% (17/377)			Predictive value of negative test = 38% (42/110) (reassurance value) False negative = 62% (68/110)			84%/71%
	Total	CAD +	CAD −	Total	CAD +	CAD −	Total	CAD +	CAD −	
Probable angina	443	295	148	241	211	30	202	84	118	
	Prevalence coronary artery disease = 67% (295/443)			Predictive value of positive test = 88% (211/241) False positive = 12% (30/241)			Predictive value of negative test = 58% (118/202) (reassurance value) False negative = 42% (84/202)			72%/80%
	Total	CAD +	CAD −	Total	CAD +	CAD −	Total	CAD +	CAD −	
Nonangina	203	44	159	53	20	33	150	24	126	
	Prevalence coronary artery disease = 22% (44/203)			Predictive value of positive test = 38% (20/53) False positive = 62% (33/53)			Predictive value of negative test = 84% (126/150) (reassurance value) False negative = 16% (24/150)			45%/79%

(Adapted with permission from Weiner, DA, et al: Exercise stress testing. Correlations among history of angina, ST segment response, and prevalence of coronary artery disease in the coronary artery surgery study (CASS). N Engl J Med 301:230–235, 1979.)

*All patients included in this table had resting ECGs with normal ST and T waves.

Definitions:

†CAD + (coronary artery disease positive) indicates the presence of greater than or equal to 70 per cent luminal narrowing of at least one coronary vessel.

$$\text{Prevalence} = \frac{\text{no. patients with disease}}{\text{no. patients studied}}$$

$$\text{Sensitivity} = \frac{\text{True positives}}{\text{True positives} + \text{False negatives}}$$

$$\text{Specificity} = \frac{\text{True negatives}}{\text{True negatives} + \text{False positives}}$$

$$\text{Predictive value positive} = \frac{\text{True positives}}{\text{True positives} + \text{False positives}}$$

$$\text{Predictive value negative (reassurance value)} = \frac{\text{True negatives}}{\text{True negatives} + \text{False negatives}}$$

Table continued on opposite page

positive test but the less reassuring is a negative test; the lower the prevalence of disease, the more reassuring is a negative test but the less predictive is a positive test. Notice, however, that in all groups in which disease prevalence is intermediate, a positive test does raise the likelihood of CAD and a negative test does lower the likelihood of CAD.

EXERCISE TESTING FOR INDIVIDUAL PATIENTS

The difficulties inherent in applying such population-based probabilities (Table 13–19) to one individual with chest pain—*my patient*—can be seen

TABLE 13–19. CORRELATIONS AMONG CLINICAL HISTORY OF CHEST PAIN, ECG EXERCISE TEST RESULTS, AND CORONARY ARTERIOGRAPHY IN MEN AND WOMEN *(Continued)*

	PREVALENCE OF CORONARY ARTERY DISEASE (DEFINED ARTERIOGRAPHICALLY)†			EXERCISE TEST POSITIVE*			EXERCISE TEST NEGATIVE			EXERCISE TEST SENSITIVITY %/ SPECIFICITY %
Females	Total	CAD +	CAD −	Total	CAD +	CAD −	Total	CAD +	CAD −	
Definite angina	67	39	28	43	31	12	24	8	16	
	Prevalence coronary artery disease = 58% (39/67)			Predictive value of positive test = 72% (31/43) False positive = 28% (12/43)			Predictive value of negative test = 67% (16/24) (reassurance value) False negative = 33% (8/24)			79%/57%
	Total	CAD +	CAD −	Total	CAD +	CAD −	Total	CAD +	CAD −	
Probable angina	153	54	99	67	36	31	86	18	68	
	Prevalence coronary artery disease = 35% (54/153)			Predictive value of positive test = 54% (36/67) False positive = 46% (31/67)			Predictive value of negative test = 79% (68/86) (reassurance value) False negative = 21% (18/86)			67%/69%
	Total	CAD +	CAD −	Total	CAD +	CAD −	Total	CAD +	CAD −	
Nonangina	175	9	166	33	2	31	142	7	135	
	Prevalence coronary artery disease = 5% (9/175)			Predictive value of positive test = 6% (2/33) False positive = 94% (31/33)			Predictive value of negative test = 95% (135/142) (reassurance value) False negative = 5% (7/142)			22%/81%

from the nether ends of the spectrum of "mistakes" in Table 13–19. The 95 per cent probability of CAD in the group of 377 men with definite angina and positive exercise tests does not help me if my patient is one of the 17 men in that group who did not have CAD. The 95 per cent probability of the absence of CAD in the group of 142 women with nonischemic pain and negative exercise tests is of no use to the 7 such women who did have CAD. Thus a few such patients will be treated unnecessarily for angina pectoris and a few others will escape detection if the clinical history and ECG exercise tests are the only methods of investigation. Many more cases will be misdiagnosed in the intermediate probability groups.

How then can such statistical correlations among large groups of patients help in the management of the individual patient with chest pain? Several concepts are helpful:

1. The individual patient's *history* is the critical factor in deciding not only how to interpret the exercise stress test but whether (and why) to perform the test in the first place. Why is this?

As we have seen above, disease prevalence is the critical factor in interpreting exercise tests in a population. But the concept of disease prevalence in one individual patient is spurious—the patient either does or does not have CAD. Analogous to the concept of disease prevalence, however, is that of "pretest likelihood," i.e., the likelihood of disease being present in a particular patient before any tests are performed. As indicated

TABLE 13–20. PRETEST LIKELIHOOD OF CORONARY-ARTERY DISEASE IN SYMPTOMATIC PATIENTS ACCORDING TO AGE AND SEX*

AGE Yr	NONANGINAL CHEST PAIN		ATYPICAL ANGINA		TYPICAL ANGINA	
	Men	Women	Men	Women	Men	Women
30–39	5.2 ± 0.8	0.8 ± 0.3	21.8 ± 2.4	4.2 ± 1.3	69.7 ± 3.2	25.8 ± 6.6
40–49	14.1 ± 1.3	2.8 ± 0.7	46.1 ± 1.8	13.3 ± 2.9	87.3 ± 1.0	55.2 ± 6.5
50–59	21.5 ± 1.7	8.4 ± 1.2	58.9 ± 1.5	32.4 ± 3.0	92.0 ± 0.6	79.4 ± 2.4
60–69	28.1 ± 1.9	18.6 ± 1.9	67.1 ± 1.3	54.4 ± 2.4	94.3 ± 0.4	90.6 ± 1.0

(From Diamond, GA, and Forrester, JS: Analysis of probability as an aid in the clinical diagnosis of coronary artery disease. Reprinted by permission of the New England Journal of Medicine 300:1350–1358, 1979.)

*Each value represents the per cent ± 1 standard error of the per cent.

in Table 13–20, the pretest likelihood of CAD varies directly with the patient's age, sex, and clinical symptoms[131]—in short, the patient's history. The importance of this pretest likelihood—the patient's history—can be exemplified by comparing Table 13–20 with Table 13–21, which indicates the likelihood of CAD after stress tests have been performed, i.e., the post-test likelihood. Consider, for example, the 60-year-old man with typical angina. An exercise stress test will not help in diagnosing (or excluding) CAD in such a patient because the pretest likelihood is so high. (Remember: This

TABLE 13–21. POST-TEST LIKELIHOOD AFTER AN ECG STRESS TEST ACCORDING TO AGE, SEX, SYMPTOM, AND DEPRESSION OF ST SEGMENT*

AGE Yr	ASYMPTOMATIC		NONANGINAL CHEST PAIN			ATYPICAL ANGINA		TYPICAL ANGINA	
	Men	Women	Men	Women		Men	Women	Men	Women
					≥2.5				
30–39	43.0 ± 24.9	10.5 ± 9.9	68.1 ± 22.1	23.9 ± 19.5		91.8 ± 7.7	63.1 ± 24.5	98.9 ± 1.1	93.1 ± 6.8
40–49	69.4 ± 21.3	28.3 ± 20.8	86.5 ± 11.8	52.9 ± 25.8		97.1 ± 2.8	85.7 ± 12.5	99.6 ± 0.4	98.0 ± 2.1
50–59	80.7 ± 15.6	56.3 ± 24.9	91.4 ± 7.9	78.1 ± 17.3		98.2 ± 1.7	94.9 ± 4.9	99.8 ± 0.2	99.3 ± 0.7
60–69	84.5 ± 13.1	76.0 ± 18.4	93.8 ± 5.8	89.9 ± 9.2		98.8 ± 1.2	97.9 ± 2.1	99.8 ± 0.2	99.7 ± 0.3
					(2.0,2.5]				
30–39	17.7 ± 10.3	3.2 ± 2.4	37.8 ± 16.6	8.2 ± 5.9		76.0 ± 12.8	32.7 ± 16.7	96.2 ± 2.6	79.4 ± 12.6
40–49	39.2 ± 16.5	10.1 ± 6.5	64.5 ± 16.0	24.2 ± 13.5		90.5 ± 6.0	63.0 ± 17.1	98.7 ± 0.9	93.2 ± 4.7
50–59	54.3 ± 17.1	26.8 ± 13.8	75.2 ± 13.0	50.4 ± 17.7		94.1 ± 3.9	84.2 ± 9.4	99.2 ± 0.5	97.7 ± 1.6
60–69	60.9 ± 16.4	47.3 ± 17.3	81.2 ± 10.6	71.7 ± 14.2		95.8 ± 2.8	93.0 ± 4.5	99.5 ± 0.4	99.1 ± 0.6
					(1.5,2.0]				
30–39	7.5 ± 5.0	1.2 ± 1.0	18.7 ± 10.9	3.3 ± 2.5		54.5 ± 17.8	15.5 ± 10.1	90.6 ± 6.1	59.3 ± 18.9
40–49	19.6 ± 11.1	4.1 ± 2.8	40.8 ± 17.1	10.8 ± 7.2		78.2 ± 12.0	39.1 ± 17.7	96.6 ± 2.3	83.8 ± 10.2
50–59	31.0 ± 15.0	12.2 ± 7.6	53.4 ± 17.6	27.8 ± 14.4		85.7 ± 8.6	66.8 ± 15.9	98.0 ± 1.4	94.2 ± 3.9
60–69	37.0 ± 16.4	25.4 ± 13.4	62.1 ± 16.7	48.9 ± 17.8		89.5 ± 6.6	83.3 ± 9.8	98.6 ± 1.0	97.6 ± 1.7
					(1.0,1.5]				
30–39	3.9 ± 0.9	0.6 ± 0.2	10.4 ± 2.2	1.7 ± 0.7		37.7 ± 5.2	8.5 ± 2.8	83.0 ± 3.2	42.4 ± 9.4
40–49	11.0 ± 1.7	2.1 ± 0.5	25.8 ± 3.8	5.8 ± 1.7		64.4 ± 4.2	24.5 ± 5.6	93.6 ± 1.1	72.3 ± 6.2
50–59	18.5 ± 2.6	6.5 ± 1.3	36.7 ± 4.5	16.3 ± 3.1		75.2 ± 3.3	50.4 ± 5.4	96.1 ± 0.7	89.1 ± 2.2
60–69	22.9 ± 3.1	14.7 ± 2.3	45.3 ± 4.7	32.6 ± 4.6		81.2 ± 2.7	71.6 ± 3.9	97.2 ± 0.5	95.3 ± 0.9
					(0.5,1.0]				
30–39	1.7 ± 0.6	0.3 ± 0.1	4.8 ± 1.6	0.7 ± 0.4		20.7 ± 5.5	3.9 ± 1.6	67.8 ± 7.4	24.2 ± 8.4
40–49	5.1 ± 1.5	0.9 ± 0.3	13.1 ± 3.7	2.6 ± 1.0		43.9 ± 7.7	12.3 ± 4.3	86.3 ± 3.7	53.0 ± 10.0
50–59	9.0 ± 2.5	2.9 ± 0.9	20.1 ± 5.1	7.8 ± 2.4		56.8 ± 7.6	30.5 ± 7.1	91.3 ± 2.5	77.9 ± 5.8
60–69	11.4 ± 3.1	6.9 ± 2.0	26.4 ± 6.2	17.3 ± 4.7		65.1 ± 7.0	52.2 ± 7.9	93.8 ± 1.8	89.8 ± 2.9
					(0,0.5]				
30–39	0.4 ± 0.1	0.1 ± 0.0	1.2 ± 0.4	0.2 ± 0.1		6.1 ± 1.7	1.0 ± 0.4	24.5 ± 6.6	7.4 ± 2.9
40–49	1.3 ± 0.3	0.2 ± 0.1	3.6 ± 0.9	0.7 ± 0.2		16.4 ± 3.5	3.4 ± 1.2	61.1 ± 6.3	22.0 ± 6.2
50–59	2.4 ± 0.6	0.8 ± 0.2	5.9 ± 1.5	2.1 ± 0.6		24.7 ± 4.8	9.9 ± 2.5	72.5 ± 5.2	46.9 ± 7.2
60–69	3.1 ± 0.8	1.8 ± 0.6	8.2 ± 2.0	5.0 ± 1.3		31.8 ± 5.5	21.4 ± 4.5	79.1 ± 4.3	68.8 ± 5.9

(From Diamond, GA, and Forrester, JS: Analysis of probability as an aid in the clinical diagnosis of coronary artery disease. Reprinted by permission of the New England Journal of Medicine 300:1350–1358, 1979.)

*Each symbol (x,y] represents depression of the ST segment in millimeters.

does not mean that a stress test is useless in such a patient—it may be very helpful in overall management—but only that it is not particularly helpful in *diagnosis*.) Similarly, the young woman with nonanginal chest pain is so unlikely to have CAD (the pretest likelihood is so low) that any exercise test result is not likely to help diagnostically. (Again, this does not mean that a stress test is always useless in such patients. A negative test may be more reassuring to that patient than the clinician's clinical impression, for example.)

The point here is that in certain clinical circumstances one should hesitate before performing the exercise test for diagnostic purposes. This need to hesitate derives from a second important concept:

2. When an individual patient's history indicates that the pretest likelihood of CAD is very low, a critical corollary is that the pretest likelihood of nonischemic chest pain must be very high. From an "either/or point of view" the individual patient's chest pain must be caused *either* by CAD *or* by something else. Thus, when the pretest likelihood of CAD is very slight, the first practical priority then becomes looking for the probable cause (chest-wall pain, esophagitis, anxiety—see text proper) rather than exhaustively excluding the highly improbable cause (CAD). As page 694 and Figure 13–5 suggest, some such patients do require exercise testing or coronary arteriography. However, when the clinical (pretest) probability of ischemic chest pain is very low, an exercise test should be used for diagnostic purposes only after a careful search for nonischemic causes of chest pain is unrevealing (barium swallow, esophageal manometry, chest-wall maneuvers, for example). Whether this approach (Fig. 13–5) would actually improve the statistical accuracy of the exercise test in patients with atypical or compatible chest pain is unknown. It seems likely, however, that the number of exercise tests performed, and thus the number of false-positive exercise tests, would be reduced.

3. Exercise tests are not simply positive or negative. The standard criterion for a positive exercise test is the development of horizontal or down-sloping ST depression greater than or equal to 1 mm (Fig. 13–30) for at least 0.08 second after the J point. When more stringent criteria are used to define positive (for example, 2-mm depression), the positive test will be more specific (false positives will be fewer) but less sensitive (more patients with CAD will have negative tests). As Table 13–22 suggests, certain clinical situations are likely to produce false-positive and false-negative exercise tests, and these must always be considered before initiating the test.

The "degree of positivity" of an exercise test *is* diagnostically helpful. For example, the 55-year-old woman with nonanginal chest pain (very unlikely to have CAD—pretest likelihood is under 10 per cent in Table 13–20) is very likely to have CAD if the exercise test is *very* positive (depression greater than or equal to 2.5 mm suggests a post-test likelihood of almost 80

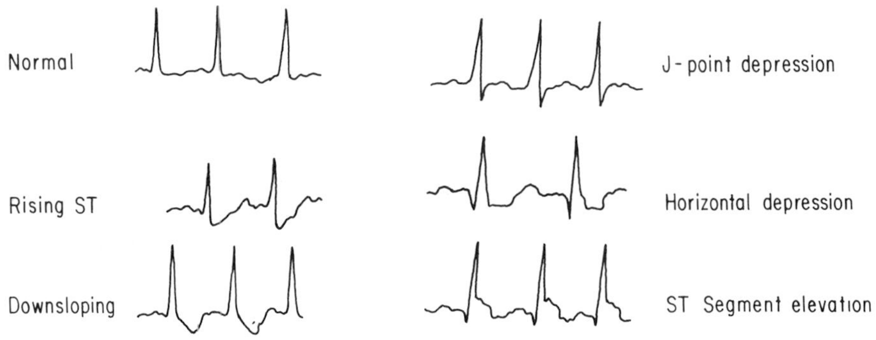

Normal   J-point depression

FIGURE 13–30. Electrocardiographic ST changes.

Rising ST   Horizontal depression

Downsloping   ST Segment elevation

TABLE 13–22. CAUSES OF FALSE-POSITIVE AND FALSE-NEGATIVE EXERCISE TESTS

FALSE-POSITIVE EXERCISE TESTS	FALSE-NEGATIVE EXERCISE TESTS
Left bundle-branch block	Left bundle-branch block
Left ventricular hypertrophy	Nitrates
Hypokalemia	Beta blockers
Glucose ingestion	Prior myocardial infarction
Diuretics	Poor exercise tolerance
Phenothiazines	Test stopped at low heart rate
Lithium	Test stopped at low work load
Digitalis	Inadequate number of ECG leads
Antihypertensives	
Mitral valve prolapse	
Cardiomyopathy	
Asymmetric septal hypertrophy	
Severe hypertension	
Hyperventilation	

per cent in Table 13–21). In such a patient, CAD is not likely if the test is "barely positive" (1.0 to 1.5 mm ST depression gives a post-test likelihood of less than 20 per cent in Table 13–21).

A "very positive" stress test thus improves the test's specificity. Such a result also may correlate with the severity of CAD (and thus ultimately the prognosis—Table 13–11.) This has important implications. As noted in the text proper, coronary artery surgery will improve prognosis in patients with left main coronary disease[64] (and probably "left main equivalent" coronary disease[62]), and thus even if such patients had stable angina, surgery would be considered. While the absence of a "very positive" test in no way excludes such severe disease[132] several findings on exercise testing may correlate with the extent of coronary disease (Fig. 13–31).

1. The magnitude of ST depression: ST depression greater than 2.5 mm suggests severe disease.

2. Time of onset of ST depression: ischemic ST changes that develop during the first 3 minutes of the exercise test suggest severe disease.

3. Duration of ST depression: persistence of ischemic changes for more than 8 minutes into the recovery period after exercise testing suggests severe disease.

4. ST segment configuration: down-sloping ST depressions or ST elevations during exercise correlate best with extent of disease.

5. Hypotension during exercise (especially at low work loads) is also ominous.

Conversely, a negative exercise test may be helpful or misleading, depending on what "negative" means.

As we have seen, false negative tests will be relatively more common in patients with a high pretest likelihood of CAD, but a negative result in such a patient at least allows an estimate of the patient's exercise capacity, which is useful in overall patient management.

Occasionally the stress test will be negative, but the patient will nonetheless experience classic angina pectoris during the test[133]—such patients usually *do* have CAD. Thus, observation of the patient during the stress test is as important as observation of the ECG—the stress test is, in a sense, an

I	AVR	V1	V4
II	AVL	V2	V5
III	AVF	V3	V6

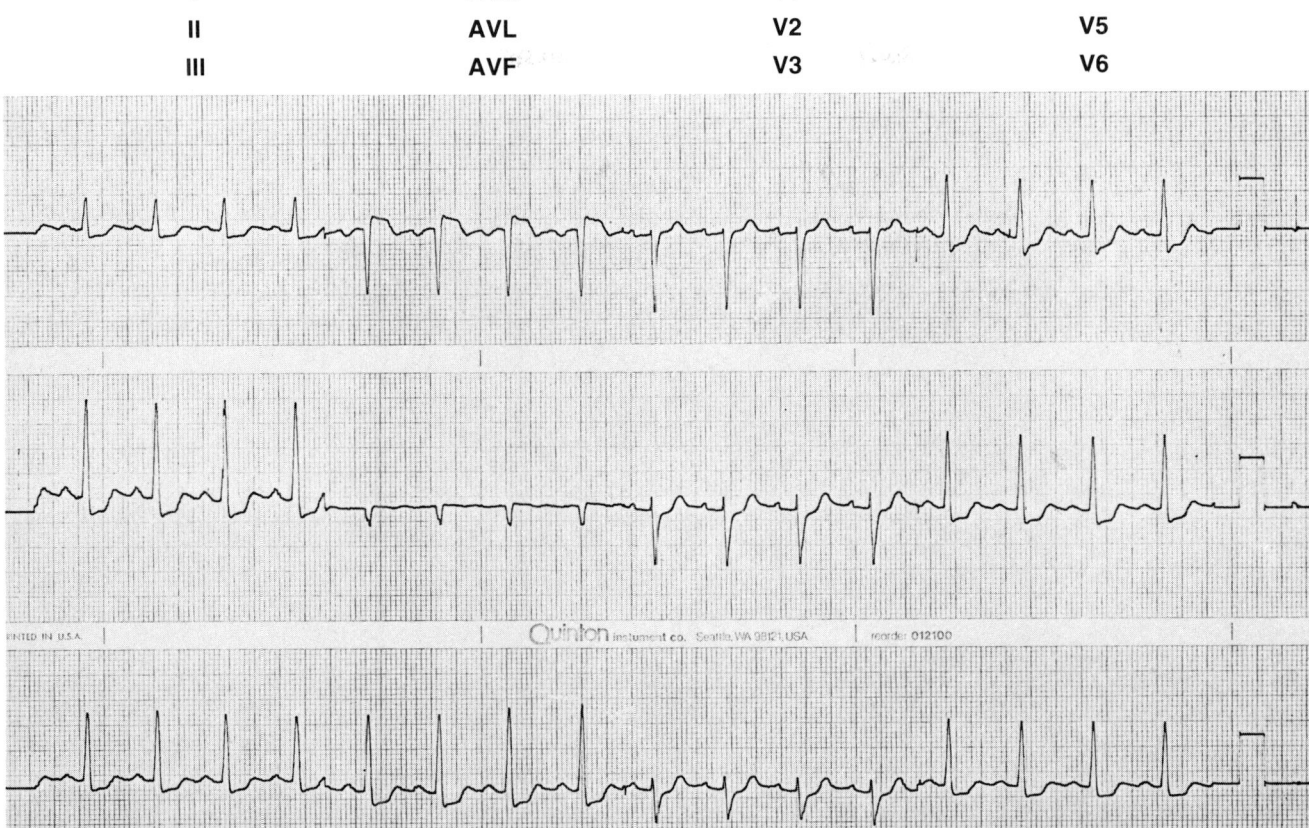

FIGURE 13–31. This 66-year-old woman described exertional angina, precipitated by simple household activities. The resting electrocardiogram and physical examination were normal. The electrocardiographic exercise test demonstrates horizontal ST depressions in leads I, II, III, AVF, and the lateral precordial leads. These changes occurred (in association with typical angina) after only 1 minute of exercise, at a heart rate of 120 beats/min, and after only 2 METS of exercise. In addition, the patient's preexercise blood pressure (140/84) fell to 115/70 at this time, and ST depression persisted for 10 minutes after stopping exercise. This is an "ominous" exercise test result. The patient was admitted to hospital, where coronary arteriography demonstrated severe three-vessel disease with 80 per cent stenosis of the left main coronary artery. Coronary bypass surgery resulted in dramatic improvement.

extension of the clinical history. When the patient develops his or her typical chest pain during a "negative" stress test and the pain is clearly recognized by the physician as nonanginal (page 687), this test result is also extremely helpful.

As noted in Table 13–21, a completely normal exercise test (no ST depression at all even at high exercise levels) tends to be reassuring in problem patients—those whose history is atypical or peculiar and whose pretest likelihood of CAD is intermediate or low.

How, then, does one use exercise tests in individual patients?

1. Patients with typical angina. As we have seen, exercise testing in most such patients is more useful in management than in diagnosis.*

---

*As suggested by Table 13–21, the exception here is the young (especially female) patient with symptomatically "typical angina." A normal exercise test in such patients makes CAD very unlikely. A positive exercise test will be diagnostically helpful, depending on degree of positivity. (As we have seen, false-positive tests are very common in this group.)

Documentation of exercise tolerance helps the patient to confidently undertake exercise programs and helps educate the patient about the nature of the problem. (The physician can then explain to the patient, "When you get *that chest pain,* sit down and take nitroglycerin. If you get *that* chest pain more frequently or if it lasts a long time, call me.")

"Ominous" findings on ECG stress testing may suggest left main coronary disease or multivessel disease, and coronary arteriography is often performed on the basis of such findings. (Remember that the absence of such findings in no way excludes such severe disease.)

Sometimes it is helpful to follow the angina patient's progress with serial exercise tests to document the effectiveness of pharmacologic therapy, exercise programs, and overall patient management.

2. Patients with nonanginal chest pain. In general, stress tests should be deferred in such patients, pending investigation of other causes of chest pain (see above).

When exercise tests are performed in such patients, a normal exercise test is usually very reassuring, but abnormal exercise tests require further investigation (radionuclide studies or arteriography or both). The specific

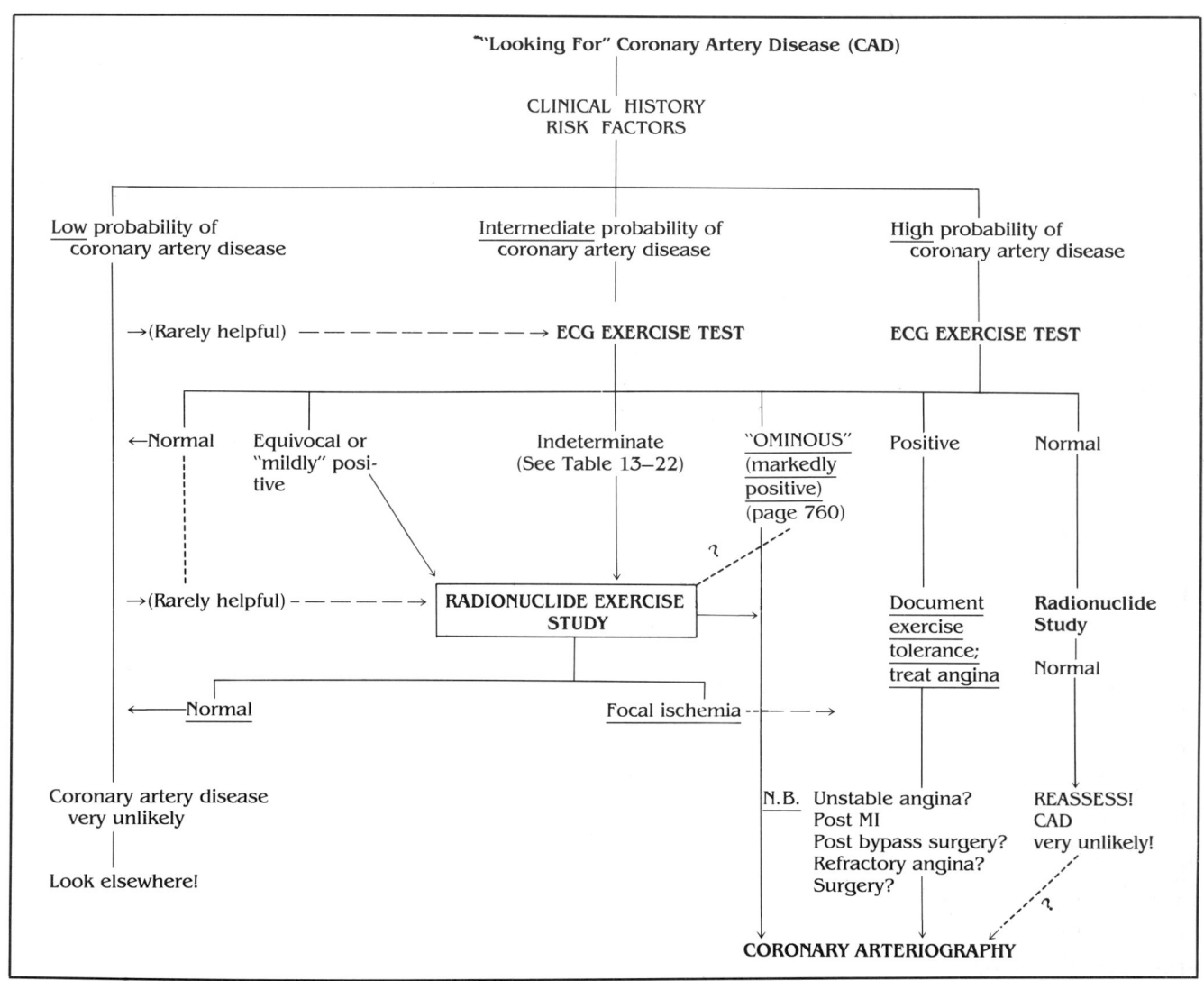

FIGURE 13–32.

approach to such patients must be individualized, depending on the patient's age, coronary risk factors and how positive the exercise test is. The 50-year-old man with greater than 2.5-mm ST depressions at only 3 minutes of exercise will usually require arteriography to exclude "surgical disease," however peculiar is his chest pain. The 35-year-old female with 1.5-mm ST depressions at maximal exercise will usually benefit from corroborative testing (see below) before any treatment is considered.

3. Patients with compatible chest pain. The most important factor here is the pretest likelihood of CAD, i.e., how atypical of angina is the patient's compatible chest pain and is the patient low risk or high risk? When pain is extremely atypical of CAD and the patient is otherwise at low risk, the approach is similar to that for nonanginal chest pain: look elsewhere first. When this search is unrevealing and the history remains at least compatible with angina, an exercise test is worthwhile (Fig. 13–32).

In these circumstances, when the exercise test is very positive (ST depressions greater than or equal to 2.5 mm), CAD is very likely. When the test is completely normal, CAD is unlikely. When exercise test results are intermediate between these two extremes (for example, ST depressions of 1.5 mm at maximal exercise levels), further conclusions are less well founded. Consider, for example, the 40-year-old male with atypical angina. Before any testing, the likelihood of CAD is intermediate—perhaps somewhere between 20 and 50 per cent (46 per cent in Table 13–20), depending on how atypical the pain is and whether he is a smoker, has hypertension, or has a positive family history of CAD (i.e., "risk factors"). If this patient's exercise ECG reveals ST depressions of 1.0 to 1.5 mm, the likelihood of CAD remains intermediate (about 60 per cent in Table 13–21).

This "gray zone" (the mildly positive exercise test in the patient with compatible but atypical chest pain) illustrates the potential importance of corroborative testing procedures, especially radionuclide exercise tests, as a means of improving the probability estimate provided by one test alone.

CONSIDER

NUCLEAR STRESS TESTING

While radionuclide cineangiography and myocardial perfusion imaging may be more sensitive and specific than ECG exercise testing[134–137] and may be more predictive of the extent of disease[137]—the relative accuracies of electrocardiographic and radionuclide stress tests (as well as other noninvasive techniques)[138, 162] remain controversial[139] and will vary in different medical centers—these tests are also imperfect and their interpretation requires similar qualifications to those discussed above. Again, these tests assess probabilities. Since these corroborative tests are not universally available and are expensive, they can be used most cost effectively when viewed as second-line tests. Figure 13–33 illustrates how the "gray zone" can be made more "black and white" by the use of multiple tests. Consider again our hypothetical 40-year-old male with atypical angina (pretest likelihood 46 per cent in Table 13–20) whose ECG stress test is positive (1.5-mm ST depressions)—we can now assign him an updated pretest likelihood of CAD of 60 per cent (because of the positive exercise test). If now a thallium exercise myocardial

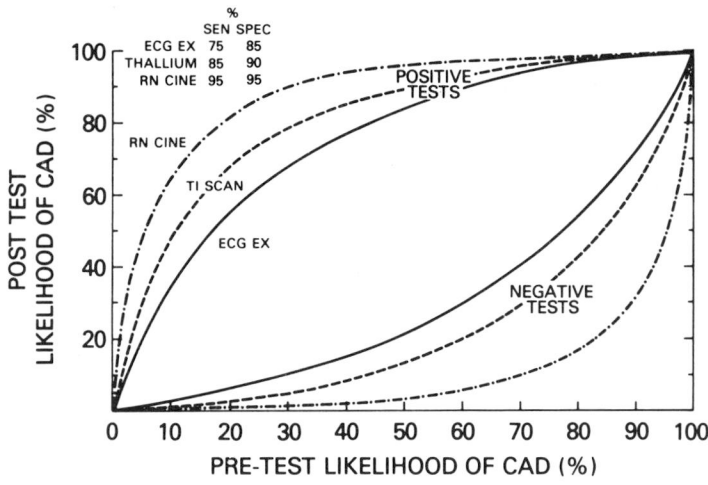

FIGURE 13–33. Probability of coronary artery disease (CAD). Comparison of electrocardiographic exercise testing (ECG EX), thalium perfusion scanning (TI scan), and radionuclide cineangiography (RN CINE). (Sensitivity [SEN] and specificity [SPEC] values are approximations derived from published series.) (Reproduced with permission from Epstein, SE: Implications of probability analysis on the strategy used for noninvasive detection of coronary artery disease. Am J Cardiol 46:496, 1980.)

perfusion scan is performed, a positive scan that corroborates the positive ECG exercise test will raise the likelihood of CAD to almost 90 per cent (from 60 per cent), while a normal thallium scan will greatly lower that likelihood. (Corroborative tests <u>must measure different and independent variables</u> to apply such statistical analyses.)

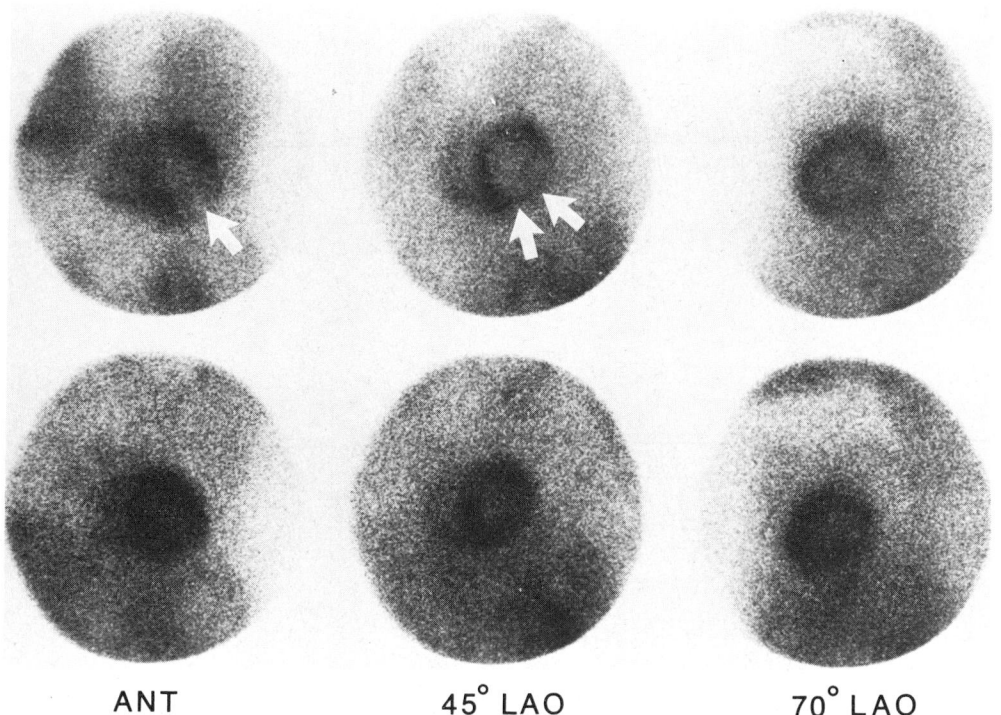

FIGURE 13–34. This 42-year-old diabetic woman described peculiar episodic chest pains that were not felt to be anginal on the basis of the history. An electrocardiographic exercise test, however, demonstrated 3-mm ST depressions in the anterolateral leads. This thallium exercise test corroborates findings of ischemia in the left coronary circulation. The upper row of images are those obtained during exercise—anterior, 45-degree left anterior oblique (LAO), and 70-degree LAO views are shown. The bottom row of images are those obtained after exercise. During exercise, the apex and lateral wall of the left ventricle *(arrows)* do not perfuse—after exercise, the perfusion defects disappear.

Coronary arteriography documented severe two-vessel disease, with prominent involvement of the left anterior descending.

Thus, corroborative testing may be useful when:

1. A false-positive exercise tolerance test is thought likely, for example, in the patient with a low clinical probability of CAD in whom the ECG exercise test is positive (Fig. 13–34).

2. A false-negative exercise tolerance test is thought likely, for example, in the patient with classic angina pectoris but a normal ECG exercise test.

3. When the ECG exercise test cannot be performed or when the ECG exercise test is difficult to interpret (Table 13–22).

4. When the combination of clinical findings and ECG exercise test results remains indeterminate—for example, in the patient with "compatible" chest pain, intermediate risk factors, and a mildly positive ECG exercise test.

5. When coronary spasm is suspected—ergonovine-stimulated nuclear testing may help here.

A few patients with compatible chest pain will have chest pain that is not related to exercise but is otherwise suspicious of angina pectoris—variant angina or coronary artery spasm must be considered here.[2, 7, 8, 11] Exercise testing may not be as helpful as ECG monitoring[35] (Fig. 13–8), especially if chest pain occurs frequently enough that 24 to 48 hours of ECG monitoring will record the ECG during a bout of chest pain.

Ultimately, when absolute certainty is required, so is coronary arteriography. Even this gold standard of diagnostic tests for coronary artery disease must be interpreted carefully.[140] In general, as discussed in the text proper, coronary arteriography is usually reserved for patients in whom surgery is contemplated (for whatever reasons). Only uncommonly should it be necessary to diagnose or exclude CAD by arteriography. An exception, however, involves the situation in which angina is felt very unlikely clinically, but the history of chest pain would imply serious and even life-threatening disease if the chest pain were in fact ischemic in origin. Another exception is the patient with "peculiar" chest pain in whom ergonovine-stimulated angiography may be necessary to exclude coronary spasm.

In some such patients, the normal coronary arteriogram can have a beneficial *therapeutic* effect and may even be economically cost effective.[141] Normal coronary arteriography in such circumstances is almost always associated with a benign prognosis.[9, 10]

APPENDIX II

Esophageal Chest Pain

Esophagitis[142-144] usually causes typical heartburn—a hot, acid discomfort in the lower retrosternal area that commonly spreads up the chest (or back) into the jaw, interscapular area, or throat. Frequently, acid brash accompanies heartburn—this is a disagreeable bitter taste in the mouth and throat that, like heartburn, is likely to occur after heavy meals, while bending over or lying supine, and is usually relieved by standing upright or swallowing antacids. Most patients with esophagitis present with a diagnostic history: Further diagnostic studies are often not indicated, especially since most patients will respond to simple conservative management as outlined in phase I of Table 13–23.

At other times, the history in the patient with esophagitis is much less specific. Episodic substernal chest pain, qualitatively different from heartburn and only inconsistently related to meals, may radiate to the neck or arms and very closely mimic angina pectoris or even myocardial infarction (depending on the severity and duration of the pain). Usually, however, there is some clue that suggests esophagitis: the relation to body position (especially bending over or lying down); associated acid brash; relief with antacids; vague intermittent swallowing trouble; nocturnal cough, or (rarely) aspiration. Nevertheless, *proof* that a patient's pain is due to esophagitis may be difficult to establish. Consider:

1. Various tests commonly used to diagnose reflux esophagitis in fact only detect gastroesophageal reflux. Not all patients with reflux have esophagitis. The barium swallow that reveals a hiatus hernia or free gastroesophageal reflux neither proves that the patient has esophagitis nor that the patient's pain is causally related. Similarly a normal barium swallow by no means excludes esophagitis. The barium swallow (with liquid barium and a "barium pill"—"hang-up" of the latter may occasionally detect a stricture, ring, or web that is inapparent otherwise) is very helpful in excluding esophageal stricture, achalasia, vigorous achalasia,[145] and esophageal carcinoma. These disorders are usually suspected, however, when the patient complains of *dysphagia,* not chest pain—endoscopy is often then required, whatever the results of the barium swallow.

Other tests that may document reflux include esophageal pH monitoring (acid reflux test) and newer radionuclide imaging procedures.[143]

2. Esophagitis can only be proven by endoscopic esophageal biopsy—even then, histologic esophagitis does not prove that the patient's chest pain is esophageal in origin. A more dynamic test involves the acid infusion (Bernstein) test, with or without simultaneous pH monitoring. Figure 13–35 illustrates the variable results of this procedure in which saline and 0.1 normal hydrochloric acid are alternately instilled into a nasogastric tube to perfuse the patient's esophagus. Only repeatedly reproducible and exact simulation of the patient's pain constitutes a positive test. A negative test is of no more diagnostic value than an uninterpretable test, since not all patients with esophagitis-caused chest pain will have a positive acid perfusion test.

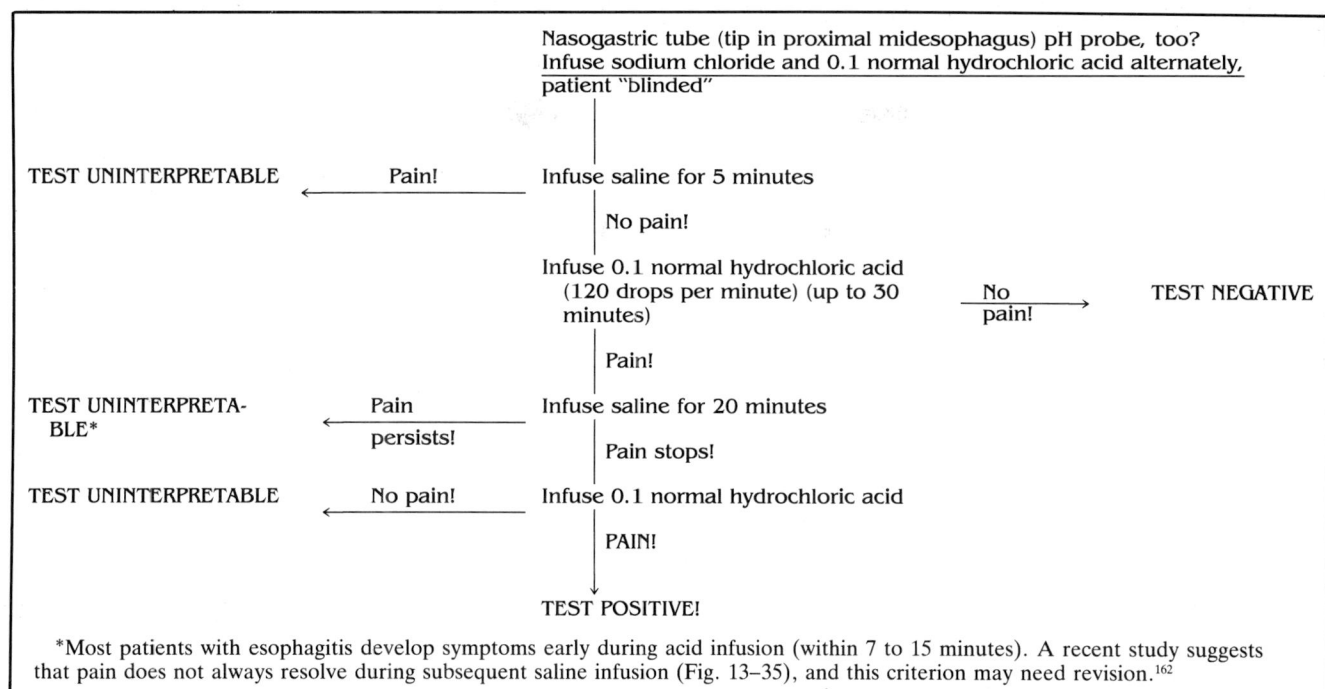

FIGURE 13-35. Acid infusion (Bernstein) test.

3. Usually a therapeutic trial is the most helpful "test." Simple, conservative treatment (phase 1, Table 13–23) is usually highly successful. Occasionally, additional pharmacologic therapy is necessary (phase 2). Antacids, cimetidine (or ranitidine), and bethanechol are most useful, in that order.

TABLE 13–23. TREATMENT OF REFLUX ESOPHAGITIS

PHASE 1
Dietary modification
    Avoid fat, chocolate, coffee, citrus juices, tomato products (the base of many spicy foods), peppermint and spearmint (in many liqueurs), alcohol, peppers, and onions

Stop smoking

Avoid certain drugs, when possible
    Theophylline, progesterone, anticholinergics, diazepam (Valium) meperidine hydrochloride (Demerol)

Antacid therapy (See Appendix, Abdominal Pain)
    As needed when symptoms are infrequent; 1 hour after meals and at bedtime when symptoms are frequent; 1 and 3 hours after meals when symptoms are severe and frequent

General measures
    Lose weight; elevate head of bed; three meals per day; no food within 3 hours of retiring

PHASE 2: PHASE 1 PLUS
Cimetidine 300 mg qid × 6 to 8 weeks; ranitidine 150 mg bid × 4 to 6 weeks; or bethanechol 25 mg qid × 4 to 6 weeks; or metoclopramide 10 mg qid × 6 to 8 weeks; or (possibly) carbenoxolone/alginic acid

PHASE 3
Consultation; consider antireflux surgery

When medical therapy (phases 1 and 2 in Table 13–23) fails, surgery is sometimes necessary.[146] Definitive proof of symptomatic esophagitis must always be documented in these (unusual) circumstances—a combination of endoscopy, esophageal biopsy, and a pH-monitored Bernstein test is probably the most specific diagnostic approach and should always be performed before surgery is considered.

Esophageal spasm is probably much less common than esophagitis (although the two may coexist), but it is more often a puzzling diagnostic problem. The pain of esophageal spasm is usually substernal and constricting, often radiates to the throat, jaw, back, and arms and usually lasts for a few minutes (simulating angina pectoris), but pain may last as long as several hours (simulating many types of acute severe chest pain—see page 727). In most patients,[147–148] there is some history of swallowing problems: either the pain immediately follows deglutition (especially of cold or carbonated substances) or there is a history of (intermittent) dysphagia (often for liquids as well as solids). In some patients, however, pain is inconsistently related to eating, may be precipitated by emotional stress (or even physical exertion), and nitroglycerin sometimes will relieve the pain.[149] Thus, when pain is (sometimes) exertional, unrelated to meals, not associated with swallowing or dysphagia or heartburn, or is relieved with nitroglycerin, cardiac (and other) causes of pain must be excluded.

The precise diagnosis of esophageal spasm may be difficult, in part because esophageal spasm may result from a variety of different disorders (diffuse esophageal spasm,[148] achalasia, vigorous achalasia,[145] the hypertensive lower esophageal sphincter syndrome[150]) all of which are incompletely understood and which may require esophageal manometry[151] for differentiation. Figure 13–36 illustrates a general approach to patients whose chest pain is suggestive of esophageal spasm. First obtaining a barium swallow x-ray always helps because it may occasionally reveal the classic "corkscrew esophagus" associated with advanced diffuse esophageal spasm, or sometimes other less specific findings (tertiary contractions, asymmetric esophageal

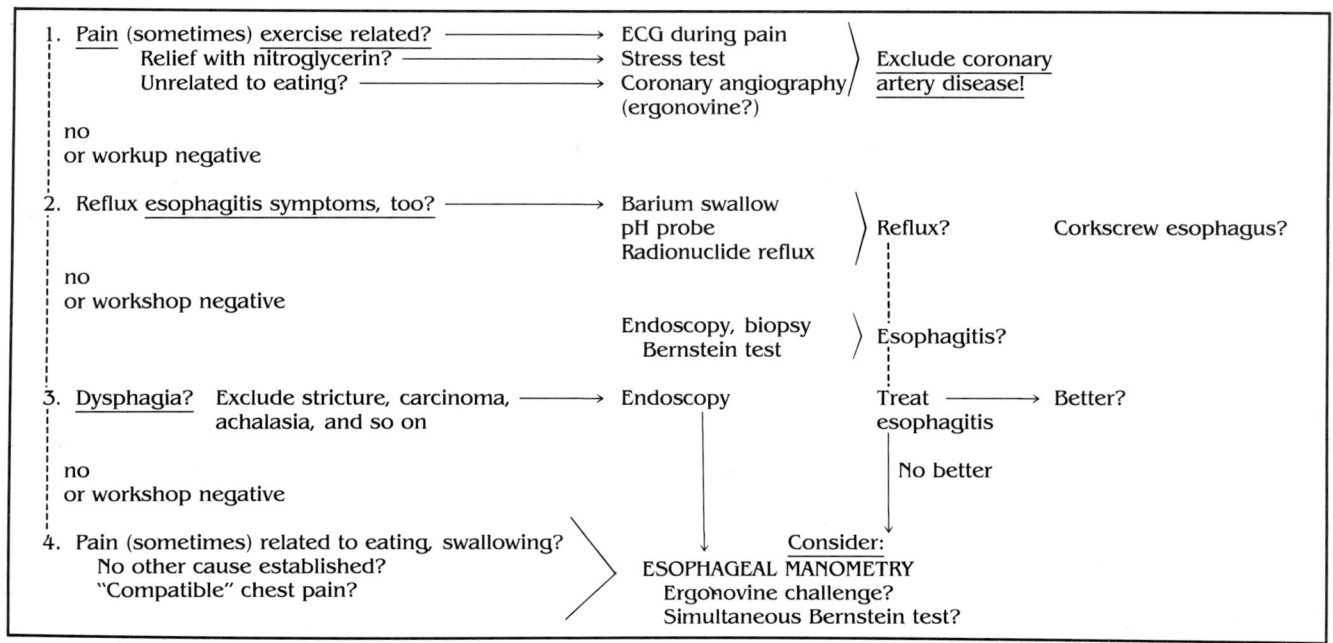

FIGURE 13–36. Esophageal spasm?

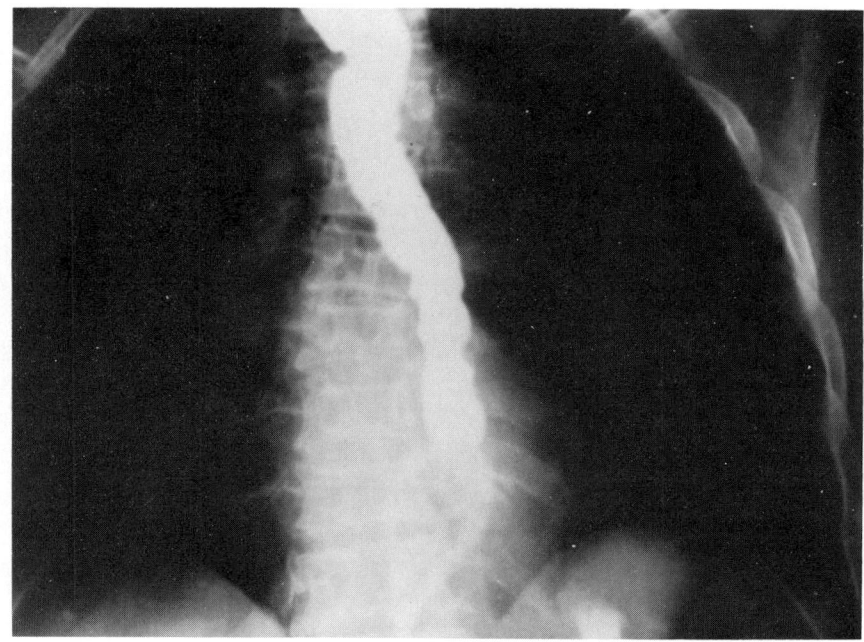

FIGURE 13–37. This 68-year-old man described episodic severe substernal chest pain usually precipitated by swallowing cold carbonated beverages. The barium swallow demonstrates disorganized esophageal contractions, but it is nondiagnostic. Esophageal manometry documented findings typical of diffuse esophageal spasm.

motility) (Fig. 13–37). These x-rays and/or endoscopy are *always* indicated in patients with dysphagia.

Sometimes documentation of reflux esophagitis and treatment of that disorder (Table 13–23) will alleviate the problem, since in some patients, reflux esophagitis may "trigger" spasm. More often, though, esophageal manometry is necessary to confirm the diagnosis. Ergonovine challenge[86] or acid perfusion during the manometry procedure may be useful in some patients.

When spasm is documented, treatment for some patients merely requires reassurance about the absence of more serious disease and some simple advice (eat slowly, avoid cold and carbonated foods, for example). Pharmacologic therapy is not usually successful (or necessary) but sublingual nitroglycerin, daily long-acting nitrates (Table 13–8), anticholinergics, oil of peppermint, and perhaps calcium channel blockers can be tried. (Note that the last three substances may *worsen* reflux esophagitis, and the coexistence of reflux esophagitis with esophageal spasm is thus sometimes a problem.)

Peroral esophageal dilatation may help some of these patients. Surgical therapy is a last resort, and only rarely necessary.[151]

Psychosomatic Chest Pain

There are several psychiatric conditions that may "cause" puzzling chest pains. In some patients, these disorders can be assumed to cause the chest pains only when exhaustive studies have excluded all other organic disease. Since the physical pain of psychologic disability may be as real as the psychologic distress associated with physical pain, the diagnostic problem may be very complicated, especially when psychiatric and organic disease coexist. Nevertheless, the history and physical examination will often suggest the major problem.

I. Anxiety, with or without hyperventilation, is the most common cause of psychosomatic chest pain.

Voluntary hyperventilation (as described in Chapter 10, "Dizziness") should always be performed in patients with atypical, confusing chest pain, since chest pain may be the only manifestation of hyperventilation (although usually a variety of other symptoms coexist). When chest pain is not exactly reproduced by hyperventilation, a few other clues may help:

A. Often there will be one or more symptom characteristics that imply definite nonangina:

The duration of pain is most often helpful—pains that are highly variable in duration, that last for hours, that are "always there when I think about it" or that flit momentarily across the chest "in a second" (or a "quick stab") are common.

B. Some such patients demonstrate the all-or-none phenomenon:

Everything the clinician asks about or attempts to simulate causes the pain, or nothing does.

C. Symptoms are often complex, very variable, or diffuse.

They may be presented by the patient with an emotional flood of language quite different from the usually straightforward and simple description of organic symptoms (for example, the patient with angina says: "I get a tight feeling in my chest when I walk up a hill").

D. Ask the patient to point to the pain.

The patient who places one fingertip at the site of pain often has psychosomatic or chest-wall pain. Pain consistently in the axilla or beneath the breast ("over my heart") is usually not cardiac.

E. Unexplained variations in pain pattern are common.

Pain that occurs only at work, only at home, only on weekends, "only when it's quiet" or that temporarily disappears on vacations, when distracted by other diversions, or after visits to a reassuring physician, is suspicious.

II. Hypochondriasis may cause pain, and many of the clues described above apply here as well.

Usually there are many other simultaneous complaints (the "positive review of systems") or there is a prior history of other unexplained peculiar symptoms that may wax and wane or cyclically reappear, depending upon the patient's "need" for symptoms of physical disability at a given time. Often the physician will sense a disparity between the subjective severity of these patients' symptoms and the disability their symptoms apparently impose. For example, chest pain is described as unbearably severe but does not interfere with daily activities (or, conversely, is described rather dispassionately with "la belle indifference"). Chest pain may be "ruining my life" in spite of its subjective mildness. (Questioning friends or family members is often very informative.) Sometimes, a role model is available: a close relative with severe heart disease, for example.

III. Depression is cause for great concern among patients with chest pain.

This is because depressive illness is as likely to be secondary to physical illness as the reverse, and because depression may so alter the patient's sense of self-worth and self-interest that a life-threatening illness (for example, unstable angina) may be minimized by the patient and thus masked by the depression. The patient with new or progressive chest pain, however atypical or variable, who also shows evidence of advanced depressive illness (vegetative symptoms, weight loss, anorexia, insomnia) deserves extremely careful attention (and often hospitalization for closer observation and testing).

IV. Cardiac neurosis refers to a debilitative concern about heart disease; recurrent chest pain is a common "substrate" for this problem.

It must be emphasized that cardiac neurosis may occur in patients with and without heart disease. In the former case, inadequate patient education, failure to foster a sense of self-reliance in coping with cardiac disease, and allowing the passive personality to become more and more dependent on family, medications, and physician are common pitfalls of which the clinician should be aware if "understandable" cardiac neurosis is to be avoided or minimized. In the patient without heart disease, all efforts should be made to exclude cardiac disease definitively so that fears can be clearly designated inappropriate. Often these patients have learned so well the symptoms of organic cardiac disease—through prior medical training or employment, exposure to relatives with cardiac disease, popular reading, or interactions with well-intentioned physicians—that cardiac disease is virtually certain on the basis of the history alone. This is one circumstance, i.e., the patient who has sought many different opinions about his or her chest pain, in which the clinical history may be very misleading and technologic testing (including coronary arteriography) often becomes mandatory. Among such patients, second opinions should be encouraged, but "doctor shopping" should be bluntly condemned. Holistic therapeutic efforts—physical exercise, periodic reassurance examinations, behavioral modification, and even group psychotherapy—are needed but treatment is difficult.

True malingering is an unusual cause of chest pain but must be considered when job disability, insurance compensation, or other secondary gains are major concerns, especially when the patient's disability is clearly disproportionate to objective evidence of disease, as indicated by coronary arteriography or other diagnostic tests.

Lung Scans and Pulmonary Embolism

The performance and interpretation of lung scans involves three steps. First, the perfusion lung scan is performed—radiolabeled albumin is injected intravenously, and gamma camera images then demonstrate functional pulmonary blood flow as the radionuclide perfuses the pulmonary capillary bed. When the perfusion scan is completely normal, pulmonary embolism within the previous 48 to 72 hours can be confidently excluded. Timing is important, not only because complete resolution of emboli within a few days has been reported[152] (a rare event[153]) but because, while the lung scan usually remains abnormal for days or weeks after embolization, a high probability scan may become indeterminate or low probability as resolution proceeds gradually (see below).

When the perfusion scan is abnormal, the perfusion defects are categorized according to their bronchial anatomy: an entire lung, lobe, segment, or subsegments may thus be poorly perfused. Next, the abnormal perfusion scan is compared with the patient's chest x-ray. When all perfusion defects correspond with abnormal areas on the chest x-ray (infiltrates, masses, effusions, atelectasis), the scan is *indeterminate,* i.e., no definite conclusion can be drawn. In these circumstances, only pulmonary arteriography can decide whether emboli are present (see below).

The third step is performed when perfusion defects correspond with areas that are radiographically normal; then the ventilation scan is performed. Here, the patient inhales a radioactive inert gas (usually xenon-133) and the gamma camera images its relative concentration in the lung after that first breath. Then the camera images the rate and uniformity of gas disappearance from the lung during 5 minutes of normal breathing. When the defects on perfusion scan correspond with areas of poor ventilation, these defects are termed ventilation-perfusion $(\dot{V}/\dot{Q})$ matches; when perfusion defects are found in areas where ventilation is normal, the defects are termed $\dot{V}/\dot{Q}$ mismatches.

Because most patients with pulmonary embolism will have multiple large (segmental or larger) perfusion defects (Tables 13–25 and 13–26, pages 776 and 777) that are well ventilated ($\dot{V}/\dot{Q}$ mismatches), such a scan result is traditionally termed "high probability" for pulmonary embolism (Fig. 13–38). Conversely, since relatively few patients with pulmonary embolism (Table 13–25) will have a single defect (Fig. 13–39), multiple small (subsegmental) perfusion defects, or perfusion defects that are all poorly ventilated ($\dot{V}/\dot{Q}$ matches) (Fig. 13–40), such scan results are traditionally termed "low probability" for pulmonary embolism.

These test results are described in terms of "probability" for good reason: no abnormal scan result of any type is definitively diagnostic or exclusive of pulmonary embolism. Only pulmonary arteriography can provide such definitive premortem information. Since other cardiopulmonary diseases (especially asthma, emphysema, or congestive heart failure) can produce high-probability perfusion scans in the absence of pulmonary embolism, since

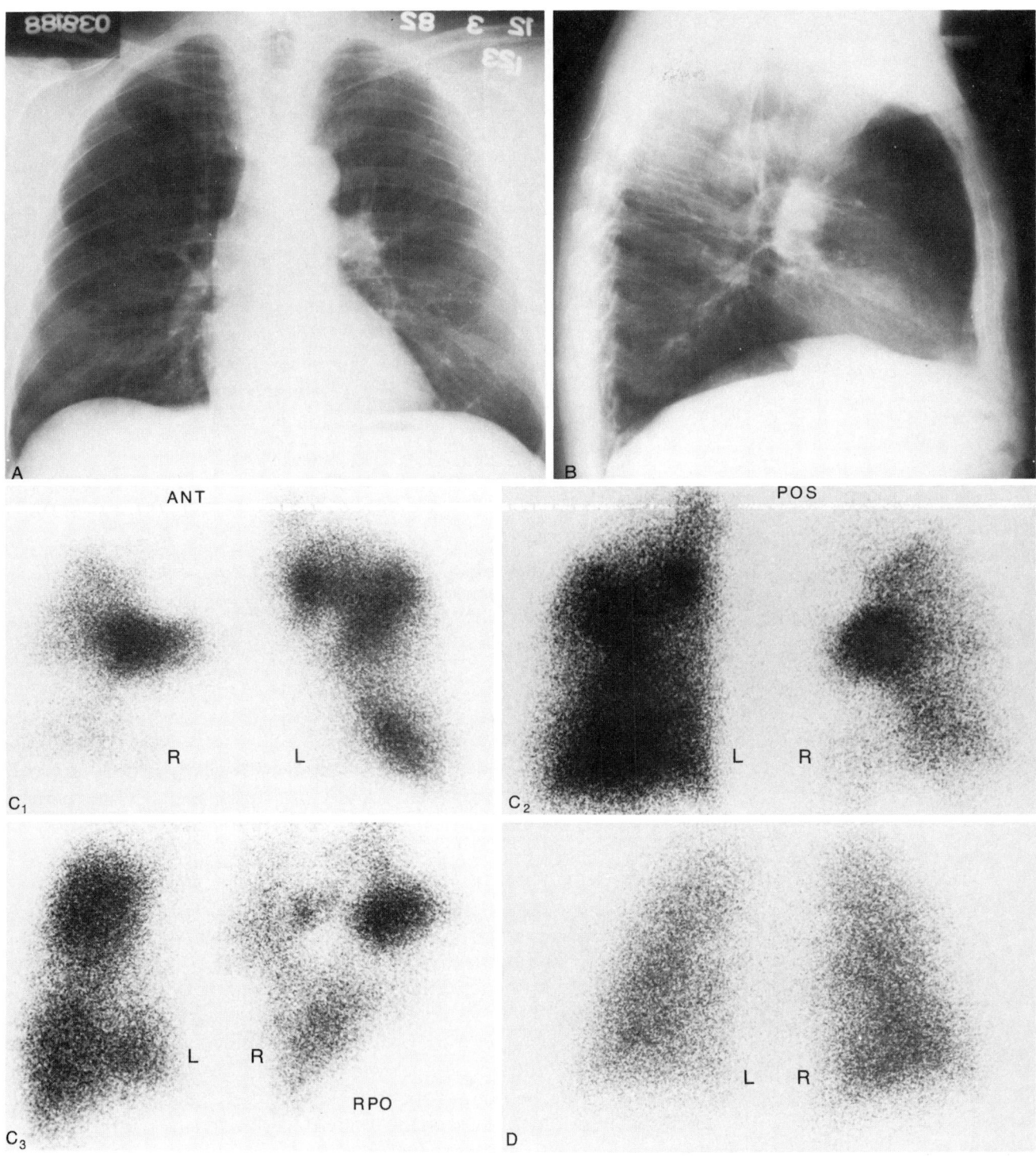

FIGURE 13–38. This 65-year-old man described sudden onset of lightheadedness, shortness of breath, and right pleuritic chest pain 2 weeks after discharge from the hospital following prostate surgery. Except for tachypnea and hypotension (90/60), examination was unremarkable. The chest x-ray *(A, B)* is normal except for a questionable prominence of both pulmonary arteries. A lung scan *(C)* reveals multiple segmental perfusion defects of both lungs (only the anterior, posterior, and RPO views are shown). The ventilation scan *(D)* was normal. (Only the "equilibrium phase" is shown, illustrating uniform ventilation throughout.)

Pulmonary arteriography confirmed the presence of multiple pulmonary emboli. The clinical picture and scan findings are sufficiently diagnostic in this case. Arteriography was performed to render the diagnosis absolutely certain, since the patient's clinical condition warranted the use of intravenous streptokinase.

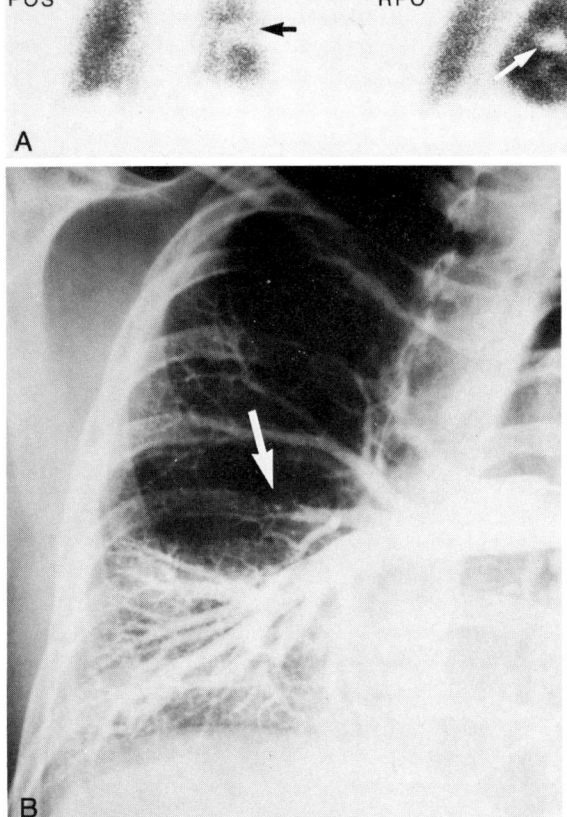

A

B

FIGURE 13–39. This perfusion lung scan demonstrates a single perfusion defect in the superior segment of the right lower lobe *(arrows)*. This is the lung scan *(A)* of the 35-year-old man described in Figure 13–24. (Only the anterior, posterior, and right posterior oblique views are shown here. Six views are performed.) Such a single perfusion defect is usually an "indeterminate" scan result (Tables 13–27 and 13–28). In this case, however, the clinical findings were highly suspicious, and a ventilation scan was completely normal, i.e., the single segmental defect is a V/Q mismatch. Selective (right lower lobe) pulmonary arteriography *(B)* documented a single pulmonary embolus to the superior segment of the right lower lobe.

definite pulmonary embolism can be associated with a low-probability scan, and since indeterminate scans (see above) are aptly named, the clinician must decide whether the clinical information and scan information are together sufficient to forgo pulmonary arteriography in the diagnostic process. This decision depends on three factors:

I. The particular patient involved.

There are two important considerations here:

A. Does the patient have underlying cardiopulmonary disease?

Whatever the radiographic interpretation of the lung scan(s), the clinician must consider: Does this patient have (nonembolic) disease that could account for an abnormal perfusion or ventilation scan(s)? If so, the high-probability scan may be very misleading. This is especially a problem in the patient with asthma, emphysema, or congestive heart failure in whom only a perfusion lung scan is performed (see below).

B. What is the clinical probability of pulmonary embolism in this particular patient?

The nuclear radiologist's interpretation of the scan(s) as high, low, or indeterminate probability must be further refined by the clinician's interpretation of the specific clinical events. For example, when the clinical probability of pulmonary embolism is overwhelming, a low-probability scan will not be sufficiently reassuring (a *normal* scan will be). Or, when the clinical probability of pulmonary embolism is very low, an indeterminate scan result might be disregarded.

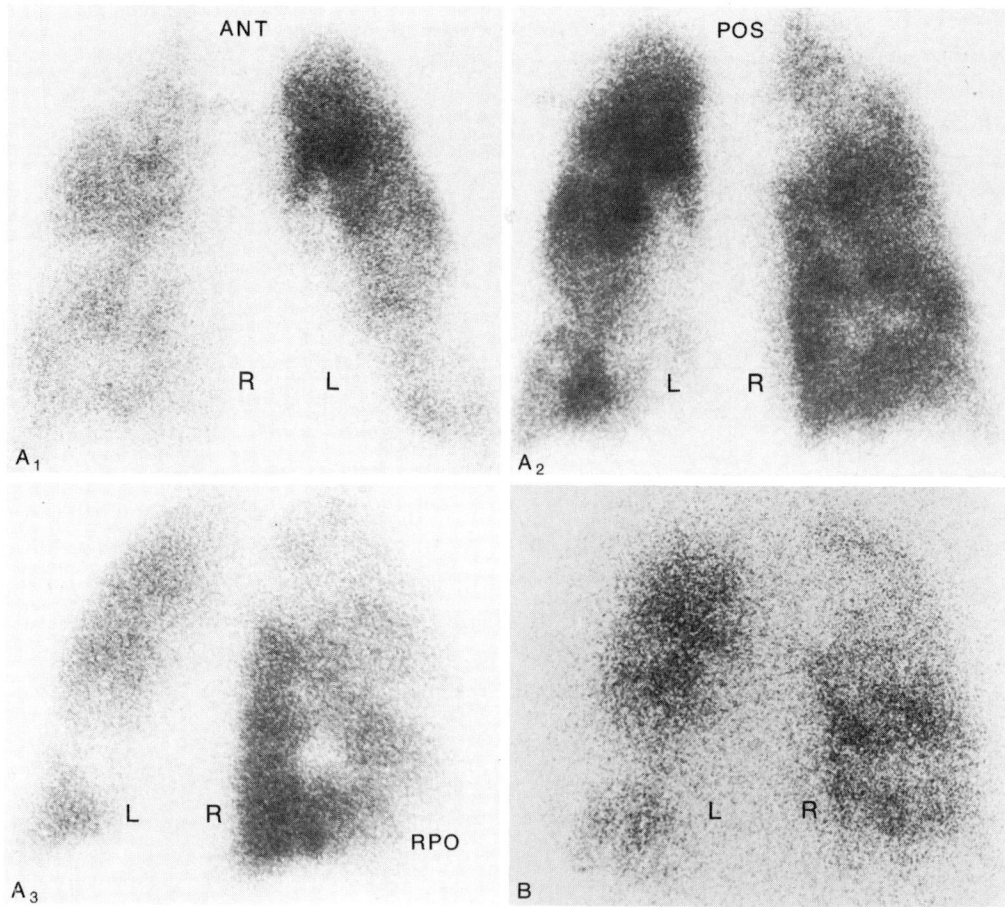

FIGURE 13–40. This 60-year-old man with longstanding emphysema described intermittent, respirophasic chest pains that were difficult to diagnose on the basis of the history. Chest x-ray was normal. A perfusion lung scan *(A)* reveals multiple segmental and subsegmental perfusion defects most prominent in the right upper and the left lower lobes. A ventilation scan, however, demonstrates impaired ventilation of these very same areas *(B)*. This is an example of matching ventilation-perfusion defects, which are "low probability" for pulmonary embolism. Subsequent arteriography was not performed. The patient's chest pain was ultimately attributed to degenerative arthritis of the thoracic spine.

Only when the radiographic and clinical probabilities *agree* (or when the perfusion scan is *normal*) are further decisions simplified.

When the clinical situation is uncomplicated—for example, in the healthy young adult with acute pleuritic chest pain—the radiologist's interpretation of the scan is the critical diagnostic factor.[98] Consider Table 13–24, which lists the results of lung scans in 97 healthy young adults (without previous cardiopulmonary diseases) who complained of acute pleuritic chest pain. Notice that in 42 patients the lung scan was normal—as we have noted, this *excludes* pulmonary embolism. In 15 patients, the perfusion abnormality corresponded with an abnormality on chest x-ray—these scans are then indeterminate, and other factors must be considered in deciding about further diagnostic or therapeutic efforts (see below). In the remaining 40 patients, all patients with a high-probability scan had pulmonary embolism documented by arteriography, while none with low-probability scans were diagnosed as having pulmonary embolism (although not all the latter patients underwent arteriography). In such a patient population (healthy young adults), then, the predictive or diagnostic value of the low-probability scan and the high-probability lung scan is excellent.

TABLE 13–24. SCINTIGRAPHIC FINDINGS IN 97 PATIENTS WITH PLEURITIC CHEST PAIN

	PULMONARY EMBOLISM (20)	ANOTHER DIAGNOSIS (77)
Normal scan	0	42
Abnormal scan interpretation:	(20)	(35)
"Low probability" of pulmonary embolism	0	23
"High probability" of pulmonary embolism	17	0
"Indeterminate"	3	12

(Reproduced with permission from McNeil, BJ, et al: Measures of clinical efficacy; the value of the lung scan in the evaluation of young patients with pleuritic chest pain. J Nucl Med 17:163, 1976.)

Unfortunately, many patients suspected of pulmonary embolism are neither young nor healthy. The diagnostic value of a high-probability lung scan in an elderly patient with congestive heart failure or emphysema is much less predictive. This does not mean that the lung scan is worthless but only that the clinician must be mindful of both the clinical context and:

II. The type of lung scan performed.

Tables 13–25 and 13–26 show the results of lung scans in 169 patients suspected strongly enough of pulmonary embolism to undergo arteriography.[154] Forty per cent had arteriographically documented emboli. This patient population is a more heterogeneous group (in terms of age, underlying disease, and clinical presentation) than the group in Table 13–24. Two facts stand out: First, *there are very few normal scans* (this is understandable since the scan result is a major determinant in the decision to perform arteriography); second, *fewer than one half of the patients underwent both ventilation and perfusion scans.* (All patients had

TABLE 13–25. DISTRIBUTION OF PERFUSION PATTERNS AMONG 169 PATIENTS STUDIED FOR PULMONARY EMBOLISM

SCAN PATTERN	PULMONARY EMBOLISM POSITIVE	PULMONARY EMBOLISM NEGATIVE
(1) Normal	0	2
(2) Indeterminate	13	22
(3) Single defect		
(a) Lung	1	2
(b) Lobe	2	2
(c) Segment	1	4
(d) Subsegment	0	6
(4) Many defects, largest being		
(a) Lung	3	2
(b) Lobe	22	5
(c) Segment	22	16
(d) Subsegment	3	41
Totals	67 (40%)	102 (60%)

(Reproduced with permission from McNeil, BJ: Ventilation-perfusion studies and the diagnosis of pulmonary embolism: concise communication. J Nucl Med 21:321, 1980.)

TABLE 13–26. DISTRIBUTION OF VENTILATION-PERFUSION (V̇/Q̇) PATTERNS AMONG 72 PATIENTS SUSPECTED OF PULMONARY EMBOLISM

SCAN PATTERNS	PULMONARY EMBOLISM POSITIVE	PULMONARY EMBOLISM NEGATIVE
V̇/Q̇ mismatch		
(1) Single perfusion defect		
(a) Lung	1	0
(b) Lobe	1	0
(c) Segment	0	4
(d) Subsegment	0	0
(2) Many perfusion defects		
(a) Lung	2	0
(b) Lobe	16	0
(c) Segment	19	1
(d) Subsegment	2	6
V̇/Q̇ match	0	13
V̇/Q̇ match and mismatch	3	4
Totals	44	28

(Reproduced with permission from McNeil, BJ: Ventilation perfusion studies and the diagnosis of pulmonary embolism: concise communication. J Nucl Med 21:321, 1980.)

perfusion scans; only 72 of the 167 total patients also had ventilation scans.) This latter fact is crucial for two reasons:

A. The ventilation scan cannot always be performed.

While ventilation scans are available in most medical centers now, they are not available everywhere.

When available, a ventilation scan requires that a patient hold the breath for 10 to 15 seconds—not all patients (who are sick, dyspneic, elderly, or uncooperative) can do this.

B. When performed, the ventilation scan adds specificity to the perfusion scan.

For example, patients in Table 13–25 with multiple segmental perfusion defects—a high-probability scan result in the healthy young adults described in Table 13–24—were almost as likely not to have pulmonary embolism (16 of 38) as to have pulmonary embolism (22 of 38). However, when the ventilation scan was also performed (Table 13–26), the finding of multiple segmental V̇/Q̇ mismatch defects was indeed a high-probability result (19 of 20 had proven emboli). In other words, what is a high-probability perfusion scan in a healthy young adult is much less reliable in a sick patient with other cardiopulmonary disease. The ventilation scan adds critical additional information.

Ventilation scans may or may not help in the patient with indeterminate perfusion scans. One large study[155] has suggested that, when the perfusion defect is substantially larger than the corresponding x-ray abnormality *and* the scan defect is a V̇/Q̇ mismatch, pulmonary embolism is likely. When the radiographic abnormality is larger than or equal in size to the perfusion defect, pulmonary embolism is unlikely. Nevertheless, these scan results must be considered indeterminate.

Ventilation scans with xenon cannot adequately resolve small areas of perfusion defects. Many patients have subsegmental defects on perfusion scan (a low-probability result in Tables 13–25 and 13–26), but the ventilation scan does not reliably specify which few of these patients (2 of 8 with subsegmental $\dot{V}/\dot{Q}$ mismatches) do have emboli.

Ultimately, then, clinical decisions will depend on the type of lung scan performed and the clinical status of the particular patient.[156] Rather than rely entirely on the radiographic categorization of the nuclear image as high, low, or indeterminate probability, the clinician must evaluate the clinical probabilities and then ask:

III. What is the precise result of the lung scan(s)?

Tables 13–27 and 13–28 indicate interpretation of scan results both when ventilation scans are performed (Table 13–28) and when ventilation scans are not available or cannot be performed (Table 13–27) in the patient suspected of pulmonary embolism who has had a chest x-ray and a perfusion lung scan. The major difference between healthy patients and "complicated patients" is the relative nonspecificity of multiple segmental perfusion defects in the "complicated patient" (Tables 13–25 and 13–26). Conversely, when both ventilation and perfusion scans are available, even the complicated case will usually be correctly diagnosed by considering the chest x-ray and both lung scans. Venography or impedance plethysmography of the legs may also be very helpful.[166]

TABLE 13–27. INTERPRETATION OF RESULTS WHEN ONLY PERFUSION LUNG SCANS AND CHEST X-RAYS ARE AVAILABLE

YOUNG, HEALTHY PATIENT (NONSMOKER, NO CARDIOPULMONARY DISEASE)	INTERPRETATION	COMPLICATED CASE*
Normal scan (common) $\longrightarrow$	Pulmonary embolism excluded	$\longleftarrow$ Normal scan (uncommon)
Subsegmental defect(s) OR Indeterminate scan— perfusion defect smaller than chest x-ray abnormality ($\dot{Q}$ < chest x-ray)† $\longrightarrow$	Pulmonary embolism very unlikely Arteriography usually unnecessary	$\longleftarrow$ Subsegmental defect(s) OR Indeterminate scan where $\dot{Q}$ < chest x-ray†
Single defect, segmental or larger OR Indeterminate scan where $\dot{Q}$ = chest x-ray† or $\dot{Q}$ > chest x-ray† $\longrightarrow$	Pulmonary embolism possibility intermediate Arteriography usually necessary	$\longleftarrow$ Single defect, segmental or larger OR Indeterminate scan where $\dot{Q}$ = chest x-ray† or $\dot{Q}$ > chest x-ray† OR Multiple segmental defects
Multiple segmental (or larger) defects $\longrightarrow$	Pulmonary embolism very likely Arteriography usually not necessary	$\longleftarrow$ Multiple defects, lobar and segmental

*For example, chronic obstructive pulmonary disease, congestive heart failure, asthma.
†$\dot{Q}$ < chest x-ray means perfusion defect *smaller* than chest x-ray abnormality.
$\dot{Q}$ = chest x-ray means perfusion defect is equal in size to area of chest x-ray abnormality.
$\dot{Q}$ > chest x-ray means perfusion defect is larger than area of chest x-ray abnormality.

TABLE 13–28. INTERPRETATION RESULTS WHEN VENTILATION-PERFUSION (V̇/Q̇) LUNG SCANS AND CHEST X-RAYS ARE AVAILABLE

RESULTS	INTERPRETATION
Normal scan	Excludes pulmonary embolism
Single or multiple defects, <u>all</u> V̇/Q̇ matches Small subsegmental defects Indeterminate, where Q̇ < chest x-ray*	Pulmonary embolism unlikely Arteriography *usually* unnecessary
Single V̇/Q̇ mismatch defect, segmental or larger Multiple segmental defects, some V̇/Q̇ match, some V̇/Q̇ mismatch Indeterminate, where Q̇ = chest x-ray* or Q̇ > chest x-ray*	Pulmonary embolism possibility intermediate Arteriography *usually* necessary
Multiple V̇/Q̇ mismatches, segmental or larger	Pulmonary embolism likely Arteriography *usually* unnecessary

*Q̇ < chest x-ray means perfusion defect *smaller* than chest x-ray abnormality.
Q̇ = chest x-ray means perfusion defect is equal in size to area of chest x-ray abnormality.
Q̇ > chest x-ray means perfusion defect is larger than area of chest x-ray abnormality.

Again, the interpretations in Tables 13–27 and 13–28 are only probabilities: Ultimately the decision to perform or withhold angiography depends on both the analysis of these probabilities and the relative need for diagnostic certainty in individual cases. This can be a complicated decision analysis,[157] depending on the clinical status of the patient. Is anticoagulation contraindicated or especially dangerous in this patient? Has the suspected embolus occurred despite anticoagulation? Is arteriography especially risky in this patient? Nevertheless, <u>when absolute diagnostic certainty is necessary, only the arteriogram will answer the question.</u> Usually, however, analysis of the radiographic results in Tables 13–27 and 13–28 in specific clinical circumstances allows prompt decisions about the need for arteriography (Fig. 13–41).

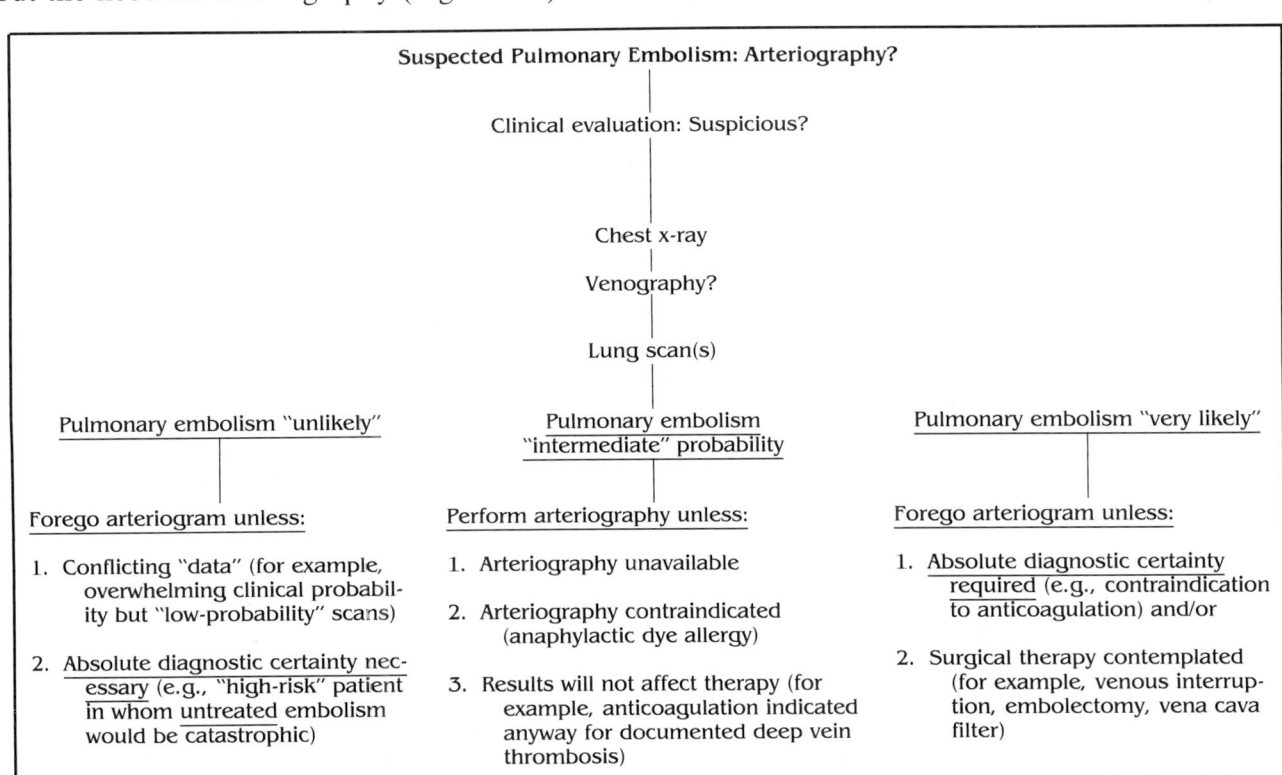

FIGURE 13–41.

REFERENCES

1. Constant, J: Recognizing nonanginal chest pain. Primary Cardiol. 87–89 (Sept) 1978.
2. Prinzmetal, M., et al.: Angina pectoris. I. A variant form of angina pectoris. Preliminary report. Am J Med 27:375–388, 1959.
3. Gazes, PC, et al.: Preinfarctional (unstable) angina—a prospective study: Ten-year follow-up. Circulation 48:331–336, 1973.
4. Unstable Angina Pectoris: National Cooperative Study Group to Compare Medical and Surgical Therapy: I. A report of protocol and patient population. Am J Cardiol 37:896–902, 1976.
5. Krauss, KR, et al.: Acute coronary insufficiency—causes and follow-up. Circulation 45,46 (Suppl 1):1–66, 1–77, 1972.
6. Segal, BL, et al.: Coronary risk factors and anginal pain patterns. Postgrad Med 61:102–107, 1977.
7. Hillis, LD, Braunwald, E: Coronary artery spasm. N Engl J Med 299:695–702, 1978.
8. Braunwald, E: Coronary artery spasm. Mechanisms and a clinical relevance. JAMA 246:1957–1959, 1981.
9. Day, LJ, Sowton, E: Clinical features and follow-up of patients with angina and normal coronary arteries. Lancet 2:344–337, 1976.
10. Waxler, EB, et al.: The fate of women with normal coronary arteriogram and chest pain resembling angina pectoris. Am J Cardiol 28:25–32, 1971.
11. Selzer, A, et al.: Clinical significance of variant angina with normal coronary arteriogram. N Engl J Med 295:1343–1347, 1976.
12. Heberden, W: Commentaries on the History and Cure of Diseases. Boston: Wells and Lilly, 1818, p. 292.
13. Riseman, J, Brown, M: An analysis of the diagnostic criteria of angina pectoris. A critical study of 100 proved cases. Am Heart J 14:331–351, 1937.
14. Master, AM: The spectrum of anginal and noncardiac chest pain. JAMA 187:894–899, 1964.
15. Harrison, TR: Some problems in the diagnosis, management, and pathophysiology of angina pectoris. Arch Intern Med 117:323–329, 1966.
16. French, EB, Robb, WAT: Biliary and renal colic. Br Med J 3:135–138, 1964.
17. Glenn, F: Pain in biliary tract disease. Surg Gynecol Obstet 122:495–508, 1966.
18. Gunn, A, Keddie, N: Some clinical observations in patients with gallstones. Lancet 2:239–241, 1972.
19. Dworkin, H, et al.: Subdiaphragmatic reference of pain from the colon. Gastroenterology 22:272, 1952.
20. Evans, DW, Lum, LC: Hyperventilation: An important cause of pseudoangina. Lancet 1:155–157, 1977.
21. Evans, DW, Lum, LC: Hyperventilation as a cause of chest pain mimicking angina. Practical Cardiol 7:131–139, 1981.
22. Shaw, RA, et al.: Pulmonary embolism presenting as coronary insufficiency. Arch Intern Med 141:651, 1981.
23. Wehrmacher, WH: The painful anterior chest wall syndromes. Med Clin North Am 42:111–119, 1958.
24. Allison, DR: Pain in the chest wall simulating heart disease. Br Med J 1:332–336, 1950.
25. Epstein, SE, et al.: Chest wall syndrome. A common cause of unexplained cardiac pain. JAMA 241:2793–2797, 1979.
26. Mendolowitz, M: Strain of the pectoralis minor muscle, an important cause of precordial pain in soldiers. Am Heart J 30:123–125, 1945.
27. Myers, G, et al.: Cervicoprecordial angina: Diagnosis and management (abstract). Am J Cardiol 39:287, 1977.
28. Heinz, GJ, Zowala, DC: Slipping rib syndrome. Diagnosis using the "hooking maneuver." JAMA 237:794–295, 1977.
29. Kayser, HL: Teitze's syndrome. A review of the literature. Am J Med 21:982–989, 1956.
30. Nachlas, W: Pseudo-angina pectoris originating in the cervical spine. JAMA 103:323–325, 1934.
31. Blackman NS: Slipping rib syndrome, with review of related anterior chest wall syndromes. NY State J Med 63:1670–1675, 1963.
32. Miller, AJ, Texidor, TA: "Precordial catch," a neglected syndrome of precordial pain. JAMA 159:1364–1365, 1955.
33. McElroy, JB: Angina pectoris with coexisting skeletal chest pain. Am Heart J 66:296–300, 1963.
34. Finegam, RE, et al.: Aortic stenosis in the elderly: Relevance of age to diagnosis and treatment. N Engl J Med 281:1261, 1969.
35. Stern, A, et al.: Diagnostic accuracy of ambulatory ECG monitoring in ischemic heart disease. Circulation 52:1045–1049, 1975.
36. Newburger, JW, et al.: Noninvasive tests in the evaluation of heart murmurs in children. N Engl J Med 308:61–64, 1983.
37. Gracie, WA, Ransohoff, DF: The natural history of silent gallstones. The innocent gallstone is not a myth. N Engl J Med 307:798–800, 1982.
38. Abrams, J: Nitroglycerin and long-acting nitrates. N Engl J Med 302:1234–1236, 1980.
39. Symposium: Beta blockade in the 1980's. Primary Cardiology Supplement No. 1, 1983.
40. Frishman, WH: Beta adrenoreceptor antagonists: New drugs and new indications. N Engl J Med 305:500–506, 1981.
41. Stern, MP: The recent decline in ischemic heart disease mortality. Ann Intern Med 91:630–640, 1979.
42. Beta Blocker Heart Attack Study Group: The beta blocker heart attack trial. JAMA 246:2073–2074, 1981.
43. Gorlin, R (ed.): Prevention of myocardial reinfarction: What is the role of beta blockers? Primary Cardiol (suppl) 1–52, (Nov 1) 1982.

44. Miller, RR, et al.: Propranolol-withdrawal rebound phenomenon. Exacerbation of coronary events after abrupt cessation of antianginal therapy. N Engl J Med 293:416–418, 1975.
45. Shand, D: Propranolol withdrawal. N Engl J Med 293:449–450, 1975.
46. Antman, E, et al.: Nifedipine therapy for coronary artery spasm. Experience in 127 patients. N Engl J Med 302:1269–1270, 1980.
47. Mueller, HS, Chahure, RA: Interim report of multiple center double-blind, placebo-controlled studies of nifedipine in chronic stable angina. Am J Med 71:645–657, 1981.
48. Dargie, JH, et al.: Nifedipine and propranolol: A beneficial drug interaction. Am J Med 71:676–682, 1981.
49. Gerstenblith, G, et al.: Nifedipine in unstable angina. A double-blind randomized trial. N Engl J Med 306:885–889, 1982.
50. Zelis, R: Calcium-blocker therapy for unstable angina pectoris. N Engl J Med 306:926–928, 1982.
51. Piepho, RW: The calcium antagonists. Mechanism of action and pharmacologic effects. Drug Ther 13(1):69, 1983.
52. Feldman, RL: Using calcium antagonists in rest and effort angina. Drug Ther 13(1):89, 1983.
53. Winniford, MD, Hillis, LD: Calcium antagonists and angina at rest. Cardiovasc Rev Rep 4(1):105, 1983.
54. Humphries, J: Selection of therapy for angina pectoris: Medical versus surgical. Cardiovasc Med 1097–1105, 1977.
55. Lesch, M, Gorlin, R: Bypass surgery in chronic stable coronary artery disease. Primary Cardiol 87–91, (Nov/Dec) 1978.
56. Lesch, M, Gorlin, R: Bypass surgery in chronic stable coronary artery disease. Primary Cardiol 92–101, (Jan) 1979.
57. Kloster, FE, et al.: Coronary bypass for stable angina. A prospective randomized study. N Engl J Med 300:149–157, 1979.
58. Aronow, WS: Indications for surgical treatment of stable angina pectoris. Arch Intern Med 139:690–692, 1979.
59. Carr, KW, et al.: Do coronary artery bypass operations prolong life? West J Med 136:295–308, 1982.
60. Epstein, SE, et al.: Strategy for evaluation and surgical treatment of the asymptomatic or mildly symptomatic patient with coronary artery disease. Am J Cardiol 43:1015–1025, 1979.
61. Cohn, PF, Braunwald, E: Chronic coronary artery disease. In Braunwald E (ed.): Heart Disease. Philadelphia: W. B. Saunders, 1980, pp. 1418–1428.
62. Akins, CW, Austen, WG: Aortocoronary bypass surgery in the management of coronary artery disease. In Johnson RA, et al. (eds.): The Practice of Cardiology. Boston: Little, Brown, 1980, pp. 370–399.
63. Hurst, JW, McIntosh, HD: Controversies in cardiology. Hosp Pract 17:106A, (Aug) 1982.
64. Plotnick, GD, et al.: Clinical indicators of left main coronary artery disease in unstable angina. Ann Intern Med 91:149–153, 1979.
65. Oberman, A, Pitt, B: Controversies in cardiology: Does exercise reduce the risk of coronary atherosclerosis? Hosp Pract 94A, (Oct) 1982.
66. Graboys, TB, Lown, B: Angina pectoris. In Branch, W (ed.): Office Practice of Medicine. W. B. Saunders, 1981, pp. 117–129.
67. Ornish, D, et al.: Effects of stress management training and dietary changes in treating ischemic heart disease. JAMA 249:54–59, 1983.
68. Neill, WA, et al.: Acute coronary insufficiency. Coronary occlusion after intermittent ischemic attacks. N Engl J Med 302:1157–1162, 1980.
69. Unstable Angina Pectoris: National Cooperative Study Group to Compare Surgical and Medical Therapy. Am J Cardiol 42:839–848, 1978.
70. Podrid, PJ, et al.: Prognosis of medically treated patients with coronary artery disease with profound ST, segment depression during exercise testing. N Engl J Med 305:1111–1116, 1981.
71. Hutter, AM, DeSanctis, RW: The evaluation and management of patients with angina pectoris. In Johnson, RA, et al. (eds.): The Practice of Cardiology. Boston: Little, Brown, 1980, pp. 281–309.
72. Theroux, P, et al.: Prognostic value of exercise testing soon after myocardial infarction. N Engl J Med 301:341–345, 1979.
73. Julian, DG: Myocardial infarction. In Beeson, PB, McDermott, W, and Wyngaarden, JB (eds.): Cecil Textbook of Medicine. 15th ed. Philadelphia: W. B. Saunders Company, 1979.
74. Wagner, GS: Optimal use of serum enzyme level in the diagnosis of acute myocardial infarction. The perspective in 1980. Arch Intern Med 140:317–319, 1980.
75. Irving, RG, et al.: Acute myocardial infarction and MB CPK. Relationship between onset of symptoms of infarction and appearance and disappearance of enzymes. Arch Intern Med 140:329–334, 1980.
76. Werner, JA, et al.: Acute myocardial infarction. Clinical application of technetium 99m stannous pyrophosphate infarct scintigraphy. West J Med 127:464–478, 1977.
77. Slater, E, DeSanctis, RW: The clinical recognition of dissecting aortic aneurysm. Am J Med 60:625–633, 1976.
78. Slater, E, DeSantis, RW: Dissection of the aorta. Med Clin North Am 63:141–154, 1979.
79. Spodick, DH: Acute Pericarditis. New York: Grune & Stratton, 1959.
80. Spodick, DH: Differential diagnosis of acute pericarditis. Prog Cardiovasc Dis 14:192–209, 1971.
81. Munsell, WP: Pneumomediastinum. JAMA 202:689, 1967.
82. Brown, RH, Cohen, PS: Nonsurgical management of spontaneous esophageal perforation. JAMA 240:140–142, 1978.
83. Vernon, SE, Carmichael, GP: Unsuspected esophageal perforation. JAMA 240:2568–2569, 1978.
84. Kaye, MD: Recognizing and managing esophageal spasm. Drug Ther 12:137–148 (Mar) 1982.
85. Fleshler, B: Diffuse esophageal spasm. Gastroenterology 52:559–564, 1967.

86. Kaye, MD: Ergonovine challenge in the diagnosis of esophageal spasm. Intern Med Specialist 3(9):97–106, 1982.
87. Ferry, DR, Crawford, MH: The limitations, sensitivity and specificity of the electrocardiogram in diagnosing acute myocardial infarction. Practical Cardiol 8:72 (Dec) 1982.
88. Madigan, WP: The clinical course, early prognosis, and coronary anatomy of subendocardial infarction. Am J Med 60:634–641, 1976.
89. Fabricious-Bjerre, N, et al.: Subendocardial and transmural infarction. A five-year survival study. Am J Med 66:986–990, 1979.
90. Fuchs, R, Scheidt, S: Improved criteria for admission to coronary care units. JAMA 246:2037–2041, 1981.
91. Rose, SD, et al.: Cardiac risk factors in patients undergoing noncardiac surgery. Med Clin North Am 63:1271–1288, 1979.
92. Kantor, FS, Hsiung, GD: Pleurodynia associated with echo virus type 8. N Engl J Med 266:661–663, 1962.
93. Finn, JJ, et al.: Epidemic pleurodynia: Clinical and etiologic studies based on 114 cases. Arch Intern Med 83:305–321, 1949.
94. Moser, KM: Pulmonary embolism. Am Rev Respir Dis 115:829–852, 1977.
95. Rosenow, EC, et al.: Pulmonary embolism. Mayo Clin Proc 56:161–178, 1981.
96. Dalen, JE, et al.: Pulmonary embolism, pulmonary hemorrhage, and pulmonary infarction. N Engl J Med 296:1431–1435, 1977.
97. Wenger, NK, et al.: Massive acute pulmonary embolism. The deceivingly nonspecific manifestations. JAMA 220:843–845, 1972.
98. McNeil, BJ, et al.: Measures of clinical efficacy. III. The value of the lung scan in the evaluation of young patients with pleuritic chest pain. J Nucl Med 17:163–169, 1976.
99. Spodick, DH: Diagnostic ECG sequence in acute pericarditis: Significance of PR segment and PR vector changes. Circulation 48:575–580, 1973.
100. Spodick, DH: ECG in acute pericarditis: Distribution of morphologic and axial changes by stages. Am J Cardiol 33:470–474, 1974.
101. Spodick, DH: Pericardial rub. Prospective, multiple observer, investigation of pericardial friction in 100 patients. Am J Cardiol 35:357–362, 1975.
102. Vignola, P, et al.: Pericardial disease. In Johnson, RA, et al. (eds.): The Practice of Cardiology. Boston: Little, Brown, 1980.
103. Spodick, DH: Differential characteristics of the ECG in early repolarization and acute pericarditis. N Engl J Med 295:523–526, 1976.
104. Fowler, NO, Manitsas, GT: Infectious pericarditis. Prog Cardiovasc Dis 16:323, 1973.
105. Fine, NL, et al.: Frequency of pleural effusion in mycoplasma and viral pneumonias. N Engl J Med 283:790–793, 1970.
106. Miller, WT, Talman, EA: Subphrenic abscess. Am J Roentgenol 101:961–969, 1967.
107. Magilligan, DJ: Suprahepatic abscess. Arch Surg 96:14–19, 1968.
108. Dressler, W: The postmyocardial infarction syndrome. A report on 44 cases. Arch Intern Med 103:28, 1959.
109. Winslow, WA, et al.: Pleuritis in SLE: Its importance as an early manifestation and diagnosis. Ann Intern Med 49:70–88, 1958.
110. Harvey, AM, et al.: SLE: Review of the literature and clinical analysis of 138 cases. Medicine 33:291–437, 1967.
111. Light, RW, et al.: Pleural effusion: The diagnostic separation of transudates and exudates. Ann Intern Med 77:507–513, 1972.
112. Ryan, CJ, et al.: The outcome of patients with pleural effusion of indeterminate cause at thoracotomy. Mayo Clin Proc 56:145–149, 1981.
113. Stevens, E, Templeton, AW: Traumatic nonpenetrating lung contusion. Radiology 85:247, 1965.
114. Berger, HW: Tuberculous pleurisy. Chest 63:88–94, 1973.
115. Black, LF: The pleural space and pleural fluid. Mayo Clin Proc 47:493–506, 1972.
116. Salyer, WR, et al.: Efficacy of pleural needle biopsy and pleural fluid cytopathology in the diagnosis of malignant neoplasm involving the pleura. Chest 67:536–539, 1975.
117. Snider, GL, Saleh, SS: Empyema of the thorax in adults: Review of 105 cases. Dis Chest 65:410–415, 1968.
118. Geha, AS: Pleural empyema. Changing etiologic, bacteriologic, and therapeutic aspects. J Thorac Cardiovasc Surg 61:626–635, 1971.
119. Simmons, EM, et al.: Review of nontuberculous empyema at the University of Missouri Medical Center from 1957–1971. J Thorac Cardiovasc Surg 64:578–585, 1972.
120. Varkey, B, et al.: Empyema thoracis during a ten-year period. Analysis of 72 cases and comparison to a previous study (1952–1967). Arch Intern Med 141:1771–1776, 1981.
121. Taryle, DA, et al.: The incidence and clinical correlate of parapneumonic effusion in pneumococcal pneumonia. Chest 74:170–173, 1978.
122. Potts, DE, et al.: Pleural fluid pH in parapneumonic effusion. Chest 70:328–331, 1976.
123. Barbour, GL, Juniper, K: A clinical comparison of amebic and pyogenic abscess of the liver in 66 patients. Am J Med 53:323–334, 1972.
124. Sabbaj, J, et al.: Anaerobic pyogenic liver abscess. Ann Intern Med 77:629–638, 1972.
125. Lazarchick, J, et al.: Pyogenic liver abscess. Mayo Clin Proc 48:349–355, 1973.
126. Rosenow, EC: The spectrum of drug-induced pulmonary disease. Ann Intern Med 77:977–991, 1972.
127. Ellestad, MH, et al.: Stress testing: Clinical applicability and predictive capacity. Prog Cardiovasc Dis 21:431–460, 1979.
128. Epstein, SE: Implications of probability analysis on the strategy used for noninvasive detection of coronary artery disease. Role of single or combined use of exercise ECG testing, radionuclide cineangiography, and myocardial perfusion imaging. Am J Cardiol 46:491–499, 1980.

129. Weiner, DA, et al.: Exercise stress testing. Correlations among history of angina, ST segment response, and prevalence of coronary artery disease in the coronary artery surgery study (CASS). N Engl J Med 301:230–235, 1979.
130. Epstein, SE: Limitation of ECG exercise testing. N Engl J Med 301:264–265, 1979.
131. Diamond, GA, Forrester, JS: Analysis of probability as an aid in the clinical diagnosis of coronary artery disease. N Engl J Med 300:1350–1358, 1979.
132. Borer, JS, et al.: Limitation of the ECG response to exercise in predicting coronary artery disease. N Engl J Med 293:367–371, 1975.
133. Weiner, DA, et al.: The predictive value of anginal chest pain as an indicator of coronary disease during exercise testing. Am Heart J 96:458–462, 1978.
134. Bodenheimer, MB, et al.: Extent and severity of coronary heart disease. Determination by thallous chloride T1 201, myocardial perfusion scanning, and comparison with stress electrocardiography. Arch Intern Med 139:630–634, 1979.
135. Bodenheimer, MB, et al.: Nuclear cardiology. II. The role of myocardial perfusion imaging using thallium-201 in diagnosis of coronary heart disease. Am J Cardiol 45:674–684, 1980.
136. McKillop, JH: Thallium-201 scintigraphy. West J Med 133:26–43, 1980.
137. Wainwright, RJ, et al.: Segmental quantitative analysis of digital thallium-201 myocardial scintigrams in diagnosis of coronary artery disease. Comparison with rest and exercise ECG and coronary arteriography. Br Heart J 46:478–485, 1981.
138. Christie, LG, Conti, CR: Periodic chest pain: Is it myocardial ischemia? Primary Cardiol 9:163 (Jan) 1983.
139. Forrester, JS, et al.: How to assess the risk of coronary artery disease. A round table discussion. Pract Cardiol 8:39 (Dec) 1982.
140. Whittle, JL, Murphy, ML: Limitation of the coronary angiogram in the evaluation of the patient with ischemic heart disease. Pract Cardiol 8(3):126–132, 1982.
141. Faxon, DP, et al.: Therapeutic and economic value of a normal coronary arteriogram. Am J Med 73:500–505, 1982.
142. Hutcheon, DF, Hendrix, TR: Esophageal reflux. Diagnosis and therapy. Postgrad Med 61:131–137, 1977.
143. Johnson, LF: New concepts and methods in the study and treatment of gastroesophageal reflux disease. Med Clin North Am 65:1195–1222, 1981.
144. Richter, JE, Castell, DO: Drugs, food, and other substances in the cause and treatment of reflux esophagitis. Med Clin North Am 65:1223–1234, 1981.
145. Sanderson, DR, et al.: Syndrome of vigorous achalasia: Clinical and physiologic observations. Dis Chest 52:508, 1967.
146. Woodward, ER: Surgical treatment of reflux esophagitis and stricture. Postgrad Med 61:143–150, 1977.
147. Moersch, HJ, Camp, JD: Diffuse spasm of the lower part of the esophagus. Ann Otol Rhinol Laryngol 43:1165–1173, 1934.
148. DiMarino, AJ, Cohen, S: Characteristics of lower esophageal sphincter function in symptomatic diffuse esophageal spasm. Gastroenterology 66:1–6, 1974.
149. Orlando, RC, Bozyinski, EM: Clinical and manometric effects of nitroglycerin in diffuse esophageal spasm. N Engl J Med 289:23–25, 1973.
150. Berger, K, et al.: Hypertensive lower esophageal sphincter: A clinical and manometric entity. Gastroenterology 80:1109, 1982.
151. Waters, PF, DeMeester, TR: Foregut motor disorders and their surgical management. Med Clin North Am 65:1235–1268, 1981.
152. James, WS, et al.: Rapid resolution of a pulmonary embolism in man. West J Med 128:60–64, 1978.
153. Dalen, JE, et al.: Resolution rate of acute pulmonary embolism in man. N Engl J Med. 280:1194–1199, 1969.
154. McNeil, BJ: Ventilation-perfusion studies and the diagnosis of pulmonary embolism: Concise communication. J Nucl Med 21:319–323, 1980.
155. Biello, DR, et al.: Interpretation of indeterminate lung scintigrams. Radiology 133:189–194, 1979.
156. McNeil, BJ: A diagnostic strategy using ventilation-perfusion studies in patients suspected of pulmonary embolism. J Nucl Med 17:613–616, 1976.
157. Pauker, SG, Kassirer, JP: Clinical application of decision analysis: A detailed illustration. Semin Nucl Med 8:324–335, 1978.
158. Zarling, EJ, et al: Failure to diagnose acute myocardial infarction. JAMA 250:1177–1181, 1983.
159. Toomey, F, et al: Pitfalls in radiologic diagnosis of pneumothorax. Hosp Med 200–223 (Aug) 1983.
160. Kirshenbaum, HD, et al: The spectrum of coronary artery spasm. The variable variant. JAMA 246:354–359, 1981.
161. Rozanski, A, et al: The declining specificity of exercise radionuclide ventriculography. N Engl J Med 309:518–522, 1983.
162. Winnan, GR, et al: Interpretation of the Bernstein test: A reappraisal of criteria. Ann Intern Med 96:320–322, 1982.
163. Braunwald, E: Effects of coronary artery bypass grafting on survival. N Engl J Med 309:1181–1184, 1983.
164. CASS Principal Investigators: Coronary Artery Surgery Study (CASS): A randomized trial of coronary artery bypass surgery: "Quality of life" in randomized subjects. Circulation 68:951–960, 1983.
165. CASS Principal Investigators: Coronary Artery Surgery Study (CASS): A randomized trial of coronary artery bypass surgery: Survival data. Circulation 68:939–950, 1983.
166. Hull, RD, et al: Pulmonary angiography, ventilation lung scanning, and venography for clinically suspected pulmonary embolism with abnomal perfusion lung scan. Ann Intern Med 98:891–899, 1983.

INDEX

Page numbers in *italic* indicate illustrations. Page numbers followed by t indicate tables.

Abdomen, auscultation of, 540
  distention of, 542–543, *542*
    causes of, 542, 543t
  examination of, patient's position in, 540, *540*
  masses of, lower, 580t
    upper, 605t
  pain in. See *Abdominal pain.*
  palpation of, 541–542
    correct vs. incorrect, *541*
  percussion of, 540, *541*
  x-rays of, in evaluation of abdominal pain, 549–551, 550t, 556t
Abdominal pain, 528–627
  acute, 530–575
    abrupt onset of, 534
    clinical setting in, 538t
    constipation preceding, causes of, 536–537, 537t
    consultation with surgeon for, 617t
    diarrhea with, 536
    differential diagnosis of, 544t–545t
    duration of, 535
    extra-abdominal physical findings in, 550t
    follow-up examination for, 557
    gradual onset of, 535
    heme-positive stool with, causes of, 549t
    high fever with, 538–539
    history in, 530–539
    location of, 530–534
    menstrual history in, 567
    nontraumatic, diagnostic approach to, *558–559*
    parietal, 530–531
      causes of, 531, *532*
      location of, 531, *532*
      signs of, 539–542, 539t
    peritoneal. See *Abdominal pain, acute, parietal.*
    radiation of, 533–534
    right lower quadrant, 560–568
      causes of, 560t–561t, 562–568
      differential diagnosis of, 560–562, 560t–561t
    right upper quadrant, 568–575
      causes of, 569–572, 570t–571t
      clinical setting in, 572–575
      differential diagnosis of, 570t–571t
      physical examination of, 569
      symptoms of, 568–569
    severity of, 535–536
    shocky patient with, 539

Abdominal pain *(Continued)*
    acute, somatic. See *Abdominal pain, acute, parietal.*
    timing of, 534–535
    types of, 530–531
    urinary tract infection and, 537
    vaginal bleeding with, 567
    visceral, 530–533
      causes of, 531–533
      localization of, *531*
      referred, 531–533
    visceral vs. parietal, 530–534
    vomiting with, 537, 538t
  chronic, 575–608
    diagnosis of, 599–608
    diagnostic approach to, *600–601*
    elderly patient with, 604
    epigastric, 599, 602
    gastrointestinal, 602–603
    lower, 577–594
      abdominal mass with, 579
      causes of, 576t, 586t–587t, 592t–593t
      clinical findings in, 581
      diagnosis of, 578–581
        presumptive, 583
      diagnostic approach to, *582*
      heme-positive stool with, 579
      history in, 579
      location of, 578
      pelvic mass with, 579
      physical examination of, 579
      tests for, 577
      timing of, 578
      types of, 578
      vaginal bleeding with, 579
      weight loss with, 579
    postprandial, 603
    radicular, 603
    upper, 594–608
      causes of, 594t–595t, 610t–611t
      chest-wall disorders and, 602
      tests for, 606–607
  emergency room evaluations of, *529*
  hyperamylasemia with, 613t
  physical examinaton of, 539–549
  recurrent. See *Abdominal pain, chronic.*
  severe central, 608–618
    causes of, 614–616, *616*
    diagnosis of, 609–614
    distention with, 613
    history in, 609
    location of, 609
    peritonitis with, 609, 612–613
    referred, 612

Abdominal pain *(Continued)*
    severe central, symptoms of, 609, 612–624
      timing of, 609, 613
      tests for, 549–557, 556t
  Abdominal viscus, ruptured, and referred shoulder pain, 389
  Abdominal wall, disorders of, and chronic lower abdominal pain, 587t
    tests for, 587t
    treatment for, 587t
    examination of, diagnosis of abdominal pain, 547
  Abortion, threatened, and acute right lower quadrant pain, 560t–561t
    signs of, 560t
    symptoms of, 560t
    tests for, 561t
    treatment of, 561t
  Abscess, chronic, and chronic lower abdominal pain, 592t–593t
    intrahepatic, and acute pleuritic chest pain, 743t
    intranephric, and acute pyelonephritis, 302
    perinephric, and fever, 376
    peritonsillar. See *Peritonsillar abscess.*
    periurethral, 360
    prostatic, 376
    retropharyngeal. See *Retropharyngeal abscess.*
    subhepatic. See *Subphrenic abscess.*
    subphrenic. See *Subphrenic abscess.*
    tubal. See *Tubal abscess.*
  Acetaminophen, for low back pain, 21
    for migraine, 203
  Acetazolamide, for altitude headache, 182
  Acid infusion test, in diagnosis of esophagitis, 766–767
  Acid phosphatase, in diagnosis of low back pain, 18t
  Aci-Jel vaginal jelly, for trichomoniasis in pregnant patient, 325
  Acoustic neuroma, and vertigo, 494t, 496
  Acromegaly, and carpal tunnel syndrome, 434
  Acromioclavicular joint, palpation of, 398, *399*
  Acromion, palpation of, 398, *398*
  Actifed, for acute bronchitis, 639t
  Acyclovir, for herpes genitalis, 343t
    for herpes simplex infection, *315*
  Adenitis, mesenteric, and acute right lower quadrant pain, 560t–561t
    signs of, 560t

Adenitis *(Continued)*
mesenteric, symptoms of, 560t
tests for, 561t
treatment of, 561t
Adenovirus, and nonbacterial pneumonia, 646t
Adhesions, postoperative, and abdominal pain, *553*
Adhesive capsulitis. See *Frozen shoulder.*
Adson maneuver, in diagnosis of thoracic outlet syndromes, 451, *452*
Aerobic capacity, in diagnosis of angina pectoris, 684
Afferent arc, in human locomotion, 463, *464*
Albuterol, for acute bronchitis, 640t
Alcohol, and acute cerebellar disease, 466
and chronic abdominal pain, 604
and disequilibrium, 465
and headache, 183
and nystagmus, 513
and orthostatic hypotension, 477t
Alkaline phosphatase, in diagnosis of low back pain, 18t
Alterna GEL, for duodenal ulcer, 620t
Altitude headache, 182
Alupent, for acute bronchitis, 640t
Alveolar cell carcinoma, and cough, *654*
Alveolitis, fibrosing, and cough, *655*
Amaurosis fugax, and acute headache, 178t
Ambulatory illness, patient anxieties in, 672–673
Amikacin, for acute pyelonephritis, 301
Aminoglycosides, and labyrinthitis, 497
for acute prostatitis, 376
for acute pyelonephritis, 301
for bacterial pneumonia, 648t
for chronic prostatitis, 371t
Amitriptyline, for migraine, 206t
for tension headache, 211
Amoxicillin, for gonococcal urethritis, 354, 354t
for urinary tract infection, 286t
Amphiarthrodial joints, location of, 61
Amphojel, for duodenal ulcer, 620t
Ampicillin, and acute diarrhea, 116
for acute diverticulitis, 586t
for acute proctitis, 146t
for acute prostatitis, 376
for acute pyelonephritis, 301
for bacterial diarrhea, 113t
for bacterial pneumonia, 649t
for bacterial urinary infection, 364
for epididymitis, *347*
for epiglottitis, 84
for Fitz-Hugh-Curtis syndrome, 575
for *Gardnerella vaginalis* in pregnant patient, 337
for gonococcal urethritis, 354, 354t
for *Hemophilus influenzae* pneumonia, 622t
for pelvic inflammatory disease, 312, 563
for shigellosis, 117
for urinary tract infections, 286t
Amyloid, and orthostatic hypotension, 477t
Amyloidosis, and carpal tunnel syndrome, 434
and referred shoulder pain, 393
Anaerobes, and epiglottitis, 84
and pelvic inflammatory disease, 312, 562
and peritonsillar abscess, 83
Analgesics, for dysmenorrhea, 586t
for headache, 202
for low back pain, 21
for mittelschmerz, 587t

Analgesics *(Continued)*
for ovarian cysts, 587t
for periarticular shoulder disorders, 416
for primary dysmenorrhea, 585
for rib fractures, 699
for tension headache, 211
for uterine myomas, 587t
potential hazards of, 202
Anemia, severe, and orthostatic hypotension, 477t
Anesthesia, local, for periarticular shoulder disorders, 417
infiltration, for fibrositis, 699
topical, for aphthous stomatitis, 75
Aneurysm, abdominal aortic, and chronic abdominal pain, 592t–593t, 610t–611t
signs of, 592t, 610t
symptoms of, 592t, 610t
tests for, 593t, 611t
treatment of, 593t, 611t
and acute headache, 179t
Angina, exertional. See *Angina pectoris.*
intestinal, and chronic abdominal pain, 592t–593t, 610t–611t
signs of, 592t, 610t
symptoms of, 592t, 610t
tests for, 593t, 611t
treatment of, 593t, 611t
Ludwig's, 88–89
Vincent's, 73, *73*
Angina decubitus, 688
Angina pectoris, and chronic sore throat, 92
and cough, 631
and epigastric pain, 602
and episodic chest pain, 681, *706*
and syncope, 484, 485t
causes of, 686
classification of, 712t
diagnosis of, 682–686
exercise tests in, 712, *761*
drug therapy for, 713–718
duration of, 685
exercise for, *722, 724*
history in, 683–686
hospitalization for, 725–726
location of, 683
management of, 713–727
alterations in life, style for, 724–725
exercise tests in, 761–762
patient education in, 720–725
nonangina vs., 680t
physical exertion and, 683–685
referral to cardiologist, indications for, 725–726
rest for, 685
symptoms of, 683–686, 684t
timing of, 685
treatment of, 725t
typical, 682–686
characteristics of, 680t
description of, 681
diagnostic approach to, *686*
physical examination of, 695
walk program for, *722, 724*
Angiography, visceral, in evaluation of abdominal pain, 556t
Ankylosing spondylitis, and chronic low back pain, 43
Antacids, and diarrhea, 102
dose effectiveness of, 619–620
for duodenal ulcer, 619, 620t
for duodenitis, 595t
for esophagitis, 767t

Antacids *(Continued)*
for functional dyspepsia, 595t, 599
for gastric ulcer, 623
Antiarrhythmic drugs, for cardiac arrhythmias, 484t
Antibiotics, and diarrhea, 102, 116
for acute diarrhea, 113t, 198–109
for acute diverticulitis, 586t, 590
for acute proctitis, 147
for acute prostatitis, 376
for acute pyelonephritis, 286, 297t, 301
for bacterial prostatitis, 369
chronic, 371, 371t
for bacterial urinary infection, 364
for bile acid deficiencies, 139
for chronic diarrhea, 134t
for chronic pelvic inflammatory disease, 593t
for diphtheria, 86
for disseminated gonococcemia, 377
for dysuria-pyuria syndrome, 281
for epididymitis, *347*
for Ludwig's angina, 89
for pelvic inflammatory disease, 312
for periodontal infection, 75
for pneumonia, 657, 662t
for pyelonephritis, 376
for recurrent vaginal candidiasis, 329–330
for retropharyngeal abscess, 86
for septic bursitis, 230
for Shigella enteritis, 108
for streptococcal pharyngitis, 78, 80–81
for toxic shock syndrome, 312
for upper tract bacteriuria, 366
for urethral syndrome, 280
for urinary tract infections, 280–282, 286t
in high-risk patient, 287, 287t
for Vincent's angina, 73
parenteral, for acute pyelonephritis, 300
prophylactic, in recurrent urinary tract infections, 297–299
single-dose, for urinary tract infections, 285
susceptibility of, in treatment of urinary tract infections, 289–290
Antibody coated bacteria test, for localizing urinary tract infection, 304
Anticholinergics and headache, 183
for esophageal spasm, 769
for functional dyspepsia, 599
for prostatosis, 369t
Anticoagulants, and cerebellar hemorrhage, *169*
and low back pain, 56
Anticonvulsants, and acute cerebellar disease, 466
and nystagmus, 513
Antidepressants, and orthostatic hypotension, 477t
for diffuse fibrositis, 699
Antidiarrheal agents, for irritable bowel syndrome, 584
Antiemetics, for acute diarrhea, 111
Antifungal agents, for candida infection, 360
Antigas drugs, for functional dyspepsia, 599
Antihypertensives, and diarrhea, 102
and orthostatic hypotension, 477t
Anti-inflammatory drugs, and chronic abdominal pain, 604
and diarrhea, 102
for acute pericarditis, 748
for bicipital tendinitis, 412
for bursitis, 230
for cervical spine disease, 700

Anti-inflammatory drugs *(Continued)*
  for costochondritis, 699
  for fibrositis, 699
  for ischial bursitis, 10
  for low back pain, 21–22, 22t
  for migraine, 203
  for pectoralis major syndrome, 702
  for periarticular shoulder disorders, 417–
    418
  for primary dysmenorrhea, 585
  for spondylosis, 49
Antimotility drugs, for acute diarrhea, 110,
    110t
Antiprostaglandin agents, for
    dysmenorrhea, 586t
Antipsychotics, and orthostatic
    hypertension, 477t
Antipyretic medications, for pharyngitis, 79
Antispasmodics, for low back pain, 21
  for irritable bowel syndrome, 584, 586t
Antistaphylococcal drug, for Ludwig's
    angina, 89
  for retropharyngeal abscess, 86
Antivert, for vertigo, 499t
Anulus fibrosus, pain sensitivity of, 65
Anxiety, and chest pain, 770
  and chronic hyperventilation, 504, 505,
    506
  in well patient, 672–673
Aortic dissection, and acute severe chest
    pain, *736*
  and nonpleuritic chest pain, 728t
  and severe central abdominal pain, 615
Aortic stenosis, valvular, and syncope, 484,
    485t
  systolic murmurs in, 704t
Aortoiliac claudication, and chronic lower
    abdominal pain, 592t–593t
  neurogenic claudication vs., 49
  signs of, 592t
  symptoms of, 592t
  tests for, 593t
  treatment of, 593t
Apley's compression test, in diagnosis of
    knee pain, 224, 249, *250*
Apraxia, frontal lobe, and disequilibrium,
    465, 468t
Appendicitis, 564–566
  and abdominal pain, *552*
  and acute right lower quadrant pain,
    560t–561t
  diagnosis of, 564–566
  retrocecal, and right upper quadrant
    pain, 571t
  signs of, 560t
  symptoms of, 560t, 564
  tests for, 561t
  treatment of, 561t
Appendix, anatomic location of, 564, *565*
Arachnoiditis, and back pain, 36t
  and shoulder pain, 392
Aristospan, for bursitis, 230
Arm, motor weakness of, analysis of, 435,
    436t, 437t, 438t
ART, for detection of syphilis, 378
Arterial claudication, and knee pain, 217
Arterial stenosis, and referred shoulder
    pain, *391*
Arteriography, abdominal, 556t
  cerebral, in diagnosis of headache, 200
    in diagnosis of subarachnoid
      hemorrhage, 168
  coronary, in diagnosis of chest pain,
    705t, 765
    indications for, 719
    results of, correlations in, 756t–757t

Arteriography *(Continued)*
  pulmonary, indications for, 774–776, *779*
Arteritis, giant cell, 173
  temporal. See *Temporal arteritis.*
Artery(ies), biopsy of, in diagnosis of
    temporal arteritis, 173
  infarction of, internal auditory, and
    vertigo, 494t, 496
  popliteal, palpation of, 227
  superior mesenteric, embolus in, and
    abdominal pain, *554*
Arthritis, bacterial, and shoulder pain, 405t
  degenerative, and knee pain, 217
    and disequilibrium, 464
    and monoarthritis of knee, 259t, *260*
    and shoulder pain, 405t
    of glenohumeral joint, *404*
    sciatica vs., 35
    synovial fluid analysis of, 258
    swelling in, location of, *236*, 236t
    tenderness in, location of, *236*, 236t
  gonococcal, and septic arthritis, 258
    hospitalization for, 377
  inflammatory, and shoulder pain, 405t
  rheumatoid, and carpal tunnel syndrome,
    434
    and chronic low back pain, 43
    and monoarthritis of knee, 262, *262*
    and popliteal cysts, 230
    and shoulder pain, 405t, *406*
    synovial fluid analysis of, 258
  septic, gonococcal arthritis and, 258
  shoulder, 391
    synovial fluid analysis of, 258
Arthrocentesis, in diagnosis of septic
    shoulder pain, 391, *392*
  in diagnosis of swollen knee, 256–258
  in diagnosis of traumatic knee pain, 249–
    251
Arthrography, in diagnosis of meniscal
    knee injury, 253, *253*
  in diagnosis of popliteal cysts, 231, *231*
  in diagnosis of rotator cuff rupture, 415–
    416, *415*
  in diagnosis of shoulder pain, 425
Arthroscopy, in diagnosis of meniscal knee
    injury, 253
  in diagnosis of shoulder pain, 425
Articular processes, location of, 63
Ascaris lumbricoides, and parasitic
    diarrhea, 117t
Aspiration, and bacterial pneumonia, 649t,
    651
  and cough, 630
Aspirin, and chronic abdominal pain, 604
  for acute knee injury, 252
  for chondromalacia, 240
  for low back pain, 21, 22t
  for migraine, 193, 203
  for periarticular shoulder disorders, 418
  for tension headache, 191–192
Asthma, bronchial, and acute pleuritic
    chest pain, 748–749
    and chest pain, 696
    and cough, 630
Asystole, and syncope, 483, 484t
Ataxia, cerebellar. See *Cerebellar disease.*
  sensory, and disequilibrium, 467, 468t
Atenolol, for angina pectoris, 716t
Atherosclerotic arterial disease, thoracic
    outlet syndrome vs., 453
Atrial myxoma, and syncope, 485t
Atrioventricular block, and syncope, 483
Atrophy, diffuse cortical, and frontal lobe
    apraxia, 465
Atropine, for irritable bowel syndrome, 584

Audiometry, pure tone, in diagnosis of
    hearing loss, 522
Auditory brain stem evoked response, in
    diagnosis of hearing loss, 523
Auditory testing, in diagnosis of dizziness,
    519–527
Automated reagent test, for detection of
    syphilis, 378
Axillary nerve, lesions of, and shoulder
    pain, 433t, 435
Azulfidine, for Crohn's disease, 593t

Bacillus cereus, and food poisoning, 149t
Back, examination of, in diagnosis of
    abdominal pain, 547
  how to care for, 24–25
  lateral flexion of, in testing range of
    motion of, 8
  low, anatomy of, 61–65
    movements of, 64–65
    pain-sensitive structures of, 65, *65*
  range of motion of, 7–8, *7*
Back exercises, for spondylosis, 49
  in therapy of low back pain, 22, 23t, 25
Back extension, in testing range of motion
    of, 8
Back flexion, effect on spinal structures,
    64–65
Back manipulation, for low back pain, 27
  indications for, 66
  procedure for, 66–67
Back pain, low, 1–70
  acute, 1–16
    chronic vs., 2, 42
    diagnosis of, 1–5, *2*
    point tenderness vs. local
      tenderness, 9
    simple mechanical, examinations for,
      27
  and patient's attitude, 7
  causes of, 2
  chronic, 42–53
    acute vs., 2, 42
    causes of, 47
    diagnosis of, 43–51
    history in, 43–44
    surgical indications for, 53
    systemic diseases and, 43
    treatment of, 51–53
  dangerous indications in, 54–56
  examination of, 2
  feigned, tests for determining, 52–53
  history in, 2
  in cancer patient, 55–56
  laboratory tests for, 18–20, 18t
  mechanical, 4–42
    indications of, 5
    nonmechanical vs., 2–4
    subsets of, 4
  neurologic, 29–42
    neurologic examination for, 14–16
    nonmechanical, 2–4, 3t
    observing patient with, 6–7
    OMINOUS, 4–5
    physical examination of, 5
    practical neurology of, 29–34
    radicular, 29–42
      atypical findings in, 38–40
      diagnosis of, 34–42
      indications of, 5
      referred muscular vs., 11
      treatment of, 34–42
      true, 35–37
      types of, *35*

Back pain *(Continued)*
  low, simple mechanical, 16–28
    acutely painful stage of, 20–23
    clinical diagnosis of, 16–18
    preventive stage in, 26–29
    recovery stage in, 23–26
    treatment for, 20–29
Bacterial endocarditis, low back pain and, 54
Bacterial overgrowth, ileal resection and, 154
Bacterial overgrowth syndromes, and lactose intolerance, 119
Bacteriuria, in patient with indwelling urinary catheter, 287
  in pregnant women, 278
  nonpharmacologic prevention of, 298
  renal failure with, 278
  upper tract, and recurrent urinary tract infections, 366
    clinical characteristics of, 278t
    cystitis vs., 277, 278t
    lower tract vs., 295
    prolonged antibiotic therapy for, 291
Baker's cysts. *See Popliteal cysts.*
Balanitis, diagnosis of, 345t
  treatment of, 345t
Barbiturates, and acute cerebellar disease, 466
  and disequilibrium, 465
  and orthostatic hypotension, 477t
  for status migraine, 207
  for tension headache, 211
Barium enema, in diagnosis of diverticulosis, 590
  in evaluation of abdominal pain, 556t
Barium studies, in diagnosis of chronic diarrhea, 136
  indications for, 106, 107t
Barium swallow, in diagnosis of chest pain, 705t
  in diagnosis of esophageal spasm, 768
  in diagnosis of esophagitis, 766
Bartholin's cysts, *316*
Behçet's disease, and pharyngeal ulcers, 75
Bed, rising from, technique of, 23t
Bed exercises, in therapy of low back pain, 22–23, 25
Bedrest, and OMINOUS mechanical low back pain, 5
  and referred low back pain, 5
  for disc herniation, 40
  for low back pain, 20–21
Bellergal, for migraine, 204t
Benadryl, for vertigo, 499t
Bernstein test, in diagnosis of acute severe chest pain, 741
  in diagnosis of esophagitis, 766–767, *767*
Beta blockers, contraindications to, 716
  for angina pectoris, 715–717, 716t
  side effects of, 716–717, 716t
Bethanechol, for esophagitis, 767t
Biceps, knee, location of, *268*
Biceps femoris, palpation of, 225, *226*
Biceps tendon, acute rupture of, and shoulder pain, 412
  palpation of, 398, *398*
Bicozamycin, for turista, 151
Bile acid, deficiencies in, causes of, 139
Bile acid breath test, in diagnosis of bile acid deficiencies, 139
Biliary colic, and acute right upper quadrant pain, 570t–571t, *573*
  and chest pain, 693

Biliary colic *(Continued)*
  and chronic upper abdominal pain, 595t, 598
  and nonpleuritic chest pain, 729t
  location of pain in, *693*
  signs of, 570t
  symptoms of, 570t, 595t, 598
  tests for, 570t, 595t
  treatment of, 570t, 595t
Biliary scan, in evaluation of abdominal pain, 556t
Bilirubinuria, in diagnosis of abdominal pain, 554
Bladder, needle aspiration of, for urine culture, 288
Bladder stones, and recurrent urinary tract infections, *297*
Bladder washout procedure, for localizing site of urinary tract infections, 303, 303t
Blocadren, for angina pectoris, 716t
Blood, occult, in diagnosis of acute diarrhea, 103–140
Blood count, in diagnosis of acute severe chest pain, 733, 735
  peripheral, in diagnosis of infectious mononucleosis, 75
  white cell, in diagnosis of bacterial pneumonia, 652
    in evaluation of abdominal pain, 555–556, 556t
Blood culture, in diagnosis of acute pyelonephritis, 300
  in diagnosis of pneumonia, 663
Blood pressure, postural, in diagnosis of orthostatic hypotension, 478
Blood tests, in diagnosis of headache, 196
  in diagnosis of malabsorption, 135
Bone, biopsy of, in diagnosis of osteopenia, 59–60
  neoplasms of, and referred shoulder pain, 392
Bone disease, metabolic, and chronic low back pain, 43
Bone scan(s), abnormal, causes of, 19t
  in diagnosis of femoral condyle osteonecrosis, 238
  in diagnosis of low back pain, 18t
  isotope, for vertebral metastases, 56
  for vertebral osteomyelitis, 54, *55*
Bonine, for vertigo, 499t
Boric acid, for candidiasis vaginitis, 328
Bornholm's disease. *See Pleuritis, viral.*
Borrelia vincentii, and Vincent's angina, 73
Bowel, disease of, and chronic low back pain, 43
  inflammatory, irritable bowel syndrome vs., 584
  obstruction of, and chronic lower abdominal pain, 586
  causes of, 543t
  hernias and, 546
  low vs. high, 543t
  surgery for, 586t
  tests for, 586t
BPV. *See Vertigo, benign positional.*
Brachial plexus, *429*
  disorders of, and shoulder pain, 402
    and shoulder/hand syndrome, 427t, 428
  lesions of, and shoulder pain, 431t
  neoplasms in, and shoulder/hand syndrome, 429
  neuritis of, and shoulder/hand syndrome, 430

Bradycardia, and syncope, 483, 484t
Brain tumor(s), and acute headache, 179t
  and nocturnal headache, 184
Branhamella catarrhalis, and pneumonia, 645
Breast, disorders of, and chest-wall pain, 698
  neoplasm of, and referred shoulder pain, 392
Breast carcinoma, metastatic, x-rays of, *45*
Brethine, for acute bronchitis, 640t
Bricanyl, for acute bronchitis, 640t
Bronchial asthma. *See Asthma, bronchial.*
Bronchial irritants, and cough, 631
Bronchiectasis, and chronic cough, *668*
Bronchitis, acute, clinical features of, 637t
  smoker with, 640–641
  symptoms of, 637
  treatment of, 638–642
  auscultatory findings in, 632–634, *634*
  chronic, nonsmoker with, 667
  smoking and, 667
  pneumonia vs., 631–632
  symptoms of, 631–632
Bronchodilators, for acute bronchitis, 640t
Bronchoscopy, in diagnosis of chronic cough, 670
Bronkodyl, for acute bronchitis, 640t
Bronkometer, for acute bronchitis, 640t
Brudzinski's sign, in diagnosis of meningitis, *177*
Bull neck, 88, *89*
  acute sialadenitis vs., 90
  dental abscesses vs., 90
Bursae, knee, swellings of, *229*
Bursal fluid aspiration, in diagnosis of septic bursitis, 230
Bursitis, and localized swelling of knee, 229–231
  calcific, diagnosis of, 412–413, 416t
  infrapatellar, causes of, 229
  ischial, 9–10
  pes anserine, causes of, 229
  prepatellar, causes of, 229
  sciatica vs., 35
  septic, symptoms of, 230
  subacromial. *See Tendinitis, calcific.*
  subdeltoid. *See Tendinitis, calcific.*
  swelling in, location of, 236t
  tenderness in, location of, 236t
  treatment of, 230
  trochanteric, 10
    and knee pain, 217
Bypass surgery, cardiac, indications for, 718

CAD. *See Coronary artery disease.*
Cafergot, for migraine, 204t
Caffeine, and headache, 183
Calan, for angina pectoris, 718t
Calcium, for osteoporosis, 59
  phosphate, in diagnosis of low back pain, 18t
Calcium channel blockers, for angina pectoris, 717–718, 718t
  for esophageal spasm, 769
  side effects of, 718, 718t
Calculus, ureteral, and acute right lower quadrant pain, 560t–561t
  signs of, 560t
  symptoms of, 560t
  tests for, 561t
  treatment of, 561t

Calendars, in diagnosis of headache, 194t, 195t, 196
Caloric testing, in diagnosis of dizziness, 462
  in diagnosis of vestibular disease, 516–518, *517*
Campylobacter, and acute invasive diarrhea, 113t
  and acute dysentery, 101, 111
  and fecal leukocytes, 103
  and food poisoning, 149t
Campylobacter enteritis, treatment of, 108
Campylobacter jejuni, and acute invasive diarrhea, 113t
  and dysentery, 111
  and urethritis, 358
    recurrent, 360
  cultures for, in diagnosis of vaginitis, indications for, 320t, 323
  KOH preparation in diagnosis of, 319, *319*
Candida albicans, and vaginitis, 316t, 317
Candidiasis, chronic atrophic, symptoms of, 75
  diagnosis of, 345t
  isolated vulvar, and vulvar pruritus, 334
  location of, *345*
  oral symptoms of, 75
  treatment of, 345t
  vaginal, recurrent, 329–333
    antibiotic treatment of, 329–330
    intestinal candida and, 330
    predisposing conditions in, 329
    venereal transmission of, 330
  symptoms of, 326
  treatment of, 327–329, 328t
Canker sores, symptoms of, 74, *74*
Cantharidin, for molluscum contagiosum, 344t
Capillaria philippinensis, and parasitic diarrhea, 117t
Carbamazepine, for trigeminal neuralgia, 190
Carbenicillin, for acute pyelonephritis, 301
Carbenoxolone/alginic acid, for esophagitis, 767t
Carbidopa/levodopa, for dizziness, 480
Cardiac arrhythmias, and syncope, 483, 484t, 509–511
  characteristics of, 484t
  treatment of, 484t
  types of, 484t
Cardiac enzyme, in diagnosis of myocardial infarction, 740
Cardiac ischemia, and syncope, 484, 485t
Cardiac neurosis, and chest pain, 771
Cardilate, for angina pectoris, 715t
Cardiopulmonary disease, and chest pain, 694
  pneumonia with, 659
Cardizem, for angina pectoris, 718t
Carotid sinus massage, in diagnosis of dizziness, 462
Carotidynia, and headache, 177
Carpal tunnel syndrome, and shoulder pain, 433–434, 433t
  causes of, 434
  thoracic outlet syndrome vs., 453
Caruncle, urethral, *316*
Cataracts, and disequilibrium, 464
Catheter, indwelling, and recurrent urinary tract infection, 366
Catheterization, ureteral, for localizing site of urinary tract infection, 303

Cauda equina lesions, lateral, symptoms of, 37, *38*
  midline, symptoms of, 37
Cauda equina syndrome, *42*
  types of, 37, *38*
Cecal volvulus, and abdominal pain, *554*, 560t–561t
Cefaclor, for *Hemophilus influenzae*, 662t
Cefamandole, for bacterial pneumonia, 649t
Cefoxitin, for gonococcal urethritis, 355, 355t
Celiac axis syndrome, and chronic abdominal pain, *603*, 610t–611t
  signs of, 610t
  symptoms of, 610t
  tests for, 611t
  treatment of, 611t
Celiac sprue, and lactose intolerance, 119
Cellular casts, red cell, in diagnosis of abdominal pain, 555
Cellulitis, peritonsillar, diagnosis of, 84
  pharyngeal, diagnosis of, 84
Central nervous system disorders, trigeminal neuralgia vs., 191
Cephalexin, for epididymitis, *347*
  for pneumococcal pneumonia, 662t
Cephalosporins, for acute prostatitis, 376
  for acute pyelonephritis, 301
  for bacterial diarrhea, 113t
  for bacterial pneumonia, 648t
  for streptococcal pharyngitis, 80
Cerebellar disease, and disequilibrium, 466, 468t
  causes of, 466–467
Cerebrovascular disease, and syncope, 483, 482t
Cervical root syndromes, and shoulder pain, 392–393, 402
Cervical spine disease, and chest-wall pain, 700
  and headache, 177
  and nonpleuritic chest pain, 729t
  simultaneous shoulder/hand pain in, 427, 427t
  tension headache vs., 210
Cervical spine films, in diagnosis of exertional headache, 182
Cervical spondylosis, and shoulder hand syndrome, 427t, 428, *428*
  tension headache vs., 210
  thoracic outlet syndrome vs., 453
Cervicitis, acute, causes of, *320*
  chronic, signs of, *317*
  vaginal discharge and, 315
Cervix, bimanual palpation of, in diagnosis of vulvovaginal disorders, 315
  carcinoma of, signs of, *317*
  cultures of, in diagnosis of vaginitis, 319–321, 320t
  disorders of, and vaginal discharge, 315
    appearance of, *317*
  dysplasia of, trichomonas infection and, 332
  polyps of, signs of, *317*
  secretions of, 310
Chancroid, diagnosis of, 343t
  location of ulcerations of, *342*
  treatment of, 343t
Chemonucleolysis, for disc herniation, 40
Chemotherapeutic drugs, and diarrhea, 102
Chest, auscultation of, in diagnosis of pneumonia, 635–636
Chest pain, 677–783

Chest pain (*Continued*)
  atypical, diagnosis of, 681
  clinical history in, correlations in, 756t–757t
  clinical presentation of, diagnostic emphasis of, 678t
  "compatible," 693–694
  diagnosis of, exercise tests in, 754–765. See also *Stress tests*.
  episodic, 678–698
    causes of, 679t
      cardiopulmonary, 696
    chest wall causes of, 696–698
    diagnosis of, 681–682
      exercise testing in, 710–711
    diagnostic tests in, 680
    gastrointestinal causes of, 696
    generalizations in, 679–681
    history in, 689–693
    innocent ejection murmur with, 704t
    ischemia and, *764*
    physical examination for, 694–698
    systolic murmurs with, 703, 704t
    types of, 681–682, *682*
  esophageal, 766–769
  malingering in, 771
  nonpleuritic, causes of, 728t–729t
  nonspecific, 693–694
    description of, 681
    diagnosis of, exercise tests in, 763
    diagnostic approach to, 695
    gastrointestinal causes of, 693
  pleuritic, 741–753
    causes of, 742t–743t
    clinical setting in, 750
    diagnosis of, 750–753
    diagnostic approach to, *749*
    drug induced, 743t
    nonpenetrating chest trauma and, 742t
    perfusion defects with, *773*, *774*
    physical examination of, 750
    pleural effusion with, *744*, *745*
    pulmonary embolism and, 742t, 744–746
    scintigraphic findings in, 776t
  psychogenic, hyperventilation and, 696
  psychosomatic, 770–771
  recurrent, 678–698. See also *Chest pain, episodic*.
  severe, 727–741
    categories of, 735–738
    diagnostic tests for, 732–735, *739*, *740*
    history in, 727–731
    location of, 727, 730
    physical examination of, 731–732
    quality of, 730
    symptoms of, 727–732
    timing of, 730
    triggers of, 730–731
  tests for, 705–713, 705t
Chest wall, abnormalities of, palpable, *698*
  examination of, 696–697
  palpation of, 696–697
Chest-wall maneuvers, in diagnosis of chest-wall syndromes, *701*
Chest-wall syndromes, 698–703
  and acute pleuritic chest pain, 742t, 748
  categories of, 698–702
  diagnosis of, 702–703
Chest x-ray, diagnostic, for chest pain, 705t, 733, 750–751
  for cough, 635–636, *636*, 669
  for hemoptysis, 642
  for pneumonia, 649–652, 665

Chest x-ray *(Continued)*
  diagnostic, for pulmonary embolism, *744,
      745, 745*
Chiasmal tumor, and acute headache, 178t
Chlamydia psittaci, and nonbacterial
      pneumonia, 647t
Chlamydia trachomatis, and pneumonia,
      645
  and urethritis, 357
  diagnosis of, 343t
  treatment of, 343t
Chlamydiae, and pelvic inflammatory
      disease, 312, 562
  and urethritis, 349
Chloramphenicol, for bacterial diarrhea,
      113t
  for bacterial pneumonia, 649t
  for epiglottitis, 84
  for *Hemophilus influenzae* pneumonia,
      662t
Chlordiazepoxide, for irritable bowel
      syndrome, 584, 586t
  for tension headache, 211
Chlorpheniramine, for postnasal drip, 668
Chlorpromazine, and orthostatic
      hypotension, 477t
  for status migraine, 207
Chlor-Trimeton, for postnasal drip, 668
Cholecystectomy, and postoperative
      diarrhea, 153
Cholecystitis, and nonpleuritic chest pain,
      729t
  and right upper quadrant pain, 570t
  diagnosis of, 572–573
  gallstones and, 572
  signs of, 570t
  symptoms of, 570t, 572
  tests for, 570t, 573
  treatment of, 570t
Cholecystogram, oral, in diagnosis of
      chronic upper abdominal pain, 606
  in diagnosis of chest pain, 705t
Cholesteatoma, and vertigo, 494t, 495
Cholestyramine, for acute proctitis, 146t
  for bacterial diarrhea, 113t
  for chronic diarrhea, 134t
Chondromalacia, and knee pain, 233–234,
      233t
  differential diagnosis of, 234–236, 233t
  mechanism of, *234*
  swelling in, localization of, *236*
Chondromatosis, synovial, and
      monoarthritis of knee, 262, *263*
Chromophobe adenoma, headache patient
      with, *199*
Ciguatoxin, and food poisoning, 149t
Cimetidine, for duodenal ulcer, 619, 620t
  for esophagitis, 767t
  for gastric ulcer, 623
  for pancreatic enzyme replacement, 158t
  side effects of, 619
Claudication, aortoiliac vascular vs.
      neurogenic, 49
Clidinium bromide, for irritable bowel
      syndrome, 584, 586t
Clindamycin, and diarrhea of
      pseudomembranous colitis, 102
  for bacterial pneumonia, 649t
  for peritonsillar abscess, 83
  for pneumococcal pneumonia, 662t
  for streptococcal pharyngitis, 80
Clinoril, for low back pain, 22t
Clonidine, for orthostatic hypotension,
      477t, 480
Clostridium botulinum, and food poisoning,
      149t

Clostridium difficile, and acute invasive
      diarrhea, 113t
  and pseudomembranous colitis, 115
Clostridium perfringens, and food
      poisoning, 149t
Clotrimazole, for erythrasma, 335
  for tinea cruris, 335
  for vaginal candidiasis, 327, 328t
  for vaginal trichomoniasis in pregnant
      patient, 325
Cluster headache, 188–189
  and nocturnal headache, 184
  characteristics of, 185t
  differential diagnosis of, 188
  location of, *188*
  therapy for, 188–189
  trigeminal neuralgia vs., 188, 190
Coccydynia, 9
  sciatica vs., 35
Coccyx, and low back pain, 9
Cochleovestibular dysfunction, and
      disequilibrium, 464
Codeine, for acute bronchitis, 638–639,
      639t
  for low back pain, 21
  for migraine, 203
  for rotator cuff tendinitis, 421
Codman's pendulum exercise, for
      periarticular shoulder disorders, 418,
      419
Cogan's syndrome, and vertigo, 494t
Coital headache, 182
Cold, topical, for low back pain, 21
Colitis. See also *Irritable bowel syndrome.*
  ischemic, 132, *132*
  ulcerative, *130*
    amebic enterocolitis vs., 131
    and chronic bloody diarrhea, 129
    and chronic lower abdominal pain,
        592t–593t
    Crohn's disease vs., 131
    Yersinia vs., 131
Collagenase, injection of, for disc
      herniation, 40
Collateral ligament, palpation of, 224, 225,
      226
  strains of, swelling in, location of, *236,*
      236t
  tenderness in, location of, *236,* 236t
Colon, distal, disease of, 124
  diverticular disease of, 588–590, *589*
    and chronic lower abdominal pain,
        586t
    and referred shoulder pain, 389
  proximal, disease of, 124
  rectosigmoid, function of, 124
  spastic. See *Irritable bowel syndrome.*
Colorectal carcinoma, and chronic lower
      abdominal pain, 592t–593t
  common locations of, *580*
  irritable bowel syndrome vs., 584
Compazine, for vertigo, 499t
Compression fractures, and low back pain,
      57–60
Conduction disease, syncope with, 509
Condylomata acuminata, *314, 344*
  syphilitic condylomata lata vs., *314*
  treatment of, *314,* 344t
Condylomata lata, syphilitic, *314, 315*
  condylomata acuminata vs., *314*
Consciousness, loss of. See *Syncope.*
Constipation, habitual, and chronic lower
      abdominal pain, 586t
  and irritable bowel syndrome, 584–585
  noncathartic prophylaxis of, 585t
  tests for, 586t

Constipation *(Continued)*
  habitual, treatment of, presumptive,
      586t
Contraceptives, oral, and chronic
      abdominal pain, 604
  and headache, 183
  for dysmenorrhea, 585, 586t
Conus lesions, symptoms of, 37, *38*
Corgard, for angina pectoris, 716t
Coronary artery disease, and episodic chest
      pain, 679–680
  and nonpleuritic chest pain, 728t
  development of, probability of, 720t–721t
  diagnosis of, exercise tests in, *762, 763*
    evaluation of, 759–761
    indications for, 756–759
    value of, 755–756
  high risk factors in, 703
  probability of, 758t, *764*
  risk-factor analysis of, 710
  risk-factor modification of, 721–724
  surgery for, 718–719
  treatment of, nonsurgical, mortality
      after, 719t
Corticosteroids, and chronic abdominal
      pain, 604
  for acute pericarditis, 748
  for acute proctitis, 146t
  for bicipital tendinitis, 412
  for bursitis, 230
  for chronic diarrhea, 129, 134t
  for Crohn's disease, 132, 593t
  for disc herniation, 40
  for epidural metastases, 56
  for frozen shoulder, 423
  for infectious mononucleosis, 70
  for periarticular shoulder disorders, 417,
      418
  for reflex sympathetic dystrophy
      syndrome, 427
  for status migraine, 207
  for temporal arteritis, 173
Corynebacterium diphtheriae, and
      diphtheria, 86
  and pharyngitis, 90
Corynebacterium genitalium and urethritis,
      357
Corynebacterium minutissimum, and
      erythrasma, 335
Corynebacterium vaginale. See *Gardnerella
      vaginalis.*
Costochondritis, and chest-wall pain, 699
Costoclavicular maneuver, in diagnosis of
      thoracic outlet syndromes, 452, *452*
Costoclavicular syndrome, 451–452
Cotazyme, for pancreatic enzyme
      replacement, 158t
Cough, 628–676
  acute, 629–667
    associated symptoms with, 632
    diagnostic approach to, 635
    infectious vs., noninfectious, 630–631
    initial approach to, 629–631
    physical examination of, 632–634
    phases of, 628–629
  causes of, 629t
  chronic, 667–671
    bronchiectasis and, *668*
    physical examination of, 669
  complications of, 638t
  psychogenic, 671
Cough reflex arc, innervation of, *628*
Cough suppressants, for acute bronchitis,
      638–639, 639t
Coxiella burnetti, and nonbacterial
      pneumonia, 647t

Coxsackie virus, and hand, foot, and mouth disease, 73
and herpangina, 73
and pleuritis, 741
CPK isoenzymes, in diagnosis of myocardial infarction, 740
Crabs, pubic. See pediculosis pubis.
Crackles, in physical examination of cough, 634
Cranial neuralgia, characteristics of, 185t
Craniovertebral anomalies, tension headache vs., 210
Crohn's disease, 130, 131
and chronic lower abdominal pain, 592t–593t
and lactose intolerance, 119
diagnosis of, 132
signs of, 592t
symptoms of, 131–132, 592t
tests for, 593t
treatment of, 132, 593t
ulcerative colitis vs., 131
Yersinia enterocolitis vs., 132
Crowing rooster maneuver, in diagnosis of chest-wall maneuvers, 700, 701
Cryptosporidiosis, 117t
CT scan(s), diagnostic, for cerebellar hemorrhage, 168
for chronic upper abdominal pain, 607
for diffuse cortical atrophy, 465
for disc herniation, 41–42
for epidural metastases, 56
for exertional headache, 182
for headache, 197, 200
for low back pain, 18t
for spinal stenosis, 49, 49
for subarachnoid hemorrhage, 168
Culdocentesis, in diagnosis of ectopic pregnancy, 567
Cyclizine, for vertigo, 499t
Cyclobenzaprine HCl, for low back pain, 21
Cyproheptadine, for migraine, 206t
Cyst(s), meniscal. See Meniscal cysts.
nabothian, signs of, 317
ovarian, and chronic lower abdominal pain, 587t
popliteal. See Popliteal cysts.
Cystic masses, and paroxysmal headache, 182
Cystitis, clinical characteristics of, 278t
interstitial, oxychlorosene sodium for, 292
types of, 273t
upper tract bacteriuria vs., 277, 278t
Cystoceles, vaginal, 316
Cystourethritis, symptomatic, antibiotics for, 286
Cytomegalovirus infection, and heterophil negative mononucleosis, 76
infectious mononucleosis vs., 76

Darier's disease, and vulvar pruritus, 336
Darvon, for headache, 202
Deafness, and disequilibrium, 464
Decadron, for disc herniation, 40
Dehydration, and orthostatic hypotension, 102
Delcid, for duodenal ulcer, 620t
Deltoid muscle, function of, 443, 444
palpation of, 399
Demyelinating diseases, trigeminal neuralgia vs., 191
Dental abscess, bull neck vs., 90

Dental infections, and headache, 177
Dental procedures, and retropharyngeal abscess, 86, 87
Depression, and chest pain, 771
and chronic hyperventilation, 504–507
in headache sufferers, 210–211
Dermatitis, and vulvar pruritus, 335–336
Dexamethasone, for disc herniation, 40
Dextromethorphan, for acute bronchitis, 639t
Diabetes, and chronic abdominal pain, 604
and orthostatic hypotension, 477t
and referred shoulder pain, 392
Diabetic neuritis, and acute headache, 179t
Diabetics, impaired bladder function in, 279
urinary tract infections in, 280
treatment for, 287, 287t
Diarrhea, 100–163
acute, 100–120
abdominal pain with, 102, 536
antibiotic therapy for, 108–109
causes of, 100, 100t
diagnosis of, 100–106, 105
drug-induced, 102
food poisoning and, 103, 148–150
in homosexuals, 102, 145–147
parasitic causes of, 116, 117t
persistent, 115–119
diagnostic approach to, 118
symptoms of, 100–106
treatment of, 108–111
viral gastroenteritis and, 100
chronic, 121–144
bloody, 129–133
causes of, 121t
diagnosis of, 121–129, 128, 129
dietary treatment for, 134t
osmotic, causes of, 143
secretory, causes of, 144
secretory vs. osmotic, 143
systemic diseases and, 122–123, 123t
tests in evaluation of, 122t
therapeutic trials for, 133, 134t
diagnostic tests for, 106–107, 107t
food-borne, 148–151
invasive bacterial, 113t
large-stool, causes of, 124
nocturnal, 127
parasitic, 117t
postoperative, 152–154
small-stool, causes of, 124
traveler's, 151
Diarthrodial joints, location of, 62–63
Diazepam, for low back pain, 21
for tension headache, 211
for vertigo, 499t
Dichloracetic acid, for condylomata acuminata, 146t
Dicloxacillin, for septic bursitis, 230
Diet(s), 155–157
100-gram fat, 155, 155t
Dihydroergotamine, for orthostatic hypotension, 477t, 480
Diiodohydroxyquin, for chronic diarrhea, 134t
for parasitic diarrhea, 117t
Dilanozide furonate, for parasitic diarrhea, 117t
Diltiazem, for angina pectoris, 718t
Dimenhydrinate, for vertigo, 499t
Dimetane, for acute bronchitis, 639t
Diphenoxylate hydrochloride, for irritable bowel syndrome, 584
Diphenylhydantoin, for trigeminal neuralgia, 190

Diphenhydramine, for vertigo, 499t
Diphtheria, and complicated sore throat, 86
Disability, employment, chronic low back pain and, 52–53
Disc, components of, 61, 61
degeneration of, 62
location of, 61–62
Disc bulges, 17
Disc disease, relapsing illness in, 42
Disc herniation(s), 42
acute, 16–18
and lumbosacral root disease, 12
and radicular low back pain, 8, 35–37
classification of, 17
hospitalization vs. surgery for, 41
in elderly, 17–18
therapy for, 40–42
Disc prolapses, 17
Disc space narrowing, 48, 49
Disequilibrium, 463–471
causes of, 465–467, 468t
definition of, 458
multiple sensory deficits and, 464, 468t
psychogenic, 467, 468t
treatment of, 464–465, 468
Diuretics, and labyrinthitis, 497
and orthostatic hypotension, 477
for premenstrual syndrome, 587t
Diverticulitis, and chronic bloody diarrhea, 133
and chronic lower abdominal pain, 586t, 590
irritable bowel syndrome vs., 584
treatment of, 586t, 590
Diverticulosis, in elderly, 590
painful, and chronic lower abdominal pain, 586t
treatment of, 586t, 590
Dizziness, 456–527
classification of, 456–461
diagnosis of, 460, 461
overlapping symptoms in, 458
peripheral vestibular disease and, 494t
physical examination of, 459–461
simulation tests in diagnosis of, 459–463, 460t
symptoms of, 457–458
tests for, costs of, 524
Douches, for vaginal trichomoniasis in pregnant patient, 325
Doxycycline, for chronic prostatitis, 371t
Drainage, surgical, for peritonsillar abscess, 83
Dramamine, for vertigo, 499t
Dressler's syndrome, and acute pleuritic chest pain, 743t
Drugs, and disequilibrium, 465, 468t
and headache, 182–183
and orthostatic hypotension 477t, 479
Dumping syndrome, and postoperative diarrhea, 152
diet for, 156
Duodenitis, and upper abdominal pain, 595t, 596
Dura mater, pain sensitivity of, 65
D-xylose excretion test, in diagnosis of pancreatic insufficiency, 140
Dysautonomia, and orthostatic hypotension, 477t, 479
Dysentery, 111–119
causes of, 101, 111–112
diagnostic approach to, 112
diagnostic tests for, 114
symptoms of, 101, 111
Dysmenorrhea, and acute right lower quadrant pain, 560t

Dysmenorrhea *(Continued)*
  and chronic lower abdominal pain, 585,
    586t
  primary, 585
  secondary, 585
  symptoms of, 585
  tests for, 586t
  treatment of, 585, 586t
Dyspepsia, functional, and chronic upper
    abdominal pain, 595t, 598–599
  symptoms of, 595t, 598
  tests for, 595t
  treatment of, 595t, 599
Dysphagia, severe chest pain with, 731
Dyspnea, severe chest pain with, 731
Dysuria, external vs. internal, 312
Dysuria-pyuria syndrome, antibiotic
    therapy for, 281

Ear, nose and throat disorders, trigeminal
    neuralgia vs., 191
Ectropion, cervical, signs of, *317*
Eczema, and vulvar pruritus, 336
Efferent arc, in human locomotion, 463,
    464
Effort headache, 182
Effusion(s), bursal, and localized swellings
    around knee, 229–230
  hemarthrosis vs., in knee injury, 245
Elderly, disequilibrium in, 465
Electrocardiography, diagnostic, for acute
    severe chest pain, 732–733
  for cardiac arrhythmias, 509–511, *510,
    511*
  for chest pain, 705t, 707–709
  for heart murmurs, 709
  for myocardial infarction, 740
  for syncope, 473, 484, 485t
  ST changes in, 759–760, *759*
Electroencephalography, in diagnosis of
    epilepsy, 483
Electromyography, in diagnosis of disc
    herniation, 42
Electronystagmography, in diagnosis of
    vestibular disease, 518
Elixophyllin, for acute bronchitis, 640t
Embolism, pulmonary. See *Pulmonary
    embolism.*
Emphysema, and chest pain, 696
Empyema, and acute pleuritic chest pain,
    743t
  Hemophilus influenzae and, *661*
  pneumonia with, 659–660, 659t, *660, 661*
  Streptococcus pneumoniae and, *660*
  subdural, epidural abcess vs., 54
  thoracostomy drainage of, 659–660
Endocarditis, bacterial, low back pain and,
    54
  untreated gonorrhea and, 356
Endocrine diseases, and chronic low back
    pain, 43
Endolymphatic hydrops, and vertigo, 494t,
    495–496
Endometrial carcinoma, and chronic lower
    abdominal pain, 592t–593t
Endometriosis, 585, 588
  and acute right lower quadrant pain, 560t
  and chronic lower abdominal pain, 587t
  and chronic low back pain, 44
  location of, 588, *588*
  symptoms of, 588
  tests for, 587t
  treatment of, 587t, 588

Endometrium, secretions of, 310
Entamoeba histolytica, and amebic
    dysentery, 114
  and parasitic diarrhea, 117t
Enterobius vermicularis and parasitic
    diarrhea, 117t
Enterococcus, and urinary tract infections,
    289
Enterocolitis, amebic, ulcerative colitis vs.,
    131
Ephedrine, for orthostatic hypotension, 480
Epicondyle, knee, location of, *268*
Epididymis, location of, *347*
  palpation of, *347*
Epididymitis, and recurrent urethritis, 361
  diagnosis of, *347*
  treatment of, *347*
Epidural abscess, and low back pain, 54
Epidural metastases, and low back pain, 56
Epidural venography, in diagnosis of disc
    herniation, 42
Epigastric pain, causes of, 530
Epiglottis, swollen, visualization of, *85,* 88
Epiglottitis, *85*
  and trismus, 82
  causes of, 84
  diagnosis of, 84
  lingual tonsillitis vs., 88
Epilepsy, and syncope, 481–483, 482t
  petit mal, characteristics of, 481, 482t
Epstein-Barr virus, and infectious
    mononucleosis, 76
Equilibrium system, components of, 463–
    464, *464*
ERCP, in diagnosis of chronic upper
    abdominal pain, 607
Ergomar, for migraine, 204t
Ergonovine, for migraine, 206t
Ergostat, for migraine, 204t
Ergot dependence, ergotamine use and,
    205
Ergotamines, and headache, 182
  contraindications to, 205
  for cluster headache, 189
  for migraine, 204t, 206t
  side effects of, 205
Ergotism, ergotamine use and, 205
Erythema multiforme, and pharyngeal
    ulcers, 75
Erythrasma, and vulvar pruritus, 334–335
  diagnosis of, 345t
  location of, *345*
  treatment of, 345t
Erythrityl tetranitrate, for angina pectoris,
    715t
Erythromycin, and acute diarrhea, 116
  for acute proctitis, 146t
  for bacterial diarrhea, 113t
  for bacterial pneumonia, 648t–649t
  for campylobacter infection, 108, 117
  for chlamydial infection in pregnancy,
    286
  for chronic prostatitis, 371t
  for diphtheria, 86
  for dysentery, 111
  for gonococcal urethritis, 355, 355t
  for mycoplasma pneumonia, 661, 662t
  for nonbacterial pneumonia, 646t
  for nongonococcal urethritis, 358, 358t
  for streptococcal pharyngitis, 80
  for unexplained vaginitis, 338
Escherichia coli, and acute invasive
    diarrhea, 113t
  and food poisoning, 149t
  and prostatitis, 367

Escherichia coli (Continued)
  and turista, 102
  and urinary infections, 289, 363
Esophagitis, and chest pain, 693
  and chronic upper abdominal pain, 594–
    595, 595t
  and heartburn, 766
  and nonpleuritic chest pain, 729t
  diagnostic tests for, 766–767
  history in, 766
  symptoms of, 594, 595t
  tests for, 595t
  treatment of, 767–768, 767t
Esophagogastroduodenoscopy, in diagnosis
    of chronic upper abdominal pain, 606
Esophagus, endoscopic biopsy of, in
    diagnosis of esophagitis, 766–767
  manometry of, in diagnosis of chest pain,
    705t
  rupture of, and acute severe chest pain,
    738
    and nonpleuritic chest pain, 729t
  spasm of, and chest pain, 693
    and episodic severe chest pain, *769*
    and nonpleuritic chest pain, 729t
    causes of, 768
    diagnostic approach to, *768*
    symptoms of, 768
    treatment of, 769
Estrogens, and headache, 183
  for atrophic vaginitis, 333, 333t
  for osteoporosis, 59
Exercise, for back, 24–25, 42
Exercise tests, in evaluation of chest pain.
    See *Stress tests.*
Exertional headache, 182
Exocervix, appearance of, *317*
Exophthalmos, and acute headache, 179t
Expectorants, for acute bronchitis, 639
Extensor muscle group, location of, 64
Eye strain, and headache, 170, 170t

Facet joints, location of, 62–63
  pain sensitivity of, 65
  sclerosis of, *48, 49*
Facet tropism, definition of, 63
Facial pain, atypical, trigeminal neuralgia
    vs., 191
Fainting. See *Syncope.*
Fallopian tubes, abscess of. See *Tubal
    abscess.*
  secretions of, 310
Fascia lata, contracted, pelvic tilting and,
    50
Fat absorption, physiologic processes
    responsible for, 138–139
  stages of, 138, *138*
Fat digestion, stages of, 138, *138*
Fat pads, painful, and knee pain, 232
  swelling in, location of, *236,* 236t
  tenderness in, location of, 236, 236t
Fecal leukocytes, bacterial causes of, 103
  in diagnosis of acute diarrhea, 103–104
  staining for, 103, *104*
Feldene, for low back pain, 22t
Femoral condyle, aseptic necrosis of,
    swelling in, localization of, *236*
  lateral, palpation of, 225
  location of, *268*
  medial, palpation of, 224
  osteonecrosis of, description of, 237–238,
    238
Femoral epicondyle, palpation of, 224–225

Femoral neuropathy, peripheral nerve lesions and, 32
Fenoprofen calcium, for low back pain, 22t
Fever, acute severe chest pain with, 732
  headache with, 175, 177
  low back pain with, 54
  urinary symptoms with, 375–377, 375
Fibrositis, and chest-wall pain, 699
  and shoulder pain, 401–402
Fibula, head of, location of, 268
Fiorinal, for headache, 202, 211
Fistula test, in diagnosis of dizziness, 462
Fitz-Hugh-Curtis syndrome, and acute right upper quadrant pain, 570t, 575
Flagyl, for vaginal trichomoniasis, 324–325, 328t
Flexeril, for low back pain, 21
Flexion, of back, 8
  of lumbar spine, 7
Flexor muscle group, location of, 64
Flip sign, in diagnosis of low back pain, 12, 12, 52
Floor touch test, in diagnosis of chronic low back pain, 52, 52
Fludrocortisone acetate (Florinef), for orthostatic hypotension, 477t, 479
Fluid(s), oral replacement of, 109, 109t
Fluid wave sign, in examination of knee, 222, 222
Fluorescent treponemal antibody absorption, for detection of syphilis, 379
Fluoride, for osteoporosis, 59
Folic acid, for tropical sprue, 142
Food(s), and headache, 183
Food intolerance, types of, 150
Food poisoning, 148–150
  and acute diarrhea, 103, 148–150
Foot, motor functions of, 29, 30
  nerve supply of, 29, 30
Foraminal narrowing, 48, 49
Fortification spectra, in classic migraine, 186, 187
Fox-Fordyce disease, and vulvar pruritus, 336
Frozen shoulder, diagnosis of, 423
  exercise therapy for, 423
  treatment of, 423
FTA-ABS, for detection of syphilis, 379
Fungal infection, and acute pyelonephritis, 302
Furamide, for parasitic diarrhea, 117t
Furosemide, and orthostatic hypotension, 477t
  for altitude headache, 182
Fusobacterium nucleatum, and Vincent's angina, 73

Gaenslen's test, 13–14, 13
Gallbladder, carcinoma of, and chronic upper abdominal pain, 610t–611t
  disease of, site of pain in, 599
  ultrasound of, in diagnosis of chronic upper abdominal pain, 606
Gallium scan, diagnostic, for low back pain, 18t
  for vertebral osteomyelitis, 54
Gallstones, and abdominal pain, 552
  and acute cholecystitis, 572
  and chest pain, 693
Gamma benzene hexachloride, for genital infestations, 334, 346t

Gardnerella, clue cells of, 319, 323
  cultures for, in diagnosis of vaginitis, indications for, 320t, 323
Gardnerella vaginalis, and vaginitis, 316t, 317
  nonspecific, 337
  appearance of, 318
  cultures for, 338
  sexual transmission of, 337
  symptoms of infection with, 316t, 318
Gardnerella vaginitis. See Gardnerella vaginalis.
Gargles, for pharyngitis, 79
Gastrectomy, and lactose intolerance, 119
Gastric carcinoma, and chronic upper abdominal pain, 595t, 596, 598
Gastric hypersecretion, small-bowel resection and, 154
Gastritis. See Duodenitis.
Gastrocolostomy, and postoperative diarrhea, 152
Gastroenteritis, food-borne, diagnosis of, 149t
Gastroileostomy, and postoperative diarrhea, 152
Gastrointestinal disorders, and low back pain, 3t
Gastroparesis diabeticorum, and chronic upper abdominal pain, 610t–611t
Gelusil, for duodenal ulcer, 620t
Genitalia, examination of, in diagnosis of abdominal pain, 548
  female, bulges of, 316
    bumps of, 314
    infestations of, 334
    normal external, 313
    rashes of, 334–336
  male, bumps of, 343, 344, 344t
    infestations of, 343, 346, 346, 346t
    normal external, 342
    rashes of, 345, 345t
    ulcerations of, 342, 343, 343t
Genitourinary infection(s), 341–385. See also Urinary tract infection(s).
  reasons for urologic consultation in, 372–373, 372t
  signs of, 342–349
  symptoms of, 342–349
Gentian violet, topical, for vaginal candidiasis, 328
Genu recurvatum, and monoarthritis of knee, 259t
Giardia lamblia, and chronic diarrhea, 122
  and parasitic diarrhea, 117t
Giardiasis, and lactose intolerance, 119
  gastric surgery and, 153
Gingivostomatitis, necrotizing ulcerative, 73, 73
Glaucoma, acute, and headache, 170, 170t, 178t, 184
Glenohumeral joint, degenerative arthritis of, 404
  dislocation of, hand pain with, 426
  exercise therapy for, 418–421, 419, 420
  motion of, assessment of, 396–397, 396
  sepsis of, 391
  subluxation of, apprehension test for, 424, 424
Glenohumeral mechanism, analysis of, 442–444
  during shoulder abduction, 442–443
Glossopharyngeal neuralgia, and chronic sore throat, 92
  trigeminal neuralgia vs., 190
Gluten-restricted diet, 156, 157t

Glycosuria, in diagnosis of abdominal pain, 554
Goiter, and episodic chest pain, 710
Gonococcal infection, and monoarthritis of knee, 259t
  and pelvic inflammatory disease, 312, 562
Gonococcemia, disseminated, and fever, 377
  untreated gonorrhea and, 356
Gonococcus, penicillin resistance to, 382–383
Gonorrhea. See also Urethritis, gonococcal.
  and urethral syndrome, 276
  and urethritis, 349
  cultures for, follow-up, 355–356
    in diagnosis of acute proctitis, 145
    in diagnosis of vaginitis, 320–321, 323
  treatment of, 354t, 345t
Gout, and monoarthritis of knee, 259t
  and shoulder pain, 405t
  synovial fluid analysis of, 258
Gram's stain, in diagnosis of urethritis, 350–352, 351
  in sputum, in diagnosis of bacterial pneumonia, 652–655, 653
Gravity traction, for disc herniation, 40
Groin, rashes of, 343, 345, 345t
Guanethidine, and orthostatic hypotension, 477t
Guillain-Barré syndrome, and orthostatic hypotension, 477t
Gynecologic disorders, and low back pain, 3t
Gyne-Lotrimin, for vaginal candidiasis, 327, 328t
  for vaginal trichomoniasis in pregnancy, 325
Gynergen, for migraine, 204t

Hailey-Hailey disease, and vulvar pruritus, 336
Haloprogin (Halotex), for erythrasma, 335
  for tinea cruris, 335
Hamstring muscles, medial, palpation of, 225
Hamstring tendons, lateral, palpation of, 225
Hand, motor weakness of, 435, 436t, 437t, 438t
Head, structures of, 72
Head trauma, and vertigo, 494t
Headache, 164–215. See also specific types.
  acute, 165–175
    causes of, 178–181, 178t, 179t
    classification of, 165t
    clinical analysis of, 166
    diagnostic approach to, 180
    homonymous hemianopia with, 179t
    ophthalmoplegia with, 179t
    pupillary asymmetry with, 179t
    timing of, 166
    visual loss with, 178t
  altitude and, 182
  arteriosclerotic, diagnosis of, 174
  chronic, 184–196
    characteristics of, 185t
    diagnostic approach to, 183, 196
    tension vs. migraine, 184–185
  cluster. See Cluster headache.
  coital, 182
  diagnostic tests in, 196–202
    sensitivity/reassurance value of, 198t

Headache (Continued)
  drug-induced, 182–183
  effort, 182
  emotional conflicts and, 201
  exertional, 182
  fever with, 175, 177
  hypertension and, 174
  infectious, diagnosis of, 175
  in special circumstances, 181–184
  in the elderly, 173–175, 173t
  low back pain and, 54
  lumbar puncture and, 181–182
  metabolic causes of, 197t
  migraine. See Migraine.
  neoplasm and, 174
  new. See Headache, acute.
  nocturnal, 183–184
  ocular, 169–173
    causes of, 170, 170t
  orgasmic, 182
  otologic causes of, 177
  paroxysmal, 182
  periorbital, 171
  photophobia with, 171
  physical examination of, 176–181
  post-traumatic, 172–173, 172t
  progressive, 186
  recurrent. See Headache, chronic.
  selected patients with, diagnosis of, 200t
  sleep, 183–184
  stiff neck with, 175
  systemic causes of, 175t, 197t
  tension. See Tension headache.
Hearing loss, cochlear vs. retrocochlear,
    523
  conductive vs. sensorineural, 519
  tests for, bedside, 519–522, 520
    technologic, 522–523
Heart, bypass surgery of, 718
Heart failure, congestive, and cough, 631
Heart rate, recording of, 723
Heartburn, esophagitis and, 766
Heat, topical, for low back pain, 21
Heavy metals, and acute cerebellar disease,
    466
  and food poisoning, 149t
Hedge clipper maneuver, in diagnosis of
    chest-wall syndromes, 701, 702
Hemarthrosis, in knee injury, causes of,
    245t
  effusion vs., 245
Hematologic disorders, and chronic
    abdominal pain, 604
Hematoma, epidural, symptoms of, 172
  subdural, diagnosis of, 173, 174
Hematuria, microscopic, in diagnosis of
    abdominal pain, 551
Hemicrania, chronic paroxysmal, cluster
    headache vs., 188
Hemophilus ducreyi, and genital
    ulcerations, 343t
Hemophilus influenzae, and bacterial
    pneumonia, 645, 649t, 661
  treatment of, 662t
  and epiglottitis, 84
  and peritonsillar abscess, 83
Hemophilus vaginalis. See Gardnerella
    vaginalis.
Hemoptysis, 642–643
  acute pleuritic chest pain with, 745
  causes of, 642t
  history in, 642
  physical examination of, 643
Hemorrhage, cerebellar, and severe
    headache, 169

Hemorrhage (Continued)
  cerebellar, anticoagulants and, 169
    symptoms of, 168
  intracranial, and headache, 166–169
  subarachnoid, and severe headache, 167,
    168
    symptoms of, 167–168
Hepatic congestion, and nonpleuritic chest
    pain, 729t
  and right upper quadrant pain, 570t
Hepatic flexure syndrome, and chronic
    upper abdominal pain, 610t–611t
Hepatitis, and right upper quadrant pain,
    570t
Hepatocellular adenoma, and chronic
    upper abdominal pain, 610t–611t
Hepatocellular carcinoma, and chronic
    upper abdominal pain, 610t–611t
Hernia(s), and bowel obstruction, 546
  and chronic lower abdominal pain, 587t
  location of, 546
  strangulation of, 546
    and acute right lower quadrant pain,
      560t–561t
  types of, 546, 546
Herpangina, symptoms of, 73
Herpes, and urethritis, 358
Herpes genitalis, diagnosis of, 343t
  location of lesions of, 342
  treatment of, 343t
Herpes simplex, diagnosis of, 343t
  genital, 314
    recurrent, 315
    symptoms of, 314–315
  peritonsillar abscess vs., 73
  streptococcal tonsillitis vs., 73
  symptoms of, 73, 74
  treatment of, 343t
Herpes zoster, and chest-wall pain, 699
  and low back pain, 3t
Heterophil agglutination test, in diagnosis
    of mononucleosis, 75
High-fiber diet, 156
High-fiber foods, 156t
High ten maneuver, in diagnosis of chest-
    wall syndromes, 700, 701
Hip disorders, pelvic tilting and, 50
Hip flexor stretch, in therapy of low back
    pain, 23t
Holter monitor, in diagnosis of chest pain,
    705t
Home therapy, in treatment of low back
    pain, 20–29
Homonymous hemianopia, acute headache
    with, 179t
Homosexuals, male, diarrhea in, 102, 145–
    147
  pharyngitis in, 90
  proctitis in, acute, 145–147
  urethritis in, diagnosis of, 353
  venereal enteric infections in, 102
Hooking maneuver, in diagnosis of chest-
    wall syndromes, 700, 701
Hoover test, for chronic low back pain, 52,
    53
Hormonal therapy, for endometriosis, 587t,
    588
Horner's syndrome, and acute headache,
    179t
Hospitalization, for acute dysentery, 112
  for acute pyelonephritis, 286, 287t, 300
  for angina pectoris, 725–726
  for chronic diarrhea, 129, 142–143, 143
  for diphtheria, 86
  for gastric ulcer, 623

Hospitalization (Continued)
  for low back pain, 20
  for Ludwig's angina, 89
  for peripheral vestibular disease, 498
  for pneumonia, 657–660, 658t
  for pulmonary embolism, 752–753
Humerus, anterior dislocation of, 448
  aseptic necrosis of, and shoulder pain,
    405t, 406
Humidification, for acute bronchitis, 639
Hycodan, for acute bronchitis, 639t
Hycomine, for acute bronchitis, 639t
Hydrophilic colloid preparation, for
    irritable bowel syndrome, 584, 586t
Hydralazine, and headache, 182
  and orthostatic hypotension, 477t
Hydrarthrosis, and monoarthritis of knee,
    259t
Hydrocele, testicular, 348
Hydrocephalus, and acute headache, 179t
Hydrocodone, for acute bronchitis, 638–
    639, 639t
Hydronephrosis, bilateral, vesicoureteral
    reflux and, 279
Hyperabduction maneuver, in diagnosis of
    thoracic outlet syndrome, 452, 452
Hyperabduction syndrome, 452
Hyperplastic dystrophy, and vulvar
    pruritus, 335
Hypertension, and headache, 174
  intracranial, and acute headache, 178t
  pulmonary, and syncope, 485t
Hyperthyroidism, and chronic low back
    pain, 43
Hypertrophy, asymmetric septal, and
    syncope, 485t
  right ventricular, exertional angina with,
    709
Hyperventilation, acute, symptoms of, 503,
    503t
  and light-headedness, 503–508
  and syncope, 472t
  breathing exercises for, 506
  chronic, causes of, 504
    symptoms of, 503–504, 503t
  emotional stress and, 507
  organic diseases vs., 504
  treatment of, 506
  voluntary, in diagnosis of dizziness, 461
    in diagnosis of light-headedness, 505
Hypoaldosteronism, and orthostatic
    hypotension, 477t
Hypochondriasis, and chest pain, 770–771
  and hyperventilation, 507
Hypogastric pain, causes of, 530
Hypoglycemia, and disequilibrium, 465,
    468t
  and light-headedness, 504
  and syncope, 482t, 483
  episodic, and acute headache, 178t
Hypoglycemic agents, oral, and headache,
    182
Hypophosphatemia, and spinal disease, 58t
Hypotension, acute, severe chest pain with,
    731
  orthostatic, 477t, 478–480
    and syncope, 472t
    causes of, 477t, 479
    dehydration and, 102
    elastic stockings for, 477t, 479
    intravascular volume depletion and,
      477t, 479
    neurologic diseases and, 477t
    salt supplements for, 477t, 479
    signs of, 478

Hypotension (Continued)
  orthostatic, treatment of, 477t, 479–480
  postural. See Hypotension, orthostatic.
Hypothyroidism, and carpal tunnel
    syndrome, 434
  and disequilibrium, 465, 468t
Hysteria, and hyperventilation, 507

Ibuprofen, for low back pain, 22t
  for migraine, 203
  for primary dysmenorrhea, 585
Ileal resection, and postoperative diarrhea,
    153
Iliac crest biopsy, in diagnosis of
    osteopenia, 59
Iliacus muscle, location of, 64
Iliolumbar ligament, location of, 64
Iliotibial band, contracted, pelvic tilting
    and, 50
  location of, 227
  palpation of, 227
Iliotibial band syndrome, and knee pain,
    232
  swelling in, location of, 236, 236t
Ilozyme, for pancreatic enzyme
    replacement, 158t
Impingement syndrome, diagnosis of, 423
Inderal, for angina pectoris, 716t
Indomethacin (Indocin), and headache, 182
  for low back pain, 22t
  for migraine, 203
  for orthostatic hypotension, 447t, 480
  for primary dysmenorrhea, 585
Influenza, and nonbacterial pneumonia,
    646t, 647
Inguinal adenopathy, diagnosis of, 344t
  location of, 344
  treatment of, 344t
Interspinal ligaments, location of, 63
Intertrigo, and vulvar pruritus, 336
Intervertebral foramina, location of, 62
Intestines, biopsy of, in diagnosis of lactose
    intolerance, 119
  mucosal disorders of, 139, 140
  obstruction of, causes of, 543t
    low vs. high, 543t
Intoxication, and acute cerebellar disease,
    466
  and disequilibrium, 465
Intracranial mass lesions, tension headache
    vs., 210
Intrahepatic abscess, and acute pleuritic
    chest pain, 743t
Intranephric abscess, and acute
    pyelonephritis, 302
Iritis, and headache, 170, 170t, 178t
Irritable bowel syndrome, 583–585
  and chronic lower abdominal pain, 586t
  clinical findings in, 125–126
  colorectal cancer vs., 584
  diagnosis of, 125
  diverticular disease vs., 584
  history in, 583
  inflammatory bowel disease vs., 584
  lactose intolerance vs., 584
  physical examination of, 583
  symptoms of, 125, 583
  tests for, 586t
  treatment of, presumptive, 584, 586t
Ischemia, cardiac, and syncope, 484, 485t
  transient, and acute headache, 178t, 179t
  vertebrobasilar, and syncope, 476, 482t,
    483

Ischial tuberosity, and low back pain, 10
Ischium, bursitis of, 9–10
  sciatica vs., 35
Isoetharine, for acute bronchitis, 640t
Isometric exercises, for chondromalacia,
    240
  for patellofemoral syndromes, 239
Isoniazid, and shoulder pain, 393
Isoproterenol, for acute bronchitis, 640t
Isoptin, for angina pectoris, 718t
Isordil, for angina pectoris, 715t
Isosorbide dinitrate, for angina pectoris,
    714–715, 715t
Isotonic exercises, for chondromalacia, 241
  types of, 241
Isuprel, for acute bronchitis, 640t

Jarisch-Herxheimer reaction, and fever, 377
Joint(s), amphiarthrodial, location of, 61
  glenohumeral. See Glenohumeral joint.
  hypermobile, and monoarthritis of knee,
    259t
  patellofemoral, function of, 265
  sacroiliac, x-rays of, 46
  shoulder, 441
  tibiofemoral, function of, 265
    plane motion of, 268
    screw home motion of, 268–269, 269
Jumper's knee, and knee pain, 233t, 234
  swelling in, localization of, 236

Keflex, for epididymitis, 347
  for urinary tract infections, 286t
Kenalog, for aphthous stomatitis, 74
Kenny-Howard sling, for dislocation of the
    acromioclavicular joint, 449
Keratosis follicularis, and vulvar pruritus,
    336
Kernig's sign, in diagnosis of meningitis,
    177
Ketonuria, in diagnosis of abdominal pain,
    554
Kidney. See also under Renal.
  neoplasms of, and referred shoulder
    pain, 392
  ultrasound examination of, in diagnosis
    of acute pyelonephritis, 302
Kidney stones, and abdominal pain, 553
Klebsiella, and female urinary tract
    infections, 289
Klebsiella pneumoniae, and bacterial
    pneumonia, 648, 648t
Knee, anatomy of, functional, 265–270
  internal, 268–270, 268
  buckling of, 219
  bursae of, swellings of, 229
  clicking of, 218, 219
  deformities of, 221
  effusion of. See Knee, swelling of.
  extensor mechanism of, function of, 265,
    265
  flexion of, description of, 269
  inspection of, 222
  locking of, 218, 219
    manipulation of, 254
  palpation of, orientation points for, 224
  physical examination of, 221–229
  range of motion of, 222–223, 223
    testing of, 249
  structures of, lateral, 226
    medial, 225
    palpable, 224–229

Knee (Continued)
  swelling of, aspiration techniques in, 256
    clinical approach to, 255–256
    diagnostic approach to, 257
    intra-articular, 222, 222
    localized, 229–232, 236, 236t
    synovial fluid analysis of, 256–258, 259t
  tenderness in, localized, 229–232, 236,
    236t
Knee pain, 216–271
  age of patient in diagnosis of, 219
  associated symptoms in, 218–219
  degenerative conditions and, 220
  disorders of meniscus and, 219
  disorders of patella and, 219
  history in, 216–221, 220
  inflammatory conditions and, 220
  mechanical use and, 216–217
  nonmechanical, 217–218, 217
  patellofemoral syndromes and, 219
  referred, 217
  traumatic, 241–254
    diagnostic approach to, 252
    effusion vs. hemarthrosis in, 245
    extensor apparatus disruption and, 243
    hemarthrosis and, 243
    immediate treatment for, 252
    ligament damage and, 242
    torn meniscus and, 242
Knee pain syndromes, swelling in,
    localization of, 236, 236t
  tenderness in, localization of, 236, 236t
KOH preparation, in diagnosis of Candida,
    319, 319
Kwell, for genital infestations, 334, 346t
  for scabies, 334
Kyphoscoliosis, pelvic tilting and, 50
Kyphosis, lumbar, angular, 9

Labyrinthine apoplexy, and vertigo, 494t
Labyrinthine disease, and disequilibrium,
    464
Labyrinthitis, acute, nystagmus in, 514
  and vertigo, 488t, 489, 494t, 497
  drug-induced, 497
  trauma and, 497
Lactose, avoidance of, for acute diarrhea,
    109
  foods containing, 156t
  tolerance test for, 119–120, 120
Lactose intolerance, acute diarrhea with,
    109
  causes of, 119
  diagnosis of, 119–120
  gastric surgery and, 153
  irritable bowel syndrome vs., 584
  symptoms of, 119
Lactose-free diet, for acute diarrhea, 120,
    156
Laguerre's test, 13, 13
Laparoscopy, in diagnosis of endometriosis,
    588
Laparotomy, in diagnosis of endometriosis,
    588
Laryngoscopy, in diagnosis of complicated
    sore throat, 90
Lateral flexion, in testing range of motion
    of, 8
Laxatives, abuse of, and diarrhea, 102, 122
LDH isoenzymes, in diagnosis of
    myocardial infarction, 740
L-Dopa and orthostatic hypotension, 477t
  for Parkinson's disease, 468

Leg(s), measuring length of, *50*
  practical neurology of, 29–34
  unequal length of, pelvic tilting and, 50
Legionella pneumophila, and bacterial
    pneumonia, 649, *650*
Legionnaires' disease, and bacterial
    pneumonia, 649t, *650*
Leukocytosis, abdominal pain with, 555–
    556
  acute severe chest pain with, 735
  appendicitis with, 564
Leukopenia, metronidazole and, 325
Leukoplakia, and vulvar pruritus, 335
Levine's sign, in diagnosis of angina
    pectoris, 683, *683*
Librax, for irritable bowel syndrome, 584,
    586t
Lice, pubic, and pruritus, 334, *346*
Lichen planus, and vulvar pruritus, 336
  diagnosis of, 344t
  treatment of, 344t
Lichen sclerosus et atrophicus, and vulvar
    pruritus, 335
Lidocaine, for aphthous stomatitis, 75
Ligament(s), knee, function of, 270, *270*
  injury to, description of, 243–244
    diagnosis of, 251t
    mechanisms of, *243*
    tests for, *247,* 248–249
    location of, 268
    severe sprain of, *244*
  longitudinal, location of, 63
  sacroiliac, location of, 64
  sacrospinal, location of, 64
  sacrotuberal, location of, 64
  spinal, location of, 64
    pain sensitivity of, 65
  supraspinal, location of, 63
Ligamentum flavum, location of, 63
Light-headedness, 502, 508
  definition of, 458
  differential diagnosis of, 502
  exertional, 504
  postural, 504
  presyncope vs., 502
  simulation testing for, 502, 505
Lincomycin, and diarrhea of
    pseudomembranous colitis, 102
Lipid profile, in diagnosis of chest pain,
    705t
Lithium, for cluster headache, 189
Liver enzymes, in diagnosis of chronic
    upper abdominal pain, 607
Locomotion, human, components of, 463,
    464
  integrative mechanism of, 463, *464*
Lomotil, for irritable bowel syndrome, 584
Lopressor, for angina pectoris, 716t
Lordosis, lumbar, *6*
Lotrimin, for erythrasma, 335
  for tinea cruris, 335
Low back stretch, in therapy of low back
    pain, 23t
Lower extremity, nerve supply of, 29, *30*
  sensory loss in, 32
Ludwig's angina, 88–89
  surgical drainage for, 89
Lumbar disc disease, long-term results in
    treatment of, 40t
Lumbar puncture, in diagnosis of
    headache, 196–197
  in diagnosis of subarachnoid hemorrhage,
    168
Lumbar puncture headache, 181–182

Lumbar spine, facets in, *64*
  lordosis of, *6*
Lumbar vertebrae, functional unit of, *61*
  location of, 61
Lumbosacral radiculopathy, and knee pain,
    217
Lumbosacral root disease, disc herniation
    and, 12
Lumbosacral spine, location of, 61–65
  palpable structures of, *8*
  x-ray of, abnormal, in diagnosis of
    chronic low back pain, 46t
    normal, in diagnosis of chronic low
    back pain, 44t
Lumbosacral spondylosis, in the elderly,
    12–13
Lumbosacral vertebrae, compression
    fractures of, 57–58
Lung. See also under *Pulmonary.*
  neoplasms of, and referred shoulder
    pain, 392
  topography of, *633*
Lung scan, in diagnosis of chest pain, 705t
  in diagnosis of pulmonary embolism, 752,
    772–779
  interpretation of, 772–774, 778–779,
    778t, 779t
  perfusion, results of, 776t
  types of, 776–778
  ventilation, indications for, 777–778
    results of, 777t
Lupus erythematosus, and acute pleuritic
    chest pain, 743t
  and pharyngeal ulcers, 75
  synovial analysis of, 258
Lymphangiectasia, intestinal, and lactose
    intolerance, 119
Lymphocytosis, atypical, in patients with
    mononucleosis, 75
Lymphogranuloma venereum, and genital
    ulcerations, 343t
Lymphomas, systemic, and low back pain,
    56

Maalox, for duodenal ulcer, 620t
Macrodantin, for female urinary tract
    infections, 286t
Malabsorption, and chronic low back pain,
    43
  diagnostic approach to, *141*
  indications of, 135
  screening tests for, 135–137
Malingering, and hyperventilation, 507
  and low back pain, 52
Mandelamine, for female urinary tract
    infections, 286t
MAO inhibitors, and orthostatic
    hypotension, 477t
Marezine, for vertigo, 499t
McBurney's point, in diagnosis of
    appendicitis, 564
McMurray test, in diagnosis of knee pain,
    224, 249, *250*
Measles, and nonbacterial pneumonia, 647t
Mebendazole, for parasitic diarrhea, 117t
Meckel's diverticulum, and chronic lower
    abdominal pain, 592t–593t
Meclizine, for vertigo, 499t
Meclofenamate sodium (Meclomen), for
    low back pain, 22t
Median nerve, lesions of, and shoulder
    pain, 433, 433t

Median nerve *(Continued)*
  peripheral entrapment of, *434*
Medrol Dosepak, for periarticular shoulder
    disorders, 418
Mefenamic acid, for primary
    dysmenorrhea, 585
Mellaril, for tension headache, 211
Meniere's disease, and vertigo, 494t, 495–
    496
Meningeal carcinomatosis, and low back
    pain, 56
Meningeal infiltration, in cancer patient, 56
Meningismus, absence of, 177
  headache with, 175
  signs of, 177
Meningitis, and headache, 175, 177–178
  and low back pain, 54
  and meningismus, 175, 177
  types of, 175
  viral, lumbar puncture in diagnosis of,
    179–181
Meniscus(i), anatomy of, *246*
  cysts of, description of, 231–232
    location of, *231*
    swelling in, location of, *236,* 236t
    tenderness in, location of, *236,* 236t
  disorders of, and knee pain, 219
  function of, 269
  injury to, description of, 244–245
    diagnosis of, 251t
    mechanisms of, *245*
    rotatory tests for, 249, *250*
    surgical exploration of, 253
  location of, *265, 268*
  medial, palpation of, 224
  tears of, examples of, *246*
    swelling in, location of, *236,* 236t
    tenderness in, location of, *236,* 236t
  tibiofemoral rotatory testing of, 223–224
Menopause, and vulvovaginal disorders,
    312
Mental status, impairment of, low back
    pain and, 54
  testing of, of headache patient, 176t
Meprobamate, for tension headache, 211
Meralgia paresthetica, peripheral nerve
    lesions and, 32
Mesenteric ischemia, and severe central
    abdominal pain, 615
  causes of, 615
  symptoms of, 615
Metabolic bone disease, and chronic low
    back pain, 43
Metabolic disturbances, and disequilibrium,
    465, 468t
Metamucil, for chronic diarrhea, 134t
  for diverticulosis, 590
  for irritable bowel syndrome, 584, 586t
Metaproterenol (Metaprel), for acute
    bronchitis, 640t
Methicillin, for bacterial pneumonia, 648t
Methocarbamol, for low back pain, 21
Methyldopa, reserpine and orthostatic
    hypotension, 477t
Methylphenidate hydrochloride, for
    orthostatic hypotension, 480
Methysergide, for cluster headache, 189
  for migraine, 206t
Metoclopramide, for esophagitis, 767t
Metoprolol tartrate, for angina pectoris,
    716t
Metronidazole, and leukopenia, 325
  for chronic diarrhea, 133, 134t
  for *Gardnerella vaginalis,* 337

Metronidazole (Continued)
  for giardiasis, 117
  for parasitic diarrhea, 117t
  for trichomonas infection, 360
    vaginal, 324–325, 328t
Miconazole nitrate, for erythrasma, 335
  for tinea cruris, 335
  for vaginal candidiasis, 327, 328t
Midodrine, for orthostatic hypotension,
    477t, 480
Midrin, for migraine, 203
Migraine, basilar, 187
  characteristics of, 185t
  classic, 186–187
    prodomes of, 186–187
    vertebrobasilar symptoms of, 187
  cluster headache vs., 188
  common, characteristics of, 192t
    locations of, 192
    symptoms of, 193
    tension headache vs., 191–196
  complicated, 187
  endogenous triggers of, 203
  exogenous triggers of, 203
  hemiplegic, 187
  intractable, hospitalization for, 207
  nonpharmacologic therapy for, 202–203
  ophthalmoplegic, 187
  pharmacologic therapy for, 203–209
  prophylactic therapy for, 205–209, 206t
  status, treatment for, 207
  symptomatic treatment of, 203–205
  treatment of, 202–209
  types of, 185t
  typical calendar of, 194t
Migral, for migraine, 204t
Minocycline, for chronic prostatitis, 371t
  for nongonococcal urethritis, 358, 358t
Minoxidil, and orthostatic hypotension,
    477t
Mitral valve prolapse, and chest pain, 696
  and orthostatic hypotension, 477t
  systolic murmurs in, 704t
Mittelschmerz, and acute right lower
    quadrant pain, 560t
  and chronic lower abdominal pain, 587t
Molluscum contagiosum, 314, 315
  diagnosis of, 344t
  location of, 344
  treatment of, 344t
Mondor's syndrome, and chest-wall pain,
    699–700
Monistat, for erythrasma, 335
  for tinea cruris, 335
  for vaginal candidiasis, 327, 328t
Monoamine oxidase inhibitors, and
    headache, 183
Monoarthritis, of knee, 258–264
  causes of, 259t
  chronic infection in, 262
  crystalline disorders and, 259t
  differential diagnosis of, 255t
  mechanical disorders and, 259t, 264
  symptoms of, 258
  systemic diseases and, 259t
Mononucleosis, and bilateral tonsillar
    swelling, 84
  bacterial tonsillitis vs., 84
  infectious, and recurrent sore throat, 92
    symptoms of, 75
    treatment of, 76
Monosodium glutamate, and food
    poisoning, 149t
Monospot test, in diagnosis of infectious
    mononucleosis, 75

Motrin, for dysmenorrhea, 590
  for low back pain, 22t
  for migraine, 203
  for primary dysmenorrhea, 585
Mouth, structures of, 72
Mouthwashes, for Vincent's angina, 73
Multifidis muscle, location of, 64
Multiple myeloma, headache patient with,
    198
Multiple sclerosis, and acute headache,
    179t
Murphy's sign, in diagnosis of acute
    cholecystitis, 572
Muscle(s). See also specific muscles.
  spinal, location of, 64
    pain sensitivity of, 65
Muscle groups, of lower extremity, nerve
    supply of, 29
Muscle relaxants, for low back pain, 21
Muscle spasm, paravertebral, palpable, 9,
    10
Muscle weakness, and chronic low back
    pain, 50–51
  and disequilibrium, 464
Muscular dystrophy, and referred shoulder
    pain, 393
Mushroom toxin, and food poisoning, 149t
Mycelex-G, for vaginal candidiasis, 327,
    328t
Mycobacterium tuberculosis, and cough,
    656
Mycolog, for vaginal candidiasis, 328
Mycoplasma infections, and acute
    bronchitis, 637
Mycoplasma pneumoniae, and pneumonia,
    645, 646, 646t
Mycostatin, for oral candidiasis, 75
  for vaginal candidiasis, 327, 328t
Myelitis, acute transverse, and low back
    pain, 55
  and shoulder pain, 392
Myelography, diagnostic, for disc
    herniation, 41
  for epidural abscess, 54
  for epidural metastases, 56
  for low back pain, 18t
  for spinal stenosis, 49, 49
Mylanta-II, for duodenal ulcer, 620t
Myocardial infarction, and nonpleuritic
    chest pain, 728t
  and syncope, 484, 485t
  anterior, and acute severe chest pain,
    734, 735
  diagnostic tests for, 740
  inferior, and acute severe chest pain, 733
  prior, and episodic chest pain, 707
  subendocardial, and acute severe chest
    pain, 736
Myocardial perfusion imaging, in diagnosis
    of chest pain, 763
Myodynia, and chest-wall pain, 699
Myomas, uterine and chronic low back
    pain, 43
Myopathies, inflammatory, and referred
    shoulder pain, 393

Nadolol, for angina pectoris, 716t
Nafcillin, for bacterial pneumonia, 648t
  for Ludwig's angina, 89
Nalfon, for low back pain, 22t
Nalidixic acid, for female urinary tract
    infections, 286

Naprosyn, for low back pain, 22t
  for primary dysmenorrhea, 585
Naproxen, for low back pain, 22t
  for primary dysmenorrhea, 585
Narcotics, for low back pain, 21
  for periarticular shoulder disorders, 417
  for status migraine, 207
Nasopharyngeal carcinoma, and acute
    headache, 179t
  trigeminal neuralgia vs., 191
Nausea, acute severe chest pain with, 731
Necator americanus, and parasitic diarrhea,
    117t
Neck, abscesses of, deep, and headache,
    177
  asymmetric adenopathy of, 83
  disorders of, and referred shoulder pain,
    388
  range of motion of, 390, 403
  structures of, 72
Neck traction, for cervical spine disease,
    700
Needle aspiration, for vertebral
    osteomyelitis, 54, 55
Neisseria gonorrhoeae, and pelvic
    inflammatory disease, 562
  and pharyngitis, 90
Neisseria meningitidis, and pharyngitis, 90
  and pneumonia, 645
Neoplasm(s), and acute pleuritic chest
    pain, 743t
  and chronic low back pain, 43
  and headache, 174, 179t, 200
  and pharyngeal ulcers, 75
  metastatic, and monoarthritis of knee,
    264
  nasopharyngeal, and headache, 177
  of pelvic bones, 9
Nerve(s), conduction studies of, in
    diagnosis of disc herniation, 42
  dorsal scapular, entrapment of, 400
  peripheral. See Peripheral nerves.
  suprascapular, entrapment of, 400
Nerve roots, anatomical course of, 33
  cervical, and shoulder pain, 431–435
  compression of, and shoulder/hand
    syndromes, 428
    spondylosis and, 47
  lesions of, and knee pain, 217
    and shoulder pain, 432t, 433
    motor examination for, 29–31
    neurologic findings in, 31t
    single vs. multiple, 29–31
Neuralgia, cranial, characteristics of, 185t
  glossopharyngeal, and syncope, 472t
  postherpetic, trigeminal neuralgia vs.,
    190
  prepatellar. See Prepatellar neuralgia.
  trigeminal, cluster headache vs., 188, 190
Neuritis, brachial, and shoulder/hand
    syndrome, 430
  optic, and headache, 170, 170t, 178t
Neurogenic claudication, aortoiliac vascular
    claudication vs., 49
Neurologic abnormalities, with headache,
    176–177
Neuronitis, vestibular, and vertigo, 488t,
    489, 494t, 497
Neuropathy(ies), and acute headache, 178t
  peripheral, and disequilibrium, 464, 468t
Neurosurgeon, referral to, 53
NGU. See Urethritis, nongonococcal.
Nifedipine, for angina pectoris, 717, 718t
Nitrates, and orthostatic hypotension, 477t
  for angina pectoris, 713–715, 715t

Nitrates *(Continued)*
  for esophageal spasm, 769
  side effects of, 714, 715t
Nitro-Bid, for angina pectoris, 715t
Nitrofurantoin, for urinary tract infections, 286t, 299
Nitrogen, liquid, for condylomata acuminata, *314,* 344t
Nitroglycerin, for angina pectoris, 713–714, 715t
  for esophageal spasm, 769
  test dose of, 714
Nitro-Disc, for angina pectoris, 715t
Nitro-Dur, for angina pectoris, 715t
Nitrol, for angina pectoris, 715t
Nitrong, for angina pectoris, 715t
Nitrospan, for angina pectoris, 715t
Nitrostat, for angina pectoris, 715t
Nocturnal headache, 183–184
Nonangina, 687–693
  and episodic chest pain, 681
  angina pectoris vs., 680t
  characteristics of, 680t
  description of, 681
  diagnosis of, exercise tests in, 762–763
  duration of, 687
  factors in, precipitating, 687–688
    relieving, 688
  history in, 687–688
  location of pain in, 688
  quality of pain in, 688
  symptoms of, 687–688
  timing of, 687
Norgesic, for headache, 202
Novahistine, for acute bronchitis, 639t
Nuclear tests, in diagnosis of chest pain, 705t
Nucofed, for acute bronchitis, 639t
Nylen-Bárány test, in diagnosis of vestibular disease, 515–516, 515t
Nystagmus, causes of, 512–513
  central, *490, 491*
  evaluation of, 512–515
  extraocular muscle weakness and, 512–513
  pendular, 512
  peripheral, 488, *488, 489*
  positional, 515t
  testing for, 512, *512*
  trauma and, 513
Nystatin, for vaginal candidiasis, 327, 328t

Ober's test, *51*
Obturator sign, in diagnosis of abdominal pain, 547, *547*
Occipital lobe disease, and acute headache, 179t
Occipital neuralgia, trigeminal neuralgia vs., 190
Ocular disease, tension headache vs., 210
Omni-Tuss, for acute bronchitis, 639t
Ophthalmoplegia, acute headache with, 179t
Orchitis, diagnosis of, *348*
Orgasmic headache, 182
Orphenadrine citrate, for headache, 202
Ornithosis, and nonbacterial pneumonia, 647t
Orthopedic disorders, and disequilibrium, 464
Orthopedist, referral to, 53
Orthostatic hypotension. See *Hypotension, orthostatic.*

Osgood-Schlatter's disease, and knee pain, 233t, 234
  swelling in, localization of, *236*
  traction epiphysitis and, *235*
Osteoarthritis, patellofemoral, and knee pain, 233t, 235
Osteoarthropathy, hypertrophic, description of, 237
  diffuse interstitial pneumonitis and, *238*
  swelling in, location of, *236,* 236t
  tenderness in, location of, *236,* 236t
Osteochondritis dissecans, synovial fluid analysis of, 258
Osteomalacia, classification of, 58t
  diagnosis of, 59
  x-rays of, *57*
Osteomyelitis, and monoarthritis of knee, 259t, *261*
  vertebral, and chronic low back pain, 43, 54, *55*
Osteonecrosis, femoral condyle, description of, 237–238
  flattening of inferior border of, *238*
  swelling in, location of, *236,* 236t
  tenderness in, location of, *236,* 236t
Osteopenia, and low back pain, 57–60
  diagnosis of, 59–60
  x-rays of, *57*
Osteophytosis, *48, 49*
Osteoporosis, and low back pain, 57–60
  classification of, 59t
  diagnosis of, 59
Otitis, and vertigo, 494t, 495
Ova, stool examination for, 106, 107t
Ovary, carcinoma of, and acute pleuritic chest pain, *752*
  and acute pyelonephritis, *301*
  and acute right lower quadrant pain, 560t
  and chronic lower abdominal pain, 592t–593t
  cyst on, rupture of, and acute right lower quadrant pain, 560t–561t
Oxacillin, for bacterial pneumonia, 648t
Oxychlorosene sodium, for interstitial cystitis, 292
Oxycodone, for low back pain, 21
Oxygen, for migraine, 203

Pacemaker, for cardiac arrhythmias, 484t
Paget's disease, and shoulder pain, 405t, *406*
  headache patient with, *199*
  x-ray findings in, *45*
Pancoast tumor, and referred shoulder pain, 392
  and shoulder/hand syndrome, 429, *430*
  thoracic outlet syndrome vs., 453
Pancreas, calcifications of, *137*
  carcinoma of, and chronic upper abdominal pain, *607,* 610t–611t
  enzyme replacement in, 134t, 158–159, 158t
  insufficient enzyme activity in, 139
  pseudocyst of, and chronic upper abdominal pain, 610t–611t
Pancrease, for pancreatic enzyme replacement, 158t
Pancreatitis, acute, and chronic upper abdominal pain, 607
  and nonpleuritic chest pain, 729t

Pancreatitis *(Continued)*
  acute, and severe central abdominal pain, 614–615
    causes of, 614t
    symptoms of, 614
  chronic, and chronic upper abdominal pain, 610t–611t
    signs of, 610t
    symptoms of, 610t
    tests for, 611t
    treatment of, 611t
Papaverine, for migraine, 206t
Paraparesis, back manipulation and, 27
Parasellar disease, and acute headache, 179t
Parasites, stool examination for, 106, 107t
Paraspinal structures, palpation of, 8–10
Parkinsonism. See *Parkinson's disease.*
Parkinson's disease, and disequilibrium, 466, 468t
  and orthostatic hypotension, 477t
Parotid tumors, trigeminal neuralgia vs., 191
Paroxysmal headache, 182
Partial sit-up, in therapy of low back pain, 23t
Past pointing, in diagnosis of dizziness, 462–463, *463*
Patella, dislocation of, recurrent, and knee pain, 233t, 235
  disorders of, and knee pain, 219
  function of, *266, 267*
  location of, *265, 268*
  manipulation of, 223, *223*
  muscle pull upon, *266*
  palpation of, 224
  patellofemoral articulation of, *266*
Patellar apprehension test, in diagnosis of knee pain, *235*
Patellar tendinitis, and knee pain, 233t, 235
  swelling in, localization of, *236*
Patella-tendon ratio, measurement of, *267*
Patellofemoral complex, examination of, 224
Patellofemoral syndromes, and knee pain, 223–241, 233t
  causes of, 223
  treatment of, 239–241
Patellotibial tendon, palpation of, 224
Pathogens, enteric, venereal transmission of, 145
Patient, physician relationship with, 672–673
Patrick's test, 13
Pectoralis major syndrome, and chest-wall pain, 702
Pectoralis minor syndrome, and chest-wall pain, 702
Pectoris dolor, 683
Pedicles, location of, 62
Pediculosis pubis, diagnosis of, 346t
  location of, *346*
  treatment of, 346t
Pellegrini-Stieda syndrome, 237
  swelling in, location of, *236,* 236t
  tenderness of medial femoral epicondyle and, *237*
Pelvic bones, and low back pain, 9
Pelvic inflammatory disease, 562–564
  and acute right lower quadrant pain, 560t–561t
  and chronic lower abdominal pain, 592t–593t
  antibiotic treatment for, 312
  causes of, 312, 562

Pelvic inflammatory disease (Continued)
diagnosis of, 563–564
gonococcal vs. nongonococcal, 562–563
signs of, 560t, 592t
symptoms of, 312, 560t, 562, 592t
tests for, 561t, 593t
treatment of, 561t, 563, 593t
Pelvic tilt, in therapy of low back pain, 23t, 50
Pelvis, disease of, and chronic low back pain, 43
disorders of, sciatica vs., 35
examination of, diagnostic, for abdominal pain, 548, 548
for endometriosis, 588
for low back pain, 10
for urinary tract infections, 283
for vulvovaginal disorders, 313
palpable structures of, 8
tilting of, and chronic low back pain, 23t, 50
Pemphigoid, and pharyngeal ulcers, 75
Pemphigus, and pharyngeal ulcers, 75
and vulvar pruritus, 336
Penicillin, for acute proctitis, 146t
for bacterial pneumonia, 648t–649t
for chronic diarrhea, 134t
for diphtheria, 86
for disseminated gonococcemia, 377
for Fitz-Hugh-Curtis syndrome, 575
for gonococcal urethritis, 354, 354t
for Ludwig's angina, 89
for peritonsillar abscess, 83
for pneumococcal pneumonia, 660, 662t
for primary syphilis, 343t
for retropharyngeal abscess, 86
for streptococcal pharyngitis, 80
gonococcal resistance to, 382–383
Penis, carcinoma of, 344, 344t
normal anatomy of, 342
rashes of, 343, 345t
ulcerations of, 342, 343, 343t
venereal edema of, 345t
Pentaerythritol tetranitrate, for angina pectoris, 715t
Pentazocine, for low back pain, 21
Peppermint, for esophageal spasm, 769
Peptic ulcer. See Ulcer, peptic.
Pepto-Bismol, for turista, 151
Percodan, for low back pain, 21
Percussion tenderness, abdominal, 540, 541
Pericardial friction rubs, in diagnosis of pericarditis, 747
Pericardial tamponade, and syncope, 485t
Pericarditis, and acute pleuritic chest pain, 742t, 746–748
and compatible chest pain, 696
and nonpleuritic chest pain, 728t
causes of, 747t
stages of, 746
treatment of, 748
Pericoronitis, symptoms of, 75
Perihepatitis, gonococcal. See Fitz-Hugh-Curtis syndrome.
Perineal sensation, testing of, 31
Perinephric abscess, and acute pyelonephritis, 302
Periodontal infection, symptoms of, 75
Peripheral nerves, anatomical course of, 33
lesions of, and shoulder pain, 402, 433–435, 433t
neurologic findings in, 31t
location of, 434
Peritonitis, and acute abdominal pain, 532
Peritonsillar abscess, and trismus, 82

Peritonsillar abscess (Continued)
complications of, 83
herpes simplex vs., 73
peritonsillar cellulitis vs., 84
symptoms of, 83, 83
treatment of, 83
Peritonsillar cellulitis, diagnosis of, 84
Peritrate, for angina pectoris, 715t
Periumbilical pain, causes of, 530
Periurethral abscess, 360
Peroneal nerve, palpation of, 227
Peroneal nerve entrapment, peripheral nerve lesions and, 32
swelling in, location of, 236, 236t
tenderness in, location of, 236, 236t
Perphenazine, for vertigo, 499t
Pes anserine tendon, palpation of, 225
Phalen sign, in diagnosis of shoulder pain, 428, 433
Pharyngeal cellulitis, diagnosis of, 84
Pharyngitis, bacterial pathogens in, 90
diagnosis of, 71–76
psychogenic, and chronic sore throat, 93
sore throat vs., 71
streptococcal, and rheumatic fever, 80–81, 95–96
definition of, 94–95
diabetic with, 79
diagnosis of, 77–79
duration of, 80
nonstreptococcal pharyngitis vs., 76–79
rheumatic fever with, 79
rheumatic heart disease with, 79
symptoms of, 77, 77t
treatment of, cost vs. benefit of, 95–97
schedule for, 80
symptoms of, 71
treatment of, 79–82
value of, 95–96
uncomplicated, 78
Pharyngotonsillitis, and headache, 177
Pharynx, irritants of, and chronic sore throat, 93
structures of, 72
Phenazopyridine hydrochloride, for symptomatic cystourethritis, 286
Phenergan, for acute bronchitis, 639t
for vertigo, 499t
Phenytoin, for trigeminal neuralgia, 190
Pheochromocytoma, and nocturnal headache, 184
and orthostatic hypotension, 477t
symptoms of, cluster headache vs., 188
Photophobia, headache with, 171
Phthirus pubis, and vulvar pruritus, 334
Physician, patient relationship with, 672–673
PID. See Pelvic inflammatory disease.
Pindolol, for angina pectoris, 716t
Piperacillin, for acute pyelonephritis, 301
Piroxicam, for low back pain, 22t
Pituitary mass lesions, tension headache vs., 210
Pleuritis, idiopathic, and acute pleuritic chest pain, 741–744, 742t
viral, and acute pleuritic chest pain, 741–744, 742t
Plumb line test, in determining pelvic tilt, 50
Pneumocystis carinii, and pneumonia, 645
Pneumoencephalography, in diagnosis of headache, 200
Pneumomediastinum, and acute severe chest pain, 737
and nonpleuritic chest pain, 728t

Pneumonia, adjuvant therapy of, 663–664
and acute pleuritic chest pain, 742t, 748
and nonpleuritic chest pain, 729t
aspiration, and bacterial pneumonia, 649t, 651
auscultatory findings in, 632–634, 634
bacterial, and cough, 648, 650, 651
causes of, 645, 648t–649t
diagnosis of, 648t–649t
symptoms of, 644
treatment of, 648t–649t
bronchitis vs., 631–632
chronic cardiopulmonary disease with, 659
community-acquired, differential diagnosis of, 644t
complications in, 664–665
diagnosis of, 643–657
follow-up examination for, 664–667
mycoplasma, duration of, 664
treatment of, 662t
nonbacterial, and cough, 646, 647
causes of, 646t–647t
diagnosis of, 646t–647t
symptoms of, 645
treatment of, 646t–647t
pneumococcal, duration of, 664
treatment of, 662t
poorly resolving, causes of, 666–667, 666t
symptoms of, 631–632
treatment of, 657–663
Pneumonitis, hypersensitivity, and cough, 655
Pneumothorax, and acute severe chest pain, 737
and nonpleuritic chest pain, 728t
Podophyllin, for acute proctitis, 146t
for condylomata acuminata, 314, 344t
Polyarthritis, of knee, differential diagnosis of, 255t
Polymyalgia rheumatica, and chronic low back pain, 43
and shoulder pain, 393
Ponstel, for primary dysmenorrhea, 585
Popliteal artery, palpation of, 227
Popliteal cysts, 230–231
popliteal aneurysms vs., 230
rheumatoid arthritis and, 230
ruptured, 231
popliteal thrombophlebitis vs., 230–231
swelling in, location of, 229, 236, 236t
tenderness in, location of, 236, 236t
Popliteal space, examination of, 227
Popliteal thrombophlebitis, ruptured popliteal cysts vs., 230–231
Popliteus muscle, location of, 226
Popliteus tendinitis, and knee pain, 232
swelling in, location of, 236, 236t
tenderness in, location of, 236, 236t
Popliteus tendon, palpation of, 225–227
Porphyria, and orthostatic hypotension, 477t
Postbronchitic bronchospasm, 641
Postconcussion syndrome, symptoms of, 172
Posterior fossa tumors, trigeminal neuralgia vs., 191
Posterior spinous processes, location of, 62
Postganglionic disease, and orthostatic hypotension, 477t
Postherpetic neuralgia, trigeminal neuralgia vs., 190
Postnasal drip, and chronic cough, 667–668
and recurrent sore throat, 92
treatment of, 668

Postpericardiotomy syndrome, and acute pleuritic chest pain, 743t
Posture, and lordosis, 6
  correct vs. incorrect, 24–25
  disorders of, and chronic low back pain, 43
  chronic, 50–51
  imbalance of, and chronic low back pain, 47–51
  poor, and chronic low back pain, 50
Post-thoracotomy pain, and acute pleuritic chest pain, 742t
Post-traumatic syndromes, tension headache vs., 210
Postvagotomy diarrhea, 152
Prazosin, and orthostatic hypotension, 477t
Precordial catch syndrome, and chest-wall pain, 700
Prednisone, for cluster headache, 189
  for disc herniation, 40
  for infectious mononucleosis, 76
  for rotator cuff tendinitis, 421
  for status migraine, 207
  for temporal arteritis, 173
Preganglionic disease, chronic, and orthostatic hypotension, 477t
Pregnancy, and orthostatic hypotension, 477t
  chlamydial infection with, erythromycin for, 286
  ectopic, pain in, 389, 560t–561t, 565, 566
    signs of, 560t, 566, 566t
    symptoms of, 560t, 566, 566t
    tests for, 561t, 567
    treatment of, 561t
  tests for, in evaluation of abdominal pain, 556t, 567–568
  urinary tract infections with, treatment for, 286, 286t, 287t
  vaginal trichomoniasis in, treatment of, 325
Premarin, for atrophic vaginitis, 333, 333t
Premenstrual syndrome, and chronic lower abdominal pain, 587t
Prepatellar neuralgia, traumatic, 237
  swelling in, location of, 236, 236t
  tenderness, in, location of, 236, 236t
(Pre)syncope. See Syncope.
Probenecid, for Fitz-Hugh-Curtis syndrome, 575
Procardia, for angina pectoris, 718t
Prochlorperazine, for vertigo, 499t
Proctitis, acute, 145–147
  causes of, 146t
  diagnosis of, 146t
  in homosexuals, 145–147
  proctoscopic findings in, 146t, 147
  symptoms of, 145
  treatment of, 146t, 147
  venereal causes of, laboratory testing for, 145–147
Proctocolitis, acute, symptoms of, 102
Proctoscopy, for acute proctitis, 146t, 147
  for pseudomembranous colitis, 115
Proctosigmoidoscopy, diagnostic, for acute dysentery, 114
  for acute proctitis, 145
  for acute proctocolitis, 102
  indications for, 106, 107t
Progressive headache, 186
Promethazine, for vertigo, 499t
Propranolol, for angina pectoris, 716, 716t
  for migraine, 206
  for orthostatic hypotension, 477t
Propoxyphene, for headache, 202, 203

Prostate, abscess of, and fever, 376
  surgical drainage of, 376
  carcinoma of, and low back pain, 3t
    and referred shoulder pain, 392
  disease of, and chronic low back pain, 44
  examination of, in diagnosis of abdominal pain, 548
Prostatitis, 366–374
  acute, and fever, 376
  and low back pain, 3t, 44
  and recurrent urethritis, 361
  chronic bacterial, antibiotics for, 371, 371t
    recurrence of, 372
    treatment of, 371–372
      prophylactic, 373
  diagnosis of, 366–367
    localization studies in, 367–368, 367
    prostatosis vs., 369
Prostatosis, and urethritis, 369, 369t
  prostatitis vs., 369
Proteinuria, in diagnosis of abdominal pain, 554
Proteus, and urinary tract infections, 289
Proteus mirabilis, and recurrent urinary tract infections, 296
Proventil, for acute bronchitis, 640t
Pruritus, persistent, causes of, 331
  vulvar, 334–336
    causes of, 334t
    primary dermatologic conditions of, 335–336
    psychogenic causes of, 336
Pseudoephedrine, for postnasal drip, 668
Pseudogout, and monoarthritis of knee, 259t, 261
  and shoulder pain, 405t
  synovial fluid analysis in, 258
Pseudomembranous colitis, diarrhea of, causes of, 102
  proctoscopy for, 115
Pseudomonas, and urinary tract infections, 289
Pseudosciatica, radicular low back pain and, 34–35
Pseudoseizures, and syncope, 476
Psittacosis, and nonbacterial pneumonia, 647t
Psoas muscle, location of, 64
Psoas sign, in diagnosis of abdominal pain, 547, 548
Psoriasis, and vulvar pruritus, 336
Psychiatric disorders, and tension headache, 210–211
Psychosis, and hyperventilation, 507
Puffer fish toxin, and food poisoning, 149t
Pulmonary embolism, and acute pleuritic chest pain, 742t, 744–746
  and cough, 631
  and nonpleuritic chest pain, 728t
  and syncope, 485t
  diagnosis of, lung scans in, 772–779
  recurrent, and chest pain, 696
Pulmonary function tests, in diagnosis of chronic cough, 669–670
Pulmonary infiltrates, and cough, 657
Pulmonic stenosis, and syncope, 485t
  systolic murmurs in, 704t
Pulse, counting of, technique for, 722
Pyelography, intravenous, in evaluation of abdominal pain, 556t
Pyelonephritis, 300–302
  and acute right lower quadrant pain, 560t–561t
  and ovarian carcinoma, 301

Pyelonephritis (Continued)
  antibiotic therapy for, 301
  clinical characteristics of, 278t
  diagnosis of, 375–376
  perinephric abscess and, 302
  recurrent, urologic investigation of, 302
  signs of, 560t
  symptoms of, 276, 300, 560t
  tests for, 561t
  treatment of, 286, 287t, 561t
  urologic investigation of, 297
  xanthogranulomatous, 302
Pyloroplasty, and lactose intolerance, 119
Pyrantel pamoate, for parasitic diarrhea, 117t
Pyridium, for symptomatic cystourethritis, 286
Pyridoxine, for premenstrual syndrome, 587t
Pyrvinium pamoate, for parasitic diarrhea, 117t
Pyuria, detection of, 282–284
  microscopic, in diagnosis of abdominal pain, 551
  quantitation of, counting chamber method for, 284, 284
  sterile, tuberculosis with, 292
  unexplained, indications of, 291
    tetracycline for, 291

Q angle, function of, 267, 267
  location of, 267
Q fever, and nonbacterial pneumonia, 647, 647t
Quadratus lumborum, location of, 64
Quadriceps disorders, and knee pain, 233t, 235–236
Quadriceps exercises, types of, 240
Quadriceps muscle, function of, 265–267, 266
  location of, 265, 266
  setting of, in treatment of patellofemoral syndromes, 239
Quadriceps tendinitis, swelling in, localization of, 236
Quadriceps tendon, palpation of, 224
Questran, for bacterial diarrhea, 113t
Quinacrine, for chronic diarrhea, 134t
  for giardiasis, 117
  for parasitic diarrhea, 117t
Quinsy. See Peritonsillar abscess.

Racing dive maneuver, in diagnosis of chest-wall syndromes, 701, 702
Radial nerve, lesions of, and shoulder pain, 433t, 435
Radiation therapy, for epidural metastases, 56
Radicular pain, with disc disease, 8
Radionuclide imaging, of biliary tract, in diagnosis of acute cholecystitis, 573–574, 574
  of brain, in diagnosis of headache, 197
  of chest, in diagnosis of chest pain, 763
Rales, in physical examination of patient with cough, 634
Range of motion, of back, testing of, 7–8
  of cervical spine, 390
  of knee, 222–223, 223
    testing of, 249
  of neck, 390, 403

Range of motion *(Continued)*
  of shoulder, 393–397, *395*
    active vs. passive, *396*
Ranitidine, for duodenal ulcer, 620t
  for esophagitis, 767t
Rapid plasma reagin, for detection of
    syphilis, 378
Raynaud's phenomenon, thoracic outlet
    syndrome vs., 453
Recruitment, in diagnosis of hearing loss,
    523
Rectoceles, *316*
Rectum, biopsy of, diagnostic, for acute
    proctitis, 147
      for amebic dysentery, 114
      for Crohn's disease, 114
      for ulcerative colitis, 114
    indications for, 106, 107t
  disorders of, sciatica vs., 35
  examination of, diagnostic, for
    abdominal pain, 549
    for low back pain, 10
Reflex(es), deep tendon, testing of, 403,
    403
  testing of, 32
Reflex sympathetic dystrophy syndrome,
    427, 427t
Rehydration, oral, for acute diarrhea, 109
Reiter's syndrome, and chronic low back
    pain, 43
  and fever, 377
  and pharyngeal ulcers, 75
  and recurrent urethritis, 361
  symptoms of, 342
Renal failure, female urinary tract
    infections with, treatment for, 286t,
    287, 287t
Renal function, unexplained impaired,
    urologic investigation of, 297
Renal parenchymal disease, and acute
    pyelonephritis, 302
Reserpine, and headache, 182
Respiratory disorders, upper, and cough,
    630
Respiratory infections, in immuno-
    compromised host, 652t
Retroperitoneal disorders, and low back
    pain, 3t
Retroperitoneal hemorrhage, and low back
    pain, 56
Retropharyngeal abscess, and trismus, 82
  dental procedures and, 86, 87
  diagnosis of, *88*
  intensive care for, 86
  surgical drainage of, 86
  symptoms of, 86
Retropharyngeal space, measurement of,
    88, *89*
Retrotracheal space, measurement of, 88,
    89
Rheumatic fever, prevention of, 80, 95–96
  untreated streptococcal pharyngitis and,
    95–96
Rheumatoid arthritis. See *Arthritis,
    rheumatoid.*
Rhinitis, and headache, 177
Rhomboid muscles, palpation of, 399
Rhonchi, in physical examination of patient
    with cough, 634
Rib, fractures of, and chest-wall pain, 698
Rickets, classification of, 58t
Rifampin, for bacterial pneumonia, 649t
  for nongonococcal urethritis, 358, 358t
Rinné test, for hearing loss, 521
Riopan Plus, for duodenal ulcer, 620t

Ritalin, for orthostatic hypotension, 480
Robaxin, for low back pain, 21
Robitussin, for acute bronchitis, 639t
Romberg testing, in diagnosis of dizziness,
    462, *462*
Rotator cuff, and traumatic shoulder pain,
    449
  function of, *443*, 444
  rupture of, diagnosis of, 414–416
    surgery for, 416
    tear vs., 414
  tear of, diagnosis of, 413–414, 416t
RPR, for detection of syphilis, 378
RSDS. See *Reflex sympathetic dystrophy
    syndrome.*

Sacral sensation, testing of, 31
Sacroiliac joints, x-rays of, 46
Sacroiliac ligament, location of, 64
Sacrospinal ligament, location of, 64
Sacrospinalis muscle, location of, 64
Sacrotuberal ligament, location of, 64
Salicylates, and labyrinthitis, 497
Salmonella, and acute diarrhea, 113t
  and acute dysentery, 101, 111
  and fecal leukocytes, 103
  and food poisoning, 149t
  and postoperative diarrhea, 153
Salmonella enteritidis, and acute invasive
    diarrhea, 113t
Salmonella gastroenteritis, treatment of,
    108
Salmonella heidelberg, and acute invasive
    diarrhea, 113t
Salmonella newport, and acute invasive
    diarrhea, 113t
Salmonella typhimurium, and acute
    diarrhea, 113t
Saphenous nerve entrapment, and knee
    pain, 217
  swelling in, location of, *236*, 236t
  tenderness in, location of, *236*, 236t
Salpingitis, untreated gonorrhea and, 356
Sarcoma, osteogenic, and monoarthritis of
    knee, *264*
  synovial, and monoarthritis of knee, 262
Sarcoptes scabiei, and vulvar pruritus, 334,
    346, 346t
Sartorius, location of, *268*
Scabies, and vulvar pruritus, 334, *346,* 346t
Scalenus anticus syndrome, 451
Scapula, muscles of, testing of, 403, *403*
  palpation of, 399, *400*
  spurs of, *400*
  syndromes of, *400*
Scapulocostal syndrome, *400*
Scapulothoracic mechanism, analysis of,
    444–446, *445*
  during shoulder abduction, *442–443*
Scarlet fever, 79
Schilling test, in diagnosis of bile acid
    deficiencies, 139
Schöber testing, in diagnosis of chronic low
    back pain, *43*
Sciatic nerve, anatomical course of, *33*
Sciatic notch, and low back pain, 10
Sciatica, differential diagnosis of, 34–37
Scissors maneuver, in diagnosis of chest-
    wall syndromes, 700, *701*
Scoliosis, of lumbar spine, *6*
  pelvic tilting and, 50
Scombrotoxin, and food poisoning, 149t
Scopolamine, for vertigo, 499t

Scrotum, normal contents of, *347*
Sedatives, and disequilibrium, 465
  and nystagmus, 513
  and orthostatic hypotension, 477t
Sedimentation rate, in diagnosis of low
    back pain, 18t
Seizures, akinetic, characteristics of, 482–
    483, 482t
  and syncope, 476
  grand mal, phases of, 481–482, 482t
  signs of, 476
Senile gait, and disequilibrium, 466, 468t
Sensory examination, for radicular low
    back pain, 31
Sensory loss, peripheral nerve lesions vs.
    nerve root lesions in, 32
Septal defect, atrial, systolic murmurs in,
    704t
Septal hypertrophy, asymmetric, exertional
    angina with, *708*
  systolic murmurs in, 704t
Serratia, and urinary tract infections, 289
Serratus anterior muscle, testing of, 403,
    403
Serum amylase, in diagnosis of abdominal
    pain, 556t, 607
Serum gastrin level, elevated, causes of,
    622t
Serum protein electrophoresis, in diagnosis
    of low back pain, 18t
Shellfish allergies, and labyrinthitis, 497
Shellfish toxin, and food poisoning, 149t
Shigella, and acute dysentery, 101, 111
  and acute invasive diarrhea, 113t
  and fecal leukocytes, 103
  and food poisoning, 149t
Shigella enteritis, treatment of, 108
Shigella flexneri, and acute invasive
    diarrhea, 113t
Shigella sonnei, and acute invasive
    diarrhea, 113t
Shoulder, abduction of, analysis of, *395,*
    441
  acromioclavicular dislocations of, 447,
    449
  anatomy of, 441–446
  arthrocentesis of, *392*
  biomechanics of, 441–446
  disorders of, articular, 405t
    bony, 405t
    periarticular, 407–426
      causes of, 410
      chronic, 423–426
      diagnosis of, 410–416
      exercise therapy for, 418–421, *419,
        420*
      injection therapy for, *417,* 418
      musculotendinous, 416t
      teatment of, 416–422
  joints of, *441*
  mobility of, impairment of, causes of,
    446
  signs of, *422*
  motor weakness of, analysis of, 435,
    436t, 437t, 438t
  muscles of, origins and insertions of, *401*
    testing of, 403, *403*
  muscular weakness of, causes of, 425
  pain in. See *Shoulder pain.*
  palpation of, 397–398, *398*
  range of motion of, 393–397, *395*
    active vs. passive, *396*
  sepsis of, and shoulder pain, 391
  sternoclavicular dislocations of, 447
  tenderness of, palpable areas of, *410*

Shoulder/hand syndromes, 427–428, 427t
Shoulder pain, 387–455
  acute, diagnosis of, *394*
    mechanical, 404
    periarticular, diagnosis of, *421*
  chronic, 391
    disability with, 391
  drugs and, 393
  examination of patient with, 393–397,
    395
  hand pain with, 426–431
  history of trauma in, 392
  initial approach to, 387–388
  muscle weakness and, 402
  muscular disorder and, 396
  neoplasms and, 405t, *407*
  neurologic complaints with, 431
  neurologic examination in, 402–403
  neuromuscular disorders and, 425
  orthopedic consultation for, 426
  postural disorders and, 402
  referred, causes of, 388t
    disorders of neck and, 388
    locations of, *389*
    neoplasms and, 392
    systemic disorders and, 392–393
  sensory examination in, 403
  signs of, 388–407
  symptoms of, 388–407
  traumatic, 405t, 447–450
    mechanism of, 448–449
    orthopedic consultation for, 447
    throwing injuries and, 449–450, *450*
Sialadenitis, acute, bull neck vs., 90
Sigmoid volvulus, and abdominal pain, *555*
Simethicone, for functional dyspepsia, 599
Sinding-Larsen-Johansson's disease, and
    knee pain, 233t, 234
  swelling in, localization of, *236*
Sinemet, for dizziness, 480
Sinoatrial arrest, and syncope, 483, 484t
Sinus disease, and acute headache, 179t
  tension headache vs., 210
Sinusitis, and headache, 177
  and vertigo, 494t, 495
  cluster headache vs., 188
  location of pain in, 171, *171*
  types of, 171
Sleep headache, 183–184
Slipping rib syndrome, and chest-wall pain,
  700
Slo-Phyllin, for acute bronchitis, 640t
Small bowel, cultures of, in diagnosis of
    bile acid deficiencies, 139
  resection of, and lactose intolerance, 119
    and postoperative diarrhea, 153
Smoking, and chronic cough, 667
  and chronic sore throat, 92
Sodium, for orthostatic hypotension, 477t,
  479
Sorbitrate, for angina pectoris, 715t
Sore throat, 71–99. See also specific types.
  acute, clinical approach to, *91*
    noninfectious causes of, 91
  causes of, 72, 72t
  chronic, causes of, 92–93
  clinical approach to, 71–76
  complicated, 82–92
    clinical findings in, 82–86
    evaluation of, 86–90, *87*
    physical abnormalities in, 86–90
    respiratory symptoms with, 84
  head and neck disorders and, 72t
  mediastinal disorders and, 72t
  pharyngitis vs., 71

Sore throat *(Continued)*
  recurrent, causes of, 92–93
  systemic diseases and, 72t
Spastic colon. See *Irritable bowel
  syndrome.*
Spectinomycin, for acute proctitis, 146t
  for gonococcal urethritis, 355, 355t
  for nongonococcal urethritis, 358, 358t
Speech discrimination, in diagnosis of
  hearing loss, 523
Spermatocele, testicular, *348*
Sphenopalatine neuralgia, cluster headache
  vs., 188
Spina bifida, 9
Spinal canal, cross-sectional outlines of, *48*
  location of, 62
Spinal cord, lesion of, thoracic outlet
  syndrome vs., 453
Spinal stenosis, 48, 49
  spondylosis and, 47
Spine. See also *Back.*
  cervical, disease of. See *Cervical spine
    disease.*
    range of motion in, *390*
  disease of, degenerative, and chronic low
    back pain, 47–49
  disorders of, OMINOUS, 4–5
  epidural hematoma of, and low back
    pain, 56
  manipulation of, for low back pain, 27
  neoplasms of, and shoulder pain, 392
  palpation of, 8–10
Splenic flexure syndrome, and chronic
    upper abdominal pain, 610t–611t
  and referred shoulder pain, 389
Splint, in treatment of acute knee injury,
  252–253
  posterior knee, 253, *253*
  wrist, for carpal tunnel syndrome, 440
Spondylitis, ankylosing, and chronic low
  back pain, 43
Spondyloarthropathies, and chronic low
  back pain, 43
Spondylolisthesis, 9
  with spondylosis, x-ray of, *47*
Spondylosis, and clinical syndromes, 47–49
  cervical. See *Cervical spondylosis.*
  chronic postural disorders and, 50
  degenerative, and chronic low back pain,
    43, *48*
  lumbosacral, intervertebral disc
    degeneration and, 47
  radiographic findings in, *48, 49*
  with spondylolisthesis, x-ray of, *47*
Sprue, celiac, and lactose intolerance, 119
  tropical, and lactose intolerance, 119
Sputum, Gram's stain of, in diagnosis of
  bacterial pneumonia, 652–655, *653*
Staphylococcus, and epiglottitis, 84
  and Ludwig's angina, 89
Staphylococcus aureus, and bacterial
    pneumonia, 648t, *651*
  and food poisoning, 149t
  and low back pain, 54, *55*
  and monoarthritis of knee, 259t
  and peritonsillar abscess, 83
  and septic bursitis, 230
  and toxic shock syndrome, 312
Staphylococcus saprophyticus, and urinary
    tract infections, 289
Steatorrhea, 138–142
  and postoperative diarrhea, 153
  causes of, 138, *138*
    pancreatic, 139
  diagnosis of, 139–142

Sterility, female, untreated gonorrhea and,
  356
Sternoclavicular disorders, and chest-wall
  pain, 702
Sternoclavicular joint, palpation of, 399
Sternocleidomastoid muscle, palpation of,
  399
Steroids, for infectious mononucleosis, 76
  for traumatic prepatellar neuralgia, 237
  topical, for aphthous stomatitis, 74
    for lichen planus, 344t
Stimson maneuver, in treatment of acute
  shoulder dislocations, 447, *448*
Stokes-Adams attack, and syncope, 483,
  484t
Stomatitis, aphthous, symptoms of, 74, *74*
  denture, symptoms of, 75
Stool, alkalinization of, 136
  cultures of, in diagnosis of acute
    proctitis, 147
    indications for, 106, 107t
  examination of, for fat, 135, *136*
    for ova and parasites, 106, 107t
  microbiologic studies of, accuracy of,
    115–119
Straight leg raising, in diagnosis of low
    back pain, 10–13. *10*
  interfering factors in, 11
  negative, 12–13
  positive, 11
  resisted, in treatment of patellofemoral
    syndromes, 240
  unresisted, in treatment of patellofemoral
    syndromes, 239–240
Strep throat. See *Pharyngitis, streptococcal.*
Streptococcus, and epiglottitis, 84
  and Ludwig's angina, 89
  and peritonsillar abscess, 83
  and pharyngitis, 78. See *Pharyngitis,
    streptococcal.*
  carriers of, 81
Streptococcus pneumoniae, and bacterial
    pneumonia, 648t, *660*
Streptococcus pyogenes, and pneumonia,
  645
Streptomycin, for chancroid, 343t
Stress, emotional, and angina pectoris, 685
  hyperextension, and ligamentous knee
    injury, 244
  rotational, and meniscal knee injury, 244
  valgus, and ligamentous knee injury, 244
  varus, and ligamentous knee injury, 244
Stress tests, conditions contraindicating,
  754t
  evaluation of, 759–761
  false-negative, causes of, 760t
  false-positive, causes of, 760t
  in diagnosis of chest pain, 705t
  in diagnosis of coronary artery disease,
    757–759, 758t
  indications for, 754t, 756–759
  nuclear, in diagnosis of chest pain, 763–
    765
    indications for, 765
  results of, correlations in, 756t–757t
Strongyloides stercoralis, and parasitic
    diarrhea, 117t
Subacromial area, of shoulder, palpation
    of, 398, *398*
Subarachnoid hemorrhage, low back pain
    and, 54
Subhepatic abscess. See *Subphrenic
  abscess.*
Subphrenic abscess, and acute pleuritic
    chest pain, 743t, *751*

Subphrenic abscess *(Continued)*
and right upper quadrant pain, 571t
Sucralfate, for duodenal ulcer, 619, 620, 620t
Sulfasalazine, for chronic diarrhea, 129, 134(t)
for Crohn's disease, 132
Sulfisoxazole, for nongonococcal urethritis, 358, 358t
for urinary tract infections, 286t
Sulfonamides, for urinary tract infections, 280
Sulindac, for low back pain, 22t
Superior mesenteric artery syndrome, and chronic abdominal pain, *602, 610t–611t*
Superior vena cava obstruction, and acute headache, 179t
Suprahumeral joint, structures of, 407–409, *408*
Supraspinal ligaments, location of, 63
Sympathectomy, and orthostatic hypotension, 477t
Syncope, 471–486
bradycardia with, 476
cardiac arrhythmia and, 509–511
carotid sinus, 472t
categories of, 480–481
causes of, 471–473, 472t
cardiac, 483–486, 484t, 485t
neurologic, 481–483, 482t
clinical analysis of, *474–475*
cough, 472t
definition of, 457–458
diagnosis of, differential, *470, 471*
laboratory tests in, 473
during ECG monitoring, 509–511, *510*
equivocal, 480–481
iatrogenic, 472t
micturition, 472t
observation of, 476
prodromal symptoms of, 476
recurrent, evaluation of, 511, *511*
typical benign, 472t, 480
vasovagal, causes of, 471, 472t
Synovitis, pigmented villonodular, and monoarthritis, 262, *263*
Syphilis, and acute headache, 178t, 179t
and fever, 377
and pharyngeal ulcers, 75
cultures for, in diagnosis of acute proctitis, 147
primary, chancre of, *314, 315, 342*
diagnosis of, 343t, 379–380
sequence of testing in, *380*
treatment of, 343t
secondary, 314–315
diagnosis of, 380–381
tests for, 378–381, *378*
screening, 380–381, *381*
serologic, 378–379
treatment of, 378–381
types of, 378
Syringomyelia, and shoulder pain, 392
Systolic murmurs, in evaluation of chest pain, 703, 704t

Tachyarrhythmias, and syncope, 483–484, 484t
Tachycardias, and syncope, 484t
Talwin, for low back pain, 21
Tegretol, for trigeminal neuralgia, 190
side effects of, 190

Temporal arteritis, cluster headache vs., 188
diagnosis of, 173
tension headache vs., 210
Temporomandibular disorders, and headache, 177
Tendinitis, acute, inflammation of contiguous structures in, *409*
bicipital, diagnosis of, 411–412, 416t
testing for, *411*
treatment of, 412
calcific, and shoulder pain, *413*
diagnosis of, 412–413, 416t
treatment of, 413
rotator cuff, chronic, 423
diagnosis of, 413–414, 416t
therapy for, 414
scapulocostal, *400*
Tendons, knee, location of, *268*
Tenormin, for angina pectoris, 716t
Tension headache, characteristics of, 185t, 192t
common migraine vs., 191–196
locations of, 191, *192*
organic disorders vs., 210
symptoms of, 191
treatment of, 209–213
typical calendar of, 195t
Tension/vascular headache, clinical features in, 193
Terbutaline, and headache, 182
for acute bronchitis, 640t
Terpin hydrate, for acute bronchitis, 639t
Testis, location of, *347*
palpation of, *347*
torsion of, diagnosis of, *348*
tumors of, *348*
Testosterone propionate, for atrophic vaginitis, 333, 333t
Tetracycline, for acute diverticulitis, 586t
for acute proctitis, 146t
for aphthous stomatitis, 74
for bacterial diarrhea, 113t
for bacterial urinary infection, 364
for *Campylobacter* enteritis, 108
for chancroid, 343t
for chlamydial urethritis, 285–286, 291
for chronic diarrhea, 134t
for chronic prostatitis, 371t
for epididymitis, *347*
for gonococcal urethritis, 291, 354, 354t
for mycoplasmal pneumonia, 661, 662t
for nonbacterial pneumonia, 646t–647t
for nongonococcal urethritis, 357–358, 358t
for pelvic inflammatory disease, 312, 563
for primary syphilis, 343t
for prostatosis, 369t
for tropical sprue, 142
for turista, 117, 151
for unexplained pyuria, 291
for unexplained vaginitis, 338
for urinary tract infections, 280, 286t
for Vincent's angina, 73
Tetralogy of Fallot, and syncope, 485t
Thallium scan, in diagnosis of chest pain, 705t, 764
Theoclear, for acute bronchitis, 640t
Theo-Dur, for acute bronchitis, 640t
Theolair, for acute bronchitis, 640t
Theophylline, and headache, 182
for acute bronchitis, 640t
Thiabendazole, for parasitic diarrhea, 117t
Thiazides, and orthostatic hypotension, 477t

Thigh, posterior muscles of, location of, *228*
sensory loss of, 32
Thioridazine HCl, and orthostatic hypotension, 477t
for tension headache, 211
Thoracentesis, in diagnosis of empyema, 659
Thoracic disease, and right upper quadrant pain, 571t
tests for, 571t
treatment of, 571t
Thoracic outlet syndromes, 451–453
and chest-wall pain, 700, 702
and shoulder/hand pain, 427t, 428–429
differential diagnosis of, 453
location of, 451
shoulder girdle exercises for, 453, 453t
signs of, 451, 571t
symptoms of, 451, 571t
types of, 451–452
Thoracic spine disease, and nonpleuritic chest pain, 729t
and respirophasic chest pain, *775*
Thoracostomy, for empyema, 659–660
Thorax, manipulation of, in diagnosis of chest pain, 697–698
Throat, Sore, 71–99. See also *Sore throat* and specific types.
Throat cultures, clinical findings in, 77t
indications for, 77–79, *78*
procedures for, 94
Throat lozenges, for pharyngitis, 79
Thrombophlebitis, popliteal, and knee pain, 217, *218*
Thumb print sign, in diagnosis of epiglottitis, *85*
Thyroid, diseases of, and referred shoulder pain, 392
neoplasms of, and referred shoulder pain, 392
Thyroiditis, and chronic sore throat, 92
and headache, 177
Tibia, popliteal surface of, location of, *268*
Tibial plateau, palpation of, 224, 225
Tibial tubercle, palpation of, 224
Tic douloureux. See *Trigeminal neuralgia.*
Ticarcillin, for acute pyelonephritis, 301
Tietze's syndrome, and chest-wall pain, 699
Tigan, for vertigo, 499t
Timolol, for angina pectoris, 716t
Tinactin, for erythrasma, 334
for tinea cruris, 334
Tinea cruris, and vulvar pruritus, 334–335
diagnosis of, 345t
location of, *345*
treatment of, 345t
Tinel sign, in diagnosis of leg pain, 31
in diagnosis of shoulder pain, 428, 433
Tobacco, and labyrinthitis, 497
Toe flexion test, for chronic low back pain, 52
Tolectin, for low back pain, 22t
Tolmetin sodium, for low back pain, 22t
Tolnaftate, for erythrasma, 334
for tinea cruris, 334
Tolosa-Hunt syndrome, and acute headache, 179t
Tone decay, in diagnosis of hearing loss, 523
Tonsil(s), asymmetric swelling of, 83
bilateral swelling of, mononucleosis and, 84
Tonsillar exudate, *78*
Tonsillectomy, for peritonsillar abscess, 83

Tonsillitis, bacterial, mononucleosis vs., 84
  chronic, and recurrent sore throat, 92
  lingual, epiglottitis vs., 88
  streptococcal herpes simplex vs., 73
Torsion, in testing back range of motion, 8
Toxic megacolon, *130*
Toxic shock syndrome, antistaphylococcal
    antibiotics for, 312
  hemodynamic support for, 312
  symptoms of, 312
Tracheotomy, for diphtheria, 86
  for epiglottitis, 84
  for Ludwig's angina, 89
Traction maneuvers, in diagnosis of low
    back pain, 10–14
Tranquilizers, and disequilibrium, 465
  for tension headache, 211
Transderm-Nitro, for angina pectoris, 715t
Transderm-V, for vertigo, 499t
Transtracheal aspiration, in diagnosis of
    pneumonia, 657, *658*
Transverse processes, location of, 62
Trapezius, testing of, 403, *403*
Treponema pallidum, and genital
    ulcerations, 343t
Triamcinolone acetonide, for aphthous
    stomatitis, 74
Triamcinolone hexacetonide, for bursitis,
    230
Triaminic, for acute bronchitis, 639t
Trichloroacetic acid, for condylomata
    acuminata, *314*, 344t
Trichomonas, and cervical dysplasia, 332
  and urethritis, 358, 360
  cultures for, in diagnosis of vaginitis,
    indications for, 321–323, 320t
Trichomonas vaginalis, and vaginitis, 316t,
    317
  wet mount in diagnosis of, 319, *319*
Trichomoniasis, vaginal, causes of, 313
  pregnant patient with, 325
  treatment of, 324–327
Trichuris trichiura, and parasitic diarrhea,
    117t
Tricyclic antidepressants, and fibrositis, 52,
    402
  and orthostatic hypotension, 477t
  for migraine, 206t
  for tension headache, 212
Trigeminal neuralgia, 189–191
  cluster headache vs., 188, 190
  differential diagnosis of, 190–191
  pain of, location of, *189*
Trigger points, in mechanical low back
    pain, 9
Trilafon, for vertigo, 499t
Trimethobenzamide, for vertigo, 499t
Trimethoprim-sulfamethoxazole, for acute
    diverticulitis, 586t
  for bacterial diarrhea, 113t
  for bacterial pneumonia, 649t
  for bacterial urinary infections, 364
  for chancroid, 343t
  for chronic diarrhea, 134t
  for chronic prostatitis, 371t
  for gonococcal urethritis, 354, 355t
  for *Hemophilus influenzae* pneumonia,
    662t
  for prostatitis, 370
  for shigellosis, 117
  for turista, 117, 151
  for urinary tract infections, 280, 286t, 299

Trismus, 82, *82*
Trochanteric bursitis, 10
Tropical sprue, and lactose intolerance, 119
Tubal abscess, and acute right lower
    quadrant pain, 560t–561t
  signs of, 560t
  symptoms of, 560t
  tests for, 561t
  treatment of, 561t
Tuberculosis, and acute pleuritic chest
    pain, 742t
  and acute pyelonephritis, 302
  and pharyngeal ulcers, 75
  miliary, and chronic cough, *670*
Tuberosity, greater, palpation of, 398, *398*
  lesser, palpation of, 398, *398*
Turista, 151
  Escherichia coli and, 102
Tussend, for acute bronchitis, 639t
Tussionex, for acute bronchitis, 639t
Tylox, for low back pain, 21
Tyramine, for orthostatic hypotension, 477t

Ulcer(s), duodendal, and chronic upper
    abdominal pain, 595–596, 595t
  perforated, and abdominal pain, *552*
    and acute right lower quadrant pain,
      560t–561t
    and referred shoulder pain, *390*
    signs of, 560t
    symptoms of, 560t
    tests for, 561t
    treatment of, 561t
  symptoms of, 595, 595t
  tests for, 595, 596
  treatment of, 619, 623
    follow-up procedure for, 621–622,
      621
  gastric, and chronic upper abdominal
    pain, 595t, 596, *597*
  documentation of healing of, 623
  hospitalization for, 623
  symptoms of, 596
  tests for, 595t, 596
  treatment of, 622–623, *623*
  mouth, types of, 73–75
  peptic, ambulatory treatment of, 619–623
    and nonpleuritic chest pain, 729t
    perforated, 571t
    surgery for, 622t
  perforated, and nonpleuritic chest pain,
    729t
  pharyngeal, systemic diseases and, 75
    types of, 71–75
Ulcer operations, and postoperative
    diarrhea, 152
Ulcerative colitis. See *Colitis, ulcerative*.
Ulnar nerve, entrapment of, thoracic outlet
    syndrome vs., 453
  lesions of, and shoulder pain, 433t, 434–
    435
  peripheral entrapment of, *434*
Ultrasound, abdominal, diagnostic, for
    abdominal pain, 556t, 606
  for chest pain, 705t
Upper extremity, practical neurology of,
    431–440
Upper GI series, diagnostic, for abdominal
    pain, 556t

Upper GI series *(Continued)*
  diagnostic, for chest pain, 705t
    for chronic abdominal pain, 606
Upper respiratory disorders, and cough,
    630
Urethra, dilatation of, for recurrent urinary
    tract infections, 297
  female, caruncle of, *316*
  male, cultures of, 352–353
    diverticulum of, 360
    obtaining specimens from, *350*, 351
    strictures of, 360–361
    stripping of, 349, *349*
Urethral stenosis, and recurrent urinary
    tract infections, *296*
Urethral syndrome, 273, *274*
  antibiotics for, 280
  gonorrhea and, 276
Urethritis, 349–363
  causes of, 292
  chlamydial, tetracycline for, 285–286
  clinical characteristics of, 278t
  gonococcal, diagnosis of, 350–353
    nongonococcal vs., 350–353
    symptoms of, 350
    treatment of, 353–357
  nongonococcal, recurrent, 360–361
    symptoms of, 350
    treatment of, 357–359
      antimicrobial spectrum of, 358t
  sources of, determination of, *359*
  traumatic, 360
  urethral discharge and, 349
  tetracycline for, 291
  types of, 273t
Urinalysis, diagnostic, for abdominal pain,
    551–553, 556t
  for acute pyelonephritis, 300
  for female urinary tract infections,
    280–283
  for pyuria, 282–284
  results of, 281t
Urinary symptoms, fever with, 375–377,
    375
Urinary tract infection(s), 272–309. See
    also *Genitourinary infection(s)*.
  acute, persistent, 290–292
    pelvic examination for, 292
    treatment of, follow-up after, 293
  and acute right lower quadrant pain,
    560t–561t
  antibiotics for, 280–282, 286t
  bacterial, 363–365
    diagnosis of, 363
    pathogens in, 289
    symptoms of, 361
  catheter-acquired, treatment for, 287,
    287t
  complicated, treatment for, 286–288,
    287t
    uncomplicated vs., *365*
  complicated situations in, 273t
  diagnosis of, *362*, 365
  documentation of relapse in, 304
  economics of, 305, 305t
  empiric approach to, 280–282, *282*
  female, 272–309
  in high-risk patients, 278t
    treatment for, 286t, 287, 287t
  individualized approach to, 282–285, *283*
  initial treatment of, 285
  localizing site of, 303–304

Urinary tract infection(s) *(Continued)*
  male, 365–374
  recurrent, 293–299, 365–374
    bladder stones and, *297*
    prophylactic antibiotics for, 297–299
    prostatic calculi and, *373*
    reinfections vs. relapses, 293–294, *294*
    staghorn calculus and, *289*
    treatment for, 287t, 288
    types of, 366
    urethral stenosis and, *296*
    urologic investigation of, 296–297
  signs of, 560t
  single-dose antibiotics for, 285
  site of infection in, 276
  symptoms of, 276, 560t
  syndromes of, 275–280, *277*
    clinical characteristics of, 278t
    specific tests for, 277
  tests for, 364, 561t
  traditional approach to, 272–275, *274*
    flaws in, 274–275
  treatment of, 561t
  types of, 273t
Urine, clean catch, for culture, 288
  Gram's stain of, in diagnosis of acute
    pyelonephritis, 300
  in-and-out catheterization of, for culture,
    288
  percutaneous needle aspiration of, 288
  pigmented, in diagnosis of abdominal
    pain, 555
Urine culture(s), collection techniques for,
    288
  diagnostic, for acute pyelonephritis, 300
    for persistent urinary tract infections,
      291t
    for prostatitis, 367–368
    for recurrent nongonococcal urethritis,
      360
  in empiric approach to urinary tract
    infections, 280–282
  in individualized approach to urinary
    tract infections, *283*
  in traditional approach to urinary tract
    infections, 272–273, *274*
  indications for, 285t
  interpretation of, 288–290
  positive, criterion for, 273
  results of, 281t
Urolithiasis, recurrent, bilateral staghorn
  calculi and, *279*
Urologic disease, female urinary tract
  infections with, treatment for, 287,
    287t
Urologic disorders, and recurrent urinary
  tract infections, 297, 366
Urorenal disease, and right upper quadrant
  pain, 571t
Uterine myomas, and chronic low back
  pain, 43
  and chronic lower abdominal pain, 587t
  tests for, 587t
  treatment of, presumptive, 587t
Uterus, carcinoma of, and acute right lower
  quadrant pain, 560t
UTI. See *Urinary tract infection(s).*
Uveitis, and headache, 170, 170t, 178t

Vagina, bulges of, *316*
  cultures of, in diagnosis of vaginitis, 319–
    321, 320t

Vagina *(Continued)*
  discharge of, causes of, 311t
    cervical disorders and, 315
    culture of, 319–320
    diagnostic approach to, *322*
    normal vs. abnormal, 310–311
Vaginitis, atrophic, symptoms of, 331–332
    treatment of, 333, 333t
  candidal, appearance of, 318
    symptoms of, 316t, 317
    causes of, 316t
    diagnosis of, 316t
  Gardnerella. See *Gardnerella vaginitis.*
  infectious, 318–333
    treatment of, 328t
  multiple simultaneous infections in, 327
  nonspecific, 337–338
  sexually acquired, 321
  specimens in diagnosis of, 318–321
  symptoms of, 276, 312, 315
  Trichomonas, appearance of, *318*
    sexual intercourse and, 324
    symptoms of, 316t, 317
  types of, 273t
Vagotonia/Valsalva mechanisms, and
  syncope, 472t
Valium, for low back pain, 21
  for vertigo, 499t
Valsalva maneuvers, voluntary, and
  syncope, 472t
  in diagnosis of dizziness, 461
Vancomycin, for acute proctitis, 146t
  for acute prostatitis, 376
  for bacterial diarrhea, 113t
  for bacterial pneumonia, 648t
Varicella, and nonbacterial pneumonia,
  647t
Varicocele, testicular, *348*
Varicose veins, and orthostatic
  hypotension, 477t
Vas deferens, location of, *347*
Vascular claudication, sciatica vs., 35
Vascular occlusion, and headache, 170,
  170t
Vasculitic arterial disease, thoracic outlet
  syndrome vs., 453
Vasodilators, and headache, 182
VDRL, for detection of syphilis, 378
Venereal disease, and vulvovaginal
  disorders, 313
  anorectal manifestations of, 145
  public problems of, 382–383
  signs of, *342*, 343, 343t
Venereal enteric infections, in
  homosexuals, 102
Ventolin, for acute bronchitis, 640t
Ventricular fibrillation, and syncope, 483,
  484t
Ventricular hypertrophy, exertional angina
  with, *708*
Verapamil, for angina pectoris, 718t
Vertebral biopsy, for vertebral
  osteomyelitis, 54
Vertebral bodies, pain sensitivity of, 65
Vertebral metastases, and low back pain,
  56
  and ominous back pain, 56
Vertebral osteomyelitis, and chronic low
  back pain, 43, 54, *55*
  types of, 54
Vertebrobasilar ischemia, and syncope, 476
Vertigo, 486–502
  benign positional, 488t, 489, 494t, 497

Vertigo *(Continued)*
  central, causes of, 488t, 489–491
    symptoms of, 488t, 491
  clinical analysis of, 492
  definition of, 457
  drug-induced, 491
  drugs for, 499t
  intermittent, 493
  peripheral, causes of, 488t, 489
    central vs., 486–493, 488t
    symptoms of, 488, 488t
  positional, 497
  psychogenic, 493
  subsets of, 491–493
  symptoms of, 486
Vesicoureteral reflux, and bilateral
  hydronephrosis, *279*
Vestibular disease, peripheral, 493–502
  adaptation exercises for, 500t
  and vertigo, 494t
  drug therapy for, 498
  treatment of, 494t
Vestibular disorders, atypical, and
  disequilibrium, 465, 468t
Vestibular function, evaluation of, 512–518
Vestibular system, dysfunction of, and
  vertigo, 486
  central, 488t, 489–491
  peripheral, 488–489
  reflex pathways of, *487*
Vestibular-ocular interaction, 513–514, *513*
Vibrio cholerae, and food poisoning, 149t
Vibrio parahaemolyticus, and acute invasive
  diarrhea, 113t
  and food poisoning, 149t
Vincent's angina, symptoms of, 73, *73*
Viokase, for pancreatic enzyme
  replacement, 158t
Visceral disease, and syncope, 472t
Vision, impairment of, and disequilibrium,
  464
Visken, for angina pectoris, 716t
Visual loss, headache with, 178t
Vitamin A intoxication, and headache, 183
Vitamin D, deficiency of, 58t
  for osteoporosis, 59
Volvulus, cecal, and acute right lower
  quadrant pain, 560t–561t
Vomiting, acute severe chest pain with, 731
Von Bekesy tests, in diagnosis of hearing
  loss, 523
Vulva, carcinoma of, and vulvar pruritus,
  335
  infectious lesions of, *314, 315*
  itching of. See *Pruritus, vulvar.*
  secretions of, 310
Vulvar dystrophy, and vulvar pruritus, 335
Vulvovaginal disorders, 310–340
  complicating factors in, 311
  differential diagnosis of, 313–318
  initial approach to, 311–313
  physical findings in, 313–318
  sexual activity and, 313
  signs of, 310–311
  symptoms of, 310–311
Vulvovaginal pruritus, causes of, 311

Warts, genital, *314,* 344, 344t. See also
  Condylomata acuminata.
Watch tick test, for hearing loss, 519, *521*
Weaver's bottom, 9

Weber test, for hearing loss, 522
Wegener's granulomatosis, and chronic
    cough, *669*
Wernicke's disease, and orthostatic
    hypotension, 477t
Wet mount, in diagnosis of *Trichomonas
    vaginalis,* 319, *319*
Whiplash, tension headache vs., 210
Whipple's disease, and lactose intolerance,
    119
Wigraine, for migraine, 204t
Wolff-Parkinson-White syndrome, syncope
    with, 509
Worried well, 672–673

Xiphoidalgia, and chest-wall pain, 698
X-rays, chest. See *Chest x-rays.*

X-rays *(Continued)*
    diagnostic, abdominal, for abdominal
        pain, 549–551, 550t, 556t
    for chronic diarrhea, 137
    for complicated sore throat, 90
    for epiglottitis, 84
    for headache, 197
    for knee pain, 238
    for low back pain, 10, 18–20, 18t, 54,
        55
    chronic, 44–49
    indications for, 19–20
    radicular, 37
    for retropharyngeal abscess, *87,* 88, *88*
    for traumatic knee pain, *242*
    for traumatic shoulder pain, 447
    for vertebral metastases, 56
Xylocaine, for aphthous stomatitis, 75

Yeoman's test, 13
Yergason's test, in diagnosis of bicipital
    tendinitis, 411–412, *411*
Yersinia enterocolitica, and acute invasive
    diarrhea, 113t
Yersinia enterocolitis, Crohn's disease vs.,
    132
    ulcerative colitis vs., 131

Zollinger-Ellison syndrome, gastric surgery
    and, 153